W9-DHH-687

Nursing in the Community

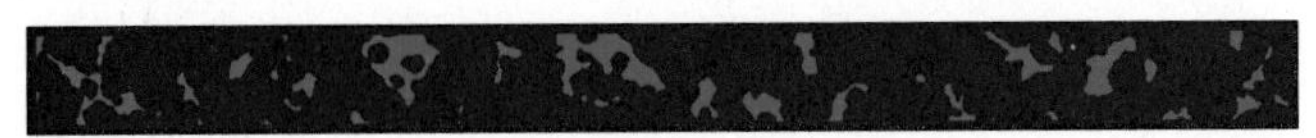

Mary Jo Clark, RN, MSN, PhD
Assistant Professor
Philip Y. Hahn School of Nursing
University of San Diego
San Diego, California

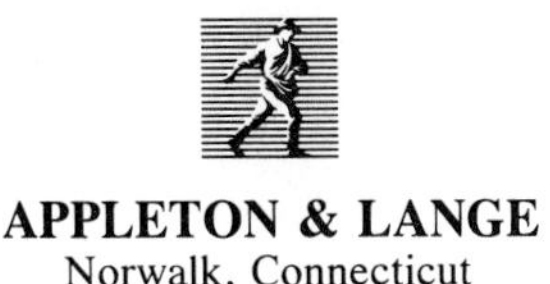

APPLETON & LANGE
Norwalk, Connecticut

Executive Editor, Nursing: William Brottmiller
Nursing Developmental Editor: Mark F. Wales
Managing Editors: Eileen Burns; John Williams
Copy Editor: James Tully
Indexer: Phil James
Art Director: Steve Byrum
Designers: Janice Barsevich and Michael J. Kelly
Manufacturing Buyer: Alexis Heydt

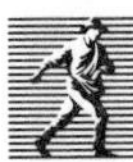

92 93 94 95 96 / 10 9 8 7 6 5 4 3 2 1

Prentice Hall International (UK) Limited, *London*
Prentice Hall of Australia Pty. Limited, *Sydney*
Prentice Hall Canada, Inc., *Toronto*
Prentice Hall Hispanoamericana, S.A., *Mexico*
Prentice Hall of India Private Limited, *New Delhi*
Prentice Hall of Japan, Inc., *Tokyo*
Simon & Schuster Asia Pte. Ltd., *Singapore*
Editora Prentice Hall do Brasil Ltda., *Rio de Janeiro*
Prentice Hall, *Englewood Cliffs, New Jersey*

Library of Congress Cataloging-in-Publication Data

Nursing in the community / [edited by] Mary Jo Clark.
p. cm.
Includes index.
ISBN 0-8385-1362-X
1. Community health nursing—United States. I. Clark, Mary Jo Dummer.
[DNLM: 1. Community Health Nursing. 2. Nursing Process.
WY 106 N97552]
RT98.N88 1991
610.73'43—dc20
DNLM/DLC
for Library of Congress 91-33428

ISBN 0-8385-1362-X
90000
9 780838 513620

PRINTED IN THE UNITED STATES OF AMERICA

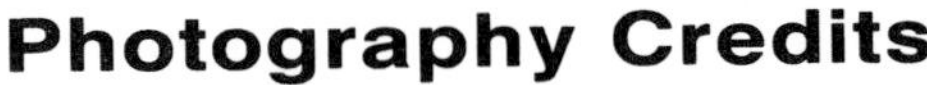

Photography Credits

Pages 6, 34, 54, 75, 78, 100, 142, 178, 196, 218, 239, 242, 264, 280, 342, 367, 370, 394, 420, 601, 604, 652, 676, 727, 730, 808, 838, 864, 898, and A–1
Pat Watson Photography
Poughkeepsie, New York

Pages xxiv, 2, 18, 74, 126, 160, 238, 366, 452, 490, 522, 548, 600, 624, 726, 938, and 942
Courtesy of the Visiting Nurse Service of New York
New York, New York

Pages 3, 582, and 939
Pat Watson Photography, in association with the Visiting Nurse Service of New York

Page 696
Courtesy of the American Red Cross
Washington, DC

We gratefully acknowledge the cooperation of the following individuals and their organizations in obtaining photographs:

Lyle Churchill
Vice President for Development
Visiting Nurse Service of New York
New York, New York

Diane Davies, RN, BSN
Director of Patient Services
Ulster Home Health Services, Inc.
Kingston, New York

Patricia S. Stumpf, RN, MS
Director of Public Health Nursing
and
Katherine Graff, RN, MS
Assistant Director of Public Health Nursing
Dutchess County Health Department
Poughkeepsie, New York

Cover Art
Community, by Barry d'Alabama Johnston, is executed in bronze, 17″ by 52″ high, and expresses the idea of interdependency and mutual support. Comprised of eight individuals, one set apart, the sculpture aspires for team enlightenment and excellence. *Community* won First Place in the National Open Sculpture Competition sponsored by Sculpture House in 1989.

CONTRIBUTORS

Norma E. Anderson, RNC, MPH
Associate Professor, Community Health Nursing
St. Louis University School of Nursing
St. Louis, Missouri
From the Community: A Nurse's Voice
"An Unbroken Process of Caring"

Susan M. Basta, RN, MS, MA
Nursing and Health Education Coordinator
University of Cincinnati Area Health Education Center Program
Georgetown, Ohio
Clinical Assistant Professor
College of Nursing and Health
University of Cincinnati
Cincinnati, Ohio
From the Community: A Nurse's Voice
"Just What *Do* You Do?"

Patricia Caudle, RN, DNSC
Lecturer
Philip Y. Hahn School of Nursing
University of San Diego
San Diego, California
Chapters 18, 21

Susan Chen, RN, BSN
Naval Hospital
Oakland, California
Chapter 21

Diane Davies, RN, BSN
Director of Patient Services
Ulster Home Health Services, Inc.
Kingston, New York
From the Community: A Nurse's Voice
"Where My Heart Is"

Susan Grover, RN, PhD
Assistant Professor
Department of Professional Roles/Mental Health Nursing
East Tennessee State University
Johnson City, Tennessee
Chapter 18

Charlene M. Hanson, RN, EdD, FNP-C
Associate Professor of Nursing
Director, Graduate Program in Nursing
Georgia Southern University
Statesboro, Georgia
Chapter 28

Kathleen Heinrich, RN, PhD
Assistant Professor
Philip Y. Hahn School of Nursing
University of San Diego
San Diego, California
Chapter 32

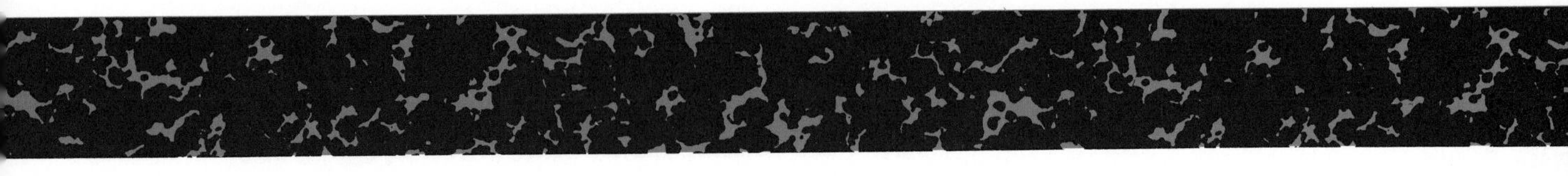

Edward A. Herzog, RNC, MSN
Assistant Professor of Clinical Nursing
College of Nursing and Health
University of Cincinnati
Cincinnati, Ohio
Chapter 22

Maxine B. Jones, RN, DSN
Associate Professor of Nursing
School of Nursing
University of Alabama at Birmingham
Birmingham, Alabama
From the Community: A Nurse's Voice
"We Learn, We Influence"

Brighid Kelly, RNC, PhD
Associate Professor of Nursing
College of Nursing and Health
University of Cincinnati
Cincinnati, Ohio
From the Community: A Nurse's Voice
"Beyond Labels"

Margaret Lockwood, RNC, MSN, EdD
Assistant Professor of Nursing
College of Nursing and Health
University of Cincinnati
Cincinnati, Ohio
From the Community: A Nurse's Voice
"Going the Distance"

Patricia P. Ruff, RN, BSN
Home Health Nurse
Department of Health
The County of Dutchess
Poughkeepsie, New York
From the Community: A Nurse's Voice
"Let Me Tell You a Story . . ."

Margaret Myers Sereda, RN, MSN
Consultant
Home Health Care Education Resources
San Diego, California
Chapter 25

Elizabeth Harper Smith, RN, MSN
Assistant Professor
Department of Professional Roles
East Tennessee State University
Johnson City, Tennessee
Chapter 12

REVIEWERS

Janet Gardner Alexander, RN, MSN
Assistant Professor
School of Nursing
University of Alabama at Birmingham
Birmingham, Alabama

Norma E. Anderson, RNC, MPH
Associate Professor, Community Health Nursing
St. Louis University School of Nursing
St. Louis, Missouri

Susan M. Basta, RN, MS, MA
Nursing and Health Education Coordinator
University of Cincinnati Area Health Education Center Program
Georgetown, Ohio

Clinical Assistant Professor
College of Nursing and Health
University of Cincinnati
Cincinnati, Ohio

Donna M. Behler, RN, MSN, C-FNP
Assistant Professor of Clinical Nursing
Field Service Assistant of Family Medicine
College of Nursing and Health
University of Cincinnati
Cincinnati, Ohio

Nancy J. Brown, RN, PhD
Assistant Professor
Communities and Organizations Division
School of Nursing
University of Colorado
Denver, Colorado

Jean Brim Cahall, RN, MSN, EdD
Associate Professor of Nursing
College of Nursing and Health
University of Cincinnati
Cincinnati, Ohio

Arthur Ree Campbell, RN, EdD
Associate Professor
School of Nursing
University of Alabama at Birmingham
Birmingham, Alabama

Jan E. Christopher, RN, MSN
Instructor
School of Nursing
University of Alabama at Birmingham
Birmingham, Alabama

Helen M. Clark, RNC, PhD
Associate Professor
College of Nursing and Health
University of Cincinnati
Cincinnati, Ohio

Doris B. Clement, RN, MEd, EdD
Faculty
College of Nursing and Health
University of Cincinnati
Cincinnati, Ohio

Linda Sue Davis, RN, PhD
Assistant Professor
College of Nursing and Health
University of Cincinnati
Cincinnati, Ohio

Sandra M. Davis, RN, MSN
Assistant Professor
School of Nursing
University of Alabama at Birmingham
Birmingham, Alabama

Kathleen M. Driscoll, RN, MS, JD
Associate Professor
Interim Department Head, Community Health Nursing
College of Nursing and Health
University of Cincinnati
Cincinnati, Ohio

Janice M. Dyehouse, RN, PhD
Associate Professor
College of Nursing and Health
University of Cincinnati
Cincinnati, Ohio

Evelyn Fitzwater, RNC, MSN
Assistant Professor of Clinical Nursing
College of Nursing and Health
University of Cincinnati
Cincinnati, Ohio

Susan Fraser, RN, MSN, CEN
Staff Nurse, Emergency Department
University Hospital
University of Alabama at Birmingham
Birmingham, Alabama

Mildred L. Hamner, RNC, EdD
Professor
School of Nursing
University of Alabama at Birmingham
Birmingham, Alabama

Edward A. Herzog, RNC, MSN
Assistant Professor of Clinical Nursing
College of Nursing and Health
University of Cincinnati
Cincinnati, Ohio

Maxine B. Jones, RN, DSN
Associate Professor of Nursing
School of Nursing
University of Alabama at Birmingham
Birmingham, Alabama

Brighid Kelly, RNC, PhD
Associate Professor
College of Nursing and Health
University of Cincinnati
Cincinnati, Ohio

Barbara A. Lloyd, RN, EdD
Associate Professor
School of Nursing
University of Alabama at Birmingham
Birmingham, Alabama

Margaret Lockwood, RNC, MSN, EdD
Assistant Professor of Nursing
College of Nursing and Health
University of Cincinnati
Cincinnati, Ohio

Charlene McKaig, RNC, EdD, SNP
Associate Professor, Graduate Programs
School of Nursing
University of Alabama at Birmingham
Birmingham, Alabama

Karen Davidson Newman, DSN, CRNP
Assistant Professor
School of Nursing
University of Alabama at Birmingham
Birmingham, Alabama

Billie R. Rozell, RN, DSN
Associate Professor
School of Nursing
University of Alabama at Birmingham
Birmingham, Alabama

Mary Kirk Wolterman, RN, MSN, EdD
Assistant Professor of Nursing
College of Nursing and Health
University of Cincinnati
Cincinnati, Ohio

CONTENTS IN BRIEF

CONTENTS IN DETAIL

4: Community Health Nursing 54

UNIT TWO: PROCESSES IN COMMUNITY HEALTH NURSING 74

5: The Nursing Process 78

6: The Epidemiologic Process 100

9: The Discharge Planning and Referral Processes 160

10: The Research Process 178

11: The Change, Leadership, and Group Processes 196

14: Ethical Influences on Community Health 264

15: Cultural Influences on Community Health 280

28: Care of Clients in Rural Settings 676

Charlene M. Hanson

29: Care of Clients in Disaster Settings 696

33: Substance Abuse 864

34: Violence 898

UNIT SEVEN: OTHER MODELS FOR COMMUNITY HEALTH NURSING 938

35: Nursing Models for Community Health Practice 942

This book is lovingly dedicated
to my husband Phil and my son Philip,
who provided help and support and
who waited (usually patiently) while I wrote this book,
to my mother
who would have made a good community health nurse, and
to my father
who has learned a lot about community health
in the last few years.

PREFACE

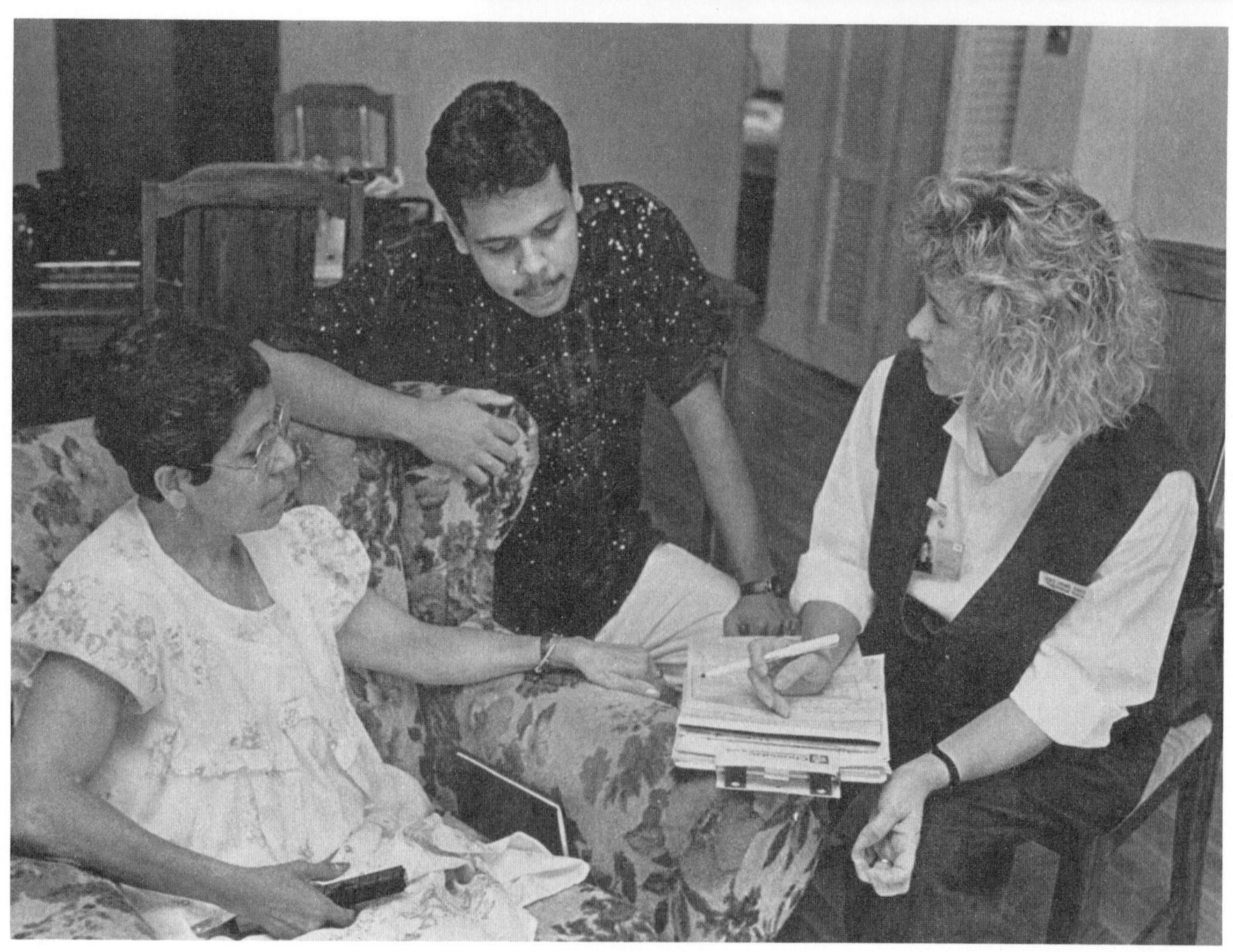

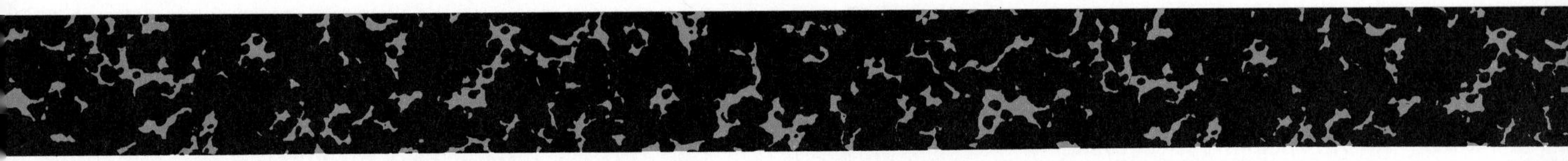

This book is the product of almost 100 years of community health nursing in the United States. 1993 marks the hundredth anniversary of the founding of the Henry Street Settlement, the beginning of modern American community health nursing practice. From 1893 to the present, the work of community health nurses, those famous and those unsung, has led to lasting improvements in the health of individuals, families, and population groups. In this book, my contributors and I have tried to distill the wisdom and expertise of a century of community health nursing practitioners to guide and direct future generations of community health nurses.

Because of the specialty's singular breadth and depth, community health nurses need to have a wide knowledge base. Community health nurses need to know something about everything—from the ethics and economics of health-care resource allocation, to the influence of culture on health, to the best means of promoting health, preventing the spread of communicable diseases, or even dealing with constipation in a newborn. The nurse's knowledge must be theoretically and scientifically sound yet practical and applicable to ever changing professional demands. This book has been written to give students a strong, balanced foundation for community health nursing practice.

Nursing in the Community is intended for use by baccalaureate nursing students in courses related to community health nursing. It is designed to provide a thorough introduction to all aspects of community health nursing, from health promotion to care of existing illness, and from care of individuals and their families to care of population groups. This book is designed to prepare a *nurse generalist* who can function in any setting where community health nurses practice.

THE APPROACH

A unique feature of *Nursing in the Community* is its use of a model designed to facilitate community health nursing practice. This model, the *epidemiologic prevention process model,* incorporates principles of public health science and nursing. The basic framework for practice is the five-step nursing process. Within the nursing process, however, assessment of health needs is based on an epidemiologic perspective derived from G. E. Alan Dever's epidemiologic model of health policy analysis. Dever's model examines health and illness from the perspective of four epidemiologic factors: human biology, environment, life-style, and the health system. In this text, each of these four factors of Dever's model are used to provide a consistent and structured approach to community health nursing assessment.

The second step of the epidemiologic prevention process model is using the diagnostic reasoning process to derive nursing diagnoses related to a client's state of health. This step of the model directs the reader to derive statements of client conditions, both positive and negative, that warrant nursing intervention. Because of the difficulty of adapting nursing diagnoses developed by NANDA or by other groups to community health nursing practice, formalized diagnostic statements have not been used. Readers are encouraged, however, to use the diagnostic reasoning process and derive diagnostic statements that describe a client's health status and contributing factors.

In the epidemiologic prevention process model, the planning, implementation, and evaluation steps of the nursing process are approached from the perspective of the three levels of prevention. Nurses are shown how to plan, implement, and evaluate nursing interventions at the levels of primary, secondary, and tertiary prevention.

The epidemiologic prevention process model is introduced in Chapter 6 and is used in subsequent chapters to structure the discussion of community health nursing practice. Each of the remaining chapters begins with a general discussion of the topic in question followed by presentation of the topic from the perspective of the model. In the chapter on cultural influences on health, for example, general principles of transcultural nursing are discussed. The model is then applied to the tasks of cultural assessment and planning, implementing, and evaluating culturally sensitive community health nursing care.

Through consistent use of the epidemiologic prevention process model, *Nursing in the Community* encourages readers to apply the principles of both public health science and professional nursing to community health nursing practice. The model helps readers to see and understand the melding of these two disciplines that is characteristic of community health nursing and prepares them to use the principles of both in practice.

ORGANIZATION

Nursing in the Community is organized in seven units:

- Contexts
- Processes
- Influences
- Clients
- Settings
- Problems
- Models

The first three units address general concepts related to community health nursing practice, while units four, five, and six examine the practice of community health nursing with specific client groups, in specialized settings, and in solving commonly encountered health problems. The final unit presents other nursing models applicable to community health nursing.

Unit One, The Community Health Nursing Context, examines the historical basis and current dimensions of community health nursing practice. Because the health of groups of people is the underlying purpose of all community health nursing activity, the importance of the community context for community health nursing practice is addressed in the first chapter. Readers are introduced to the concept of communities or population groups, rather than individuals or families, as the recipients of nursing care. The historical development of public health practice and community health nursing are addressed in Chapter 2, and the structure of the American health-care system is described in Chapter 3. The unit concludes by examining the roles and functions performed by community health nurses.

Unit Two, Process and Community Health Nursing, introduces readers to the professional processes most commonly used by community health nurses in their practice. Chapter 5 surveys the nursing process as it applies to community health nursing, whereas Chapter 6 presents fundamental concepts of epidemiology. Both processes are synthesized and then combined with the levels of prevention presented earlier in Chapter 1 to create the epidemiologic prevention process model used throughout the remainder of the book. Chapter 6 concludes with the application of the model to health promotion in the community.

Health education is an important facet of community health nursing practice. Accordingly, readers are introduced to the health education process in Chapter 7. The remaining chapters in Unit Two present other processes essential to community health nursing—the home visit process; the discharge planning and referral processes; the research process; the change, leadership, and group processes; and the political process. Each process is discussed as it specifically applies to community health nursing and in relation to the epidemiologic prevention process model.

In *Unit Three,* Influences on Community Health, readers are introduced to social and environmental factors that influence the health of population groups and the practice of community health nursing. In order to assist clients to gain access to health-care services, for example, community health nurses need to understand mechanisms for financing those services. In Chapter 13, readers are introduced to how economic factors influence health and illness and to various current and projected modes of health-care financing.

Chapter 14 examines the ethics of health-care delivery. Although the modes of ethical decision making presented in the chapter are applicable to ethical dilemmas related to providing nursing care for individuals, families, or groups of people, emphasis is placed on ethics as it relates to the care of population groups, the hallmark of community health nursing.

Culture and the physical environment also significantly influence the health of communities. General principles of transcultural nursing are reviewed in Chapter 15, and the epidemiologic prevention process model is applied to providing community health nursing care to clients from other cultures. Special emphasis is placed on the care of clients from Native

American, Asian, Black, Latino, and Appalachian cultures. Chapter 16 addresses environmental issues of concern in community health and applies the epidemiologic prevention process model to formulating nursing interventions designed to modify adverse environmental effects on health.

In *Unit Four,* Care of Clients, the emphasis shifts from general concepts and principles of community health to the application of those principles to special target populations. In Chapters 17 through 19, readers are guided in applying the epidemiologic prevention process model to the care of individuals, families, and communities or target groups. The remaining chapters in this unit examine the application of the model to the care of children, women, men, the elderly, and the homeless.

Community health nurses practice in almost any setting where health-care services are provided. Although the principles of practice are the same across settings, each setting modifies the way in which these principles are applied. *Unit Five,* Care of Clients in Specialized Settings, examines the use of the epidemiologic prevention process model in providing care to individuals, families, and groups of people in a variety of community health practice settings. Settings addressed include the home, the school, the work setting, the rural setting, and disaster settings.

Community health nurses are confronted by a wide variety of health problems and need a sound knowledge base related to several categories of problems commonly encountered in practice. *Unit Six,* Common Community Health Problems, provides students with background information and nursing interventions related to communicable diseases, chronic physical and mental health problems, substance abuse, and problems of violence.

Finally, some community health nurses might find that other nursing models may be better suited to their style of practice or to a given situation. For this reason, *Unit Seven,* Models for Community Health Nursing, presents several other nursing models adapted for use in community health nursing. The models addressed are those of Roy, Levine, Orem, Johnson, Neuman, and Pender. In Chapter 35, each of the models is applied to the care of individuals, families, and communities.

As noted earlier, the consistent use of a model based on principles of both public health and nursing science unifies the coverage in Units Two through Six. In addition, the book examines several of the processes used in nursing from a distinct community health perspective. Other chapters present in-depth material that may be scantily covered or not addressed in other texts. The chapters on disaster nursing and on care of men, for example, are unique to this book, and the extensive coverage of topics such as cultural influences on health, communicable disease, and both chronic physical and mental health problems provides students with the knowledge needed to function effectively as community health nurses.

SPECIAL FEATURES

Nursing in the Community includes several special features that make it an ideal textbook for baccalaureate nursing students in community health nursing. The book includes numerous tables and boxes that summarize information, highlighting for the reader the critical concepts presented in each chapter. An especially useful feature is the inclusion of resource tables providing names and addresses of agencies where readers can obtain additional information and support on a variety of topics from family violence, to international health, to health program planning.

Nursing in the Community is intended to provide students with a realistic view of community health nursing as it is practiced by real community health nurses. To this end, each unit begins with a feature entitled "From the Community: A Nurse's Voice." Each is a brief "letter from the heart" by a practicing community health nurse concerning his or her profession. Through their thoughts, feelings, and recommendations, the nurses reveal an abiding commitment to community health nursing and the clients they serve.

The breadth of clinical examples used in the text is another feature that assists readers in applying theoretical principles to everyday practice. In each chapter, examples are provided to elucidate the application of community health principles to the care of individuals, families, and population groups. Examples also convey a sense of the breadth of practice, from the care of an abusive family to preventing sexually transmitted diseases, to promoting health in a pregnant woman. Whether a community health course addresses the care of individuals and families or of community aggregates, readers will be able to apply the principles of community health nursing presented in this book.

LEARNING RESOURCES

Nursing in the Community includes a variety of resources designed to facilitate student learning. Each chapter contains:

- Learning objectives
- A topic outline
- Key terms
- Chapter highlights
- Review questions
- An application and synthesis exercise
- References
- Recommended readings
- Numerous boxes and tables

Additional learning resources include a comprehensive index and a series of carefully selected appendices that contain assessment tools for students to use in practice.

The topic outline allows readers to develop an overall picture of a chapter's organization. The outline also facilitates assigning selected portions of chapters prior to a particular class. In addition, the outline and index allow students to rapidly locate specific material for review.

Each chapter is followed by a series of resources that assist students in synthesizing key concepts and applying them to practice. Resources provided at the end of each chapter include *chapter highlights,* a set of review questions, an *application and synthesis* exercise, an extensive reference list, and several recommended readings. The chapter highlights summarize important points and assist students to review the material presented, whereas the review questions are designed to assist students to synthesize chapter concepts for application in practice. Review questions are intended to stimulate thought as well as to review content presented in the chapter.

Application and synthesis exercises offer readers the opportunity to apply the concepts presented in a chapter to a situation that might be encountered in practice. Faculty can use these exercises as a point of departure for class discussion or as a means of evaluating comprehension. Each exercise includes a case description from community health nursing practice and questions focusing on the application of the epidemiologic prevention process model to the situation. Readers are also encouraged to incorporate concepts specific to the chapter topic within the context of the model. Answers to both the application and synthesis questions and the chapter review questions are provided in the instructor's guide that accompanies the text.

Nursing in the Community also includes a set of appendices containing assessment tools that can be used by students in clinical practice. Each tool is adapted to the epidemiologic prevention process model and reflects the principles of community health nursing discussed in the text. Assessment tools are provided for health risk appraisal, health education, the home setting, discharge planning, the school setting, and for the care of individuals, families, communities, target groups, children, adults and the elderly. Each tool provides the initial guidance needed to apply the model and the principles of community health nursing to the actual care of clients. Alternatively, each can serve as the basis for class discussion or clinical learning experiences.

TEACHING SUPPORT

In addition to the teaching support provided within the text itself, *Nursing in the Community* is accompanied by an instructor's guide that will facilitate implementing the text in a variety of community health curricula and maximize student learning. Features of the instructor's guide include:

- An introduction to the use of the guide
- Individual chapter coverage that includes:
  - A complete outline
  - Key terms
  - Learning objectives
  - Suggestions for building lecture notes
  - Answers to review questions
  - Answers to application and synthesis exercises
  - Test questions
- A guide to text appendices and their use
- Transparency masters

The building lecture notes section includes recommendations on points to highlight when presenting content in class as well as suggestions for potential teaching strategies. This assistance should prove helpful to new faculty members and to those nursing educators wanting to explore fresh approaches to familiar topics.

Answers to the application and synthesis questions are provided as a guideline for faculty. The answers provided may stimulate thought or provide a point of departure for a more complex consideration of a case. The answers will also help faculty familiarize themselves with the epidemiologic prevention process model prior to introducing it to students.

Suggestions are also provided for the use of the appendices to facilitate student learning. Assessment tools included in the appendices can be used in conjunction with case studies to facilitate class discussion or in clinical experiences to assist students in applying the epidemiologic prevention process model to actual practice.

The instructor's guide also contains transparency masters of all the figures included in *Nursing in the Community*. These masters are intended to aid faculty in presenting concepts covered in the book.

ACKNOWLEDGMENTS

In writing this book, I have tried to create a text that will serve as a reference for readers both during their community health nursing courses and in the future. It is my hope that this book will induce readers to feel the excitement and enthusiasm for community health that has always been a part of my own practice. A number of people have assisted me in that endeavor, and I would like to take this opportunity to thank:

- William Brottmiller, Executive Editor, Nursing, who had faith in this book
- Linda B. Nold, Nursing Acquisitions Editor, whose enthusiasm led to the creation of the epidemiologic prevention process model
- Mark F. Wales, Nursing Developmental Editor, whose attention to detail, logic, and coherence has made this a much better book
- My contributors, who shared their special expertise and enthusiasm with our readers
- My reviewers, who helped to polish and refine the book to meet the needs of community health nursing students and educators
- Donald P. O'Connor, who is responsible for the book's beautifully executed line art
- The Visiting Nurse Service of New York for their assistance in selecting the wonderful historic photographs that highlight unit and chapter openers
- Wayne Furman, Director of the Office of Special Collections of the New York Public Library, for the use of Lillian Wald's inspirational comments
- Patrick Watson, whose photographs convey the spirit of community health nursing
- The design and production staff at Appleton & Lange for their superlative work in transforming reams of typed pages into a cohesive and attractive book
- All my current and former students, who have taught me as much as I taught them.
- And, most importantly, Phil and Philip, who folded clothes, did the shopping, and generally put their lives on hold while I wrote and rewrote.

Mary Jo Clark

UNIT ONE

The Community Health Nursing Context

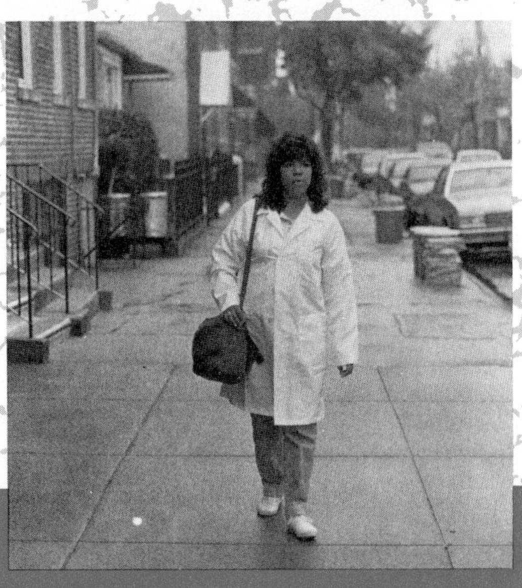

Over the years, community health nurses have been engaged in efforts to improve the health of the public. Frequently, these efforts have been directed toward changes in societal factors detrimental to health. Community health nurses have been crusaders in bringing health care to those most in need. Our history has been one of service and advocacy for underserved populations.

Social and historical influences have shaped our practice and continue to do so. Community health nursing occurs within the context of a health-care system influenced by social factors, past and present. As we will see in Chapter 3, that health-care system has been minimally responsive to the health needs of the total population. Change is needed, and community health nurses can be prime movers in this change.

To bring about change, however, we must understand our client and the needs of our client, as well as the factors that led to the current health-care crisis. For community health nurses, the *client* is a group of people or a community, and our goal is to improve the health of the total population. Communities are defined by characteristics reflecting collective action for the common good. Community health nurses guide that action toward a common goal of optimal health for the group and its members.

The historical overview provided in Chapter 2 traces the development of concern for the health of population groups that is the focus of community health. It also presents major historical events influencing the development of the health-care system, community health, and community health nursing practice. In knowing where we have been and how we got there, we can profit by past successes and failures to improve health status and health-care delivery. It is hoped that by identifying past mistakes we can avoid similar mistakes in the future. We can also identify factors that have promoted population health and learn to capitalize on these factors. Through an understanding of both positive and negative influences on health, we can pinpoint those societal forces that can, and should, be manipulated to gain our ultimate goal—better health for all people.

Community health nursing occurs in the context of a health-care delivery system plagued by inequity, inefficiency, and lack of response to societal needs. Working within this system, community health nurses can initiate changes that promote quality health care for all. To do so, however, we need to understand the current system and identify areas where change is needed. Exploration of the organization, focus, and function of various components of the health-care system provides that understanding. Armed with this knowledge, we can engage in systematic efforts to initiate change.

In this unit we will set the stage for our exploration of community health nursing as a unique field of nursing practice. We begin in Chapter 1 by defining our clientele, the community, and our goal—namely community health. In Chapter 2 we explore the historical influences on community health and community health nursing. Then, in Chapter 3, we will examine the health-care system in which we practice. These three chapters create the context in which community health nursing occurs. The unit culminates with an introduction to community health nursing, defining the field and exploring the roles and functions performed by community health nurses.

From the Community: A Nurse's Voice

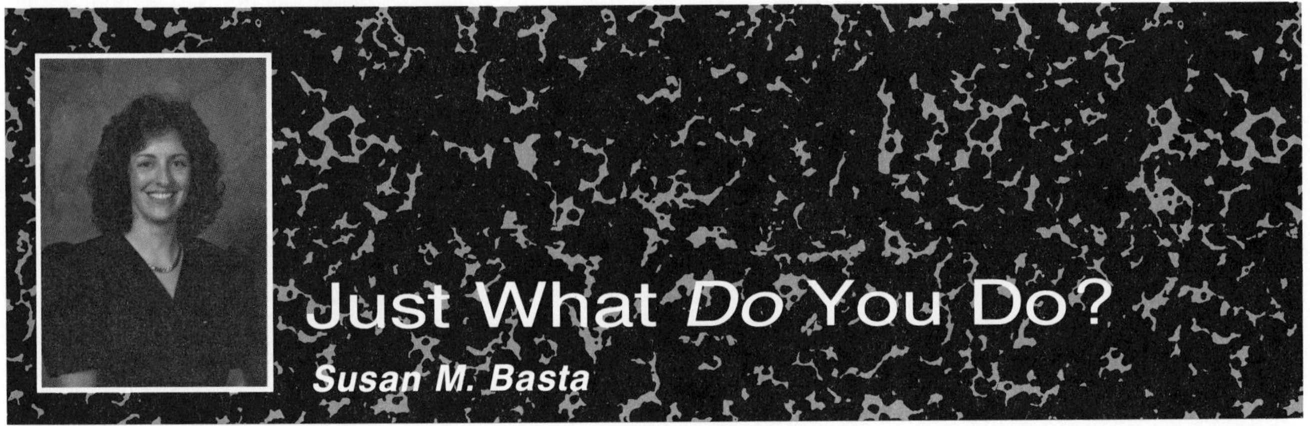

Just What *Do* You Do?

Susan M. Basta

The woman on the other end of the telephone line, who happened to be my mother, was saying, "I was talking with your grandmother the other day, and had trouble explaining what you do at work. Just what *do* you do?" I really couldn't blame her for not knowing, because I realized that my job is very different from the "typical" nursing position as perceived by the public.

As a community health nurse employed by a university-based area health education center and practicing in a rural region, I generally have whole communities or groups, rather than individuals, as my clients. And I see a great deal of diversity in the people whom I serve, the settings in which I practice, and in my nursing roles.

In my current position I have worked with school-aged children, adolescents, and adults of all ages. I've been involved with children in the local 4-H program, farmers, displaced homemakers, and community-based ambulatory older adults. I've been asked to conduct programs at summer camps, in public schools, at a community-action agency, and in senior citizen nutrition centers.

I would be hard pressed to describe my "typical" day, because I don't really have typical days at work! My daily roles can include teaching older adults about various aspects of health promotion; writing grant proposals for new projects; organizing a teen sexuality and pregnancy prevention training workshop for local school teachers; and coordinating a consortium of local agency representatives that is devising a county plan for health promotion/disease prevention in accordance with the *Year 2000 Health Objectives for the Nation.*

All of this diversity has, in one sense, shaped my identity as a nursing *generalist* rather than a *specialist.* Yet I do specialize in one activity and philosophy that is a constant in my practice: *prevention.* The "apples and oranges" character of my job can, at times, be overwhelming. But my position is also challenging and rewarding, and I seldom—if ever—feel as if I'm in a professional rut!

CHAPTER 1

The Community Context

KEY TERMS

aggregates
community
community health
community of interest-orientation
community of problem ecology
community of solution
feeling community
geopolitical communities
group orientation
health promotion
levels of health care
levels of prevention
prevention of disease
preventive medicine
primary prevention
public health practice
relational-bond communities
secondary prevention
territorial-bond communities
tertiary prevention
therapeutic medicine

This book is about community health nursing. That does not mean, though, that we are going to dwell exclusively on the practice of nursing in community settings as opposed to hospitals or other institutions. When we talk about the "community context" of community health nursing, we mean that our primary client is the community itself rather than its individual members.

Sometimes our practice involves care to individuals and families within the community, but our primary focus is improving the health of the total population group. We want to create healthy communities. When we say that the community is our client, what does this mean? What exactly is a "community"? How can we tell if a community is healthy or unhealthy? What kind of activities will result in a healthy community? The answers to these and similar questions are the focus of this chapter.

LEARNING OBJECTIVES

After reading this chapter you should be able to:

- Describe three critical attributes that define a community.
- Distinguish between communities with territorial bonds and those with relational bonds.
- Differentiate among the goals of therapeutic medicine, preventive medicine, and public health practice.
- Discuss the significance of the National Health Objectives.
- Describe the three levels of prevention related to community health.
- Discuss the relationship of the levels of prevention to the National Health Objectives for the Year 2000.
- Discuss five categories of intervention designed to promote community health and prevent illness.

DEFINING COMMUNITY

There are many definitions of community. Some definitions focus on functions performed by communities. For example, a community has been defined as "a system of formal and informal groups characterized by interdependence and whose function is to meet the collective needs of group members."[1] Another functional definition described communities as "wherever the needs of the individual are being met."[2]

Other definitions use locale as the basis for community. For instance, a community is defined as "a social system, a place, and a people."[3] Community is also defined operationally as a group of people in a specific time and place who have a common purpose, the "who," "where and when," and "why and how" of community.[4]

The use of place as a defining attribute for community is somewhat problematic, though, if we wish to address certain groups of people as communities. Certainly it would be impractical to consider the aspect of place in defining military veterans as a community, yet we can apply principles of community health to meet the health needs of this group.

In some definitions, the focal point is the existence of commonalities among members of the community. A community has been referred to as "a collection of people who share some important features of their lives." Similarly, a community has been defined as "a social unit in which there is a transaction of a common life among the people making up the unit."[5] Other authors take the more eclectic view that community can be "defined either in terms of geography or special interests."[6]

CRITICAL ATTRIBUTES OF COMMUNITIES

Despite the diversity in definitions of community, analyzing the previous examples reveals certain common elements. These elements are a group orientation, a bond between individuals, and human interaction. These three elements are the critical attributes that define a group of people as a community.

GROUP ORIENTATION

Humans form communities because it is advantageous to do so. Through group membership, an individual gains access to skills, services, necessities, and amenities of life that one cannot provide on one's own. For the community to continue to provide these services, it must safeguard its survival. For this reason, communities adopt a ***group orientation*** in which the goals of the group take priority over those of individual members. Because of this group orientation, communities take collective action in regard to common concerns. For example, it may be to an individual's advantage to speed through town. However, it is not in the interest of the local residents and their children who may have to cross busy streets. Through collective action, in the interest of the overall good, the community acts to erect a stoplight at the intersection, slowing traffic and ensuring safe crossing for all citizens.

BOND BETWEEN INDIVIDUALS

The second defining attribute of a community is some form of bond between individual members. This bond may take many forms. In some communities, the bond is a life-style held in common. The bond may be shared ethnicity or culture, or the fact of living in a specific geographic location. In other instances, the bond assumes the form of similar interests, goals, or occupations. As we will see later, the type of bond between members determines the type of community that exists.

HUMAN INTERACTION

The third critical attribute of a community is some type of human interaction. There must be significant social interaction between individuals in order for a community to exist. To illustrate, a number of people may live side by side in an apartment building. They have a bond in their way of life as apartment dwellers and in their common residence, but they cannot be considered a community unless there is some form of social interaction between them. Without social interaction they remain a collection of isolated individuals rather than a community. Such interaction might include visiting back and forth, cooperative babysitting, or unified action on some common grievance.

A WORKING DEFINITION OF COMMUNITY

Bearing in mind these critical attributes of communities, the following definition can be derived for use in community health nursing. A ***community*** is a group of people who share some type of bond, who engage in interaction with each other, and who function collectively regarding common concerns.

Using this definition, a variety of groups or aggregates encountered by community health nurses can be viewed as "communities." ***Aggregates*** are groups of people with some characteristic in common. Aggregates may or may not be communities depending on the presence of the defining attributes. For example, all the people in town with arthritis constitute an aggregate. They have a common bond in their shared disease, but, because they do not interact with each other or take collective action on common concerns, they are not a community. However, if they form an association to work for handicapped access to public buildings, the aggregate becomes a community. The activities of community health nurses are not confined to a specific locale but are directed to any group or aggregate with health needs.

Our working definition of community also helps to decrease a frequently encountered tendency to define community health nursing responsibility in terms of specific cases. The entity served by the community health nurse is the total group or aggregate, not just those individuals or families referred for services.

TYPES OF COMMUNITIES

As mentioned previously, the type of bond between group members is a major determinant of the type of community. Two basic categories of bonds unite communities—territorial bonds and relational bonds.

COMMUNITIES WITH TERRITORIAL BONDS

Territorial-bond communities are those with specifically defined boundaries that may be either spatial or temporal, or both. Such bonds reflect the "where" and "when" dimension of the definition of community discussed earlier. Inmates of a county jail, their jailers, and ancillary personnel would be a community bound by specific spatial boundaries, namely the walls of the jail. Likewise, the graduates of Nurse University from 1975 to 1990 comprise a community bound by time relationships. The boundary here excludes graduates from Nurse University prior to 1975, graduates of the class of 1991, and graduates from other programs.

Several subtypes of communities exist within the territorial-bond category. These include geopolitical communities, communities of problem ecology, and communities of solution.

GEOPOLITICAL COMMUNITIES

Geopolitical communities are probably most familiar to us and are communities with defined geographic and jurisdictional boundaries such as towns, cities, counties, and so on. A city is defined by its boundaries, the city limits. One either lives within the city limits or one does not, so it is easy to decide whether or not one is a member of that particular community. A school of nursing could also be considered a geopolitical community because it typically has specific physical boundaries as well as enrollment boundaries.

COMMUNITIES OF PROBLEM ECOLOGY

The second and third types of territorial-bond communities are not quite so well defined in terms of specific boundaries but are closely related to each other. A ***community of problem ecology*** is the locale within which a particular problem exists. We are using the word *ecology* here in terms of the interrelated factors that contribute to a health problem rather than in its usual meaning related to the natural environment. A community of problem ecology would be the area that encompasses any type of health problem and its contributing factors. This type of community frequently cuts across territorial bounds of one or more geopolitical communities. For example, pollution of a river may arise from chemicals dumped by an industry in one state but affect drinking water in a large city in another state. The area in which the problem and its contributing factors exist is the community of problem ecology, and in this case it includes both states.

COMMUNITIES OF SOLUTION

The ***community of solution*** is the area in which the resources necessary to solve a problem are found. As with the community of problem ecology, the community of solution does not always coincide with the boundaries of a specific geopolitical community. It may coincide with the community of problem ecology, but frequently does not. In the case of the polluted river, the solution may not lie within the affected area but may require the assistance of the federal Environmental Protection Agency (EPA) and the federal courts.

Figure 1–1 represents the three types of territorial-bond communities for the water pollution example. The areas bounded by solid lines in the figure represent four geopolitical communities, in this instance four neighboring states. City C is also a geopolitical community. The broken line encompasses the portions of two states involved in the water pollution problem. This area constitutes the community of problem ecology for *this* problem. The dark area represents the community of solution or the area in which the resources necessary to solve the problem are to be found. In this instance, the community of solution goes beyond the boundaries of the states affected by the problem and involves the federal government.

COMMUNITIES WITH RELATIONAL BONDS

The second major category of communities, ***relational-bond communities,*** includes groups in which the bond between individuals exists in the form of a

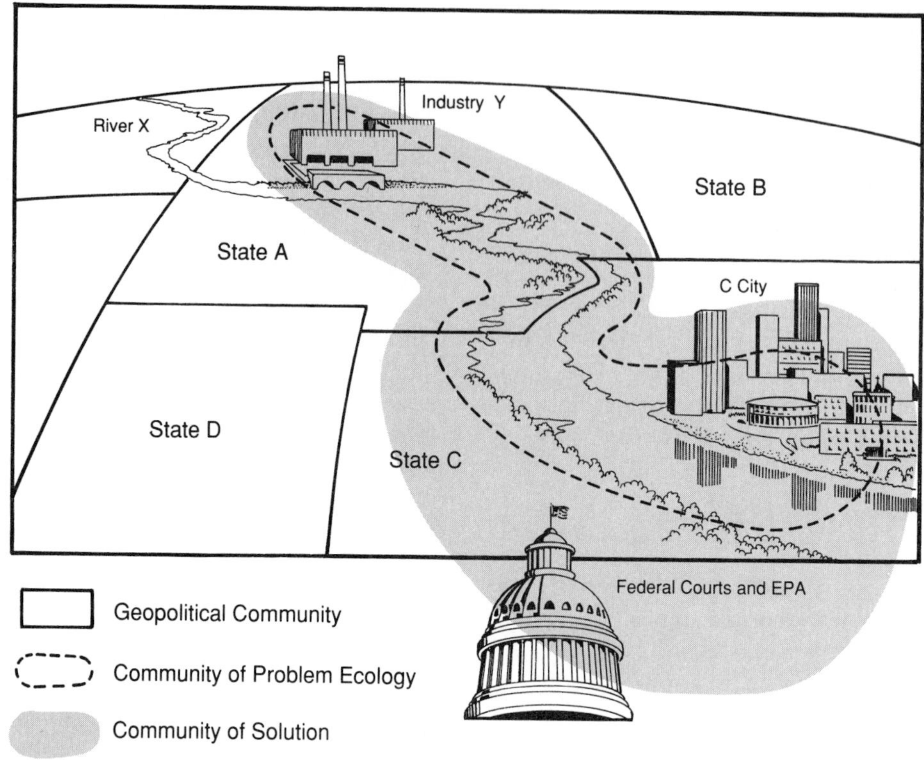

Figure 1–1. The relationship among geopolitical communities, a community of problem ecology, and a community of solution.

common relationship rather than specific boundaries. There are two types of relational-bond communities—communities of interest-orientation and feeling communities.

COMMUNITIES OF INTEREST-ORIENTATION

In the *community of interest-orientation,* the relational bond is one of shared interests or goals. Examples of this type of community could be a professional organization such as the state nurses' association, an ostomy support group, or a right to life group. In each instance, members of the group share a common interest or concern, and they use the group as a means of advancing that interest.

FEELING COMMUNITIES

A *feeling community* is one in which the relational bond is an emotional feeling of belonging or camaraderie. One feels at home in one's "neighborhood" or with one's own ethnic group. This is the community in which one has "roots." Your nursing class may be an example of a feeling community. Members of the class are bound together by certain emotional ties or feelings of closeness that arise from shared experiences.

None of the types of communities discussed here are mutually exclusive. Any group may simultaneously represent more than one type of community. Take, for example, members of your own nursing class. Certainly you are all part of a community of interest-orientation with a common interest in nursing and, more specifically, in graduating from nursing school. At the same time, you are part of a feeling community with emotional attachments resulting from shared experiences. You are also part of a geopolitical community that has specific spatial and temporal boundaries.

DEFINING COMMUNITY HEALTH

The goal of nursing in any form is to maintain or improve the health of the client. In community health nursing, the primary client is the community itself. What does the health of a community entail? What is "community health"?

Health "implies maintaining a balance between the demands on us as biologically delimited, socially created beings and our capacity to meet them individually and collectively."[7] The health status of a community is a composite of the health of individuals, families, and groups that comprise the community. Community health, however, is not just the sum of the health status of all community members. More than this, there is an aspect of community health that relates to the community as a unique entity, a totality in itself.

What are the health problems of the community as a whole? Obviously, problems for the community at large will also be problematic for certain members of the community. However, the reverse is not necessarily true. While arthritis, for example, may be a problem for some individuals, it may not pose a problem for the entire community. In community health one focuses on the health status of a group of people as a collective entity rather than as individuals.

A decided shift is evident in definitions of community or public health over the last few decades. In 1923 community health was defined in terms of longevity and absence of disease.[8] More recently, community health has been defined as "the common attainment of the highest level of physical, mental, and social well-being consistent with available knowledge and resources at a given time and place"[9] or as successful adaptation to the environment that allows people to live a life relatively free of disease and to achieve successfully their "biological, psychological, and chronological potential."[10]

Community health has also been viewed as competence in carrying out community responsibilities.[1] Florence Nightingale[11] defined health as "not only to be well, but to use well every power that we have." This definition can be applied both to communities and to individuals. A healthy community, then, is one that uses well its powers for the benefit of its members.

In comparing these definitions of community health, one notes a subtle change in emphasis. Earlier definitions dealt with preventing disease and prolonging life, while later ones speak first of attaining the highest possible level of well-being. Outside of nursing, there has been a change in focus over the years from preventing specific diseases to enhancing the quality of life and a greater tendency to deal with death as a part of life. As demonstrated by Florence Nightingale's definition, nursing has always focused on high-level wellness. Given the current emphasis on wellness, ***community health*** can be defined as the attainment of the greatest possible biological, psychological, and social well-being of the community as an entity and its individual members.

A healthy community displays evidence of biological, psychological, and social well-being in itself. For example, a healthy community is economically stable, unpolluted, and is able to provide for the needs of its members at adequate levels. In addition, individual members of the community are able to achieve their greatest physical, mental, and social potential.

GOALS OF COMMUNITY HEALTH PRACTICE

Therapeutic medicine, preventive medicine, and public health practice differ in terms of their respective goals.[9] ***Therapeutic medicine*** is aimed at diagnosing and treating disease. ***Preventive medicine*** consists of three aspects: (1) preventing disease by biological means (for example, through immunizations, vitamins, etc.); (2) preventing consequences of preventable or treatable chronic diseases (for example, preventing complications of syphilis through early diagnosis and treatment); and (3) preventing consequences of nonpreventable and noncurable diseases (for example, preventing contractures in arthritic clients). Both therapeutic and preventive medicine have a negatively stated goal, namely absence of disease.

Public health practice, on the other hand, has as its goal the promotion of health and the development of maximum potential of individuals, families, and communities. Recently the Institute of Medicine[12] stated the goal of public health practice as "assuring conditions in which people can be healthy."

The goal of public health practice was delineated more specifically in several objectives for improving the health of Americans by the year 1990. These objectives were established in 1980 in the publication *Promoting Health/Preventing Disease: Objectives for the Nation*[13] and relate to areas of preventive health services, health protection, and health promotion. A subsequent set of national health objectives has been established with a target date for the year 2000.[14] Objectives for preventive health services include those related to hypertension control, family planning, pregnancy and infant health, immunization, and sexually transmitted diseases. Health protection objectives deal with toxic agent control, occupational safety and health, accident prevention and injury control, surveillance and control of infectious diseases, and fluoridation and dental health. Objectives in the area of health promotion relate to smoking and health, misuse of alcohol and drugs, physical fitness and exercise, control of stress and violent behavior, and nutrition. Finally, several additional objectives were established dealing with disability, birth defects, and death.

Within each subcategory of national objectives are objectives related to improvement of health status, reduction of relevant risk factors, and increased public and professional awareness of health problems. Also included are objectives dealing with improvement of services and protective activities and improvement or establishment of surveillance and evaluation systems. In later chapters of this book we will address specific objectives among those set for 1990 and discuss the extent to which they have been achieved.

LEVELS OF HEALTH CARE

The national goals noted above can be achieved through health care at four distinct levels. The four ***levels of health care*** are health promotion, disease prevention, diagnosis and treatment, and rehabilitation. National health goals will be achieved primarily through activity at the first two levels, promotion and prevention.

HEALTH PROMOTION

The first level of health care, that of ***health promotion,*** involves activities designed to improve or maintain health status. Examples of health promotive activities with individual clients may include ensuring adequate rest for a toddler, designing an exercise program for a mother, or enhancing the self-image of an adolescent. The family as a unit may be the recipient of health promotion measures in the form of education for parenting, whereas health promotion activities for the community as client might include provision of well-child and family planning services and educational programs related to basic nutrition or physical fitness. As noted earlier, a number of national objectives are related specifically to health promotion. These include objectives for enhancing childhood growth and development, retention of natural teeth, and physical fitness and exercise.

DISEASE PREVENTION

The second level of health care includes specific measures aimed at the ***prevention of disease*** or disability. Immunizing a child is an example of preventive health care for an individual client. In working with families, providing a support group for teenage parents may be a preventive measure that will decrease the potential for child abuse. At the community level, prevention could take the form of fluoridation of the community water supply. As has already been mentioned, the majority of the national health status objectives reflect the preventive level of health care.

DIAGNOSIS AND TREATMENT

At the diagnosis and treatment (restoration) level of health care, the emphasis is on early recognition of and therapy for health problems that have occurred. Previously, diagnosis and treatment were areas left almost exclusively to the realm of therapeutic medicine. Now, however, diagnosis and treatment are becoming part of community health practice, although both receive far less emphasis than do the two previous levels of health care. Treatment of an adolescent for sexually transmitted disease is an example of this level of health care directed toward the individual. With families, providing counseling for marital problems may be considered treatment, while providing access to contraceptive services may be used to "treat" the problem of teenage pregnancy at the community level. The national health objective related to control of hypertension is another example of activity at this level of health care.

REHABILITATION

The fourth level of health care, rehabilitation, involves attempts to limit the incapacitation caused by health problems and to prevent recurrences. Assisting the arthritic individual to prevent contractures is an example of a rehabilitative activity. Similarly, the family may be assisted in dealing with chronic debilitation of the primary wage earner. Finally, the community may be "rehabilitated" through plans to provide services to children born to teenage parents thereby preventing further health problems in the population. Few of the national health status objectives reflect this level of health care; this is because promotion and prevention of health problems are the desired goals, as opposed to dealing with problems once they develop.

LEVELS OF PREVENTION

The four levels of health care focus on all aspects of health-care delivery. The intent at the first two levels is the promotion of health and the prevention of illness. At the third and fourth levels, the intent is to prevent serious consequences arising from health problems that cannot, in themselves, be prevented. The focus in community health practice, however, remains on prevention. This focus provides the basis for the three ***levels of prevention***—primary, secondary, and tertiary—emphasized in community health practice.[15]

PRIMARY PREVENTION

Primary prevention was defined by the originators of the term as "measures designed to promote general

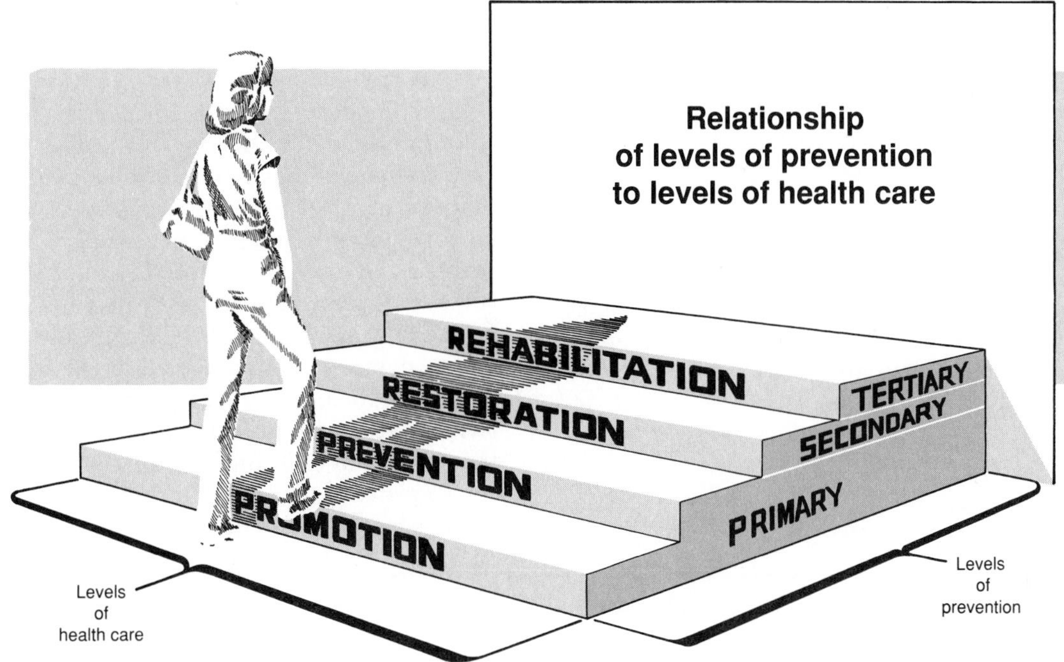

Figure 1–2. Relationship of primary, secondary, and tertiary prevention to levels of health care.

optimum health or . . . the specific protection of man against disease agents."[16] Primary prevention is action taken to prevent the occurrence of health problems and encompasses activities related to the first two levels of health care—health promotion and disease prevention. Primary prevention activities might focus on the health of individuals, families, and groups or communities; these activities occur prior to the onset of a problem. Eating nutritious foods and having routine immunizations are both examples of primary prevention.

SECONDARY PREVENTION

Secondary prevention focuses on the early identification and treatment of existing health problems[16] and occurs after the health problem has arisen. In community health practice at this stage, the primary emphasis is on preventing serious consequences of the problem, whenever the problem itself has not been prevented. Secondary prevention encompasses those activities involved in the third level of health care—the diagnosis and treatment level. Screening for glaucoma is an example of secondary prevention. Secondary prevention would also include the actual diagnosis and treatment of a person with glaucoma.

TERTIARY PREVENTION

Tertiary prevention is activity aimed at returning the client to the highest level of function possible following the occurrence and correction of a health problem.[15] In community health nursing, tertiary prevention also focuses on preventing recurrences of the problem. Tertiary prevention correlates with the fourth, or rehabilitative, level of health care. For example, placing a client on a maintenance diet after the loss of a desired number of pounds constitutes tertiary prevention. The levels of prevention and their relationship to the four levels of health care are depicted in Figure 1–2.

A particular nursing intervention may be viewed as a primary, secondary, or tertiary preventive measure in terms of its relationship to the occurrence of a problem. Take, for example, nutrition education as a particular nursing intervention. Nutrition education is a primary preventive measure when the nurse is teaching concepts of good nutrition in an effort to promote health and prevent overweight. The intervention is employed prior to the occurrence of a problem. Nutrition education for the client who is already overweight is a secondary preventive measure. The problem has already occurred and the education program is designed to help the client lose weight. Nutrition education may also be a tertiary preventive measure when the client goes on a "maintenance diet" after the weight loss has occurred.

HEALTH INTERVENTION

The developers of the national objectives for health promotion and disease prevention suggested five categories of promotion and prevention measures that would lead to the achievement of the objectives. These measures include education and information; service; technologic; legislative and regulatory; and economic measures.

EDUCATION AND INFORMATION MEASURES

Education and information measures involve education and counseling of individuals, families, groups, and the general public to promote health and prevent illness. National campaigns to educate the public on the hazards of smoking or high cholesterol levels are examples of such measures. The federal government's recent mass mailing of information on AIDS to all homes in the country is one example of a measure to inform and educate the public regarding health matters.

SERVICE MEASURES

The category of service measures includes efforts to provide access to health-care services needed to promote health and to prevent illness. Past federal subsidizing of immunization services, family planning services, emergency care, and so on are examples of service measures. Other attempts to provide access to care include the initiation of the National Health Service in 1979. This program is intended to meet the needs of underserved areas of the country for health-care providers.

TECHNOLOGIC MEASURES

Technologic measures are those that employ the use of scientific technology in health promotion and illness prevention. Efforts to develop a vaccine to prevent AIDS and the work done on various forms of contraceptives are examples of technologic measures to prevent health problems. Similarly, use of a condom is a technologic measure designed to prevent both pregnancy and sexually transmitted diseases.

LEGISLATIVE AND REGULATORY MEASURES

Legislation and regulation can also serve as measures to promote health and prevent illness. In this case, laws are passed that mandate behaviors or conditions that enhance health or prevent illness. For example, laws regulating professional medical and nursing practice are intended to protect the public from incompetent practitioners. In the same way, legislation mandating seat belt use are intended to limit injuries in the event of motor vehicle accidents. Other examples of such measures are statutes regulating food substances and medications, environmental conditions, and safety in the workplace.

Legislative and regulatory measures may also be used to enhance service measures. For example, in 1973, Congress passed the Health Maintenance Organization Act to provide funds for the development of health maintenance organizations and, thereby, increase access to care for underserved populations. Legislation at both the federal and state level has also provided funds for maternal-child services, mental health facilities, emergency services, and so forth.

ECONOMIC MEASURES

Economic measures are those that use economic incentives and sanctions to motivate healthy behavior. For example, high taxes on cigarettes in Great Britain have contributed to a decline in the number of people who smoke. Similarly, reduced life insurance rates for nonsmokers may motivate some persons to quit smoking.

Activities in each of the above five categories can result in the promotion of health and prevention of

TABLE 1–1. CATEGORIES OF HEALTH INTERVENTION

Intervention Measure	Effect
1. Education and information	Acquaints people with healthy behaviors
2. Services	Provides access to needed health-care services
3. Technologic	Uses scientific technology to protect and promote health
4. Legislative and regulatory	Mandates healthy behavior and promotes a safe and healthful environment
5. Economic	Uses financial incentives and penalties to motivate healthy behavior

illness, the major foci of community health practice. Efforts thus far have contributed to partial achievement of the national health objectives for 1990 and can contribute to accomplishment of the objectives for the year 2000 as well. Categories of health-care interventions are summarized in Table 1–1. Involvement of community health nurses in these activities will be described throughout this book.

CHAPTER HIGHLIGHTS

- A community is a group of people characterized by some type of bond, interaction, and collective activity regarding common concerns.
- Communities differ in terms of the type of bond between members. The two major categories of communities are territorial-bond and relational-bond communities.
- Territorial-bond communities are of three types: (1) geopolitical communities with specific temporal or spatial boundaries, (2) communities of problem ecology or the locale in which a problem exists, and (3) communities of solution in which are found the resources needed to resolve a problem.
- Relational-bond communities include communities of interest-orientation in which members are bound by a shared interest, and feeling communities where the bond is an emotional attachment.
- The health status of a community is both separate from and greater than the health status of its members. Community health is the attainment of the highest possible biological, psychological, and social well-being of the community as an entity and of the individual members of that community.
- The goals of community health practice differ from those of therapeutic and preventive medicine in that they are positively stated to reflect health promotion rather than disease prevention.
- Health care takes place at four levels: health promotion, disease prevention, diagnosis and treatment, and rehabilitation. These four levels of health care are translated into three levels of preventive activity: primary, secondary, and tertiary prevention.
- Primary prevention takes place before a health problem occurs and may take the form of health promotion or disease prevention. Secondary prevention involves action during the acute stage of a problem and includes diagnosis and treatment, whereas tertiary prevention is aimed at rehabilitation and preventing a recurrence of the problem.
- Health promotion can take place via education and information measures, service measures, technologic measures, legislative and regulatory measures, or economic measures.

Review Questions

1. What are the three critical attributes that define a group of people as a community? Give an example of each. (p. 8)
2. Distinguish between communities with territorial bonds and those with relational bonds. Give examples of each type of community. (pp. 9–10)
3. How do the goals of public health practice differ from those of therapeutic medicine and preventive medicine? (p. 11)
4. What is the significance of the National Health Objectives? (p. 11)
5. What are the three levels of prevention in community health practice? Give examples of each related to the health of individuals, families, and communities. (pp. 12–14)
6. What is the relationship between the levels of prevention and the National Health Objectives for the Year 2000? (pp. 12–13)
7. What are the five categories of health interventions designed to promote community health and prevent illness? Give an example of a nursing activity related to each. (p. 14)

APPLICATION AND SYNTHESIS

Over the years, several people who have become disenchanted with the modern world have relocated to a small valley in the hills of Tennessee. Residents of the surrounding towns refer to this valley as "Hermit Hollow." The people who live there each raise their own fruits and vegetables in small gardens. Many of them make craft items to trade for other items they need in the nearby towns. The "hermits" are relatively solitary individuals and rarely speak to each other. In fact, they tend to build their cabins so that they can neither see nor be seen by their neighbors. Each family tends to its own concerns and works to meet the needs of family members.

If assistance is needed (that is, medical care), it is usually sought outside the valley in one of the surrounding towns. Recently, when flooding threatened the homes in the valley, residents packed up their valuables and family members to stay with friends or family outside the area. There are no schools, churches, or stores in the valley itself. Those families that do not educate their children themselves take them to school in one of the surrounding towns.

A number of health problems are common to residents of the valley. These include pinworms and anemia in the children, and tetanus among the working adults (particularly men working in the gardens). Many adults are also obese and have hypertension.

1. Would you consider the residents of Hermit Hollow a community? Why?
2. If Hermit Hollow constitutes a community, what type(s) of community does it represent? If it is not a community, what critical attributes would be needed to view this group of people as a community? If these attributes were present, what type(s) of community would you have?
3. What types of primary, secondary, and tertiary preventive measures would be appropriate for this group of people? Why?

REFERENCES

1. Goeppinger, J., Lassiter, P. G., & Wilcox, B. (1982). Community health is community competence. *Nursing Outlook, 30,* 464–467.
2. Wigley, R., & Cook, J. R. (1975). *Community health: Concepts and issues.* New York: D. Van Nostrand.
3. Josten, L. E. (1989). Wanted: Leaders for public health. *Nursing Outlook, 37,* 230–232.
4. Shamansky, S., & Pesznecker, B. (1981). A community is . . . *Nursing Outlook, 29,* 182–185.
5. Green, L. W., & Anderson, C. L. (1986). *Community health.* St. Louis: Times Mirror/Mosby.
6. Williams, C. A. (1988). Population-focused practice. In M. Stanhope & J. Lancaster (Eds.), *Community health nursing: Process and practice for promoting health* (2nd. ed.). St. Louis: C. V. Mosby.
7. Milio, N. (1983). *Primary care and the public's health: Judging impacts, goals, and policies.* Lexington, MA: Lexington Books.
8. Winslow, C. E. (1923). *The evolution and significance of the modern public health campaign.* New Haven, CT: Yale University Press.
9. Hanlon, J. J., & Pickett, G. E. (1984). *Public health: Administration and practice* (8th ed.). St. Louis: Times Mirror/Mosby.
10. Banta, J. E. (1979). Definition of community health. In *Community health for today and tomorrow.* New York: National League for Nursing.
11. Nightingale, F. (1860). *Notes on nursing: What it is and what it is not.* London: Harrison.
12. Institute of Medicine. (1988). *The future of public health.* Washington, DC: National Academy Press.
13. United States Department of Health and Human Services. (1980). *Promoting health/preventing disease: Objectives for the nation.* Washington, DC: Government Printing Office.

14. United States Department of Health and Human Services. (1990). *Healthy people 2000: National health promotion and disease prevention.* Washington, DC: Government Printing Office.
15. Shamansky, S., & Clausen, C. (1980). Levels of prevention: Examination of the concept. *Nursing Outlook, 28,* 104–108.
16. Leavell, H. R., et al. (1965). *Preventive medicine for the doctor in his community* (3rd ed.). New York: McGraw-Hill.

RECOMMENDED READINGS

Archer, S. E. (1982). Synthesis of public health science and nursing science. *Nursing Outlook, 30,* 442–446.

Discusses the aspects of public health science that should be included in baccalaureate nursing programs to produce graduates able to function as community health nurses and to go on to graduate study. Also addresses the need for synthesis of public health and nursing content into a unified whole to form a basis for community health nursing practice.

Salmon, M. E. (1989). Public health nursing: The neglected specialty. *Nursing Outlook, 37,* 226–229.

Focuses on potential conflict of values between public health practice and nursing and the problems inherent in preparing nurses for community health practice due to these value conflicts. Also details the changes that are needed in nursing education to prepare public health leaders.

Schultz, P. R. (1987). Clarifying the concept of "client" for health care policy formation: Ethical implications. *Family and Community Health, 10*(1), 73–82.

Stresses the importance of redefining client in terms of groups of people so as to deal adequately with "ethical dilemmas of the aggregate." Differentiates between aggregates and groups and addresses ethical decision making related to population groups.

Schultz, P. R. (1987). When client means more than one: Extending the foundational concept of person. *Advances in Nursing Science, 10*(1), 71–86.

Examines the nursing concept of person in the light of aggregate groups that are the client for such nursing specialty areas as community health and nursing administration. Addresses the concept of aggregate in the light of related concepts such as family, group, and community and in its relationship to the other components of the nursing paradigm—environment, health, and nursing.

Shirreffs, J. H. (1982). *Community health: Contemporary perspectives.* Englewood Cliffs, NJ: Prentice-Hall.

Presents an overview of community health practice including its social, epidemiological, and organizational foundations. Also addresses contemporary challenges for community health in the context of the health-care delivery system.

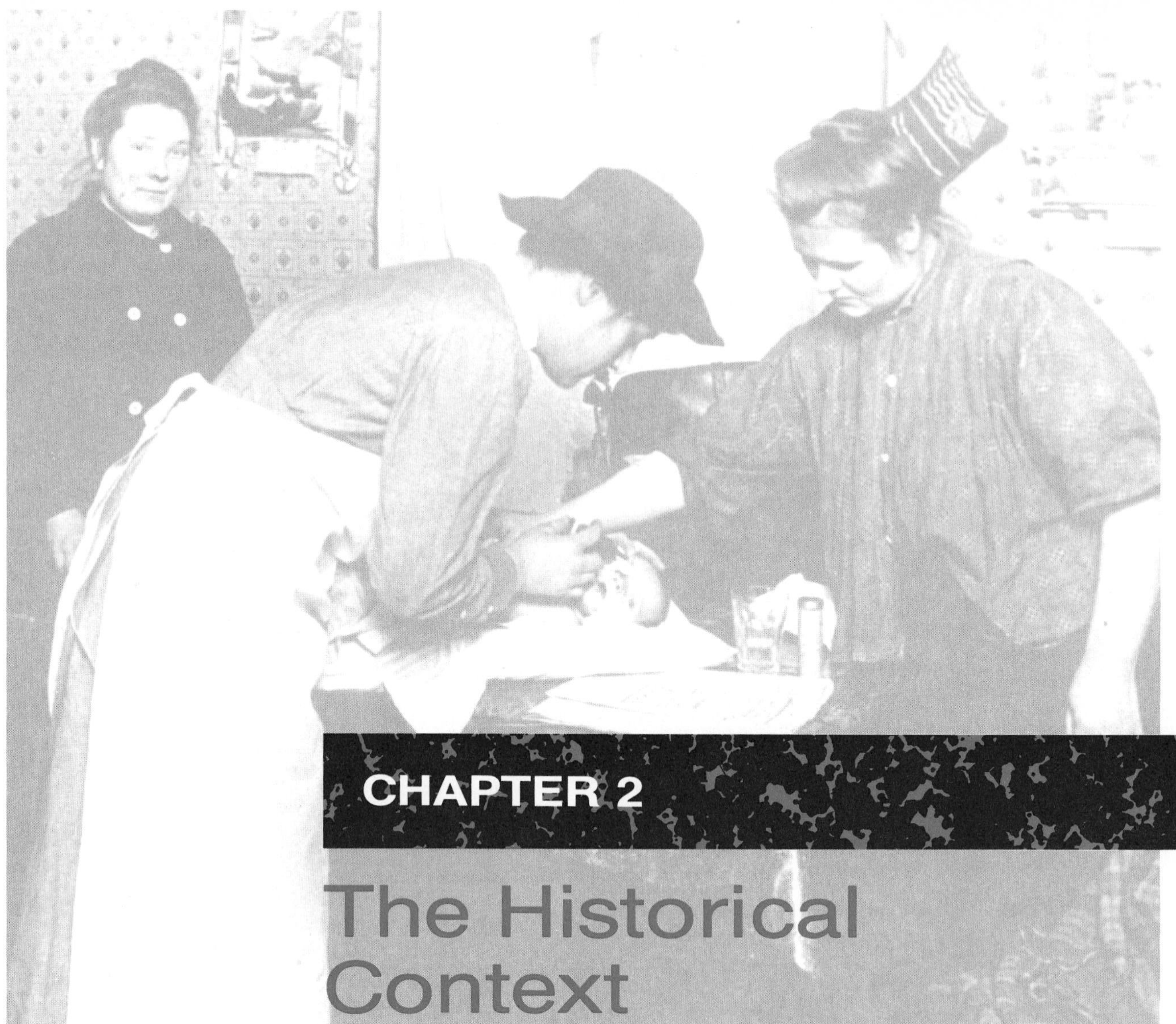

CHAPTER 2

The Historical Context

KEY TERMS

American Red Cross
Brown Report
Center for Nursing Research
diagnosis related groups
Florence Nightingale
Goldmark Report
Henry Street Settlement
Industrial Revolution
Lillian Wald
missionary nurses
National League for Nursing (NLN)
National Organization for Public Health Nursing (NOPHN)
Rural Nursing Service
Report of the Massachusetts Sanitary Commission
Social Security Act
Tax Equity and Fiscal Responsibility Act (TEFRA)
United States Public Health Service (USPHS)
visiting nurse associations

Unless community health nurses are aware of the road taken to reach their current position in the health-care delivery system, they run the risk of making wrong turns similar to those made in the past. As stated in an early work on the history of community health nursing, the "task of the true historian is to so relate the past with the present that our future work is more clearly outlined in the light of former mistakes or seemingly feeble beginnings."[1] Knowledge of past social and political events that have shaped the present allows us to identify factors that promote or undermine the health of the public. Such historical awareness also gives us a sense of the direction that community health nursing should take to achieve its goal—improved health for all people. Historical events that gave rise to a concern for the health of population groups influenced the development of both community health science and community health nursing. This chapter will examine some of these events with an eye toward understanding the development of community health nursing.

LEARNING OBJECTIVES

After you read this chapter you will be able to:

- Identify the contributions of Florence Nightingale and Lillian Wald to the development of community health nursing.
- Discuss the report that prompted creation of the forerunner of the modern board of health.
- List significant historical events in the development of community health nursing in the United States.
- Describe the influence of diagnosis related groups on community health nursing.
- Describe evidence for a shift in public health policy toward greater emphasis on health promotion.

HISTORICAL ROOTS

The roots of modern community health and community health nursing practice go far back in history. Early historical records provide evidence of concern for health and prevention of disease in several ancient civilizations. As early as 2000 B.C., Hammurabi, king of Babylonia, codified the laws of that land. Portions of the *Code of Hammurabi* specified health practices and regulated the conduct of physicians.[2]

In ancient Egypt there was a well-developed system of sewage disposal, and personal hygiene measures were encouraged, while Hebrew Mosaic law addressed many aspects of health. Hebrew segregation of lepers and proscriptions against eating pork are examples of early community health measures. Other aspects of Mosaic law specified personal and community responsibilities for maternal health, communicable disease control, fumigation, decontamination of buildings, protection of food and water supplies, waste disposal, and sanitation of campsites.[2]

The early Greeks were more concerned with personal than with community health, but they practiced many health-promoting behaviors that are encouraged today. These included emphasis on a healthy diet, exercise, and hygiene. Ancient Rome, on the other hand, emphasized the welfare of the total population and developed a number of regulations related to community health. Roman concern for public sanitation was evident in systematic efforts at street cleaning and rubbish removal and in the construction of elaborate water and sewage systems. The Romans also regulated building construction, ventilation, and heating, and mandated nuisance prevention and destruction of decaying goods. In 494 B.C., the Roman Office of Aedile was created to supervise health concerns.[3] This official was the forerunner of today's state or county health officer.

Nursing of the sick at this period in history was the function of the women of the family. In the case of large and wealthy households, the matron of the family cared for the health needs of both family members and servants and slaves. The care provided, however, was primarily palliative in nature and was only slightly related to today's concept of nursing.

THE INFLUENCE OF CHRISTIANITY

THE EARLY CHURCH

The advent of Christianity brought with it a concept of personal responsibility for the corporal and spiritual welfare of others. Care of the sick was seen as one means of fulfulling this responsibility, and early Christians exercised their time and monetary wealth ministering to the sick. Such efforts were intended to provide comfort and material goods to the sick and suffering[4] and bore little resemblance to modern community health nursing. Such services, although lacking an emphasis on prevention and health promotion or cure, did serve to bring about an awareness of illness within the population.

With the growth of Christianity and charitable giving by Christians, the wealth of the early Christian Church began to accumulate. A large portion of this wealth was used for organized care of the sick and needy through almshouses, asylums, and hospitals rather than through personal visitation of the sick. Hospitals or hospices of this time were not designed exclusively for care of the sick but ministered to all in need, including the sick, the poor, and travelers or pilgrims. The first hospital exclusively for the care of the sick was the Nosocomia or "house for the sick" established by the Roman matron Fabiola in the fourth century A.D.[4]

THE MIDDLE AGES

The mystical tradition of Christianity during the Middle Ages (A.D. 500–1500) led to a decline in community and personal health status. Castigation and neglect of the body to purify the soul resulted in a number of health problems. During this time, many of the health-promotive activities of antiquity were abandoned in favor of fasting and the wearing of sackcloth and ashes. The need for healthy warriors to fight in the Crusades sparked a slight renewal of interest in health and led to the development of military orders such as the Ancient Order of the Knights of Malta. The function of this order and similar groups was not only military service but also to care for the sick and wounded.[5] It is believed that the majority of casualties suffered in the Crusades were the result of illness rather than battle wounds.

During this same era, other religious orders were formed to look after the sick. Groups of monks and nuns established hospitals to care for the ill. In many instances, particular orders would focus on the care of specific groups or illnesses. For instance, the Knights Templar cared for pilgrims, travelers, and soldiers, whereas the Lazarists emphasized care of those with leprosy, smallpox, and pustular fevers.[4] As we can see, the concept of specialization among health-care providers is not as recent as one might believe.

In addition to the religious orders, groups of laypeople also cared for the sick. One such group was the Beguines, an order of lay women who tended the sick in both the hospital and the home. The Beguines were an early forerunner of modern visiting nurse associations. The Beguines also provide an early example of political influence by nurses. Because they refused to accept rules for cloistered orders, they were often at odds with the Church hierarchy and were periodically excommunicated. Their exemplary service to their communities, however, allowed them to enlist the aid of wealthy and influential patrons who prevented the Church from disbanding the order.[4] The focus of nursing care remained the easing of distress rather than therapeutic or preventive activity.

The concept of quarantine, developed in response to repeated epidemics of bubonic plague, was one of the few advances in public health science during the Middle Ages. In 1377, the quarantine was first used by the Sicilian city of Ragusa. Travelers were detained outside the city for two months. At the end of that time, they were allowed to enter if they appeared free of disease. Quarantine was officially legislated in Marseilles in 1383.[2]

THE EUROPEAN RENAISSANCE

From A.D. 1500 to 1700, Europe experienced a period in its history characterized by the rebirth of intellectual inquiry. This age saw the examination of various phenomena and gave rise to the beginnings of scientific thought. The intellectual inquiry characteristic of the Renaissance also led to the development of a social conscience and dawning recognition of social responsibility for the health and welfare of the population. England enacted the first *Poor Law* in 1601 making families financially responsible for the care of the aged and disabled and creating publicly funded almshouses for those with no families.

For most of the population, nursing was performed by family members. However, in 1633, St. Vincent De Paul founded the order of the Sisters of Charity to care for the needs of the sick poor in France. The activities of this order approximated those of a modern visiting nurse service and incorporated the use of field supervisors for sisters making home visits.[4]

A NEW WORLD

THE COLONIAL PERIOD

While new avenues of scientific thought were being opened in Europe, some of the ideas generated were being translated into a new way of life on a new continent. In the early colonial period in America, the health status of those living in the colonies was good compared to that of their European counterparts, and longevity at this time approached today's figures for life expectancy. The relative good health of the population was due primarily to low population density and, interestingly, poor transportation. Communities remained relatively isolated, and the spread of communicable diseases, the major health problem of the era, was curtailed by lack of movement between population groups.[6]

Because doctors were few, health care was primarily a function of the family. Nursing care was provided by the women of the family, with assistance from neighbors where this was possible.

EARLY PUBLIC HEALTH EFFORTS

The growth of population centers led to concern for sanitation and vital statistics, the foci of early public health efforts in the colonies. In 1639, both Massachusetts and Plymouth colonies mandated the reporting of all births and deaths, instituting the official reporting of vital statistics in what would later become the United States. Environmental health and sanitation were also of concern in the early colonies. Evidence of such concern is legislation in 1647 prohibiting pollution of Boston Harbor.[2]

Control of communicable disease was also of concern as populations increased in size. In 1701, Massachusetts passed legislation regarding isolation of smallpox victims and quarantine of ships in Boston Harbor. For the most part health was seen as a personal responsibility with little governmental involvement. Temporary boards of health were established in response to specific health problems, usually epidemics of communicable disease, and these were disbanded after the crisis had passed. The first such board of health was established in Petersburg, Virginia, in 1780. Similar temporary state boards of health were established in New York and Massachusetts in 1797.[7]

Recognition of the need for a consistent and organized approach to health problems was growing, however, and in 1797, the state of Massachusetts granted local jurisdictions legal authority to establish health services and regulations. The following year, the Marine Hospital Service was established to provide health care to merchant marines. The service also adopted a systematic approach to quarantine of seaports as one of the first efforts to deal with health problems at a national, rather than a state or local, level.

Nursing during this period remained a function of the family. As was true in the past, the care given was primarily palliative in nature, although the women of the house might also engage in some health-promotive practices, such as regular purging with castor oil. Treatment tended to rely on home remedies, and the literature of the era is replete with housewives' recipes for use in a variety of ailments.

In 1813, the Ladies' Benevolent Society of Charleston, South Carolina, was established. This was the first organized approach to home nursing of the sick in America. This organization was initiated in response to a yellow-fever epidemic and was completely nondenominational and nondiscriminatory in an era characterized by widespread racial discrimination. Care was provided to the sick in their homes by upper-class women. Because these women had no background in nursing, care focused on relieving suffering and providing material aid.[4] With the exception of a 20-year period during and after the Civil War, the Ladies' Benevolent Society provided services until the 1950s.

Another early attempt at home-care nursing also saw upper-class women visiting the homes of indigent women during delivery. The Lying-in Charity for Attending Indigent Women in Their Homes was established in 1832. The purpose of this organization was to assist poor women during and after delivery. Because of their lack of training, the services provided by these women emphasized social and emotional support for the woman in labor and assistance to her after delivery.

THE INDUSTRIAL REVOLUTION

The ***Industrial Revolution*** profoundly influenced health in both Europe and the United States. Movement from an agricultural to an industrial economy led to the development of large industrial centers and the need for a large work force to labor in unhealthy conditions in mines, mills, and factories. The demand for manufactured goods and the necessity to get goods to market prompted advancements in transportation that increased mobility and the potential for spreading communicable diseases. In the United States, rural-urban migration and the presence of large contingents of poor immigrants, come to escape the poverty of their homelands, created crowded living conditions that further enhanced the potential for disease.

The poor were overworked and underpaid. Poor nutrition contributed to increased incidence of a variety of diseases, particularly tuberculosis. The use of children in the work force, coupled with low wages, inadequate food, and hazardous working conditions, led to many preventable illnesses and deaths among the children of the poor.

The nineteenth century saw a beginning recognition of the effects of these social and economic conditions on health, and the concept of social responsibility for public health began to take root. The growth of this concept was fostered by the publication in the mid-1800s of several landmark reports. The first of these publications was C. Turner Thackrah's treatise on occupational health, *The effects of Arts, Trades, and Professions . . . on Health and Longevity*. In this document, Thackrah described the effects of working conditions on health. In 1842, Edwin Chadwick's *Inquiry into the Sanitary Conditions of the Labouring Population of Great Britain* was published to provide additional fuel for reformers' efforts to change working and social conditions that contributed to disease.

While Thackrah and Chadwick addressed the effects of working conditions on health and instigated reforms to prevent disease, Henry W. Rumsey focused on health promotion. Rumsey's *Essays on State Medicine* emphasized health promotion and illness prevention as social obligations of government. His description of the functions of a proposed district medical officer embodied most aspects of modern community health programs.[8]

Similar documents were published in the United States. The Massachusetts Sanitary Commission was established in response to concern for the effects of crowded living conditions, poverty, and poor sanitation on health. In 1850, Lemuel Shattuck drafted the commission's findings, aptly titled the ***Report of the Massachusetts Sanitary Commission.*** The report included recommendations for establishing state and local health departments, systematic collection of vital statistics, sanitation inspections, and the institution of programs for school health and control of mental illness, alcohol abuse, and tuberculosis. Other recommendations included public education regarding sanitation, control of nuisances, periodic physical examinations, supervision of the health of immigrants, and the construction of model tenements. In addition, the report recommended improved education for nurses and the inclusion of content on preventive medicine and sanitation in medical school curricula.

Publication of the *Report of the Massachusetts Sanitary Commission* marks the beginning of community health practice as we know it today. Recommendations of the report form the basis for much of the present work of official state and local public health agencies. The eventual effect of the commission's report was the establishment of the Massachusetts State Board of Health in 1869, nearly 90 years after the advent of the first temporary boards of health and 19 years after publication of Shattuck's report. This first permanent board, similar to modern boards of health, emphasized six aspects of community health practice: inspection of housing, public education in hygiene, investigation of disease, regulation of slaughterhouses, regulation of the sale of poisons, and health care for the poor.[2]

During this period, great strides were being made in the fledgling science of epidemiology. In 1856, without knowledge of the nature of the causative organism, John Snow determined the source of a London epidemic of cholera to be something in the water of the Broad Street pump. However, it was not until 1877 that Louis Pasteur and Robert Koch, working independently, identified specific bacteria. These and other epidemiologic findings allowed more scientific measures to be applied to the control of communicable disease and contributed greatly to the armamentarium of later community health nurses in preventing disease.

DISTRICT NURSING IN ENGLAND

The "three great revolutions" of the late eighteenth and early nineteenth centuries—the intellectual revolution, the French and American political revolutions, and the Industrial Revolution—set the stage for the development of community health nursing. In England, the same spirit that motivated industrial and prison reform led to concern for the health of large urban populations and development of nursing practices to address these concerns.

In addition to being the acknowledged founder of modern hospital nursing, ***Florence Nightingale*** was instrumental in the development of community health or district nursing. Miss Nightingale received her training in nursing at the school for deaconesses established by Theodor Fliedner. Fliedner's second wife, Caroline Bertheau, conceived the idea of extending the nursing services offered in the hospital to the sick in their homes. This concept influenced Florence Nightingale, who endorsed the idea of "health nursing" as well as home care for illness.[9]

In 1859, Miss Nightingale assisted William Rathbone to form the first district public health nursing association in England. The organization was funded by philanthropic citizens and hired trained nurses who were assigned to specific districts in London. Each nurse was responsible for the health needs of the people in her district. The nurses were viewed as social reformers as well as providers of care for the sick, evidence of the early development of the advocacy role of the community health nurse.

The need to standardize community health nursing services was recognized early in the development of the district nursing associations. The East London Nursing Society was established for this purpose but proved ineffective. Subsequently, investigation of the district nursing system revealed a need for a national association. As a result, the Metropolitan and National Nursing Association for Providing Trained Nurses for the Sick Poor was established in 1875. This group fostered employment of educated women in public health nursing as a step toward the professionalization of nursing.

One of the first activities of the association, which was headed by Florence Lees, a protege of Miss Nightingale's, was a study of the needs for public health nursing, the personnel available, and the training needed and work done by district nurses. Results of the study of 115 district nurses employed by various organizations throughout London indicated that the work done by those nurses who were trained was effective. Unfortunately, over half of those studied had no training in public health and were found to be insufficiently prepared for their role in the unsupervised care of the sick. Hospital training was found to be inadequate for district nursing and a recommendation was made that district nurses receive 3 months of training in public health in addition to their year of hospital training.[4]

The district nursing associations embodied three of the principles of modern community health nursing. The first of these, as noted above, was the need for special training for nurses working in the community. By 1889, this need for special preparation for community health nursing had been widely recognized. At that time, monies donated to Queen Victoria's Jubilee fund were allocated to Queen Victoria's Jubilee Institute for Nursing. The institute was established to prepare nurses for community health practice and to extend community health nursing throughout the British Empire. A program was instituted to provide an additional 6-month educational experience for community health nurses following the initial 3 years of training in the hospital.[10]

The second principle of modern community health nursing embodied in the district nursing associations was the separation of nursing care from the provision of material goods. As noted earlier, many early efforts at visiting the sick focused on dealing with material needs through the distribution of money, food, or clothing. The district nursing concept eliminated such charitable activities from the role of the nurse and focused on the provision of nursing care per se.

The third principle was the prohibition of religious proselytizing by the nurses. Again, because much prior visiting of the sick had been done in the name of Christian charity, visits had been used as an opportunity to encourage supposed sinners to mend their evil ways. Much of this type of activity derived from convictions that poverty, illness, and suffering were punishment for one's sins and that repentance was needed.

VISITING NURSES IN AMERICA

In the United States, proselytizing was also part of the role of nurses who provided early home care to the sick poor. However, efforts had been made to incorporate the provision of *nursing care* in addition to proselytizing and providing for material needs. In 1877, the Women's Branch of the New York City Mission employed Frances Root as the first salaried American nurse to visit the sick poor. Her role and that of many ***missionary nurses*** to follow her was to provide nursing care and religious instruction for the sick poor.[4]

In 1878, the Ethical Culture Society of New York employed four nurses in dispensaries, inaugurating the ambulatory care role of the community health nurse. These nurses worked under the supervision of a physician and emphasized health teaching as well as illness care.[4] In the next few years, ***visiting nurse associations*** were established in Buffalo (1885), and in Boston and Philadelphia (1886). The Philadelphia agency was the first to institute a nurse's uniform, a fee for services, and the community nursing supervisor. The Boston Instructive Visiting Nurse Association emphasized the community health nurse's educative function as well as her role in the care of the sick, signaling the beginning of the health promotion emphasis that now characterizes community health nursing. By 1890, visiting nurse services were available in 21 American cities.[11]

NURSING AND THE SETTLEMENT HOUSES

The settlement movement was based on beliefs espoused by Arnold Toynbee that educated persons could promote learning, morality, and civic responsibility in the poor by living among them and sharing certain aspects of their poverty. Groups of students from Oxford and Cambridge, acting on these beliefs, "settled" in homes in the London slums with the idea that their poor neighbors would learn through watching their behavior.[12]

In the United States, the settlement idea was adapted by nurses such as ***Lillian Wald,*** who believed that the most effective way to bring health care to the poor immigrant population was for nurses to live and work among them. Accordingly, Miss Wald and several associates established the ***Henry Street Settlement*** in New York City in 1893.

The Henry Street Settlement is usually considered the first American community health agency because of its incorporation of modern concepts of community health nursing. The nurses of the Henry Street Settlement were involved in more than visiting the sick in their homes. Health promotion and disease prevention were heavily emphasized, as was political activism. Miss Wald herself was a prime example of the political activist, supporting many changes in social conditions that would benefit the health of the public.[13]

Other nursing settlement houses patterned on the Henry Street model were established. One particularly inspiring example was the Nurse's Settlement established in Richmond, Virginia, by the graduating class of Old Dominion Hospital in the year 1900. These nurses had been exposed to the needs of Richmond's poor during student experiences with the Instructive Visiting Nurse Association of Richmond. The settlement they founded differed from the Henry Street Settlement in that it did not have any wealthy patrons to provide support and was initiated with the limited resources of the graduates themselves. Like Henry Street, the Richmond settlement focused on health promotion and education as well as care of the sick.[12]

EXPANDING THE FOCUS ON PREVENTION

The effectiveness of community health nurses in preventing sickness and death among the poor was recognized and became the basis for visiting nurse services offered by the Metropolitan Life Insurance Company.[4] This program was begun at the instigation of Lee Frankel and Lillian Wald. Miss Wald convinced the Metropolitan board that providing nursing services to its policyholders would improve the public image of an industry tarnished by economic scandal. The telling argument, though, was evidence that community health nursing reduced mortality and would limit the benefits paid by the company. Services were begun on an experimental basis in 1909 with one of the Henry Street nurses.

The 3-month experiment was such a success that the program was extended and continued to provide services until 1953. This association with the business world was an education for community health nurses who had no conception of marketing or economic bases for programs. The program was finally discontinued because of nursing's failure to grasp economic realities and the realization of diminishing returns by the insurance company.[14]

The emphasis of community health nursing on health promotion began with health in the home during visits to the poor in large cities. Gradually, however, the concepts of health promotion and illness prevention were expanded to other population groups to include services to mothers and young children, school-age youngsters, employees, and the rural population.

Concern for the health of mothers and children was growing, and the nurses of Henry Street Settlement and other similar programs spent a large portion of their time in health promotion for this group of clients. They recognized, however, that services to individual families would not overcome the effects of poverty, and they worked actively to improve social conditions affecting health. Because of the efforts of Lillian Wald and other social activists, the first White House Conference on Children was held in 1909. As a result of the conference, the U.S. Children's Bureau was established in 1912 to develop programs to promote the health of youngsters.

School nursing, another arena for health promotion, actually began in London in 1892 and was introduced in the United States by Lillian Wald, of the Henry Street Settlement. The initial impetus for school health nursing was the high level of school absenteeism due to illness. In New York City in 1902, 15 to 20 children per school were being sent home daily. In response, Miss Wald assigned nurses from the Henry Street Settlement to four New York City schools in a pilot project in school nursing. Because of the overwhelming success of the project, the New York Board of Health absorbed the program and hired additional nurses to continue the work.[15]

The concept of school nursing spread to other parts of the country. In 1904 Los Angeles became the first of many municipalities to employ nurses in the schools.[10] Early school nursing focused on preventing the spread of communicable diseases and treating ailments related to compulsory school life. By the 1930s, however, the focus had shifted to preventive and promotive activities including case finding, integrating health concepts into school curricula, and maintaining a healthful school environment.[16]

The first rural nursing service was established in 1896 in Westchester County, New York, by Ellen Morris Wood and was followed in 1906 with the initiation of a nursing service for both the poor and the well-to-do of Salisbury, Connecticut. Despite her usual sphere of activity in the city, Lillian Wald was also involved in the growth of rural community health nursing. It was she who convinced the ***American Red Cross,*** founded in 1881, to direct its peacetime attention to expanding community health services in rural America. In 1912, the Red Cross established the ***Rural Nursing Service*** (later the Town and Country Nursing Service) to extend community health nursing services to rural areas.[4]

Occupational health nursing provides another avenue for health promotion by community health nurses. This specialty area began in 1895 when Vermont's Governor Proctor employed nurses to see to the health needs of villages where employees of his Vermont Marble Company lived.[11] In 1897, the Employees' Benefit Association of John Wanamaker's department store in New York City hired nurses to visit employees' homes. These nurses soon expanded their role to include first aid and prevention of illness and injury in the work setting. The number of firms employing nurses increased rapidly from 66 in 1910 to 871 by 1919.[4]

STANDARDIZING PRACTICE

The need to standardize community nursing practice was recognized in both the United States and England. Early American attempts to standardize visiting nursing services included publications related to public health nursing and the development of a national logo by the Cleveland Visiting Nurse Association (VNA). This logo, or seal, was made available to any visiting nurse organization that met established standards. Both the Chicago (1906) and Cleveland (1909) VNAs published newsletters titled *Visiting Nurse Quarterly* to aid attempts to standardize care.[4]

In 1911, a joint committee of the American Nurses' Association and the Society for Superintendents of Training Schools for Nurses met to consider the need for standardization. The result was a second meeting held in 1912. Letters inviting representation were sent to 1,092 organizations employing visiting nurses at that time. These organizations included VNAs, city and state boards of health and education, private clubs and societies, tuberculosis leagues, hospitals and dispensaries, businesses, settlements and day nurseries, churches, and charitable organizations. A total of 69 agencies responded with their intent to send a representative to the meeting. The result of this second meeting was the formation of the ***National Organization for Public Health Nursing*** (NOPHN).[4] The objectives of this organization were to provide for stimulation and standardization of public health nursing. This was the first professional body in the United States to provide for lay membership.

The NOPHN was influential in maintaining public health nursing services at home during World War I and in the organization of the Division of Public Health Nursing within the United States Public Health Service in 1944. NOPHN also provided advisory services regarding postgraduate education for public health nursing in colleges and universities. NOPHN was incorporated into the ***National League for Nursing*** (NLN) in the 1952 restructuring of professional nursing organizations.

EDUCATING COMMUNITY HEALTH NURSES

During the 1920s nursing education was under study. The ***Goldmark Report,*** *Nursing and Nursing Education in the United States,* published in 1923, dealt with nursing education in general and pointed out the need for advanced preparation for community health nursing. The report recommended that nursing education take place in institutions of higher learning. As a result, the Yale University School of Nursing and the Frances Payne Bolton School of Nursing at Western Reserve University opened in 1923. The curricula of both programs included community health nursing content.[17]

Prior to the education of nurses in university settings, special postgraduate courses in public health nursing had been established by various agencies. The first of these was undertaken by the Instructive District Nursing Association of Boston in 1906. In 1910, Teachers' College of Columbia University offered the first course in public health nursing in an institution of higher learning.[4] In 1929, NOPHN developed criteria for evaluating courses in public health nursing.[17]

In addition to witnessing the movement of community health nursing education to institutions of higher learning, the 1920s saw a shift in employment of public health nurses. Prior to this time, most public health nursing services were provided by voluntary agencies such as the Red Cross and similar organizations. During the 1920s, however, public health nursing services began to be taken over by official governmental agencies such as local and state health departments.[18]

The ***Brown Report*** of 1948, *Nursing for the Future,* reemphasized the need for nurses to be educated in institutions of higher learning so as to prepare them to meet community health needs.[19] In 1964 the American Nurses' Association (ANA) formally defined the public health nurse as a graduate of a baccalaureate program in nursing. Today, in states such as California, only graduates from baccalaureate programs in nursing can be certified as public health nurses. Moreover, today there are master's and doctoral programs with a community health nursing focus.

FEDERAL INVOLVEMENT IN HEALTH CARE

For most of its history the federal government has left health matters to the states. It wasn't until 1858 that the United States established a National Board of Health in response to a yellow-fever epidemic. This board continued to function until 1888 when it was dissolved. In 1912, the need for a permanent national agency responsible for the country's health was recognized, and the ***United States Public Health Service*** (USPHS) was created out of the reorganization of the Marine Hospital Service. In that same year, federal legislation was passed creating the office of the Surgeon General and mandating federal involvement in health promotion. It was not until 1953, however, that the need for advisement on health matters at the cabinet level was recognized in the creation of the Department of Health, Education, and Welfare. This department was reorganized in 1980 to create the present Department of Health and Human Services (DHHS).

Since the turn of the century, the federal government has become progressively more involved in health-care delivery. Unfortunately, this involvement has been rather haphazard, dependent upon the interests and concerns of differing administrations. In the early years of the twentieth century, the health needs of specific segments of the population began to be recognized, resulting in federal programs designed to enhance the health of mothers and children, the poor, those with sexually transmitted diseases, the mentally ill, and so on. Recognition of the need for federal support of health-care research to address the health needs of these and other specialty groups led to the development of the National Institutes of Health in 1930.

As a result of the Great Depression of the 1930s, the federal government became even more active in health and social welfare programs. Jobs were created to employ thousands of the unemployed. Nurses were also employed at this time to meet the health needs of the population. The first public health nurse was employed by USPHS in 1934.

Recognition of the economic plight of the elderly led to passage of the ***Social Security Act*** in 1935. This act established the Old Age Survivors Insurance Program (OASI, better known as "Social Security") to improve the financial status of the elderly. In 1966, the Social Security Act was amended to create the Medicare program to fund health care for older Americans. Medicaid, a program that funds health care for the indigent, was instituted in 1967.[20] These two programs contributed to increased demands for health-care services and resulted in rapid increases in the cost of health care.

World War II also influenced health-care delivery. During the war, some 15 million American servicemen were exposed to quality health care, some for the first time in their lives. Afterwards, these veterans began to demand the same quality of care for themselves and their families in the civilian sector. This increased demand for care led to new arrangements for financing health care and a subsequent burgeoning of the health insurance industry. The growth in health insurance was further influenced by the 1954 inclusion of premiums as legitimate tax deductions.[21] This development led to the use of insurance benefits as a tax-deductible substitute for higher wages in business and industry. Because such benefits were tax exempt for employees, they were readily accepted in lieu of salary increases by unions and other bargaining agents.

Increased demands for services also led to a lack of adequate facilities, especially in nonurban areas. In 1946, pressured by U.S. Public Health Service officials, Congress responded with passage of the Hill-Burton Act to finance hospital construction in underserved areas.[22] Hospital construction and insurance coverage for care provided in the hospital further strengthened the national emphasis on curative rather than preventive care. Hospitals became a major focus for health and illness care. During this same period, the first hospital-based home care program was established at Montefiore Hospital,[23] setting a precedent for the burgeoning home care industry of today. This development has also led to the growing need for community health nurses to provide home health services.

Acknowledging the growing demand for health care and recognizing the differing abilities of certain areas of the country to meet those needs, the federal government responded with the Comprehensive Health Planning Act of 1966 and the National Health Planning and Resources Development Act of 1974. Both pieces of legislation were attempts to organize the planning of health-care delivery to meet differing needs throughout the country.[24] Unfortunately, both efforts failed. One positive effect of the 1974 act was recognition of the contribution of nurse practitioners to the health status of the public.[25]

The Child Health Act of 1967 and the Health Maintenance Organization Act of 1973 also recommended use of nurses in extended roles. The 1971 publication of a report entitled *Extending the Scope of Nursing Practice* provided additional support for the use of nurses in expanded capacities. The nurse practitioner movement began as a community health movement with the institution of the first pediatric nurse practitioner course at the University of Colorado in 1965.[26] Subsequent legislation has led to the increased use of nurse practitioners in a variety of settings. Over the last few years there has been increased use of community health nurses with advanced educational preparation as nurse practitioners providing primary care to selected populations.

Federal legislation has also influenced community health nursing in other ways. For example, several manpower training acts have provided funds for advanced training in community health nursing. The ***Tax Equity and Fiscal Responsibility Act*** of 1982 (TEFRA) has had a profound effect on health care and community health nursing. This act, passed in an effort to reduce Medicare expenditures, led to the development of ***diagnosis related groups*** or DRGs as a mechanism for prospective payment for services provided under Medicare.[27] Basically, prospective payment means that health-care institutions are paid a flat fee set in advance for the care of clients under Medicare. The fee is based on the client's diagnosis. The effect of this legislation has been earlier discharge of sicker clients and greater demand for home health and community health nursing services. Diagnosis related groups and their effects have changed the role of community health nurses, who may need to return to the earlier role of care of the sick in their homes, in addition to their health-promotive and illness-preventive roles.

THE PRESENT AND THE FUTURE

In the last few years, economic difficulties, inaccessibility of health care, and the energy crisis have also changed the role of the community health nurse. Community health nurses with advanced preparation are being used to a greater extent in expanded roles as nurse practitioners. Some traditional services, such as home visits, are being curtailed in favor of more cost-effective approaches to health care. Nursing services are still not reimbursable through third-party payments except in certain instances (for example, for some services provided under Medicare and Medicaid). Health-promotive and illness-preventive activities by nurses are generally not reimbursable.

A recent report on the status of the nation's public health system, *The Future of Public Health*, described a system in disarray. The report concluded that major reforms will be required to promote and protect the health of the public. This report may or may not in-

TABLE 2–1. HISTORICAL EVENTS INFLUENCING THE DEVELOPMENT OF COMMUNITY HEALTH NURSING

Date	Event
1601	First "Poor Law" enacted in Great Britain
1639	Massachusetts and Plymouth colonies mandate reporting of births and deaths
1647	Massachusetts enacts regulations regarding pollution of Boston harbor
1701	Massachusetts laws enacted regarding quarantine of ships and isolation of persons with smallpox
1780	First local board of health in the United States established at Petersburg, Virginia
1797	Temporary State Boards of Health established in Massachusetts and New York
	Massachusetts grants local jurisdictions the authority to establish local health services
1798	National Quarantine Act passes providing a systematic national approach to quarantine of seaports
1813	* Ladies Benevolent Society organized in South Carolina as the first home nursing service in the United States
1831	Thackrah's treatise on occupational health published
1832	* Lying-in Charity for Attending Indigent Women in Their Homes established
1842	Publication of Chadwick's *Inquiry into the Sanitary Conditions of the Labouring Population of Great Britain*
1850	Publication of Shattuck's *Report of the Massachusetts Sanitary Commission*
1856	Rumsey's *Essay on State Medicine* published, arguing for government responsibility for public health
	Snow's historic epidemiologic study of cholera conducted
1858	National Board of Health established in the United States
1869	First modern State Board of Health established in Massachusetts
1875	* Metropolitan and National Nursing Association for Providing Trained Nurses for the Sick Poor established in England
1877	Pasteur and Koch independently identify specific bacteria
	* Women's Branch of the New York City Mission first employed trained nurses for home visiting
1878	* Ethical Culture Society of New York City places four nurses in dispensaries
1881	* American Red Cross founded
1885–6	* Visiting nurse associations established in Buffalo, Boston, and Philadelphia
1892	* First school nurse employed in London
1893	* Henry Street Settlement founded by Lillian Wald
1895	* Vermont Marble Company employed first occupational health nurse
1896	* First rural nursing service established (Westchester County, New York)
1900	* Richmond, Virginia, nurses' settlement house founded
1902	* First school nursing program in the United States established by Henry Street Settlement
1903	* Henry Street Settlement school nursing program absorbed by New York City Department of Health
1904	* First school nurse employed by a municipality (Los Angeles, California)
1906	* First publication of the *Visiting Nurse Quarterly* (Chicago)
	* First postgraduate course in public health nursing established by Instructive District Nursing Association of Boston
1909	First meeting of White House Conference on Children
	* Metropolitan Life Insurance Company offered visiting nurse services to policyholders
1910	* First postgraduate course in community health nursing in an institution of higher learning established at Columbia University
1912	Children's Bureau set up to foster child health
	Passage of first law empowering Surgeon General to promote health
	Marine Hospital Services became United States Public Health Service (USPHS)
	* National Organization for Public Health Nursing (NOPHN) established
	* Red Cross Town and Country Nursing Service established
1923	* Goldmark Report published recommending education for nurses in institutions of higher learning and additional preparation for community health nursing
1929	* NOPHN established criteria and procedures for grading courses in public health nursing, initiating the accreditation process
1930	National Institutes of Health set up to fund and conduct health research
1934	* First public health nurse employed by USPHS
1935	Social Security Act passed establishing Old Age Survivor's Insurance Program (OASI)
1944	* Division of Nursing established in USPHS
1946	Hospital Survey and Construction (Hill-Burton) Act passed providing funds for hospital construction in underserved areas
1948	* Brown Report published reemphasizing the need to educate nurses in institutions of higher learning and to include community health nursing content in curricula
1952	* NOPHN absorbed into National League for Nursing (NLN)
1953	United States Department of Health, Education, and Welfare created

(*continued*)

TABLE 2–1. (*Continued*)

Date	Event
1954	Health insurance premiums first allowed as tax deductions
1964	* Public health nurse defined by ANA as a graduate of a baccalaureate program in nursing
1966	Passage of Comprehensive Health Planning and Public Health Services Act Medicare program instituted to fund health care for the elderly
1967	* Child Health Act passed recommending use of nurse practitioners in the care of children Medicaid program instituted to fund health care for the indigent
1974	National Health Planning and Resources Development Act passed in an attempt at systematic health-care planning
1980	Department of Health, Education, and Welfare reorganized, creating the Department of Health and Human Services First national health objectives developed
1982	Tax Equity and Fiscal Responsibility Act (TEFRA) passed
1983	Prospective payment system based on DRGs instituted under Medicare
1988	Institute of Medicine report, *The Future of Public Health*, published recommending changes in the U.S. health-care system * National Center for Nursing Research established

* Events affecting nursing directly.

fluence community health nursing. Unfortunately, the report did not address at all the contribution of community health nursing to the health of the public. This, in itself, may be ominous. Community health nursing may not survive as an area of specialty practice if it is not seen as contributing to public health.[28]

There are a few bright spots in recent events, however. Growing evidence indicates a shift to greater emphasis on health promotion and illness prevention in public health policy. The national health objectives, first published in 1980 and discussed in Chapter 1, are one sign of this shift. A second bit of evidence is the 1988 creation of the ***Center for Nursing Research*** within the National Institutes of Health. One of the reasons given in Senate testimony favoring the center was the health promotion and illness prevention focus in much of nursing research.

In this chapter we have seen how community health nursing grew to its present state. Some of the events influencing its development are summarized in Table 2–1. The future direction of community health nursing will be determined by the community health nurses of today and tomorrow. Let us learn from the past as we move into the future.

CHAPTER HIGHLIGHTS

- Ancient civilizations such as the Egyptians, Hebrews, Greeks, and Romans were concerned about public health and enacted laws and engaged in activities to protect the health of the general public.
- Concern for health care, which declined with the mysticism of the Middle Ages, experienced a resurgence with the concern over the fighting capacity of the Crusaders. Health care was provided primarily by religious and military orders.
- The Renaissance, marked by the rise of a social conscience, also saw a resurgence of concern for the health of the general public. Advances in scientific thought set the stage for the development of the science of epidemiology.
- Epidemics of communicable disease were often the impetus for health-related laws and government activities such as the institution of quarantine laws and the creation of boards of health.
- The influence of social and economic conditions on health began to be widely recognized during the Industrial Revolution, and the idea of government responsibility for the health of its citizens began to gain sway.

(*continued*)

- Shattuck's *Report of the Massachusetts Sanitary Commission* is considered the beginning of modern community health practice. This report led to the creation of the forerunner of modern boards of health.
- Community health nursing in the United States began with the establishment of the Ladies Benevolent Society in South Carolina. Gradually, community health nurses began to expand their arena of practice into schools and industry as well as the home, and greater emphasis was placed on educating people for healthier lives.
- Florence Nightingale and Lillian Wald were key figures in the development of modern community health nursing. Miss Nightingale fostered the concept of health nursing and helped William Rathbone establish the first district nursing association in England.
- The prototype of the modern community health nursing service was the Henry Street Settlement founded by Lillian Wald in 1893. Miss Wald was also instrumental in the development of school and rural health nursing and in the creation of the U.S. Children's Bureau and the visiting nurse services of the Metropolitan Life Insurance Company.
- It was not until 1912 that a permanent national agency responsible for health was created in the United States. This agency was the U.S. Public Health Service.
- The National Organization for Public Health Nursing was instituted to oversee the standardization of community health nursing education and practice and was the first professional organization to incorporate lay membership. NOPHN later became the National League for Nursing with the 1952 reorganization of professional nursing organizations.
- The Goldmark Report in 1923 and the Brown Report in 1948 emphasized the need for higher education for nurses and the need for specific preparation in community health nursing.
- In the twentieth century, attention has focused on the health needs of specific population groups including mothers and children, the elderly, the mentally ill, and the mentally handicapped, to name a few.
- The institution of health insurance and subsequent designation of health insurance premiums as an income tax deduction started the spiraling rise in health-care costs seen today. This rise was a result of increased demand for services, further compounded by the creation of the Medicare and Medicaid programs.
- Legislation such as the Child Health Act of 1967 and the Health Maintenance Act of 1973 influenced the expansion of the community health nurse's role in the provision of primary care. The 1971 report *Extending the Scope of Nursing Practice* also emphasized the need for expanded practice by nurses.
- Prospective reimbursement in the form of diagnosis related groups (DRGs) was instituted in an attempt to curb federal expenditures for health care under the Medicare program.
- Recently, attention has been focused on the need for health promotion and disease prevention rather than illness care. Development of the first national health objectives and the creation of the Center for Nursing Research are indicators of this change in focus.

Review Questions

1. Describe the contributions made by Florence Nightingale to the development of community health nursing. (p. 23)
2. Describe the contributions of Lillian Wald to the development of community health nursing in the United States. (pp. 24–25)
3. What report led to the creation of the forerunner of the modern board of health? List at least five recommendations from this report. (pp. 22–23)
4. List at least four major historical events in the development of community health nursing in the United States. (pp. 22, 24–26)
5. How have DRGs influenced community health nursing practice? (p. 27)
6. Describe evidence for a shift in public health policy toward greater emphasis on health promotion. (p. 29)

APPLICATION AND SYNTHESIS

LILLIAN WALD—"BEST HELPS TO THE IMMIGRANT THROUGH THE NURSE"—1907

The following is an excerpt from a typed manuscript of comments made by Lillian Wald, founder of the Henry Street Settlement.

. . . District nursing today follows the tradition of its earliest conception. It has been used since the beginning of its history to carry propaganda as there has been always an enthusiastic belief in the possibility of the nurse as teacher in religion, cleanliness, temperance, cooking, housekeeping, etc. My argument loses none of its force, I think, if much of this education has seemed to her lost energy because with greater knowledge and wider experience she has learned that the individual is not so often to blame, as she at first supposed. That while the district nurse is laboring with the individual she should also contribute her knowledge towards the study of the large general conditions of which her poor patient may be the victim.

Many of these conditions seem hopelessly bad but many are capable of prevention and cure when the public shall be stimulated to a realization of the wrong to the individual as well as to society in general if (they) are permitted to persist. Therefore her knowledge of the laws that have been enacted to prevent and cure, and her intelligence in recording and reporting the general as well as the individual conditions that make for degradation and social iniquity are but an advance from her readiness to instruct and correct personal and family hygiene to giving attention to home sanitation and then to city sanitation, an advance from the individual to the collective interest. The subject is tremendously important, even exciting, and adds the glamor of a wide patriotic significance to the daily hard work of the nurse. The prevalence of tuberculosis, for instance, brings attention directly to conditions of industry and housing, next to hours of work, to legal restrictions, to indifference to the laws, to possible abuse of the weaker for the benefit of the stronger.

It is splendid vindication of the value of comprehensive education and stimulated social conscience that the district nurses who have had this vision have been the most faithful and hard working and zealous in their actual care of the sick . . . [The] wider vision [of the district nurse] makes for thoroughness as an all important educational, social and humanitarian necessity where the patients are concerned.

These opportunities . . . bear the closest relationship to the immigrants, because they are the most helpless of our population and the most exploited; the least informed and instructed in the very matters that are essential to their happiness. The country needs them and uses them and it is obviously an obligation due them as well as safe guarding of the country itself to give them intelligent conception and education of what is important to their and our interests. . . .

1. Based on this excerpt, what do you think was Lillian Wald's perception of the primary focus of community health nursing practice?
2. What kinds of roles does Lillian Wald envision for community health nurses?
3. Lillian Wald speaks of European immigrants as those most in need of community health nurses' services and advocacy. What groups today take the place of these immigrants in their need for assistance?
4. What do you think would be Miss Wald's perception of the modern world? Would she think it had changed for the better or worse? In what ways? Is there still a need for the type of role that she describes for the community health nurse?

REFERENCES

1. Foley, E. L. (1985). Introduction. In A. M. Brainard, *The evolution of public health nursing* (pp. i–vii). New York: Garland. Reprinted from A. M. Brainard (1922), *The evolution of public health nursing*. Philadelphia: W. B. Saunders.
2. Anderson, C. L., Morton, R. F., & Green, L. W. (1978). *Community health* (3rd ed.). St. Louis: C. V. Mosby.
3. Winslow, C. E. (1923). *The evolution and significance of the modern public health campaign*. New Haven, CT: Yale University Press.
4. Brainard, A. M. (1985). *The evolution of public health nursing*. New York: Garland. Reprinted from A. M. Brainard (1922), *The evolution of public health nursing*. Philadelphia: W. B. Saunders.
5. Kelly, L. Y. (1981). *Dimensions of professional nursing* (4th ed.). New York: Macmillan.
6. Grob, G. N. (1983). Disease and environment in American history. In D. Mechanic (Ed.), *Handbook of health, health care, and the health professions* (pp. 3–22). New York: Free Press.
7. Smolensky, J. (1982). *Principles of community health* (3rd ed.). Philadelphia: W. B. Saunders.
8. Rosen, G. (1974). *From medical police to social medicine: Essays on the history of health care*. New York: Science History Publications.
9. Fitzpatrick, M. L. (1975). *The National Organization for Public Health Nursing, 1912–1952: Development of a practice field*. New York: National League for Nursing.
10. Gardner, M. S. (1952). *Public Health Nursing* (3rd ed.). New York: Macmillan.
11. Novak, J. C. (1988). The social mandate and historical basis for nursing's role in health promotion. *Journal of Professional Nursing, 4*(2), 80–87.
12. Erickson, G. (1987). Southern initiative in public health nursing. *Journal of Nursing History, 3*(1), 17–29.
13. Coss, C. (1989). *Lillian Wald: A progressive activist*. New York: Feminist Press.
14. Hamilton, D. (1989). The cost of caring: The Metropolitan Life Insurance Company's Visiting Nurse Service, 1909–1953. *Bulletin of the History of Medicine, 63*, 414–434.
15. Buhler-Wilkerson, K. (1985). Public health nursing: In sickness or in health. *American Journal of Public Health, 75*, 1155–1161.
16. Igoe, J. B. (1980). Changing patterns in school health and school health nursing. *Nursing Outlook, 28*, 486–492.
17. Tinkham, C. W., & Voorhies, E. F. (1977). *Community health nursing evolution and practice*. New York: Appleton-Century-Crofts.
18. Bigbee, J. L., & Crowder, E. L. M. (1985). The Red Cross Rural Nursing Service: An innovative model of public health delivery. *Public Health Nursing, 2*, 109–121.
19. Benson, E. R., & McDevitt, J. Q. (1976). *Community health and nursing practice*. Englewood Cliffs, NJ: Prentice-Hall.
20. McCarthy, C., & Thorpe, K. E. (1986). Financing for health care. In S. Jonas (Ed.), *Health care delivery in the United States* (3rd ed.) (pp. 272–312). New York: Springer.
21. Ginzberg, E. (1985). *American medicine: The power shifts*. Totowa, NJ: Rowman & Allanheld.
22. Thompson, F. J. (1984). *Health policy and the bureaucracy: Politics and implementation*. Cambridge, MA: MIT Press.
23. Jonas, S., & Rosenberg, S. (1986). Ambulatory care. In S. Jonas (Ed.), *Health care delivery in the United States* (3rd ed.) (pp. 125–165). New York: Springer.
24. Sofaer, S. (1988). Community health planning in the United States: A postmortem. *Family Community Health, 10*(4), 1–12.
25. Barhydt-Wezenaar, N. (1986). Nursing. In S. Jonas (Ed.), *Health care delivery in the United States* (3rd ed.) (pp. 166–183). New York: Springer.
26. Ford, L. C., & Silver, H. K. (1967). The expanded role of the nurse in child care. *Nursing Outlook, 15*(9), 43–45.
27. Harris, M. D. (1988). The changing scene in community health nursing. *Nursing Clinics of North America, 23*(3), 559–568.
28. Salmon, M. E. (1989). Public health nursing: The neglected speciality. *Nursing Outlook, 37*, 226–229.

RECOMMENDED READINGS

Buhler-Wilkerson, K. (1987). Left carrying the bag: Early experiments in visiting nursing, 1877–1909. *Nursing Research, 36*, 42–47.

Describes the development of the visiting nurse movement in terms of its origin, sponsorship, variation, and appeal.

Buhler-Wilkerson, K. (1988). Public health nursing: A photographic study. *Nursing Outlook, 36*, 241–243.

Analyzes the use of photographs to publicize the work of early visiting nurse associations. Provides a delightful look at community health nursing of the past.

Coss, C. (1989). *Lillian Wald: A progressive activist*. New York: Feminist Press.

Provides a provocative look at the life and work of Lillian Wald, foundress of the Henry Street Settlement. Contains the play Lillian Wald: At Home on Henry Street *as well as excerpts from the letters and speeches of Lillian Wald.*

Erickson, G. (1987). Southern initiative in public health nursing: The founding of the Nurses' Settlement and Instructive Visiting Nurse Association of Richmond, Virginia, 1900–1910. *Journal of Nursing History, 3*(1), 17–29.

Examines the founding of a southern nurses' settlement house similar to the Henry Street Settlement House in New York City, by a group of recent graduates. Describes differences and similarities between the two organizations and the situational factors influencing each.

Frachel, R. R. (1988). A new profession: The evolution of public health nursing. *Public Health Nursing, 5*(2), 86–90.

Describes the life and times of Lillian Wald as one of the early pioneers of community health nursing in the United States.

Hamilton, D. (1989). The cost of caring: The Metropolitan Life Insurance Company's Visiting Nurse Service, 1909–1953. *Bulletin of the History of Medicine, 63,* 414–434.

Looks at the societal events that led to the incorporation of visiting nursing into services provided to premium holders of the Metropolitan Life Insurance Company. Also details the differences in perspective between business and nursing that led to the project's demise in 1953.

Monteiro, Lois A. (1987). Insights from the past. *Nursing Outlook, 35*(2), 65–69.

Reviews two fictional nurses created by public health nursing historian Mary Gardner. Discusses past and current issues that surface in the stories and their implications for community health nursing then and now.

Sofaer, S. (1988). Community health planning in the United States: A postmortem. *Family and Community Health, 10*(4), 1–12.

Discusses the reasons for the demise of regional health planning and health systems agencies in the U.S. and the lessons to be learned for future efforts at systematic planning for health-care delivery.

Young, E. E. (1989). A quiet day: A peep at some of the varied homes visited by a district nurse in the course of one "quiet day." *Public Health Nursing, 6*(1), 43–44. Reprinted from *The Public Health Nurse,* February 1923.

Provides an idea of some of the activities performed and clients served by early community health nurses.

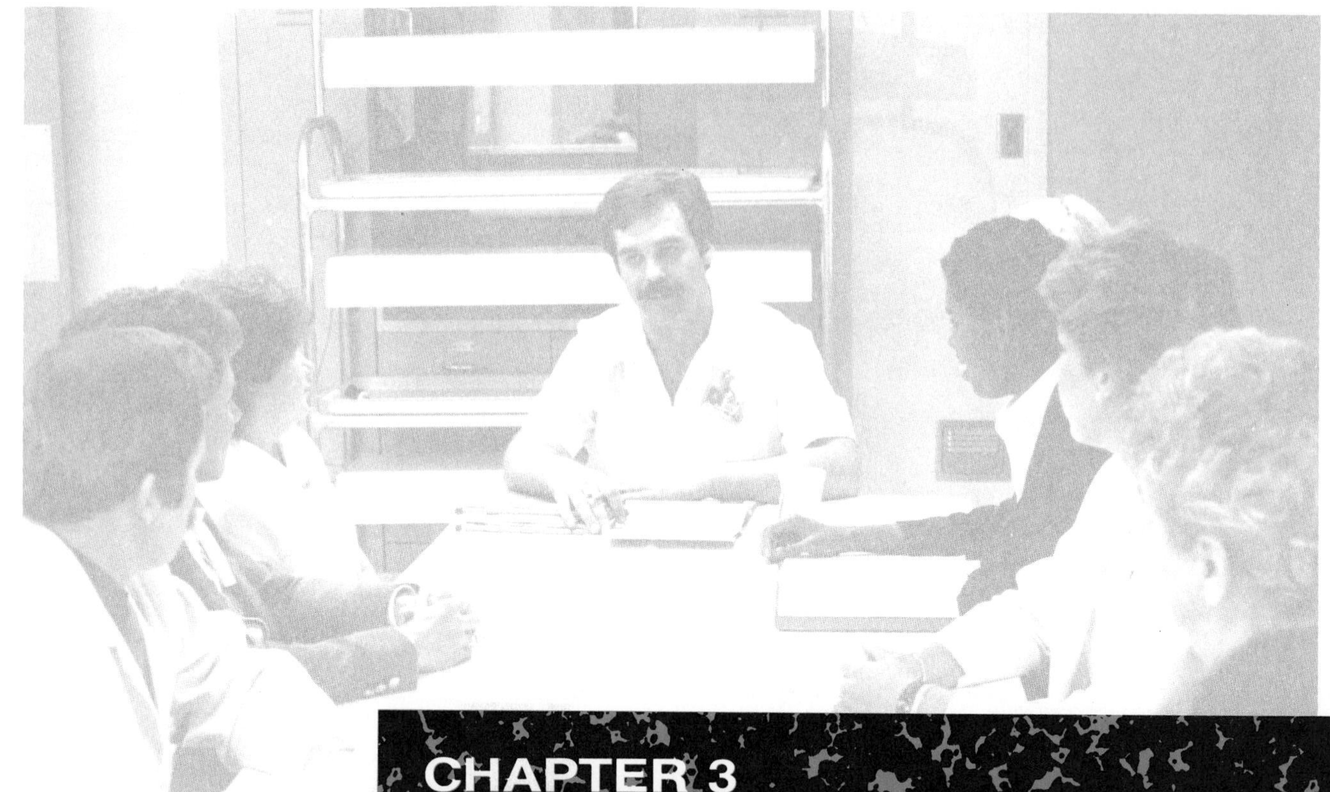

CHAPTER 3

The Health-Care Context

KEY TERMS

Alcohol, Drug Abuse, and Mental Health Administration
bilateral agencies
Centers for Disease Control
community health-care sector
Department of Health and Human Services
fragmentation
Food and Drug Administration
health-care system
Health Resources and Services Administration (HRSA)
Health Care Financing Administration (HCFA)
multicentric
multilateral agencies
National Institutes of Health
Office of Human Development Services
official health agencies
Pan American Health Organization
popular health-care subsystem
personal health-care sector
pluralism
scientific health-care subsystem
Social Security Administration
traditional health-care subsystem
United States Public Health Service
voluntary health agencies
World Health Organization

one single system, such as found in Great Britain, Canada, Australia, and elsewhere, many independent systems provide scientific health care in the United States. Personal health-care services are separated from community health services, and care may be provided by either public or private organizations.

MULTICENTRICITY

The U.S. scientific health-care subsystem is also ***multicentric***—that is, decisions regarding health care arise at many points within the system. No single agency is totally responsible for determining health-care goals and activities for the nation. The multicentric nature of the American health-care system often results in conflicting health-care goals and little concerted effort to consolidate resources or apply them in an effective and efficient manner.

FRAGMENTATION

The third characteristic of the U.S. scientific health-care subsystem, ***fragmentation,*** arises out of the first two. Because there are multiple foci for decision making, health-care delivery is fragmented, resulting in duplication in some services and gaps in others. Concerted planning efforts have decreased, but not entirely eliminated, fragmentation. A recent report by the Institute of Medicine (IOM) indicated that the nation's health-care system is ineffective in meeting the needs of the public. The report included findings of a total lack of any local public health-care facility in some parts of the nation and ineffective use of resources in all areas. According to the report, health-care crises, such as the high cost of health care and the growing AIDS epidemic, are consistently addressed on a short-term basis without considering long-term solutions. There is also inequity in the way in which health-care resources are distributed and a lack of response by health officials to the needs of the population. The report concluded that, because of the weaknesses of a fragmented health-care system, unnecessary deficits in the public's health continue to exist.[4]

COMPONENTS OF THE SCIENTIFIC HEALTH-CARE SUBSYSTEM

The scientific health-care subsystem consists of two sectors that differ primarily in terms of their focus of care. These sectors are the personal health-care sector and the community health-care sector.[1]

THE PERSONAL HEALTH-CARE SECTOR

The focus of care in the ***personal health-care sector*** is the health of the individual. The primary emphasis in this sector is cure of disease and restoration of health, although individuals may also receive some health-promotive and illness-preventive services. Personal health services are provided in office settings, clinics, hospitals, and other places where care is dispensed to individual clients. Institutions, such as hospitals and clinics, that provide personal health care may be either privately or publicly funded. For example, both private hospitals and publicly funded community hospitals are part of the personal health-care sector.

THE COMMUNITY HEALTH-CARE SECTOR

Although health-care services may be provided to individual clients in the ***community health-care sector,*** the primary focus of this sector is on the health of populations. Care provided usually centers on promoting health and preventing disease, although some curative care does occur in this sector. Emphasis is on designing health-care programs that meet the needs of population groups. Health-care services in this sector may be provided by official or voluntary agencies.

Official Health Agencies

Official health agencies are agencies of local, state, and national governments that are responsible for the health of the people in their jurisdiction. Official agencies are supported by tax revenues and other public funding. They are accountable to the citizens of their jurisdiction, usually through an elected or appointed governing body. Many of the activities conducted by official agencies are mandated by law. For example, local health departments are required by state law to report cases of certain diseases. We will discuss the functions of official agencies at local, state, and national levels in more detail later in this chapter.

Voluntary Health Agencies

Voluntary health agencies are organizations that are formed by groups of people because of their interest in a particular health concern, such as diabetes, child abuse, or environmental pollution. Voluntary agencies are funded primarily by donations. They are accountable to their supporters, and their activities are determined by supporter interest, rather than legal mandate. Their primary emphasis lies in the areas of research and education, although they may provide a few direct health-care services.

Voluntary agencies can be categorized on the basis of their source of funding. The first category consists of agencies supported by citizen contributions, such as the American Cancer Society. The second category consists of foundations established by private philanthropic contributions. An example of this type of voluntary organization would be the Kellogg Foundation that provides funding for health-care research. The third category of voluntary agency is funded by member dues. The American Public Health Association and the American Nurses' Association are examples of this type of agency. Integrating agencies, such as the United Way, coordinate the fund-raising activities of several voluntary agencies. The final category of voluntary health agency is the commercial organization that engages in health-care activities. For example, the American Dairy Association provides literature and visual aids for nutrition education. Similarly, health insurance companies often put out literature on health promotion and illness prevention.

Voluntary agencies perform eight basic functions within the scientific health-care subsystem. The first of these is *pioneering* activities. Voluntary agencies explore areas that are underserved by the other components of the health-care system. For example, research that culminated in the development of a vaccine for polio was the early focus of the March of Dimes. Now, polio immunization is largely a function of official agencies.

The second function of voluntary agencies is *demonstration* of pilot projects in health-care delivery. For instance, the Planned Parenthood Association instituted clinics for contraceptive services long before most official health agencies became involved in this area of service. *Education* of the public and health professionals is the third function of voluntary agencies. For example, the American Cancer Society has spearheaded educational campaigns on the hazards of smoking. The fourth function of voluntary health agencies is *supplementation* of services provided by official health agencies. For instance, some voluntary agencies provide transportation to clinics, respite care, special equipment, and other ancillary services.

Fifth, voluntary health agencies engage in *advocacy* for the public's health. For example, a voluntary agency may campaign against reduction of health-care services due to budget cuts. The sixth function, promoting *legislation* related to health, is a closely related function. In Tennessee, for example, the Fraternal Order of Police and the Tennessee Nurses' Association were instrumental in getting child car restraint legislation passed.

The seventh function of voluntary agencies relates to health *planning and organization.* Voluntary agencies often assist official agencies in determining health-care needs in the population and in planning programs to address those needs. The final function of voluntary agencies is *assisting official agencies* in developing well-balanced community health programs. For example, voluntary agencies often provide services that fill gaps in services available from official agencies.

LEVELS OF HEALTH-CARE DELIVERY

Health-care delivery in the United States takes place on local, state, and national levels. Each level has certain responsibilities with respect to the health of the population. Both official and voluntary agencies exist at each level, but official agencies will be the focus of this discussion.

The Health Services Extension Act of 1977 mandated the development of standards for official community preventive health services. This mandate led to the creation of a Model Standards Work Group composed of representatives of the American Public Health Association (APHA), the Association of State and Territorial Health Officials, the National Association of County Health Officers, and the Centers for Disease Control (CDC). This work group developed the document *Model Standards for Community Preventive Health Services,* first published by APHA in 1979. A second edition of this document was prepared and published in 1985.[5]

The model standards identified 34 areas of responsibility for preventive health services by official public health agencies. These areas range from responsibilities for program administration to providing care for special population groups such as the elderly, the poor, and mothers and children. Official agencies are also responsible for environmental and occupational health; control of specific types of health problems such as chronic and communicable disease; and substance abuse, animal control, health-promotion and illness-preventive services.

THE LOCAL LEVEL

The official agency at the local level is usually the *local health department.* The health department's authority is derived, in part, from responsibilities delegated by the state for certain functions. For example, the state delegates to the local level the responsibility for collecting statistics on births and deaths. Because this responsibility has been legally delegated, the local health department has the authority to ensure that death certificates are filed for every death that occurs. The local agency also derives authority from local health ordinances. For instance, local government might pass an ordinance requiring all residential rental units to have functioning smoke detectors. Enforcement of this ordinance might then become the responsibility of the local health department.

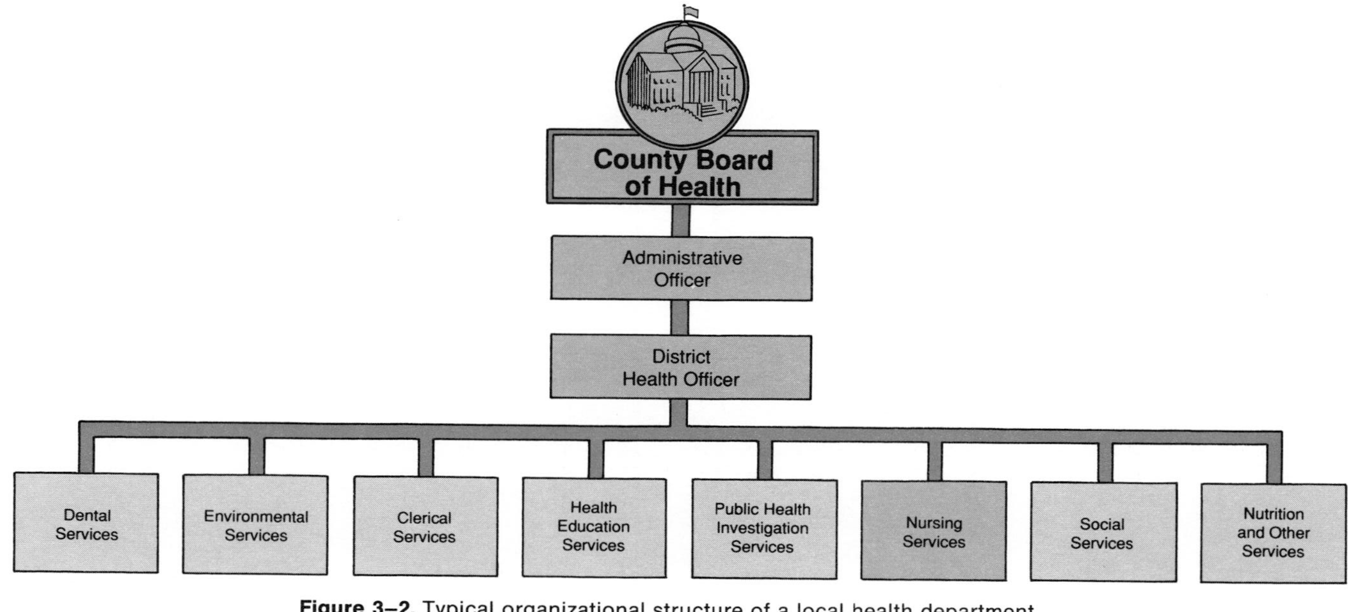

Figure 3–2. Typical organizational structure of a local health department.

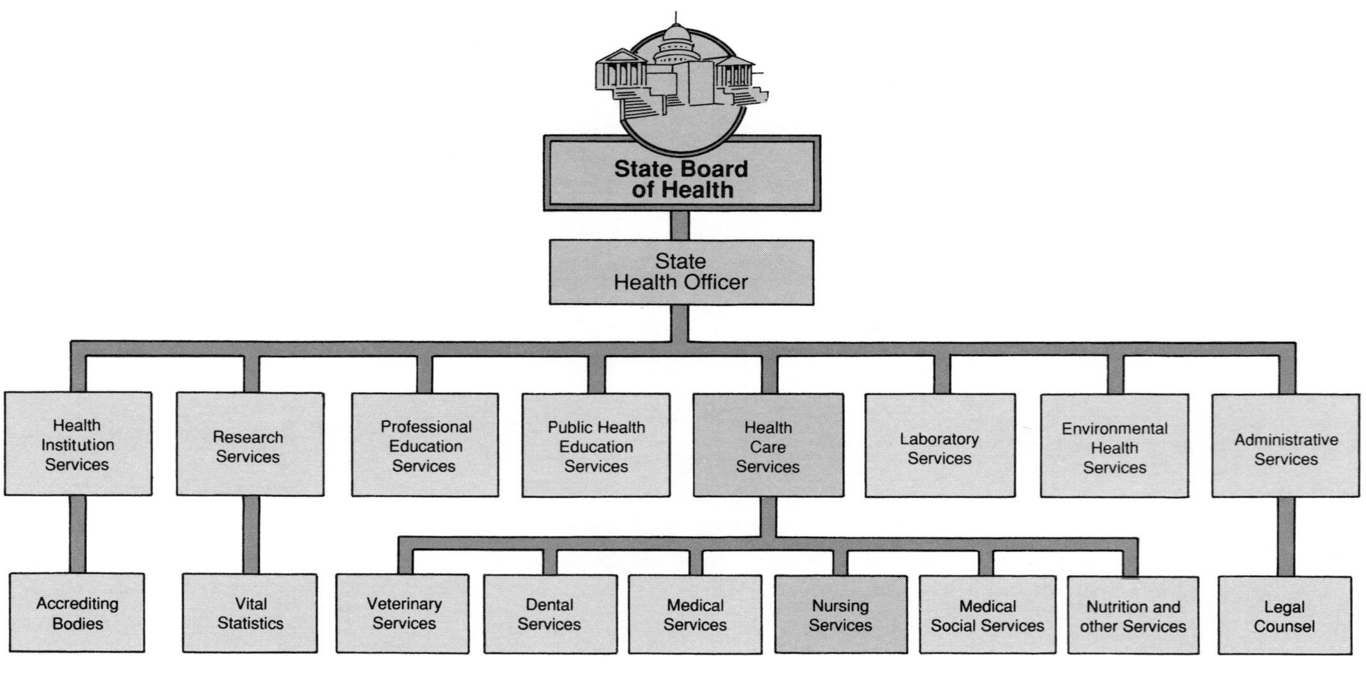

Figure 3–3. Typical organizational structure of a state health department.

Funding at the local level comes from both local taxes and state and federal subsidies. Figure 3–2 depicts the typical organizational structure of a local health department. The staff and programs included will vary from place to place. In some areas, the district health officer might also fulfill the role of administrative officer. Small counties and districts may not be able to afford the full-time services of some types of personnel, and the services of nutritionists, social workers, dentists, and other personnel might be shared by several counties. Nurses and clerical staff would be found in almost any health department. Other personnel who may be available include environmental specialists, physical therapists, psychologists, laboratory and X-ray technicians, and pharmacists.

Because delegation of specific responsibilities to local jurisdictions is the function of the state, the responsibilities assumed will vary from state to state. Local responsibilities may also vary within regions of a particular state depending upon the local jurisdiction's capabilities and resources. In general, local health agencies perform four primary functions. These functions include disseminating health information, providing leadership in local health-care planning, promoting the use of area health resources, and providing direct services as designated by the state. The local government health agency is responsible for identifying and monitoring health problems in the population and ensuring the availability of services to resolve those problems.[5]

THE STATE LEVEL

The official agency at the state level has traditionally been a state department of health. The state, as opposed to the federal government or the local jurisdiction, has primary authority in matters relating to health. This authority is derived from the sovereign powers reserved to the states under the U.S. Constitution. This being the case, the state retains the ultimate responsibility for the health of the public and possesses essential power to make laws and regulations regarding health.

The state health department derives funding from state tax revenues and may also receive monies from the federal government. A general organizational schema for a state department of health is depicted in Figure 3–3. The various divisions coordinate services at the state level and provide assistance to the local level.

In general, state health agencies have four major functions. These include leadership in health planning and programming, financial and technical assistance to local agencies, establishment and enforcement of health standards, and provision of certain direct services. A 1977 survey of health laws in the 50 states identified 44 specific functions mandated by state laws.[6] These functions can be grouped into several categories relating to (1) regulation, inspection, and licensure, (2) personal health services, (3) control of communicable disease, (4) environmental health, (5) laboratory and hospital services, (6) health education, (7) resource planning, and (8) collection of vital statistics. Specific functions related to each category are presented in Table 3–1.

THE NATIONAL LEVEL

Because the Constitution makes no reference to any responsibilities of the federal government regarding health, the federal government has no direct authority to regulate health-related matters. The powers of the federal government with respect to health are derived indirectly from three constitutional powers. The first of these is the *power to regulate foreign and interstate commerce.* For example, because most cosmetics are transported across state lines, the federal Food and Drug Administration (FDA) has the authority to establish standards of purity for the manufacture of cosmetics.

The second constitutional source of authority over health matters is the *power to levy taxes and pro-*

TABLE 3–1. FUNCTIONS OF OFFICIAL STATE AGENCIES AND RELATED ACTIVITIES

Functional Category	Related Activity
Regulation, inspection, and licensure	• Inspect housing, food, milk, and restaurants • License health-care facilities • Register health-care personnel • Monitor occupational health
Personal health services	• Provide nutrition programs for selected populations • Provide medical treatment services • Provide dental services • Provide school health services • Provide community health nursing services • Provide family planning services

(*continued*)

TABLE 3–1. ***(Continued)***

Functional Category	Related Activity
	• Provide treatment for substance abuse • Provide services for handicapped persons • Provide programs for control of chronic diseases • Provide ambulatory and emergency medical services • Provide screening for specific diseases
Control of communicable diseases	• Control rabies • Conduct surveillance and report incidence and prevalence of communicable diseases • Initiate quarantine measures • Diagnose and treat specific communicable diseases (including sexually transmitted diseases and tuberculosis)
Maintenance of environmental health	• Monitor environmental conditions • Prevent or reduce pollution • Control nuisances • Provide for refuse and toxic waste disposal • Control vectors • Monitor and control radiation levels
Laboratory and hospital services	• License and monitor biological testing laboratories • License and inspect hospitals • Provide laboratory services for selected tests • Monitor results of specific laboratory tests (e.g., tests for syphilis)
Health education	• Provide public education on health promotion and disease prevention • Provide public education related to secondary and tertiary prevention of selected disorders
Resource planning	• Assess state health needs • Assess state health resources • Plan health programs to meet state health needs
Collection of vital statistics	• Collect vital statistics and health statistics • Summarize and publish state vital statistics

mote the general welfare. For instance, it can be argued that such programs as Medicaid and Medicare promote the general welfare and are, therefore, within the authority of the federal government. The *power to make treaties* is the third source of federal power in matters relating to health. For example, a treaty with Mexico could specify that the Mexican government would take specific steps to control the shipment of illicit drugs into the United States.

The official health agency at the national level is the ***Department of Health and Human Services*** (DHHS) created in 1980 with the division of the former Department of Health, Education, and Welfare into two separate departments. The head of the agency is the secretary for Health and Human Services who fills a cabinet post and acts in an advisory capacity to the president in matters of health.

Figure 3–4 depicts part of the organizational structure of this department. The health component of the Department of Health and Human Services is the ***United States Public Health Service*** (USPHS). The USPHS consists of five agencies. The ***Food and Drug Administration*** (FDA) is responsible for establishing and enforcing standards for the manufacture and processing of food, drugs, and cosmetics. It is also responsible for ascertaining the safety of new drugs and other health-related products, such as food additives and medical devices. The ***Centers for Disease Control*** (CDC) investigates causes of communicable disease and establishes policies and standards for the diagnosis and treatment of communicable disease as well as establishing immunization schedules and recommendations. The CDC also now houses the National Center for Health Statistics, previously a part of the Office of the Assistant Secretary for Health. The ***National Institutes of Health*** (NIH) conducts health-related research and provides some direct service to individuals in the course of that research.

The ***Health Resources and Services Administration*** (HRSA) was created by the merging of the previous Health Services Administration and Health Resources Administration. This combined agency is responsible for training and utilization of health professionals and health resources planning and utilization. This agency is also responsible for the administration of the Indian Health Service, the Bureau of Prisons, the National Health Service Corps, the Bureau of Health Maintenance Organizations and Resources Development, and programs for maternal and child health, family planning, rural and migrant health, community health centers, and emergency medical services. One additional bureau within this agency of interest to community health nurses is the Bureau of Health Professionals, which houses the Division of Nursing.

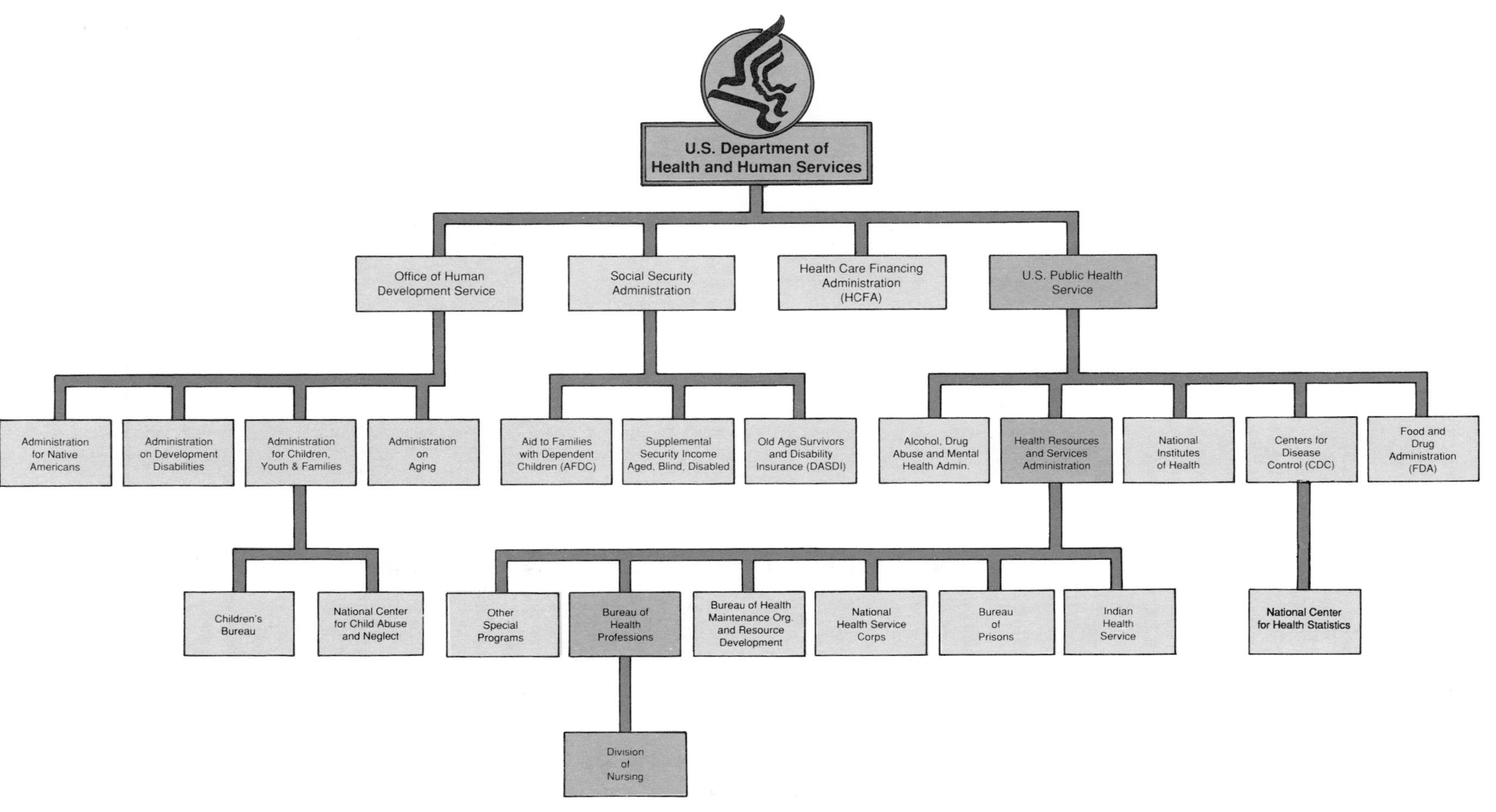

Figure 3–4. Partial organizational structure of the U.S. Department of Health and Human Services.

The last of the agencies under USPHS, the ***Alcohol, Drug Abuse, and Mental Health Administration,*** coordinates programs in these areas. This administration includes the National Institute on Alcohol Abuse and Alcoholism, the National Institute on Drug Abuse, and the National Institute of Mental Health.

The ***Health Care Financing Administration*** (HCFA) is responsible for federally funded programs under Medicare, Medicaid, and the Civilian Health and Medical Program of the Uniformed Services (CHAMPUS). This agency is responsible for reimbursement under these programs and sets reimbursement rates under the DRG system discussed earlier. The HCFA is also responsible for quality and utilization control for the programs under its jurisdiction.

The ***Social Security Administration*** handles the Social Security program, more properly titled the Old Age, Survivors and Disability Insurance program (OASDI). This agency is also responsible for the administration of the Supplemental Security Income for the Aged, Blind, and Disabled program (SSI) and has recently become the administrative agency for the program of Aid to Families with Dependent Children (AFDC).

The last major component of the Department of Health and Human Services is the ***Office of Human Development Services.*** Under the aegis of this agency

TABLE 3–2. FEDERAL HEALTH-RELATED AGENCIES AND THEIR FUNCTIONS

Agency or Organization	Functions
Alcohol, Drug Abuse, and Mental Health Administration 5600 Fisher's Lane Rockville, MD 20857 (301) 443-4797	Coordinate programs for mental health research, information
Centers for Disease Control 1600 Clifton Rd. Atlanta, GA 30333 (404) 329-3291	Conduct research on prevention Conduct disease-prevention programs
Food and Drug Administration 5600 Fisher's Lane Rockville, MD 20857 (301) 443-2410	Prevent adulteration of food, drugs, and other products
Health Care Financing Administration 200 Independence Ave, S.W. Washington, DC 20201 (202) 245-6726	Fund federal health programs
Health Resources and Services Administration 5600 Fisher's Lane Rockville, MD 20857 (301) 443-2216	Educate health personnel Administer Native American health maternal-child, prison, health maintenance organization, family planning, and other programs
National Institutes of Health 9000 Rockville Pike Bethesda, MD 20892 (301) 496-4000	Conduct and fund health-related research
Office of Human Development Services 200 Independence Ave, S.W. Washington, DC 20201 (202) 472-7257	Administer funds for services to special populations such as the aged, children, the disabled, etc.
Public Health Service 200 Independence Ave, S.W. Washington, DC 20201 (202) 245-7694	Coordinate federal health programs
Social Security Administration 6401 Security Bldg. Baltimore, MD 21235 (301) 594-3120	Administer Social Security and Medicare programs
U.S. Department of Health and Human Services 200 Independence Ave, S.W. Washington, DC 20201 (202) 245-6298	Formulate and implement national health policies

are programs for a variety of social and health services for populations with special needs. Agencies within the office include the Administration on Aging, the Administration for Children, Youth, and Families (which houses the Children's Bureau and the newly created National Center on Child Abuse and Neglect), the Administration on Developmental Disabilities, and the Administration for Native Americans. The components of the Department of Health and Human Services and their functions are summarized in Table 3–2. The address and phone number of each agency is provided for those who wish to obtain further information on specific services.

Agencies at the federal level provide assistance to state and local agencies in the form of health resources and professional education. Agencies also assist in improving health-care delivery, and they conduct, support, and disseminate findings of health-related research. Additional federal responsibilities related to health include protecting the public against unsafe food and drugs, controlling communicable diseases, and functioning as liaison between the United States and international health organizations or with other countries. Federal agencies also provide direct services to certain population groups such as Native Americans and military personnel, retirees, and dependents.

INTERNATIONAL HEALTH CARE

Because of the interdependence among nations and the ability that people now have to travel to any place in the world in a matter of hours, there is increasing concern for international health. Increased mobility means increased potential for the spread of disease from nation to nation. This remains true of communicable diseases traditionally spread by travelers from infected to noninfected areas. In addition, increased global communication and mobility have led to changes in life-style that bring the attendant risks of many life-style related chronic illnesses. For example, dietary changes that occur as many developing countries are exposed to Western culture have contributed to a rise in heart disease. Adoption of new life-styles in many parts of the world have also contributed to the development of stress-related disorders.[7] Increased travel and import/export opportunities have also increased the potential for trafficking in illegal substances and increased drug use around the world. Alcoholism is another growing concern worldwide.[8] Finally, environmental concerns are now international, rather than local, in scope.

HEALTH-CARE SYSTEMS IN OTHER COUNTRIES

The health-care delivery systems of many other countries differ greatly from the U.S. system of health care. These systems can be categorized on the basis of their economic structure and the political system governing their operation. Economic features include a system's source of funding and its payment mechanisms, whereas political considerations reflect the extent to which government is involved in the health-care delivery process. The five categories of health systems are: (1) the free-enterprise system, (2) the welfare system, (3) the transitional system, (4) the underdeveloped system, and (5) the socialist system.[9]

FREE-ENTERPRISE SYSTEMS

The free-enterprise system is exemplified by the United States. In this type of system, health services are primarily delivered in an open market with comparatively little governmental intervention or control over supply, demand, or cost of services. A free-enterprise system usually operates on a fee-for-service basis, although the fee may not be paid directly by the person receiving care. As we will see in Chapter 13, Economic Influences on Community Health, very little health care in the United States is paid for directly by the consumer.

WELFARE SYSTEMS

The welfare system emphasizes equal services for all members of the population and is usually financed by some form of social insurance contributions. There is considerable governmental involvement in the delivery of health care, and the government may actually provide the bulk of available health-care services. Welfare systems of health-care delivery are found in the United Kingdom, France, Canada, Sweden, Norway, and Germany.

In the United Kingdom, the National Health Service provides basic health care to all citizens. Services are relatively comprehensive, with about 85 percent of health-care costs financed by general revenues, 10 percent by social insurance, and only 5 percent by out-of-pocket expenditures by consumers.[10] All hospitals are operated by the government through the British Ministry of Health. Physicians are of two primary types—general practitioners and specialists. General practitioners are paid a basic salary plus a per capita allotment for the number of clients served. Specialists are salaried employees of the hospitals, though many specialists also maintain a part-time, fee-for-service practice. In most cases, hospitalization or specialist services require a referral from a general practitioner.

The Canadian health-care system shares many features of the British system, but it also has some features in common with the American model. In Canada, there is an approximately equal sharing of financial costs between the federal and provincial governments derived from comprehensive health insurance plans. For provinces to be eligible for cost-sharing, the provincial health-care system must cover all medically required physician and hospital services, provide equal coverage for all citizens (despite risk), cover clients while traveling in other provinces, and be managed on a nonprofit basis by a public agency. Coverage does not include drugs or dental care nor does it pay for some extended-care and rehabilitation services; for example, nursing home services are not covered.

Canadian hospitals have not been nationalized as is the case in Great Britain; they do, however, submit budgets to the government to cover their operating costs. The Canadian system of payment for physicians also differs from the British system. In Canada, as in the United States, most physician services are reimbursed on a fee-for-service basis rather than salary. Fee schedules are negotiated between medical associations and the government of each Canadian province.

TRANSITIONAL SYSTEM

Transitional systems exist in countries where much of the population is poor and rural and where there is a modest government-run structure for providing basic health services coexisting with a growing private fee-for-service health-care sector for the affluent. There may be a rudimentary program of social insurance for health care for workers and their families. Many Latin American and Middle Eastern countries have transitional health-care systems.

Peru has a transitional health system in which approximately 50 percent of health-care funding comes from private payments. Other sources of funding include general revenues, social security contributions, and charity. As is the case in many transitional systems, the majority of expenditures go to provide care for the affluent and beneficiaries of the social insurance system. The majority of physicians care for the poor on a salaried basis and for the rich in fee-for-service private practices.[9]

Another transitional system is found in India where there is a plurality of sources of health care and of funding. The Ministry of Health controls a centralized health-care system that provides basic services throughout the country. These services are supplemented, however, by those provided on a fee-for-service basis by a variety of practitioners of both Western and traditional medicine. Government physicians are salaried and are usually educated at government expense. Following their education, they are usually expected to serve in a rural location within the official system for several years before they are free to establish a private practice.

UNDERDEVELOPED SYSTEMS

Underdeveloped countries have poorly organized systems of health-care delivery, particularly in rural areas. There is little government involvement in health care and little funding available for services. In many instances, the health care that is available is provided by missionary groups and other humanitarian organizations. Many African nations have underdeveloped systems.

SOCIALIST SYSTEMS

Socialist systems are characterized by almost complete government control of health-care delivery. Examples of such systems are found in the Soviet Union, throughout Eastern Europe, and in the People's Republic of China.

In the Soviet Union, funding is derived from general revenues with services nominally available to all. In reality, people in metropolitan areas and individuals in high government circles receive higher-quality care than others. All facilities are government-owned and operated, and physicians are salaried employees. In Poland, health care is free to all citizens, and hospitals have been nationalized. Physicians are salaried but are permitted to engage in private practice. However, private practice accounts for only approximately 2 percent of office and home visits.[11] The system is centralized and provides comprehensive care.

In China, despite revolutionary tenets of health care as a right, services are not free. China's health-care system is funded by a health insurance fund titled the Cooperative Medical Service (CMS). Citizens are organized in collectives or work units that control much of everyday life in China. These production units collect and administer health insurance funds, and basic health-care services are provided at the production-unit level. More specialized services may be provided at regional or metropolitan levels. Contributions to the fund are made on a yearly basis by each participant with a per capita contribution from the welfare fund of the production unit. There is also some co-payment for services. Physicians are salaried and health-care facilities are government-owned and operated.

As can be seen from the discussion in the preceding paragraphs, there is a great deal of variety in national health-care delivery systems. Table 3–3 compares the primary features of the health-care systems of several nations to the U.S. health-care system.

TABLE 3–3. COMPARISON OF U.S. AND OTHER NATIONAL HEALTH-CARE SYSTEMS

		Economic Features				Government Involvement		
System Type	**Country**	***Source of Funding***	***Set Fee Schedule?***	***Physician Payment***	***Client Payment***	***Locus of Control***	***Hospitals***	***Comprehensive Services?***
Free enterprise	U.S.	Multiple sources	No	Fee-for-service	Variable	Pluralistic	Public and private, profit and nonprofit	No
Welfare	United Kingdom	General revenues and social insurance	N/A	Capitation and/or salaried	Some co-payment	Centralized	Nationalized	Yes
	Canada	Provincial health insurance	Yes	Fee-for-service	—	Decentralized	Government-supported	No
	Sweden	Health insurance taxes	N/A	Salaried	Some co-payment	—	—	Yes
	Norway	Social insurance and general revenues	Yes	Salaried and fee-for-service	Some co-payment	Centralized	Nationalized	No
	Germany	Sick-fund contributions	Yes	Fee-for-service and salaried	Some co-payment	Decentralized	Government support and per diem negotiated with sick-fund	Yes
Transitional	Peru	General revenues, Social Security, charity, private pay	No	Fee-for-service and salaried	Variable	Decentralized	Variable	No
	India	General revenues, charity, private pay	No	Fee-for-service and salaried	Variable	Pluralistic	Public and private	No
Socialist	Soviet Union	General revenues	N/A	Salaried	—	Centralized	Nationalized	Yes
	Poland	General revenues	No	Salaried and fee-for-service	None	Centralized	Nationalized	Yes
	People's Republic of China	Health insurance fund	N/A	Salaried	Some co-payment	Decentralized	Nationalized	

INTERNATIONAL HEALTH AGENCIES

On the global level the organization of health services is somewhat less structured than in the national systems discussed above. A number of organizations and agencies are concerned with international health. These agencies can be described as either bilateral or multilateral.[12] ***Multilateral agencies*** are those that involve several countries in joint activities related to health, while ***bilateral agencies*** usually involve only two countries in any single project.

MULTILATERAL AGENCIES

The primary agency dealing with health concerns at the international level is the ***World Health Organization*** (WHO), a multilateral agency. A specialized agency attached to the United Nations by formal agreement, but not subordinate to the U.N., WHO is funded through subscription by member nations and is responsible for monitoring the incidence of disease throughout the world and for setting international standards for sanitation, biological products, laboratory techniques and procedures, and the manufacture of drugs. The World Health Organization supports graduate study and research efforts and assists member nations in controlling disease. A further responsibility is monitoring environmental pollution levels through a program called "Earthwatch" and providing assistance to underdeveloped countries to prevent or eliminate pollution.

The ***Pan American Health Organization*** (PAHO) is another multilateral health organization of particular interest. This agency deals with health-related concerns in the Americas and provides an avenue for collective efforts to promote the health status of people in all nations in the Western Hemisphere.

One of PAHO's current programs provides profiles of the health assessment efforts of international agencies. This is the Health Situation and Trend Analysis Program. The intent of this program is the development of health profiles of member nations as part of a continuing effort to identify factors influencing health. National profiles include information on the health status of citizens, the health system within the country, and the environmental context in which the society is evolving.[13] This information will provide direction for programs to enhance health status in member nations. Recent research in Tijuana, Mexico, has also been aimed at obtaining reliable health status data.[14]

Other multilateral agencies include the health components of the North Atlantic Treaty Organization (NATO) and the Southeast Asia Treaty Organization (SEATO). The United Nations International Children's Emergency Fund (UNICEF) and the United Nations Educational, Scientific, and Cultural Organization (UNESCO) are two other agencies within the United Nations that provide assistance with matters of international health. The Food and Agricultural Organization (FAO) is also a multilateral organization designed to enhance the world's food supply. Finally, the World Bank provides both funding and technical assistance in dealing with health problems around the world.

BILATERAL AGENCIES

A number of bilateral organizations with health concerns exist throughout the world. Virtually all developed countries provide some form of health-related aid to underdeveloped countries, with the contribution of some countries far in excess of that provided by the United States. This section will focus on the bilateral organizations found in the United States. Such organizations may be either governmental or nongovernmental. One of the federal agencies that is concerned with international health is the Agency for International Development (AID), which administers all federally financed projects for foreign development, including those that are health-related. AID is housed in the U.S. State Department.

The Department of Health and Human Services includes the Office of International Health, which is also concerned with cooperative projects for improving international health. The Fogarty International Center is housed in the National Institutes of Health (NIH) and focuses on international health. Other branches of NIH (for example, the Geographic Medicine Branch of the Institute of Allergy and Infectious Diseases) are involved in activities that are international in focus, as is the Centers for Disease Control (CDC). ACTION is the volunteer organization of the federal government that houses both the domestic assistance programs of VISTA (Volunteers in Service to America) and the international programs of the Peace Corps, many of which have a health focus. Federally chartered institutions such as the Institute of Medicine (IOM) and the National Science Foundation are also concerned with problems of international health, as well as with domestic problems.

As of 1977, there were more than 120 registered nongovernmental voluntary agencies in the United States[12] that provide health-related assistance to other countries. Examples of these agencies include CARE and Project HOPE. In addition, there are more than 50 private philanthropic foundations such as the Rockefeller Foundation that are actively involved in international health programs. Finally, there are numerous missionary groups that provide health care in developing countries as well as in underserved areas in developed nations. Names and addresses of several of the multilateral and bilateral health organizations are included in Table 3–4 for those who wish to obtain further information.

CONCERNS IN INTERNATIONAL HEALTH

The health of third-world countries is of particular concern to international health agencies. In these countries, many health problems that are of minor concern in the United States and other developed nations continue to have devastating effects on citizens. In the 40 poorest countries of the world, life expectancy at birth is only 46 years, mortality in children under age 5 is 22 percent, and 31 percent of children suffer some form of malnutrition. Even in neighboring areas of Mexico, the infant mortality rate is 92 per 1000 live births.[14]

Throughout the world, approximately 4.5 million children die each year from diarrheal diseases, while communicable diseases of all kinds remain a serious problem despite raising immunization levels for childhood diseases from 5 percent to 50 percent of the world's population in the last 10 years. Cholera, yellow fever, plague, Hansen's disease (leprosy), typhoid, parasitic diseases, pneumonia, hepatitis B, sexually transmitted diseases, and tuberculosis remain prevalent in most underdeveloped countries.[15–18] Although immunization programs save the lives of an estimated 1.5 million children each year, still only half of the world's children under 1 year of age are adequately immunized[19] and polio, tetanus, diphtheria, measles, and pertussis continue to be prevalent.[20]

AIDS is a serious problem not only in the United States but globally. Nutrition is another primary problem in most of the world. Wasting, resulting from acute dietary insufficiency, occurs in less than 5 percent of children in the United States compared to more than 30 percent in places like India. Similarly, the average number of calories per day available to U.S. citizens is more than 3200, while that in some parts of the world is less than 2000. The diets of people in countries like India and much of Africa are particularly deficient in vitamin A, while population segments in most countries, including the United States, have diets deficient in iodine.[21]

Environmental concerns are drawing greater attention in international health than ever before. For years there has been concern with safe water, yet today safe water supplies are available to less than 60 percent of the population of many countries and less than 20 percent of the population of Bangladesh and some parts of Africa. There is a distinct difference in the availability of safe water in urban versus rural areas. In the United States, for instance, 93.6 percent of the urban population has access to safe water compared to 42.5 percent of the rural population. In Africa, with the poorest water situation, 66.5 percent have access to safe water in urban areas compared to only 27.6 percent in rural areas.[21]

More recent environmental issues include global concern over radiation,[22] destruction of the ozone layer, air pollution, lead poisoning, and chemical con-

TABLE 3–4. HEALTH-RELATED INTERNATIONAL AGENCIES

Agency or Organization	Services
Concern/America 2024 N. Broadway P.O. Box 1790 Santa Ana, CA 92702	Provides hunger relief and development
Direct Relief International P.O. Box 41929 Santa Barbara, CA 93140-0820	Provides hospital and clinic care Emergency relief
International Association for Maternal and Neonatal Health Kurberstrasse 1 CH 8049 Zurich, Switzerland	Projects to improve maternal and neonatal health in developing countries
International Organization for Cooperation in Health Care Postbus 1547 NL-6501 BM Nijmegen, Netherlands	Provides socio-medical information on emerging nations, technical assistance
International Planned Parenthood Federation 18–20 Lower Regent Street London, SWIY 4PW, England	Promotes family planning services, research, and education Sex education

(*continued*)

TABLE 3–4. (*Continued*)

Agency or Organization	Services
International Rescue Committee 386 Park Ave South New York, NY 10016	Provides feeding programs, emergency relief, and clinic services Clinics
International Union Against Tuberculosis 3 rue Georges Ville F 75116 Paris, France	Aids government efforts at TB control Provides training, drugs, equipment, and transport
International Women's Health Coalition P.O. Box 8500 New York, NY 10150	Program development and women's health clinics
National Council for International Health 1101 Connecticut Ave, N.W. Suite 605 Washington, DC 20036 (202) 833-5900	Supports U.S. involvement in international health
Pan American Health Organization 525 23rd St., N.W. Washington, DC 20037 (202) 861-3200	Coordinates and funds health-care programs in the Americas
Parachute Medical Rescue Service P.O. Box 693 Boulder, CO 80306	Relief operations in natural disasters in remote areas
Peace Corps P-301 Washington, DC 20526 or Recruitment Office 806 Connecticut Ave. N.W. Washington, DC 20526	Primary health care and nutrition programs
Project Hope Milwood, VA 22646	Health care and education
Task Force for Child Survival Carter Presidential Center One Copenhill Ave Atlanta, GA 30307 (404) 688-8855	Assists with immunizations
United Nations International Children's Emergency Fund (UNICEF) United Nations New York, NY 10017 (212) 754-1234	Assists health programs in developing countries Provides health education
U.S./Mexico Border Health Association 6006 N. Mesa, Suite 600 El Paso, TX 79912 (915) 581-6645	Improves border health care Keeps health statistics
World Health Organization Avenue Appia CH-1211 Geneva, 27, Switzerland	Coordinates worldwide health efforts
WHO Collaborating Center on AIDS c/o Centers for Disease Control 1600 Clifton Rd., N.E. Atlanta, GA 30333 (404) 329-3311	Coordinates worldwide efforts related to AIDS
World Medical Relief 11745 Rosa Parks Blvd. Detroit, MI 48206 (313) 866-5333	Provides equipment, supplies, medication

tamination of food supplies.[23] In 1988, the United States signed the first international agreement to limit the production of materials that work to deplete the earth's ozone layer, and efforts have been instituted via such groups as Earthwatch to deal with other environmental health hazards.

Adolescent pregnancy is another area of growing concern around the world. In the United States, nearly a million girls aged 15 to 19 become pregnant each year in addition to 30,000 females under the age of 15. In Latin America, 20 percent of all pregnancies involve girls under 18 with similar statistics occurring in the Caribbean region.[24] The median age range for first sexual encounter in Europe and North America is 16–20 years, while in Africa the median range is 14–15 years.[15]

Chronic diseases and mental health problems are also of international concern. Recent news coverage has highlighted alcoholism in the Soviet Union and in other parts of the world. Mental disorders are frequently thought to be primarily a problem of developed countries, yet a WHO report indicated that epidemiologic studies show no significant difference in the prevalence of mental disorders throughout the world and that roughly 10 percent of the world's population will experience some form of mental disorder.[25]

A final concern in international health is that of human response to disasters. One can hardly pick up a newspaper without reading of natural or manmade disasters that affect large numbers of people. Those in recent memory include the near meltdown of the nuclear reactor at Three Mile Island in Pennsylvania in 1979; the toxic chemical leak in Bhopal, India, in 1985; the nuclear disaster at Chernobyl in 1986; destruction caused by several hurricanes in 1988; and devastating earthquakes in China and San Francisco in 1990. International efforts coordinated by WHO and the International Red Cross have led to the development of disaster planning groups throughout the world.[26] These groups or collaborating centers provide information, services, research and training in support of international disaster response.[27] One group in the United States designated as a WHO collaborating center is the Center for Emergency Preparedness and Response at the Centers for Disease Control. The function of this group is to coordinate disaster response and to conduct field research related to disasters. Disaster preparedness and the community health nurse's role in disaster will be addressed in some detail in Chapter 30, Care of Clients in Disaster Settings.

Past experience has indicated that international cooperation and effort can make a difference in the health status of the population of the world. The classic example of the benefits of such cooperation is the eradication of smallpox. It took just 13 years of global effort to wipe out a disease that was taken for granted by the populations of two millennia.[18] Similar concerted international efforts in other areas can influence the health of population groups throughout the world.

CHAPTER HIGHLIGHTS

- The U.S. health-care delivery system is composed of three subsystems: the popular subsystem, the folk or traditional subsystem, and the scientific subsystem.
- The scientific health-care subsystem is characterized by pluralism, multicentricity, and fragmentation.
- The scientific health-care subsystem is comprised of personal and community health-care sectors. The community health-care sector contains both voluntary and official agencies.
- Voluntary agencies perform eight functions: pioneering; demonstrating pilot projects; public and professional education; supplementing official agency efforts; advocacy for public interests; promoting legislation; contributing to planning and implementation of health-care programs; and assisting the work of official agencies.
- Official agencies in the United States operate at three levels: local, state, and national. Authority for health matters is one of the sovereign powers reserved to the states because the Constitution does not specify any direct federal government responsibility for health.
- The official agency at the local level is usually a local health department. At the state level, it is usually a state board of health. Responsibility for health at the national level is assumed by the Department of Health and Human Services.
- Health-care systems in some other nations differ greatly from the U.S. health-care delivery system. Types of health-care delivery systems found throughout the world include free enterprise systems, welfare systems, transitional systems, underdeveloped systems, and socialist systems.

Review Questions

1. Diagram the organizational structure of the U.S. health-care delivery system. (pp. 36–38, 43)
2. What are the three major characteristics of the U.S. scientific health-care subsystem? Give an example of each characteristic. (pp. 36, 37)
3. Compare and contrast voluntary and official health agencies. (pp. 37–38)
4. Describe five functions performed by voluntary health agencies. Give an example of each. (p. 38)
5. What level of official health agencies has primary responsibility for the health of the American public? Why? (p. 41)
6. What type of health-care delivery system exists in the United States? (p. 45)
7. Describe three alternative types of national health-care delivery systems. Identify at least one national health-care system that exemplifies each type. (p. 45)

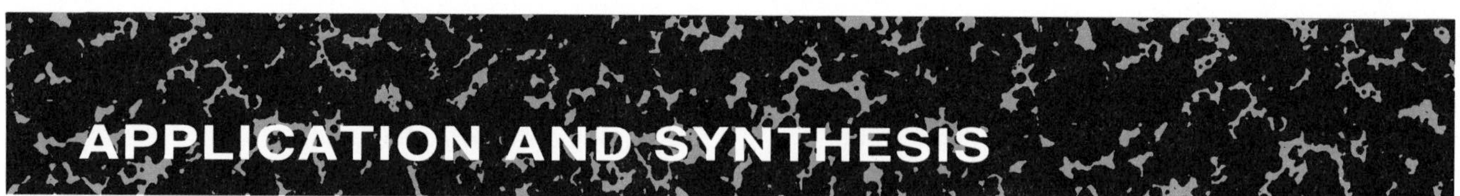

Design a health-care delivery system that would meet the health needs of the American public. Diagram the organizational structure of the system, making sure that your system addresses all types of health needs in some way. Address the following questions:

1. What features (if any) would you incorporate from the health-care delivery systems summarized in Table 3–3?
2. How would you address the responsibilities of official health agencies discussed in the chapter?
3. How would you fund your system? Would health-care providers operate on a fee-for-service basis or be salaried employees of the system? Why?
4. Would you offer comprehensive health-care services? Why or why not?
5. How would you address the three levels of prevention in your health-care delivery system? Would one level receive priority over the others? If so, why?
6. What changes would be required in the United States for your proposed system to be implemented?

REFERENCES

1. Banta, D. (1986). What is health care? In S. Jonas (Ed.), *Health care delivery in the United States* (3rd ed.). New York: Springer.
2. Sofaer, S. (1988). Community health planning in the United States: A postmortem. *Family and Community Health, 10*(4), 1–12.
3. Chrisman, N. J., & Kleinman, A. (1983). Popular health care, social networks, and cultural meaning. In D. Mechanic (Ed.), *Handbook of health, health care and the health professions* (pp. 569–590). New York: Free Press.
4. Institute of Medicine. (1988). *The Future of Public Health.* Washington, DC: National Academy Press.
5. Model Standards Work Group. (1985). *Model standards: A guide for community preventive health services* (2nd ed.). Washington, DC: American Public Health Association.
6. Raffel, M. W. (1980). *The U.S. health system: Origins and functions.* New York: Wiley.
7. Diekstra, R. (1988, June). City lifestyles. *World Health,* pp. 18–19.
8. Martynov, A. (1988, June). Battles won—but not yet the war! *World Health,* pp. 26–27.
9. Roemer, M. I. (1977). *Systems of health care.* New York: Springer.

10. Bloomquist, A. (1979). *The health care business.* London: Frazer Institute.
11. U.S. Department of Health and Human Services. (1988). Hospital use in Poland and the United States. *Comparative International Vital and Health Statistics,* Series 5(2), 6–9.
12. Joseph, S. C., Koch-Weser, D., & Wallace, N. (1977). *Worldwide overview of health and disease.* New York: Springer.
13. Research on health profiles. (1988). *Epidemiological Bulletin,* 9(2), 1–3.
14. Valenzuela, H. R., & Vasquez, R. A. L. (1988, September). Mortality in the city of Tijuana, B.C. in 1987. *Border Health,* pp. 46–51.
15. Leslie-Harwit, M., & Meheus, A. (1988, July). Information may be their only defense. *World Health,* pp. 16–17.
16. Jilg, W., & Deinhardt, F. (1988, July). Hepatitis B: Eradicable? *World Health,* pp. 10–12.
17. Monath, T. P. (1988, July). Yellow fever gains ground. *World Health,* pp. 20–23.
18. Torrigiani, G., & Parra, W. (1988, July). Communicable diseases. *World Health,* pp. 3–4.
19. WHO estimates immunization is saving 1.5 million children a year. (1988, December). *The Nation's Health,* p. 3.
20. *EPI Newsletter.* (1988, April).
21. Viedma, C. (1988, May). A health and nutrition atlas. *World Health,* pp. 1–31.
22. Abramov, V. (1988, June). One man's meat, another man's becquerel. *World Health,* pp. 12–13.
23. Kjellstrom, T. (1988, June). Measuring the harm. *World Health,* pp. 2–5.
24. Chelala, C. A. (1988, June). Teenage pregnancy in the Americas. *World Health,* pp. 22–23.
25. Warner, M. M. (1988). Decanting a psychiatric hospital: Development of a patient assessment methodology. *Bulletin of the Pan American Health Organization, 33,* 292–302.
26. *Disaster Preparedness in the Americas.* (1988, July). Washington, DC: Pan American Health Organization.
27. WHO collaborating centers. (1988, July). *Disaster Preparedness in the Americas,* pp. 1, 7.

RECOMMENDED READINGS

Institute of Medicine. (1988). *The future of public health.* Washington, DC: National Academy Press.

Reports the findings of an extensive study on the state of the public health-care system in the United States.

Jonas, S. (1986). *Health Care Delivery in the United States* (3rd ed.). New York: Springer.

Describes the past and present health-care delivery system in the United States. Addresses current issues in health-care delivery.

Lamm, R. D. (1990). The ten commandments of health care. In P. R. Lee & C. L. Estes (Eds.), *The nation's health* (3rd ed.) (pp. 124–133). Boston: Jones and Bartlett.

Provides direction for development in health-care delivery based on current trends and future predictions.

Litman, T. J. (1990). Government and health: The political aspects of health care—a sociopolitical overview. In P. R. Lee & C. L. Estes (Eds.) (3rd ed.) (pp. 140–153). Boston: Jones and Bartlett.

Discusses the past and present role of government in health-care delivery in the United States. Also provides recommendations for future directions in health care.

McCreight, L. (1989). The future of public health. *Nursing Outlook, 37,* 219–225.

Examines the Institute of Medicine report in terms of its implications for community health and community health nursing practice. Addresses the essential responsibilities of public health agencies and barriers to public health action.

McKeown, T. (1990). Determinants of health. In P. R. Lee & C. L. Estes (Eds.), *The nation's health* (3rd ed.) (pp. 6–13). Boston: Jones and Bartlett.

Evaluates the inappropriate direction of health-care delivery in the past and factors that have contributed to decreased mortality and increased longevity. Proposes a revised concept of health with increased emphasis on behavioral and environmental changes to facilitate health.

Rice, D. P. (1990). The medical care system: Past trends and future projections. In P. R. Lee & C. L. Estes (Eds.), *The nation's health* (3rd ed.) (pp. 72–93). Boston: Jones and Bartlett.

Describes past and current trends in health-care delivery and health status in the United States and factors influencing both. Also reviews policy issues related to reimbursement, access, long-term care, and corporate medicine.

Shirreffs, J. A. (1982). Organization and administration of public health. In J. A. Shirreffs, *Community health: Contemporary perspectives* (pp. 47–71). Englewood Cliffs, NJ: Prentice-Hall.

Presents a model for examining community health organization. Concepts of the model are based on the functions of a health-care system.

Ward, D. (1989). Public health nursing and "The Future of Public Health." *Public Health Nursing, 6,* 163–168.

Discusses the absence of any discussion of community health nursing and its contribution to community health in the IOM report. Also addresses the implications of this absence for community health nursing.

White, M. S. (1982). Construct for public health nursing. *Nursing Outlook, 30,* 527–530.

Defines public health and the priorities for public health practice as well as three general categories of public health intervention.

CHAPTER 4

Community Health Nursing

KEY TERMS

advocate
case finding
case manager
change agent
client-oriented roles
collaboration
community care agent
community health nursing
coordination
counseling
delivery-oriented roles
discharge planning
education
group-oriented roles
index of suspicion
leadership
liaison
primary care
researcher
referral
role model

Community health nursing practice takes place not only in the community but also in the historical and health-care contexts described in the last three chapters. Community health nursing is a specialty area with unique characteristics that set it apart from other fields of nursing. Community health nurses provide an array of services to a wide variety of clients, always with the goal of improving the health of the overall population. In this chapter we will explore those features that make community health nursing a unique field of practice and examine the roles and functions of community health nurses.

(continued)

LEARNING OBJECTIVES

After reading this chapter you should be able to:

- Define community health nursing.
- Identify at least five attributes of community health nursing.
- Describe the primary focus of community health nursing practice.
- Summarize the ANA standards for community health nursing practice.
- Distinguish among client-oriented, delivery-oriented, and group-oriented community health nursing roles.
- Describe at least five client-oriented roles performed by community health nurses.
- Describe at least three delivery-oriented roles performed by community health nurses.
- Describe at least four group-oriented roles performed by community health nurses.

Group-oriented Roles

Case Finder

Leader

Change Agent

Community Care Agent

Researcher

CHAPTER HIGHLIGHTS

DEFINING COMMUNITY HEALTH NURSING

Community health nurses, other health-care providers, and the public are confused about the definition of community health nursing. There is also debate whether the term "community health nursing" or "public health nursing" best describes the field. Many authors and much of the literature within and outside of nursing use the terms interchangeably.

On the other hand, participants in the Consensus Conference on the Essentials of Public Health Nursing Practice and Education[1] made a distinction based on education rather than practice setting. In the view of the conference members, community health nurses possess a standard array of nursing competencies, but they practice nursing in community, rather than institutional, settings. Public health nurses have had specific educational preparation and have received supervised clinical experience in a public health setting. The public health nurse may or may not function in an official public health agency but has the qualifications to do so. An example of this distinction might be the home health nurse who provides care to clients in a community setting, but the care provided is focused on the individual with no concern for the health of the total population. According to the conference participants, this nurse is a community health nurse, not a public health nurse. The public health nurse, on the other hand, may provide care to individuals and families, but the primary focus is the health of the larger population group.

Other authors suggest that community health nursing is more than just nursing carried out in nonhospital settings. For example, community health nursing has been described as "an area of professional nursing and public health practice characterized by the systematic application of selected nurturing, medico-technical, educational, or social-action skills for the analysis and amelioration of personal or community situations inimical to preserving health."[2] In other words, community health nursing is a synthesis of nursing and public health practice applied to population groups.

In 1980, the Public Health Nursing Section of the American Public Health Association (APHA) adopted a new definition of public health nursing.

> The speciality of public health nursing is professional nursing directed toward a total community or population group. Consideration is given to environmental, social, and personal health factors affecting health status. Its practice includes identification of subgroups or aggregates within the community who are at higher risk of illness or poor recovery and targeting its resources toward those groups and the families and individuals who comprise them. Emphasis is placed on planning for the community as a whole rather than on individual health care. Its purpose . . . is achieved by working with and through community leaders, health-related groups, groups at risk, families, and individuals and by becoming involved in relevant social action.[3]

This definition purposefully used the older term *public health nursing*, recognizing that this specialty is a "synthesis of public health science and professional nursing theories."[3]

The American Nurses' Association (ANA) presented a similar definition, but used the term *community health nurse*, in the introduction to *Standards of Community Health Nursing Practice.*[4]

> Community health nursing practice promotes and preserves the health of populations by integrating the skills and knowledge relevant to both nursing and public health. The practice is comprehensive and general, and is not limited to a particular age or diagnostic group; it is continual, and is not limited to episodic care. . . . While community health nursing practice includes nursing directed to individuals, families, and groups, the dominant responsibility is to the population as a whole.[4]

A number of similar elements are to be noted in both the ANA and APHA definitions of public health nursing or community health nursing. These definitions speak to the combination of elements from nursing science and public health science, and both view population aggregates as the primary focus of care. Both definitions emphasize promoting health and preventing illness. The essential elements of a satisfactory definition of community health nursing or public health nursing describe the relationship between nursing and public health practice, the focus of care, the goal of care, and the methods of achieving those goals.

For our purposes, the terms *community health nurse* and *public health nurse* will be used interchangeably within the context of the following definition of community health nursing. ***Community health nursing*** is a synthesis of nursing knowledge and practice and the science and practice of public health, implemented via systematic use of the nursing process and other processes, designed to promote health and prevent illness in population groups. The focus of care is the aggregate. The goal of care is the promotion of health and the prevention of illness. Health promotion and illness prevention in the population may be achieved through interventions directed at the total population or at individuals, families, and groups that constitute its members. The mode of achieving this goal is the application of principles of both public health and nursing science in the use of the nursing process with clients at all levels—individual, family, group, or community. Community health nursing, as used in this text, is not merely the performance of nursing activities in a community setting.

ATTRIBUTES OF COMMUNITY HEALTH NURSING

Community health nursing is characterized by a constellation of attributes that make it a unique field of nursing practice. These attributes are an orientation to health, a population focus, autonomy, continuity, collaboration, interactivity, public accountability, and a sphere of intimacy.

ORIENTATION TO HEALTH

The Institute of Medicine report[5] noted that the mission of public health is that of "fulfilling society's interest in assuring conditions in which people can be healthy." Promotion of health has also been a nursing function from as far back as the first school of nursing established by Florence Nightingale. At that time, a full year of the nursing curriculum was devoted to the promotion of community health.[6]

In other nursing specialties, health promotion is a facet of care, but one that is, of necessity, frequently given lower priority than health restoration needs. In community health nursing, on the other hand, the emphasis is on health promotion and maintenance rather than the cure of disease or disability. Although community health nurses frequently help clients resolve existing health problems, their major goal is to promote clients' highest level of physical, emotional, and social well-being.

POPULATION FOCUS

As stated in the definition of community health nursing presented earlier, the primary concern of community health nurses is the health of the general public rather than that of individuals or families. Community health nursing practice is designed to gather and interpret data on the health status of groups of people in an effort to identify and resolve health problems common to the population as a whole or to certain subgroups within the population.[7,8] When care is provided to individuals and families, it is done so primarily as a means of enhancing the health status of the total population. Consequently, it is the needs of the population that determine which individuals or families are to be served.[4] In other words, the scope of practice of the community health nurse "extends from a one-to-one nursing intervention to a global perspective of world health."[9]

From its earliest days in the United States, community health nursing has focused on the health of population groups. Even while they provided care to individuals and families, the nurses of the Henry Street Settlement and other similar organizations had as their goal the improved health of the immigrant population, school children, and the working poor. The continued prominence of a population focus was demonstrated in a recent study of community health nursing activities. Study findings indicated that family and community continued to be "basic units of service and thus confirmed the communitywide orientation to public health nursing demonstrated and advanced by Wald and her associates."[10]

AUTONOMY

Autonomy, or self-direction, is a twofold attribute of community health nursing. Both the community health nurse and the client tend to be more self-directed than either might be in an institutional health-care setting. Although all clients have the right and responsibility to make decisions about their health care, their autonomy in this regard tends to be eroded by the way health-care institutions operate.

Because community health nursing care is typically provided in the client's home or neighborhood, the client is more likely to demand an active role in health-care decision making, a situation the community health nurse should anticipate and foster.

Community health nurses also exercise a considerable degree of professional autonomy. In some situations, community health nurses may be the only providers of health care available. They must then rely on their own judgment to choose an appropriate course of action, usually without the guidance of a physician or supervisor. In this sense, the community health nurse is more autonomous in practice than is the institution-based nurse.

CONTINUITY

Continuity of care is another hallmark of community health nursing.[6] Whatever the setting in which community health nurses work, relationships between nurse and client tend to be of relatively long duration. Community health nurses usually have the flexibility to work with most clients until both feel that services are no longer needed. Because of the extended nature of the relationship, community health nurses are able to evaluate long-term as well as short-term effects of nursing interventions. They are also able to provide care for a wider range of client needs than is usually possible in acute care nursing. Problems not addressed today can be dealt with in subsequent meetings, and changing circumstances can be evaluated over time.

COLLABORATION

Because of the autonomy discussed earlier and the fact that interaction occurs in settings familiar to clients, nurse and client interact on a more equal footing than might otherwise be the case. This equality increases the potential for a truly collaborative relationship between nurse and client.

There is also greater opportunity for interaction and collaboration with other providers of client services linked directly or indirectly to health. In the acute care setting, nurses frequently interact with other health and social services providers. These opportunities for collaboration also arise in community health nursing. In addition, community health nurses have the opportunity to collaborate with a variety of nonhealth-related personnel. Examples of others with whom a community health nurse might collaborate include teachers, police and fire personnel, religious leaders, and government officials, to name a few.

INTERACTIVITY

The community health nursing attribute of interactivity reflects the community health nurse's perspective on factors that contribute to client health problems. Because community health nurses see clients in their own setting, they are able to identify a wide range of factors and interrelationships between factors that lead to health problems. The community health nurse is aware of the fact that health and illness are not isolated events in human existence. Both health and illness result from a complex interaction of multiple factors. This multiplicity of influences must be explored and dealt with if the nurse is to have any impact on the health status of the community. This awareness of interactivity also means that the nurse is cognizant of factors that will influence potential solutions to identified client problems.

PUBLIC ACCOUNTABILITY

Community health nursing also differs from other nursing specialties in the level of accountability involved. Like all nurses, community health nurses are morally and legally accountable to clients for the adequacy of care provided and for reasonable outcomes of care. Community health nurses, as with their acute-care counterparts, are also accountable to employers and to the nursing profession for the quality of care provided. However, unlike most other nurses, community health nurses are also accountable to society for the overall health of the public.

Because of their focus on the health of population groups, community health nurses need to deal with the public health problems they encounter. This is true whether or not the nurse is employed by a public agency or institution. For example, the community health nurse working in a well-child clinic who sees the multiple problems that homelessness creates for some of these children needs to work to resolve the problems of homelessness in addition to dealing with the specific needs of children seen in the clinic. Community health nurses are accountable, as well, for providing health-promotive and illness-preventive care that emphasizes community participation in health planning.[6]

The source of legal authority for nursing practice is another facet of public accountability. The legal authority for nursing actions in the hospital setting is based on institutional policy and the applicable nurs-

BOX 4–1

Attributes of Community Health Nursing

Health orientation
Emphasis on health promotion and disease prevention rather than cure of illness

Population focus
Emphasis on health of population groups (aggregates) rather than individuals or families

Autonomy
Greater control over health-care decisions by both nurse and client than in other settings

Continuity
Provision of care on a continuing, comprehensive basis rather than a short-term, episodic basis

Collaboration
Interaction between nurse and client as equals; greater opportunity for collaboration with other segments of society

Interactivity
Greater awareness of interaction of a variety of factors with health

Public accountability
Accountability to society for the health of the general population

Sphere of intimacy
Greater awareness of the reality of client lives and situations than is true of other areas of nursing

ing practice act. Authority to perform medically delegated tasks derives from the client's personal physician who closely oversees these dependent functions of the nurse.

Legal authority for the practice of the community health nurse also arises from state nursing practice acts in addition to health-related laws and regulations of a particular jurisdiction. The local health department has the legal responsibility for the health of the community and is one source of the community health nurse's authority. Medical authority is more indirect and, in many cases, clients may not be under the care of a physician at all.

SPHERE OF INTIMACY

Another difference between community health nursing and other areas of nursing practice is the sphere of intimacy that typifies community health practice settings. Hospitals and other institutional health-care environments often modify a client's behavior, thus affecting the accuracy of the nurse's observations of clients, their families, and their problems. Practicing in the community setting, however, the nurse can get a more accurate picture of the factors that affect the client's health. The community health nurse may also become more intimately aware of everyday details of the client's normal life and environment. For example, the community health nurse might discover evidence of spouse abuse that might not be uncovered in other health-care settings.

All of these attributes are evidence of the unique status of community health nursing, which uses principles of both nursing and public health to prevent or alleviate health problems of groups of people as well as individual members of society. The attributes of community health nursing are summarized in Box 4–1.

STANDARDS FOR COMMUNITY HEALTH NURSING PRACTICE

One of the hallmarks of a profession is the establishment of standards of practice. Nursing, like other health-related professions, has set up standards for nursing practice and nursing service. The standards for nursing practice are further delineated in standards established for each of several specialty areas in nursing. Among these, and of particular interest to community health nurses, are the American Nurses' Association *Standards of Community Health Nursing Practice.*

Why does a profession need standards? According to the ANA, "standards are developed to characterize, to measure, and to provide guidance in achieving excellence in care."[4] A set of standards for practice provides a means by which one can evaluate the quality of nursing service provided. The standards for community health nursing practice have been developed within the framework of the nursing process. They relate to the areas of assessment, diagnosis, planning, implementation or action, and evaluation. Additional standards deal with the use of theory as a basis for practice, quality assurance, and professional development, collaboration, and research. The ANA standards for community health nursing practice are summarized below and in Box 4–2.

BOX 4–2

ANA Standards for Community Health Nursing

1. The nurse applies theoretical concepts as a basis for decisions in practice.
2. The nurse systematically collects data that are comprehensive and accurate.
3. The nurse analyzes data collected about the community, family, and individual to determine diagnoses.
4. At each level of prevention, the nurse develops plans that specify nursing actions unique to client needs.
5. The nurse, guided by the plan, intervenes to promote, maintain, or restore health, to prevent illness, and to effect rehabilitation.
6. The nurse evaluates responses of the community, family, and individual to interventions to determine progress toward goal achievement and to revise the data base, diagnoses, and plan.
7. The nurse participates in peer review and other means of evaluation to assure quality of nursing practice. The nurse assumes responsibility for professional development and contributes to the professional growth of others.
8. The nurse collaborates with other health-care providers, professionals, and community representatives in assessing, planning, implementing, and evaluating programs for community health.
9. The nurse contributes to theory and practice in community health nursing through research.

The first standard asserts the need to base community health nursing practice on a sound theoretical foundation. The theoretical concepts underlying community health nursing are derived from nursing, public health, and the physical, social, and behavioral sciences.

The second and third standards address client assessment. Data collection (second standard) regarding the health status of individuals, families, and communities should be systematic, continuous, and accessible, and should be recorded in a way that facilitates communication with others. Data pertinent to individuals and families include health history and physical assessment, growth and developmental data, and information on mental and emotional status and family dynamics. Other individual and family assessment data include economic, legal, political, and environmental factors influencing health; cultural and religious factors; knowledge of and motivation toward health; strengths; and health risk factors. Community-related data to be obtained include information on community resources and power structure, demographics and vital statistics, community dynamics, and socioeconomic, cultural, and environmental characteristics.

The third standard states that nursing diagnoses should be derived from the data collected. Nursing diagnosis includes identification of client needs as well as availability of resources and patterns of health-care delivery. A complete nursing diagnosis also necessitates identifying the client's potentials and limitations. The concept of nursing diagnosis will be dealt with in more detail in Chapter 5.

The fourth standard directs planning to meet client health needs. Plans for nursing intervention should be based on the nursing diagnoses derived from the data collected and should include measurable goals and objectives. Plans should also be based on sound theoretical concepts and should identify an appropriate sequence of activities for achieving the goals specified. Finally, the plan of care should list resources required for its implementation and reflect consideration of the costs involved.

The fifth standard addresses plan implementation. Achieving desired outcomes requires client participation. The client should be provided with sufficient information to make informed decisions regarding health-related activities and the selection of appropriate health-care services. During the intervention phase of the nursing process, the community health nurse may serve as direct care-giver, supervisor of other care-givers, coordinator, advocate, educator, and modifier of plans.

Client participation is also required to achieve the outcomes of the sixth standard, which deals with evaluating interventions and their results. Evaluation involves comparing baseline and current data regarding the status of health problems diagnosed by the nurse. Evaluative data must be interpreted and the results of nursing interventions documented. Finally, data must be used to revise priorities, goals, and interventions as needed.

The seventh standard describes the nurse's responsibility for assuring quality care and participating in professional development. In meeting this standard the nurse evaluates the quality of care provided, updates personal knowledge and that of others, and incorporates new knowledge into community health practice.

The eighth standard directs the nurse to engage in collaborative and consultative activities with professional colleagues and community representatives. These activities include joint goal setting, planning interventions, teaching, and research, as well as communicating nursing and public health knowledge to others.

The final standard describes the nurse's responsibility with respect to research. The community health nurse is expected to be a critical consumer of research. He or she should also be involved in identifying researchable problems in community health and should participate in the investigation of these problems.

The ANA also developed criteria to measure the degree to which each of the standards has been achieved. These are divided into structural, process, and outcome criteria. Structural criteria describe the environment and resources required for achieving the standard. For example, a structural criterion related to the standard for use of theory states that resource materials discussing conceptual bases for practice must be available to the nurse. Process criteria describe the activities or processes in which the nurse engages to meet the standards. For instance, a process criterion dealing with data collection details the manner in which the nurse records data. Outcome criteria describe the expected result of the nurse's activities—for example, that data are accurate and current.

The ANA standards for community health nursing apply general principles of nursing to the unique practice of community health. The standards delineate the means by which the nursing process can be incorporated into community health nursing. They provide a mechanism and criteria for evaluating the quality of care given and can be applied throughout the tri-level focus of community health nursing: care of individuals, families, and groups or communities. Applying the ANA standards to client assessment, diagnosis, planning, implementation, and evaluation of nursing interventions with respect to the individual, family, and community client will be addressed in Chapter 17, Care of the Individual, Chapter 18, Care of the Family, and Chapter 19, Care of the Community or Target Group.

ROLES AND FUNCTIONS OF COMMUNITY HEALTH NURSES

The role of the community health nurse has evolved over the last few years, and it remains in transition, evolving as societal needs change. This evolution has been referred to as the "form-follows-function perspective" of community health nursing,[11] meaning that the form of the overall role is dictated by the functions performed in meeting the changing needs of society.

Some authors have expressed concern about the proliferation of various specialties that diminish the role of community health nurses.[6] Some examples of this phenomenon are the advent of the "health educator" and the use of nurse practitioners to provide primary care, a function that has historically been part of the community health nurse role. Similar concern has been voiced in England regarding the diminished role of the health visitor,[12] the British counterpart of the community health nurse. On both sides of the Atlantic, the point is made that there is no need to create new specialties to meet new societal health problems, but only for community health nurses as a group to reassert the fullness of their role.

The roles most commonly performed by community health nurses are categorized on the basis of their orientation as client-oriented roles, delivery-oriented roles, and group-oriented roles. Because the needs of specific population groups with which they work differ, not all community health nurses engage in each of the roles mentioned here. Some nurses may perform several of the roles and functions discussed, while others restrict their activities to a few, depending upon the situation and setting.

CLIENT-ORIENTED ROLES

Client-oriented roles involve direct provision of client services. These include the roles of care-giver, educator, counselor, referral resource, role model, advocate, primary care provider, and case manager.

CARE-GIVER

The care-giver role involves applying the principles of epidemiology and the nursing process to the care of clients at any level—individual, family, group, or community. Some of the functions entailed in this role include assessing client needs and planning appropriate nursing intervention. Implementing the plan of care may involve performing technical procedures or assuming one or more of the other client-oriented roles. Evaluating nursing care and its outcomes is another function performed in the care-giver role. This role is basic to all client encounters, and its functions are performed whether or not any of the other community health nursing roles are assumed.

EDUCATOR

Education is the process of providing someone with the knowledge and skills needed to make appropriate choices among alternative courses of action. In the educator role, the community health nurse provides clients and others with information and insights that allow them to make informed decisions on health matters. The educator role may be performed at any client level. Community health nurses, for example, educate individuals and their families about adequate nutrition. At the same time, they may educate the general public regarding the harmful effects, say, of a high cholesterol, low-fiber diet.

In performing the educator role, the nurse engages in a variety of different functions or activities that parallel those of the care-giver role, but are specific to the role of educator. The first of these functions is assessing the client's need for education and motivation for learning. A second function is developing and presenting a health lesson. A final function is evaluating the effects of health education. We will discuss these functions in greater detail in Chapter 7, The Health Education Process.

Although the educator role is primarily a client-oriented role, the community health nurse may also serve as an educator for his or her peers or other professionals. The nurse may be involved, for example, in educating student nurses or students in other health-related disciplines. On occasion, the nurse may be called upon to educate other health professionals as well. For example, it has been the responsibility of community health nurses in Los Angeles County to assist in educating private physicians regarding appropriate diagnostic, treatment, and reporting procedures for sexually transmitted diseases.

COUNSELOR

Many people do not distinguish between counseling and education. They *are* different, however. ***Counseling*** is the process of helping the client to choose viable solutions to health problems. In educating, one is presenting facts. In counseling, one is *not* telling people what to do but helping them to engage in the problem-solving process and to decide on the most appropriate course of action. In the role of counselor, community health nurses explain the problem-solving process and guide clients through each step. In this way, the nurse is not only helping the client to solve the immediate problem but also assisting in the development of the client's problem-solving abilities. This is true whether the client is an individual, a family, or a community.

Counseling is a process that involves several steps on the part of the community health nurse. The first step is to assist the client to identify and clarify the problem to be solved. The nurse and client together examine factors contributing to a problem and those that may enhance or impede problem resolution.

At the second step of the counseling process, the community health nurse helps the client identify alternative solutions to the problem. If, for example, the client's problem is lack of money for food, one could suggest applying for food stamps, getting a second job, or establishing a budget.

Assisting the client to develop criteria for an acceptable solution to the problem is the third step in the counseling process. For example, an acceptable solution to the problem of poor nutrition would need to fit the client's budget and might need to conform to cultural dietary patterns.

Next, the community health nurse would assist the client to evaluate each of the alternative solutions in terms of criteria established for an acceptable solution. The most appropriate of the alternatives is the one that best meets the acceptability criteria. This alternative is then implemented. Evaluation is the fifth step of the problem-solving process. If the alternative selected solves the problem, fine! If not, the process begins again. The steps of the problem-solving process are depicted in Figure 4–1.

REFERRAL RESOURCE

Referral is the process of directing clients to resources needed to meet their needs. These resources may be other agencies that can provide necessary services or sources of information, equipment, or supplies that the client needs and the community health nurse cannot supply. Referral is one of the key functions of community health nurses. A distinction must be made, however, between the functions of referral and consultation. In a referral, the client is directed toward another source of services. In consultation, on the other hand, the nurse may seek assistance or information needed to help the client, but the client does not receive services directly from the consultant.[13]

Referral is an important part of the role of the community health nurse in any practice setting. It is

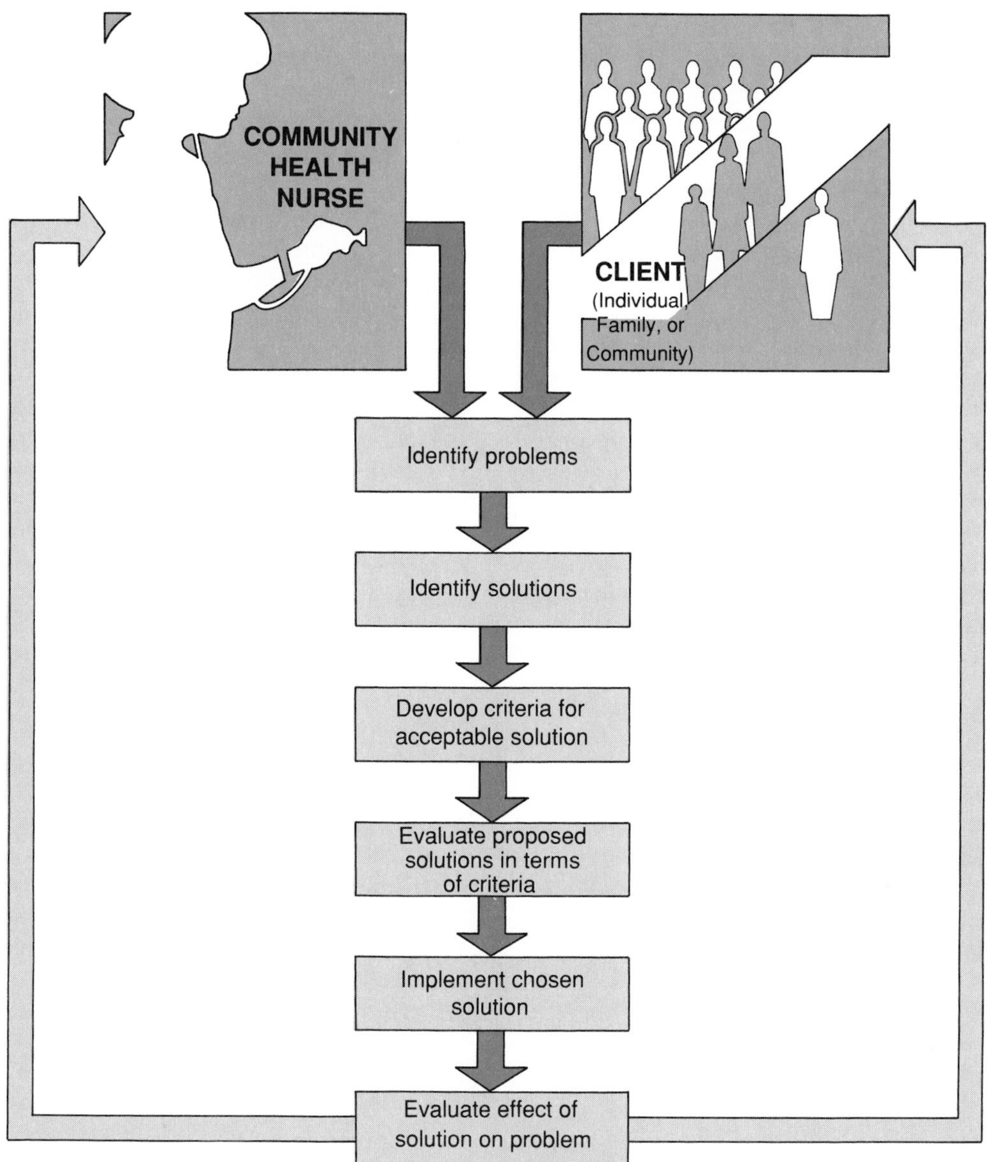

Figure 4–1. Steps of the problem-solving process.

the nurse's responsibility to explore available resources and direct clients to them as appropriate. The degree of intervention required in a specific referral will vary with the type of referral and the client situation. Sometimes it is sufficient to let a client know that a certain resource exists. On other occasions, the particular agency may require a written referral from the nurse or from a physician.

In some instances, the client may not be capable of following through on a referral. For example, the depressed client may not have the energy to phone for an appointment at the local mental health center, but may be able to keep an appointment made by the nurse. The nurse must determine in each situation the degree of dependence or independence needed by that client at that time, with the goal, of course, of gradually increasing the client's ability to function independently. Specific functions of the community health nurse in the referral role include determining the need for referral, identifying the appropriate referral resources, and making and following up on the referral. The referral process will be discussed in more detail in Chapter 9, The Discharge Planning and Referral Processes.

ROLE MODEL

A ***role model*** is someone who consciously or unconsciously demonstrates behavior learned by others who will perform a similar role. Community health nurses serve as role models for a variety of people with whom they come in contact. Through their own behavior, nurses influence the behavior of others.[14] For instance, the community health nurse's ability to deal with crisis without panic provides direction for clients to do the same.

The community health nurse's role as a model is not confined solely to influencing the health-related behavior of clients. The nurse also serves as a role model for other health professionals. One of the areas in which the role-modeling function is of primary importance is in the educational preparation of student nurses. The way the community health nurse treats clients, the type of activity in which the nurse engages, and the level of competence displayed may all influence students' attitudes and practice. This influence can be either positive or negative.

ADVOCATE

An ***advocate*** is someone who speaks on behalf of those who, for whatever reason, cannot speak for themselves. Client advocacy is another of the roles of the community health nurse that may take place at the individual, family, or community level. The nurse may serve as an advocate for the individual client in explaining the client's needs to the family or to other health-care providers. For example, the parents of a handicapped child may tend to be overprotective, refusing to allow the child to engage in normal activities out of fear for the child's safety. The nurse can serve as an advocate for the child by explaining to the parents that their behavior is actually detrimental to the child's development. The nurse is intervening here to prevent the child from developing a further handicap—a psychological one—and is speaking for the child who cannot speak for himself or herself.

Community health nurses also engage in advocacy when they act to resolve difficulties encountered by clients in dealing with the health-care system. Insisting that a case worker reevaluate a family's application for food stamps because their financial status has changed is an example of advocacy at the family level.

Advocacy also takes place at the community level. The commitment of community health nursing to improving the health of population groups necessitates "advocacy for the aggregate."[9] As mentioned in Chapter 2, The Historical Context, this level of advocacy was a primary concern of the early leaders in community health nursing. Helping communities organize and present grievances to the city council is an example of advocacy for aggregates in today's world. Other forms of advocacy at this level include nurses' involvement in political activity at local, state, and national levels. Advocacy via the political process will be discussed in Chapter 12, The Political Process.

As an advocate, the community health nurse engages in a number of activities or functions. The first of these is determining the need for advocacy and factors that prevent clients from acting on their own behalf. Such factors can be quite varied. Some clients, for example, may not know how to go about making their needs known. Fear of reprisal might be another reason why clients do not speak for themselves. Other factors include apathy, feelings of hopelessness, or even language barriers.

A second function of the nurse as advocate is determining the point at which advocacy will be most effective. For example, should the nurse raise concerns of safety violations in rental housing with the landlord, with the housing authority, or with the media? Answers to such questions might be derived from knowledge of what has been tried previously and the effects of prior action. Related questions involve how the case should be presented. Should one ask, for example, for a meeting with interested parties or stage a demonstration?

Collecting facts related to the problem is another advocacy-related function. An advocate is considerably less effective when he or she does not have all the facts about a situation. A community health nurse advocate should get a detailed chronological account of events related to the problem for which advocacy is needed. The nurse should also try to validate or verify the information obtained to support the claim that a problem exists and action is needed.

The fourth task in advocacy is presenting the client's case to the appropriate decision-makers. This function requires tact and interpersonal skill. Threatening or confrontational behavior should be avoided whenever possible as both set up an adversarial relationship, rather than a collaborative one, that may be detrimental to the client's cause. When other avenues fail, threats may have to be employed, but nurse and client must be committed to acting on them. For example, if the nurse threatens to report a landlord for safety code violations unless action is taken to remove hazards, he or she should actually be prepared to make the report.

The final function of the nurse as an advocate is to prepare clients to speak for themselves. The activities and functions of advocacy should not be carried out by the nurse alone, but should be a collaborative effort between nurse and client. In this way, clients learn how to develop and present a forceful argument for their own needs and may, in the future, be able to act without nursing intervention.

Advocacy necessitates involvement and commitment. The effective community health nurse cannot be content with the attitude that "I'd like to help, but my hands are tied." Advocacy is not a popular concept. It frequently means frustration and argument. It is the antithesis of complacency and is essential to the practice of effective community health nursing. Community health nurses must speak for those who cannot speak for themselves and articulate their needs to those in power. Nurses must also assist members of the community to learn how to speak for themselves rather than remain dependent upon the nurse. Advocacy is a twofold obligation to take the part of others and, in time, to prepare them to stand alone.

PRIMARY CARE PROVIDER

Many community health nurses have assumed roles as nurse practitioners providing primary care to a variety of clients.[6,8] ***Primary care*** is defined as essential care made universally accessible to all.[15] It consists of initial care provided to clients at their point of entry into the health-care system. The primary care function of most community health nurses involves health-promotive and illness-preventive interventions such as routine prenatal assessments, well-child care, immunizations, and so on. Community health nurses also routinely deal with minor health problems such as constipation, diarrhea, and so forth.

Other community health nurses, with advanced educational preparation, provide primary care as nurse practitioners. These nurses have assumed diagnostic and treatment services that were once the exclusive province of physicians. There has been some concern that incursions into medical practice by nurse practitioners might detract from the emphasis placed by community health nurses on health promotion and illness prevention.[12] Although this is sometimes the case early in a nurse practitioner's career, most practitioners regain their nursing perspective fairly rapidly[6] and provide both curative and health-promotive services.

There are five key elements of primary care: accessibility, comprehensiveness, coordination, continuity, and accountability.[6] The elements of continuity and accountability are identified attributes of community health nursing discussed earlier. As we will see later in this chapter, coordination is an aspect of the community health nurse role even when the nurse does not engage in primary care. Accessibility refers to health care obtainable by all members of the population whatever their attributes or characteristics, while comprehensiveness refers to the degree to which care includes preventive, promotive, curative, and rehabilitative services.[6] Performance of the primary care role by community health nurses enhances the accessibility and comprehensiveness of health-care services available to the general public.

CASE MANAGER

The final client-oriented role to be discussed here is that of the ***case manager.*** Case management is "the process of ensuring that the services provided are appropriate for the client's needs."[16] The case manager role is similar to, but different from, the delivery-oriented coordination role discussed later in this chapter. The role of the coordinator focuses on the delivery of efficient care with minimal waste of resources and maximum benefit for the client. The focus in the case manager role is on meeting the needs of the client, rather than on the efficiency of health-care delivery.

The case manager is responsible for designing the plan of care for meeting client needs and for overseeing the implementation of that plan by others.[17] As we will see later, in the coordinator role, the nurse does not plan aspects of care provided by other health-care professionals, but organizes the care in such a way that the client's needs are met as efficiently and competently as possible. The coordinator does not, however, necessarily assume primary responsibility for the client's care.

Functions of the case manager include assessment and identification of client needs and the design of a plan of care to meet those needs. The case manager also directs implementation of the plan of care by others and evaluates the outcomes of intervention. Areas that might be addressed by the case manager include physical needs for care, counseling needs, assistance with homemaking and other activities of daily living, nutritional needs, legal and financial assistance, transportation, and housing. Other areas to be considered and planned for include spiritual assistance, medical treatment, health education, dental care, and so on.[16] Nursing functions in the case manager role and other client-oriented roles are summarized in Table 4–1.

DELIVERY-ORIENTED ROLES

The ***delivery-oriented roles*** of community health nurses are those designed to enhance the operation of the health-care delivery system, resulting in better care for clients. Roles in this category include coordinator, collaborator, liaison, and discharge planner.

TABLE 4–1. CLIENT-ORIENTED COMMUNITY HEALTH NURSING ROLES AND RELATED FUNCTIONS

Role	Function
Care-giver	• Assess client health status • Derive nursing diagnoses • Plan nursing intervention • Implement the plan of care • Evaluate the outcome of nursing intervention
Educator	• Assess client's need for education • Develop health education plan • Present health education • Evaluate outcome of health education
Counselor	• Identify and clarify problem to be solved • Help client identify alternative solutions • Assist client to develop criteria for solutions • Assist client to evaluate alternative solutions • Assist client to evaluate effects of solution • Make client aware of steps of problem-solving process
Referral resource	• Obtain information on community resources • Determine the need for and appropriateness of a referral • Make the referral • Follow up on the referral
Role model	• Perform the behavior to be learned by clients or others
Advocate	• Determine the need for advocacy • Determine the appropriate avenue for advocacy • Obtain facts related to the situation • Present the client's case to decision-makers • Prepare clients to stand alone
Primary care provider	• Assess client health status and identify problems • Plan and provide treatment for problems • Introduce other supportive services as needed • Teach and supervise others • Modify care plan as required • Teach clients self-care • Coordinate health-care services • Serve as liaison between client and system
Case manager	• Assess and identify client health needs • Design plan of care to meet needs • Oversee implementation of care by others • Evaluate outcome of care

COORDINATOR

Community health nurses frequently care for clients who are receiving services from a variety of sources. Because of their awareness of the needs of the client as a whole being, community health nurses are in an ideal position to serve as coordinators of care. ***Coordination*** is a process of organizing and integrating services to best meet client needs in the most efficient manner possible.

It is the community health nurse who most frequently enters the home or community and sees firsthand how the client is responding to a physical therapy program or how effective a roach-control program has been. It is also the nurse who is in the best position to transmit to other providers information regarding client needs, attitudes, and progress. The community health nurse is also best able to interpret to the client, in language he or she can understand, the purposes and procedures involved in programs instituted by other health-care providers.

The community health nurse serving as a coordinator of client care performs a variety of functions. The first function involves determining who is providing care to the client, where services overlap, and where gaps in care may be occurring. The second function is to communicate with other providers regarding the particulars of the client situation and needs. Communication includes informing providers of other persons and agencies dealing with the client. Except in certain circumstances (for example, child abuse or threat of harm to self or others), communication should be undertaken *only* with the consent of the client.

A simple example of coordinating services might involve arranging for appointments in a prenatal clinic and a child health clinic on the same day, when both services are provided at the same location. Coordinating appointments in this way will assist a pregnant woman with a 2-year-old and limited transportation to obtain needed health care for herself and her child without a second bus trip.

One additional function of the community health nurse in a coordinator role might be arranging a case conference to include nurse, client, and other providers of services. For example, the school nurse might arrange a meeting that would include not only the nurse but also the child, parents, teachers, and the school psychologist to discuss the child's behavior problems in school.

COLLABORATOR

Collaboration is a process of joint decision making by two or more people. As a collaborator, the community health nurse engages in joint decision making regarding action to be taken to resolve client health problems. Collaboration should always take place between nurse and client or a significant other. Collaborative efforts, however, may also include other providers.

Collaboration is frequently confused with the nurse's coordination role. Coordination is essentially a management function, and involves making sure that efforts to provide services are consistent and occur without gaps or overlaps. Collaboration, on the other hand, entails joint decision making. Both collaboration and coordination, of course, necessitate working with clients and other professionals (and nonprofessionals) who contribute to the health care of clients. This contribution by others may be directly related to the client's health status, as in the case of physicians, physical therapists, nutritionists, and other health-care personnel. It may also be indirectly related to the client's health status, as are the services of police and firefighters, sanitation collectors, and city officials.

Collaboration is not a matter of each health-care worker designing and providing a program in his or her area of expertise with a certain amount of coordination between efforts. Rather, it is a joint effort on the part of health-care providers *and clients* to set mutual goals and to arrive at a mutually acceptable plan for achieving them. Collaboration is a relatively new function for most nurses and cannot take place without a mutual feeling of respect and collegiality among health team members.

The two primary functions of the community health nurse in a collaborative role are communication and joint decision making. In communicating, the nurse conveys to other team members his or her perceptions of client needs, factors influencing those needs, and ideas for problem resolution. In decision making, the community health nurse participates in joint problem-solving efforts, using the problem-solving process with the care team to identify and evaluate alternative solutions to client problems and to select an appropriate alternative. Collaboration may also extend to joint activity to implement solutions selected and to evaluate the outcome.

LIAISON

The liaison role of the community health nurse incorporates facets of the coordinator and referral resource roles and may even incorporate the advocacy role depending upon the client situation. A ***liaison*** provides a connection, relationship, or intercommunication. The community health nurse working with clients and dealing with multiple health and social agencies may serve as that connection or liaison. In the referral resource role, the community health nurse may function as the initial point of contact between client and agency. The liaison role might involve continued communication between client and other providers via the nurse. Sometimes this communication includes the additional function of interpretation and reinforcement of provider recommendations to the client or advocacy for the client with the provider agency.

DISCHARGE PLANNER

Discharge planning is the process of determining and planning to meet client needs following release from a health-care facility. Discharge planning is a role usually equated with nursing in an institutional setting. A concept of nursing discharge has been advanced in which the hospital nurse continues to provide needed acute-care services after the client's discharge from the hospital (institutional discharge).[18] The acute-care nurse continues to follow the client until the client is deemed recovered enough to be discharged by the nurse (the nursing discharge) to the care of a "traditional" community health nurse for health-promotion and maintenance services. This concept, however, assumes either that clients' only needs at the time of hospital discharge relate to their acute problems, or that the hospital nurse has an adequate grasp of community resources and the processes required to meet additional needs. Neither condition is found to exist in the majority of hospital discharges.

More and more health-care professionals are realizing that community health nurses need to be involved in discharge planning from the beginning and not just as a recipient of a referral for community health nursing care when the client is discharged. Plans for a client's release back to the home or other agency have traditionally been based on the client's medical diagnosis and needs related to that diagnosis. Needs other than those related to the client's medical condition, however, can and do impinge on the client's health status. For example, plans for financial assistance for the client who is an amputee and the sole support of a family must be part of the discharge plan as well as plans for his or her physical rehabilitation. Or, plans may need to be made to convert a home to accommodate use of a wheelchair. It is the community health nurse who is most likely to be aware of these additional needs. Thus, the nurse must be involved in discharge planning to meet these needs.

The community health nurse is also likely to be more aware of resources available to the client than other members of the health-care team. The nurse may know what agencies can provide a pair of crutches or a hospital bed to a client who cannot rent or purchase them. Or, the nurse may know of an ostomy support group that can help the client with a colostomy deal with changes in self-image as well as other practical concerns.

Discharge planning involves a number of related activities or functions. The first of these activities is the identification of client needs. This will frequently entail a visit to the client's home prior to discharge and an exploration of home and family conditions that will affect the client's ability for self-care. A second function of the community health nurse as a discharge planner is the identification of resources available to meet client needs. As noted earlier, the community health nurse is the one member of the discharge planning team most likely to be aware of community resources and services.

Linking the client to available resources through referral is the third function of the discharge planner. Again, care must be taken that referrals are appropriate to the client situation. The community health nurse may make arrangements for services or have the client or a significant other make them depending on their ability to follow through with a referral.

The final function in discharge planning is to plan for follow-up related to the discharge plan and its execution as well as the client's health status after discharge. Plans should be made to see that the client is able to function effectively after discharge and that discharge planning was adequate to meet client needs. For example, plans for follow-up might include a home visit or telephone call by the nurse or scheduling a clinic visit shortly after discharge. A summary of delivery-oriented roles and related functions is presented in Table 4–2.

TABLE 4–2. DELIVERY-ORIENTED COMMUNITY HEALTH NURSING ROLES AND RELATED FUNCTIONS

Role	Function
Coordinator	• Determine who is providing care to client • Communicate with other providers regarding client situation and needs • Arrange case conferences as needed
Collaborator	• Communicate with other health team members • Participate in joint decision making • Participate in joint action to resolve client problems
Liaison	• Serve as initial point of contact between client and agency • Facilitate communication between client and agency personnel • Interpret and reinforce provider recommendations • Serve as client advocate as needed
Discharge planner	• Identify client needs • Identify resources available to meet client needs • Link client to available resources • Follow up on client progress after discharge

GROUP-ORIENTED ROLES

The client-oriented and delivery-oriented roles of community health nurses usually occur in relation to the care of specific clients. At times these roles may be extended to the care of groups of people or communities. For example, the role of coordinator may be applied to the organization of several services provided to groups of people, as when a community health nurse occupies the position of clinical services coordinator for a county health department. More often, though, client-oriented and delivery-oriented roles focus on providing services to specific clients.

As noted throughout this text, community health nurses are primarily concerned with the health of the population, and they perform a number of roles that are exclusively group-oriented. ***Group-oriented roles*** are those of case finder, leader, change agent, community care agent, and researcher.

CASE FINDER

Case finding has been described as one of the "basics of public health nursing."[6] ***Case finding*** by the community health nurse involves identifying individual cases or occurrences of specific diseases or other health-related conditions requiring services. Why, then, is this considered a group-oriented role? Despite the fact that case finding involves location of individual cases of a condition, the primary intent of this role is the assessment and protection of the health of the general public. As we will see in Chapter 31, Communicable Disease, case finding is an important strategy in preventing the spread of communicable diseases in large population groups. Case finding is also a means of monitoring the health status of a group or community. For example, identifying more instances of child abuse may be an indication of a community health problem.

Community health nurses have a relatively close and usually prolonged association with clients and have the opportunity to note changes in health status or early signs of health problems. During a community health nurse's visit to a hypertensive client, for example, the nurse may discover that the client's teenage daughter is pregnant and in need of prenatal care. Or, the nurse may observe that members of a number of families who obtain water from a common source have had recent episodes of vomiting and diarrhea. If the nurse is dealing with clients as unified entities (whether they are individuals, families, or communities), he or she is in a position to detect potential or actual health problems early and intervene as rapidly as possible. The abilities of recently educated community health nurses to conduct physical examinations have enhanced their case-finding abilities by giving them another avenue for detecting the presence of disease or disability.[8]

Case-finding responsibilities include developing an index of suspicion, identifying instances of disease or other health-related conditions, and providing follow-up services. An ***index of suspicion*** is an estimation of the likelihood that a disease or problem may exist and is based on a broad foundation of knowledge of the signs and symptoms of a variety of health problems and factors contributing to them. For example, to assess a case of tuberculosis, the nurse must be familiar with the signs and symptoms of TB. The nurse should also be aware of factors that are associated with TB. When the community health nurse encounters a client from Asia (where the incidence of tuberculosis is relatively high) who complains of a chronic cough with hemoptysis, weight loss, and night sweats, a suspicion of a possible case of TB is developed.

The case-finding role necessitates the use of the diagnostic reasoning process to identify potential cases of disease or instances of other health-related conditions (such as pregnancy or the need for immunizations) based on relevant cues present in the situation. This diagnostic processing of relevant signs and symptoms into a probable diagnosis of the disease is the second function of the community health nurse as a case finder.

The third community health nursing function related to case finding is the provision of follow-up care to the person with a specific condition. This usually entails referral for further diagnostic services and for treatment if needed. In the case of nurse practitioners, community health nurses might provide these services themselves.

LEADER

Leadership in the community health nursing context has been described as "a requisite 'clinical' intervention aimed at mobilizing multiple and diverse people and organizations."[11] The leadership role of the community health nurse may be enacted both with individual clients or families and with groups and communities. However, because this role demands knowledge of group dynamics as well as interpersonal skills, we will deal with leadership as a group-oriented role.

Leadership is the ability to influence the behavior of others. Community health nurses may assume a leadership role with a variety of individuals, including clients, other health professionals, members of other disciplines, public officials, the general public, and so on. Because of the number of different types of followers that may be involved, the community health nurse as leader must be able to adapt a leadership style to fit the needs of the moment.

Community health nurse functions in the leadership role include identifying the need for action and leadership, assessing the leadership needs of followers, and selecting and executing a style of leadership appropriate to both the followers and the situation. The leadership process and the functions involved are discussed in greater detail in Chapter 11, The Change, Leadership, and Group Processes.

CHANGE AGENT

Community health nurses also fill the role of change agent. A ***change agent*** is one who initiates and brings about change. Frequently this role is performed in conjunction with the leadership role.[11] Change is an unavoidable part of human existence, but when change is systematically planned it can be controlled and used to enhance rather than undermine health. Specific functions of the community health nurse in the change-agent role include recognizing the need for change, making others aware of the need for change, motivating others to change, and initiating and directing the desired change.

Community health nurses may serve as change agents working with individuals, families, groups and communities, or in health-care delivery. For example, change may be required in the dietary patterns of individual clients or families. Or, there may be a need for alteration in the way a community deals with the homeless or approaches sex education in the schools. Similar changes might be needed in the health-care system. For example, services might need to be redesigned to meet the needs of ethnic minority groups moving into the area. A recent study of community health nursing activity in official health departments[10] raised some concern about the extent to which the change-agent role at the aggregate level is played by community health nurses. A large proportion of the agencies studied indicated that no changes in funding allocations or services were needed in their jurisdictions. These findings were interpreted as evidence of a lack of proactivity (activism) by community health nurses in the change-agent role. Work toward changes in health-care delivery to meet evolving societal needs has been an area of strength throughout the history of community health nursing in the United States. If we are to continue to enact our full role as community health nurses and achieve our purpose of improved health for all, we must renew our efforts as change agents at the aggregate level. The change process and its implications for community health nursing will be discussed in greater detail in Chapter 11, The Change, Leadership, and Group Processes.

COMMUNITY CARE AGENT

Earlier, we discussed the primary care role of community health nurse practitioners with individuals and families. There is also a group-related role as community care agents in which community health nursing clinical specialists perform an expanded role working with communities as clients. In this role, the health problems of population groups or communities are diagnosed and treated much like the nurse practitioner diagnoses and treats the health problems of individuals and families. The ***community care agent*** is the person who provides care at an expanded level to communities as clients.

Community diagnosis requires an understanding of the wide variety of factors that impinge on the health of the community. Only a nurse with the theoretical background necessary for community assessment can delineate the interrelationships of these factors and use the information to plan for solutions to community problems. There is a need for "nurses who can diagnose community health problems and institute measures to protect, advance, and monitor the health of populations as a whole."[19]

Because of recent changes in the educational preparation of community health nurses, a community health nurse is emerging who is capable of gearing extended practice to the needs of communities in general rather than individuals or families. The Pan American Health Organization delineated four functions that are part of the community care agent role of the community health nurse. These functions include:

1. diagnosis of the level of health of the community;
2. decision making regarding solutions to health problems diagnosed;
3. preparation of the community to identify and meet health needs; and
4. evaluation of health-care delivery.[20]

The concept of the community as the recipient of health care will be discussed in detail in Chapter 19, Care of the Community or Target Group.

TABLE 4–3. GROUP-ORIENTED COMMUNITY HEALTH NURSING ROLES AND RELATED FUNCTIONS

Role	Function
Case finder	• Develop knowledge of signs and symptoms of health-related conditions and contributing factors • Use diagnostic reasoning process to identify potential cases of disease or other health-related conditions • Provide follow-up care to identified cases
Leader	• Identify the need for action • Assess situation and followers to determine appropriate leadership style • Motivate followers to take action • Coordinate group member activities in planning and implementing action • Assist followers to evaluate the effectiveness of action taken • Facilitate adaptation of group members • Represent the group to outsiders
Change agent	• Identify driving and restraining forces operating in change situation • Assist in unfreezing and creating motivation for change • Assist in implementation of change • Assist group to internalize change
Community care agent	• Diagnose the community's level of health • Develop solutions to identified community health problems • Prepare the community to identify and meet health needs • Evaluate health-care delivery
Researcher	• Critically review research findings • Apply research findings to practice as appropriate • Identify researchable problems • Design and conduct nursing research • Collect data • Disseminate research findings

RESEARCHER

A ***researcher*** explores phenomena observed in the world with the intent of understanding, explaining, and ultimately controlling them. The research role of the community health nurse is a relatively recent one and may be carried out at any of several levels. Responsibilities of the community health nurse related to research include critical review of relevant research and its application to practice. Other functions that may be carried out by community health nurses include identifying researchable problems, designing and conducting research studies, data collection, and dissemination of research findings. The research role in community health nursing will be discussed in greater depth in Chapter 10, The Research Process. Functions related to the role of researcher and other group-oriented community health nursing roles are summarized in Table 4–3.

CHAPTER HIGHLIGHTS

- Community health nursing is a synthesis of nursing and public health science designed to promote health and prevent illness in population groups.
- Community health nursing is characterized by an orientation to health, a population focus, autonomy, continuity, collaboration, interactivity, public accountability, and a sphere of intimacy not found in other nursing specialties.
- Community health nursing is practiced in accord with the American Nurses' Association *Standards of Community Health Nursing Practice,* based on the nursing process.
- Community health nursing roles are categorized as client-oriented roles, delivery-oriented roles, and group-oriented roles.
- Client-oriented roles involve providing direct care to clients and include the care-giver, educator, counselor, referral resource, role model, advocate, primary care provider, and case-manager roles.
- Delivery-oriented roles are designed to enhance the delivery of health-care services and include the coordinator, collaborator, liaison, and discharge-planner roles.
- Group-oriented roles focus on the health needs of groups of people and include case-finder, leader, change-agent, community-care-agent, and researcher roles.

Review Questions

1. Define community health nursing. (p. 57)
2. Describe at least five attributes of community health nursing. Give an example of each attribute. (p. 57)
3. What is the primary focus of community health nursing? (p. 57)
4. Summarize the ANA standards for community health nursing practice. (p. 60)
5. Distinguish among client-oriented, delivery-oriented, and group-oriented community health nursing roles. (p. 61)
6. Describe at least five client-oriented community health nursing roles. Give an example of the performance of each role. (p. 61)
7. Describe at least three delivery-oriented community health nursing roles. Give an example of the performance of each role. (p. 65)
8. Describe at least four group-oriented community health nursing roles. Give an example of the performance of each role. (p. 68)

APPLICATION AND SYNTHESIS

Miss Brown is a community health nurse who has received a request to visit Mrs. Jones to inform her of a class II Pap smear from her last visit to family-planning clinic. On her record, Miss Brown notes that Mrs. Jones is 45 years old, married, and has three children. When Miss Brown arrives at the home and explains the reason for her visit, Mrs. Jones tells her that Mr. Jones is unemployed and they have no health insurance. She doesn't know how she will be able to afford to have a repeat Pap smear now.

Mrs. Jones is also concerned because she has not had a period for two months. She has been on birth control pills for several years and has had no problems with missed periods until now. Her periods have become rather scanty in the last few months. She has no complaints of urinary frequency or breast tenderness.

Mrs. Jones states that she has been very irritable lately and can hardly stand to be around her older daughter, a 15-year-old, because she and her daughter argue all the time. The problem with her daughter has strained Mrs. Jones's relationship with her husband because he thinks she is being too hard on the daughter. Mrs. Jones suspects this daughter might be pregnant, because she has been very moody and has gained several pounds in the last few months. However, when she asks her daughter what is wrong, the girl changes the subject.

1. What community health nursing roles will Miss Brown probably perform in caring for Mrs. Jones and her family? Why are these roles appropriate to this situation?
2. Give examples of some specific activities that Miss Brown might carry out in performing each of these roles.

REFERENCES

1. United States Department of Health and Human Services. (1985). *Concensus conference on the essentials of public health nursing practice and education.* Rockville, MD: Bureau of Health Professions, Division of Nursing.
2. Freeman, R. B., & Heinrich, J. (1981). *Community health nursing practice* (2nd ed.). Philadelphia: W.B. Saunders.
3. Public Health Nursing Section of the American Public Health Association. (1980). *The definition and role of public health nursing in the delivery of health care.* Washington, DC: American Public Health Association.
4. American Nurses' Association. (1986). *Standards of community health nursing practice.* Kansas City, MO: American Nurses' Association.
5. Institute of Medicine. (1988). *The future of public health.* New York: The Academic Press.
6. Laffrey, S. C., & Page, G. (1989). Primary health care in public health nursing. *Journal of Advanced Nursing, 14,* 1044–1050.
7. Josten, L. E. (1989). Wanted: Leaders for public health. *Nursing Outlook, 37,* 230–232.
8. Riner, M. B. (1989). Expanding services: The role of the community health nurse and the advanced nurse practitioner. *Journal of Community Health, 6,* 223–230.
9. White, M. S. (1982). Construct for public health nursing. *Nursing Outlook, 30,* 527–530.
10. Erickson, G. P. (1987). Public health nursing initiatives: Guideposts for the future. *Public Health Nursing, 4,* 202–211.
11. Salmon, M. E. (1989). Public health nursing: The neglected specialty. *Nursing Outlook, 37,* 226–229.
12. Fatchett, A. B. (1990). Health visiting: A withering profession? *Journal of Advanced Nursing, 15,* 216–222.
13. Luker, K. A., & Chalmers, K. I. (1989). The referral process in health visiting. *International Journal of Nursing Studies, 26*(2), 173–185.
14. Lee, H. A., & Frenn, M. D. (1987). The use of nursing diagnoses for health promotion in community practice. *Nursing Clinics of North America, 22*(4), 981–987.

15. World Health Organization. (1978). *Primary health care: Report of the International Conference on Primary Health Care.* Geneva: World Health Organization.
16. Ryndes, T. (1989). The coalition model of case management for care of HIV-infected persons. *Quality Review Bulletin, 15,* 4–8.
17. Birmingham, J. J. (1987). The wellness frontier: The community. *Nursing Administration Quarterly, 11*(3), 14–18.
18. Peters, D. A. (1989). A concept of nursing discharge. *Holistic Nursing Practice, 3*(2), 18–25.
19. Mahler, H. (1988). Present status of WHO's initiative, "Health for all by the year 2000." *Annual Review of Public Health, 6*(2), 92–102.
20. Pan American Health Organization. (1977). *The role of the nurse in primary care.* Geneva: World Health Organization.

RECOMMENDED READINGS

Fagin, C. M. (1990). The visible problems of an "invisible" profession: The crisis and challenge for nursing. In P. R. Lee & C. L. Estes (Eds.), *The nation's health* (3rd ed.) (pp. 190–202). Boston: Jones and Bartlett.

Addresses factors contributing to the current nursing shortage and the impact on nursing of changes in the health-care system. Also presents potential needs for nursing in the health-care system of the future.

Fatchett, A. B. (1990). Health visiting: A withering profession? *Journal of Advanced Nursing, 15,* 216–222.

Provides a glimpse at some of the concerns surrounding community health nursing as practiced in England, concerns that parallel those of the specialty here in the United States.

Gulino, C., & LaMonica, G. (1986). Public health nursing: A study of role implementation. *Public Health Nursing, 3*(2), 80–91.

Presents the findings of a study on the components of the community health nurse role performed by nurses employed in one official health department.

Pesznecker, B., Draye, M. A., & McNeil, J. (1982). Collaborative practice models in community health nursing. *Nursing Outlook, 30,* 298–302.

Describes the interplay of the roles of the community health nurse and the family nurse practitioner in providing comprehensive health care for communities.

Rothman, N. L. (1990). Toward description: Public health nursing and community health nursing are different. *Nursing & Health Care, 11,* 481–483.

Sets forth arguments for differentiating public health nursing from community health nursing.

Ryndes, True. (1989). The coalition model of case management for care of HIV-infected persons. *Quality Review Bulletin, 15,* 4–8.

An excellent application of the principles of case management to the care of clients with HIV infection. Describes a coalition model that fosters effective case management for these clients. The model would also be applicable to case management in other settings and with other clients.

Tansey, E. M., & Lentz, J. R. (1988). Generalists in a specialized profession. *Nursing Outlook, 36,* 174–178.

Describes some of the barriers to educating effective community health nurses in a world that glorifies technology and insists upon measurable outcomes. Stresses the contribution of community health nursing content and experience in the education of the baccalaureate-prepared graduate.

U.S. Department of Health and Human Services. (1990). Secretary's Commission on Nursing, Executive summary, Final report. In P. R. Lee & C. L. Estes (Eds.), *The nation's health* (3rd ed.) (pp. 175–180). Boston: Jones and Bartlett.

Examines the findings and recommendations of the Secretary's Commission on Nursing regarding the causes of, and potential solutions to, the nursing shortage. Discusses changes needed in the use of nursing resources, compensation, recognition of nurse decision making, and development and maintenance of nursing resources.

UNIT TWO

Processes in Community Health Nursing

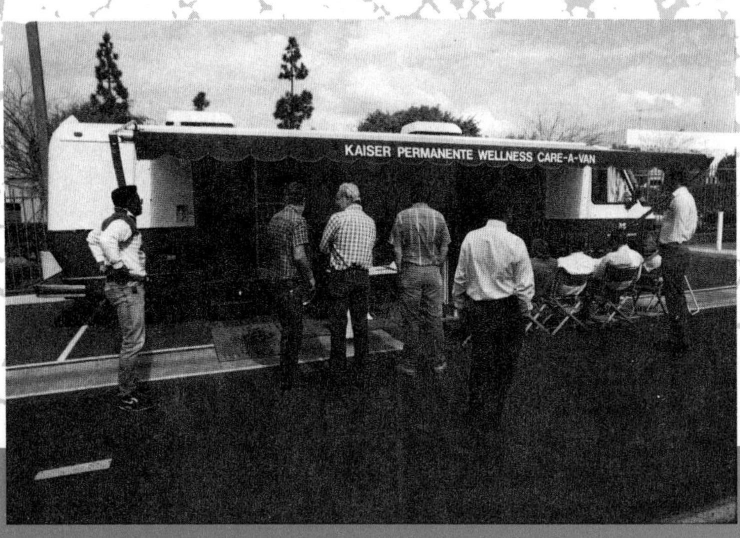

Community health nurses perform a wide variety of roles and functions in their efforts to promote and safeguard the health of the public. Effective performance in these roles involves the use of several systematic processes including the nursing process; the epidemiologic process; the health education process; the home visit process; discharge planning and referral processes; the research process; change, leadership, and group processes; and the political process. In this unit, each of these processes is discussed as it applies to community health nursing.

The nursing process (discussed in Chapter 5) is the basis for all nursing care, including care provided by community health nurses. The nursing process directs the community health nurse in providing care to meet clients' health needs, whether the client is an individual, a family, a group, or a community. The nursing process does not, however, delineate the kind of data that the nurse should collect about clients in determining their health status, so community health nurses use the epidemiologic process to direct data collection and to identify the health-care needs of clients. They also use the concept of levels of prevention discussed in Chapter 1, The Community Context, to plan nursing intervention appropriate to clients' needs. The combination of the nursing process, the epidemiologic process, and levels of prevention results in a model to direct community health nursing practice. This "epidemiologic prevention process model," described in Chapter 6, The Epidemiologic Process, can be used to guide community health nurses in performing their many roles.

When community health nurses encounter clients with educational needs, they use the process described in Chapter 7, The Health Education Process, to meet those needs. Health education is more than providing information on health. It is a systematic approach to the creation of a firm foundation of knowledge and attitudes that permits clients to make choices that enhance and protect their health. Use of a process based on scientific principles of teaching and learning enables the community health nurse more effectively to influence clients toward healthy behaviors.

Home visits are a traditional approach to providing community health nursing services. Too often, though, the potential benefits of this approach are unrealized, because the home visit is unfocused and the objectives to be achieved are not well delineated. Using the systematic process described in Chapter 8, The Home Visit Process, the community health nurse can plan and execute interventions in clients' homes that are focused on meeting identified health needs.

Community health nurses frequently encounter clients moving from one segment of the health-care system to another. This movement can be facilitated by use of the two processes discussed in Chapter 9, The Discharge Planning and Referral Processes. In discharge planning, the community health nurse assists in identifying and planning to meet clients' continuing needs for health care when they are discharged from one component of the health-care system to care by another agency or provider, by family members, or by themselves.

Community health nurses, no matter how dedicated, may find that they cannot meet all clients' needs themselves, either at discharge or in other situations. When this is the case, the nurse engages in the referral process linking the client with other sources of necessary services. Unless both discharge planning and referral are approached systematically, clients' needs for care may go unrecognized and unmet.

With everything else that they do, how can community health nurses also be involved in research? Not all community health nurses will conduct research, but all should incorporate research findings in the care of clients as appropriate. Research on the outcomes of community health nursing is needed to document its effectiveness and to justify its existence as a unique field of nursing. Community health nurses can generate research questions that will document their effectiveness and may be involved in conducting studies to that end. Even those who do not actually conduct research need an understanding of the research process to examine studies critically and to see their applicability to community health nursing practice. For this reason, the research process and its application to community health nursing are presented in Chapter 10, The Research Process.

Some of the problems with the U.S. health-care system discussed in Chapter 3, The Health-Care Context, indicate a need for change. Community health nurses can use the three processes described in Chapter 11, The Change, Leadership, and Group Processes, and Chapter 12, The Political Process, to facilitate these changes. Throughout their history, community health nurses have been involved in shaping society and the health-care delivery system to meet the needs of their clients. Without knowledge of the change, leadership, group, and political processes, community health nurses of the future will not be able to uphold this heritage of leadership in health-care delivery. Too often, nurses tend to see societal factors affecting client health and health-care delivery as beyond their sphere of influence. However, by judicious use of these four processes, community health nurses can contribute to changes in the fabric of society that will promote health and prevent illness.

Knowledge of the processes discussed in this unit provides community health nurses with the tools needed for effective performance of their many roles. The community health nurse who learns and applies these processes well will be an effective force for community health.

From the Community: A Nurse's Voice

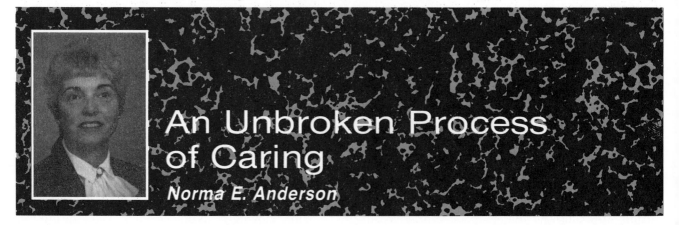

An Unbroken Process of Caring

Norma E. Anderson

When I began my public health nursing career in Wake County, North Carolina, I had already been in nursing practice for 12 years, with psychiatric, surgical, and pediatric staff nursing in my background. I had enjoyed my student experience in public health in Columbus, Ohio, and found that Wake County offered similar opportunities. Our six-nurse team was responsible for all nursing services—public health, home health care, school and clinic services—in a mostly rural southwestern section of the county. I was "different" from the other nurses on my team because I "talked funny," as one of my elderly patients commented to me. I was a "Yankee."

Most of my assigned families were very poor socioeconomically and were nonwhite—either black or American Indian families. Many of the families worked in tobacco fields as a whole family, and I found myself learning about tobacco farming as I sometimes made my visits with them in the fields. I was still seeking acceptance from these people when I received a referral to visit a young woman in our small town who had a grade–III Pap test report and had failed to respond to telephone messages and a letter from the clinic asking her to follow up on this report with further testing.

When I arrived at the family home, located in a poor neighborhood, I did not find the woman there. However, her mother, who had answered the door, asked me in. As it happened, the woman's younger daughter was confined to a reform school for girls in the western mountains near Asheville and had given birth to an infant 2 weeks earlier. Several days prior to my visit, the grandmother and other family members had driven to the institution and brought the baby home with them. At that time inmates were not allowed to keep their youngsters with them. Grandmother was concerned that the baby seemed to be "spitting up" excessively and, since I was there, asked me to examine the infant.

At that time I was not yet a nurse practitioner, but I had examined many newborn infants and I knew that this baby was not well. His color and skin turgor were poor. According to the grandmother, his intake was inadequate and he was not wetting many diapers. Rather than merely telling the grandmother to call the county hospital pediatric clinic and request an appointment, I called the clinic myself from the home and explained the situation and my findings and insisted upon an immediate appointment. Grandmother was told to take the baby to the hospital immediately and the clinic staff would see the infant as soon as possible. I knew the grandmother would not have been able to get an appointment that afternoon if she had called herself because all of the clinic appointments were booked.

Later the grandmother phoned to thank me. The baby had been admitted to an intensive care unit at the hospital and treated for lactose intolerance and dehydration. The grandmother was very grateful; however, I considered it a lucky thing that I had been requested to visit that home on that day. What did this lucky event do for me? It gained me complete acceptance with this community and credibility as a caring, helpful nurse. From that day, whenever I came back to my car in that neighborhood, I seldom failed to find someone waiting for me there with a question, a sick child, or a request for a referral. I also found that most of the families in our district seemed to be related. By helping this one family, I gained entry into all of the relatives' homes and the homes of their friends, because word spread rapidly about the nurse from "up North." I was very fortunate to have made the right decision in this situation, because it solidified my role as the public health nurse in the area.

Several years later I had major surgery at one of the Raleigh hospitals. Each day, one nurse's aide hovered around my room, changing water, straightening my bed, and doing whatever she could to make me comfortable. She looked vaguely familiar, and I asked one day if I didn't know her from somewhere. A huge smile crossed her face as she told me, "Oh yes, Miz Anderson, you were my nurse and my sister's nurse when we had our babies!" She told me her full name then, and I recalled her farm home where I had beeped my car's horn as I drove in so a family member would handle the large dogs as I got out of the car. Both teenagers had new babies. I had visited both of them before and after their deliveries and helped the girls get into a WIN educational program for young welfare mothers. This young woman had studied to become a nurse assistant and now supported herself and her child. She was very happy to have the opportunity to help me because I had helped her. The day of my discharge she proudly pushed my wheelchair to our family car. I was as thrilled as she was that this young woman was able to return my caring.

I've told these two stories to a number of my students over the years. To me the stories exemplify the caring and continuity of community health nursing. Community health nurses often cannot see the immediate results of their work—but weeks, months, or even years later, families may be in better circumstances because a nurse touched their lives. Sometimes my students become frustrated with the lack of immediate results, and I remind them that perhaps down the road another nurse will see the results of their involvement with a family. Sometimes, too, good luck, as well as skill and intuition, may play a role in our successes. Either one of these stories is inspiration enough for me *never* to give up; we really can't know how significant a role we may play in any of our clients' lives.

CHAPTER 5

The Nursing Process

KEY TERMS

affective aspect
assessment
cognitive aspect
data base
diagnostic hypothesis
etiology
evaluation
goals
health status summary
implementation
initial plan of care
nursing diagnosis
nursing orders
nursing process
objective data
objectives
outcome evaluation
planning
positive nursing diagnoses
problem-focused nursing diagnoses
process evaluation
progress notes
psychomotor aspect
status-oriented record
subjective data

Community health nurses, like nurses in other practice areas, use the nursing process as a framework for nursing care. As we shall see, however, community health nurses use the nursing process from a slightly different perspective, incorporating knowledge and principles derived from public health science. Community health nurses, however, also apply the nursing process to provide nursing care to communities and other client aggregates. Community health nurses work with both sick and well individuals and with people of all ages, applying the nursing process to meet the needs of these different clients. This chapter reviews the attributes and steps of the nursing process.

(*continued*)

LEARNING OBJECTIVES

After reading this chapter you should be able to:

- Discuss the components of the nursing process in the context of community health nursing.
- Describe the activities involved in developing nursing diagnoses.
- Write nursing diagnoses reflecting client health needs, incorporating appropriate descriptors and etiologic factors.
- Describe four tasks of the planning stage of the nursing process.
- Write nursing orders incorporating cognitive, affective, and psychomotor aspects of care.
- Describe five tasks in implementing the nursing plan of care.
- Differentiate between process and outcome evaluation and develop evaluative criteria for each.
- Identify the components of a SOAP note.

ATTRIBUTES OF THE NURSING PROCESS

The ***nursing process*** has been described as "an efficient method of organizing thought processes for clinical decision making and problem solving."[1] This systematic decision-making process is characterized by cognition, client-centeredness, and goal direction. In addition, the nursing process consists of a planned series of steps and is circular, cyclic, and sequential.[2] The nursing process is cognitive in that it requires systematic thought rather than intuition. It is goal-directed in that all of the activities involved are geared toward achieving specific client-centered goals for health promotion or restoration.

Use of the nursing process involves the planned execution of a series of steps. In 1967, these steps were delineated as *assessment, planning, implementation,* and *evaluation.*[2] *Diagnosis* was incorporated as a fifth step, between assessment and planning, prior to 1980.[3] These steps are performed sequentially and each step depends upon adequate performance of prior steps. The process itself is cyclic, and evaluative findings become assessment data in subsequent cycles of the process. All five steps of the process are incorporated in its use, but may overlap to a certain extent.

CLIENT ASSESSMENT

Client assessment is the first step of the nursing process. Prior to initiating action, the nurse assesses the client to determine the client's health status and the need for nursing intervention. In community health nursing, client needs are many and varied, affecting the biological, psychological, and social well-being of the community and its members.

Assessment is "the act of reviewing a human situation from a data base in order to affirm the wellness state and diagnose potential client problems; to affirm an illness state, diagnosing the client's prevailing problems; determining the potential for problems and identifying the wellness aspects of the ill client."[4] As indicated in this definition, assessment is not only a determination of a client's health *problems* but also the identification of strengths and weaknesses and the client's state of *health.*

Assessment consists of data collection for the purpose of identifying client health status. The types of data collected may be subjective or objective, current or historical.[5] ***Subjective data*** are reported by the client or a significant other, and cannot be validated by the nurse. ***Objective data,*** on the other hand, are observed, described, and verified by the nurse. Historical data are information about the client's past that influence current health status, while current data reflect present factors affecting health, either positively or negatively.[1]

Assessment data may be collected by several methods including interview, physical examination, review of records and diagnostic reports, and collaboration with colleagues.[6] Community health nurses tend to collect a wider array of data than do nurses in other specialty areas. For example, the school nurse may need to collect data on crime rates in the area around the school or on the employment level and tax base of the surrounding community so as to plan a school health program that adequately addresses community needs. Community health nurses are also likely to require data on groups of people as well as individuals and families. It is worth noting that the data-collection skills used by community health nurses in assessing individuals, families, groups, and communities must also be applied when assessing health policy issues, health-care financing issues, nursing research, and environmental and ethical issues to be examined in later chapters.

The client assessment performed by a community health nurse is influenced by an epidemiologic perspective. During the assessment, the nurse examines the interplay of multiple factors influencing client health. In the next chapter we will discuss incorporating this perspective into the assessment phase of the nursing process. Assessment of particular client groups will be addressed in Unit Four, "Care of Clients," while assessment in specific practice settings is explored in Unit Five, "Care of Clients in Specialized Settings."

DIAGNOSING CLIENT HEALTH STATUS

Using data obtained through various assessment procedures, the nurse identifies the client's health status and formulates nursing diagnoses. A ***nursing diagnosis*** is a statement that "describes the health status of an individual or group and the factors that have contributed to the status."[7] Nursing diagnoses reflect client conditions that require nursing intervention. Both positive and negative conditions can necessitate nursing action. Activities of the diagnostic phase of the nursing process include analyzing data and formulating diagnostic statements.[5] Relationships among these activities are depicted in Figure 5–1.

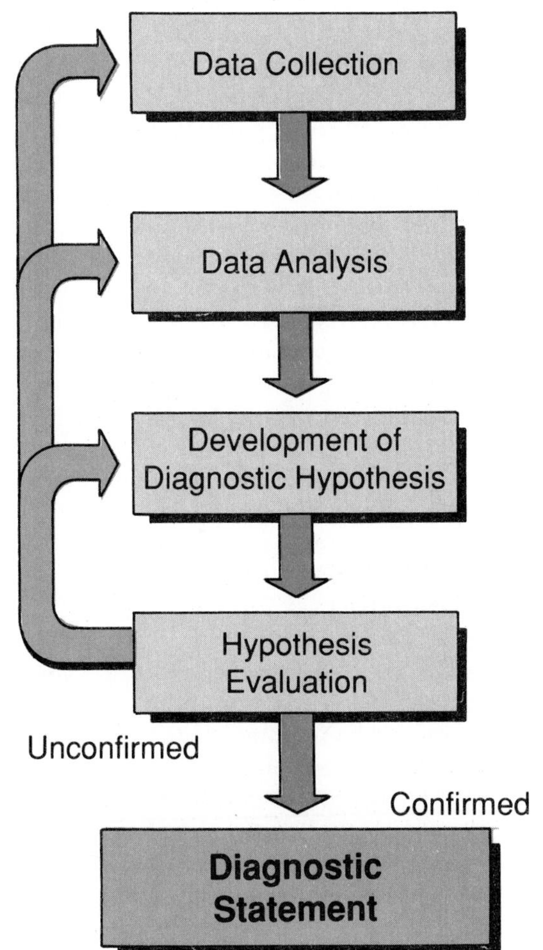

Figure 5–1. Relationships among steps of the diagnostic reasoning process.

DATA ANALYSIS

To be of value in directing nursing care, assessment data must be processed and analyzed. This analysis involves activities of classification, interpretation, and validation.[5] Data must first be classified or sorted into specific categories based on the types of data involved. For example, some data may reflect the client's physiologic health status, while other data relate to socioeconomic status. The categories used will depend on the organizing framework used by the nurse. In Chapter 6, The Epidemiologic Process, we will discuss an epidemiologic framework that can be used by community health nurses to categorize assessment data.

Once data have been classified, they must be interpreted. Data interpretation involves comparison of client-specific data with known norms and standards. For example, the community health nurse might note that a particular child has had more injuries than children of that age normally experience. Interpretation also includes recognizing patterns and trends in the data and making inferences based on the data. These inferences may be referred to as *diagnostic hypotheses.*[8]

A ***diagnostic hypothesis*** is a possible explanation for the client's condition and is generated on the basis of data patterns and trends. For example, data may include a history of questionable injuries to a young child with a teenage parent experiencing economic problems and lacking adequate social and emotional support. These data suggest a hypothesis of child abuse to explain a current broken arm.

The last aspect of data analysis is validating inferences or diagnostic hypotheses. This validation process may be referred to as *hypothesis evaluation.*[8] The hypothesis is tested by the collection of additional data that will either verify or disconfirm the diagnosis. Using the previous example, the nurse might observe parent-child interaction and question the parent and child more closely about how the broken arm occurred. The nurse might also request an investigation of the situation by the local child protective service to confirm the diagnostic hypothesis of abuse.

If additional data collected fit the diagnostic hypothesis, the hypothesis is verified and a specific diagnosis made. If not, the nurse recycles through the process, collecting data and establishing and testing hypotheses until one is confirmed. Verified hypotheses should be validated by both the client and the nurse.[2] For example, the nurse might confront the teenage parent with the suspicion of child abuse and evaluate the parent's response.

FORMULATING NURSING DIAGNOSES

Valid inferences or diagnostic hypotheses based on assessment data are formulated as diagnostic statements. Statements of nursing diagnoses may reflect strengths and positive states of health as well as health problems experienced by clients. When clients have no identified health problems, the nurse writes ***positive nursing diagnoses.***[9] Identified client health problems are the basis for ***problem-focused nursing diagnoses.***

Diagnostic statements should include a description of a client condition and its status. Underlying etiologic factors contributing to the condition are also included in the diagnostic statement.

DESCRIBING AND QUALIFYING CLIENT CONDITION

The client condition that has been identified is frequently described in terms of a general category of conditions in which it falls and may be further described by several qualifiers that specify the subtype of condition and its current status. For example, a general category describing a client condition might be "parenting." Parenting would be further described by a qualifier such as "effective" or "ineffective."

As an example, a community health nurse might find that a teenage parent is effectively meeting the needs of his or her child. The nurse might write a positive nursing diagnostic statement, reflecting "effective parenting." In this statement, the nurse is indicating that the parent is exhibiting effective parenting skills and that nursing intervention should be directed toward supporting and encouraging the parent's current behaviors.

Other qualifying descriptors of client conditions reflect the status of the condition as actual, potential, or possible.[7] An actual condition is one for which certain defining characteristics are present. Using the example of physical abuse, the victim exhibits signs of injury (i.e., fracture lines on X-ray, bruises, etc.) and there is evidence that the injury was willfully inflicted by another. The diagnostic statement would say that there is a problem of "actual physical abuse." In many diagnoses, the word "actual" is implied rather than stated, so the diagnostic statement might be "physical abuse."

Some authors recommend including the defining characteristics of an actual condition in the diagnostic statement itself, usually preceded by the phrase "as evidenced by. . . ." The diagnostic statement related to abuse would then be "physical abuse as evidenced by a history of repeated injury and parental explanations incongruent with type and location of injuries." Including the defining characteristics in the actual diagnostic statement, however, often creates a lengthy statement that does not contribute appreciably to an understanding of the client's health status. A more effective approach is to document the presence of defining characteristics using the status-oriented record discussed later in this chapter.

A potential condition is one for which defining characteristics are not evident, but which may occur without intervention.[7] For instance, child abuse is a potential problem when a parent is under stress, is coping poorly, and had abusive parents as role models. The parent has not been abusive yet, but abuse may occur without intervention. The diagnostic statement in this instance would reflect "potential for child abuse."

Only problem-focused nursing diagnoses have "potential" status. Saying that a client has "potential for adequate nutrition" implies that his or her nutritional status is currently *not* adequate. Indeed, if the client's nutrition is inadequate, the diagnosis would be stated as "inadequate iron intake" or whatever wording reflects the client's actual status.

Problem-focused nursing diagnoses also may reflect health problems that are acute, chronic, or intermittent. In a diagnosis related to child abuse, the problem may be one of chronic neglect, or it may be an acute problem in which the child is left unsupervised when mother has been hospitalized and father has to go to work. Or, the problem of neglect may be intermittent, occurring only when the parent is in the throes of periodic depression. In this case, the problem category would be qualified as "intermittent" and the diagnosis would be written as "intermittent child neglect."

DESCRIBING THE ETIOLOGY OF THE CONDITION

The examples of nursing diagnostic statements presented thus far have all been incomplete because they have not included the etiology of the condition. The ***etiology*** is the probable cause of the condition, and the etiologic component of the diagnostic statement describes the factors contributing to the condition. For example, one might write a nursing diagnosis of "potential intermittent child neglect due to maternal depression." In this diagnosis, the mother's periodic depression is described as the source of the potential for neglect. In another instance, the cause might be lack of knowledge of children's needs on the part of the parent. The diagnosis then becomes one of "potential for child abuse due to lack of knowledge of children's physical and emotional needs."

Many authors use the phrase "related to" to indicate the etiology of a health condition.[4,7] However, since etiology refers to the "actual or probable cause of the health problem,"[3] the phrase "due to" is used in this book. One circumstance might be "related to" another without any connotation of cause and effect. For example, sugar consumption has been found to be significantly related to lung cancer, but certainly does not cause the cancer. However, when one states that one event is "due to" another, one implies causality and provides direction for actions to be taken to either change or reinforce a situation. For example, a diagnosis of "ineffective parenting due to lack of parental role models" might be addressed by providing adequate role models. Similarly, when a diagnosis of "effective coping due to use of extended support system" is made, the nurse would encourage continued use of the support system to maintain this healthy state.

ACCEPTED NURSING DIAGNOSES

Several "accepted" nursing diagnoses have been developed by nursing groups throughout the nation. Such attempts to generate standardized nursing diagnoses have been criticized by a number of community health nurses because of the concentration of these diagnoses on physical health problems of individual clients and minimal attention to psychological problems. The majority of these diagnoses do not address the myriad social, environmental, and economic problems encountered in community health nursing.

Another criticism of the accepted diagnoses is the absence of diagnoses reflecting positive states of health or client strengths. For instance, the current list of nursing diagnoses approved by the *North American Nursing Diagnosis Association* (NANDA) "contains problem-oriented diagnoses useful for clients whose predominant health experience at the time of nursing care is illness."[10] There is a need for nursing diagnoses that reflect client health status as encountered by community health nurses. This need relates not only to statements of health problems but also diagnoses related to positive health states.

Some attempts have been made to develop nursing diagnoses applicable to community health nursing. One such attempt is the *Omaha Visiting Nurse Association* system, which incorporates the needs of individuals and families in four categories: environmental, psychosocial, physiologic, and health behavioral needs.[11] Unfortunately, these attempts remain problem-focused with little attention to health promotion. They also address individuals and families and do not reflect the health of groups of clients or communities served by community health nurses.

One further criticism of the current taxonomies of nursing diagnoses is their wordiness, a characteristic that may obscure, rather than clarify, meaning, particularly for clients. For example, clients will probably understand a diagnosis of "constipation." Does the precursor phrase in the related NANDA diagnosis "alteration in elimination, constipation" add clarity? Probably not. What it may do is alienate the typical client of the community health nurse. Nor does such terminology enhance communication with other health-care providers.

While the accepted nursing diagnoses generated thus far leave much to be desired, the community health nurse should make use of the diagnostic reasoning process to generate diagnoses that are meaningful in community health nursing and that accurately reflect client health status. The task is not so much to derive a diagnosis that fits accepted terminology, but to describe client health in terms that are meaningful and provide direction for action.

NURSING DIAGNOSIS AND COMMUNITY HEALTH NURSING

Community health nurses are likely to develop a broader range of nursing diagnoses than nurses in other fields. In addition to developing diagnoses related to the health of individuals, the community health nurse may also make diagnoses concerning families, groups, or communities. For example, the nurse may make a diagnosis of "inadequate financial resources due to husband's unemployment" for a family unable to afford health-care services. A related diagnosis for this family would be "inadequate provision of health care due to limited income."

In a similar vein, the nurse might diagnose health problems found in a community or group of people. A nursing diagnosis at this level might be "inadequate access to health care due to increased unemployment among community members." Such a diagnosis indicates that the problem exists, not in one family, but in a sizable portion of the population. Because the problem is widespread, its solution will be more complex. Intervention for a specific low-income family might entail referral for financial assistance, but when the problem involves a group of people, this type of intervention would rapidly deplete the community's economic resources. Effective intervention needs to be directed toward alleviating the problem of unemployment.

Each of these diagnostic statements includes information about the probable cause or etiology of the problem. This component of the diagnostic statement provides direction for problem resolution. Because we know that the family's failure to obtain adequate health care is due to financial limitations, we know what actions are likely to resolve the problem. If the underlying cause of the family's failure to seek health care is lack of motivation, referral for financial assistance will do little to resolve the problem. The same is true in the community situation. If failure to seek health care is due to a low value placed on health, dealing with unemployment will not help. The etiologic portion of the diagnostic statement, then, provides guidance in solving problems. Similarly, factors identified as contributors to positive health states indicate areas for support and reinforcement by community health nurses.

PLANNING NURSING INTERVENTION

The next step in the nursing process is planning primary, secondary, or tertiary preventive actions appropriate to the client's diagnosed health conditions. ***Planning*** is defined as "a collaborative, orderly, cyclic process to attain a mutually agreed-on desired future goal."[12] The plan of care should be developed to provide continuity of care and enhance communication among providers and with the client; to assist in determining priorities for action; and to support the documentation of effective use of the nursing process. In addition, a well-developed plan of care may serve as a learning tool for other providers and for clients in modeling the problem-solving process.[13]

Whether the client is an individual, family, group, or community, the planning component of the nursing process consists of six basic tasks: prioritizing nursing interventions; developing goals and objectives for those interventions; establishing critical criteria for potential means of achieving goals; selecting appropriate means; writing nursing orders; and planning for evaluation.

PRIORITIZING NURSING INTERVENTIONS

Because clients with whom community health nurses come in contact may have multiple health needs, nurses will usually not be able to resolve all of these needs during an initial contact. The nurse, in collaboration with the client, will need to decide which needs must be addressed now and which might be deferred until a later time.[6]

The priority given to a particular condition may be based on the degree to which it threatens health. As a simplistic example, one would certainly want to deal with hemorrhage before worrying about the psychological trauma that may result from an injury. In this respect, it is useful to consider Maslow's hierarchy of basic human needs as a way of establishing priorities among problems. Problems that impair the client's ability to meet physiologic needs would have a higher priority than those interfering with self-actualization needs.

Priority also may be assigned on the basis of the client's concern about a particular problem. Dealing first with problems of major concern to the client can help to free client energy for dealing with other problems. Addressing the client's concerns first also may improve the nurse's credibility. Clients who see their needs met as they perceive them are likely to be more willing to take action in areas that they may not see as immediate problems.

Another criterion for assigning priorities to specific problems may simply be ease of solution. If a problem can be solved with minimal effort by nurse or client, there are few reasons why that problem cannot be dealt with immediately and "gotten out of the way."

Finally, one problem may be given priority over others because it contributes to other problems. For example, a client may not have a regular source of health care and may also have the problem of unemployment. In this case, if the nurse focused on helping the client to become employed, the lack of health care might resolve itself when the client obtained health insurance through his or her employment.

DEVELOPING GOALS AND OBJECTIVES

The second aspect of planning is developing expected outcomes related to identified nursing diagnoses. This involves establishing goals and objectives for each nursing diagnosis. ***Goals*** are broad statements of outcome, whereas ***objectives*** are the specific, short-term achievements expected to result in goal accomplishment. Objectives should be stated in terms of "maintenance or change to a favorable status of the client after nursing care."[6] For example, a nurse might state that the client "will be able to correctly identify foods high in iron within one week" or "will eat at least four iron-rich foods per week" as a result of nutrition teaching. Or, "the community will show a decrease in the rate of adolescent pregnancy" following the institution of a family-planning clinic for teens. Objectives should be client-centered, clear and concise, observable and measurable, and limited in duration. Other criteria for objectives are that they are realistic and jointly established by nurse and client.[5]

Statements of objectives for nursing care usually include three components: content, modifiers, and a time for achievement.[6] The phrase *content component* is a verb and its object, which reflects what the client will be or do as a result of intervention. Using the previous examples, the verbs and their objects were "identify foods" and "eat foods." Modifiers are adjectives and adverbs that qualify the verb and its object. "Correctly," "high in iron," "four," and "iron-rich" were modifiers used in the objectives stated above. The ability to identify foods high in iron should be achieved "within one week," while the client would include four iron-rich foods "per week" as the time frame of the objectives.

ESTABLISHING CRITERIA FOR MEANS TO ACHIEVE GOALS

The next task in the planning phase of the nursing process is establishing criteria by which to evaluate potential nursing interventions. In a given situation there may be several alternative actions that could be taken to achieve the desired outcome. In deciding among these alternatives, it is helpful to have criteria for evaluating the relative merit of each option. Criteria to evaluate alternative courses of action should be jointly developed and employed by the nurse and the client. The client best understands the situation in which intervention needs to occur and the effects that specific alternatives might have. The client may, however, not be aware of the consequences of some alternatives, and these consequences may need to be pointed out by the nurse.

Examples of criteria by which to evaluate potential actions might be that the action selected must fit the client's budget and be culturally acceptable to the client. Suppose, for example, that the goal is to reduce adolescent pregnancies in the community by 50 percent over the next 3 years. Possible alternative actions might include providing sex-education programs in schools and referring sexually active teenagers to existing contraceptive services or creating contraceptive clinics in each junior and senior high school. The first alternative is less costly and more apt to be culturally acceptable to the community than the second. Based on the criteria of cost and cultural acceptability, the first alternative would be the most appropriate.

SELECTING APPROPRIATE MEANS TO GOALS

Once the nurse and client have determined the evaluative criteria to be used, they can generate potential solutions to problems or measures that have been identified so as to enhance client health status. The interventions selected might reflect primary, secondary, or tertiary levels of prevention or a combination of levels. Primary prevention would be employed to promote health and prevent illness. This level of prevention is particularly pertinent to clients without identified health problems. Secondary prevention would be warranted when clients have existing health problems, and tertiary prevention would be appropriate to prevent a recurrence of a problem or to return a client to a previous level of function.

Nurse and client evaluate each primary, secondary, and tertiary alternative generated in terms of the evaluative criteria established.[12] Alternatives that come closest to fitting the critical criteria are usually the ones selected for implementation.

For example, a community may be concerned about increased drug abuse reported in other parts of the state. Although the community does not have a drug abuse problem at present, residents may be interested in preventing such a problem from occurring. A variety of primary preventive strategies can be suggested for preventing drug abuse among young people. Those concerned with the issue would probably like to find an alternative that is not too costly, but that has a lasting effect on drug use among the young. Cost and length of effect would then be the criteria used to evaluate potential alternatives. Possible approaches might be an intensive educational program for junior high school students, an integrated drug education program throughout elementary and secondary school curricula, or increased police presence to apprehend drug dealers. The costs of the three alternatives might be approximately the same. Education at the junior high level might be effective for a while, but determined drug dealers would be likely to turn, instead, to younger children as buyers. Adding to the police force might also be effective until drug dealers learned to circumvent police efforts. The approach that best fits the criteria of lasting effect is education across all grade levels that helps children refrain from initiating drug use.

WRITING NURSING ORDERS

When an appropriate alternative has been selected, the nurse develops nursing orders related to the client condition. ***Nursing orders*** are specific statements of

BOX 5–1

Sample Nursing Orders for the Diagnosis of "Inadequate Immunization Status"

Goal

Client will be adequately protected against communicable diseases

Objective

Client will receive immunizations appropriate to age

Nursing orders

Cognitive aspect:

1. Explain to parent the need for immunizations
2. Explain legal requirement for immunization prior to school entry
3. Discuss possible side effects of immunizations
4. Explain how to deal with possible immunization side effects
5. Give parent information on immunization clinic

Affective aspect:

1. Encourage parent to express reluctance to cause child pain
2. Encourage parent to discuss concerns about potential side effects of immunizations
3. Acknowledge fears as normal
4. Praise other aspects of positive parenting to increase parent motivation to get immunizations

Psychomotor aspect:

1. Demonstrate how to take child's temperature
2. Have parent demonstrate taking temperature
3. Give positive and corrective feedback
4. Continue demonstrations and practice until parent can exhibit correct technique for taking axillary temperature and can read thermometer accurately

actions to be taken to achieve the desired outcome or stated objective.[5] Effective nursing orders are characterized by consistency with the plan of care and the nursing diagnoses derived from the client assessment and by their basis in scientific principles. Nursing orders individualize the plan of care to a specific client situation and incorporate the provision of a safe and therapeutic environment and opportunities for health teaching. Finally, nursing orders should reflect appropriate use of resources.[5]

Nursing orders should address three aspects of nursing care: cognitive aspects, affective aspects, and psychomotor aspects.[14] The ***cognitive aspect*** of nursing orders relates to the client's knowledge of health conditions and their causes. For example, the nurse may plan to explain to the client how poor hygiene has contributed to a bladder infection and how subsequent infections can be prevented. Or, plans may be made to educate intravenous drug users about the risks of needle sharing in the transmission of AIDS and how to limit their chances of exposure to infection.

The ***affective aspect*** of nursing orders involves considering the client's feelings about a health condition and planning interventions that encourage the client to explore or reduce those feelings. For instance, the nurse caring for a client whose child is to have surgery may encourage the client to discuss fears about the surgery and arrange for the client to visit the surgical unit in the hope that reducing uncertainty will help to alleviate anxiety. Similarly, if AIDS is a problem in the community, nursing orders related to the problem may focus on reducing fears about the disease as well as on preventing the spread of infection.

The ***psychomotor aspect*** of nursing orders focuses on developing skills that the client may need to meet personal health needs or those of others. For example, the new mother may need help learning how to bathe an infant.

In writing nursing orders, the nurse should address all three aspects of care in relation to a particular condition. For example, one objective of primary preventive activities with young children is that they will be adequately immunized. To accomplish this objective, the nurse may write the nursing orders presented in Box 5–1, reflecting all three aspects of nursing care.

The nursing orders in Box 5–1 consist of behaviorally stated objectives or expected client outcomes and the activities to be performed to accomplish those objectives. The nurse deals with the cognitive aspects of care by providing the parent with information about immunization. Affective aspects of care are addressed with opportunities to discuss concerns about immunization, and teaching the manual skill of taking a temperature reflects the psychomotor aspects of care.

When nursing diagnoses are positive statements as in the example in Box 5–1, nursing orders will reflect efforts to maintain a positive state. When secondary prevention is warranted, nursing orders will focus on activities that will relieve symptoms and resolve an existing health problem. Nursing orders at the tertiary prevention level will include activities designed to return the client to his or her previous state of health and prevent a recurrence of the particular health problem. In planning nursing intervention, the nurse and client together establish the expected outcomes and design activities that will lead to their achievement.

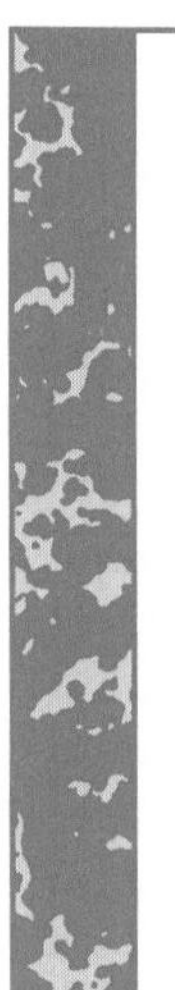

BOX 5–2

Tasks of the Planning Stage of the Nursing Process

- Prioritize nursing interventions
- Develop goals and objectives
- Establish criteria for means to achieve goals
- Select appropriate means to goals
- Write nursing orders
- Plan for evaluation

PLANNING FOR EVALUATION

The last task in the planning stage of the nursing process is planning for evaluation. Evaluation of the outcome of nursing care takes place after intervention has occurred. Planning for evaluation, however, should occur while interventions are being planned. If this does not happen, data needed for evaluation may not be available at the time the evaluation is to be conducted. For example, if the objective of an immunization program is to increase measles immunization levels among preschool children by 50 percent in 6 months, evaluation will focus on comparisons of immunization levels before and after the program. If evaluation procedures have not been planned ahead of time, data on preprogram immunization levels may not be available. If, on the other hand, those planning the program plan for evaluation as well, they will identify the need for this data and take steps to collect the data prior to starting the program.

Considerations to be addressed in planning to evaluate the outcome of nursing intervention include who should conduct the evaluation, what type of data will be needed, and how that data will be collected. Both nurse and client should be involved in evaluating nursing effectiveness, and others may be involved as well. In the case of the immunization program, evaluation might be conducted by health-care providers and community policymakers.

Decisions on the type of data to be collected should be based on the objectives established. Using the immunization example, the objective deals with immunization levels, so data on immunization levels before and after the program will be needed to determine whether or not immunization levels have increased 50 percent. Decisions on data-collection methods will depend upon the kind of data needed and potential sources of that data. A general estimate of immunization levels among preschool children, for example, might be obtained by examining immunization records in child-care facilities and reviewing a sample of client records in the offices of local pediatricians. Planning for evaluation will be discussed in greater detail in Chapter 19, Care of the Community or Target Group. Tasks of the planning stage of the nursing process are summarized in Box 5–2.

IMPLEMENTING NURSING CARE

Implementation is the fourth stage of the nursing process. ***Implementation*** involves organizing and carrying out the plan of care. Tasks involved in this stage of the nursing process include identifying requisite knowledge and skills, designating responsibility for implementation, recognizing impediments to implementation, and communicating the plan to others. Additional tasks include providing an environment conducive to implementation and actually performing the activities required for implementation.

IDENTIFYING REQUISITE KNOWLEDGE AND SKILLS

The first task of implementation is identifying the knowledge and skills needed to implement the plan. This information will aid in determining the most appropriate person for implementing a specific segment of the plan. For example, knowledge of nutrition and skill in developing menus on a limited budget are required to assist an individual client to adjust to the demands of a diabetic diet on a limited income. Knowledge of contraceptive measures and adolescent development, as well as good interpersonal skills, will be needed to implement a plan to increase contraceptive use among sexually active adolescents.

DESIGNATING RESPONSIBILITY FOR IMPLEMENTATION

The second task of implementation is designating those responsible for carrying out the planned interventions. The person or persons designated should have at least some of the required skills and knowledge to implement the plan of care. Either a nurse or a nutritionist, for example, would have the knowledge and skills needed to assist a client with a diabetic diet. Many nurses or health educators would also have the knowledge required to teach adolescents about contraceptives.

The person given responsibility for implementing a specific aspect of the intervention plan should also have the authority to perform the necessary activities. For example, it would be inappropriate (and illegal) to designate a nurse's aide as the person responsible for giving intravenous medications to a homebound client. As another example, the mayor or police chief would have the authority to initiate a community response to a disaster situation and could be assigned the responsibility for this aspect of a community disaster plan.

Responsibility for carrying out the plan of care may be assumed by the community health nurse. Certain aspects of implementation might also entail delegating responsibility to others or making a referral to another source of assistance.

DELEGATION

Delegating responsibility for implementing aspects of the plan of care to others involves three primary considerations. The first is the presence or absence of needed knowledge and behavioral skills in the person to whom the activity is being delegated. Competence improves the chances of implementing the plan as designed. The nurse may need to teach the necessary skills to the person involved. For example, the nurse may need to instruct family members or ancillary staff in the proper procedure for daily dressing changes. Or the person responsible for preparing meals for the client with hypertension might need information on low-salt recipes. It is particularly important for the nurse to remember that the development of required skills can take time. Thus, the nurse should ensure that sufficient time for learning is provided and that progress in learning is evaluated.

The second consideration in delegation is whether or not the incentives for implementing the plan are present. The nurse needs to consider whether plan implementation is consistent with the self-interest of the person to whom it is being delegated. If implementation is not in that individual's self-interest, implementation is less likely to occur. When such is the case, the nurse may need to develop the plan so the individual's self-interests are indeed served by implementing the plan. For example, if the mother of the family is budget conscious, the nurse may point out that attending the health department's immunization clinic is less expensive than visits to a private physician. Or, if a harried mother wants to enroll her children in day care, the nurse can point out that the children will need to be up-to-date on their immunizations, thus motivating the mother to bring them to clinic.

The final consideration in delegation is whether the necessary cognitive supports are present. Does the client or other concerned party firmly believe that the suggested action is necessary? Is there support for implementing the plan from significant others? The nurse may find, for example, that he or she must sell the plan to a key family member before other family members are willing to carry out activities involved. Or, if the individual implementing the plan is unconvinced of the efficacy of the proposed activities, plan implementation may be approached on a trial basis and the person convinced to give it a chance. If the persons who are to implement the plan have been involved in its development, it is more likely that the necessary cognitive supports will be present. This is another reason for including clients in developing the plan of care, since they are the ones most likely to be implementing the bulk of the plan.

REFERRAL

Referral for outside assistance is another approach that may be used in implementing planned interventions. In using this approach the nurse should be sure to consider the acceptability of the referral to the client, client eligibility for service, and any situational constraints influencing the referral. Other considerations include providing necessary information to the client and the referral agency and following up on the effectiveness of the referral in solving the client's problem. The referral process will be discussed in greater depth in Chapter 9, The Discharge Planning and Referral Processes.

RECOGNIZING IMPEDIMENTS TO IMPLEMENTATION

The community health nurse must identify any constraints that might impede implementing the plan and take steps to modify or eliminate those constraints. Ideally, limitations of the chosen intervention have been identified during the evaluation of alternative approaches to solving the problem, but it is useful to look again for any constraints that may have been overlooked during the planning stage or that may have arisen in the interim. For example, part of the plan of care might be a referral for financial assistance. At the time the plan was designed, the client may have had adequate transportation. Since that time, however, he or she might have had an accident and be without a car until repairs are completed. In such a case, the nurse would need to assist the client to find another means of transportation so as to implement the planned referral.

COMMUNICATING THE PLAN

A further task of implementation is communicating the plan to those involved. Clients should have been involved in developing planned interventions, but the nurse can remind clients of their responsibilities for implementation. Similarly, there may be a need to communicate expectations to others who are to assume responsibility for implementing certain segments of the plan. For example, specific responsibilities of health, police, and fire personnel in a disaster plan need to be adequately communicated to them.

PROVIDING AN ENVIRONMENT FOR IMPLEMENTATION

The nurse also needs to provide an environment conducive to implementation of the plan of care. This involves providing the resources needed for implementation, providing for the comfort of the client, and maintaining the client's safety during implementation. Necessary resources can include time, personnel, or equipment. If a staff member is to give a bedfast client a bath, time must be provided within the client's schedule. Or it may be necessary to engage the services of a physical therapist to implement segments of the plan. For some activities, special equipment might be required and the nurse should either obtain that equipment or assist the client to do so. For example, if preventing falls by an older client necessitates the use of a walker, the nurse can help the family obtain one.

Implementing planned interventions should also allow for both the physical and psychological comfort of the client. For instance, the client might not speak English well and might feel uncomfortable about trying to explain his or her need for financial assistance to social service workers. In this case, the nurse might contribute to the client's psychological comfort by arranging for an interpreter. Or, the plan of care may be implemented in such a way as to diminish fatigue for the older client.

Safety considerations in implementation will vary based on the client's age, level of mobility, presence or absence of sensory deficits, and level of orientation. For example, young children would not be expected to take their own medications, or the older person with impaired vision might need color-coded labels on medication bottles so as to take them correctly.

CARRYING OUT PLANNED ACTIVITIES

The final task in the implementation phase of the nursing process is actually carrying out the activities included in the nursing orders. Planned activities are executed by those assigned responsibility for them. These activities may occur at the primary, secondary, or tertiary levels of prevention depending upon the needs of the client. Tasks of the implementation stage of the nursing process are summarized in Box 5–3.

EVALUATING NURSING CARE

The last component of the nursing process is evaluation. ***Evaluation*** is a "systematic comparison of client's health status with the outcomes" projected.[5] Evaluation can take two basic forms—outcome evaluation and process evaluation. ***Outcome evaluation***

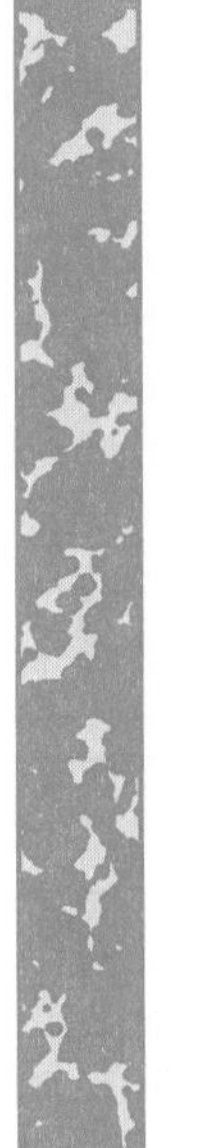

BOX 5–3

Tasks of the Implementation Stage of the Nursing Process

- Identify knowledge and skills needed for implementation
- Designate responsibility for implementation
- Recognize impediments to implementation
- Create an environment conducive to implementation
- Carry out planned activities

is the assessment of the outcome of nursing intervention. ***Process evaluation,*** on the other hand, is the examination of the quality of actions taken and the processes used to achieve that outcome. Either or both types of evaluation may be involved in evaluating the application of the nursing process to a given community health nursing situation. Evaluation involves several tasks. These tasks include conducting the evaluation itself, interpreting findings, and using evaluative findings.

CONDUCTING THE EVALUATION

Like each of the other steps of the nursing process, evaluation must be planned and executed systematically. Planning for both outcome and process evaluation occurs during the planning stage of the nursing process. Once interventions have been implemented, the planned evaluative procedures are put into effect. Data are gathered (if this has not been gathered throughout the implementation stage) and organized for analysis.

Data should be collected to evaluate both the outcome of interventions and the process used in implementing them. Outcome-related data should reflect the stated objectives or expected outcomes for care. Process-related data are obtained by examining how interventions were implemented. If the stated objective was to have the client include at least one iron-rich food in the daily diet, intervention outcomes could be evaluated by asking the client to complete a 3-day diet history and looking for the inclusion of iron-rich foods in each day's diet. Process evaluation might entail examining how well the nurse adapted dietary teaching to the client's educational level, culturally determined food practices, and economic situation.

INTERPRETING FINDINGS

Evaluation always involves the comparison of the actual outcome with some kind of standard. These standards are the evaluative criteria developed in planning for evaluation. Once data related to the evaluative criteria have been collected, they must be analyzed and interpreted in terms of the criteria. Has the client included at least one iron-rich food in his or her diet each day? If not, why not? Process evaluation data may provide possible explanations for nonachievement of objectives. In the dietary example, process evaluation may indicate that education about iron-rich foods provided by the nurse focused on foods eaten by members of the dominant cultural group and did not fit the client's food preferences. Or, the nurse may not have suggested food alternatives that were congruent with the client's economic situation. The community health nurse compares the data obtained to the evaluative criteria to determine if set standards were achieved. Judgments on the achievement of these standards form the basis for the third task of evaluation—making further care decisions.

USING EVALUATIVE FINDINGS

Findings of both outcome and process evaluation are used to make decisions about nursing care. Basically, three decisions are possible. First, the evaluation may show that intervention was effective and that objectives were met. Intervention can then be continued or terminated as needed. Second, evaluation findings may indicate that objectives were not met and another approach can be tried. Or, third, the evaluation may suggest that the implementation of the nursing plan was not up to par and the nurse (or other involved party) can make changes in the quality of performance that may lead to the intended outcomes.

Evaluation can also lead to changes in other components of the nursing process. For example, the nurse may find that interventions were not effective because they were based on an inadequate or inaccurate data base. If this is the case, the nurse will want to expand the client assessment. Or, the plan of care may not have been sensitive to the constraints of the client situation and modifications can be made in the plan. As we have already seen, evaluation findings might also indicate a need for changes in the way the plan is implemented. Tasks of the evaluation stage of the nursing process are summarized in Box 5–4.

DOCUMENTING USE OF THE NURSING PROCESS

Documentation is a critical feature of all phases of the nursing process. Community health nurses, like their

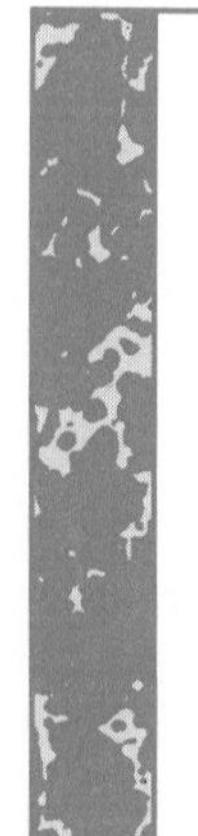

BOX 5–4

Tasks of the Evaluation Stage of the Nursing Process

- Conduct the evaluation
- Interpret data in light of evaluative criteria
- Use evaluative findings to make client care decisions

counterparts in other areas of nursing, must carefully document client data and diagnoses, plans and interventions, and their outcomes. In the assessment phase of the nursing process, documentation focuses on the data on which nursing actions are based. The written diagnostic statements derived from the data base document the use of the diagnostic reasoning process. Plans related to each nursing diagnosis are also documented, as is implementation of the plan of care. Finally, the evaluation phase of nursing process is documented in terms of the outcome of nursing interventions.

Several approaches can be taken to document the use of the nursing process. One of the most effective for use in community health nursing is an adaptation of the problem-oriented record (POR) allowing for positive as well as negative client health states. This adaptation is called the ***status-oriented record*** (SOR) because it reflects both positive and negative client health status.

The status-oriented record is an organized systematic method for recording client data, nursing diagnoses based on that data, intended outcomes of care, plans for achieving those outcomes, implementation of the plan of care, and the outcome of care. There are four basic components to the status-oriented record that allow the community health nurse to document each step of the nursing process. These components are the client data base, the health status summary, the initial plan of care, and the progress notes. Components of the SOR are depicted in Figure 5–2.

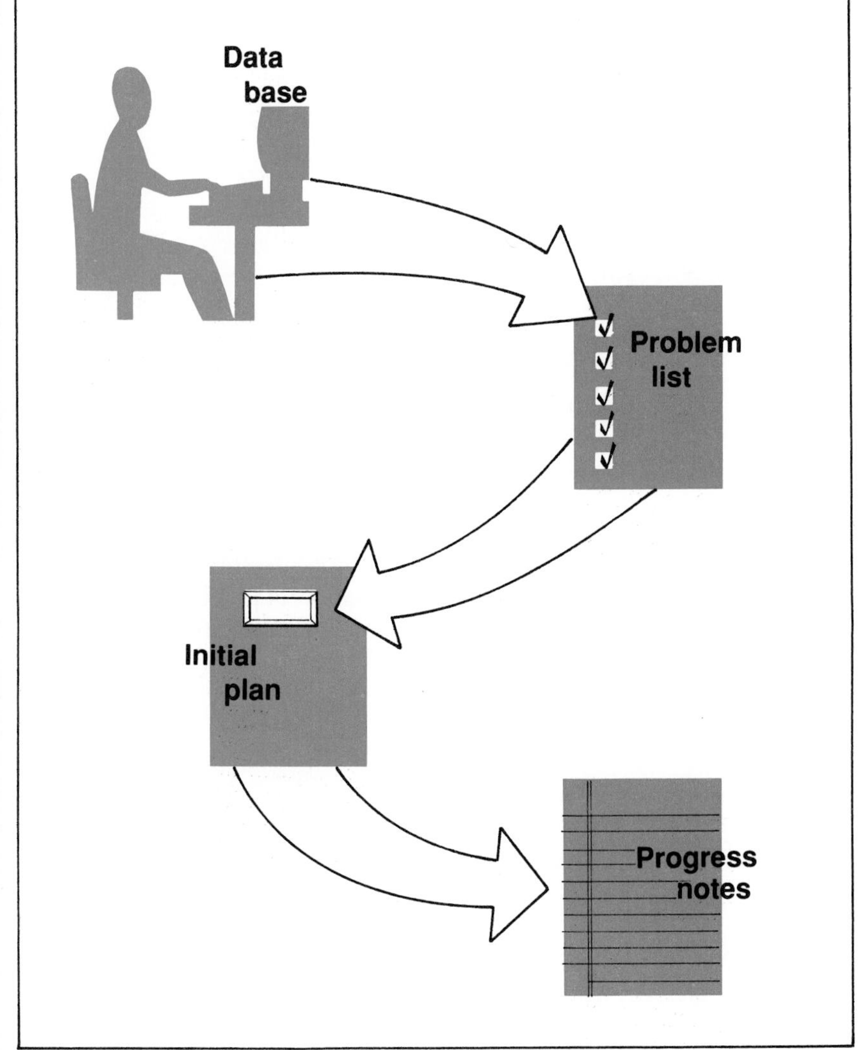

Figure 5–2. Components of the status-oriented record.

DOCUMENTING CLIENT ASSESSMENT: THE DATA BASE

The ***data base*** is a compilation of information about the client obtained in the nursing assessment. Areas included in the data base would reflect all aspects of the client's health. Specific information included will vary with client and setting. For example, the data base in a pediatric clinic would not include the client's work history, while that in an occupational setting would. The community health nurse should be involved in the determination of what information will routinely be included in the data base used in a given practice setting.

There are several reasons for documenting the data base.[5] The first reason is the most obvious; the data base provides direction for nursing diagnosis and intervention. In addition, the data base improves communication between health-care providers and provides a baseline for later evaluation of the outcome of intervention. The data base constitutes part of the client's legal record and may be used to determine legal liability for unfavorable client outcomes. Finally, the data base may serve as a source of data for later research.

The compilation of the data base is not a one-time occurrence. Information contained there should be reviewed and updated as the client's situation changes. Typical components of the data base for the individual client include a health history, a physical examination, results of various laboratory and x-ray procedures, and findings of other screening tests. Data obtained about a community client would include information on the physical environment, age composition of the population, common illnesses, social factors such as unemployment and educational level, and so on.

The data base should be written objectively, without incorporating personal bias or value judgments. Interpretation of data should be supported by specific observations, and generalizations should be avoided. The data base should thoroughly describe the client situation and should include both positive and negative findings. Finally, the data base should be documented clearly and concisely without irrelevancies, should be legible, and should use correct grammar, spelling, and appropriate abbreviations.

DOCUMENTING NURSING DIAGNOSES: THE HEALTH STATUS SUMMARY

The ***health status summary*** is a list of abbreviated nursing diagnoses derived from the data base. The diagnoses are abbreviated in the sense that etiologic factors are not included here. Complete nursing diagnoses, including the statement of etiology, are documented elsewhere in the status-oriented record. Other information included in the health status summary is the date on which a particular diagnosis was established, its assigned number, and the date on which objectives related to the diagnosis were achieved. Table 5–1 depicts a sample health status summary.

According to the health status summary in Table 5–1, four nursing diagnoses were identified on January 9, 1990. Three of the diagnoses are problem-focused, while the fourth reflects a positive health state to be maintained. Each diagnosis was given a number and a title that describes the client condition. For example, the first diagnosis was "inadequate immunization status." Diagnoses should always be referred to by both number and title in subsequent entries in the SOR. Whenever possible, problem-focused diagnoses should be stated in the client's own words.

The status of conditions should be updated on the health status summary as appropriate. As objectives are met, their accomplishment should be noted on the summary sheet. In Table 5–1, diagnosis 1 was inadequate immunization status. At the first encounter with the client, the nurse may have made a referral to an immunization clinic. If the client followed through on the referral and obtained the needed immunizations, inadequate immunization status is no

TABLE 5–1. SAMPLE HEALTH STATUS SUMMARY

Date Identified	No.	Diagnosis	Date Objectives Achieved
1-9-90	1	Inadequate immunization status	2-13-90
1-9-90	2	Overweight	
1-9-90	3	Inadequate knowledge of nutrition	
1-9-90	4	Effective coping skills	

TABLE 5–2. REDEFINITION OF A NURSING DIAGNOSIS

Date Identified	No.	Diagnosis	Date Objectives Achieved
1-12-90	3	Amenorrhea—redefined as diagnosis 5	
1-12-90	4	Conflict with parents	
1-12-90	5	Unwanted pregnancy	

longer a problem for this client. This has been noted on the summary sheet by entering the date of problem resolution in the far right-hand column.

The status of a condition may also be updated through redefinition. For example, an original diagnosis of "amenorrhea" in an unmarried adolescent may be redefined as "unwanted pregnancy" following a positive pregnancy test. In this case, the diagnosis would be given a new number and title on the summary sheet and a notation made by the original diagnosis "redefined as diagnosis 5." This is depicted in Table 5–2.

Organization of the health status summary depends on the needs of the agency using the SOR. Diagnoses may be listed either chronologically in the order of identification or organized by categories. For instance, diagnoses might be categorized on the basis of the level of prevention involved. The diagnoses presented in Table 5–1 would then fall into two categories. The diagnoses related to immunization, inadequate knowledge of nutrition and coping skills reflect the primary level of prevention, while the diagnosis of overweight reflects a need for secondary prevention.

DOCUMENTING PLANNING: THE INITIAL PLAN

The third component of the SOR is an initial plan for each nursing diagnosis. Each of the diagnoses listed on the health status summary must be addressed, either through action by the community health nurse or through referral to another source of care. The particular agency where the nurse is employed may choose not to provide care for certain types of diagnoses. These diagnoses cannot be ignored, however, and some arrangement for providing care must be made. This is essential if the client is to be treated as a whole unit.

The ***initial plan of care*** for each diagnosis includes the broad goal and specific objectives to be achieved through intervention. The plan of care is then written in the *SOAP* format taken from the problem-oriented record system. The *S* includes subjective information or data reported by the client or significant others. For example, information from the health history related to a particular diagnosis is included in the S component of the initial plan for that diagnosis. The *O* refers to objective data observable by the community health nurse. Objective data might include findings on physical examination, results of laboratory tests, observations of the home or of client interactions with others, and so on.

A refers to the community health nurse's analysis of the situation and a statement of its probable etiology—in other words, the nursing diagnosis. For example, the problem might be a temperature elevation and would be stated in the health status summary as such. The analysis would also include the probable cause, if known, since this information will make a difference in the nursing interventions employed. An expected postsurgical temperature elevation, for example, will be treated differently from a fever due to an infectious process.

The *P* reflects the plan of action or nursing orders designed to address the diagnosis and includes four components: additional diagnostic measures, treatment measures, client education, and follow-up. Box 5–5 depicts a sample plan for the diagnosis of overweight. The goal for intervention is that the client will reach a normal weight for his or her height, while the objectives are stated more specifically, "The client will lose 2 pounds per week until goal is achieved" and "The client will be eating a well-balanced, nutritious diet by the end of 6 months."

The subjective data includes information that the client has shared with the nurse about his or her weight problem, typical diet, and knowledge of nutrition. The objective data is the client's height and weight, which indicate that the client is definitely overweight for his or her height. The analysis includes the nursing diagnostic statement that the client is "Overweight due to poor eating habits and inadequate knowledge of nutrition."

The inclusion of the etiology of the problem in the diagnostic statement provides direction for the intervention plan. If the client's overweight was due to a metabolic disorder, the plan of care would be

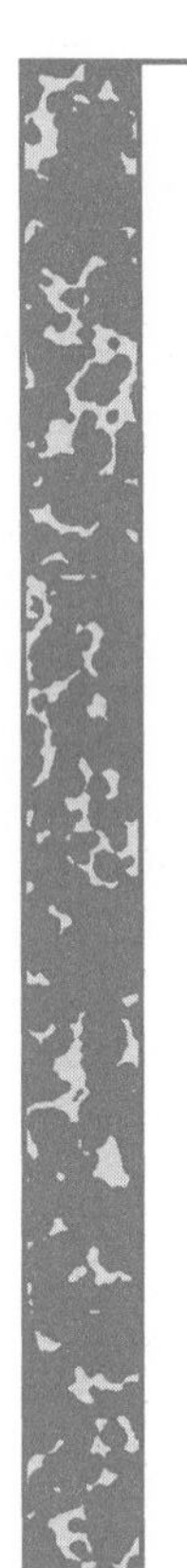

BOX 5–5

Sample Initial Plan for the Diagnosis of "Overweight"

1-9-90 Diagnosis 2: Overweight

Goal: The client will reach and maintain optimal weight for height

Objectives:
1. The client will lose 2 pounds per week until goal is achieved.
2. The client will be eating a well-balanced, nutritious diet by the end of 6 months.

S. States "I have always been fat. I just can't seem to lose weight." Description of typical day's diet indicates predominance of starches, fats, little protein or fiber. Knowledge of adequate nutrition limited.

O. Weight 263 lb. Height 5′6″

A. Overweight due to poor eating habits and inadequate knowledge of nutrition

P. Diagnostic:
1. Obtain a 3-day diet history
2. Obtain a list of food preferences

Treatment:
1. Refer to nutritionist for 1800-calorie diet
2. Assist client to plan low-calorie meals
3. Provide reinforcement of weight loss

Client education:
1. Review basic nutrition
2. Discuss hazards of obesity

Follow-up:
1. Recheck weight in 2 weeks
2. Obtain a second diet history in 2 weeks

quite different. In the situation depicted in Box 5–5, the plan of care is based on knowledge that the problem is related to dietary patterns and lack of knowledge about nutrition. Plans are made to obtain additional diagnostic information by having the client complete a 3-day diet history and provide information about food preferences. This allows the nurse to get a better understanding of the client's typical diet and to design interventions that are more likely to be acceptable to the client than might otherwise be the case.

The treatment component of the plan, in this case, involves referring the client to a nutritionist for an 1800-calorie diet and assisting the client to plan low-calorie meals that provide a balanced diet but are as consistent as possible with food preferences. Another aspect of the planned treatment is providing positive reinforcement for the client's progressive weight loss.

The plan for client education focuses on reviewing basic nutrition and discussing the hazards of obesity in terms of self-image as well as physical health. The last component of the *P* is the plan for follow-up. The nurse will recheck the client's weight in 2 weeks and obtain an updated diet history at that time.

DOCUMENTING INTERVENTIONS: PROGRESS NOTES

The last component of the SOR is the progress notes. ***Progress notes*** document the current status of health conditions, implementation of the plan, and the results of intervention. If for some reason the plan was not implemented, the reason for nonimplementation should also be documented. Progress notes are written in the SOAP format. Box 5–6 depicts a sample progress note for the diagnosis of overweight.

In the progress note in Box 5–6, subjective data obtained from the client indicates that the plan for dealing with this problem has been implemented, that she is adhering to the 1800-calorie diet, and that she has noticed some results. The nurse's observations included in the objective data also indicate that the client is eating appropriately and has lost weight. The analysis reflects the current status of the particular problem, the client is continuing to lose weight but has not yet achieved the goal of an appropriate weight for her height. At this point, the plan does not include any additional diagnostic interventions because none are needed. Nor is there a need for further educational measures. The plan now focuses

BOX 5–6

Sample Progress Notes for the Diagnosis of "Overweight"

7-11-90 Diagnosis 2: Overweight

S. States "I have gone down two whole dress sizes." Diet history indicates adherence to 1800-calorie diet. States she "uses calorie counter religiously."

O. Client visited at lunchtime. Found eating well-balanced, low-calorie meal. Weight 225 lb; 38-lb. weight loss in last 6 months; 2-lb weight loss in last week.

A. Continued weight loss

P. Diagnostic:

Treatment:
1. Praise client for continued weight loss.
2. Reinforce new self-image as "not fat."

Education:

Follow-up:
1. Return visit in 1 month to check weight.

on continuing positive reinforcement for weight lost and reinforcing a new self-image. The plan for follow-up is to check back with the client in 1 month.

Progress notes are always numbered and titled, as well as dated. Someone auditing this client's record would have no difficulty determining the status of diagnosis 2 as of July 1990. Progress notes, as well as plans, should be signed by the person making the entry.

DOCUMENTING EVALUATION

The SOR also facilitates documenting evaluation nursing care. Evaluation is documented in several of the components of the SOR discussed earlier. When objectives related to a specific nursing diagnosis have been achieved, their accomplishment is reflected in the progress notes as well as on the health status summary sheet. For example, if the overweight client has reached her desired weight, the objective data of the progress notes would include the client's current weight, and the analysis would reflect that the goal has been achieved and the problem resolved. The nurse would then indicate the date when objectives were achieved in the appropriate column on the health status summary. If the client continues to need support to maintain her weight at this level, the nurse might enter a new diagnosis on the health status summary, "maintenance of desired weight," and develop an initial plan for helping the client to maintain her weight. This diagnosis would reflect a need for tertiary preventive measures designed to prevent the recurrence of the weight problem.

Not every nursing diagnosis will be evaluated each time the client is seen. This is particularly true in the case of clients with multiple diagnoses. Therefore, progress notes for any particular client encounter may not include notations about each of the client's diagnoses. The nurse uses his or her judgment to establish priorities, dealing with the most crucial problems first and others as time permits. For example, if the client has made suicidal gestures and also needs new glasses, it is more important to evaluate the status of the emotional problem, if time does not permit exploration of both. The status of the vision problem can be explored at a later date. It is important, however, not to push these secondary problems aside indefinitely, since they need to be addressed and may be contributing factors in the major problems. Therefore, the current status of such secondary problems must be documented as often as appropriate.

When a client no longer requires services and is discharged from care, the progress notes should include a summary of the current status of all diagnoses listed on the health status summary sheet. This summary provides additional evidence of evaluation and that the client's problems are sufficiently resolved for services to be terminated.

CHAPTER HIGHLIGHTS

- Community health nurses use the nursing process with a wider variety of clients than do nurses in other specialty areas, caring for healthy and unhealthy individuals, families, groups, and communities.
- Use of the nursing process involves systematic steps of assessment, diagnosis, planning, implementation, and evaluation.
- The diagnostic phase of the nursing process involves data analysis and formulation of nursing diagnostic statements.
- Nursing diagnoses are statements describing health-related conditions in terms of the category of problem or strength involved, appropriate qualifying descriptors, and the etiologic factors contributing to the condition.
- Community health nurses formulate positive as well as problem-focused nursing diagnoses, reflecting their focus on health promotion and illness prevention.
- The planning stage of nursing process includes prioritizing needs for nursing intervention, developing goals and objectives, establishing criteria for selecting means to achieve goals, selecting appropriate means to goals, writing nursing orders, and planning for evaluation.
- Nursing orders describe specific actions to be taken by the nurse or others to achieve desired outcomes. Nursing orders address cognitive, affective, and psychomotor aspects of care.
- Tasks of the implementation stage of the nursing process include identifying knowledge and skills required, designating responsibility for implementation, recognizing and removing impediments to implementation, communicating the plan, providing an environment conducive to implementation, and carrying out the activities planned.
- Evaluation of nursing care may focus either on the outcomes of intervention or the processes used. Activities involved in evaluation include collecting evaluative data, comparing data with established evaluative criteria, and using findings to make decisions regarding care.
- All phases of the nursing process are documented. Documentation may be accomplished by means of the status-oriented record (SOR).
- Client assessment is documented in the data base of the SOR. The data base is updated as client circumstances change.
- Nursing diagnoses are documented in an abbreviated form in the health status summary. Complete diagnoses are included in the analysis component of the SOAP note delineating the initial plan of care.
- Care planning is documented in the initial plan of care for each nursing diagnosis included in the health status summary.
- Implementation is documented through progress notes written in the SOAP format.
- Evaluation of the effects of nursing intervention is documented in the progress notes of the SOR and on the health status summary sheet. When services are terminated, progress notes include a discharge summary that completes documentation of the evaluation of nursing care.

Review Questions

1. What are the components of the nursing process? Describe how the nursing process might be used somewhat differently in community health nursing than in other nursing specialties. (p. 80)
2. Describe two types of activities involved in developing nursing diagnoses. (p. 81)
3. What are the three components of a nursing diagnostic statement. Write a nursing diagnosis that incorporates these three components. (p. 82)
4. Describe at least four tasks involved in the planning stage of the nursing process. Give an example of a community health nurse performing each of these tasks. (p. 84)
5. Write a set of nursing orders for the following nursing diagnosis, "overweight due to inadequate knowledge of nutrition." Be sure to address all three aspects of nursing care in your orders. (p. 85)
6. Describe at least five tasks in implementing the plan of care. Give an example of the performance of each task. (p. 87)
7. Differentiate between process and outcome evaluation. Give examples of evaluative criteria that might be used for each. (p. 89)
8. Identify the components of a SOAP note. Write an initial plan in the SOAP format for the following nursing diagnosis, "inadequate access to health care due to financial difficulties." (p. 93)

APPLICATION AND SYNTHESIS

You receive the following request for community health nursing services:

Request for Community Health Nursing

Date: Jan. 22, 1991 Source of request: Clark Hospital

Family name: Marks

Address: 8359 Oaks Dr, Los Angeles Phone: 993-1256

Client(s): Miranda (birth date: 10-21-48)

Jason (birth date: 1-21-91)

Reason for referral: postpartum & newborn follow-up

Comments: Has two other children at home. Husband is unemployed. No prenatal care. Pregnancy, labor, and delivery uncomplicated.

When you visit the Marks family, you find that mother and baby are doing well. Mother has not yet made an appointment for a postpartum check-up because they have no health insurance, and she does not know how she will pay for the visit. Her husband is a nonunion construction worker. He has been laid off because construction is slow during the winter. He expects to be able to find work in 2 or 3 months, when the weather starts to warm up. Currently, the family is living off his unemployment compensation, which is just sufficient to pay the rent and buy food.

Mrs. Marks is concerned about her 3-year-old son who is fussy and irritable. He has had a fever for 2 days and has not been eating well. Last night he did not sleep well, and now you notice that he is pulling at his ear.

Mrs. Marks also mentions that she and her husband have been arguing about their financial situation. She would like to go back to work as a computer programmer. She feels that the family needs the money. If she were to go back to work for her former employer, the family could obtain health insurance at group rates, and her income would be more stable than her husband's. Her husband thinks that she should stay home and take care of the children.

During your visit, the 6-year-old daughter comes home from school. You note that she is somewhat overweight and looks anemic. In discussing the family's diet with Mrs. Marks, you find that they eat a lot of inexpensive starches, but eat few meats and vegetables because of the cost.

You also note that the baby seems clean, and when Mrs. Marks feeds him during your visit, she uses appropriate feeding and burping techniques. She appears to be knowledgeable about child care and discipline. Despite the fussiness of the 3-year-old, she is patient with him and succeeds in distracting him from pulling on the baby by letting him help hold the baby's bottle.

1. What diagnostic hypotheses are suggested by the data in this situation? Is there evidence of any positive nursing diagnoses in the data presented? How would you go about evaluating your hypotheses?
2. Write a health status summary including at least four nursing diagnoses appropriate to this situation. How would you prioritize your diagnoses? Why?
3. Write one objective for each of your nursing diagnoses. What alternative interventions might achieve these objectives? What criteria might you use to evaluate these alternatives?
4. Using the SOAP format, write an initial plan for addressing one of the nursing diagnoses. How would you evaluate the effectiveness of your interventions?

REFERENCES

1. Doenges, M., & Moorhouse, M. (1988). *Nurse's pocket guide: Nursing diagnosis with interventions* (2nd ed.). Philadelphia: F.A. Davis.
2. Doheny, M., Cook, C., & Stopper, C. (1987). *The discipline of nursing: An introduction* (2nd ed.). Norwalk, CT: Appleton-Century-Crofts.
3. Guzzetta, K. (1988). Nursing diagnosis. In J. M. Flynn & P. B. Heffron (Eds.), *Nursing: From concept to practice* (2nd ed.) (pp. 169–181). Norwalk, CT: Appleton & Lange.
4. Yura, H., & Walsh, M. B. (1988). *The nursing process: Assessing, planning, implementing, evaluating* (5th ed.). Norwalk, CT: Appleton & Lange.
5. Iyer, P. W., Taptich, B. J., & Bernocchi-Losey, D. (1986). *Nursing process and nursing diagnosis.* Philadelphia: W. B. Saunders.
6. Carpenito, L. J. (1989a). *Nursing diagnosis: Application to clinical practice* (3rd ed.). Philadelphia: J.B. Lippincott.
7. Carpenito, L. J. (1989b). *Handbook of nursing diagnosis, 1989–1990.* Philadelphia: J.B. Lippincott.
8. Carnevali, D. L. (1985). The diagnostic reasoning process. In D. L. Carnevali, P. H. Mitchell, N. F. Woods, & C. A. Tanner (Eds.), *Diagnostic reasoning in nursing.* Philadelphia: J.B. Lippincott.
9. Stolte, K. (1986). A complimentary view of nursing diagnosis. *Public Health Nursing, 3,* 23–28.
10. Lee, H. A., & Frenn, M. D. (1987). The use of nursing diagnoses for health promotion in community practice. *Nursing Clinics of North America, 22*(4), 981–986.
11. Simmons, D. A. (1986). Implementation of nursing diagnosis in a community health setting. In M. E. Hurley (Ed.), *Classification of nursing diagnosis: Proceedings of the sixth conference* (pp. 151–158). St. Louis: C.V. Mosby.
12. Archer, S. E., Kelly, C. D., & Bisch, S. A. (1984). *Implementing change in communities: A collaborative process.* St. Louis: C.V. Mosby.
13. Moorhouse, M. F., & Doenges, M. E. (1990). *Nurse's clinical pocket manual: Nursing diagnoses, care planning, and documentation.* Philadelphia: F.A. Davis.
14. LaMonica, E. L. (1979). *The nursing process: A humanistic approach.* Menlo Park, CA: Addison-Wesley.

RECOMMENDED READINGS

Carpenito, L. J. (1989). *Nursing diagnosis: Application to clinical practice* (3rd ed.). Philadelphia: J. B. Lippincott.

Describes nursing diagnosis and its relationship to the nursing process.

Iyer, P. W., Taptich, B. J., & Bernocchi-Losey, D. (1986). *Nursing process and nursing diagnosis.* Philadelphia: W.B. Saunders.

Examines the nursing process and its use in clinical nursing practice.

Lewis, T. (1988). Leaping the chasm between nursing theory and practice. *Journal of Advanced Nursing, 13,* 345–351.

Views the nursing care plan as the bridge between nursing theory and practice. Presents the experience of one unit in implementing the nursing process in the context of nursing theory.

Martin, K. S. (1982). Community health research in nursing diagnosis: The Omaha study. In M. J. Kim & D. A. Moritz (Eds.), *Classification of nursing diagnoses: Proceedings of the third and fourth national conferences* (pp. 167–175). New York: McGraw-Hill.

Inquires into the development of the Omaha system of nursing diagnosis for use in community health nursing. Also describes the categories of nursing diagnoses used.

NAACOG Committee on Practice. (1989). *Nursing Diagnosis.* Washington, DC: NAACOG.

Describes nursing diagnosis as the concept is used in obstetrical nursing. Includes arguments for the development of health promotion diagnoses as well as problem-focused diagnoses.

Peters, D. A. (1988). Development of a community health intensity rating scale. *Nursing Research, 37,* 202–206.

Describes the development of a tool to classify community health clients on the basis of nursing care requirements. Used in home health nursing.

Sienkiewicz, J. L. (1984). Patient classification in community health nursing. *Nursing Outlook, 32,* 319–321.

Describes a study using a patient classification scale based on Orem's self-care model as a basis for deriving nursing costs in a home health nursing agency.

Stolte, K. (1986). A complimentary view of nursing diagnosis. *Public Health Nursing, 3,* 23–28.

Presents the need for positive nursing diagnoses to reflect the health promotion emphasis of community health nursing.

Yura, H., & Walsh, M. B. (1988). *The nursing process: Assessing, planning, implementing, and evaluating* (5th ed.). Norwalk, CT: Appleton & Lange.

Introduces the concept of the nursing process and its components as applied to nursing practice.

CHAPTER 6

The Epidemiologic Process

KEY TERMS

active immunity
agent
carrier
case
causality
chronic carrier
convalescent carrier
cross-immunity
environment
epidemiologic prevention process model
epidemiologic process
epidemiology
exposure potential
health appraisal
health promotion
herd immunity
host
immunity
incidence
incubationary carrier
infectivity
intermediary
morbidity
mortality
natural history
passive immunity
pathogenicity
populations at risk
prevalence
rates of occurrence
relative risk ratio
reservoir
risk
susceptibility
target group
transient carrier
vectors
vehicle
virulence

Epidemiology is a health-related discipline that provides a systematic framework for examining states of health in terms of factors contributing to their development. The primary concern of epidemiology, like community health, is the health of groups of people. However, epidemiologic principles can also direct community health nurses in assessing health-related conditions experienced by both individuals and families. The nursing process indicates the need for client assessment, and the epidemiologic process suggests the type of data to be collected and how it can be organized to facilitate nursing intervention. In this chapter we will explore an epidemiologic perspective that can be used as a frame of reference in all aspects of community health nursing.

(*continued*)

LEARNING OBJECTIVES

After reading this chapter you should be able to:

- Describe at least two theories of disease causation.
- Identify at least three criteria for determining causality in a relationship between two events.
- Define risk.
- Distinguish between morbidity and mortality rates.
- Distinguish between incidence and prevalence.
- Identify six steps of the epidemiologic process.
- Identify the three major elements of the epidemiologic triad model.
- Describe the web of causation model.
- Describe the four major components of Dever's epidemiologic model.
- Identify the components of the epidemiologic prevention process model.
- Describe at least three strategies for promoting health.

BASIC CONCEPTS OF EPIDEMIOLOGY

Epidemiology is the study of the distribution of various states of health within the population and the environmental conditions, life-styles, or other circumstances associated with those states of health.[1] This definition encompasses two broad concepts: control of health problems through an understanding of their contributing factors, and application of epidemiologic techniques to health-related conditions other than acute communicable disease.

The purposes of epidemiology are twofold: to search for causal relationships in health and illness, and to control illness through the resultant understanding of causality. The ultimate concern of epidemiology in any of its uses is preventing disease and maintaining health. Specific uses of the epidemiologic process include:

1. Studying the contributing factors, signs and symptoms, effects, and outcomes of a single condition.
2. Diagnosing the health status of a specific group of people.
3. Evaluating the effectiveness of health programs.
4. Establishing indices of risk or the statistical probability of a particular condition occurring.

The study of factors contributing to communicable diseases was the initial focus of epidemiologic investigation. As the incidence of many communicable diseases declined, epidemiologists directed their attention to chronic disease as a focus of investigation. More recently still, epidemiologic methods have been used to identify factors that promote health.

Three basic concepts underly epidemiologic investigation of health and illness: causality, risk, and rates of occurrence. Each of these concepts finds direct application in community health nursing.

CAUSALITY

To control health problems, epidemiologists and community health nurses must have some idea of causality. The concept of ***causality*** is based on the idea that one event is the result of another event. Theories about the cause of disease have evolved over time.

THEORIES OF DISEASE CAUSATION

The first recognized attempt to attribute a cause to illness occurred during the "religious era," which extended from roughly 2000 B.C. through the age of the early Egyptian and Greek physicians to around 600 B.C. During this period, disease was thought to be caused directly by divine intervention, possibly as punishment for sins or as a trial of faith.[2]

Subsequent to the religious era, disease was often attributed to various physical forces, such as miasmas or mists. A rudimentary environmental theory of disease was developed by Hippocrates in his treatise "On Airs, Waters, and Places" about 400 B.C. The primary belief at that time was that disease was caused by harmful substances in the environment.

The bacteriologic era commenced in the late 1870s with the discovery of specific organisms as etiologic (causative) agents for specific diseases. One of the classic epidemiologic studies demonstrating the probability of some causative organism in communicable diseases was that of John Snow, who deduced that the cause of a cholera epidemic was contaminated water from a specific London well. Subsequently, actual bacteria were isolated and found to be the source of this and other infectious diseases. These discoveries gave rise to theories of a single cause for any specific disease.

Single-cause theories were further supported by the identification of other specific agents as causative elements for certain health problems. For example, lack of vitamin C was found to result in scurvy. The discovery of specific agents responsible for particular diseases did not, however, explain why one person

TABLE 6–1. HISTORICAL DEVELOPMENT OF THEORIES OF DISEASE CAUSATION

Era	Time Period	Theory of Causation Prevalent
Religious era	2000–600 B.C.	Disease caused by divine intervention, possibly as punishment for sins or test of faith
Environmental era	circa 400 B.C.	Disease caused by harmful miasmas, or mists, or other substances in the environment
Bacteriologic era	1870–1900	Disease caused by specific bacteriologic or nutritive agents
Era of multiple causation	1900 to present	Disease caused by interaction of multiple factors

exposed to an agent developed the disease, while another did not, so the evolution of disease theory entered the current era of multiple causation.

The hallmark of the era of multiple causation is the recognition of the interplay of a variety of factors in the development of health or illness. Epidemiology examines this interplay of factors with an eye toward control of a particular health condition. Prevention or control of any disease within population groups will depend on knowledge of these factors and determination of the point at which intervention will be most feasible and most effective.

The historical development of theories of disease causation is summarized in Table 6–1. It should be noted that, while the scientific community has accepted the idea of multiple causation, each of the preceding theories, which are presented in Table 6–1, continues to have support among members of the lay population.

CRITERIA FOR CAUSALITY

With the advent of single-cause–single-effect theories of disease causation, the scientific community began to look for specific causes for all health problems. Now, however, the concept of causality has become more complicated in view of the recognized interplay of a variety of factors in the development of illness. A factor may be considered causative if the health condition is more likely to occur in its presence and less likely to occur in its absence. Even when these conditions are met, however, a specific factor may not necessarily cause a particular condition. Five criteria are generally used in determining causality between associated events.[1] These criteria are the consistency and the strength of the association, its specificity, the temporal relationship between events, and coherence with other known facts.

Consistency

The first criterion for establishing a causal relationship is *consistency*. The association between the factor in question and the problem must be consistent. The condition in question must only occur when the factor is present, and not when it is absent. For example, people cannot develop measles without being exposed to measles virus. In addition, the association must always occur in the same direction. Exposure cannot result in disease in one instance, and disease result in exposure to the virus in another.

Strength of Association

The second criterion for establishing causality is the *strength of the association*. The greater the correlation between the occurrence of the factor and the health condition, the greater the possibility that the relationship is one of cause and effect. For example, not every susceptible person who is exposed to measles virus develops the disease, but most of them will. The association between exposure and disease, in this instance, is quite strong and supports the idea that the measles virus causes measles.

Specificity

Specificity is the third criterion for causality. Specificity is present when the factor in question results in one specific condition. For instance, exposure to measles virus only results in measles, not mumps, chicken pox, or any other communicable disease.

Temporal Relationship

The fourth criterion for establishing causation is the *time* (or temporal) *relationship* between the factor and the resulting condition. The factor thought to be causative should occur before the health condition appears. For example, one is always exposed to measles virus before one gets measles, not afterwards.

Coherence

Coherence with the established body of scientific knowledge is the last criterion for determining causality. The idea that one condition causes another must be logical and congruent with other known facts. For example, it is known that alcohol consumption increases reaction time for voluntary muscle movements. Therefore, it is reasonable to consider alcohol consumption as a causative factor in many accidents because this interpretation is consistent with the idea of slowed reaction time.

TABLE 6–2. CRITERIA FOR DETERMINING CAUSALITY

Criterion	Description of Criterion
Consistency	The association between the supposed cause and its effect is consistent and always occurs in the same direction
Strength of association	The greater the correlation between supposed cause and effect, the greater the possibility the relationship is a causal one
Specificity	The supposed cause always creates the same effect
Temporal relationship	The supposed cause always occurs before the effect
Coherence	The supposition of one event causing another must be coherent with other existing knowledge

All of the criteria for causality must be met for a particular factor to be considered causative for a specific health problem. Criteria for determining causality are summarized in Table 6–2.

RISK

In addition to establishing the causes of health-related conditions, epidemiologists are interested in estimating the likelihood that a particular condition will occur. ***Risk*** is the probability that a given individual will develop a specific condition. One's risk of developing a particular condition is affected by a variety of physical and emotional factors, environmental factors, life-style factors, and so on. When epidemiologists speak of ***populations at risk,*** they are referring to groups of people who have the greatest potential for developing a particular health problem because of the presence or absence of certain contributing factors.

The basis for risk may lie in one's susceptibility to a condition or potential for exposure to causative factors. ***Susceptibility*** is one's ability to be affected by factors contributing to a particular health condition. For example, very young unimmunized children are susceptible to, and comprise the population at risk for, pertussis (whooping cough). In this case, the basis for increased risk lies in the increased susceptibility of this group. Persons over the age of 10 and children who have been immunized against pertussis are unlikely to develop the disease and so are not part of the population at risk. Another example of risk based on susceptibility is found in the population of sexually active women of child-bearing age who are at risk for pregnancy. Men, children, and older women are not susceptible to pregnancy and, therefore, are not considered part of the population at risk.

Exposure potential is another factor in one's risk of developing a particular condition. ***Exposure potential*** is the likelihood that one will be exposed to factors that contribute to the condition. For example, those most at risk for sexually transmitted diseases are adolescents and young adults. In this instance, the basis of risk is not increased susceptibility, as in the case of pertussis, but an increased potential for exposure due to more frequent and less selective sexual activity. Another population at risk through increased chance of exposure includes individuals whose occupation brings them in contact with toxic substances.

Members of a population at risk have a greater probability of developing a specific condition than those persons who are not affected by factors known to contribute to the condition. This difference in the probability of developing a given condition is known as the ***relative risk ratio.***[1] This ratio is derived by comparing the frequency of occurrence of the condition in a group of people with known risk factors to that among individuals without these factors. For example, if 50 percent of smokers develop heart disease versus only 5 percent of nonsmokers, smokers have a risk of heart disease 10 times greater than their nonsmoking counterparts. The relative risk ratio is useful in identifying those areas where preventive interventions will have the greatest impact on the occurrence of disease.

The population at risk becomes the target group for any intervention designed to prevent or control the problem in question. The ***target group*** is comprised of those individuals who would benefit from an intervention program and at whom the program is aimed. Using one of the previous examples, the target group for an immunization campaign against pertussis would include unimmunized children under the age of 10.

RATES OF OCCURRENCE

The rate of occurrence of a health-related condition is also of concern to community health nurses. ***Rates of occurrence*** are statistical measures that indicate the extent of health problems in a group. Rates of occur-

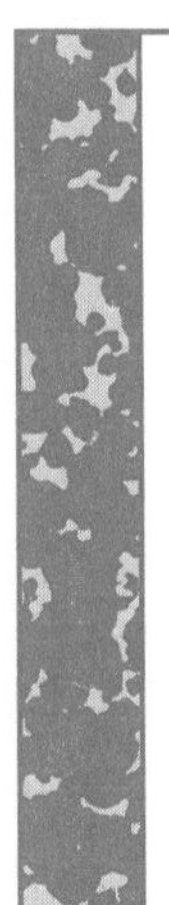

BOX 6–1

Basic Formula for Calculating Statistical Rates

$$\text{Rate} = \frac{\text{Number of events over a period time}}{\text{Population at risk at that time}} \times 1000 \text{ (or 100,000)}$$

Example: In a community with a population of 10,000 females aged 13 to 18 years, there were 200 teenage pregnancies in 1991.

$$\text{Rate of teenage pregnancy} = \frac{\text{200 pregnancies in females 13–18 during 1991}}{\text{10,000 females aged 13–18 in the population at midyear}} \times 1000$$

$$= \text{20 pregnancies per 1000 females}$$

rence also allow comparisons between groups of different sizes with respect to the extent of a particular condition. For example, a community with a population of 1000 may report 50 cases of syphilis this year, while another community of 100,000 persons may report 5000 cases. On the surface, it would seem that the second community has a greater problem with syphilis than the first. However, both communities have experienced 50 cases per 1000 population. In other words, both have a problem with syphilis of a comparable magnitude.

Computing the statistical rates of interest in community health nursing involves dividing the *number of instances of an event* during a specified period of time (for example, the number of teenage pregnancies that occurred last year) by the *population at risk* for that event (the number of adolescent girls in the community) and *multiplying by 1000* (or 100,000 if the numbers of the event are so small that the result of the calculation using a multiplier of 1000 would be less than 1). This calculation is represented by the formula in Box 6–1.

Both morbidity and mortality rates are of concern in community health nursing. ***Mortality*** is the ratio of the number of deaths in various categories to a given population, whereas ***morbidity*** is the ratio of the number of cases of a disease or condition to a given population. Mortality rates describe deaths; morbidity rates describe cases of disease that may or may not result in death. For example, the number of people in a particular group who die as a result of cardiovascular disease is reflected in the mortality rate. However, the number of people experiencing cardiovascular disease is indicated by morbidity rates.

MORTALITY RATES

Mortality rates that are of interest in community health nursing include the overall or "crude" death rate, cause-specific death rates, infant and neonatal mortality rates, fetal and perinatal mortality rates, and maternal death rate. Formulae for calculating each of these mortality rates are provided in Box 6–2. Each rate is calculated from the number of events during a specified time period and the average population at risk during that same period.

Rates are reported in terms of the multiplicative factor used to calculate them. For example, cancer deaths occur in fairly large numbers, so a cause-specific death rate for cancer would be calculated using 1000 as the multiplier. If community A, with a population of 50,000, had 100 cancer-related deaths, the cause-specific death rate for cancer would be reported as 2 deaths per 1000 population. Deaths from pancreatic cancer, on the other hand, occur relatively infrequently, so 100,000 would be the multiplier used to calculate the pancreatic cancer death rate. For instance, if there were 6 deaths from pancreatic cancer in Community B last year, and Community B has a population of 500,000 people, the annual pancreatic cancer mortality rate would be reported as 1.2 deaths per 100,000 population. Calculation of these rates is shown in Box 6–3.

Age-adjusted mortality rates can be calculated to account for differences in age distribution between groups. This allows one to make more accurate comparisons of mortality between groups with widely different age distributions. For example, Community A might have a considerably higher crude death rate for influenza than Community B. However, if Community A also has a higher proportion of elderly persons in the population, more influenza deaths would be expected, because older people are more vulnerable to this condition. Age-adjusted mortality rates for influenza, on the other hand, allow the community health nurse to compare the effects of influenza on Community A and Community B as if they had sim-

BOX 6–2

Formulae for Calculating Selected Mortality Rates

$$\text{Crude death rate} = \frac{\text{Total number of deaths during year}}{\text{Total population at midyear}} \times 1000$$

$$\text{Cause-specific annual death rate} = \frac{\text{Number of deaths from specific cause during year}}{\text{Total population at midyear}} \times 1000$$

$$\text{Annual infant mortality rate} = \frac{\text{Number of deaths during year (birth to 1 year of age)}}{\text{Number of live births during year}} \times 1000$$

$$\text{Annual neonatal mortality rate} = \frac{\text{Number of deaths during year (birth to 28 days of age)}}{\text{Number of live births during year}} \times 1000$$

$$\text{Annual fetal death rate} = \frac{\text{Number of fetal deaths during year (20 to 28 weeks' gestation)}}{\text{Number of live births plus fetal deaths during year}} \times 1000$$

$$\text{Annual perinatal death rate} = \frac{\text{Number of perinatal deaths during year (20 weeks' gestation to 1 week of age)}}{\text{Number of live births plus fetal deaths during year}} \times 1000$$

$$\text{Annual maternal death rate} = \frac{\text{Number of maternal deaths during year}}{\text{Number of live births during year}} \times 100{,}000$$

BOX 6–3

Sample Mortality Rate Calculations Using Multipliers of 1000 and 100,000

Community A

$$\text{Cancer mortality rate} = \frac{\text{100 deaths due to cancer, 1991}}{\text{50,000 population at midyear}} \times 1000$$

$$= \text{2 cancer deaths per 1000 population}$$

Community B

$$\text{Pancreatic cancer mortality rate} = \frac{\text{6 deaths from pancreatic cancer, 1991}}{\text{500,000 population at midyear}} \times 100{,}000$$

$$= \text{1.2 deaths due to pancreatic cancer per 100,000 population}$$

ilar proportions of elderly in the population. If Community A's influenza death rate remains higher when adjusted for age, the nurse would look for other factors in the community to explain this difference.

MORBIDITY RATES

Morbidity rates reflect the number of cases of particular health conditions in a group or community. Morbidity is described in terms of incidence or prevalence rates. ***Incidence*** rates are calculated on the basis of the number of *new* cases of a particular condition identified during a specified time period. ***Prevalence*** is *the total number* of people affected by a particular condition at a specified point in time.

To illustrate the concepts of incidence and prevalence, consider a town with a population of 30,000 in which 15 new cases of hypertension were diagnosed in June. This is an indication of the incidence of hypertension. People who were diagnosed as hypertensive prior to June and who still live in the town still have hypertension. These additional cases of hypertension, however, are not reflected in the hypertension incidence rate for June, but are included in the prevalence, the total number of people in the community affected by hypertension. Formulae for calculating annual incidence and prevalence rates are presented in Box 6–4. Again, the results of the calculations are reported in terms of the rate per 1000 population.

Other rates that may be of interest to community health nurses include marriage and divorce rates, illegitimacy rates, employment rates, utilization rates for health-care services and facilities, and rates for alcohol and drug use and abuse.

Community health nurses use morbidity and mortality data in assessing the health status of a community. Community morbidity and mortality rates that are generally high or higher than state or national rates indicate health problems that require nursing intervention. For example, the nurse may note that local morbidity rates for childhood illnesses such as measles and rubella are twice those of the rest of the state. These differences indicate that there is a significant portion of the local child population that is unimmunized. The nurse then uses these data to begin an investigation of the factors involved in the problem and to plan for a solution. Is it a matter of inaccessibility of immunization services, lack of education on the need for immunization, or poor surveillance of immunization levels in the schools? The solution to the problem must be geared to the cause. Statistical data merely serve to indicate the presence of a problem; they do not delineate its specific nature.

Low morbidity and mortality rates do not indicate the absence of health problems in the community, as biostatistics are only one indicator of the health status of a locality. Many health problems are not reported statistically and their presence in the community will not be reflected in morbidity and mortality rates. The nutritional status of the population is one example of an area not addressed by biostatistics such as morbidity and mortality rates. Other indicators that the community health nurse employs in assessing a community's health status will be discussed in Chapter 19, Care of the Community or Target Group.

THE EPIDEMIOLOGIC PROCESS

Epidemiologists use a systematic process to study states of health and illness in an effort to control disease and promote health. The steps of this ***epidemiologic process*** include defining the condition for study, determining the natural history of the condition, identifying strategic points of control, and designing, implementing, and evaluating control strategies. These steps are listed in Box 6–5. Determining the natural history of the condition is analogous to the assessment and diagnosis phases of the nursing process. Identifying strategic points of control and designing control programs reflect the planning aspects

BOX 6–4

Formulae for Calculating Annual Incidence and Prevalence Rates

$$\text{Annual incidence rate} = \frac{\text{Number of new cases of a condition last year}}{\text{Total population at risk at midyear}} \times 1000$$

$$\text{Annual prevalence rate} = \frac{\text{Total number of cases of a condition last year}}{\text{Total population at risk at midyear}} \times 1000$$

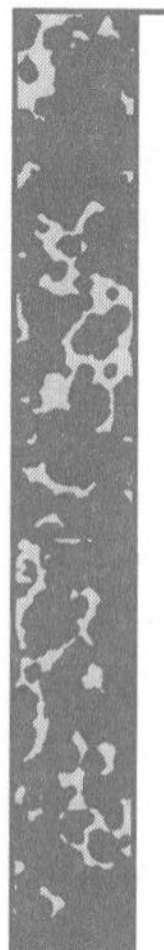

BOX 6–5

Steps in the Epidemiologic Process

- Defining the condition
- Determining the natural history of the condition
- Identifying strategic points of control
- Designing control strategies
- Implementing control strategies
- Evaluating control strategies

of the nursing process, while the implementation and evaluation steps are equivalent to similar steps in the nursing process.

DEFINING THE CONDITION

The first step in the epidemiologic process is defining the health condition requiring intervention. As we will see later, the epidemiologic process can be applied to conditions of health as well as illness. In either case, it is necessary to define the state or condition for which intervention is required. Taking a health promotion focus, one needs to define health. With respect to a specific disease or health problem, one must clearly define what is and is not an instance of the problem. For example, to study the factors contributing to suicide, one must be able to differentiate suicide from accidental death. Similarly, one must be able to differentiate cases of measles from cases of rubella so as to study and control either of these diseases.

DETERMINING THE NATURAL HISTORY OF THE CONDITION

The ***natural history*** of a disease or condition is a description of the events that precede its development and occur during its course, as well as a description of its outcomes. Determining the condition's natural history involves identifying factors that contribute to its development, its signs and symptoms, its effects on the human system, and its typical outcomes and factors that may affect those outcomes. For example, crowded living conditions, lack of immunization, and exposure to influenza virus are some of the factors involved in the development of influenza. The typical course of influenza includes a short incubation period and the rapid onset of respiratory and/or gastrointestinal symptoms. Most cases of influenza resolve after several days, but the eventual outcome depends on such factors as the individual's overall health, age, nutritional status, personal habits such as smoking, and so on. All of these bits of information are part of the natural history of influenza.

The description of the natural history also incorporates information on the frequency of occurrence, severity of outcomes, and geographic distribution of the condition. Information is also obtained on time relationships and trends related to the condition. Time relationships refer to the occurrence of the condition at specific times or during particular seasons. For example, influenza occurs primarily in the winter, and the incidence of suicide rises around holidays. Trends refer to patterns of occurrence for the condition. Incidence of hepatitis A, for example, is declining, while patterns of occurrence for family violence indicate increasing incidence.

The natural history of a condition is usually divided into four stages. The first of these is the *pre-exposure stage* when factors contributing to the development of the condition are present. When exposure to causative factors has occurred, but no symptoms have appeared, the condition is in the *preclinical stage.* The third stage is the *clinical stage,* which begins with the onset of signs and symptoms characteristic of the disease or condition. The final stage is the *resolution stage,* in which the condition culminates in a return to health, death, or continuation in a chronic state. These stages are depicted in Figure 6–1.

Determining the factors involved in the natural history of a condition is usually undertaken using a specific epidemiologic model. Three such models will be discussed later in this chapter.

IDENTIFYING STRATEGIC POINTS OF CONTROL

Knowledge of the natural history of a disease or condition allows epidemiologists to identify strategic points of control. One might, for example, design interventions to eliminate or modify factors contributing to a condition to prevent its occurrence. Similarly, knowledge of factors affecting a condition's course may lead to interventions designed to minimize its effects.

Strategic points of control may involve interventions at the primary, secondary, or tertiary levels of prevention. Primary prevention takes place before the problem occurs, during the pre-exposure and preclinical stages of its natural history. Secondary pre-

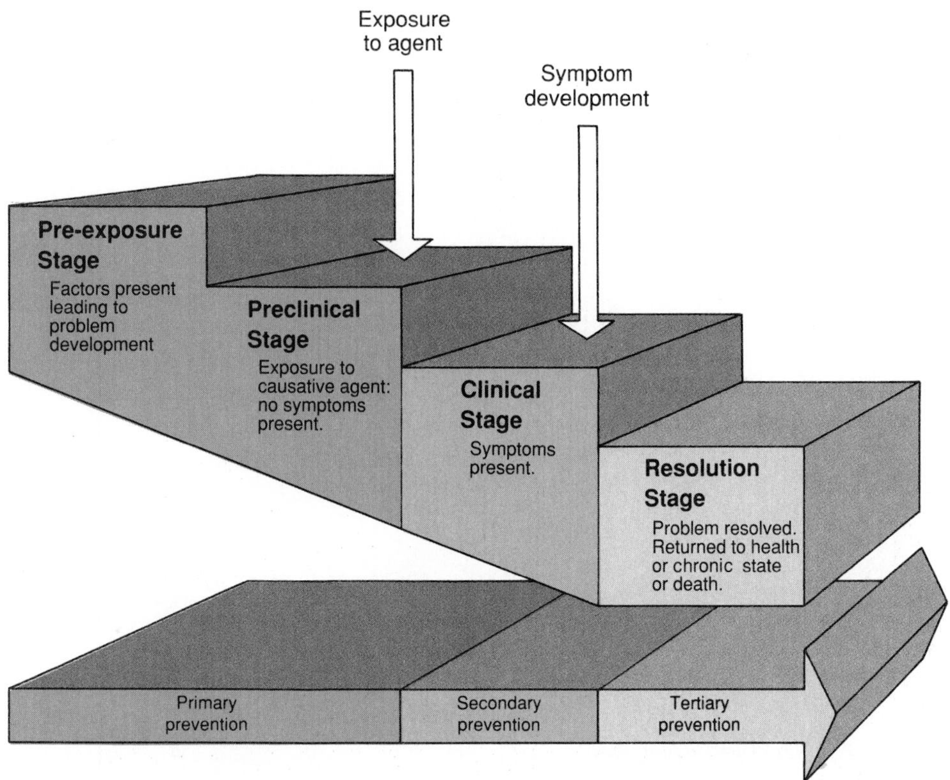

Figure 6–1. Stages of the natural history of a condition and their relationship to primary, secondary, and tertiary levels of prevention.

vention occurs once the problem appears, during the clinical stage, while tertiary prevention may be required during the resolution stage either to prevent lasting effects or prevent a recurrence of the problem. Figure 6–1 depicts the relationship of levels of prevention to the stages of the natural history of a health-related condition.

DESIGNING, IMPLEMENTING, AND EVALUATING CONTROL STRATEGIES

Once strategic points of control for a specific condition have been identified, health-care programs can be designed to prevent it or minimize its effects on the health of the population. Programs are then implemented and evaluated in terms of their effects on the occurrence of the particular condition. These steps of the epidemiologic process parallel similar components of the nursing process and will be discussed in relation to health-care programming in Chapter 19, Care of the Community or Target Group.

EPIDEMIOLOGIC MODELS

Both nurses and epidemiologists use the epidemiologic process to direct interventions to control health-related conditions. Determining the natural history of a health condition and identifying control strategies involve collecting large amounts of data about multiple factors that may be contributing to the condition. For this reason it is helpful to have a model or framework to direct the collection and interpretation of these data. We will explore three such models: the epidemiologic triad, the web of causation model, and Dever's epidemiologic model.

THE EPIDEMIOLOGIC TRIAD

Traditionally, epidemiologic investigation has been guided by the epidemiologic triad. In this model, data are collected with respect to a triad of elements: host, agent, and environment. The interrelationship of these elements results in a state of relative health or illness.[3] The relationship of host, agent, and environment and specific considerations under each are depicted in Figure 6–2.

HOST

The ***host*** is the client system affected by the particular condition under investigation. Community health nursing is concerned with the health of human beings, so, for our purposes, mankind is the host. A

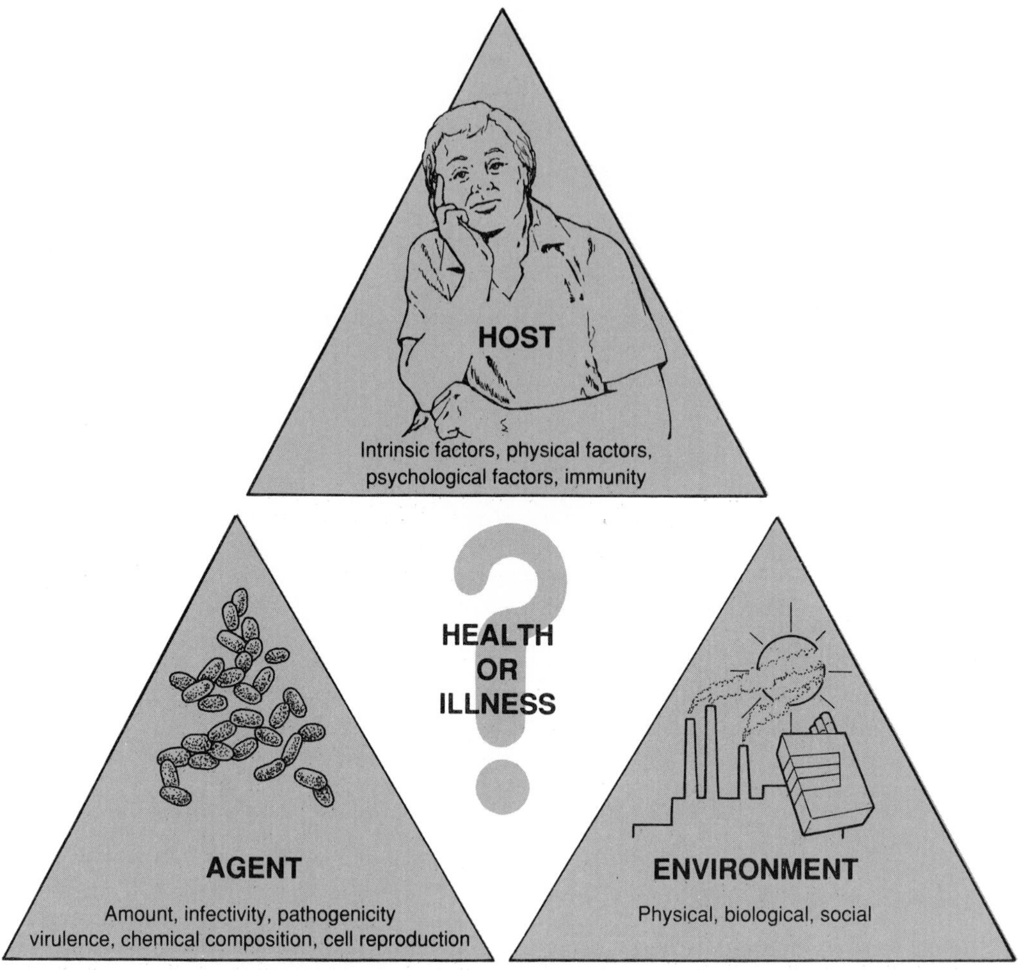

Figure 6–2. Elements of the epidemiologic triad model.

variety of factors can influence the host's exposure, susceptibility, and response to an agent. Host-related factors include intrinsic factors (for example, age, race, and sex), physical and psychological factors, and the presence or absence of immunity. These factors will be addressed in more detail in the discussion of Dever's epidemiologic model.

AGENT

The ***agent*** is the primary cause of a health-related condition. The causes of some health problems may be so complex that no single agent can be identified. The concept of agent, however, remains useful for exploring many health problems.

Agents can be classified into five basic types: physical agents, chemical agents, nutritive elements, infectious agents, and psychological agents. Physical agents include such things as heat, trauma, and genetic mutation. Genetically determined diseases, for instance, are the result of physical changes in gene structure, whereas heat is an agent in such conditions as burns and heat exhaustion. Chemical agents include various substances to which people may develop untoward reactions. Some plants such as poison ivy or ragweed can be considered chemical agents since they cause a chemical reaction resulting in an allergic response.

An absence or an excess of a variety of nutritive elements is known to result in disease, as does the presence of and exposure to a number of infectious agents that cause communicable diseases. Finally, psychological agents such as stress can produce a variety of stress-related conditions. The types of agents and examples of health conditions to which they contribute are presented in Table 6–3.

An agent's characteristics influence whether a given individual develops a particular health-related condition. These characteristics vary somewhat depending upon the type of agent involved.

TABLE 6–3. AGENTS AND SELECTED HEALTH PROBLEMS TO WHICH THEY CONTRIBUTE

Type of Agent	Example	Problems
Physical	Heat	Burns, heat stroke
	Trauma	Fractures, concussion, sprains, contusions
	Genetic change	Down syndrome, Turner's syndrome, etc.
Chemical	Medications	Accidental poisoning, suicide
	Chlorine	Poisoning, asphyxiation (in gas form)
	Poison ivy	Rash and pruritus
Nutritive	Vitamin C	Scurvy (in absence of vitamin C)
	Iron	Anemia (in absence of iron)
	Vitamin A	Poisoning (in excess)
Infectious	Measles virus	Measles, encephalitis
	HIV	AIDS
	Varicella virus	Chickenpox
	Influenza virus	Influenza
Psychological	Stress	Ulcerative colitis, heart disease, suicide, asthma, alcoholism, drug abuse, violence

Characteristics of Infectious Agents

Characteristics that influence the effects of infectious agents include the extent of one's exposure to the agent and the agent's infectivity, pathogenicity, and virulence. Additional characteristics of infectious agents include chemical composition and structure and cell reproduction. The *extent of exposure* to a disease-causing microorganism or the "infective dose" will affect the outcome of the exposure. For instance, the person exposed to a few mycobacteria tuberculosis is unlikely to develop tuberculosis (TB). The greater the number of these microorganisms inspired, however, the greater the likelihood of developing TB.

Infectivity is the ability of an agent to invade the host system. Measles virus, for example, has a higher infectivity than does tetanus bacillus. The measles virus enters the body quite easily through the respiratory system, whereas tetanus gains entry through a break in the skin, usually a deep puncture wound. ***Pathogenicity*** is the ability of the agent to cause disease. In terms of infectious agents, measles virus will cause disease in most susceptible infected individuals. *Mycobacterium tuberculosis,* on the other hand, produces disease in only a small portion of individuals infected. Therefore, the measles virus has a higher pathogenicity than *M. tuberculosis.*

Virulence is a term used to describe the severity of the health problem caused by the agent. Roseola has a low virulence since uncomplicated measles is not a serious illness. Tetanus, on the other hand, is extremely virulent because it results in fatality unless treatment is instituted. The virus that causes AIDS is another infectious agent with a very high virulence. Virulence is frequently confused with pathogenicity, but the two terms refer to different agent characteristics. For example cold viruses that cause disease in infected individuals are highly pathogenic, but have a low virulence because the diseases caused are relatively minor.

The *chemical composition and structure* of a microorganism can also influence the effects of an infectious agent on a host. It is the composition of bacterial cell walls, for instance, that makes penicillin and similar antibiotics effective against several microorganisms. Similarly, the composition of many viruses makes it necessary for them to attach to specific protein structures in human cells in order to gain entry.

Another important factor that influences the effect of an infectious agent is its *reproductive cycle.* The rate at which an infectious agent reproduces can influence the body's ability to kill invading organisms before they are able to overwhelm bodily defense mechanisms. Organisms' reproductive cycles can also affect their ability to cause disease or prompt interventions to control them, both of which affect the natural history of disease. It was knowledge that the reproductive cycle of the *Plasmodium* occurs in the Anopheles mosquito, for instance, that prompted efforts to control malaria by eradicating this mosquito. These and other factors influencing infectious agents will be addressed in more detail in Chapter 31, Communicable Disease.

Characteristics of Noninfectious Agents

Noninfectious agents share some of the characteristics of infectious agents. For example, the extent of exposure to the agent affects its ability to cause health problems. Ingesting moderate amounts of alcohol or aspirin, for instance, does not cause problems, while excessive consumption does. The amount of stress to which one is exposed can also affect the development of stress-related illness.

The concept of infectivity can also be applied to other types of agents, although the term was developed in relation to communicable diseases. For example, asbestos, which can be inhaled, has a higher "infectivity" than an overdose of aspirin, which must be ingested. Stress, as an agent of illness, also has a high infectivity since it is an everyday factor impinging on people. All of us are "infected" by stress.

Stress can also be viewed in terms of its ability to cause disease. Although everyone experiences some degree of stress, not all people develop stress-related illnesses. Stress, therefore, has a relatively low pathogenicity. Noninfectious agents may vary in terms of their virulence as well. Stress can produce a mild stomach upset in some individuals and drive others to suicide. In the first instance, stress has a low virulence, while it has a high virulence in the second.

Chemical composition is a relevant factor for many noninfectious agents. For example, it is the chemical composition of a poisonous substance that produces chemical reactions in the human body that result in poisoning. Similarly, it is the chemical composition of poison ivy that causes a pruritic rash.

ENVIRONMENT

The third element of the epidemiologic triad includes factors in the physical, biological, and social ***environment*** that contribute to health-related conditions. The physical environment consists of such factors as weather, terrain, buildings, and so on. A variety of physical environmental factors can influence health. For example, air pollution contributes to respiratory disease as well as other physiologic and psychologic effects in human beings. Similarly, the temperature and humidity of tropical areas is associated with increased incidence of hyperthyroidism.

The biological environment, in the triad model, consists of all living organisms, other than man. Components of the biological environment include plants and animals as well as microorganisms, all of which can influence health.

The social environment includes factors related to social interaction that may contribute to health or disease. For example, cultural factors, which are part of the social environment, can influence health behaviors. In a similar fashion, social norms may influence health and illness. For example, societal views of alcoholism and drug abuse as character weaknesses have hampered efforts to control these problems.

THE WEB OF CAUSATION MODEL

The "web of causation" is a second model for understanding the influence of multiple factors on the development of a specific health condition. In this model, factors are explored in terms of an intricate interplay of factors, in which both direct and indirect causes of the problem are identified.[4] The web of causation approach allows the epidemiologist to map out the interrelationships among factors contributing to the development (or prevention) of a particular health condition. This approach also assists in determining areas where efforts at control will be most effective.

The web of causation for the problem of adolescent pregnancy is depicted in Figure 6–3. It is obvious from the complexity of Figure 6–3 that multiple factors contribute to adolescent pregnancy. The interplay of these factors determines whether or not the problem occurs. The most direct causes are those linked directly to the pregnancy outcome: sexual activity and inconsistent or no use of contraceptives. Numerous other factors, however, contribute to the adolescent's decision to engage in sexual activity without effective contraception.

Factors influencing sexual activity and contraceptive use include motivation, perceptions regarding sexuality, knowledge, and factors related to contraceptive services. The motivation to engage in sexual activity without adequate contraception, and even intentionally to become pregnant, may derive from still other factors. The teen may be motivated by a desire to get away, by a desire to love and be loved (either by the partner or by a child), by peer pressure, or by low personal aspirations. Desires to get away and for someone to love may be influenced by a poor home situation and a poor self-concept, both of which have their roots in family interaction patterns and other factors depicted in Figure 6–3.

Perceptions regarding sexuality in general are the result of perceptions about sexual activity, perceptions of pregnancy and parenthood, and perceptions of contraception and abortion. Sexual activity may be seen as a way to interact with others (particularly for the teen with a poor self-concept), a means of demonstrating "adulthood," or as what one does to be popular. Similarly, the teen may have unrealistic perceptions of pregnancy and parenthood, expecting both to be rewarding experiences devoid of frustration or problems. The adolescent may also perceive contraceptives as dangerous, a nuisance, or as evidence of immorality. Or, the adolescent may see abortion as an easy way out if pregnancy does occur.

These perceptions arise out of a number of other factors and are influenced by peer communication, family exposure to pregnancy and parenting roles, and media messages. These factors, in turn, are influenced by community attitudes to adolescent sexual activity, which will also affect factors influencing the teenager's knowledge.

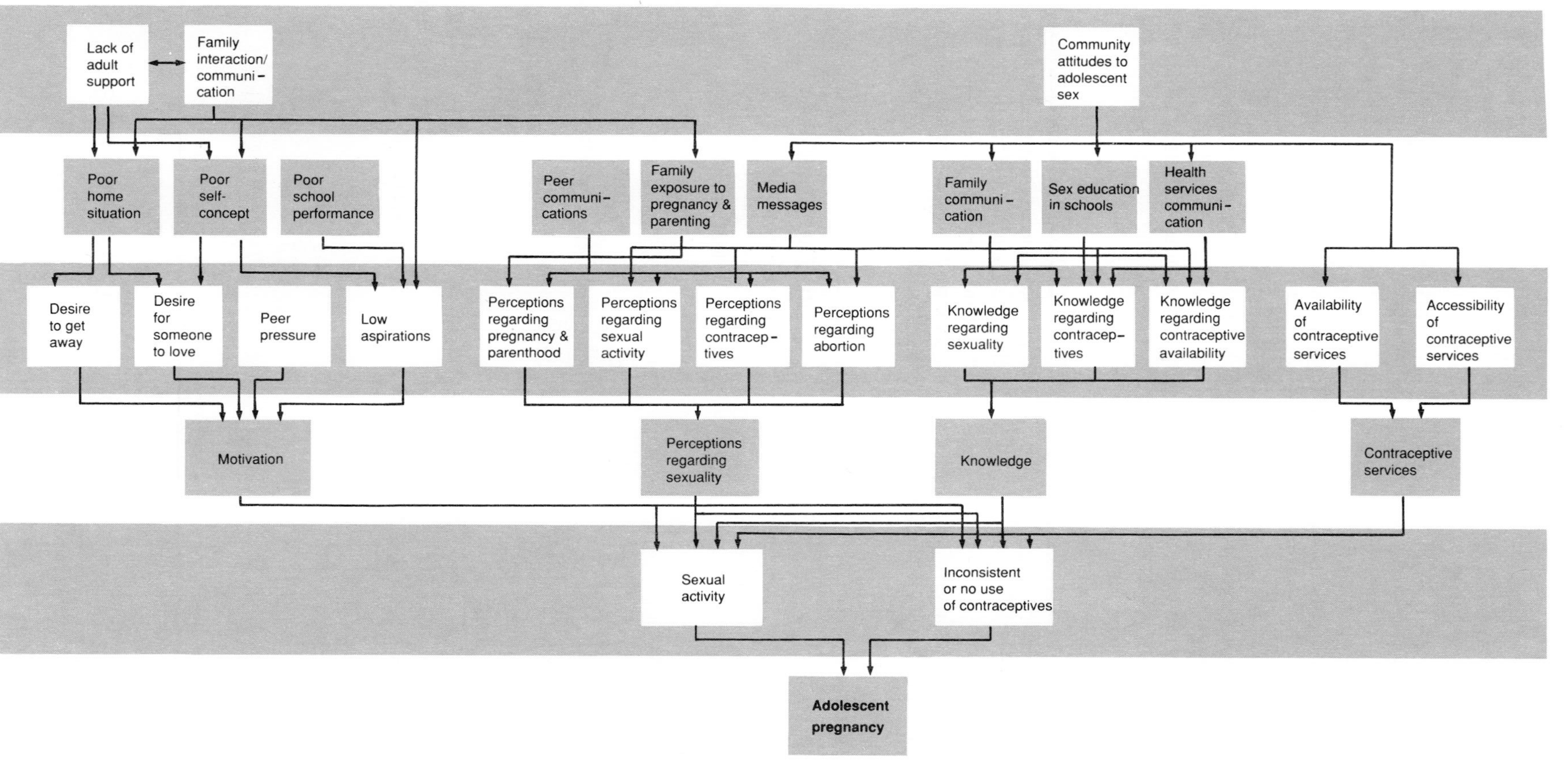

Figure 6–3. The "web of causation" for adolescent pregnancy indicating the interplay between multiple direct and indirect causative factors.

Knowledge factors influencing sexual activity and contraceptive use include information about sexuality and its consequences, knowledge regarding contraceptive methods, and knowledge of contraceptive availability and accessibility. All of these are influenced by family communication, health services communications, and the extent and openness of sex education at home and in the schools. These, in turn, are influenced by community attitudes to sexuality and to adolescent sexual activity. Community attitudes also influence the availability and accessibility of contraceptive services for adolescents, the last major factor in decisions to engage in unprotected sexual activity. For example, a community that perceives provision of contraceptive services to teens as condoning sexual activity will resist such services. When this occurs, contraceptives may not be available even to those teens who would use them.

DEVER'S EPIDEMIOLOGIC MODEL

Dever's epidemiologic model provides a third approach to conceptualizing the interplay of factors involved in the development of a particular condition. The model was developed as an approach to formulating health-care policy for the State of Georgia and was used to determine health-care priorities and to design programs to address those priorities. G. Alan Dever was a health-policy analyst with the Georgia State Department of Health at the time of the model's development. The model itself consists of four basic elements—human biology, environment, life-style, and the health-care system.[5] The elements of Dever's model and specific considerations related to each are depicted in Figure 6–4. As we shall see, several general epidemiologic concepts such as immunity, reservoirs, carriers, and so on have been incorporated into the model.

HUMAN BIOLOGICAL FACTORS

Human biological factors in Dever's model are similar to the host-related factors of the epidemiologic triad and include genetic inheritance, the functioning of complex physiologic systems, and factors related to maturation and aging.

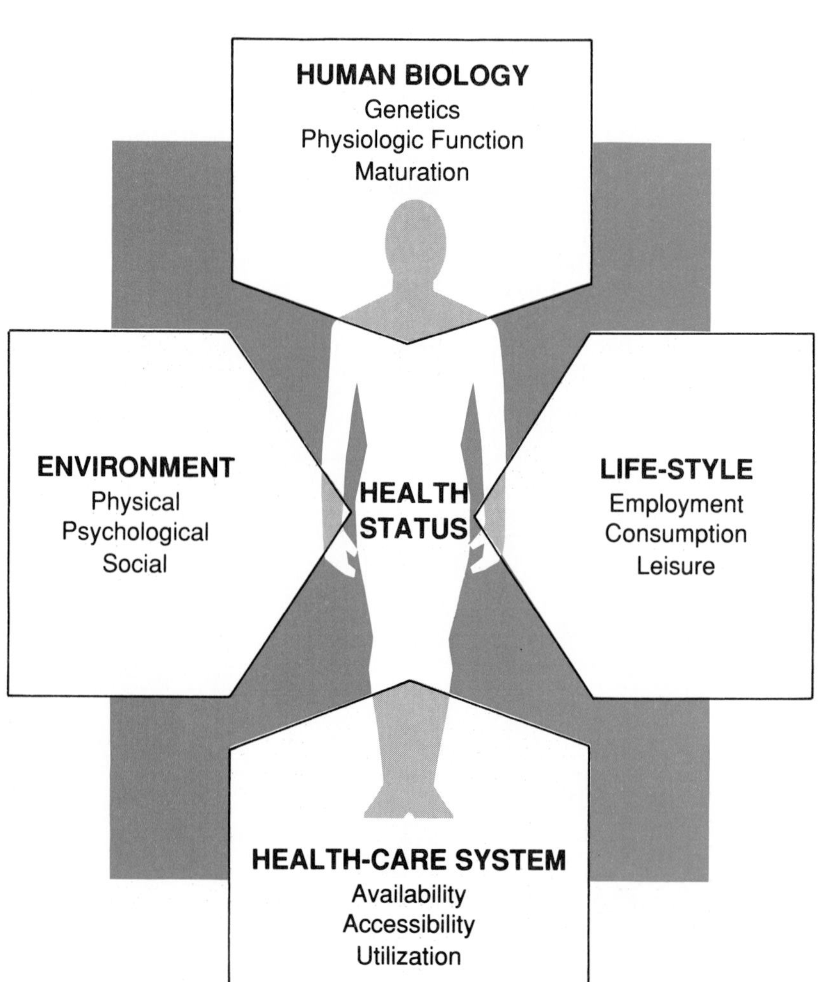

Figure 6–4. Elements of Dever's epidemiologic model.

Genetic Inheritance

As a biological factor, genetic inheritance encompasses sexual and racial characteristics as well as the specific gene pattern transferred by one's parents. Certain health problems are more frequently associated with some sex or racial groups than with others. With respect to sex as a biological factor, pregnancy obviously affects only females, while hemophilia occurs primarily among males. The classic example of race as a biological factor in a specific illness is, of course, sickle cell anemia among blacks. Blacks have traditionally had a higher incidence of hypertension as well. However, there is evidence to suggest that hypertension among blacks may be a by-product of the stresses resulting from lower socioeconomic status rather than a racial influence.[6]

The presence of certain genetically transmitted diseases also increases one's risk of developing some health problems. For example, genetic inheritance is known to play a significant part in the development of diabetes, heart disease, and cancer and may be implicated in alcoholism and other forms of substance abuse.

Complex Physiologic Function

Factors related to complex physiologic function as a biological factor include one's basic state of health as it affects one's probability of developing other health problems. Considerations in this area would include the presence or absence of other disease states. For example, infection with human immunodeficiency virus (HIV) will increase one's chances of developing tuberculosis, while obesity contributes to a variety of health problems including heart disease, diabetes, and stroke. Returning to our teenage pregnancy example, failure to ovulate because of hormonal imbalance will prevent pregnancy from occurring.

Another aspect of complex physiologic function involves the concept of physiologic ***immunity.*** Immunity is one's ability to resist the influence of an infectious agent and its effects. Immunity can be either general or specific in nature. General immunity consists of the body's normal defenses against the invasion of an agent. Such defenses include an intact skin, the normal pH of gastric secretions, or the presence of adequate coping mechanisms. Specific immunity can be either physiological as in the case of antigen-antibody responses, mechanical as that produced by the use of protective clothing, or psychologic as in the development of specific mechanisms for dealing with stress.

Physiologic immunity can be passive or active in nature depending upon the role of the host in developing antibodies to specific antigens. In ***active immunity*** the host is exposed to the antigen, either through having the disease or via immunization with active antigens (for example, DPT vaccine). Active immunity is relatively long-lasting. In ***passive immunity,*** externally produced antibodies are provided to the host either by way of immunization (for example, hepatitis immune globulin) or transfer (for example, across the placental barrier).

Another type of immunity is termed cross immunity. ***Cross immunity*** occurs when immunity to one agent also confers immunity to a related agent. It can be either passive or active in nature. This type of immunity was the basis for Edward Jenner's original concept of vaccination for smallpox. He noted that milkmaids who developed cowpox seemed immune to smallpox. The concept of cross immunity is also used when contacts to Hansen's disease (leprosy) are given BCG, an antituberculin agent, to prevent the development of the disease. BCG creates limited immunity to tuberculosis and cross immunity to the related microorganism causing Hansen's disease.

Another concept related to host immunity that has relevance for groups of people is that of herd immunity. ***Herd immunity*** is the proportion of the population who are immune to a particular disease. When herd immunity is high, the incidence of the disease is reduced because there are fewer susceptible individuals in the population. High levels of herd immunity also mean that unimmunized individuals have less risk of exposure to the disease. Suppose, for example, that there are 100 children in a particular preschool and that 99 of them are adequately immunized against measles. The risk of exposure for the unimmunized child is greatly reduced because none of his schoolmates will develop measles and give it to him.

Maturation and Aging

Maturation and aging also affect one's risk of developing specific health problems. For example, pertussis, or whooping cough, is usually confined to unimmunized children under the age of 10, while sexually transmitted diseases are more prevalent among adolescents and young adults. The elderly are more susceptible to complications and death due to influenza than are people in other age groups. Similar differences in the probability of disease based on age are noted for chronic health problems as well. Accidents are a serious source of morbidity and mortality for both the young and the elderly, whereas obesity is a common problem in all age groups.

ENVIRONMENTAL FACTORS

The environmental component of Dever's model consists of physical, psychological, and social environments. These categories are comparable to the concepts of physical and social environment and host psychological factors included in the epidemiologic triad model.

Physical Environment

The physical environment consists of such factors as weather, geographic locale, soil composition, terrain, temperature and humidity, and hazards posed by poor housing, unsafe working conditions, and so forth. For example, the presence of a physical environmental factor such as many swimming pools in a community increases the risk of drowning accidents among young children. Similarly, high noise levels in the work environment contribute to hearing loss, while the presence of ragweed in the environment contributes to hay fever in susceptible individuals.

Another aspect of the physical environment is the presence of pathogenic microorganisms such as viruses and bacteria. The influence of such biologic agents on health is dependent on a number of factors including the amount of the agent, its infectivity, pathogenicity, and virulence, and other factors discussed earlier in this chapter. Other important environmental considerations are the presence of reservoirs and intermediaries for infectious agents.

A ***reservoir*** is the habitat in which a microorganism exists and multiplies.[1] A reservoir does not merely transmit the agent but is actually infected by the agent. For example, humans can acquire bovine tuberculosis from cows, or rabies from dogs or other diseased animals. In the first instance, the reservoir is the cow; in the second it is the dog or other rabid animal. An organism that merely transmits the agent is not a reservoir but an intermediary. The mosquito merely transfers the *Plasmodium* from an infected person to an uninfected person, so the reservoir for malaria is humans, not the mosquito.

Reservoirs can be human, animal, or environmental. Diseases acquired from animals are called "zoonoses." Examples of diseases acquired from animal reservoirs include ringworm from cats, anthrax from sheep, and rabies and bovine tuberculosis as previously mentioned.

Human reservoirs may be divided into two categories—cases and carriers. A ***case*** is an individual who actually has the disease (for example, the person with a cold who coughs in your face). A ***carrier*** is an individual who harbors the agent without actually having symptomatic disease at the time. Carriers may be classified as incubationary, convalescent, chronic, or transient.

Incubationary carriers are individuals who are in the process of developing the disease. Thus, the susceptible person exposed to chicken pox is an incubationary carrier prior to the development of symptoms. People recuperating from communicable diseases who continue to harbor the agent for a period of time after clinical symptoms have subsided are ***convalescent carriers.*** Convalescent carriers continue to be capable of transmitting the disease to others.

Occasionally, a convalescent carrier continues to harbor the agent beyond the usual convalescent period. These people become ***chronic carriers*** who persist in carrying the infectious agent and may communicate it to others over a prolonged period of time. Chronic carriers are usually restricted from certain forms of employment, called sensitive occupations, based on the mode of transmission for the particular disease. The concept of sensitive occupations will be discussed in greater detail in Chapter 31, Communicable Disease. Chronic carriers are frequently associated with staphyloccal and streptococcal illness or typhoid.

The last category of human carrier to be considered is the ***transient carrier.*** This is the person who carries the agent for a limited period of time but never exhibits any signs or symptoms of the illness. For example, someone who has a "subclinical case" of a disease is a transient carrier.

A third type of reservoir involves free-living agents. Hookworm is an example of a free-living agent for which soil is the reservoir. Plants may also be considered free-living agents of health problems.

As noted earlier, an ***intermediary*** provides the means of transmitting certain agents from reservoir to host. Intermediaries can be either living or nonliving. Living intermediaries are ***vectors.*** An example of a vector is the flea that transmits *Yersinia pestis,* the bacterium that causes bubonic plague, from infected rats (the reservoir) to humans (the host). As previously mentioned, the Anopheles mosquito functions as an intermediary in malaria, transmitting the *Plasmodium* from infected to uninfected individuals.

A nonliving intermediary is called a ***vehicle.*** Another term that may be used for this type of intermediary is a "fomite." Scabies is frequently transmitted by means of a vehicle. Clothing worn by the infested person contains eggs of the mite. When the clothing is worn by another person, the eggs hatch and infest the other person as well. Food and water also serve as common vehicles for several communicable diseases.

Psychological Environment

The psychological environment can be influenced by factors internal or external to the individual. Depression and poor self-image are two factors in one's internal psychological environment that contribute to a variety of health problems including suicide, substance abuse, family violence, obesity, and so on. Internal psychological factors can even contribute to such problems as sexually transmitted diseases if sexual behavior is used as a primary mode of interpersonal interaction.

External psychological factors can also influence the development of health problems. For instance, when one has a great deal of emotional support in a time of crisis, suicide is less likely to result than when one faces a crisis without such support. Stress is another factor in the external psychological environment that is associated with a variety of health problems. One's ability to cope with stress, on the other hand, is a factor in one's internal psychological environment.

Social Environment

Social factors comprise the third environmental element in Dever's model. The social environment includes such factors as social structure, accepted modes of behavior, social norms, and family structure. Another important factor in the social environment is prevailing social attitudes toward the problem under investigation. For example, the fear and stigma attached to AIDS may seriously hamper efforts to control the disease. Alcoholism, drug abuse, mental illness, and adolescent pregnancy are other examples of health problems in which social attitudes contribute to the problem or hamper the solution.

The social environment can also contribute to the development of health problems in other ways. Congregating in large groups, particularly indoors during the winter, enhances the spread of certain diseases such as colds and influenza. Media portrayals of a variety of healthy and unhealthy behaviors are another way in which the social environment influences health and illness. For example, the communication media's graphic coverage of suicides and other forms of violence are thought to lead to imitative behavior, whereas media presentation of smoking, drinking, and sexual activity as desirable behaviors may contribute to the incidence of lung cancer, heart disease, alcoholism, and sexually transmitted diseases.

LIFE-STYLE FACTORS

Dever contended that life-style factors are the greatest contributors to most health problems and provide the best avenue for control of those problems.[5] Life-style factors include employment, consumption patterns, and leisure activity and associated risks.

Employment or Occupation

Employment or occupation can influence health in a number of ways. Some occupational groups are more likely than others to encounter specific health hazards. For instance, the potential for accidental injury is greater for people employed in construction than those who work in offices. Conversely, occupational stress levels are likely to be higher for white-collar than for blue-collar occupations. One's employment can also affect other aspects of one's health status. Those in high-paying jobs are more likely to be able to afford health care than can those in low-paying jobs. Some occupational groups do not receive health insurance as a benefit of employment. For example, part-time employees or migrant workers are unlikely to have health insurance.

Consumption Patterns

Consumption patterns and similar life-style behaviors also influence health and illness. Nutritional habits can either enhance or undermine health. Adequate nutrition promotes health, while both leanness and obesity predispose one to several health problems. Exercise patterns also influence health status as do smoking, drinking, and drug use.

Leisure and Other Life-Style Factors

Other life-style factors that influence health status include leisure activities, the use of safety precautions, and sexual activity. Engaging in certain sports such as skiing or hang gliding increases the risk of serious accidental injury. Similarly, failure to wear seat belts or motorcycle helmets increases one's potential for serious injury; increased numbers of sexual partners puts one at greater risk for sexually transmitted diseases.

HEALTH SYSTEM FACTORS

Health system factors include the availability, accessibility, adequacy, and use of health-care services at all three levels of prevention. Health system factors can influence health status either positively or negatively. For example, immunization services that are available and easily accessible to all community members promote control of such diseases as measles, polio, tetanus, and so on. On the other hand, lack of adequate emergency services in rural areas increases the risk of death from heart attack or accident.

Some health system contributions to health problems stem from the economics of health-care delivery. The high cost of health services limits the ability of many to take advantage of them. In other instances, inappropriate actions on the part of health-care providers may actually contribute to health problems. For example, inappropriate use of antibiotics has contributed to the development of antibiotic-resistant strains of gonorrhea and syphilis. Failure of health-care providers to recognize and intervene with persons at risk for suicide, substance abuse, and family violence has also led to increased incidence of such problems.

Each of the three epidemiologic models presented here can be used to organize information related to client health status, to identify health problems, and to direct intervention. The epidemiologic triad is the most familiar of the three models, but may be somewhat difficult to use in describing health problems that have no identifiable agent or that arise from the complex interaction of multiple factors. The web of causation model addresses the complexity of factors influencing health and illness, but its very complexity may limit its utility. In using the model, one could potentially go on at length examining causative factors. This model is useful, however, in identifying points at which intervention is likely to eliminate or control a health problem. Neither of these two models acknowledges the influence of the health-care system on the health of populations, nor do they highlight life-style factors that are some of the greatest influences on health and illness. For these reasons, Dever's model, rather than either of the other two models, has been incorporated in a model to guide community health nursing practice.

THE EPIDEMIOLOGIC PREVENTION PROCESS MODEL

Community health nurses use the nursing process somewhat differently from nurses in other areas of practice. This difference in use arises, in part, from the variety of clients that community health nurses serve—individuals, families, and groups or communities. More fundamentally, however, community health nurses use the epidemiologic perspective[7] provided by Dever's model and the three levels of prevention within the accepted nursing process framework. In essence, community health nurses practice according to an ***epidemiologic prevention process model*** of nursing care. This term reflects the model's three components: Dever's epidemiologic perspective, the levels of prevention, and the nursing process. The components of this model are depicted in Figure 6–5.

The model's epidemiologic perspective is derived from Dever's epidemiologic model, the four basic components of which are human biology, environment, life-style, and the system of health-care organization. In the epidemiologic prevention process model, these components serve to organize the community health nurse's assessment of client needs and identification of health-related conditions and factors contributing to them.

Although primary prevention is the major emphasis in community health nursing, community health nurses engage in activities related to primary, secondary, and tertiary prevention. For this reason, all three levels of prevention are incorporated in the epidemiologic prevention process model. The nurse may plan and implement interventions at all three levels depending on client needs. In addition, he or she evaluates the outcome of interventions in terms of the level of prevention involved. For example, outcome criteria for primary prevention would reflect improved health status and the absence of specific health problems. Evaluation of secondary preventive measures would focus on the extent to which existing problems have been resolved, while evaluative criteria for tertiary preventive measures would reflect return of the client to a prior level of function or prevention of recurrent problems.

Throughout most of the rest of this book, the epidemiologic prevention process model will be used as a framework to examine issues influencing the practice of community health nursing and the care of a variety of clients in a variety of settings.

AN "EPIDEMIOLOGY OF HEALTH"

To this point, epidemiology has been discussed primarily in relation to problems of ill health. In addition to considering factors that contribute to or prevent specific problems, community health nurses should investigate and identify those factors that promote health. It has been suggested that the health-care professions should focus on an "epidemiology of health."[8] Members of the nursing profession in particular have been urged to focus on health promotion.[9]

From its beginning, community health nursing has been engaged in health promotion, and this should remain a primary focus of community health nursing practice.[10] Recently, other health-care providers have become aware of the need for promoting health in addition to treating or even preventing specific diseases. However, this recognition is coming slowly, and community health nursing has the advantage of already being the forerunner in this area.

Interest in health promotion has occurred as a result of the shift from infectious to chronic disease as the major cause of death. This shift has been accompanied by increased cost for medical care, changes in payment sources, and research indicating that individual behavior may contribute to chronic illness. These factors have encouraged consumers and funders of health-care services to turn to health promotion and behavior modification as a means of decreasing costs.[11]

Health promotion has been described as "all the measures that enhance the possibility of a full life."[12]

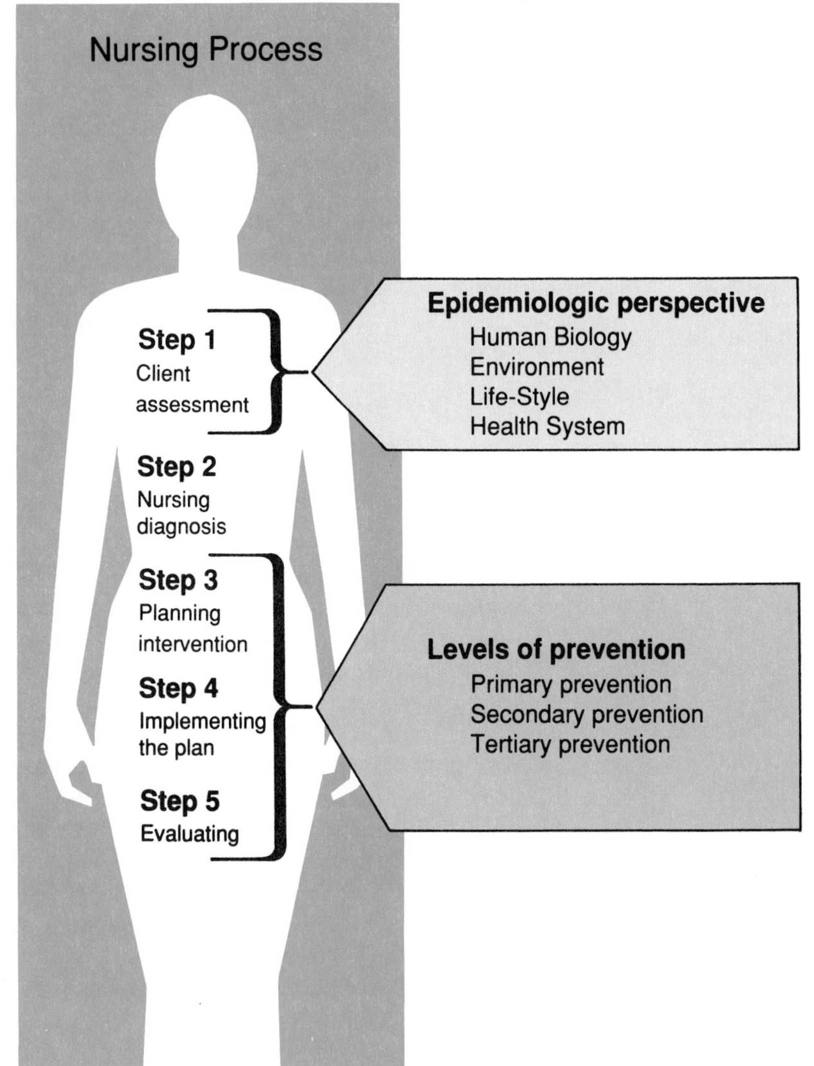

Figure 6–5. Components of the epidemiologic prevention process model.

Health promotion differs from health protection or illness prevention in that health protection is directed toward decreasing the probability of illness, whereas health promotion focuses on "sustaining or increasing the level of well-being and self-actualization of a given individual or group."[13]

Health promotion entails responsibilities for both clients and nurses. Clients need actively to pursue health and health care by means of health-related behaviors, while nurses facilitate healthy behavior by clients.[13] Community health nurses do this by preparing individuals to make behavioral choices that maximize their health potential. Such preparation may occur on a one-to-one basis or with groups of clients.[14]

There are also societal responsibilities in health promotion. One such responsibility is the provision of access to health-promotive services for all people.[15] Another societal responsibility is the creation of an environment that enhances health[12] through engineering technology and legislative enforcement.[16]

IDENTIFYING HEALTH-PROMOTION FACTORS

To promote health, the community health nurse must have a solid grasp of factors that lead to optimal health. Using the epidemiologic process with *health,* rather than a health problem, as the focus is one means of identifying these factors. Using Dever's epidemiologic perspective, community health nurses can examine the human biological, environmental, life-style, and health-system factors that promote health.

HUMAN BIOLOGY

Several biological indicators of health that may be influenced by health promotion have been identified.[12] These include anatomical, physiological, chemical, and immunologic indicators of health status. Anatomical indicators such as height and weight and physiologic indicators such as blood pressure are influenced by a variety of factors. Similarly, chemical indicators like blood cholesterol levels and immunologic indicators of immunity to disease may also be affected by health promotion. Health promotion in the biological sense involves manipulation of factors that influence physical health.

While biological factors such as age, race, and sex influence health as well as illness, they are not amenable to control and cannot be manipulated to promote health. Genetic inheritance can be manipulated only in the sense that persons with specific disorders can receive genetic counseling regarding the potential for genetic transmission of the problem to their children. Genetic counseling can promote the health of the overall population if fewer individuals with genetic disorders are born as a result.

Perhaps the most important area in which human biological factors can serve to promote health is maturation. Factors that promote normal growth and development also promote health. Promotion of growth and development can begin before birth with adequate prenatal care and prenatal nutrition. A well-balanced diet throughout life will also promote maturation and health.

ENVIRONMENT

Health promotion may alter factors in the physical, psychological, and social environments that contribute to disease.[17] Environmental factors that promote health would include such things as living and working conditions that are adequate and free of hazards, as well as an environment conducive to physical, emotional, and social development. Particularly important in this area would be the development of adequate coping skills and the ability to adapt to environmental changes without diminishing health. A social environment that emphasizes the desirability of healthy behaviors and downplays those that are unhealthful would also be conducive to health.

LIFE-STYLE

A number of life-style factors promote health.[12] Life-styles that incorporate adequate rest and exercise contribute to health,[17] as does moderate or nonuse of potentially harmful substances such as tobacco and alcohol. Adequate nutrition is another life-style factor that contributes to overall health, while consistent use of safety devices such as seat belts, hearing protection, smoke detectors, and so on also contribute their part.

HEALTH SYSTEM

Health system factors that would promote health include the availability and accessibility of health-promotive services.[11] Of special concern to community health nurses involved in health promotion is education of the general public regarding health-promoting behaviors. When the health system does not make health education a primary function of all health-care providers, that system does not promote health.

Unfortunately, although there is evidence to support the beneficial effects of many health-promotive activities related to human biology, environment, life-style, and the health system, the extent to which these activities are performed by the general public is minimal. While good nutrition for all persons is a priority of the objectives for the nation, a recent study indicated that three-quarters of state efforts with respect to nutrition are geared toward pregnant and lactating women, infants, and children.[18]

In a similar vein, the 1986 annual survey of behavioral risk factors conducted in 25 states indicated that from 48 percent to 72.2 percent of the population of these states still pursues a sedentary life-style, engaging in less than 20 minutes of leisure-time physical activity at least three times a week. Nonuse of seat belts was reported by 8.8 percent to 71.2 percent of the sample in the states surveyed. In the same study, heavier drinking (over 60 drinks per month) was reported by 3.7 percent to 10.8 percent of people in the state samples.[19] It is obvious from these figures that efforts for health promotion have a long way to go.

HEALTH-PROMOTION STRATEGIES

By their very nature, strategies to promote health occur at the primary level of prevention. There are five categories of health-promotion strategies: health education, health appraisal, life-style modification, providing a healthy environment, and developing effective coping skills. Health education will be discussed in detail in Chapter 7, The Health Education Process.

HEALTH APPRAISAL

Health appraisal is the process of identifying factors that influence the health of an individual or a group. From the perspective of health promotion, a thorough health appraisal can identify healthy behaviors to be reinforced and indicate areas in which health-promoting behaviors are not being performed. By conducting health appraisals, community health nurses can help clients identify areas for behavior change to enhance and promote health. They can also identify healthy behaviors currently performed by clients and encourage continuing these behaviors. For example, the nurse might encourage an older client to continue daily walks as a form of exercise. A tool that can be used to appraise client life-styles and health-promotive behaviors is included in Appendix A.

LIFE-STYLE MODIFICATION

The health appraisal provides direction for the next health-promotion strategy, namely life-style modification. This strategy involves action in regard to health behaviors rather than just identification provided by the health appraisal. Using this strategy, an attempt is made to motivate clients to make life-style changes that will promote health. For example, a relatively sedentary individual would be encouraged to exercise.

PROVIDING A HEALTHY ENVIRONMENT

Another health-promotion strategy—providing a healthy environment—involves consideration of a client's physical, psychological, and social environments. Safety hazards can be eliminated from the physical environment. For example, a home with small children can be "child-proofed," and safety precautions can be taken in handling hazardous substances in the workplace. Other approaches to providing a healthy physical environment include the use of protective devices such as seat belts or hearing protection in high noise levels, mandatory motorcycle helmet use, legislation and engineering efforts to curb environmental pollution, and so on.

Attention should also be given to the psychological environment. For example, many businesses are attempting to reduce employee stress levels as a means of promoting health. Interventions designed to enhance individuals' self-esteem, especially among

TABLE 6–4. RESOURCES FOR HEALTH PROMOTION

Agency or Organization	Functions
Action on Smoking & Health 2013 H. St., N.W. Washington, DC 20006 (202) 659-4310	Public advocacy related to smoking
Aerobics International Research Society 12330 Preston Rd. Dallas, TX 75230 (214) 661-3374	Research, education on exercise and fitness
American College of Preventive Medicine 1015 15th St., N.W., Suite 403 Washington, DC 20005	Information on health promotion programs
American Hospital Association Center for Health Promotion American Hospital Association 840 N. Lake Shore Dr. Chicago, IL 60611	Literature on health promotion
Participation Director of Marketing 80 Richmond St. W., Suite 805 Toronto, Ontario M5H 2A4, Canada	Information on fitness
President's Council on Physical Fitness and Sports 400 6th St., S.W., Rm 3030 Washington, DC 20201	Public information on fitness
Wellness Associates 5433-E Mill Valley, CA 94942 (707) 632-5398	Resources to improve health and life-style, public education on wellness
A Wellness Center, Inc. 15 E. 40th St., Suite 704 New York, NY 10016 (212) 532-4286	Public education for improved life-style, vocational rehabilitation, and counsel for disabled
Wellness & Health Activation Networks P.O. Box 923 Vienna, VA 22180 (703) 281-3830	Increase awareness of health rights and responsibilities, public education

children, also create a more healthful psychological environment.

Changes in the social environment can also foster health. Positive attitudes to healthy behaviors such as exercising, not drinking, not overeating, and so on, can create peer pressure to engage in such behaviors. For example, campaigns to make exercise the "in thing to do" change public attitudes to exercise and promote exercise by individuals. Social and economic changes can also enhance client access to health-promotive services. Providing exercise facilities in the workplace is another example of a social environmental change reflecting changes in employer attitudes to health promotion that influence the behavior of individual employees.

DEVELOPING COPING SKILLS

The last category of strategies for health promotion involves developing effective ways of coping with stress. People who can deal adequately with life's stresses experience fewer stress-related physical and psychological problems. Community health nurses can assist clients to identify sources of stress in their lives. Efforts can then be undertaken to identify coping strategies that allow the particular client to deal with these sources of stress. For instance, one client may be encouraged to engage in physical activity to reduce the effects of stress, while another might be taught relaxation techniques. Or, the client may be assisted to develop more positive approaches to problem solving as a way of dealing with stress.

Each of the health-promotion strategies discussed here require knowledge and expertise on the part of the community health nurse. Nurses and clients may be interested in obtaining information on various forms of health promotion. This information is available from a variety of agencies and organizations, some of whom are included in Table 6–4.

CHAPTER HIGHLIGHTS

- Epidemiology is the study of the distribution of health and illness in populations and the factors that contribute to health and illness.
- The primary purposes of epidemiology are to search for causal relationships in health and illness and to use knowledge of these relationships to control health and illness.
- The five criteria of causation are consistency of association between factors, strength of association, specificity, correct temporal relationship, and coherence with existing knowledge.
- Risk is the probability that a given individual will develop a specific health problem based on the presence or absence of certain identified risk factors. Populations at risk are groups of people most likely to develop a given health problem because of the presence of these factors.
- Morbidity refers to the extent of illness in the population, whereas mortality reflects the occurrence of death. Specific morbidity rates of interest to community health nurses are incidence and prevalence rates. Incidence reflects the number of new cases of a condition diagnosed in a specified time period; prevalence is the total number of cases of the condition existing at a certain point in time.
- Epidemiologists use the epidemiologic process to investigate health-related conditions. The steps of this process are defining the condition, determining its natural history, identifying strategic points of control, and designing, implementing, and evaluating control programs.
- Epidemiologic models are used to organize data related to a health condition. Three such models are the epidemiologic triad, the web of causation, and Dever's epidemiologic model.
- Host, agent, and environment are the three components of the epidemiologic triad. The host is the client system affected by the condition under study, whereas the agent is the condition's primary causative factor. The environment includes all other factors that influence the condition.
- The web of causation model examines direct and indirect causes of a health-related condition as well as the interplay between causative factors.
- Components of Dever's epidemiologic model are human biology, environment, life-style, and the health system.
- Human biological factors of interest in epidemiologic investigation of health and illness conditions include genetic inheritance, com-

(*continued*)

plex physiologic function, and maturation and aging.

- The environmental component of Dever's model includes the physical, psychological, and social environments.
- Life-style considerations in Dever's model include employment or occupation, consumption patterns, and leisure activities and other behaviors.
- Health system considerations include the availability of health-care resources and their influence on health and illness.
- The epidemiologic prevention process model incorporates Dever's epidemiologic model and the levels of prevention within the framework of the nursing process to provide a model to direct community health nursing practice.
- Epidemiology can be used both to promote health and to control disease. The epidemiologic prevention process model is used to plan and direct nursing care aimed at health promotion.
- Strategies used in health promotion include health appraisal, life-style modification, providing a healthy environment, and developing effective coping skills.

Review Questions

1. Describe at least two theories of disease causation. During what periods of history were these theories prevalent? (p. 102)
2. Identify at least three criteria for determining causality in a relationship between two events. Give an example of each. (p. 103)
3. Define risk. Identify at least two risk factors for cardiovascular disease. Who would be the population at risk for cardiovascular disease? (p. 104)
4. Distinguish between morbidity and mortality rates. Give an example of each. (p. 105)
5. Distinguish between incidence and prevalence rates. Give an example of each. Which would give you more information about the effects of a primary prevention program? Why? (p. 107)
6. What are the six steps of the epidemiologic process? (p. 107)
7. Describe the three major elements of the epidemiologic triad. Identify at least two considerations related to each. (p. 109)
8. Describe the web of causation model. (p. 112)
9. What are the four major components of Dever's epidemiologic model? Identify at least two considerations related to each component. (p. 114)
10. What are the components of the epidemiologic prevention process model? (p. 118)
11. Describe at least three strategies for health promotion. Give an example of each. (p. 120)

APPLICATION AND SYNTHESIS

Janie, a 14-year-old female, lives with her mother and grandmother. Janie's parents are divorced and she only sees her father during the summer because he lives in another state. Janie has been having occasional sexual intercourse with her steady boy friend, Jim, for about a year. She started having sex with him because he told her he would find another girlfriend if she didn't. Most of Janie's girlfriends are also sexually active.

Janie is not using contraceptives. She feels guilty about her sexual activity and keeps telling herself that she isn't going to have sex with Jim any more. Janie's mother and grandmother both work, so Janie is home alone from the time she arrives back from school until her mother gets home about 5 P.M. Jim usually walks Janie home from school on days when he doesn't have football practice. He frequently stays and has dinner with Janie and her family.

Last week Janie found out that she is pregnant. She is afraid to tell her mother and comes to you, the nurse at her school, for assistance.

1. What human biological factors influenced Janie's pregnancy?
2. What environmental factors contributed to Janie's pregnancy?
3. What life-style factors are involved in this situation? How have they influenced Janie's pregnancy?
4. What health system factors might be involved in this situation?
5. What primary, secondary, and tertiary prevention measures might influence this situation?

REFERENCES

1. Valanis, B. (1986). *Epidemiology in nursing and health care.* Norwalk, CT: Appleton-Century-Crofts.
2. Wigley, R., & Cook, J. R. (1975). *Community health: Concepts and issues.* New York: D. Van Nostrand.
3. Lilienfeld, A. M., & Lilienfeld, D. E. (1980). *Foundations of epidemiology* (2nd ed.). New York: Oxford University Press.
4. Friedman, G. D. (1987). *Primer of epidemiology* (3rd ed.). New York: McGraw-Hill.
5. Dever, G. E. A. (1980). *Community health analysis.* Germantown, MD: Aspen.
6. Keil, J. E. (1977). Hypertension: Effects of social class and racial admixture. *American Journal of Public Health, 67,* 634–639.
7. Josten, L. E. (1989). Wanted: Leaders for public health. *Nursing Outlook, 37,* 230–232.
8. Terris, M. (1975). Approaches to an epidemiology of health. *American Journal of Public Health, 65,* 1037–1045.
9. Hall, B. A., & Allan, J. D. (1986). Sharpening nursing's focus by focusing on health. *Nursing & Health Care, 7,* 314–321.
10. Novak, J. C. (1988). The social mandate and historical basis for nursing's role in health promotion. *Journal of Professional Nursing, 4*(2), 80–87.
11. McLeroy, K. R., Gottlieb, N. H., & Burdine, J. N. (1987). The business of health promotion: Ethical issues and professional responsibilities. *Health Education Quarterly, 14*(1), 91–109.
12. Breslow, L. (1983). The potential of health promotion. In D. Mechanic (Ed.), *Handbook of health, health care, and the health professions* (pp. 50–66). New York: Free Press.
13. Lee, H. A., & Frenn, M. D. (1987). The use of nursing diagnoses for health promotion in community practice. *Nursing Clinics of North America, 22*(4), 981–986.
14. Swinford, P. A., & Webster, J. A. (1989). *Promoting wellness: A nurse's handbook.* Rockville, MD: Aspen.

15. Birmingham, J. J. (1987). The wellness frontier: The community. *Nursing Administration Quarterly, 11*(3), 14–18.
16. White, M. S. (1982). Construct for public health nursing. *Nursing Outlook, 30,* 527–530.
17. Duffy, M. E. (1988). Health promotion in the family: Current findings and directives for nursing research. *Journal of Advanced Nursing, 13,* 109–117.
18. Kaufman, M., Heimendinger, J., Foerster, S., & Carroll, M. A. (1987). Progress toward meeting the nutrition objectives for the nation. *American Public Health Association, 77,* 299–303.
19. Behavioral risk factor surveillance—selected states, 1986. (1987). *MMWR, 36,* 252.

RECOMMENDED READINGS

Abramson, J. H. (1984). Application of epidemiology in community oriented primary care. *Public Health Reports, 99,* 437–441.

Presents the use of epidemiologic concepts in primary practice. Discusses the need for primary-care providers to focus on the health of populations, as well as individuals, served.

Brubaker, B. H. (1983). Health promotion: A linguistic analysis. *Advances in Nursing Science, 5*(3), 1–14.

Analyzes the meaning of the term health promotion *as used in community health, medical, and wellness literature. Identifies common themes in the definition of health promotion to create an encompassing definition of the term.*

Friedman, G. D. (1987). *Primer of Epidemiology* (3rd ed.). New York: McGraw-Hill.

Provides an introduction to principles of epidemiology.

Levine, S., & Lilienfeld, A. M. (1987). *Epidemiology and health policy.* New York: Tavistock.

Describes the uses of epidemiology in health policy formation in the areas of child health, nutrition, chronic and communicable disease, occupational health, and mental health.

Lilienfeld, A. M., & Lilienfeld, D. E. (1980). *Foundations of epidemiology* (2nd ed.). New York: Oxford University Press.

A basic introduction to principles and concepts of epidemiology.

McLeroy, K. R., Gottlieb, N. H., & Burdine, J. N. (1987). The business of health promotion. *Health Education Quarterly, 14*(1), 91–109.

Discusses the upsurge in interest in health promotion and some of the ethical issues deriving from that interest.

Mullan, F. (1984). Community-oriented primary care: Epidemiology's role in the future of primary care. *Public Health Reports, 99,* 442–445.

Focuses on the means of integrating epidemiologic concepts into primary care to meet community, as well as individual, health needs.

Pender, N. J. (1982). *Health promotion in nursing practice.* Norwalk, CT: Appleton-Century-Crofts.

Describes nursing strategies for the promotion of clients' health. Presents a model of health promotion to be used in practice.

Riley, J. C. (1987). *The eighteenth century campaign to avoid disease.* New York: St. Martin's Press.

Delineates the historical development of epidemiology since the eighteenth century as well as its early beginnings in Hippocratic thought. Addresses some of the major accomplishments of epidemiology in the control of disease.

Swinford, P. A., & Webster, J. A. (1989). *Promoting wellness: A nurse's handbook.* Rockville, MD: Aspen.

Presents nursing strategies for promoting wellness among clients.

Waller, J. A. (1985). The epidemiologic basis for injury prevention. *Public Health Reports, 100,* 575–576.

Describes the application of epidemiologic principles to the prevention of accidental injury.

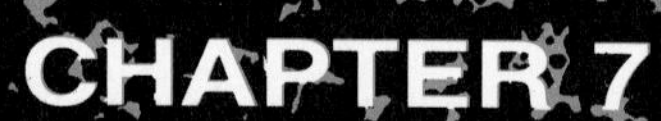

CHAPTER 7

The Health Education Process

KEY TERMS

developmental readiness
enabling factors
focusing event
formative evaluation
health education
iatrogenic health education disease
learning objectives
learning tasks
predisposing factors
reinforcing factors

Much of the practice of community health nursing involves educating people about healthier life-styles. As a primary preventive measure, health education is directed toward promoting health and preventing illness. The health education process also can be used at the secondary and tertiary levels of prevention. As a secondary prevention measure, community health nurses might teach clients about self-care related to specific health problems. Teaching clients to minimize the consequences of health problems or to prevent their recurrence is the object of health education at the tertiary prevention level. Whatever the level of prevention involved, the health education process used remains the same.

The health education process includes two components—an educational process derived from the behavioral sciences, and information content derived from the health sciences. ***Health education*** has been described as the use of a variety of learning experiences to facilitate changes to more healthful behaviors[1] and as a process that frees people to make health-related decisions based upon full knowledge of the consequences of their choices.[2] Learning experiences that free people to make appropriate decisions are created using a systematic health education process occurring within the context of the epidemiologic prevention process model.

(continued)

LEARNING OBJECTIVES

After reading this chapter you should be able to:

- Identify three types of precursors to healthy behavior.
- Describe three types of health-related decisions facilitated by health education.
- Describe at least two barriers to health education.
- Describe the steps of the health education process.
- Identify three types of learning tasks that may be involved in a health education encounter.
- Define a focusing event.
- Describe the use of formative evaluation in a health education encounter.
- Describe at least four guidelines for developing health education programs.

PRECURSORS OF HEALTHY BEHAVIOR

The ultimate expected outcome of health education is healthy behavior on the part of the client. For healthy behavior to occur, however, certain precursor conditions must be present. These precursors fall into three categories: predisposing factors, reinforcing factors, and enabling factors.[3] These factors are components of the PRECEDE model (*P*redisposing, *R*einforcing, and *E*nabling *C*auses in *E*ducational *D*iagnosis and *E*valuation) used to design and evaluate health education.

In the PRECEDE model the design of health education takes place in seven stages. The first stage involves an assessment in which major social problems are identified. Assessment continues in the second stage when health problems contributing to these social problems are identified. In the third stage, health-related behaviors associated with identified problems are delineated. These behaviors are then examined in light of the predisposing, reinforcing, and enabling factors that would promote a change to healthier behaviors. In the fifth stage, the nurse selects those factors that will be the focus of the health education encounter and, in stage 6, develops and implements a health presentation to address these factors. The final stage, stage 7, involves evaluation of the health education encounter and its effects. These stages are summarized in Box 7–1.

BOX 7–1

Stages of the PRECEDE Model

Stage 1: Identifying major social problems
Stage 2: Identifying health problems contributing to social problems
Stage 3: Identifying health behaviors associated with identified health problems
Stage 4: Identifying predisposing, reinforcing, and enabling factors involved in health behaviors
Stage 5: Selecting factors on which to focus the health education encounter
Stage 6: Developing and implementing the health education encounter
Stage 7: Evaluating the health education encounter

PREDISPOSING FACTORS

Predisposing factors are factors internal to the client that enhance or deter motivation for healthy behavior. Examples of predisposing factors are client knowledge about health and illness and client attitudes, values, and perceptions that influence behavior. Knowledge of health concerns, issues, and activities is required for action to occur. People do not decide to act unless they are aware of a need for action. One of the tasks of the community health nurse is to foster that awareness by providing information about health-related concerns. For example, a client is unlikely to attempt dietary changes designed to lower serum cholesterol unless he or she knows that a high cholesterol level increases the risk of heart disease and other problems. Similarly, clients will not use a condom to protect against exposure to human immunodeficiency virus (HIV) unless they know that AIDS can be transmitted via sexual intercourse and that condoms decrease the likelihood of HIV transmission. The client must also have knowledge of how to use a condom correctly.

Information alone is often insufficient to motivate healthy behavior. The client also must possess values and attitudes toward health that foster such behavior. For instance, even when clients understand that lowering serum cholesterol will help prevent heart disease, they might not change dietary habits unless they also believe that heart disease is undesirable and health is valuable. Similarly, decisions to use a condom will be influenced by clients' attitudes to sexual activity and condoms as well as attitudes to health. If a client thinks that condoms are a nuisance or that they diminish sexual pleasure, and the client values pleasure over health, he or she is unlikely to use them despite knowledge of their efficacy.

REINFORCING FACTORS

Reinforcing factors are forces external to the client that affect his or her motivation to act in a healthy way. Such factors may include attitudes and beliefs of significant others toward health and health behaviors. Communications from significant others in the client situation can facilitate or impede healthy behavior. For example, an adolescent may know that sexually transmitted diseases (STDs) are acquired via sexual intercourse and that condoms prevent transmission of disease. He or she may also have no strong negative feelings about condom use. However, if the sexual partner objects to their use, the teenager is unlikely to use condoms.

ENABLING FACTORS

Enabling factors are also external to the client and include other factors in a situation that influence clients' abilities to act in a healthy manner. For example, availability of condoms and money to buy them are enabling factors that promote condom use. The absence of enabling factors will deter healthy behavior. For instance, if a teenager cannot afford to buy condoms and does not know where to get them free, he or she is unlikely to use them.

PURPOSE OF HEALTH EDUCATION

The purpose of health education is to promote the presence of precursors to healthy behavior and to assist clients in making appropriate health-related decisions. Clients can make three types of decisions: decisions about personal health behaviors, decisions about use of available health resources, and decisions about societal health issues.[4]

PERSONAL HEALTH BEHAVIORS

Health education enables people to make decisions regarding personal behaviors that promote health or prevent or cure illness. Should I smoke? Should I change my diet? Should I exercise? Should I have my child immunized? How should I deal with stress? How should I discipline my child? Should I take my blood pressure medication? Should I stay off my ankle like the nurse told me to? All of these questions require decisions that can be influenced by health education.

Health education has been perceived as a means of freeing people from factors that "enslave" them to unhealthy behaviors.[2] Unhealthy behavior, in this perspective, is believed to arise from a need to conform that results from poor self-esteem, alienation, guilt, hostility, anger, low assertiveness, inability to communicate effectively, and isolation. The purpose of health education, then, is to improve self-esteem, clarify values, reduce alienation and isolation, and improve clients' understanding of their own motivations in order to free them to make appropriate health decisions. As we can see, health education involves more than imparting knowledge and skills, but includes changing and creating attitudes conducive to healthful behavior.

RESOURCE USE

The second type of health decisions that people make relates to their use of health resources. Questions that may arise in this area include: Am I sick enough to go to the doctor? Should I see a nurse practitioner or a physician? Should I use the emergency room for care or find a regular health-care provider? Health education can help people become aware of the health-care resources available to them and help them make decisions regarding what type of resources to use and when to use them.

HEALTH ISSUES

The third type of decisions that can be influenced by health education includes decisions related to societal health issues. Health education, for example, can help people determine whether they should vote for or against mandatory screening for AIDS in the general population, or whether they should contribute funds to the local heart association. Health education can also aid in decisions regarding the merits of motorcycle helmet laws, banning smoking on aircraft, or the development of a nuclear power plant. Health education can create an informed public prepared to make thoughtful decisions on major health issues.

BARRIERS TO LEARNING

Prior to planning for health education, the community health nurse must recognize that there may be barriers to learning that may make health education ineffective unless they are overcome. Barriers to learning may be either internal or external.[5] Internal barriers can be physical, social, or psychological in nature. Physical barriers include pain, fever, visual disturbances, and so on, that could interfere with clients' abilities to focus on concepts presented. Social barriers to learning include educational level, language barriers, and incongruence of client beliefs and values with those of the health system. Psychological barriers include such factors as anxiety, depression, denial, and inability to accept, or, occasionally, overacceptance of the sick role. Other psychological barriers might be previous negative experiences with illness or the health-care system and lack of readiness to learn.

External barriers to learning may arise from the learning environment (for example, noise, distractions, etc.) or from the learning situation. Factors related to the learning situation that may create barriers include the timing of educational efforts, the method of teaching used, the level of material presented, or the quality of interaction between nurse and client. In using the educational process, the community health nurse identifies potential barriers in a given client situation and circumvents these barriers by planning appropriate interventions.

One final barrier to desired behavior as a result of health education has been called iatrogenic health education disease.[2] ***Iatrogenic health education disease*** is disease or adverse response caused or made worse by health education. For example, when one teaches a client about possible side effects of medications, the power of suggestion may create those side effects. Similarly, routine education on child safety for new parents may cause them to be overprotective and hinder the child's development. The nurse should remain alert to the potential for such responses to health education and should take action to minimize or avoid this type of response.

THE EPIDEMIOLOGIC PREVENTION PROCESS MODEL AND HEALTH EDUCATION

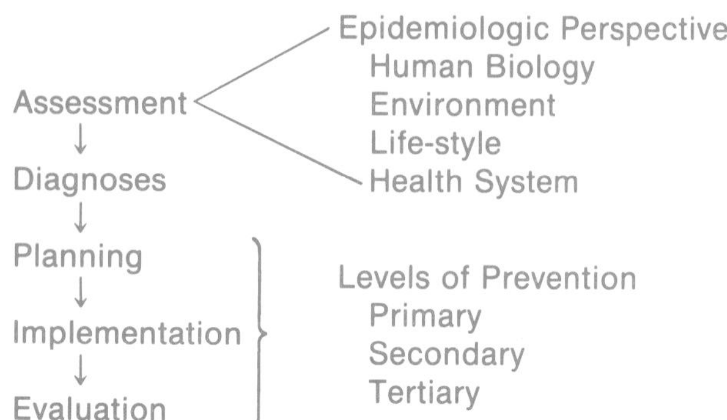

In designing a health education encounter, the community health nurse uses an educational process that parallels the epidemiologic prevention process model. The education process consists of assessing the learner and the learning setting in terms of Dever's epidemiologic perspective, diagnosing learning needs, and planning, implementing, and evaluating a health education presentation. A tool to assist in applying the educational process is included in Appendix B.

ASSESSING THE LEARNER AND THE LEARNING SETTING

The health education process begins with an assessment of the learner, his or her learning needs, and the learning environment. When the client is a group or a community, the first task in assessment is to identify the target audience for the educational effort.[6] Selection of the target audience may be based on level of need, resources available, or probability of success.[7] Assessment then proceeds to identifying characteristics of the client that influence the learning situation.[6] The assessment can be conducted in terms of the four components of Dever's epidemiologic perspective: human biology, environment, life-style, and health system.

HUMAN BIOLOGY

Human biology will influence both the learning needs and the learning capabilities of the client. Areas for consideration include skills and needs related to the client's level of maturation and the adequacy of the client's physiologic function.

Skills and Needs Related to the Level of Maturation

To learn effectively, the client needs to have the skills appropriate to his or her level of maturation. In educational terms this is called ***developmental readiness.*** For example, small children who have not yet developed abilities for abstract thought will need concrete examples of concepts to be learned. Similarly, a child who still has poorly developed eye-hand coordination will have difficulty learning insulin injection techniques, so teaching will necessarily involve parents as well.

Age or maturational level also affects the client's need for education. For instance, a preschool child does not need information about menstruation, but a preadolescent girl does. In addition, the client's maturational level may influence his or her existing knowledge of a particular subject. For example, a group of third graders will probably have a broader knowledge of nutritional concepts than preschoolers.

Physiologic Function

Assessing a clients' physiologic function may reveal special needs for health education or impediments to learning. For example, a young girl with recurrent urinary tract infections may require education on appropriate hygiene, while a diabetic client may require information and assistance with diet, exercise, medication, foot care, and other self-care measures. Inadequate physiologic function can also give rise to impediments to learning. For example, a group of hearing-impaired youngsters or visually impaired older people require specialized approaches to health education to facilitate their ability to learn.

ENVIRONMENT

Environmental factors can also influence learning needs and abilities. Environmental considerations include the physical environment, the psychological environment, and the social environment.

Physical Environment

Conditions in the physical environment often give rise to the need for health education. For example, families living in older housing painted with lead-based paint will need to be taught how to prevent lead poisoning. Similarly, a client using crutches whose apartment is upstairs will need to learn stair-climbing with crutches.

The physical environment should also be considered in terms of its effects on learning.[8] Is there adequate lighting for the tasks to be accomplished? Is there too much noise? Will clients be distracted by other activities occurring in the learning environment? During a home visit, for example, it might be wise to turn off the television before attempting to educate a hypertensive client about his or her medication.

Psychological Environment

The psychological environment can profoundly influence the client's willingness and ability to learn. Attitudes toward health and health behaviors can either enhance or detract from the motivation to learn. Among clients attending a series of parenting classes, for example, those parents who attend only because of a court mandate related to child abuse usually benefit less than do those who attend because they perceive a need for help.

Psychological factors such as stress and anxiety can also impede learning, even for those who are motivated to learn. Nurses can limit the negative effects of the psychological environment by actions designed to decrease stress and anxiety. For instance, the nurse can create a climate in which the client does not feel threatened and in which the nurse educator is seen as a source of support rather than a threat. The nurse who has children and who teaches parenting classes for abusive parents might create such a climate by beginning the first session with a description of the frustration the nurse sometimes feels as a parent.

Other psychological factors that motivate healthy client behaviors can be reinforced to enhance learning. For example, if saving money motivates a client, the nurse might focus on the cost-effectiveness of health-promotion behaviors.

Social Environment

The social environment is particularly influential in shaping attitudes about health and health-related behaviors. For example, if an adolescent's peer group thinks condom use is "dumb," health education on this subject is less likely to be effective than if peer attitudes were favorable.

Social environment can also influence one's exposure to health-related information. People with lower educational levels are less likely than those with more formal education to have been exposed to prior health education. A client's educational level will necessarily influence the nurse's choice of teaching strategies and content to be presented.

The client's primary language is another social factor that might hamper learning abilities unless the nurse allows for language differences in planning for health education. In conducting the client assessment, the nurse will determine the client's fluency in the dominant language (usually English in the United States) as well as the language usually spoken by the client. When educating clients who speak other languages, community health nurses should keep in mind that educational materials translated directly from English may not convey the intended message, or may be unintelligible to the client. Interpreters can be used, but again it is important to use interpreters who speak a form of a language familiar to the particular client.

LIFE-STYLE

Life-style factors will influence client needs for health education. For instance, the client who overeats will probably need dietary education, while those who don't use seat belts need safety education. A client's occupation is another life-style factor that can influence specific learning needs. For instance, trash collectors might require education related to body mechanics and proper techniques for lifting heavy objects, whereas nurses require information about how to handle contaminated needles and other equipment.

HEALTH SYSTEM

The degree of emphasis placed on health education by health-care providers and providers' expertise in using the health education process are health system factors that influence clients' health-related knowledge and attitudes. Health-care providers who engage in health education need a strong background in both educational principles and health content. Community health nurses designing health education offerings will assess their ability to employ principles of education and will take the steps needed to enhance that ability.

An assessment tool such as the Educational Planning and Implementation Guide, included in Appendix B, can be used to direct the community health nurse's assessment of the client and the learning situation. Completing the tool also documents assessment findings. In addition, the tool can be employed to document the other elements of the health education process discussed later in this chapter.

DIAGNOSTIC REASONING AND LEARNING NEEDS

Clients also assess their needs for health education. In many instances, clients may actively seek the assistance of the community health nurse because of recognized needs for health education. For example, a new mother may call the health department to request information and nursing assistance with breast feeding. Or, a local school may request help in educating students, teachers, and parents on a variety of health topics.

Nurse and client assessment of learning needs is used to develop nursing diagnoses. Nursing diagnoses may reflect a knowledge deficit, a lack of motivation for healthful behavior, or both. In either case, health education might be the solution of choice to improve clients' knowledge or motivation. On the positive side, nursing diagnoses may also indicate adequate health knowledge or motivation to learn in areas of knowledge deficit. For example, assessment might reveal adequate knowledge of infant nutritional needs on the part of a new teenage mother, but lack of knowledge of proper bottle-feeding techniques. The nursing diagnosis in this instance might be "knowledge deficit regarding infant feeding techniques due to lack of experience with infant care."

Assessment might also reveal adequate knowledge in an area, but poor attitudes to health behaviors. A related nursing diagnosis might be "failure to request condom use by sexual partners due to poor self-image and lack of assertiveness." In this instance, health education efforts would be directed toward attitude change and assertiveness techniques rather than knowledge of the effects of condom use on preventing STDs.

PLANNING THE HEALTH EDUCATION ENCOUNTER

Several tasks are to be accomplished in planning a health education encounter. These tasks include establishing priorities for health education, identifying goals and the level of prevention involved, identifying learning tasks to be accomplished, developing objectives, and selecting content and teaching strategies. Reviewing or developing educational materials and planning for evaluation are two additional tasks in planning a health education encounter.

PRIORITIZING LEARNING NEEDS

The first task in planning for health education is prioritizing learning needs. A client may exhibit several unrelated learning needs. Because clients can only assimilate a certain amount of information at a time, the community health nurse and client will need to decide which learning needs should be addressed first. Other needs can be addressed later, as time permits. For example, if a young wife with four children is expecting her soldier husband home next month and does not want another pregnancy, contraceptive education may have greater priority than needs for nutrition education. The reverse would be true for the pregnant teenager who is anemic and who is not due to deliver her baby for several months.

IDENTIFYING GOALS AND LEVELS OF PREVENTION

Goal identification involves specifying the broad purpose of the lesson. The goals of a presentation on AIDS, for instance, might be to broaden learners' understanding of AIDS and to decrease fears of the disease. For an educational program on parenting, the goal would be the development of good parenting skills.

Identifying goals for an educational encounter will also enable the community health nurse to identify the level of prevention to be addressed. For example, a goal of reducing the incidence of adolescent pregnancy indicates that education will be directed toward preventing teenage girls from becoming pregnant and involves primary prevention. The goal of preparing clients to give CPR in emergency situations, on the other hand, reflects secondary prevention—dealing with an existing problem—whereas an educational program directed at preventing further abuse of children by abusive parents reflects tertiary prevention.

IDENTIFYING LEARNING TASKS

Another task in planning health education is identifying specific ***learning tasks*** or types of learning that will be required to achieve the goals established. This may be referred to as "instructional analysis."[6] The six types of learning tasks that clients may need to accomplish during a health education encounter are: information acquisition, concept development, skill development, values awareness, development of communication skills, and development of problem-solving or decision-making skills.

In information acquisition, the client's task is to learn facts about health and health-related issues. When this is the case, the community health nurse focuses on providing information. For example, in a presentation on AIDS, the nurse may want clients to acquire knowledge of the ways in which HIV infection is spread.

Concept development involves creating new concepts in the mind of the client. As a result of the AIDS presentation, clients should develop concepts of "safe" and "unsafe sex." Similarly, to avoid the hazards of drug and alcohol use, learners will need to develop a concept of "substance abuse."

Skill development might be another learning task to be accomplished by clients in a particular situation. Skill development includes acquiring intellectual as well as manual or "psychomotor" skills. The ability of a mother to discriminate between circumstances when her child needs medical attention and those that can be treated at home is an intellectual skill that might be acquired through health education. The ability to put on a condom correctly is an example of a manual skill that clients might need to develop.

Values awareness tasks involve client recognition and examination of health-related attitudes and values. We said earlier that one of the goals in a presentation on AIDS might be to decrease clients' fears of the disease. To accomplish this goal, clients will need to examine their attitudes toward AIDS and emotions generated by this condition.

Development of communication skills is another type of learning that may be required to achieve the stated goals of a health education encounter. This learning task focuses on clients' abilities to interact and communicate with others. Clients who learn to communicate effectively have accomplished learning tasks related to communication skills.

The final type of learning task is developing decision-making or problem-solving skills. The focus in this task is on learning how to solve problems and make health-related decisions. For instance, clients who can evaluate the pros and cons of smoking and decide not to smoke have accomplished this type of learning task.

Identifying the type of learning tasks that need to be accomplished in a given health education encounter assists the community health nurse to identify the teaching strategies appropriate to the tasks involved. As we will see later, certain tasks are best accomplished using certain teaching methods. For example, demonstration is an effective way to teach a manual skill, whereas a lecture is less effective.

DEVELOPING LEARNING OBJECTIVES

Developing specific learning objectives is the next activity in planning for health education. ***Learning objectives*** are statements of specific behaviors the nurse expects the client to be able to perform as a result of the health education encounter. A well-constructed learning objective consists of several components.[2] The first of these is an activity in which the client will engage; for example, the client might *demonstrate* something. That "something" is the object of the activity, the second component of the objective. After a presentation on infant feeding, the nurse might expect clients to demonstrate *preparation of infant formula*.

The objective should also specify the level of performance expected. The community health nurse will presumably want clients to prepare the formula using the *correct* proportion of formula to water. Or, an objective might specify that learners will answer a certain percentage of test questions correctly after the lesson, another measure of the level of performance expected. The learning objective might also indicate the situation in which the activity is to take place. For example, one might say, "*Given a description of a hypothetical family*, the client will be able to" perform the designated activity. Finally, the objective may specify certain constraints under which the activity is to be performed. For example, the client might be expected to "identify *from memory* the two populations most at risk for AIDS."

Learning objectives reflect the types of learning tasks to be accomplished. If the learning task is information acquisition, for instance, objectives will focus on clients' abilities to demonstrate acquisition of certain facts; for instance, "the client will be able to correctly list, in writing, three of the seven danger signs of cancer." In this objective, the learning task is the acquisition of information about the warning signs of cancer. The activity is "to list" and the object of that activity is "the warning signs of cancer." The expected level of performance is only three of the seven signs and the constraint is that the learner must be able to do this in writing. In this particular objective, no specific situation is designated for the performance of the expected behavior.

SELECTING AND SEQUENCING CONTENT

The next task in planning the health lesson is selecting and sequencing the content to be presented. Because the nurse usually has greater knowledge of a particular topic than can or should be presented in a health education encounter, the nurse needs to select content that is most appropriate and relevant to clients' needs and that is most likely to result in accomplishing the stated learning objectives. Once content has been selected, it must be organized in a logical sequence so that new learning is based on previous learning. Content is also usually sequenced from simple to complex.

SELECTING TEACHING STRATEGIES

Selection of teaching strategies depends on characteristics of clients, characteristics of the nurse, the type of learning tasks and content involved,[9] and the availability of resources needed to implement specific strategies. The teaching strategies selected should be appropriate to both the age and developmental level of the audience and to their educational level. Strategies should be chosen that will maintain the interest of the learner and adequately address the content to be presented.[10] Another consideration here is clients' preferred modes of learning. Some people learn best when content is presented visually, while others tend to learn what they hear.

Certain learning tasks lend themselves to particular teaching strategies. For example, discussion and role-play are effective methods for creating awareness of personal values, while lecture is more appropriate to information acquisition.[11,12] Problem-solving skills, on the other hand, are best learned through exercises in problem resolution. Table 7–1 presents several commonly used teaching strategies and the learning tasks for which they are best suited.

PREPARING MATERIALS

Any materials needed for the health education encounter must be either developed or obtained. Materials selected should be appropriate to the client audience and to the content presented. For example, if the audience is a group of young children, a coloring book might be an effective teaching aid in a lesson on nutrition. A coloring book would not be appropriate, though, for a group of adolescents.

Nurses planning health education may use existing materials and teaching aids. This is appropriate when these materials have been thoroughly reviewed and found to be appropriate to the client audience. Materials used need to convey information at a level that can be understood by clients. They should also be sensitive to client cultural beliefs, attitudes, and values. For example, materials on sexually transmitted diseases (STDs) that picture only persons from minority groups imply that only members of these groups get STDs. Such an implication is not only erroneous but also discriminatory and offensive to members of minorities who might be part of the client audience.

Problems with written materials occur when members of the client audience have low literacy skills. Recent studies of written information on contraceptive methods, for example, indicate that most are written at reading levels above that of many clients.[13] For clients with low literacy levels, pictorial materials, videotapes, or filmstrips are more appropriate teaching aids than are written materials.

Problems also arise for audiences who are literate in other languages when materials written in English are translated literally. Again, research has shown that readers indicate minimal understanding of materials literally translated from English into their mother tongue.[14] Translated materials should be reviewed for their consistency with local idiomatic language.

Other considerations in selecting teaching aids and other materials to be used include the need for special equipment (e.g., projector and screen for filmstrips), currency of content, and ease of use. Constraints may be imposed by the type of setting in which the learning occurs. For example, if a class is to be conducted outdoors, filmstrips are inappropriate. Or, if education is being provided to a family who lack a television set, a videotape will not be useful. A final consideration in selecting visual aids is the ability of the client to see the materials. If overhead transparencies are used, for example, the print must be large enough to be read by all those in the back of the room. Similarly, when demonstration is used, all clients in the group need to be able to see what is being demonstrated.

TABLE 7–1. COMMONLY USED TEACHING STRATEGIES

Strategy	Description	Learning Task Applicability
Case study	Use of a detailed account of an actual or hypothetical situation to help learners apply principles learned or to make them aware of attitudes and values and enhance the potential for change	Values awareness Decision skill development Intellectual skill development
Computer-assisted instruction	Use of computers to present content	Information acquisition Decision skill development Concept formation
Demonstration	Teacher performance of a skill or process to be learned, usually followed by a return demonstration (see below)	Motor skill development
Discussion	Verbal exploration of an idea or concept, attitude, value, etc., with participation by learners and teacher	Concept formation Values awareness Decision skill development Communication skill development
Lecture	Formal oral presentation of information by teacher	Information acquisition Concept formation
Media	Use of auditory or visual media presentations (i.e., audiotapes, filmstrips) to present content	Information acquisition Concept formation Values awareness Motor skill development Decision skill development Intellectual skill development
Readings	Presentation of content in written form, frequently followed by discussion	Information acquisition Concept formation Values awareness
Return demonstration	Learner performance of a learned skill or process	Development of motor skills
Role modeling	Teacher performance of a behavior to be adopted (i.e., sensitivity to the needs of others)	Values awareness Communication skill development
Role-playing	Acting out the role of another to get a different perspective, usually followed by discussion	Values awareness Concept formation Communication skill development
Supervision	Teacher guided performance of desired behavior by learner	Motor skill development Decision skill development Communication skill development
Visual aids	Use of visually oriented materials to present content (i.e., pictures, posters)	Information acquisition Motor skill development Concept formation

PLANNING FOR EVALUATION

The last task of the planning stage of a health education encounter is developing a plan to evaluate the lesson. Criteria for evaluating the outcomes of health education are derived from the stated objectives for the encounter. Criteria for evaluating the performance of the nurse and the educational process used should also be developed. The nurse will also want to identify mechanisms for ***formative evaluation,*** which involves assessing the effects of the presentation as it is presented. Formative evaluation includes determining whether clients understand what is being presented and whether the presentation maintains their interest. The nurse would also be alert to cues that indicate client response to the content presented. For example, the nurse might note that description of discrimination against a person with AIDS generates anger in the listeners. If the nurse was trying to make clients aware of attitudes toward AIDS, such a response would indicate success.

Formative evaluation also reflects the quality of the presentation. For example, frenzied note-taking by learners would indicate that content is being presented too rapidly. Tasks involved in planning a health education encounter are summarized in Box 7–2.

IMPLEMENTING THE HEALTH EDUCATION ENCOUNTER

Several key points must be kept in mind in implementing a health education encounter.[15] The first is to speak the client's language. This refers not only to the use of a foreign language or an interpreter for non-English-speaking clients, but also eliminating medical

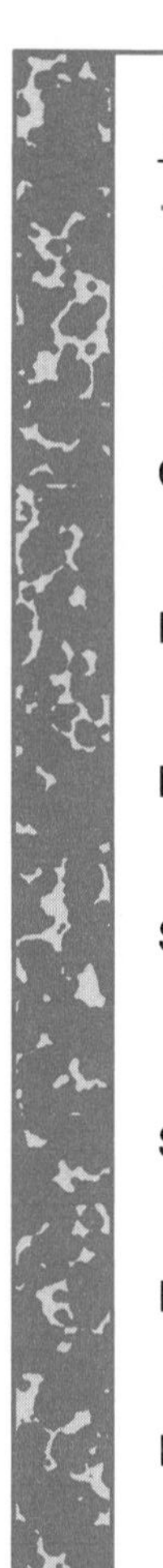

BOX 7–2

Tasks Involved in Planning a Health Education Encounter

Goal identification:
  Specifying the broad purpose to be accomplished
Identifying learning tasks:
  Describing the types of learning involved in the encounter
Developing objectives:
  Stating specific behavioral outcomes expected as a result of the encounter
Selecting and sequencing content:
  Determining what will be taught and the order in which it will be presented
Selecting teaching strategies:
  Determining approaches to be used in presenting content
Preparing materials:
  Developing any teaching aids to be used in the presentation
Planning for evaluation:
  Determining criteria and processes to be used for formative, outcome, and process evaluation

and nursing jargon. The second recommendation is to be specific; the third is to keep the message short. Key points should be presented early in the lesson for emphasis and to enhance recall. Verbal headings will help clients keep track of material presented and recognize transitions from one topic to another. Finally, repetition, particularly of important points, will enhance learning and recall.

Actually presenting the health lesson occurs in three phases. The first phase is the focusing event, the second and third phases involve presenting content and summarizing the information presented.

THE FOCUSING EVENT

The lesson itself begins with a ***focusing event,*** which is a specific strategy designed to gain the attention of the audience and to focus that attention on the material to be presented. A focusing event in a presentation on child abuse might involve showing several slides of abused children or the presentation of statistics on the incidence of child abuse in the community.

PRESENTING THE CONTENT

Following the focusing event, the lesson is presented as planned with formative checks during the course of the lesson to determine the need for on-the-spot revisions of the presentation. The presentation of content should include audience participation whenever possible. Learning theory indicates that the greater the learner's involvement with the material, the greater the learning that results. Client participation can be facilitated by such activities as group discussion, case studies, role-play, and so on. The nurse can also encourage participation by asking thought-provoking questions or questions that serve to summarize and synthesize previous content.

SUMMARIZING

The lesson should close with a summary that reinforces pertinent points. In summarizing, the community health nurse recaps and highlights the major concepts covered. He or she should also attempt to synthesize content in a few major themes that the client needs to remember. The three components of lesson plan implementation—the focusing event, content presentation, and summary—are presented in Box 7–3.

EVALUATING THE HEALTH EDUCATION ENCOUNTER

As noted earlier, evaluation takes place throughout the presentation and as the last step of the educational process. Three aspects of evaluation include forma-

BOX 7–3

Considerations in Implementing a Health Education Encounter

Focusing event:
  A teaching strategy designed to attract attention to the topic
Presentation of content:
  Actual presentation of planned content, encouraging learner participation as much as possible
Summary:
  Restatement and reinforcement of the most important points of the presentation

tive evaluation, outcome evaluation, and process evaluation.

FORMATIVE EVALUATION

During the presentation of the lesson, the community health nurse will perform periodic formative evaluations to assess the lesson and its effects as it is being presented. During formative evaluation, the nurse uses client feedback to determine whether the content of the lesson is being effectively communicated. For example, if clients' facial expressions indicate confusion, the nurse might infer that they do not understand the material being presented. Similarly, the nurse might ask questions on material offered earlier in the lesson as a formative evaluation strategy. If clients are able to answer these questions correctly, the lesson has been effective thus far. Again, formative evaluation might also include assessing client emotional responses to content presented.

OUTCOME EVALUATION

After the lesson, the nurse evaluates the presentation in terms of its outcomes. Outcomes can best be measured in terms of the degree to which the learning objectives were met. Were the learners able to perform the stated behaviors at the expected level of performance?

In evaluating outcomes, the nurse should remain alert to other outcomes of the educational program in addition to the intended outcomes or objectives. Health education may result in unlooked-for outcomes that are serendipitous in nature. These results should not be overlooked or underestimated and may be reason for continuing a program even when intended objectives are not accomplished.

PROCESS EVALUATION

The nurse also evaluates the presentation in terms of the use of the educational process. Was one as well prepared as desired? Did the lesson maintain the interest of the audience? Were the teaching strategies, materials, and content selected appropriate to the learning needs of the clients? The answers to such questions will allow the nurse to make any necessary modifications in the lesson plan for future use. Considerations in evaluating the health education encounter are summarized in Box 7–4.

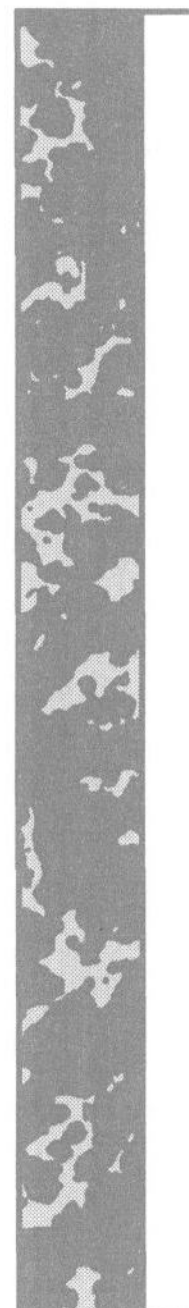

BOX 7–4

Considerations in Evaluating a Health Education Encounter

Formative evaluation:
An evaluation conducted periodically during the presentation to detect a need for immediate modification

Outcome evaluation:
Evaluating the encounter to determine whether stated learning objectives have been met

Process evaluation:
Evaluating the performance of the community health nurse in presenting the materials

DEVELOPING HEALTH EDUCATION PROGRAMS

Health education may involve single presentations to specific individuals, families, or groups. More often, however, health education by community health nurses is structured as an organized ongoing program designed to meet specific community health goals.

GUIDELINES FOR HEALTH EDUCATION PROGRAMS

An Ad Hoc Work Group of the American Public Health Association[16] issued the following guidelines for developing health promotion and health education programs:

1. Health promotion programs should address one or more carefully defined, measurable, and modifiable risk factors that are prevalent among the target group selected.
2. The program should be designed to reflect the special attributes, needs, and preferences of the target group.
3. Programs should present interventions that clearly reduce the identified risk factors and that are appropriate for the group.
4. Programs should implement interventions that make the best possible use of resources.
5. Programs should be specifically designed to allow for evaluation of program effects and operation.

EFFECTIVENESS OF HEALTH EDUCATION PROGRAMS

Health education has been shown to be effective in changing health-related behaviors and to have great promise for creating an epidemiology of health. For example, studies of the effects of school health education programs in 20 states indicated that health education programs for children resulted in increased health knowledge, improved attitudes to health, and healthier behavior.[17]

Similarly, a publicity campaign in Elmira, New York, increased seat belt use from 49 percent to a level of 60 percent 8 months after the campaign, compared to a stable figure of just over 40 percent in another nearby community.[18]

Numerous other instances can be found of the effectiveness of health education in changing health-related behaviors. Health education is an effective tool for the promotion of health. It is also one of the community health nurse's most frequently used tools, whether with individuals, families, or groups of clients. To provide effective health education, however, nurses should engage in systematic planning as described here.

Community health nurses involved in health education programs may find that they need additional sources of information on content or on the health education process. Several such sources of health education information are included in Table 7–2 for those who wish to pursue this topic further.

TABLE 7–2. RESOURCES FOR HEALTH EDUCATION

Agency or Organization	Functions
American Council for Healthful Living 439 Main St. Orange, NJ 07050 (201) 674-7476	Education on STD, aging, adult sexuality
American Physical Fitness Research Institute 654 N. Sepulveda Blvd. Los Angeles, CA 90049 (213) 476-6241	Public education regarding fitness and health promotion
Association for the Advancement of Health Education 1900 Association Dr. Reston, VA 22091 (703) 476-3440	Promotes legislation regarding health education, develops audiovisual and computer software aids
Center for Disease Control Center for Health Promotion and Education 1600 Clifton Rd. Atlanta, GA 30333 (404) 329-2838	Health education information
Center for Medical Consumers and Health Care Information 237 Thompson St. New York, NY 10012 (212) 674-7105	Educational programs on self-care; free library use
Center for Preventive Services 1600 Clifton Rd. Atlanta, GA 30333 (404) 329-1800	Programs on STD, diabetes control, TB control, immunization, dental disease, quarantine
Council on Health Information and Education 250-A Potero St. Santa Cruz, CA 95060 (408) 427-2070	Information on health, fitness, and nutrition; research
Do It Now Foundation P.O. Box 21126 Phoenix, AZ 85036 (602) 257-0797	Information on prescription and OTC drugs, alcohol and illicit drugs; literature
Health Education Resources 4733 Bethesda Ave., Suite 735 Bethesda, MD 20814 (301) 656-3178	Public health education; programs for educators
National Center for Health Education 30 E. 29th St. New York, NY 10016 (212) 689-1886	Provides programs for elementary and secondary school health education
National Health Information Clearinghouse P.O. Box 1133 Washington, DC 20013	Provides referral to federal information resources for health-related topics
U.S. Department of Health and Human Services Office of Health Education and Health Promotion Washington, DC 20203	Provides information for health education

CHAPTER HIGHLIGHTS

- Health education is a process that prepares people to make health-related decisions.
- Precursors to healthy behavior include predisposing, reinforcing, and enabling factors that must be present for healthful behavior to occur.
- The purpose of health education is to facilitate client decision making regarding personal health behaviors, use of health resources, and general health issues.
- Barriers to learning can be internal or external. Internal barriers can be physical, social, or psychological in nature. External barriers can relate to the learning environment or to the learning situation.
- Assessing the client includes identifying the target audience and client characteristics and learning needs. Client characteristics and needs are influenced by levels of maturation and physiologic function.
- Environmental factors influencing clients and learning situations include conditions in the physical, psychological, and social environments.
- Life-style factors such as occupation, consumption patterns, and other health-related behaviors may give rise to needs for health education. Health system factors may also influence health education needs.
- Planning for health education begins with prioritizing learning needs and identifying goals to be accomplished.
- The specific learning tasks involved in goal accomplishment should be identified. The six possible types of learning tasks are information acquisition, concept development, skill development, values awareness, development of communication skills, and development of abilities in problem solving and decision making.
- Learning objectives should be stated behaviorally and should include the behavior to be demonstrated, the level of performance expected, and constraints placed upon performance of the behavior.
- Teaching strategies should be selected on the basis of client characteristics, the type of learning task involved, and resources available in the learning situation. Certain strategies are better suited to specific learning tasks and situations than others.
- Health education materials should be reviewed for their appropriateness to the client audience and the content presented.
- Implementing the health education encounter begins with a focusing event to gain client attention. It concludes with a summary of important points and should be short, specific, and presented in language understood by the client. Important concepts should be presented early and repetition should be used to enhance learning.
- Evaluating the health education encounter involves formative, outcome, and process evaluation.
- Health education has been shown to be effective in changing health-related behaviors and is one of the primary role functions of community health nurses.

Review Questions

1. What are the three types of precursors necessary for healthy behavior? Give an example of each type of precursor. (p. 128)
2. What three types of health-related decisions can be facilitated by health education? Give an example of each type of decision. (p. 129)
3. Describe at least two barriers to health education. Give an example of each and describe how a community health nurse might circumvent them. (p. 130)
4. Identify and describe the steps in the health education process. (p. 130)
5. Describe three types of learning tasks that may be involved in a given health education encounter. Give an example of each. (p. 133)
6. What is a focusing event? What is the purpose of the focusing event? (p. 136)
7. Give two examples of how formative evaluation might be used in a health education encounter. (p. 137)
8. Describe at least four guidelines for developing health education programs. Give examples of programs that might meet these guidelines. (p. 137)

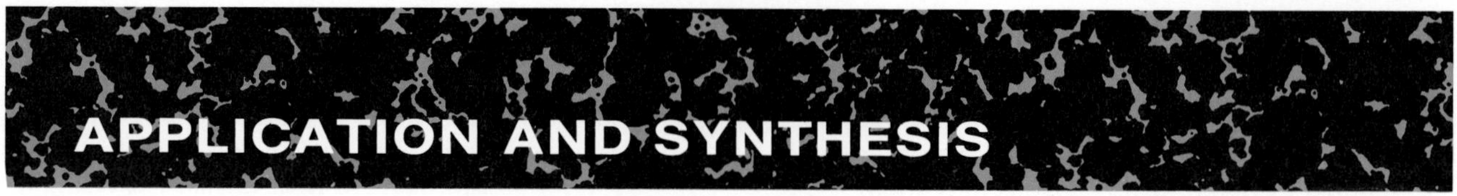

APPLICATION AND SYNTHESIS

You have been asked by a private elementary school principal to give a presentation on AIDS to the Parent/Teacher Group and, afterwards, to make a presentation to students in the seventh and eighth grades on the same topic. The school is run by a nondenominational Christian foundation. Students in the school come from an upper-middle-class neighborhood and most of their parents are professional people. The students are above the national average in all areas of standardized testing, and English is the primary language spoken by both parents and students.

Recently, in a nearby public school, there was a tremendous parental outcry when it became known that one of the children in the school had AIDS. Parental response in that school was such that the parents of the child with AIDS were finally asked to accept a home-study program for their child rather than keep him in school.

So far, similar problems have not occurred in this school, but school officials are interested in avoiding potential problems should a child with AIDS be admitted. Parents of children in this school have already begun to ask about policies related to children with AIDS.

1. Using the Educational Planning and Implementation Guide in Appendix B, document the assessment data that you have available to you. What additional assessment data might you want to obtain? How would you obtain it?
2. What are your goals for the two presentations?
3. What learning tasks are involved in the presentations? Would the learning tasks differ between the student and parent groups? Why or why not?
4. Develop two or three specific objectives that you would expect learners to accomplish as a result of your presentation.
5. Would content presented differ between your two audiences? What would you present and why? Would you sequence content any differently? Why or why not?
6. What teaching strategies might be most effective with each group? What type of teaching aids or materials would you need? Where might you obtain these teaching aids?
7. What type of focusing event would you use for the student group? For the parent group? How would you encourage learner participation in the two groups? Would you use similar or different approaches to stimulating learner participation?
8. What key points would you be sure to include in the summary of your presentation? Would these be the same or different for the two groups of learners?
9. How would you conduct formative evaluation during your presentation? How would you evaluate the presentation in terms of client outcomes and your performance?

REFERENCES

1. Green, L. W. (1984). Health education models. In J. D. Matarazzo, S. M. Weiss, J. A. Herd, N. E. Miller, & M. A. Weiss (Eds.), *Behavioral health: A handbook of health enhancement and disease prevention*. New York: Wiley.
2. Greenberg, J. S. (1989). *Health education: Learner-centered instructional strategies*. Dubuque, IA: Wm. C. Brown.
3. Green, L. W., Kreuter, M. H., Deeds, S. G., & Partridge, K. B. (1980). *Health education planning: A diagnostic approach*. Palo Alto, CA: Mayfield.
4. Dalis, G. T., & Strasser, B. B. (1977). *Teaching strategies for values awareness and decision making in health education*. London: Charles B. Stack.
5. Flynn, J. M. (1988). The teaching and learning process. In J. M. Flynn, & P. B. Heffron (Eds.), *Nursing: From concept to practice* (2nd ed.) (pp. 261–276). Norwalk, CT: Appleton & Lange.
6. DiFlorio, I. A., & Duncan, P. A. (1986). Design for successful patient teaching. *MCN, 11*, 246–249.
7. Evans, L. K. (1980). Health education from a group perspective. *Topics in Clinical Nursing, 2*(2), 45–55.
8. Redican, K., Olsen, L. K., & Baffi, C. R. (1986). *Organization of school health programs*. New York: Macmillan.
9. Frantz, R. A. (1980). Selecting media for patient education. *Topics in Clinical Nursing, 2*(2), 77–83.
10. Pohl, M. L. (1981). *The teaching function of the nursing practitioner* (4th ed.). Dubuque, IA: Wm. C. Brown.
11. Cooper, S. S. (1982a). Methods of teaching—revisited: The demonstration. *The Journal of Continuing Education in Nursing, 13*(3), 44–45.
12. Cooper, S. S. (1982b). Methods of teaching—revisited: The lecture. *The Journal of Continuing Education in Nursing, 13*(4), 39–41.
13. Swanson, J. M., Forrest, K., Ledbelter C., *et al.* (1990). Readability of commercial and generic contraceptive instructions. *Image: The Journal of Nursing Scholarship, 22*(2), 96–100.
14. Peterson, J., & Marin, G. (1988). Issues in the prevention of AIDS among black and Hispanic men. *American Psychologist, 43*, 871–877.
15. Miller, A. (1985). When is the time ripe for teaching? *American Journal of Nursing, 85*, 801–804.
16. Ad Hoc Work Group of the American Public Health Association. (1987). Criteria for the development of health promotion and education programs. *American Journal of Public Health, 77*, 89–91.
17. The effectiveness of school health education. (1986). *MMWR, 35*, 593.
18. Williams, A. F., Preusser, D. F., Blomberg, R. D., & Lund, A. K. (1987). Seat belt use law enforcement and publicity in Elmira, New York: A reminder campaign. *American Journal of Public Health, 77*, 1450–1451.

RECOMMENDED READINGS

Close, A. (1988). Patient education: A literature review. *Journal of Advanced Nursing 13*, 203–213.

Provides a review of recent literature on patient education. Discusses the need for patient education, the role of nurses as educators, barriers to education, and some of the problems encountered in patient education.

Cooper, S. S. (1980–1982). Methods of teaching—revisited. *The Journal of Continuing Education in Nursing, 11–13.*

A series of monthly articles reviewing various teaching strategies. Describes the advantages and appropriate use of strategies addressed as well as other pertinent information regarding specific teaching strategies.

Gentine, M. (1980). Methods of teaching—revisited: Self-learning packages. *The Journal of Continuing Education in Nursing, 11*(3), 57–58.

Discusses the use of self-learning packages as a teaching strategy.

Hinthorne, R. (1980). Methods of teaching—revisited: Self-instructional modules. *The Journal of Continuing Education in Nursing, 11*(4), 37–39.

Examines the use of self-instructional modules as a teaching strategy.

Hochbaum, G. M. (1980). Patient counseling vs. patient teaching. *Topics in Clinical Nursing, 2*(2), 1–7.

Differentiates between counseling and education and factors contributing to the need for client education by nurses. Describes barriers other than knowledge deficit that deter compliance with health instructions and strategies for overcoming these barriers.

Pohl, M. L. (1981). *The teaching function of the nursing practitioner* (4th ed.). Dubuque, IA: Wm. C. Brown.

Provides a sound introduction to principles of teaching and learning and the nurse's role in health education.

Redman, B. (1990). *Patient teaching in nursing*. St. Louis: C. V. Mosby.

An introduction to the teaching role in nursing. Presents an overview of teaching and learning and strategies for implementing health education.

Wise, P. S. Y. (1980). Methods of teaching—revisited: Character play and role play. *The Journal of Continuing Education in Nursing, 11*(1), 37–38.

Discusses the use of role-play as a teaching strategy in education.

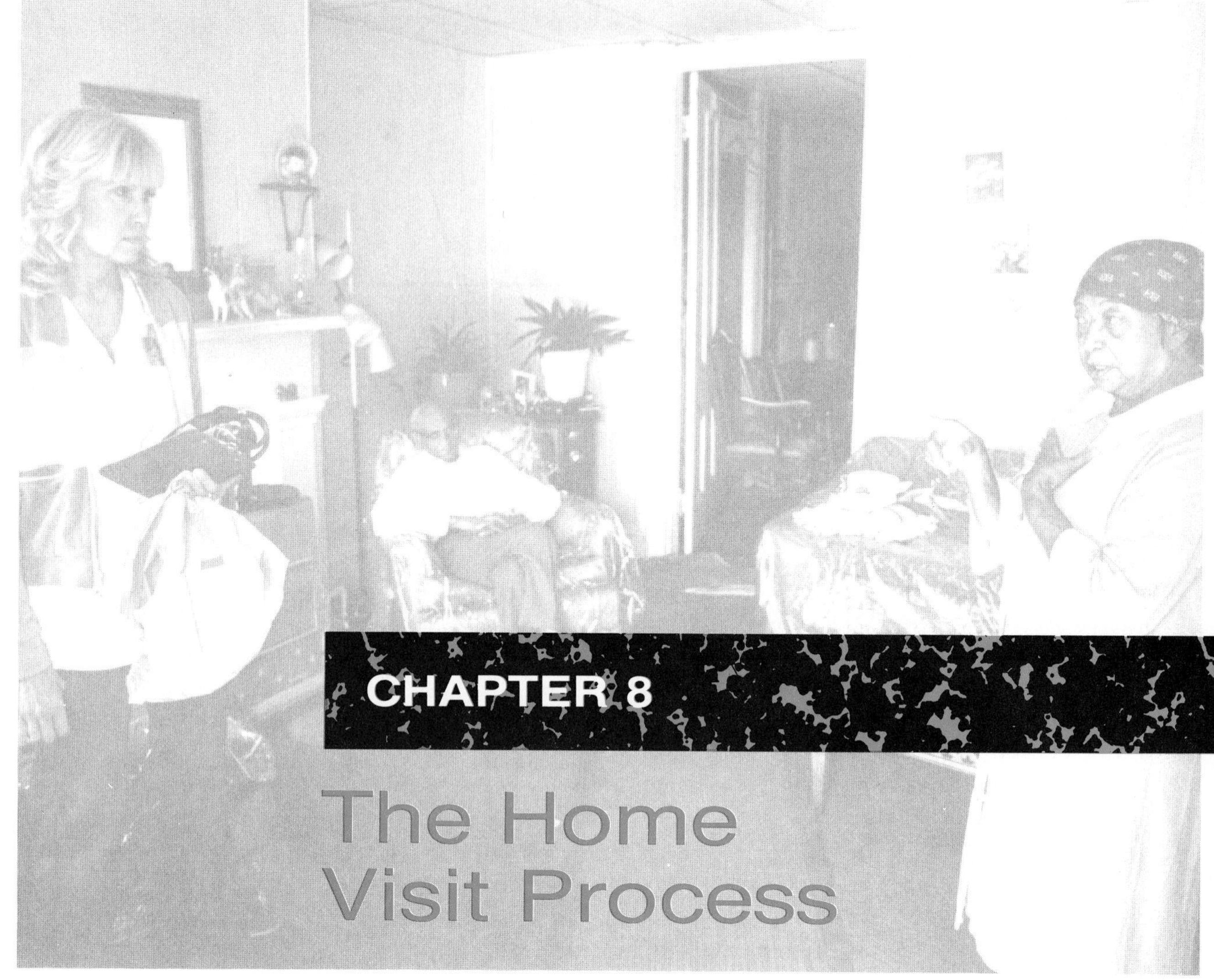

CHAPTER 8

The Home Visit Process

KEY TERMS

distractions
home visit
preparatory assessment

Historic photographs of community health nurses often show them caring for clients in their homes. In fact, home care was the initial focus of community health nursing.[1] Home visits have been shown to be an effective way to provide care for a diversity of clients[2–6] and continue to be a viable mode of practice for community health nurses.

Both community health nurses and home health nurses may visit client's homes. Some, but not all, home health nurses may be community health nurses as well. The principal distinction between the two specialties is the client focus. Only those nurses whose primary concern is the health of groups of people are community health nurses. The primary concern of those home health nurses who are not community health nurses is the health of individual clients. The second distinction between community health nurses and home health nurses is their health-care emphasis. Community health nurses are primarily concerned with health promotion and illness prevention; they provide care for existing illness as a lesser priority. Home health nurses, on the other hand, enter the home for the purpose of providing care for a specific illness.[7] Home health nursing will be addressed in greater detail in Chapter 25, Care of Clients in the Home Setting. Whether the nurse enters a client's home for purposes of health promotion or treatment of illness, that person uses the home visit process as an avenue to provide care. That process is the subject of this chapter.

LEARNING OBJECTIVES

After reading this chapter you should be able to:

- Differentiate between home visits by community health nurses and those by home health nurses in terms of client focus and health-care emphasis.
- Describe at least three advantages of a home visit as a means of providing nursing care.
- Identify at least four aspects of planning for a home visit.
- Describe at least four tasks in implementing a home visit.
- Identify three types of potential distractions during a home visit.
- Discuss the need for both long-term and short-term evaluative criteria for the effectiveness of a home visit.

A HOME VISIT

A home visit by a nurse is different from a social visit that might be made by friends or relatives. A ***home visit*** is a formal call by a nurse on a client at the client's place of residence for the purpose of providing nursing care. Home visits also differ from "technical visits" that take place in the home. Home visits are made by professionals for the purpose of providing health care; technical visits are made by professionals or nonprofessionals for purposes of technical care. A community health nurse, for example, makes a home visit, whereas a homemaker aide, physical therapist, or home health nurse makes a technical visit. The visit by the community health nurse involves consideration of all of the client's health needs—physical, psychological, and social. A technical visit, on the other hand, is made for the purpose of performing a specific activity such as changing a dressing, providing range-of-motion exercises, administering intravenous medications, and so on. Such technical activities might also be performed by the community health nurse, but only as one aspect of the home visit.

ADVANTAGES OF HOME VISITS

Why do community health nurses make home visits? It would seem to be more cost-effective for clients to come to the nurse. More clients might be seen in a given period if the nurse did not have to consider travel time or time wasted being lost in unfamiliar areas. What is there about a home visit that outweighs these obvious disadvantages? One very practical consideration is the client's ability to go elsewhere. Some clients are homebound or even bedfast and cannot come to the nurse. Others have no means of transportation available to them.

There are, however, other more important considerations in choosing to use home visits as a means of delivering care. A home visit allows the nurse to see firsthand the interplay of factors influencing the client's health status.[8] Also, a home visit provides an opportunity for monitoring, on a continuing basis, the effectiveness of nursing interventions in solving client problems. What the client may do or say in the hospital or clinic setting may or may not reflect what occurs at home. For example, the client may tell the nurse in clinic that he or she is adhering to a low-sodium diet. If the nurse visits at home, however, and finds the client munching potato chips, it is readily apparent that dietary instruction has not been as effective as desired.

Another advantage to the home visit is the client's greater autonomy. In clinic or hospital settings, the client enters the health professional's domain and is more or less constrained by the rules that apply there. In a home visit, on the other hand, the nurse is in the client's environment. The client is likely to be more at ease in familiar surroundings and may be more open to suggested interventions, particularly if the interventions are tailored to the client's specific situation.[9]

A home visit also provides the nurse with a better picture of possible resources and hazards that can influence the client's health. The interaction of family members during the visit might suggest the extent of the client's support network and the ability of family members to provide care.[9] Similarly, detecting potential health hazards in the client's home, such as seeing a number of loose throw rugs in the home of an older client, can provide impetus for health education to promote physical safety.

Seeing the client in the home setting also affords the nurse the opportunity to assess accurately the client's ability to perform activities of daily living. In addition, the costs of care provided in the home have been shown to be less expensive than health care provided in institutional settings in some instances. Finally, frequent contact in the client's home may allow the nurse to identify minor health changes for which clients would not seek help and to act to prevent major problems later on.[9]

THE EPIDEMIOLOGIC PREVENTION PROCESS MODEL AND HOME VISITS

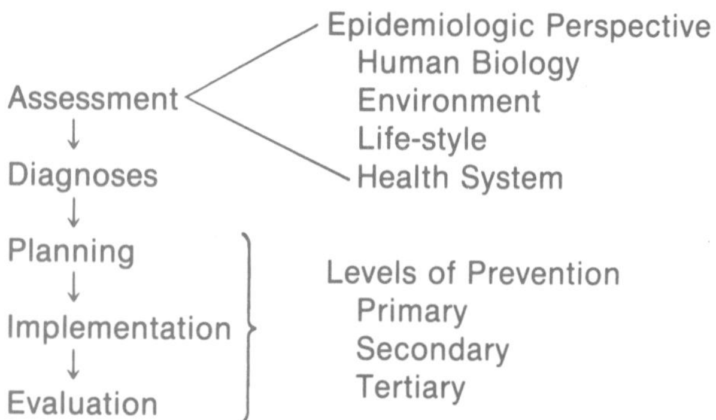

Although home visits have some distinct advantages over care provided in other settings, to be effective, home visits must be focused, purposeful events. Research has demonstrated that home visits with a specific purpose can positively influence client health.[6] Like any other nursing intervention, the home visit should be a planned event with specified goals and objectives.[2] The epidemiologic prevention process model provides a framework for systematically organizing the home visit to make it an effective nursing intervention.

INITIATING THE HOME VISIT

Home visits by community health nurses are initiated for a variety of reasons. Many times the nurse receives a request for a visit from another health-care provider or agency. Reasons for such requests include health-care needs related to specific health problems or needs for health-promotive services. For example, many hospital obstetrical units refer all first-time mothers for home visits by community health nurses in order to provide assistance in parenting and to promote a successful postpartum course and adjustment to parenthood. Or, a physician might request a home visit to educate a hypertensive client about prescribed medications.

Home visits might also be initiated by clients themselves. For example, a mother concerned about her child's recurrent nightmares may call and request a home visit by a community health nurse. Friends and family might also initiate a home visit. For instance, a neighbor might inform the nurse that he or she thinks the children next door are being abused. Or, a mother may request a home visit to help her daughter deal with the loss of a child. Finally, the community health nurse may initiate a home visit. For instance, the nurse might note that a child seen in the well-child clinic is developmentally delayed and decide to visit the home to see if there are environmental factors contributing to the delayed development.

PREPARATORY ASSESSMENT

Before the home visit the nurse conducts a ***preparatory assessment*** to review existing information about the client and his or her situation. Previously acquired client data should be reviewed and client health status defined. If the client is already known to the nurse or the agency, there is a certain amount of data available in agency records, notes from previous visits, and so on. The nurse uses such data to refresh his or her memory regarding the client's health status.

If the client is new to service, data available will most probably be limited to that received with the request for services. In such a case, the nurse will need to look for general cues that suggest client strengths and potential problems. For example, if the home visit is requested for follow-up on a newborn and his adolescent mother, the nurse knows that infant feeding, sleep patterns, maternal knowledge of child care, bonding, involution, maternal coping abilities, and family planning are areas that may need to be addressed with this family. Similarly, if the referral is for an elderly woman with uncontrolled hypertension, the nurse will identify areas related to diet, medication, safety, exercise, and so on, for investigation during the visit.

All aspects of the client's life should be reviewed to detect strengths, existing problems, and potential problems that may need to be addressed during the visit. Using Dever's epidemiologic perspective as a framework, the nurse would review available information on human biological, environmental, lifestyle, and health system factors that influence the client's health status. By assessing client factors in each of these areas, the nurse will enter the client's residence better prepared to deal with the wide variety of client needs likely to be encountered.

HUMAN BIOLOGY

A client's age and race will provide clues to health needs that might be encountered during the home visit. For example, if the client is a child, the nurse may want to assess the child's development; assessing for constipation is appropriate for both children and elderly clients. Black and other minority clients usually have less access to health care and, consequently, more health problems are apt to be encountered during the home visits.

One area of concern in any home visit is the development of the client and other family members. Are developmental tasks being accomplished? Is there evidence of developmental lag? What are possible factors involved in the lag? Table 8–1 summarizes functional, interpersonal, and psychosocial developmental tasks to be accomplished at particular stages of development. Functional tasks reflect the development of physical abilities that allow one to perform the functions and activities of everyday life. Interpersonal tasks relate to the development of abilities to interact effectively with others, and psychosocial tasks reflect development of a personal self and abilities to function effectively in the social environment.

The nurse would assess each member of the household with respect to accomplishment of expected developmental tasks and would identify needs for health promotion or problem resolution related to development. For example, if there is a toddler present in the home, the nurse might want to focus on anticipatory guidance for toilet training or the diminished appetite common in this age group. Or, if the home includes older family members, attention may be given to the older person's adjustment to retire-

TABLE 8–1. LIFE-STAGE-RELATED FUNCTIONAL, INTERPERSONAL, AND PSYCHOSOCIAL DEVELOPMENTAL TASKS

Life Stage	Functional Tasks	Interpersonal Tasks	Psychosocial Tasks
Infant (0–1 yr)	• Achieve physiologic equilibrium • Achieve increased wakefulness • Display neurologic responses appropriate to age • Vocalize • Localize sound • Develop motor skills • Develop beginning mobility	• Develop self-awareness and recognition of others • Develop feelings of trust and affection • Develop rudimentary social interactions • Begin to adjust to expectations of others • Indicate needs and wishes • Develop and resolve stranger anxiety • Begin to say few words	• Develop awareness of social environment • Understand and control physical world via exploration
Young child (2–6 yrs)	• Develop increased physical independence • Become toilet-trained • Refine motor skills • Dress self with decreasing supervision • Feed self	• Give and share affection • Interact increasingly with age-mates • Increase language use • Develop team abilities • Express emotion in healthy ways • Increase communication with a wider variety of people	• Follow directions • Learn to obey without supervision • Identify with male/female role models • Display increasing concern for others • Imitate adult behavior • Develop a routine • Function as a family member • Display initiative tempered by conscience • Lay foundations for a philosophy of life
School-age child (6–12 yrs)	• Increase motor skills • Display independence in physical hygiene • Increase neuromuscular strength	• Converse with peers and adults • Display increased need for privacy • Form peer friendships • Learn to belong • Display increased interaction with same-sex peers • Verbalize and handle emotions effectively	• Learn math, reading, writing skills, etc. • Seek heroes and role models • Begin separation from family • Accept responsibility at home • Develop a sense of humor • Give increasing attention to personal appearance • Become more self-directed in learning • Make logical decisions with help • Be influenced more by peers and less by family • Seek socially acceptable ways of earning money and saving • Develop positive attitudes to self and others and differences noted
Adolescent (13–18 yrs)	• Develop secondary sex characteristics • Develop sexual capabilities • Learn to handle a changing body	• Learn appropriate role in heterosexual relationships • Develop mutual affectional bonds with someone of opposite sex • Verbalize value conflict	• Accept self • Display strong sexual identification • Prepare self as a responsible citizen • Display increased influence by peers, then increased self-direction • Become aware of world and national events • Develop abilities to generate alternatives • Take increased financial responsibility • Increase independence from parents • Develop adult value set

(continued)

TABLE 8–1. (*Continued*)

Life Stage	Functional Tasks	Interpersonal Tasks	Psychosocial Tasks
Young adult	• Establish healthy routines of eating, rest, exercise, etc.	• Find means to express love outside sexual activity • Establish an intimate relationship	• Become financially independent • Establish a vocation • Establish and manage a home • Decide on having a family • Establish a philosophy of life and value system • Become an involved citizen • Learn a husband/wife role
Middle adult	• Maintain healthy routines • Learn new motor skills as needed for leisure and other pursuits • Accept and adjust to bodily changes of middle age	• Develop interdependence with others • Establish new ways of relating to children and grandchildren • Cultivate and maintain friendships	• Assist children to be independent • Deal with aging parents • Develop a reasonable balance of activities • Carry a socially adequate role • Develop leisure pursuits
Older adult	• Accept and adjust to decreased mobility • Adapt interests to reduced strength and energy • Develop ways to deal with physical illness and disability as needed	• Accept help graciously • Learn new affectional roles with children and grandchildren • Establish and maintain friendships • Be a good companion for an aging spouse	• Establish satisfactory living arrangements • Adjust to retirement • Adjust to reduced income • Adjust to loss of spouse and friends • Maintain social interaction • Maintain integrity and values despite disappointment • Prepare for death

ment, decreased mobility, income reduction, and so on.

The nurse will also consider information about the physiologic function of the client and other family members. Does the mother of a handicapped youngster have asthma? How has the child's problem affected the mother's health status? Does the older client have arthritis? What does this mean in terms of abilities to perform activities of daily living? Does someone in the family have other chronic health problems that may affect the health status of the client or the family? Are client or family members taking any medication? What effect, if any, does medication have on ability to function? For example, the child who takes antihistamine for allergies may exhibit poor school performance due to drowsiness.

Normal physiologic states may also give rise to a need for nursing intervention. If the client is pregnant, for example, the nurse will want to address normal physiologic changes in pregnancy, adequate nutrition, signs of impending labor, and so on.

Another consideration to be made by the nurse is the possible interplay between maturation and physiologic function. For example, it may be more difficult for an adolescent with diabetes to adhere to a diabetic diet than an older or younger client because of the pressure to conform to peer group norms, including dietary norms. Similarly, pregnancy will pose more of a risk for an adolescent or a middle-aged woman than for a young adult woman.

ENVIRONMENT

Knowledge of the client's environment—physical, psychological, and social—can provide the nurse with clues to health needs that may be encountered in the course of a home visit.

Physical Environment

Where does the client live? Is the neighborhood safe? Are there adequate services and facilities close to the client's home? For the elderly client, age, distance to shopping facilities, and lack of transportation may contribute to poor nutrition because of diminished opportunity to obtain food.

What is the condition of housing in the client's neighborhood? Is this likely to contribute to health hazards for the individual client or family members? For example, young children in a family living in an older neighborhood may be at risk for lead poisoning from lead-based paint used on older dwellings. Or, if an older client lives in an apartment, he or she may have to deal with stairs or other impediments to mobility.

Review of the client's record prior to the home visit might provide information about known safety hazards in the home. Is the home of a family with young children child-proofed? Are there loose rugs in the home of an elderly client? Community health nurses may want to complete the *home safety assessment* guides included in Appendix C when there are children or older persons living in the home the nurse plans to visit.

Psychological Environment

Knowledge of the client's psychological environment can also help to identify potential health problems. What was the client's cognitive and emotional status on previous visits? Does the client or any member of the family have a history of substance abuse or mental illness? In recent years, for example, community health nurses have received increasing numbers of requests for home visits to newborns with fetal exposure to drugs. Information regarding past maternal drug use included in the referral alerts the nurse to assess carefully the infant's development and look for evidence of neglect if the mother continues drug use.

Family dynamics also contribute to a positive or negative psychological environment. What is known about family interaction patterns? Coping skills? Is there a history of violence within the family? If the client is debilitated and requires care by family members, what emotional support is available for caretakers? Is respite care available if needed? The nurse would also look for evidence of client and family strengths. Do extended family members serve as a support system for the client?

Social Environment

Knowledge of the client's social environment assists the nurse to identify factors contributing to client health status as well as factors that will influence nursing intervention. Areas for consideration include the client's educational level, financial status, and social network. Other considerations include the influence of religious beliefs on the client's health and clients' access to transportation. Some of the considerations in these areas are summarized in Table 8–2.

LIFE-STYLE

Life-style factors to be considered include the employment status and occupation of family members, nutrition and other consumption patterns, recreation, and health practices. What are the occupations of client and family members? How do these occupations influence health?

The client record may also provide information about family nutritional practices. Are these appropriate to the growth and development needs of family members? Other considerations related to consumption patterns include the presence or absence of substance abuse problems and the influence of such problems on health.

One area of assessment that is particularly important in relation to a home visit is a functional assessment.[9] Areas to be addressed in a functional assessment include client abilities to meet needs related to mobility, cognition, eating, toileting, dressing, hygiene, shopping, cooking, and managing money. All of these areas influence client life-style. Some of the specific considerations related to life-style assessment prior to a home visit are presented in Table 8–3.

TABLE 8–2. SOME CONSIDERATIONS IN ASSESSING THE SOCIAL ENVIRONMENT

Area	Considerations
Education	• What is the client's educational level? • What is the extent of the client's health knowledge? • How does the client's educational level affect health?
Financial status	• What is the client's usual income? • Is the client's income sufficient to meet needs? • What is the client's source of income? • How does the client finance health care?
Social network	• With whom does the client interact on a regular basis? • Do these persons form a social support network for the client? • How effective is the client's social support network in assisting the client to meet his or her needs? • What are the attitudes of significant others to health and health care? • What influence do the attitudes of significant others have on the client's health?
Religion	• Does the client have a particular religious affiliation? • Does religion provide an emotional support or outlet for the client? • What influence do religious beliefs and practices have on the client's health?

TABLE 8–3. SOME CONSIDERATIONS IN ASSESSING LIFE-STYLE INFLUENCES ON HEALTH

Area of Influence	Considerations
Employment and occupation	• Is the client or other family member employed? • What kind of occupation does the client have? • Does client or family member occupation pose any health hazards? • Does employment contribute to any other health needs (for example, is there a need for child care)?
Nutrition	• What is the client's usual dietary pattern? • Does the client obtain adequate nutrition from his or her typical diet? • How are foods usually prepared? • What is the client's typical meal pattern?
Use of other substances	• Does the client drink alcohol? If yes, how much? • What medications does the client use? Are they appropriate? • Is there evidence of abuse of medications? • How much caffeine does the client consume? • Does the client smoke? If yes, how much?
Exercise	• How often does the client exercise? • Does exercise or lack of it pose any health risks? • In what forms of exercise does the client engage?
Use of safety devices	• Does the client consistently use seat belts? • Does the client use hearing protection when appropriate?
Leisure activities	• What type of leisure activities does the client pursue? • Do leisure activities pose any health risks?

HEALTH SYSTEM

Information about client interaction with the health-care system will also assist the community health nurse to prepare for an effective home visit. Where does the client/family usually receive health care? Is access to care limited by the client's financial status or lack of health insurance? What health-care providers are working with the client? Is there any coordination between provider activities?

How does the client/family interact with health-care professionals? Are they open to recommendations? Are they hostile or suspicious of the motives of providers? This and other information will assist the nurse to plan an approach to the client that will lead to rapport and a therapeutic relationship.

DIAGNOSTIC REASONING AND THE HOME VISIT

Based on the data available in the preparatory assessment, the nurse will make nursing diagnoses related to health conditions to be addressed during the home visit. These diagnoses may be either positive or problem-focused nursing diagnoses.

The process used is the diagnostic reasoning process discussed in Chapter 5, The Nursing Process. The nurse examines data available and develops diagnostic hypotheses that seem to explain the data. Hypothesis evaluation will take place when the nurse actually makes the home visit and obtains additional data to confirm or disconfirm the diagnostic hypotheses. The diagnostic hypotheses generated from the preparatory assessment, however, give the nurse some direction for planning nursing interventions to be performed during the home visit.

Positive nursing diagnoses will reflect client strengths evidenced in the preparatory assessment. For example, available data may indicate "effective coping with the demands imposed by a handicapped child due to a strong family support system." This diagnosis suggests that the nurse will reinforce family support as a factor contributing to effective coping.

Problem-focused nursing diagnoses may reflect actual problems for which there is evidence in the preparatory assessment data or potential problems. For example, an existing problem of "ineffective contraceptive use due to inadequate knowledge of contraceptive methods" may have been documented on a previous home visit. Unless there is also an indication that this problem has been resolved, the nurse will probably address it during the subsequent home visit. Preparatory assessment data may suggest potential problems as well. For instance, the request for services might indicate that the client's husband is in the Navy and is due to leave on extended sea duty. This information would suggest a nursing diagnosis of "potential for ineffective coping due to loss of spousal assistance."

Nursing diagnoses might also reflect the need for health-promotive services. For example, there will soon be a "need for routine immunizations" for a newborn child. Similarly, the mother has a "need for postpartum follow-up due to recent delivery."

PLANNING THE VISIT

Based on the preparatory assessment, the community health nurse makes plans for a home visit to address the health needs most likely to be present in the situation. Tasks to be accomplished in planning for the visit include reviewing previous interventions, prioritizing client needs, developing goals and objectives for care, and consideration of client acceptance and timing. Other tasks of this stage include delineating activities needed to meet client needs, obtaining needed materials, and planning for evaluation.

REVIEW OF PREVIOUS INTERVENTIONS

The first step in planning is to review any previous interventions related to client health needs and the efficacy of those interventions. This information allows the nurse to eliminate interventions that have been unsuccessful in the past and to identify interventions that have worked.

PRIORITIZING CLIENT NEEDS

The next task is to give priority to identified client needs. Client care needs may be prioritized on the basis of their potential to threaten the client's health, the degree to which they concern the client, or according to their ease of solution (see Chapter 5 for a more complete discussion of criteria for prioritizing health needs). It is often impossible to address all of the client's health problems in a single visit, so the nurse must decide which needs require immediate attention. For example, if the wife has been admitted to an alcohol treatment center and there is no one to care for the children while the father works, provision of child care and dealing with the children's feelings about the mother's absence may be the only things that can be accomplished on the initial visit. Other problems, such as poor nutritional habits and need for immunizations for the toddler, can be deferred until a later visit.

DEVELOPING GOALS AND OBJECTIVES

After determining which client needs will be addressed in the forthcoming visit, the nurse develops goals and objectives related to each area of need. Goals are generally stated expectations, whereas objectives are more specific. Using the previous example, the nurse's goal might be to enable the family to function adequately in the mother's absence. In this instance, an objective might be that adequate child care will be obtained so the father can return to work.

The health-care needs that will be addressed during a home visit may reflect the primary, secondary, or tertiary levels of prevention. When health-care needs occur in the realm of primary prevention, goals and objectives will reflect positive health states or absence of specific health problems as expected outcomes of care. For example, a goal for primary prevention might be "development of effective parenting skills." A related objective might be that the client "will display effective communication skills in relating to children."

Goals and objectives related to needs for secondary prevention would focus on alleviation of specific problems. For example, a goal for a hypertensive client might be "effective control of elevated blood pressure," while the related objective might be a blood pressure that is "consistently below 140/90." Similarly, goals and objectives for tertiary prevention would reflect client achievement of a prior level of function or prevention of recurrence of a health problem.

CONSIDERATIONS OF ACCEPTANCE AND TIMING

In planning a home visit, the nurse should consider the client's readiness to accept intervention as well as the timing of the visit and introduction of intervention. The nurse may find, for example, that a relatively minor problem with which the client is preoccupied must be addressed before the client is willing to deal with other health needs.

The nurse must also consider the degree of dependence or independence required by specific clients. Some clients may need initially to be very dependent on the nurse. For example, the nurse may need to make a counseling appointment for depressed clients who do not have sufficient energy to make the appointment for themselves. Other clients will be able to function more independently with only the support of the nurse.

Timing is another important consideration in planning an effective home visit. If the visit interferes with other activities important to the client, the client may not be as open to the visit as would otherwise be the case. Other activities that compete with a home visit for the client's attention might be the visit of a friend, an upcoming doctor's appointment, getting the children ready for an outing, or even something as mundane as a favorite soap opera. Prescheduling or rescheduling home visits can make the visit a more effective intervention if something else is interfering.

Timing also relates to the degree of rapport established between client and nurse. Clients need time to develop trust in the nurse before intimate issues can be addressed. For example, a pregnant adolescent may feel too uncomfortable and threatened by the nurse during early visits to admit to prior drug use and ask about its effects on the baby. The nurse should judge the appropriateness of the timing in bringing up intimate issues for discussion and wait, if possible, until there is an established rapport with the client.

DELINEATING NURSING ACTIVITIES

The next aspect of planning for the home visit is the planning of specific nursing activities for each nursing diagnosis to be addressed. The activities planned will reflect the nurse's assessment of health-care needs and the factors influencing them. For example, referral to a Head Start program may provide assistance with child care, but only if the children involved are of the right ages. If the youngsters are of school age, the appropriate nursing intervention might be to help the father explore the possibility of an afterschool program, if one is available, or having the children go home with the parents of a friend until the father can pick them up after work.

Nursing activities can focus on both health promotion and resolution of health-related problems. For example, the community health nurse might provide the parents of a toddler with anticipatory guidance regarding toilet training or assist parents to discuss sexuality with their preteen daughter. Other positive interventions might focus on providing adequate nutrition for a young child or promoting a healthy pregnancy for the pregnant female.

Specific interventions employed by the nurse can include referral, education, technical procedures, and so on. For example, the nurse might refer a family to social services for financial assistance, teach a mother about appropriate nutrition for the family, or check a hypertensive client's blood pressure. The actions selected should be geared to achieving the goals and objectives established while taking into account the constraints and supports in the individual client situation.

OBTAINING NECESSARY MATERIALS

One aspect of planning the home visit that does not apply to many of the other processes discussed in this unit is obtaining materials and supplies that may be needed to implement planned interventions. Because the nurse is going to be in the client's home, one cannot assume that necessary supplies will be available there. If the nurse plans to engage in nutrition education, he or she might want to leave a selection of pamphlets with the client to reinforce teaching. If planned activities involve weighing a premature infant, the nurse will want to take along a scale.

Equipment and supplies may also be needed for other procedures such as dressing changes, catheterizations, injections, blood pressure checks, and so on. Because the nurse frequently does a physical assessment of one or more clients, additional equipment such as a stethoscope, percussion hammer, tongue blade, flashlight, otophthalmoscope, and so on, will need to be obtained prior to setting out for the visit.

PLANNING FOR EVALUATION

As with every other process employed by community health nurses, the planning phase of the home visit process concludes with plans for evaluation. The nurse will determine criteria to be used to evaluate the effectiveness of the home visit. Criteria for evaluating client outcomes are derived from the objectives developed for the visit. Because the outcome of nursing interventions undertaken during a home visit may not be immediately apparent, the nurse will need to develop both long-term and short-term evaluative criteria. Short-term criteria are likely to be based on client response to interventions. If, for example, the nurse makes a referral for immunizations, the mother cannot follow through on the referral and receive immunizations on the spot. However, the nurse can evaluate the mother's response to the referral. Does the mother seem interested? Does she indicate that she will follow through on the referral? On subsequent visits, the nurse would employ long-term outcome criteria to evaluate the effects of interventions. In this instance, criteria would include whether the client had her child immunized.

Outcome evaluation will address the level of prevention of nursing interventions. Evaluative criteria for primary preventive measures, for instance, would reflect health promotion or the absence of specific health problems. For example, criteria for interventions to foster immunity to childhood diseases would include whether immunizations were obtained and the presence or absence of immunizable diseases such as measles. If the client develops measles, primary prevention of this disease obviously was not effective.

Evaluation of secondary preventive measures would focus on the degree to which an existing problem has been resolved. For example, a client's hypertension may have been uncontrolled because of poor medication compliance. Evaluative criteria in this instance would include the degree of compliance achieved and the client's blood pressure measurements. Criteria to evaluate tertiary preventive measures would reflect the degree to which a client has regained a prior level of health or the prevention of recurrent health problems. For example, have passive range-of-motion exercises helped a client recovering from a broken arm to regain strength and mobility?

Or, has parenting education by the nurse prevented further episodes of child abuse in an abusive family?

The nurse will also want to develop criteria to evaluate implementation of the planned home visit. For example, was the nurse adequately prepared to address the health-care needs encountered during the visit? Were the appropriate supplies available for implementing planned interventions? And so on.

IMPLEMENTING THE PLANNED VISIT

The next step in the home visit process is conducting the visit itself. Several tasks are involved in implementing the planned visit. These include validating the health needs and diagnoses identified in the preparatory assessment, identifying additional needs, modifying the intervention plan as needed, performing nursing interventions, and dealing with distractions.

VALIDATING ASSESSMENT AND DIAGNOSES

The first task in implementing the home visit is to validate the accuracy of the preparatory assessment. Problems identified from the available data may or may not exist when the nurse actually enters the home. For example, the nurse may find that the family's poor diet is not the result of lack of knowledge about nutrition, but stems from a lack of money to purchase nutritious foods. Or the nurse may find that what appeared to nurses on the postpartum unit to be poor maternal-infant bonding was not actually the case. Similarly, the nurse may discover that expected strengths or positive nursing diagnoses do not accurately reflect the client's actual health status. For example, a mother who appeared to be coping effectively with her child's handicap may really have been exhibiting denial of the condition.

IDENTIFYING ADDITIONAL NEEDS

During the visit the nurse will also collect additional data related to human biology, environment, lifestyle, and health system factors to identify additional health-care needs. For example, when the nurse arrives to visit a new mother and her infant son, he or she may find that the client's father has recently had a heart attack and been taken to the hospital. The client may be much more in need of assistance in finding child care for her new baby so she can spend time at the hospital than in discussing child care and postpartum concerns. Or, the nurse may find that, in addition to having a new baby, the client's husband is out of work and the 12-year-old has been skipping school.

MODIFYING THE PLAN OF CARE

Based on what the nurse finds in the course of the home visit, the initial plan of care may need to be modified. The nurse will share with the client the initial goals established for addressing health needs identified in the preparatory assessment, as well as additional problems identified, and engage in mutual goal setting or goal revision. In doing this, the nurse might find a need to restructure priorities based on new data and client input. For instance, if the 2-year-old has cut her arm and is bleeding profusely when the nurse arrives, this problem will take precedence over the nurse's plan to discuss with the mother the potential for sibling rivalry. In other words, the nurse can either implement interventions as planned or modify the plan as the client situation dictates.

PERFORMING NURSING INTERVENTIONS

Once the plan of care has been modified as needed, the nurse performs whatever nursing interventions are warranted by the client situation. As noted earlier, these activities may include primary, secondary, and tertiary preventive measures. For example, the nurse working with a new mother might discuss parenting skills as a means of preventing child abuse (primary prevention), give the mother suggestions for dealing with the infant's spitting up (secondary prevention), and discuss options for contraception to prevent a subsequent pregnancy (tertiary prevention).

Any or all of the three levels can be emphasized depending upon the situation encountered. For example, if the mother is inexperienced and concerned about child-care skills in feeding, bathing, parenting, and so forth, the emphasis would be on primary prevention. Conversely, if the nurse arrives to find a baby screaming with gas pains, emphasis will be placed on making the infant more comfortable and relieving the mother's anxiety. Once this has been accomplished, the nurse can then focus on suggestions to prevent a recurrence of the problem.

DEALING WITH DISTRACTIONS

One important consideration in implementing a home visit is dealing with distractions. ***Distractions*** are generally of three types: environmental, behavioral, and nurse-initiated.[10] Environmental distractions arise from both the physical and social environments and may include background noise, crowded surroundings, and interruptions by other family members or outsiders. The occurrence of such distractions during the home visit can give the nurse a clear picture of the client's environment and the way in which the client and family interact among themselves and with others. For example, if mother and child are continually yelling at one another during the visit, this suggests the existence of family communication problems. On the other hand, positive interactions between a mother and her young child provide evidence of effective parenting skills.

Despite the information that can be gleaned from these distractions, their negative effects on the interaction between client and nurse need to be minimized. Requesting that the television be turned off during the visit or moving the client to a more private area can minimize some distractions. Or, the nurse may ask an intrusive younger child to draw a picture to allow parent and nurse to talk with fewer interruptions. If there are too many distractions that cannot be eliminated or overcome, the nurse can ask the client if there is a better time for the visit, when fewer interruptions will occur, and reschedule the visit for a later date. For example, subsequent visits might be planned to coincide with the toddler's nap.

Behavioral distractions consist of behaviors employed by the client to distract the nurse from the purpose of the visit. Again, the use of such distractions can be a cue for the nurse that certain topics are uncomfortable for the client or that the client does not quite trust the nurse or may feel guilty about something. The nurse can benefit from the distraction by exploring the reasons for the client's behaviors and working to establish trust with the client.

The last category of distractions originate with the nurse. These distractions create barriers to relationships with clients. Fears, role preoccupation, and personal reactions to different life-styles can distract the nurse from the purpose of the home visit. Nurses may fear bodily harm, rejection by the client, or the lack of control that is implicit in a home visit. In today's violent society, fear of bodily harm is understandable and nurses making home visits should exercise reasonable caution. For example, it is unwise to drive an expensive car or wear jewelry when making visits. Nurses should get in the habit of locking their cars, even if they only expect to be in a client's residence for a short time. In some high-crime areas, community health nurses often visit in pairs, rather than alone, and visits are only scheduled during daylight hours. If the nurse encounters a situation that suggests possible danger (for example, arriving for a home visit at a time when illicit drugs are being sold), the wisest course is to leave and return at another time. Of course, if danger threatens others as well, the nurse has a responsibility to notify the appropriate authorities.

Community health nurses may also create distractions by being so preoccupied with their original purpose that they fail to see the need to modify the planned home visit. No planned intervention is so important that it cannot be postponed if more important needs intervene. Nurses who continue to pursue predetermined goals in the light of other client needs reduce their credibility with clients and create barriers to effective intervention. For example, the nurse who insists on talking about infant feeding when the client just had an argument with her husband and fears he will leave her is not meeting the client's needs.

Finally, community health nurses may be put off by the contrast between their own life-style and that of the clients they are visiting. In dealing with feelings engendered by such differences, it is helpful to understand that one's own attitudes are the product of one's upbringing and that clients derive their attitudes in the same way. In dealing with life-style differences, the nurse must be aware of personal feelings and their impact on nursing effectiveness. The nurse must also determine what aspects of the client's life-style may be detrimental to health and focus on those, while accepting other differences in attitude or behavior as hallmarks of the client's uniqueness. Being thoroughly informed about cultural and ethnic differences will also minimize negative reactions by the nurse to such differences. Some of these differences will be discussed in Chapter 15, Cultural Influences on Community Health.

EVALUATING THE HOME VISIT

Before concluding the visit, the nurse will evaluate the effectiveness of interventions in terms of their appropriateness to the situation and client response. This evaluation will be conducted in terms of criteria established in planning for the visit. It may not be possible, at this point, to determine the eventual outcome of nursing care. The nurse can, however, examine the client's initial response to interventions. Was mother interested in obtaining food stamps? Is it likely that she will follow through on a referral to the immunization clinic? Did the client voice an intention to reduce salt intake? Could the client accurately demonstrate the correct technique for self-breast-examination?

Evaluating the ultimate outcome of interventions may occur at subsequent visits. For example, on the next visit, the nurse might determine whether the mother applied for food stamps and whether she obtained them. If she applied, but did not obtain food stamps, the nurse would determine the reason for denial. Based on information obtained, there may be a need for advocacy on the part of the nurse. If the client did not apply for the stamps, the nurse should determine the reason for her behavior. Was the client distracted by crises that occurred in the meantime,

NURSING PROGRESS NOTES

Date

7-9-91 H.V. for routine PP & newborn eval as requested by La Paloma Hosp.

Client is 17 yo unwed Hispanic girl c̄ a normal full-term baby boy born 7-5-91. Lives c̄ parents and two sisters ages 13 & 8.

Diagnosis #1: Inadequate family income

Goal: Provide family income adequate to needs

Objective: Obtain foodstamps, AFDC, & Medicaid assistance.

S. Client states was unable to afford PN care, has no funds for PP check or well-child care. Family has no health insurance, unable to pay hospital bill

O. Ø

A. Inadequate family finances due to low income and educational level

P. 1. Determine eligibility for financial assistance programs

2. Refer for Medicaid, foodstamps, AFDC

3. Revisit in 2 wks to f-u on referrals

Eval: Referrals made, family seemed accepting. Grandmo states will apply for aid next week.

Diagnosis #2: Overprotection of 13 yo girl

Goal: Provide environment conducive to normal development

Objective: Parents will be less restrictive ofr 13 yo's activities

S. Grandmo states husb will not let 13 yo date or go out c̄ girl friends due to older sister's pregnancy. 13 yo states she is not sexually active & resents restrictions

O. 17 yo unwed mother in home

A. Potential for inadequate development of 13 yo due to father's overprotectiveness

P. 1. Explore family attitudes to unwed pregnancy, sexual activity, etc.

2. Discuss developmental tasks of adolescence with parents

3. Encourage parents to foster responsible decision-making by 13 yo

4. Follow-up discussion c̄ family in 1 mon.

Eval: Grandfather states he'll allow 13 yo to go out c̄ girl friends but not to date 'til age 16.

Diagnosis #3: Inadequate child care skills

Goal: Improved child care skills

Objective: 1. Client will be able to adquately feed, bathe, diaper, clothe child

2. Client will maintain safe environment for child

3. Client will provide adequate health care for child

S. Client states she has little experience c̄ child care, no baby-sitting experience. Grandmo states it has been a long time since there was a baby in home.

O. 17 yo girl with newborn son, asking many questions re: child care

A. Inadequate child care skills due to lack of experience

P. 1. Assess extent of child care knowledge

2. Demonstrate child care skills of feeding, burping, diapering, bathing, and clothing over next several visits

3. Discuss infant nutrition

4. Discuss infant safety & immunization

5. Discuss care of minor illnesses

6. Provide educational material on child care, immunization, growth & development, etc.

7. Suggest addtl literature from public library

8. Return vistis q 2-3 wks to continue teaching as needed

Eval: Client eager to learn, accepted educational materials to be read by next visit. Able to exhibit correct bottle-feeding & burping technique p̄ demonstration.

M. Clark, R.N., P.H.N.

Client name: Flores, Maria Record No. 567-8359

Figure 8–1. Sample documentation of a nursing home visit.

but plans to apply for assistance next week? Did she not have transportation to the social services office? Or, maybe she does not really want food stamps. If the client lacks transportation, the nurse might help her explore ways of getting transportation. If the client does not really want food stamps, the nurse can either explore why and work to change her attitude or accept the client's wishes and look for other means of improving the family's nutritional and financial status.

As noted earlier, evaluation of nursing intervention during a home visit should reflect the level of prevention involved. The nurse examines both short-term and long-term effects of interventions at the primary, secondary, and tertiary levels of prevention, as appropriate. For instance, if the home visit focused on secondary prevention, evaluation will also be focused at this level. If several levels were addressed during the visit, evaluation will focus on the effects of interventions at each level.

The nurse will also evaluate his or her use of the home visit process. Was the preparatory assessment adequate? Was there information available that the nurse neglected to review, resulting in unexpected problems during the visit itself? For example, did the nurse ask about the husband's reaction to the new baby only to be told that the client was not married, when this information was included in the client's record? Did the nurse miss cues to additional problems during the visit? Was the nurse able to plan interventions consistent with client needs, attitudes, and desires? Was the nurse able to deal effectively with distractions? If not, why not? Answers to these and similar questions will allow the nurse to improve his or her use of the home visit process in subsequent client encounters.

DOCUMENTING THE HOME VISIT

Documentation constitutes the last stage of the home visit. The nurse must accurately record the client's health status, nursing interventions employed, and the effectiveness of interventions. The nurse documents validation of diagnoses made in the preparatory assessment, as well as additional needs identified, by recording both subjective and objective data obtained during the visit. Goals and objectives established for addressing client health needs are also recorded. In addition, the nurse documents actions taken, client response to those actions, and the outcome of interventions if known. Also included in documenting the visit are future plans and recommendations for subsequent home visits. A chart entry for a nursing home visit using the status-oriented record

BOX 8–1

Elements of a Home Visit

- Preparatory assessment
  - Review available client data to determine health-care needs related to human biology, environment, life-style, and health system
- Diagnosis
  - Develop diagnostic hypotheses based on preparatory assessment
- Planning
  - Review previous interventions and their effects
  - Prioritize client needs and identify those to be addressed during the visit
  - Develop goals and objectives for visit and identify levels of prevention involved
  - Consider client acceptance and timing of visit
  - Specify activities needed to accomplish goals and objectives
  - Obtain needed supplies and equipment
  - Plan for evaluation of the home visit
- Implementation
  - Validate preparatory assessment and nursing diagnostic hypotheses
  - Identify other client needs
  - Modify plan of care as needed
  - Carry out nursing interventions
  - Deal with distractions
- Evaluation
  - Evaluate client response to interventions
  - Evaluate long-term and short-term outcomes of intervention
  - Evaluate the quality of implementation in the home visit
- Documentation
  - Document client assessment and health needs identified
  - Document interventions
  - Document client response to interventions
  - Document outcome of interventions
  - Document future plan of care

format might look like the sample presented in Figure 8–1. Client assessment and health status summary would be documented separately and are not included in the figure.

The entry reflects problems identified in a routine postpartum visit to an adolescent with a new baby. The "S" and "O" notations reflect subjective and objective assessment data, respectively. Subjective data is information provided by the client or other informant, while objective data is that observed directly by the nurse. The "A" notation refers to the nurse's analysis of the situation or the nursing diagnosis and the "P" is the plan of care for addressing the particular health need. Here a brief narrative statement evaluating the effects of intervention is provided. In subsequent visits, evaluative comments would be reflected in the subjective and objective data related to the current status of the health-care need.

The epidemiologic prevention process model provides a context for structuring home visits to provide health care to individuals and their families. The components of a home visit within the context of the model are summarized in Box 8–1.

CHAPTER HIGHLIGHTS

- Home visits are a traditional community health nursing approach to the care of individuals and families.
- Home visits have the advantage of permitting the nurse to experience, firsthand, the client's situation and factors that may influence client health. In addition, home visits permit monitoring of client health status as well as the effects of interventions and allow the nurse to assess client's abilities to function in everyday life.
- Home visits may be initiated by referrals from other health-care providers, by clients' friends or family, by clients themselves, or by community health nurses.
- Preparation for a home visit begins with a preparatory assessment of probable client needs based on available information. The assessment is conducted from Dever's epidemiologic perspective of human biology, environment, life-style, and health system.
- Diagnostic hypotheses related to client health needs are derived from assessment data.
- Tasks in the planning stage of the home visit include prioritizing client needs and determining those needs to be addressed during the visit, developing goals and objectives and levels of prevention to be addressed during the visit, delineating activities to be carried out, obtaining necessary supplies and equipment, and planning for evaluation.
- Client acceptance and timing are important considerations in planning a home visit.
- Implementing the visit begins with validation of the preparatory assessment and diagnosis of the client's needs. Based on this validation, the nurse revises diagnoses or identifies additional client needs and performs nursing interventions.
- Distractions arising from the environment, the client, or the nurse must be minimized for the home visit to be an effective intervention.
- In evaluating the home visit, the nurse assesses client response to interventions as well as the ultimate outcome of intervention. Evaluation of outcome may not be possible immediately following the visit, so the nurse may need to plan for follow-up at a later time.
- The home visit concludes with documentation of the visit and its effects. Documentation includes the client assessment, diagnoses, interventions and both their long-term and short-term effects. Documentation also includes future plans for care.

Review Questions

1. Describe the differences in client focus and health-care emphasis in home visits made by community health nurses and those made by home health nurses. (p. 143)
2. Describe at least three advantages of home visits as a means of providing nursing care. (p. 144)
3. Identify at least four aspects of planning for a home visit. Give an example of each. (p. 150)
4. Describe at least four tasks in implementing a home visit. Give an example of the performance of each task. (p. 151)
5. Identify three types of potential distractions during a home visit. Give an example of each and describe actions by the nurse that might eliminate the distraction. (p. 152)
6. Why is there a need for both long-term and short-term criteria for evaluating the effectiveness of a home visit? Give examples of the use of both types of criteria. (p. 153)

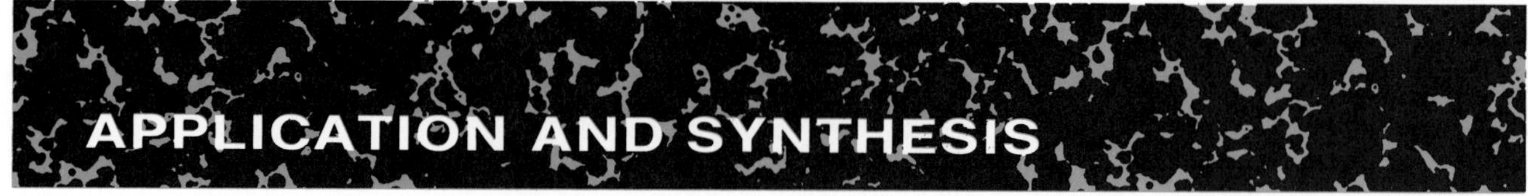

APPLICATION AND SYNTHESIS

You are a community health nurse working for the Clark City Health Department. Your supervisor took the following request for nursing services by phone and passed it on to you because the address is part of your district. You know that this address is in an older residential area with a large Hispanic population.

Clark City Health Department
Request for Nursing Services

Source of request: La Paloma Hospital Maternity Unit

Date of request: 7-7-91

Client: Maria Flores Date of birth: 10-21-74

Address: 8359 Mallboro Way, Marquetta AL 30619

Head of household: Juan Flores (client's father)

Reason for referral: Delivered 5 lb 7 oz baby boy on 7-5-91. Client had no prenatal care prior to delivery. Lives with parents and two younger sisters, ages 8 & 13. Both parents work, but family income insufficient to pay hospital bill. Family does not have insurance or Medicaid. Request routine postpartum/newborn evaluation

1. Based on the information you have, what health-care needs would you identify in your preparatory assessment? List your diagnostic hypotheses.
2. What nursing interventions would you plan for the health needs you are likely to encounter in a visit to this client? Identify your planned interventions as primary, secondary, or tertiary preventive measures.
3. What materials might you need on this home visit?
4. How would you go about validating your preparatory assessment and diagnostic hypotheses?
5. What additional assessment data would you want to obtain during your visit?
6. What evaluative criteria would you use to conduct outcome and process evaluation of care provided to this client and her family?

REFERENCES

1. Humphrey, C. J. (1988). The home as a setting for care: Clarifying the boundaries of practice. *Nursing Clinics of North America, 23*(2), 305–315.
2. Barkauskas, V. H. (1983). Effectiveness of public health nurse home visits to primarous mothers and their infants. *American Journal of Public Health, 73,* 573–580.
3. Combs-Orme, T., Reis, J., & Ward, L. D. (1985). Effectiveness of home visits by public health nurses in maternal and child health: An empirical review. *Public Health Reports, 100,* 490–499.
4. Highriter, M. E. (1984). Public health nursing evaluation, education, and professional issues. In H. H. Werley & J. J. Fitzpatrick (Eds.), *Annual Review of Nursing Research* (Vol. 2). New York: Springer.
5. Norr, K. F., Nacion, K. W., & Abramson, R. (1989). Early discharge with home follow-up: Impacts on low-income mothers and infants. *JOGNN, 18*(2), 133–141.
6. Oda, D. S. (1989). Home visits: Effective or obsolete nursing practice? *Nursing Research, 38,* 121–123.
7. Green, J. L., & Driggers, B. (1989). All visiting nurses are not alike: Home health and community health nursing. *Journal of Community Health Nursing, 6*(2), 83–93.
8. Peoples-Sheps, M. D. (1990). Perinatal home visiting returns. *Nursing Outlook, 38*(2), 54–55.
9. Hewner, S. J. (1986). Bringing home the health care: Nurses make a difference. *Journal of Gerontological Nursing, 12*(2), 29–35.
10. Pruitt, R. H., Keller, L. S., & Hale, S. L. (1987). Mastering distractions that mar home visits. *Nursing & Health Care, 8,* 344–347.

RECOMMENDED READINGS

Combs-Orme, T., Reis, J., & Ward, L. D. (1985). Effectiveness of home visits by public health nurses in maternal and child health: An empirical review. *Public Health Reports, 100,* 490–499.

Presents a review of research literature on the effectiveness of public health nursing home visits in the area of maternal and child nursing.

Freiberg, K. (1987). *Human development: A life-span approach* (3rd ed.). Boston: Jones and Bartlett.

Addresses aspects of human development from birth to death. Provides a sound review of developmental tasks and influences at each stage of the human life span.

Green, J. L., & Driggers, B. (1989). All visiting nurses are not alike: Home health and community health nursing. *Journal of Community Health Nursing, 6*(2), 83–93.

Describes differences in home visiting from the perspective of home health nurses and community health nurses.

Hewner, S. (1986). Bringing home the health care: Nurses make a difference. *Journal of Gerontological Nursing, 12*(2), 29–35.

Discusses the utility of home visits in meeting the health needs of older clients.

Lathrop, J. (1989). *Milestones: Growth and development guide.* Milwaukee: Maxishare.

Provides a quick review of developmental milestones related to motor control, communication, play, socialization, and physical growth as well as safety implications for children from birth to 18 years of age.

Murray, R. B., & Zentner, J. P. (1989). *Nursing assessment and health promotion through the life span* (4th ed.). Englewood Cliffs, NJ: Prentice-Hall.

Offers an overview of human development with emphasis on physiologic and psychosocial development. Also reviews implications for nursing interventions to foster development.

Norr, K. F., Nacion, K. W., & Abramson, R. (1988). Early discharge with home follow-up: Impacts on low-income mothers and infants. *JOGNN, 18*(2), 133–141.

Sets forth the findings of a research study on the effectiveness of home visits to low-income mothers with new infants.

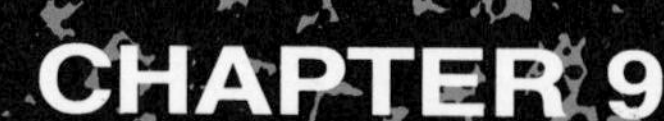

CHAPTER 9

The Discharge Planning and Referral Processes

KEY TERMS

continuity of care
discharge planning
referral
resource file
situational constraints

Some of the clients that community health nurses visit may have recently been discharged from acute-care settings. Because of DRGs, these clients tend to be sicker at the time of discharge than they might have been in the past. They have more needs and require more resources from the health-care system. Similarly, clients may be discharged from community health nursing services to other health-care agencies or to self-care. The complexity of the American health-care system may necessitate assistance in moving from one area of the system to another.[1] Clients may also need assistance in identifying and linking with needed health-care services other than those provided by the community health nurse. The two processes described in this chapter, discharge planning and referral, can provide the assistance required by clients in both of these areas.

LEARNING OBJECTIVES

After reading this chapter you should be able to:

- Identify two purposes for discharge planning.
- Describe one advantage of discharge planning for the client.
- Describe two advantages of discharge planning for the health-care providers or agencies involved.
- Discuss two reasons why community health nurses should be involved in discharge planning.
- Identify at least three activities involved in developing the discharge plan.
- Describe at least three purposes for referrals.
- Identify at least four categories of information that should be included in a resource file entry.
- Describe four considerations in assessing a specific referral situation.
- Identify at least three activities involved in planning a referral.
- Describe the two aspects of evaluation relevant to discharge planning and referral.

DISCHARGE PLANNING

Discharge planning occurs when a client will be dismissed from care by one agency or institution and will require continued care by other providers. The discharge planning process is used primarily to meet the health-care needs of individual clients, but may be used to address the needs of families as well. ***Discharge planning*** is a process in which client and family needs are identified and evaluated and responsibility for meeting those needs is transferred to the client, to significant others, or to other health-care providers.[2,3]

Discharge planning is needed to assure continuity of care as clients move from one segment of the health-care system to another. ***Continuity of care*** means that care is provided in an organized and systematic manner on a continuing basis despite its provision by several different people.[4] Continuity of care exists, for instance, when teaching on infant nutrition, begun by a pediatrician, is continued by a community health nurse, or when passive range-of-motion exercises initiated by nurses in the hospital are continued by family members at home. Without adequate planning, clients may be discharged from service by one health-care provider or agency with continuing health-care needs that go unmet.

The need for discharge planning for hospitalized clients has become more apparent since the advent of diagnosis related groups (DRGs), a system for determining reimbursement rates for hospital costs based on the client's diagnosis. Under this system, it is to a hospital's financial advantage to discharge clients as rapidly as possible. Consequently, clients are more often released with continuing needs for health-care services. Meeting these needs requires comprehensive and systematic planning that, ideally, should begin with admission to the hospital.[5] In fact, since 1986, systematic discharge planning and transfer or referral of clients for appropriate services have been required for hospital reimbursement under Medicare.[6]

PURPOSES OF DISCHARGE PLANNING

Discharge planning has two primary purposes. The first is to promote continuity of care to improve client health status. Discharge planning is used to facilitate the client's transition between components of the health-care system and to coordinate services between and among a variety of health-care providers. Through successful discharge planning, clients receive uninterrupted health-care services despite their movement from one agency to another. Discharge planning permits a plan of care begun by one agency to be continued by another. For example, teaching for the client with newly diagnosed diabetes often begins in the hospital. But, because of the typically short period of hospitalization and the amount of teaching and follow-up needed, the client will most likely need continued teaching after discharge. If this need has been considered as part of discharge planning, plans will have been made for a community health nurse or other provider to continue the educational process.

The second purpose of discharge planning is coordinating a client's needs with available resources. Discharge planning involves identifying the client's post-discharge needs and the resources needed to meet those needs. Discharge planning also includes plans for linking the client with those resources.

ADVANTAGES OF DISCHARGE PLANNING

Discharge planning has advantages for both clients and health-care agencies. The primary client advantage is improved continuity of care. Advantages for health-care agencies that engage in effective discharge planning include reductions in average length of service, resulting in lower costs, and more efficient use of resources.[7] For example, if plans for discharging a new mother from community health nursing services include referral to a parents' self-help group, community health nursing services may be discontinued earlier than would otherwise be the case.

Adequate discharge planning may also result in fewer requests for additional services, freeing up resources for use with other clients. The mother who has other resources for meeting her needs as a parent, for instance, is less likely to call the nurse with additional questions, leaving the nurse free to meet the needs of other clients. Similarly, effective discharge planning in the hospital setting may prevent or minimize hospital readmissions, freeing beds that may be needed for other clients.[8]

Discharge planning has the additional advantage of improved communication and better information on client needs and previous plan of care for the person or agency that assumes responsibility for meeting health-care needs.[9] For example, the client discharged to self-care will be more likely to receive adequate self-care instruction when effective discharge planning has taken place. Similarly, discharge planning may ensure that the community health nurse who will be visiting the client at home receives adequate information on the client and his or her needs.

COMMUNITY HEALTH NURSES AND DISCHARGE PLANNING

Discharge planning is a client-care activity that can be performed by a variety of health-care providers, including nurses, physicians, social workers, nutritionists, chaplains, and so on. Several authors have suggested that effective discharge planning is best carried out by a multidisciplinary team,[8–10] whereby members of several disciplines jointly assess individual and family post-discharge needs for health care and plan interventions to meet those needs.

Some institutions have created a special liaison or discharge planning position to coordinate discharge planning for the institution.[1,8,9] The person holding this position is responsible for identifying clients most in need of discharge planning, consulting with client caretakers within the institution to identify needs, educating staff regarding discharge planning, and coordinating discharge-planning activities.[9]

It has been suggested that the hospital nurse should continue to provide care in the client's home, particularly when the client continues to require technically skilled care.[11] This nurse would function as the discharge planner and would later discharge the client to appropriate community services. Community health nurses, however, are probably better suited than are acute-care nurses to fulfill the liaison role and assist with discharge planning.

Community health nurses' involvement in discharge planning facilitates recognition of the totality of clients' needs that may not be apparent to staff in a particular agency. For example, nurses working in a hospital may have little idea of the home situation to which a client is being discharged. For this reason, it is helpful to include community health nurses in planning for the client's discharge. Community health nurses can assess the home setting and family strengths and weaknesses prior to discharge and make situational needs known to other health-care providers. Because of their familiarity with community resources, community health nurses can assist other members of the discharge-planning team to identify resources appropriate to client needs. In addition, they can facilitate referral to community agencies and can follow up on the effectiveness of planning after client discharge from the hospital or other institution.

One study of approaches to discharge planning found that hospital nurses working as discharge planners were often unaware of community resources.[1] The same study found that these nurses tended to communicate poorly with outside agencies about clients' needs and current plan of care. When nurses with a community background worked as discharge planners, however, communication between agencies was much more effective. A similar study found that community health nurses working as discharge planners were able to identify and provide for 91 percent of client needs as perceived by the clients themselves.[3]

Community health nurses may function as discharge planners in a variety of settings. Some community health nurses, for example, are employed by hospitals to coordinate discharge-planning activities. Some nurses employed by local health departments participate in discharge-planning meetings in local hospitals. Other community health nurse entrepreneurs have started their own businesses and contract with area hospitals and other institutions to do discharge planning.

Community health nurses may also be involved in planning for clients' discharge from community health nursing services. Clients may be discharged to care by other agencies or to self-care. For example, a terminally ill client may be discharged to hospice care by a community health nurse. Or, clients may be able to function without further intervention and be discharged to self-care. In each case, the community health nurse employs the discharge-planning process to facilitate the transition.

THE EPIDEMIOLOGIC PREVENTION PROCESS MODEL AND DISCHARGE PLANNING

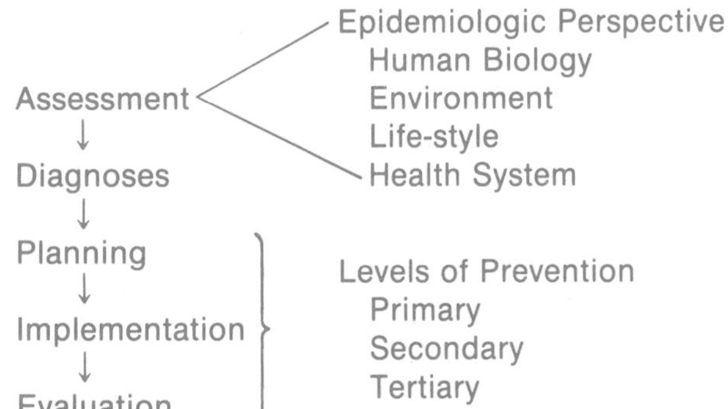

Discharge planning is a systematic activity that can be carried out in the context of the epidemiologic prevention process model. Using the model, the community health nurse assesses the client and diagnoses post-discharge health-care needs. The nurse then plans to meet those needs, implements the plan, and evaluates the outcome of discharge planning.

ASSESSING DISCHARGE NEEDS

Discharge planning should occur with all clients being discharged from any health-care service. Many

TABLE 9–1. CRITERIA FOR IDENTIFYING CLIENTS WHO NEED IN-DEPTH DISCHARGE PLANNING

Criterion	Factors Indicating a Need for In-depth Discharge Planning
Age and developmental level	• Very young clients • Elderly clients • Mentally retarded clients
Behavior factors	• Clients who have a history of noncompliance with treatment plans • Clients with a history of substance abuse
Medical factors	• Clients with recurrent health problems • Clients experiencing multiple trauma, or head or spinal cord injury • Clients with chronic health problems • Clients with degenerative or debilitating illnesses • Clients with terminal illnesses • Clients with obstetrical complications • Clients who have had joint replacements or organ transplants • Clients with nutritional problems or special diets
Nursing needs	• Clients needing continued health education • Clients needing skilled nursing care • Clients with continuing needs for primary, secondary, or tertiary preventive measures • Clients discharged with special equipment • Clients needing reassurance or emotional support
Place of residence	• Clients living alone • Clients discharged to or from nursing homes and other residential facilities • Clients who live outside of normal service areas for the discharging agency • Homeless clients
Psychological factors	• Clients with a history of emotional illness • Clients experiencing spiritual distress • Clients experiencing anxiety • Clients experiencing altered body images • Victims or perpetrators of violence to self or others
Social service needs	• Clients with financial problems • Clients with unmet housing needs • Clients needing child care or respite care • Clients with transportation problems

clients, however, need only routine discharge activities.[6] The community health nurse may need to identify those clients for whom more detailed discharge planning is required. These clients are considered at high risk for the development of serious health consequences without discharge planning. Criteria for use in identifying these clients include the client's age and developmental level, behaviors conducive to ill health, complex medical problems, continuing needs for nursing care, place of residence, psychological factors that impair health, or continuing social service needs. These criteria and examples of each are presented in Table 9–1.

For those clients who require in-depth discharge planning, the nurse would use Dever's epidemiologic perspective to identify discharge needs related to human biology, environment, life-style, and the health system. Use of the Client Discharge Inventory included in Appendix D can facilitate the community health nurse's assessment of post-discharge needs.

Human Biology

Human biological factors related to maturation and aging, genetic inheritance, and physiologic function can all influence a client's need for health-care services following discharge. Genetic factors such as mental retardation, congenital anomalies, and so on can give rise to a need for extended services that should be instituted soon after discharge.

Age can also influence needs for care after discharge. For example, an adolescent with a new baby is likely to need more extensive post-discharge follow-up than a more mature woman. Similarly, elderly clients may have more need of assistance after discharge.

Physiologic function can profoundly influence the need for care following discharge. For example, clients with chronic health problems will need periodic monitoring of their conditions. The client's compliance with his or her treatment plan and the effectiveness of that plan will also require monitoring.

Clients recently diagnosed with a chronic illness may need education regarding the condition, its effects, and its treatment that cannot be accomplished during hospitalization.

Clients with physical disabilities may need assistance with obtaining supplies and equipment or such services as occupational and physical therapy. There may also be a need for help with activities of daily living or with household chores such as cooking, cleaning, or shopping. Terminally ill clients and their significant others may need similar services after discharge as well as social and emotional support.

Moreover, problems with physiologic function can give rise to the need for technical nursing care at home or in an institutional setting. For example, there may be a need for periodic catheterization, intravenous infusion, respiratory therapy, dressing change, and so on, which necessitates a referral for home health care or nursing home placement.

Environment

Elements of the client's physical, psychological, and social environments can influence the person's health-care needs on discharge. Adjustments may be needed in the physical environment to allow the handicapped client to function independently. Or, a young mother may need help in child-proofing a home.

The psychological environment can affect the client's self-care ability or to resume role functions after discharge. A client experiencing a psychiatric disorder, for example, may require referral for continued therapy as well as social and emotional support. Depression, grief, and/or inability to cope with a home situation also necessitate plans for continued follow-up services. The confused client with Alzheimer's disease may not be able to care for himself or herself. If requirements for care place insupportable burdens on family caretakers, there may be a need for institutional placement.

Factors in the social environment, such as educational level, strength of social support systems, economic status, transportation, and so on, will also influence client care needs. Clients with lower educational levels may need more extensive health teaching than other clients, while those who live alone and have few social supports may require referral for assistance with self-care or housekeeping.

Economic status can profoundly influence clients' needs and abilities to meet those needs. Clients may require financial assistance to meet basic survival needs related to food, housing, and so on as well as requiring help with health-care needs. The client's ability to pay for needed health-care services should not be overlooked in discharge planning.

Transportation is another social factor that may influence a client's health status after discharge. Clients may not be able to avail themselves of needed services if they do not have access to transportation. For example, the mother of a handicapped child may recognize the need for medical follow-up, but lack the means to get to the physician's office or specialty clinic.

Life-style

Needs for health care after discharge can also arise from life-style factors. For example, the client may need a follow-up evaluation of his or her readiness to return to work. Or, referral might be needed to help a handicapped individual become self-supporting through work-training programs or employment assistance.

Consumption patterns related to substance abuse may necessitate referral for counseling and continued therapy. Problems of weight control or failure to thrive may require reinforcement of nutritional education, counseling, referral, and so on.

Health System

Consideration should be given in the discharge-planning process to the types of health-care services required by the client and their availability in the community. If there are needs for specialized services not found in the area, it may be necessary to transfer the client to a specialized facility elsewhere. This may necessitate arrangements for transportation, housing for the client or significant others, admission to the new facility, and so forth.

Again, the cost of specific health services within the health-care system and the client's ability to pay must be considered in discharge planning. Is there a less expensive way of providing needed care? For example, can the older client be maintained at home with frequent visits by home health nurses and homemaker aides, rather than be placed in a nursing home at greater cost?

Client attitudes to the health-care system and toward discharge-planning efforts are another important consideration in assessing discharge-planning needs.[12] Clients may feel that they do not need any additional help after discharge and, consequently, may not be interested in discharge planning. Or, the client may feel that he or she possesses the skills needed for self-care and resist even discharge planning related to self-care.

TABLE 9–2. SAMPLE NURSING DIAGNOSES IN DISCHARGE PLANNING FOR A MOTHER AND INFANT

Area of Focus	Related Nursing Diagnoses
Human biology	• Normal postpartum course • Potential for breast soreness due to breast feeding • Weakness due to abnormal blood loss during delivery
Environment	
Physical	• Potential safety hazard owing to plans for baby to sleep with parents
Psychological	• Potential for jealousy of 3-year-old sibling due to birth of baby
Social	• Inability to pay hospital bill because of inadequate income • Strong social support system stemming from close relationships with extended family members
Life-style	• Need for increased nutritional intake owing to breast feeding • Need for child care due to mother's plan to return to work • Potential for fatigue due to interruption of sleep for breast feeding
Health system	• Potential for inadequate postpartum and infant care stemming from lack of health insurance and inadequate income

DIAGNOSTIC REASONING AND DISCHARGE PLANNING

Once the client's need for and willingness to accept discharge planning have been assessed and factors influencing discharge planning needs identified, the discharge planner uses the assessment data to diagnose specific client health-care needs. The preliminary diagnosis may reflect the need for in-depth discharge planning and the factors contributing to that need. For example, the community health nurse may diagnose a "need for in-depth discharge planning due to limited self-care abilities." Secondary diagnoses would address specific areas of focus in developing the discharge plan. These areas may be related to human biological, environmental, life-style, and health-system factors influencing the client's health status. Examples of nursing diagnoses in each of these four areas for a mother and her newborn son discharged 2 days after delivery are presented in Table 9–2.

Nursing diagnoses in discharge planning may be either positive or problem-focused. Positive nursing diagnoses in Table 9–2 are those indicating a normal postpartum course and a strong social support system.

PLANNING FOR DISCHARGE

Nursing diagnoses that form the basis for discharge plans may reflect needs for primary, secondary, or tertiary prevention. For example, the diagnoses related to potential safety hazards, sibling jealousy, and inadequate health care indicate needs for primary preventive measures to prevent their occurrence. Measures directed toward adequate nutrition during breast feeding would also be primary prevention because they focus on health promotion through adequate dietary intake. Secondary prevention would be appropriate for diagnoses indicating existing problems such as weakness, the need for child care, and the inability to pay the hospital bill. Secondary prevention is also indicated for those problems for which primary prevention is not possible. For example, there is no way to prevent initial breast tenderness due to breast feeding, but the nurse can educate the mother about measures to minimize breast tenderness when it occurs. The need for tertiary preventive measures is indicated in the diagnosis of the potential for subsequent pregnancy.

The client and the community health nurse, as discharge planner, prioritize identified health-care needs and develop plans for meeting them. Planning entails developing goals and objectives for continued client care. The goals and objectives developed will reflect the level of prevention involved. Goals related to primary prevention, for example, would reflect health promotion and prevention of health problems, and would include goals of adequate health-care services for mother and child and adjustment of the 3-year-old to the presence of a newborn. Related objectives might include immunization of the infant, a routine postpartum check for the mother, dietary intake adequate to the nutritional needs of mother and baby, and incorporation of the 3-year-old in the care of the newborn.

Goals in secondary prevention would include elimination or reduction of existing problems. For example, the mother's weakness would abate, and she would obtain child care. Objectives for care related to secondary prevention might be that the mother will be able to perform her normal daily routine without undue fatigue, and that she will obtain daily child care prior to returning to work. Finally, the goal of tertiary prevention in this example would be to prevent a subsequent pregnancy, while related objectives might include the use of an effective contraceptive.

Alternative approaches to meeting client needs for primary, secondary, and tertiary prevention are generated, and services and resources best suited to accomplishing goals and objectives are selected on the basis of criteria generated by both nurse and client. Primary preventive measures selected might include referral for financial assistance in getting a crib to prevent potential safety hazards, encouraging mother to spend time with the 3-year-old and include her in the care of the baby, education about the nutritional needs of a breast-feeding mother, and so on.

Primary preventive activities would also be geared to reinforcing positive nursing diagnoses. For example, the mother might be encouraged to make use of the support of extended family members while adjusting to the presence of a new baby. Similarly, actions would be taken to promote continuation of a normal postpartum course by explaining to the mother when it will be safe to return to her prior strenuous exercise pattern and when she can safely resume sexual activity.

Secondary prevention might include referral for assistance in paying the hospital bill. Other secondary preventive measures could include encouraging extended family members to help with housework and care of the 3-year-old to permit the mother to rest and regain her strength, and educating the mother on measures to minimize breast tenderness. Referral for family planning services and education about contraceptive methods would be tertiary preventive measures aimed at preventing another pregnancy.

During the planning stage of discharge planning, the community health nurse and client also develop criteria for evaluating the effectiveness of the discharge plan.[12] These criteria are derived from established goals and objectives and reflect the level of prevention involved in specific nursing interventions. For primary preventive measures, criteria would include evidence of health promotion through adequate dietary intake, immunization, and so on, and the absence of health problems like sibling rivalry and safety hazards. Criteria related to secondary prevention would reflect elimination of existing problems. For example, if one of the objectives for secondary prevention was to obtain Medicaid coverage to pay the hospital bill, the evaluative criterion would be whether or not Medicaid coverage was obtained. Evaluative criteria for tertiary prevention would focus on whether or not health-related problems have been prevented. For example, has the client become pregnant again?

IMPLEMENTING THE DISCHARGE PLAN

The discharge plan is then implemented by communicating with the agencies and care providers who will assume continuing care of the client. Referrals are initiated, appointments scheduled, and so on. It is important to remember that good communication is essential at this stage. Outside agencies need to be apprised of client needs, previous treatment plans, and expectations for continued care as well as any other information relevant to the client's situation.

Clients and their significant others need to be informed of arrangements made and expectations of them. For example, an agency might be contacted by the community health nurse regarding the client's discharge and need for services, but the client may need to call for a specific appointment. Clients will also need to know about any payments required for services and the name of contact persons in agencies to which they have been referred.

If the discharge plan included pre-discharge education, the community health nurse may be involved in teaching the client or significant others how to meet self-care needs. Or, such education may be provided by other health-care personnel: a physician, nutritionist, or the nurse in an in-patient setting.

Implementation of the discharge plan could include activities at each level of prevention—primary, secondary, tertiary. Generally speaking, if the client has been followed by the discharging agency or provider for existing health problems, all three levels of prevention are usually involved. For example, with an adolescent diabetic hospitalized for a hypoglycemic reaction due to noncompliance with diet, insulin administration, and so on, there will probably be a continued need for secondary measures to solve the problem of noncompliance. Tertiary measures will also be needed to prevent a recurrence of the hypoglycemic reaction that precipitated hospitalization. The primary prevention needs of this client should also be addressed in implementing the discharge plan. Arrangements may be made, for instance, for the client to obtain a repeat measles immunization due at this age, or education about contraceptives may be undertaken if the client is sexually active.

For clients who have been receiving health-promotive services, measures undertaken in implementing the discharge plan may be related only to primary prevention. For example, if a postpartum mother without any existing health problems is being discharged from perinatal services, interventions will focus on promoting the health of mother and baby and may include referral for well-child care, discussion of dietary needs for mother and baby, and so on.

EVALUATING DISCHARGE PLANNING

The discharge plan should be evaluated throughout its execution, even prior to discharge. As the client's condition and circumstances change, discharge plans may need to be modified accordingly. For example, the decision may have been made to discharge an elderly man into his wife's care with periodic assistance from a home health nurse and aide. If, prior to the man's discharge, his wife has a heart attack, plans for his discharge will need to be revised.

After discharge, discharge planning is evaluated in terms of client outomes (outcome evaluation) and the effectiveness of the discharge planning process (process evaluation). Client outcomes are evaluated on the basis of the goals and objectives established, and will reflect the level of prevention involved. Have primary preventive activities actually promoted the client's health and prevented health problems from occurring? Have existing problems been resolved by the secondary preventive measures employed? Or, has tertiary prevention limited the consequences of existing problems for the client or prevented problems from recurring? If client-care objectives have not been met, what factors contributed to this lack of success? Based on this information, the community health nurse, as discharge planner, can modify the discharge plan as needed.

The second aspect of evaluation after the client is discharged is related to the use of the discharge planning process itself. Was the assessment of the client situation adequate? Were the nursing diagnoses on target? Did planning take into consideration the client's needs, available resources, and situational constraints? Were referrals made to appropriate agencies? Was communication sufficient to apprise agencies of client needs and clients of the arrangements made for them? Answers to these and similar questions will allow community health nurses to modify their use of the discharge planning process and improve the effectiveness of future discharge planning. The components of the discharge-planning process, as used by community health nurses, are summarized in Box 9–1.

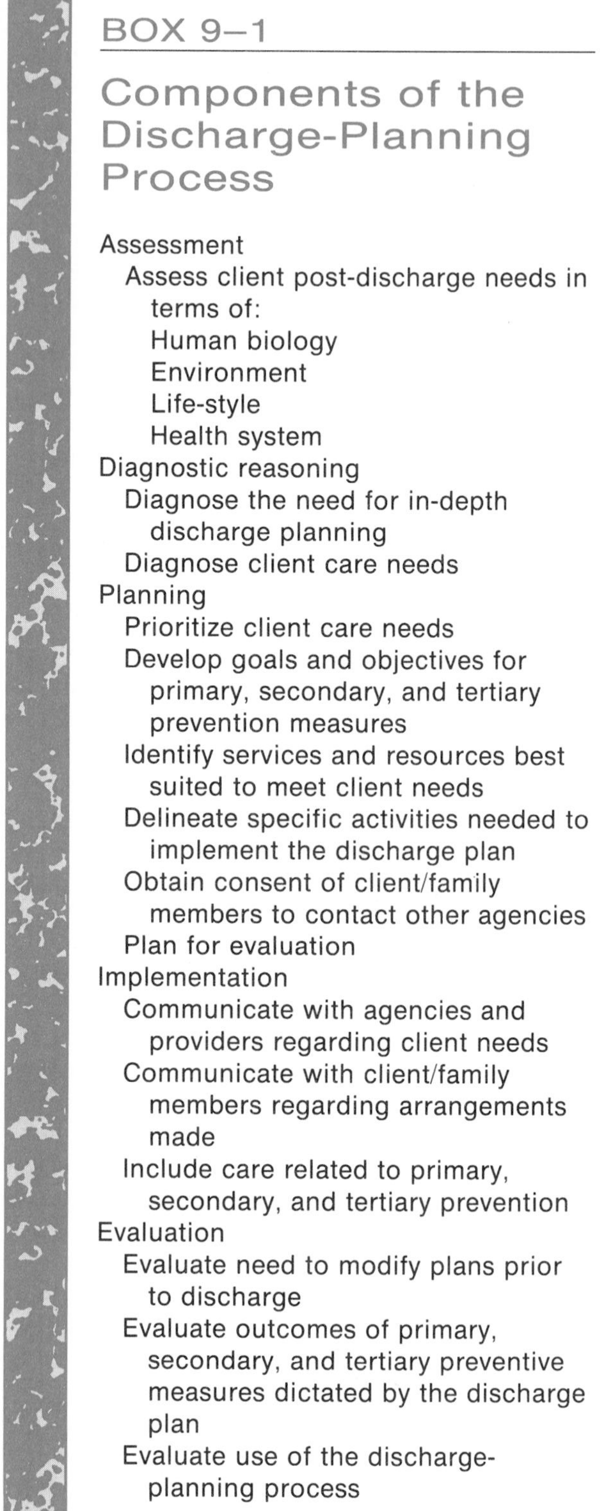

BOX 9–1

Components of the Discharge-Planning Process

Assessment
- Assess client post-discharge needs in terms of:
  - Human biology
  - Environment
  - Life-style
  - Health system

Diagnostic reasoning
- Diagnose the need for in-depth discharge planning
- Diagnose client care needs

Planning
- Prioritize client care needs
- Develop goals and objectives for primary, secondary, and tertiary prevention measures
- Identify services and resources best suited to meet client needs
- Delineate specific activities needed to implement the discharge plan
- Obtain consent of client/family members to contact other agencies
- Plan for evaluation

Implementation
- Communicate with agencies and providers regarding client needs
- Communicate with client/family members regarding arrangements made
- Include care related to primary, secondary, and tertiary prevention

Evaluation
- Evaluate need to modify plans prior to discharge
- Evaluate outcomes of primary, secondary, and tertiary preventive measures dictated by the discharge plan
- Evaluate use of the discharge-planning process

THE REFERRAL PROCESS

Referral is the process of directing a client to another source of information or assistance. Referrals to a variety of health-care and related services may be part of discharge planning for an individual client and his or her family. A community health nurse also makes referrals for other clients who have needs that the community health nurse is unable to meet.

While the discharge-planning process is used primarily with individual clients and their families, the referral process can be employed by community health nurses to meet the needs of individuals, families, groups, or communities. For example, the community health nurse might make a referral for contraceptive services for an adolescent client or refer an abusive family for counseling. Similarly, the community health nurse might refer a group or community to a source of assistance in writing a grant proposal to fund a health-care project for the homeless.

PURPOSES OF REFERRAL

Referrals to other sources of health and social services are made for a variety of reasons and with a variety of purposes. The primary purpose has already been stated—providing the client with access to health care and supportive services that cannot be provided by the nurse. Additional purposes identified include obtaining a second opinion on client problems or available courses of action, setting the stage for the next step in the plan of care, withdrawing from an untenable situation, and protecting oneself from lawsuits.[13] Community health nurses may make a referral to confirm a diagnosis or obtain a second opinion. For example, the nurse might refer a child with a rash for medical care if he or she suspects that the child has scabies but wants to have that diagnosis either confirmed or disconfirmed.

Community health nurses might also use the referral process to set the stage for further intervention. Using the previous example, if the diagnosis of scabies is confirmed, the nurse may use the opportunity to focus on the need for improved personal hygiene within the family. He or she may use the findings of the second opinion to increase credibility with the family. Similarly, the nurse may refer a teenager with amenorrhea for a pregnancy test before discussing options for dealing with a possible pregnancy. If pregnancy test results are negative, the nurse may use the opening provided by the referral and the results to discuss the issue of contraception.

Nurses may also refer clients because they have reached an impasse and do not feel able to provide further assistance to the client. The impasse may stem from lack of trust on the part of the client or from the nurse's frustration with a client's failure to follow through on recommendations. When interactions between nurse and client are such that the relationship is no longer therapeutic for the client, it is appropriate for the nurse to refer the client to another health-care provider who may be able to establish an effective helping relationship with the client. Occasionally, this also may be done when the client has become overly dependent on the nurse and the nurse needs to clear the way for increased independence. In choosing to refer clients to other sources of help in such instances, the nurse is not abandoning the client, but is providing an avenue for more effective intervention than he or she is able to provide.

Finally, community health nurses may make referrals in order to protect themselves and their employers from potential lawsuits.[13] For example, the community health nurse in a state correctional setting may be virtually certain that a particular prisoner does not have hepatitis, but may make a referral for diagnosis to prevent the possibility of exposure of other inmates and the potential for legal action in a particularly litigious population group. In this instance, the referral serves the dual purposes of either confirming or disconfirming a diagnosis and preventing expensive litigation for the state.

IDENTIFYING REFERRAL RESOURCES

To make effective referrals, the community health nurse needs to be cognizant of health-care and other support services available in the community. Information on community resources can be obtained in a number of ways. Two major sources of information are the local health department and the yellow pages. Other sources of information are neighborhood information and referral centers, local government offices and chambers of commerce, and police and fire departments. The local library is also a source of information and may even have a directory of local resources. The League of Women Voters will have information on area officials, legislators, and important issues. Officials and legislators can frequently provide other information of interest to the nurse. Additional sources of information within the community include local newspapers and television and radio stations.

It is not sufficient for the community health nurse merely to be aware of the existence of community resources. The nurse must know where these resources are located and understand the requirements for a referral to each resource. The nurse needs systematically to collect information on the type of services a referral resource provides, criteria for eligibility for services, and whether there is any fee involved. For this reason, community health nurses should establish a ***resource file*** or data base to organize information on area resources systematically. Figure 9–1 depicts a sample resource file entry. A copy of the Resource File Entry Form is included in Appendix E.

The file could be organized according to categories of resources included. An example of categorical organization of entries is included in Box 9–2. A particular agency with more than one type of service could be entered in several different categories or a cross-reference system could be used. The resource described in Figure 9–1 deals with the category of transportation.

Information about the resource's funding source

Resource category: Transportation   Funding source: voluntary

Agency name: St. Martha's Catholic Church

Address: 3710 Montebank Rd, Otenada, Mississippi

Phone number: 817-3421   Business hours: Mon–Fri 8–4

Contact person: Mrs. Jefferson   Title: receptionist / secretary

Source of referral: self or other

Eligibility: anyone without transportation – need not be members of church

Fee: none

Services: provides transportation to church services as well as other services such as Dr.'s office, grocery shopping, etc. on periodic basis

Access: call to arrange transportation

Other comments: 1.) Do not provide transportation on long-term basis, i.e., to work or to school
2) depends upon availability of volunteer drivers

Figure 9–1. Sample resource file entry.

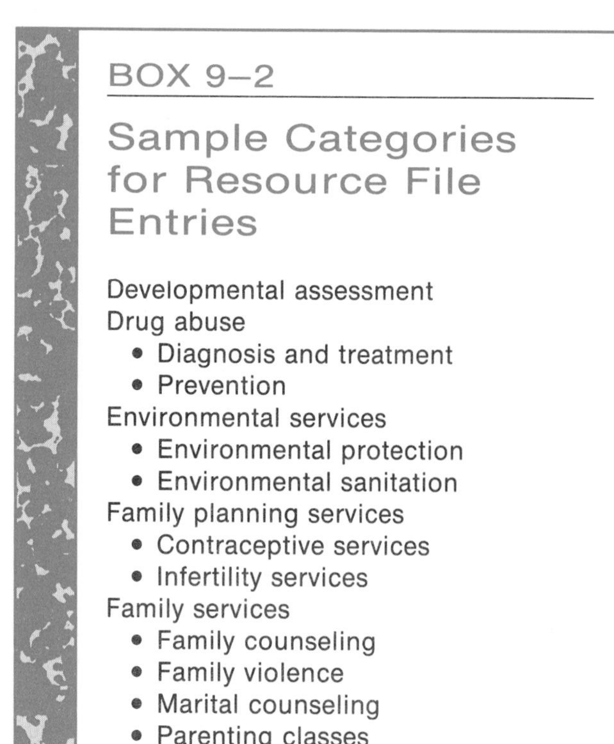

BOX 9–2

Sample Categories for Resource File Entries

Developmental assessment
Drug abuse
- Diagnosis and treatment
- Prevention

Environmental services
- Environmental protection
- Environmental sanitation

Family planning services
- Contraceptive services
- Infertility services

Family services
- Family counseling
- Family violence
- Marital counseling
- Parenting classes

can be useful. For example, if tax revenues have declined in the area, the community health nurse may need to contact agencies to determine whether services have been cut prior to making a specific referral. Also, it may be important to some clients to know that the services they receive from an agency are provided by tax dollars rather than "charity."

Of course, the resource file entry will include the referral resource's full name, address, and telephone number. The business hours notation may refer to when the agency is open or to times when a particular service is offered. For example, the entry might read "Family planning: Monday, 9–12, Prenatal: Tuesday, 1–4."

It is helpful to have the name of a contact person in the agency as well. Referrals are facilitated when agency personnel are familiar with the person making the referral. Unfortunately, it is often true that some agency employees are less inclined to offend professional colleagues than clients. When the nurse refers a client to an agency and gives that individual the name of a contact person who knows the nurse, the client can mention that he or she was referred by the nurse and they may get a more prompt response than would otherwise be the case. Having a specific contact person within an agency may also facilitate requests for services when the request is made by the nurse rather than the client.

The notation entitled "Source of referral" in Figure 9–1 refers to the preferred originator of the referral. As previously noted, some agencies accept referrals only from specific persons, usually physicians. If a professional referral is required, the nurse should specifically inquire about the acceptability of referrals from nurse practitioners, if they are available in the area. In the example in Figure 9–1, no specific referral source is required. Clients may request services on their own or be referred by anyone else.

Information related to the eligibility of clients for service is very important. To make appropriate referrals, the nurse must know who is eligible for services and who is not. This will help to minimize client frustration in being referred for services for which they do not qualify. The nurse should also be aware of how eligibility is determined. For example, clients receiving Supplemental Security Income (SSI) have, in the past, been automatically eligible for Medicaid. Eligibility for the Women, Infants, and Children's program (WIC), on the other hand, is based on evidence of nutritional need (for example, low hematocrit) as well as on age and economic status.

The importance of a notation regarding fees is obvious. Clients need to know beforehand if they will be charged for services provided by the referral resource. This information can make a difference in decisions on the use of a particular service. An additional notation here might indicate whether or not the agency can help clients with financial arrangements. For example, hospitals will frequently allow clients to pay bills in installments. The nurse should also know whether the agency expects payment at the time of service or will bill the client later. The nurse should be aware, as well, of whether the agency accepts Medicaid, Medicare, health insurance, or other third-party payments.

Notation should also be made regarding the types of services provided by the agency. The entry regarding access refers to the means by which the client gains entry to the system. In the example in Figure 9–1, the client needs to call ahead for an appointment. Additional information under this entry would indicate any supporting documentation that the client must provide to be eligible for services. Should he or she bring health insurance papers or just the policy number? Will the client need proof of residency, monthly expenditures, medical expenses, and so on?

The type of information included in the sample resource file entry allows the community health nurse to make appropriate referrals that do not waste clients' time and energy. It also allows the nurse to prepare clients for what they will encounter in following up a referral. The file should be updated on a regular basis and as circumstances in various agencies change. Having a specific contact person in each agency may help to ensure that the nurse is notified of program changes. Experiences and reactions of clients following use of a particular resource can also be used to update resource information and to evaluate the quality of service provided.

THE EPIDEMIOLOGIC PREVENTION PROCESS MODEL AND REFERRAL

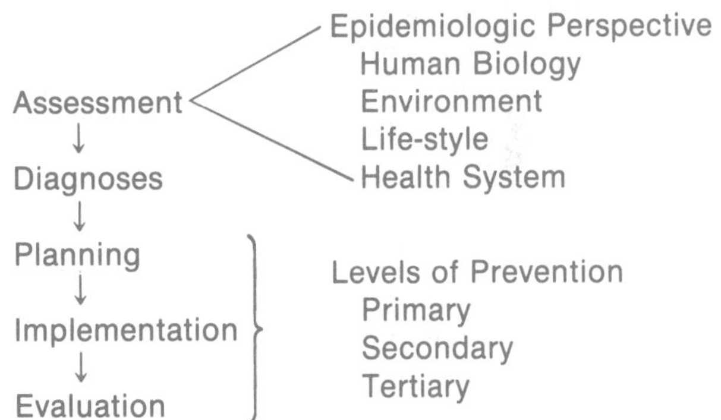

Referral is a systematic approach to directing clients to needed services. Referral can be undertaken within the context of the epidemiologic prevention process model. Like all of the other processes employed by community health nurses, referral begins with client assessment and diagnosis of health needs and progresses to the planning, implementation, and evaluation of the referral.

ASSESSING REFERRAL REQUIREMENTS

Referral begins after an assessment of client health-care needs reveals that the community health nurse is not able, for whatever reason, to meet those needs. Factors influencing the need for referral arise from each of the four components of Dever's epidemiologic perspective. For example, the nurse may make a presumptive diagnosis of gonorrhea and refer a client for treatment. Similarly, the biological fact of delayed development in an infant may prompt a referral for in-depth developmental testing.

Environmental factors can also give rise to needs for referrals. Cockroaches or rats in the physical environment indicate a need for referral to an exterminator. In the psychological environment, evidence of the potential for suicide necessitates an immediate referral for counseling. Similarly, at the group level, evidence of conflict among personnel in a business may lead to a referral for assistance with conflict resolution.

Community health nurses also make many referrals necessitated by factors in the social environment. For example, the nurse might refer a family for financial assistance or suggest that the local school district contact the area chapter of the American Cancer Society for help in designing a program to make smoking an undesirable behavior among school children.

Smoking is itself a life-style factor that may give rise to a need for referral. For instance, a smoker with emphysema may be referred to a program to help him or her quit smoking. Families might be referred to a nutritionist for education about diet, while an overweight person may be referred for a complete medical evaluation before undertaking a program of diet and exercise designed to lose weight.

Health-system factors frequently give rise to a need for referral to a source of needed health-care services. Families on Medicaid may need to be referred to health-care facilities that accept Medicaid. Or, an industry that wants to establish an in-house occupational health service may require a referral to an appropriate consultant.

In addition to assessing factors giving rise to a need for referral, there are four special considerations in assessing a potential referral situation. These include considerations of acceptability of the referral to the client, client eligibility for services, constraints operating in the situation, and community resources available.

Acceptability to the Client

The first consideration in making a referral is the acceptability of the referral to the client. Some clients may be unwilling to obtain help if they perceive it as "charity." In other cases, clients may have philosophies different from those of the referral resource. For example, a Southern Baptist client may be reluctant to accept assistance from an agency supported by the Roman Catholic Church. Similarly, members of a community may be reluctant to seek outside funding for a proposed health program because they do not want to have to adhere to requirements set by the funding agency. For instance, community members may not believe they can meet all of the federal requirements for starting a Head Start program and resist the community health nurse's suggestion that they apply for federal funding under Head Start.

Client Eligibility for Service

The second consideration in referral is the client's eligibility for the service provided. There are many types of determinants of eligibility for service. Sometimes eligibility is based on financial need, and clients will need to provide evidence of income and expenditures. In other instances, eligibility might be based on residence within a particular jurisdiction or membership in a particular group. For example, nonresidents are not usually eligible for state-supported medical assistance. Or, a particular agency may only provide services to members of a specific religious or ethnic group. Eligibility can also be based on age. As an example, senior citizens groups usually do not provide services for anyone under the age of 55. Finally, eligibility sometimes is based on the existence of a particular condition. For instance, shelter services might only be available to abused wives rather than to homeless people in general.

Similar eligibility requirements may influence referrals of communities or groups of people to outside sources of assistance. For example, some scholarship funding to educate health-care providers is tied to the proportion of minority group members included in the student body. If the community health nurse is trying to improve access to health care in a community by promoting education of indigenous health-care providers, referral to funding sources for such programs may not be appropriate if the community does not meet eligibility requirements.

Situational Constraints

The presence of any ***situational constraints,*** or factors in the client's situation that would prevent a client from following up on a referral, is the third consideration in referral. For example, does the client have transportation available to go to the appropriate office? If clients do not speak English, will they be able to find an interpreter to assist them? The nurse making the referral should identify any situational constraints present and then take action to eliminate or minimize the effects of those constraints.

Availability of Resources

The final consideration in assessing a specific referral situation is the availability of community resources to meet client needs. Once the client's needs have been identified, the community health nurse would examine entries in the resource file to see if one of the agencies listed there can meet those needs. When there is nothing in the file appropriate to the client's needs, the nurse will have to explore other agencies that may be able to provide for the client. Prior to referring the client to such services, the nurse would obtain information about these agencies, including eligibility requirements, fees, and so on. If the agency is found to be appropriate to the client's situation, the nurse can proceed with the referral. If not, the nurse would explore other avenues for providing the needed services. Finally, the community health nurse can include the information obtained in the resource file for future use with other clients.

DIAGNOSTIC REASONING AND REFERRAL

Nursing diagnosis as part of the referral process focuses on identifying a need for referral. As noted before, the community health nurse makes a determination that the client requires services that the nurse cannot provide. This determination leads to a diagnosis of a need for referral. For instance, the nurse might make a preliminary diagnosis of a "need for referral due to requirements for services not provided by the health department." The nurse will also diagnose what types of referrals are needed to meet client situation. Diagnoses of needed referrals may be derived from any of the four components of Dever's epidemiologic perspective. Examples of nursing diagnoses of referral needs related to human biology, environment, life-style, and the health system for a family with adolescent children are presented in Table 9–3.

PLANNING THE REFERRAL

Planning for a referral in a specific client situation begins with identifying goals and objectives for the referral. Goals and objectives will direct the selection of the appropriate referral resource, the second step in planning the referral. If, for example, the desired outcome of the referral is improvement in the client's marital relationship, referral for marriage counseling is appropriate. If, on the other hand, the desired outcome is a divorce, a referral for legal assistance would be more appropriate.

Selection of the appropriate referral resource is based on other considerations in addition to the expected outcome. These include the need to select a referral resource that is acceptable to the client, for which the client is eligible, and that fits the constraints of the client situation. Information obtained in the assessment stage of the process allows the nurse to select a referral resource that addresses these considerations.

Diagnosed needs for referral may reflect any of the three levels of prevention—primary, secondary, or tertiary. For instance, the sample diagnoses in Table 9–3 related to immunization and nutrition education reflect needs for primary prevention. A need for tertiary prevention is indicated by the diagnosis related to suicide prevention, while the remaining diagnoses included in the table reflect needs for secondary preventive measures.

The level of prevention indicated by the diagnosed need for a referral will help direct the selection of appropriate referral resources. For example, the first diagnosis included in Table 9–3 indicates a need for primary prevention of childhood illnessess and for a referral to an agency such as the local health department for immunization services. If, on the other hand, the need is for diagnosis and treatment of an existing illness resembling polio, the referral would be made to a physician. Similarly, if the client has suffered paralysis as a result of polio, a referral for tertiary preventive measures in the form of rehabilitation would be required.

The third aspect of planning the referral is preparation of the client. This may be referred to as "working up the client."[13] There may be a need to work with clients to enable them to recognize the need for and accept the referrals. The need to prepare clients is frequently seen in situations of substance abuse or family violence. For instance, a client might initially deny a drinking problem and refuse a referral for help. Or, an abused wife may hesitate to take advantage of a shelter referral, hoping that the abuse will stop. Community health nurses in one study frequently noted that preparing the client for the referral involved presenting the referral at the appropriate time. Referrals suggested at a time when the client has acknowledged a problem and the inability to cope with it are much more effective than referrals pre-

TABLE 9–3. SAMPLE NURSING DIAGNOSES RELATED TO REFERRAL NEEDS OF A FAMILY WITH ADOLESCENT CHILDREN

Area of Focus	Related Nursing Diagnosis
Human biology	• Need for referral for immunizations due to inadequate immune status • Need for referral diagnosis and treatment for gonorrhea due to exposure to a diagnosed case
Environment	
Physical	• Need for referral to sanitation department owing to cockroaches in home
Psychological	• Need for referral for counseling to prevent a second suicide attempt
Social	• Need for referral for financial assistance because of income inadequate to meet needs
Life-style	• Need for referral to nutritionist due to inadequate knowledge of dietary requirements of adolescents • Need for referral of father to smoking cessation program stemming from children's allergies to cigarette smoke
Health system	• Need for referral to Medicaid program because of low income and lack of a source of health care

sented when the client denies the immediacy of the problem or is otherwise unreceptive.[13] Findings of other studies also support the idea that adequate preparation of the client enhances compliance with the referral.[14]

Finally, the nurse plans for follow-up on the referral. This necessitates establishing evaluative criteria as well as plans for contacting the client to assess the outcome of the referral. Evaluative criteria would reflect the level of prevention involved in specific interventions. For example, criteria related to the diagnosed need for a referral to immunization services, a primary preventive measure, would focus on whether the client received immunizations. Evaluative criteria for a referral for assistance with existing financial problems would involve the adequacy of the client's finances after the referral. Finally, evaluation of a tertiary preventive measure such as referral for counseling to prevent a subsequent suicide attempt would focus on whether or not the client again attempted suicide.

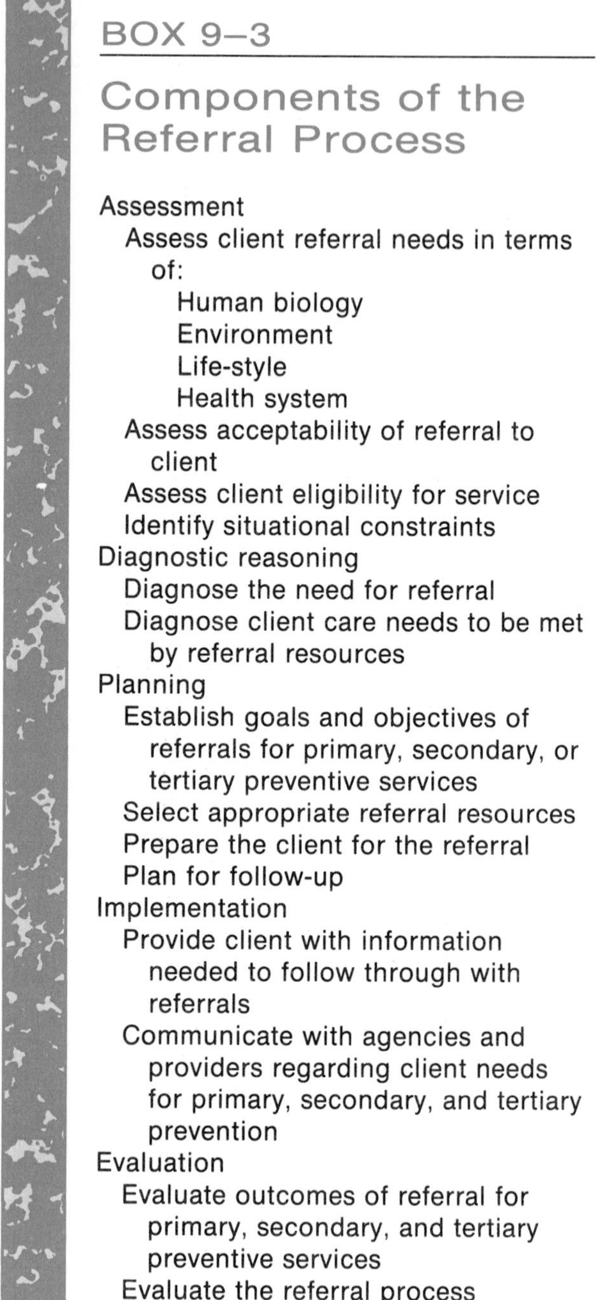
BOX 9–3

Components of the Referral Process

Assessment
- Assess client referral needs in terms of:
  - Human biology
  - Environment
  - Life-style
  - Health system
- Assess acceptability of referral to client
- Assess client eligibility for service
- Identify situational constraints

Diagnostic reasoning
- Diagnose the need for referral
- Diagnose client care needs to be met by referral resources

Planning
- Establish goals and objectives of referrals for primary, secondary, or tertiary preventive services
- Select appropriate referral resources
- Prepare the client for the referral
- Plan for follow-up

Implementation
- Provide client with information needed to follow through with referrals
- Communicate with agencies and providers regarding client needs for primary, secondary, and tertiary prevention

Evaluation
- Evaluate outcomes of referral for primary, secondary, and tertiary preventive services
- Evaluate the referral process

IMPLEMENTING THE REFERRAL

Implementing the referral entails providing the client with the information he or she will need to contact a referral resource and successfully obtain assistance. This information includes where the referral resource is located, when the client should go there, how to obtain services, what services are provided, and any fees involved. The client also needs to know what items, if any, should be taken to the agency (for example, pay stubs, medical bills, etc.), and what to expect when they follow through on the referral. For example, clients may need to know that they may have to wait all day to be seen or that the application process may take several days. When clients have a clear understanding of what to expect from a referral, they are less likely to be frustrated and more likely to follow through than if they encounter unexpected roadblocks.

The second aspect of implementing the referral involves providing the referral resource with information about the client. This information may not be strictly required, but will usually ease the client's entry into the referral system. Information can be telephoned to the agency in advance of the client's visit or can be written down for clients to take with them. Types of information that may be useful include client information (name, age, address, etc.), the source of the referral (yourself and/or your agency), and the reason for the referral. It may also be helpful to inform the referral agency of any need for feedback and how you would like to receive that feedback. For example, if the nurse calls the agency to provide information about the client and the reason for referral, the nurse might ask agency personnel to call after the client's visit, or might request a written summary of action taken.

EVALUATING THE REFERRAL

The final step of the referral process is to follow up on the results of the referral using the evaluative criteria developed in the planning stage of the process. These criteria, as noted earlier, reflect the level of prevention involved in interventions employed. Some of the questions asked might include the following: Did the client follow through on the referral? If so, what was the outcome? Were services provided or was the client rejected? If the client has not followed through, why not? What happened to prevent him or her from doing so? Were there constraints that were overlooked in your assessment of the situation or did the client just choose not to follow through? The final consideration in follow-up is whether the referral served to resolve the problem for which it was made. If not, the planning stage of the epidemiologic prevention process model begins again and other solutions are attempted.

Evaluation also focuses on the use of the referral process itself. Again, questions related to the adequacy of the assessment, the accuracy of diagnosis, and the thoroughness of planning and implementation of the referral can provide direction for modifying future use of the referral process. Components of that process are summarized in Box 9–3.

CHAPTER HIGHLIGHTS

- Discharge planning and referral facilitate client transitions between components of the health-care system and provide for continuity of client care.
- Discharge planning has the advantage of promoting continuity of care for the client. For health-care providers or agencies, discharge planning may reduce the length and cost of services provided and improve communication about client needs and plan of care.
- Discharge planning is usually employed with individuals and families as the recipients of care. Individuals, families, groups, or communities can be the beneficiaries of the referral process.
- Assessment in both processes focuses on human biological, environmental, life-style, and health-system factors that influence client health.
- Special considerations in assessing the referral situation include the acceptability of the referral to the client, client eligibility for services, situational constraints, and availability of resources to meet the client's needs.
- Information about community resources is needed in both processes. This information can be included in a resource file entry that contains data on agency funding, business hours, contact persons, how referrals are to be made, eligibility requirements, fees, and types of services provided.
- Nursing diagnoses in discharge planning and referral may indicate needs for primary, secondary, or tertiary preventive measures, and any or all of these levels of prevention may be addressed by planning in either process.
- Planning for discharge includes prioritizing client needs, developing goals and objectives, identifying appropriate sources of service, and delineating specific discharge activities. Obtaining client consent to contact outside agencies and planning for evaluation are other tasks in planning for discharge.
- Planning for referral involves establishing goals and objectives for the referral, selecting referral resources appropriate to client needs, preparing the client for the referral, and planning for evaluation of the referral.
- Implementing a discharge plan or a referral involves communicating with both the client or significant others and those individuals who will assume responsibility for the client's care.
- Evaluation of a discharge plan or a referral focuses on the achievement or nonachievement of the desired client outcome as well as on the effectiveness of the process used.

Review Questions

1. Describe two purposes of discharge planning. Give an example of each purpose. (p. 162)
2. What are the advantages of discharge planning for the client? For the health-care providers or agencies involved? (p. 162)
3. Give two reasons why community health nurses should be involved in discharge planning. (p. 163)
4. Identify at least three activities involved in developing a discharge plan. Give an example of each. (p. 166)
5. Describe at least three purposes for making a referral. Give an example of each purpose. (p. 169)
6. Identify at least four categories of information that would be included in a resource file entry. Why might each of these categories of information be needed? (p. 171)
7. Describe four considerations in assessing a specific referral situation. Give an example of the influence of each on the referral. (p. 172)
8. Identify at least three activities involved in planning a referral. Give an example of a community health nurse performing each activity. (p. 173)
9. What are the two aspects of evaluation related to both discharge planning and referral? (pp. 167 and 174)

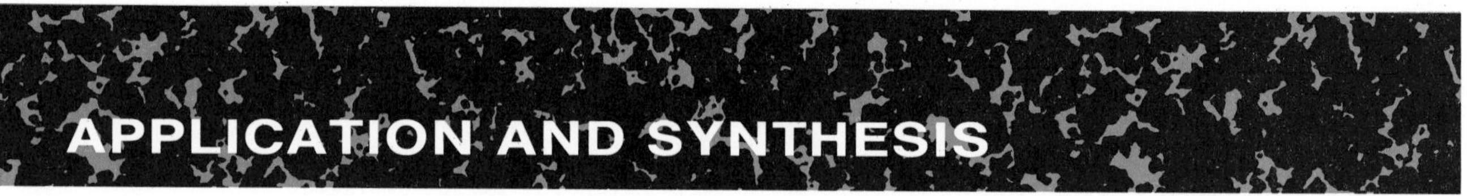

APPLICATION AND SYNTHESIS

Mrs. Smith is 67 years old. She was admitted to the hospital a week ago with a broken ankle. It is believed that she fractured her ankle stepping off a curb. Her bones are very fragile because of osteoporosis.

Mrs. Smith is retired and receives Social Security benefits. She lives with her son and 5-year-old grandson. Mrs. Smith's son is employed in heavy construction. Because of the recent rains, he has not been able to work consistently and they have little savings. Mrs. Smith confides that she doesn't know how they will pay for the portion of the hospital bill that Medicare does not cover. Mrs. Smith usually takes care of her grandson when her son is working. She also does the housework, although her son does most of the heavy work around the house.

Mrs. Smith will be ready for discharge in a day or two. She has a follow-up appointment for the orthopedist in a week, but says she doesn't know how she will get there if her son is working that day. Mrs. Smith has been taught how to use a walker and will need to continue its use for several weeks.

1. Is Mrs. Smith a candidate for in-depth discharge planning? Which criteria for in-depth discharge planning does she meet?
2. What are Mrs. Smith's discharge planning needs? How do human biological, environmental, life-style, and health-system factors influence these needs?
3. What are your goals and objectives for discharge planning in this situation? How would you involve Mrs. Smith in planning for her discharge? Who else should be involved?
4. What primary, secondary, and tertiary preventive measures are indicated for Mrs. Smith?
5. What referrals would be appropriate for Mrs. Smith? What is the expected outcome of these referrals? How would you go about making the referrals?
6. How would you evaluate the effectiveness of discharge planning and referral in the care of Mrs. Smith? What evaluative criteria would you use?

REFERENCES

1. Jowett, S., & Armitage, S. (1988). Hospital and community liaison links in nursing: The role of the liaison nurse. *Journal of Advanced Nursing, 13,* 579–587.
2. Clausen, C. (1984). Staff R.N.: A discharge planner. *Nursing Management, 15*(11), 58–60.
3. Kromminga, S. K., & Ostwald, S. K. (1987). The public health nurse as discharge planner: Patient's perceptions of the discharge process. *Public Health Nursing, 4*(4), 224–229.
4. Hartigan, E. G., & Brown, J. (1985). *Discharge planning for continuity of care.* New York: National League for Nursing.
5. Weinberger, B. (1989). Discharge planning: The sooner, the better. *Nursing 89, 19,* 75–76.
6. Hartigan, E. G. (1987). Discharge planning: Identification of high-risk groups. *Nursing Management, 18*(12), 30–32.
7. Schlemmer, B. (1989). The status of discharge planning in intensive care units. *Nursing Management, 20*(7), 88A–B, 88D, 88F, 88J, 88L, 88P.
8. Thliveris, M. (1990). A hospitalwide discharge planning program. *Dimensions, 67*(1), 38–39.
9. Packard-Hellie, M. T., & Lancaster, D. B. (1989). A vital link in continuity of care. *Nursing Management, 20*(8), 32–34.
10. Esper, P. S. (1988). Discharge planning—A quality assurance approach. *Nursing Management, 19*(10), 66–68.
11. Peters, D. A. (1989). A concept of nursing discharge. *Holistic Nursing Practice, 3*(2), 18–25.
12. Slevin, A. P., & Roberts, A. S. (1987). Discharge planning: A tool for decision making. *Nursing Management, 18*(12), 47–50.
13. Luker, K. A., & Chalmers, K. I. (1989). The referral process in health visiting. *International Journal of Nursing Studies, 26,* 173–185.
14. Jones, S. L., Jones, P. K., Katz, J., & Ring, S. (1988). Improving compliance with referrals from the emergency department. *Journal of Emergency Nursing, 14*(1), 27–29.

RECOMMENDED READINGS

Jowett, S., & Armitage, S. (1988). Hospital and community liaison links in nursing: The role of the liaison nurse. *Journal of Advanced Nursing, 13,* 579–587.

Describes three models of linkage in discharge planning. Addresses the role of the community health nurse and the effectiveness of each model.

Kromminga, S. K., & Ostwald, S. K. (1987). The public health nurse as discharge planner: Patient's perceptions of the discharge process. *Public Health Nursing, 4,* 224–229.

Presents findings of a research study on the effectiveness of discharge planning by community health nurses in addressing client-identified needs.

Luker, K. A., & Chalmers, K. I. (1989). The referral process in health visiting. *International Journal of Nursing Studies, 26,* 173–185.

Sets forth the results of a qualitative study of the reasons for and process used in referrals made by community health nurses in England.

O'Meara, R. (1986). A contractual relationship between a visiting nurse association and a hospice. *Quality Review Bulletin, 12*(5), 172–174.

Discusses the facilitation of the referral process in two agencies with a long-term contractual relationship.

Slevin, A. P., & Roberts, A. S. (1987). Discharge planning: A tool for decision making. *Nursing Management, 18*(12), 47–50.

Presents another model for directing discharge planning. A flowsheet diagram of the process provides an easy understanding of the model.

Thliveris, M. (1990). A hospitalwide discharge planning program. *Dimensions, 67*(1), 38–39.

Offers a model used for discharge planning by the Salvation Army Grace General Hospital. Also addresses standards for discharge planning.

Volland, P. J. (1988). *Discharge planning: An interdisciplinary approach to continuity of care.* New York: National Health.

Provides an overview of discharge planning by a multidisciplinary group.

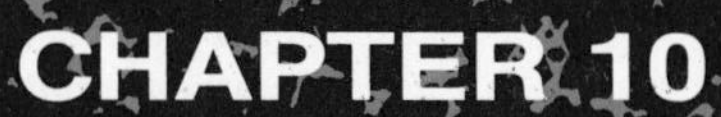

CHAPTER 10

The Research Process

KEY TERMS

analytic epidemiology
confidentiality
cross-sectional studies
dependent variable
descriptive epidemiology
ecological studies
experimental studies
extraneous variables
independent variable
informed consent
institutional review boards
hypothesis
literature review
observational studies
prophylactic trials
prospective studies
phenomena
relational studies
research
research design
research population
research sample
research problem
retrospective research
therapeutic trials
trial
triangulation

Many of the roles of community health nurses are duplicated by other health-care providers. If community health nursing is to flourish as a nursing specialty, community health nurses must prove their effectiveness in improving the health of the population. Nursing research can provide that proof.

In general, those best able to conduct research in a scientific field are those who know the field. Because community health nurses are intimately acquainted with their practice, they are in a position to identify areas in which research is needed and to study the outcomes of their practice. For this reason, community health nurses should conduct community health nursing research.

Although not every community health nurse may have the talent, inclination, or educational preparation to conduct research, each nurse has a responsibility to keep abreast of research findings in his or her areas of practice and should be prepared to review that research critically. To do this, community health nurses must have a basic understanding of the research process and its implications for community health nursing.

(*continued*)

LEARNING OBJECTIVES

After reading this chapter you should be able to:

- Identify at least seven steps of the research process.
- Describe four factors influencing research in community health nursing.
- Identify at least three research roles for community health nurses.
- Differentiate between observational and experimental studies.
- Describe three types of observational studies.
- Discuss at least four ethical concerns in community health nursing research.
- Identify three aspects of assessment related to the role of research consumer.
- Describe four considerations in planning for the use of research findings in community health nursing practice.

STEPS OF THE RESEARCH PROCESS

Research is the systematic study of observed events with the intent to expand knowledge about those events and—in a practice-oriented discipline—to control them. To use or conduct research, community health nurses need to be conversant with the research process. The steps in this process may vary somewhat depending upon the type of research conducted, but generally include the steps presented in Box 10–1.

Identifying the research problem or question is the first step of the process. In this step, the nurse researcher identifies a question derived from community health nursing practice that requires an answer. The ***research problem*** is a statement of the purpose of the research study, usually phrased as a question, and forms the basis for a research study designed to answer the question posed.

BOX 10–1

Steps in the Research Process

1. Identify the research problem or question
2. Review the literature related to the problem
3. Identify the research variables
4. Formulate research hypotheses
5. Select an appropriate research design
6. Select a representative sample for the study
7. Collect the data
8. Analyze the data
9. Communicate the findings to others

The second step in the research process is the ***literature review,*** an examination of published materials in the area of interest. In the literature review, the nurse researcher examines previous studies done on the topic, their findings, and the methods employed. He or she also examines literature on theoretical perspectives that may help to explain the phenomenon being studied.

Identifying the research variables is the third step of the process. As noted earlier, variables are conditions that change or *vary*. Variables can be of three types: independent variables, dependent variables, and extraneous variables.[1] ***Independent variables*** are the conditions that change, either via manipulation by the researcher or in the normal course of affairs, that result in changes in dependent variables. ***Dependent variables*** are the conditions that are expected to vary as a result of changes in the independent variable.[1] An independent variable may be viewed as the cause in a cause-effect relationship, while the dependent variable is the effect. ***Extraneous variables*** are other factors in the research situation that may affect the outcome or the dependent variable. Using child-abuse research as an example, the occurrence of child abuse would be a dependent variable that might change with exposure to parenting education, an independent variable. In this example, economic pressures and alcohol abuse would be extraneous variables that could also influence the occurrence of child abuse.

The fourth step in the research process is formulating hypotheses. A ***hypothesis*** is an educated guess as to the outcome of the research study. Not all research studies contain hypotheses, because the nurse researcher may be trying to determine factors involved in a phenomenon and may not know before hand what those factors are. For instance, a community health nurse might initiate a preliminary study to determine what factors contribute to the abilities of some nurses to work effectively with clients from other cultures. If there is no previous research in this area and the nurse has not identified any possible contributing factors from his or her observations, the study will not have any hypotheses. If there are some possible contributing factors suggested in the literature or observed by the nurse, the nurse might hypothesize that effective nurses have more of factors x, y, and z than do ineffective nurses.

The ***research design*** is the type of approach taken to answer a specific research question. Selection of a research design, the fifth step in the research process, is based on the type of question being asked. Research designs frequently used in community health research will be discussed in more detail later in this chapter.

Selecting a research sample is the sixth step in the research process. The ***research sample*** is the group of individuals who will participate in the research study. The sample selected needs to represent as closely as possible the larger group of people about whom the research question is asked. This larger group is usually referred to as the ***research population.***

Collecting data for the study (step seven) involves measurement of the variables of interest to the researcher. Data can be collected in a variety of ways including observation, actual instrument measurements (for example, measuring blood pressure with a sphygmomanometer), interviews, questionnaires, and so forth. Methods used should be consistent with the research question asked and the variables to be measured.

Once data have been collected, they must be analyzed (step eight in the research process) and patterns among data interpreted. What do the measurements mean in terms of the answer to the research questions posed? Finally, in step nine the findings of the research study must be communicated to others (for example, to other community health nurses who might be able to use the findings in their practice).

RESEARCH IN COMMUNITY HEALTH NURSING

Research generates knowledge and understanding of observed events. Community health nurses use knowledge derived from research to address problems of health promotion, illness prevention, and health restoration. Research is also used to develop and test theories that explain events of interest to nursing.

Community health nursing research serves several additional purposes. The first is to identify and define the scope of community health nursing. As noted in Chapter 4, Community Health Nursing, there is ongoing disagreement about the definition of this unique field of practice. Some practitioners have suggested a need for research that better defines the specialty of community health nursing,[2,3] and some studies have been undertaken for this purpose.[4–7]

An equally important goal of research is documenting the effects of community health nursing interventions. Facing cutbacks in program funding, community health nurses must provide evidence of the value of their role in the health-care system.[8] This goal is sometimes difficult to accomplish in a field where a successful intervention or outcome is frequently manifested by the *absence* of a particular condition. It is difficult, for example, to verify that the fact that an adolescent does not become an abusive parent is the result of nursing intervention rather than other factors. Outcome measures must be developed that will validate the effectiveness of community health nursing interventions.[3] Some research efforts have been undertaken to this end,[9–11] but additional work is needed.

The cost-effectiveness of community health nursing interventions also require research. Cost savings due to community health nursing care versus institutional care are somewhat easier to document than client health outcomes, and several studies have been conducted in this area.[2,3]

Research in community health nursing can also guide community health nursing education. Studies that identify societal needs or delineate the roles and functions of community health nurses provide direction for community health nursing curriculum development at baccalaureate, master's, and doctoral levels and guide the development of textbooks such as this. For example, research on the educational needs of home health nurses provided the direction for Chapter 25, Care of Clients in the Home Setting.[12]

A final purpose for community health nursing research is to provide a basis for influencing health policy formation.[13] Community health nurses can use research findings to influence institutional policymakers as well as policymakers at local, state, and federal levels in developing health policies that will contribute to wellness for all people.

FACTORS INFLUENCING COMMUNITY HEALTH NURSING RESEARCH

Many factors influence the type and extent of research conducted in community health nursing. These factors include societal needs, the extent of theory development and previous research, the educational preparation for research within the profession, and the profession's access to funding.

SOCIETAL NEEDS

In a practice-based discipline such as community health nursing, research should be guided by the health-related needs of society rather than the quest for knowledge in and of itself.[14] While the curiosity and interest of a researcher are important in motivating one to undertake a research study, they are insufficient reasons for conducting research. Community health nursing research should contribute to achievement of the profession's overall goal, namely improving the health of the public.

THEORY DEVELOPMENT AND PRIOR RESEARCH

Two reviews of nursing research literature revealed that research on community health nursing tends to lack a theoretical foundation.[2,15] This state of affairs may be due to an absence of nursing theories that adequately address the population focus of community health nursing. Valid theoretical frameworks for community health nursing research should incorporate this population focus and address the diversity of health problems that community health nurses encounter.[2] The epidemiologic prevention process model used in this book is one attempt to provide a theoretical framework that can guide both community health nursing practice and research.

The quantity and quality of previous research in a field also influences current research efforts. The majority of research related strictly to community health nursing has been descriptive in nature. Descriptive research is characteristic of disciplines, such as community health nursing, that are still defining and describing the events of interest to the profession. Once a discipline has adequately described the phenomena of interest, researchers can begin to turn to relational and experimental studies designed to understand and control those phenomena. Thus far, there have been relatively few experimental studies in community health nursing. Few studies have been replicated and most studies reflected program evaluation themes.[2]

While research on community health nursing per se is somewhat lacking, there is a large body of research in and outside of nursing that is used by community health nurses as a basis for practice. Epidemiologic research, as well as research in the physical and behavioral sciences, contributes to the interventions used by community health nurses in addressing a wide variety of societal health problems. In many of these areas, research has advanced beyond the exploratory phase and includes both experimental and quasi-experimental studies. The applicability of the findings of such research to community health nursing remains to be tested by community health nurse researchers.

EDUCATIONAL PREPARATION FOR RESEARCH

Another factor that influences research within a discipline is the educational preparation of its members relative to research. According to the American Nurses' Association Commission on Nursing Research,[16] nurses educated at the baccalaureate level should be prepared to evaluate and implement research findings in their practice. To do so, these nurses need a basic understanding of the research process. At the master's level, nurses should be prepared to participate in the design and implementation of research studies, while doctorally prepared nurses should be capable of independent research.

RESEARCH FUNDING

Access to research funding is another factor that significantly influences the research activities of a discipline. One of the many effects of the Gramm-Rudman balanced-budget legislation of 1985 is a reduction in federal funding for research in a number of fields including nursing.[17] Research can be an expensive, time-consuming endeavor, and external sources of funding are needed if nurses are to continue their research efforts.

Several approaches have been suggested for offsetting the reduced availability of federal research funds. One approach is to organize a network of nurse researchers to influence legislators to support nursing research. This strategy was effective in promoting the creation of the Center for Nursing Research.[13] Another suggestion is to seek funding avenues other than federal research grants. Private foundations and alternative funding sources could be more fully explored than they have been in the past.[17]

One source of research funding particularly appropriate to community health nursing could be business and industry.[18] The corporate sector is always interested in interventions that will limit expenditures for employee health benefits, and it is also interested in marketable health-related products. Both of these interests provide avenues for research related to community health nursing.

RESEARCH ROLES FOR COMMUNITY HEALTH NURSES

Although not every community health nurse has the educational preparation to conduct research, research *involvement* is an integral part of the community health nurse's role. This involvement in research might include any of four basic research roles: using research findings, identifying research questions, collecting data, and designing and conducting research studies.

To be of practical value to the profession, research findings must be incorporated into nursing practice. For this reason, every community health nurse should be conversant with research studies related to his or her practice setting and be able to evaluate the applicability of research findings in everyday practice. The task of evaluating research findings will be discussed in more detail later in this chapter.

The second research role for all community health nurses involves identifying research questions. These questions are derived from observations of community health nurses in their everyday practice. For example, a community health nurse working in a high school might question why some sexually active adolescents use effective methods of contraception and some do not. This question might be the catalyst for research in this area.

In community health nursing, research questions might be related to the influence of human biological, environmental, life-style, or health system factors on health or to the effectiveness of community health nursing interventions at the primary, secondary, and tertiary levels of prevention. Sample research questions related to the influence of the four components of Dever's epidemiologic perspective are presented in Table 10–1, while Table 10–2 presents potential research questions related to primary, secondary, and tertiary preventive measures.

Data collection is a third research role for every community health nurse. In this role, the nurse collects data under the direction of a researcher, using specific measurement techniques designed to obtain data needed to answer a research question. Continuing with the example of contraceptive use by some adolescents, the community health nurse might in-

TABLE 10–1. SAMPLE RESEARCH QUESTIONS RELATED TO HUMAN BIOLOGY, ENVIRONMENT, LIFE-STYLE, AND THE HEALTH SYSTEM

Area of Focus	Related Research Questions
Human biology	• To what extent does decreased physical mobility limit the interaction of elderly clients? • Is there a difference in the incidence of hypertension in black and white clients of similar education and economic background?
Environment	• Does sexuality as presented in the popular media contribute to adolescent sexual activity? • What effect does the availability of public transportation have on the extent of social isolation experienced by older clients?
Life-style	• Is there a relationship between dietary patterns throughout life and the incidence of arthritis in later years? • What is the relationship between caffeine intake and weight in middle-aged women?
Health system	• Does collaboration among health-care agencies reduce fragmentation of health care? • Are there differences in client outcomes between public and private health-care services?

TABLE 10–2. SAMPLE RESEARCH QUESTIONS RELATED TO PRIMARY, SECONDARY, AND TERTIARY PREVENTION

Level of Prevention	Related Research Questions
Primary prevention	• Does elementary school education on smoking decrease the number of persons who smoke later in life? • What effect do efforts to promote self-esteem in school-age girls have on sexual activity in adolescence? • What effect does mandatory seat belt use by children and adults have on the incidence of motor vehicle accident fatalities?
Secondary prevention	• What effect do periodic home visits by community health nurses have on client compliance with treatment for tuberculosis? • Do warm soaks prior to treatment improve the effectiveness of passive range-of-motion exercises in increasing joint mobility in clients with arthritis? • Do brown sugar dressings improve healing of decubiti in bedfast clients?
Tertiary prevention	• Does education on the use of condoms for individuals with sexually transmitted diseases reduce the incidence of subsequent infections? • Does participation in a support group for abusive parents reduce the number of instances of subsequent abuse by group members? • What is the effect of contact notification practices on the incidence of primary and secondary syphilis?

terview selected adolescents, using a particular set of questions, to elicit their reasons for using or not using contraceptives.

The methods used to collect data can be either qualitative or quantitative in nature. Qualitative methods allow the researcher to describe events in community health nursing practice in terms that are not numerically quantifiable, whereas in quantitative methods the events observed in practice are described in terms of numerical values. For example, qualitative research methods such as observations and interviews with local residents and health-care providers might be used to describe the health of a community. The community's health could also be described quantitatively in terms of numbers of specific events that occur within the community, such as the number of cases of measles that occurred last year, the number of adolescent pregnancies, and so on.

Because of the broad nature of many questions posed in community health nursing research, it has been suggested that nurse researchers engage in ***triangulation,*** or the use of several types of research methods in a single study.[19] Certainly in a study of the health needs of a population, both quantitative and qualitative methods of data collection would be appropriate.

The three research roles described to this point may be performed by community health nurses educated at the baccalaureate, master's, or doctoral level. Independent execution of the fourth role, designing and conducting research studies, requires advanced educational preparation, usually at the doctoral level. In this role, the community health nurse selects a question and designs a means of obtaining answers to that question. For example, the nurse researcher might design a study to discover factors contributing to use or nonuse of contraceptives by adolescents.

RESEARCH DESIGNS FOR COMMUNITY HEALTH NURSING

As noted earlier, the research design is the approach taken to answer the research question. The design is structured to exert as much control as possible over the study so findings can be relied upon. Because community health nursing is a synthesis of nursing and the science of public health, much of the profession's research terminology is borrowed from epidemiology. Epidemiologic research is quantitative in nature and can be either descriptive or analytic.[20]

In ***descriptive epidemiology,*** the community health nurse researcher observes and records patterns of events related to an area of interest. Questions related to factors influencing health would generally give rise to descriptive epidemiologic research. The intent of descriptive research is to describe ***phenomena,*** or occurrences relevant to community health nursing. Child abuse, for instance, is a phenomenon or an observed occurrence that is of interest to community health nurses. A descriptive study of child abuse would attempt to describe the factors associated with child abuse.

Results of descriptive studies might suggest relationships between factors and outcomes that merit further study. These relationships are tested in analytic epidemiologic studies. ***Analytic epidemiology*** tests the validity of relationships that may have been suggested by the findings of descriptive studies.[21] These studies examine the strength of statistical relationships among factors. For example, descriptive studies suggested a relationship between natural fluoride in the water and the absence of dental caries. Analytic studies of populations with and without natural fluoride in their water indicated significant differences occurred in the incidence of dental caries with lower incidence of caries in communities with fluoride in the water.

Analytic studies can be of two types—ecological or relational.[20] ***Ecological studies*** examine relationships between factors within population groups and compare the incidence of a specific event in population groups with and without a supposed causative factor. In the fluoride example, studies compared the incidence of dental caries in towns with and without fluoride in the water. The findings of ecological studies may hold up for population groups, but not necessarily for all the individuals who make up a particular group.

In ***relational studies,*** on the other hand, the relationship between the event and the supposed cause is examined within single individuals rather than in population groups. For instance, a researcher could compare the incidence of dental caries in those particular people who got their water from the local fluoride-rich water supply and those who drank bottled water that did not contain fluoride. Greater incidence of dental caries among those drinking bottled water would provide additional support for the supposed relationship between fluoride and dental caries.

Relational studies can be either observational or experimental.[22] In an ***observational study,*** the nurse researcher observes the effects of a naturally occurring event, and contrasts the outcome in those individuals experiencing the event with those who have not experienced it. For example, the community health nurse who examines the relationship between marital stress and child abuse would conduct an observational study since he or she would not create the marital stress in order to study its effects. The nurse would compare the incidence of child abuse in families experiencing marital stress with families having stable marriages.

In epidemiologic research terminology, observational studies can be retrospective, cross-sectional, or prospective depending upon the timing of subject selection in relation to exposure to the independent variable and development of the effect or dependent variable. When study subjects include people with and without the health condition in question, a ***retrospective research*** approach is used.[21] For instance, in a study of factors influencing adolescent alcohol use, groups of teenagers who drink alcohol and those who do not might be interviewed to determine what factors contributed to the decision to drink or not to drink. Retrospective research works backwards from the effect to try to establish a relationship with a suspected cause. Retrospective research studies are also called "case-control" studies.[22,23]

In ***prospective studies,*** some subjects have been exposed to the suspected causative factor, while others have not.[21] These two groups are then followed forward in time to determine the incidence of the condition of interest in individuals who were exposed versus those who were not. In a prospective study of the effect of parental smoking on children's decisions to smoke or not smoke, a group of youngsters whose parents smoke and those whose parents do not smoke would be followed for a period of years to see what proportion of each group begins to smoke. Other terms for prospective studies include "cohort" studies and "longitudinal" studies.[20,22]

Cross-sectional studies explore the relationship of a health condition to other variables of interest in a defined population at a given point in time.[24] These studies are also called "prevalence" studies because they aid in determining the prevalence of both condition and potential causative factors at any particular time. A school nurse, for example, might want to study the use of seat belts by children at different grade levels. Differences in findings among grade levels might suggest factors that influence seat belt use (for example, parents may pay more attention to seat belt use by younger children) or suggest particular groups to be targeted for educational efforts related to seat belt use.

In ***experimental studies,*** the community health nurse researcher manipulates exposure of subjects to the independent variable and looks for differences in the dependent variable among groups of people exposed to the causative factor and those who are not. Questions related to the efficacy of primary, secondary, and tertiary prevention would be answered by experimental studies. In such studies, manipulation of the independent variable involves applying an intervention. This application of an intervention by the researcher is called a ***trial.*** Trials can involve the removal of a risk factor or addition of some other factor and can be either prophylactic or therapeutic in nature depending upon the timing of the intervention.[20]

In a ***prophylactic trial,*** the intervention is designed to prevent the occurrence of a health problem. Prophylactic trials could be used to study the effectiveness of either primary or tertiary prevention. In a prophylactic trial of a primary preventive intervention, the dependent variable would be prevention of an event from occurring at all, while the dependent variable in a prophylactic trial would reflect prevention of the recurrence of a problem. Interventions designed to promote health would also be tested in prophylactic trials.

Therapeutic trials, on the other hand, investigate the effects of secondary preventive interventions. In these studies, the researcher exposes a group of subjects to an intervention designed to resolve an existing health problem.[20] Again, the intervention itself can be either positive or negative. Positive interventions add a factor to the situation being studied, whereas negative interventions reduce or eliminate causative factors. For example, one might explore the effects of teaching parenting techniques (a positive intervention) or reducing environmental stressors (a negative intervention) on the incidence of child abuse by parents who are already abusive.

Community health nurses engaged in research can use one or a combination of the research designs depicted in Figure 10–1. The selection of a particular design will depend on the research question and the extent of previous research related to the question. For example, descriptive studies are appropriate in studying topics about which little is known. In other areas where there is already evidence of possible relationships between variables, observational or experimental studies might be more appropriate. Whether an observational or an experimental design is chosen will depend primarily on whether the situation permits manipulation of variables by the researcher. In some instances, manipulation of variables is not possible, whereas in others manipulation of the variables involved would be unethical.

ETHICAL CONCERNS IN COMMUNITY HEALTH NURSING RESEARCH

Research in community health nursing, as in other fields, generates a number of ethical concerns. The ethical issue related to selection of research questions was addressed earlier in the chapter. Community

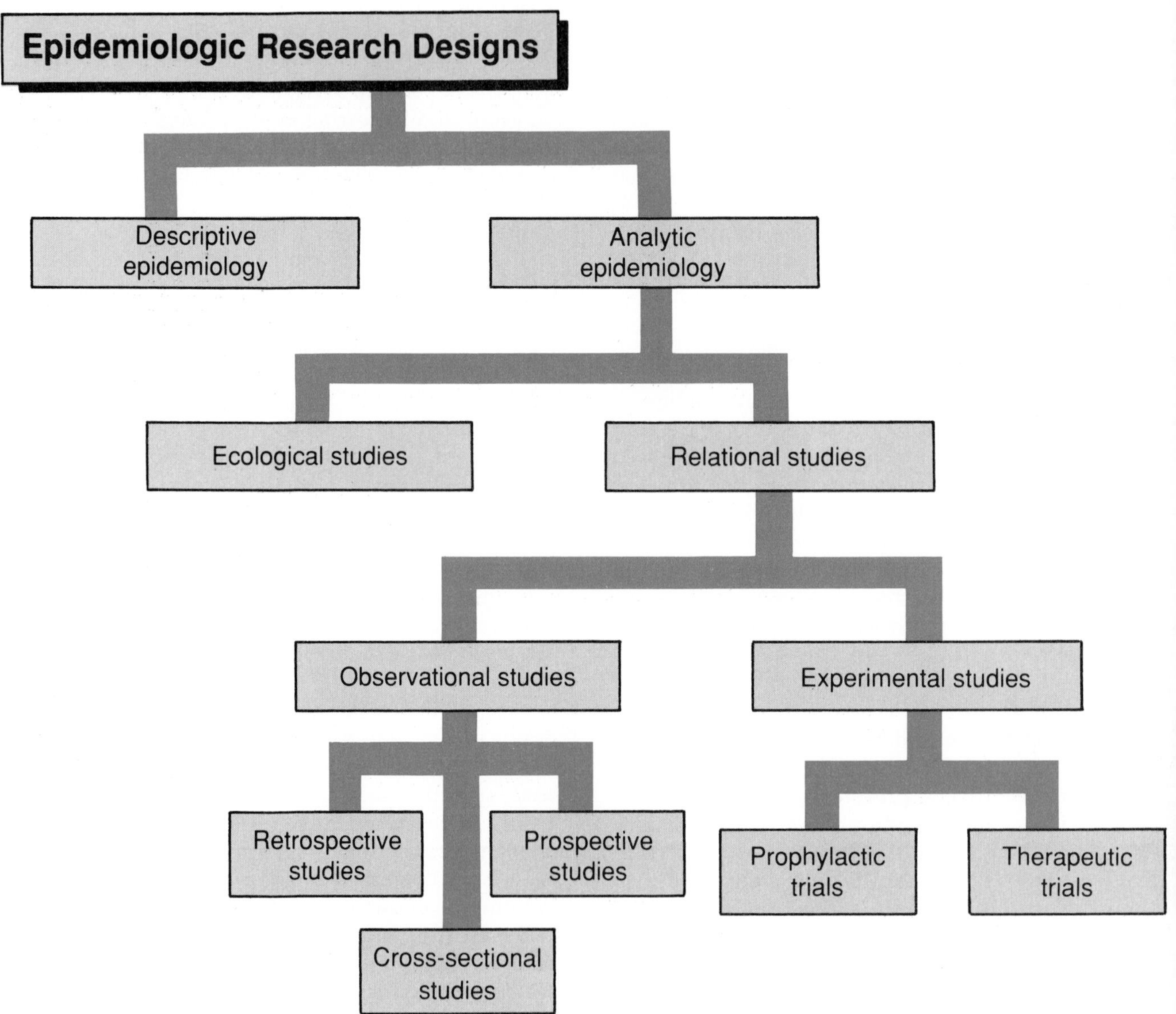

Figure 10–1. Designs used in community health nursing and epidemiologic research.

health nurses have in the public interest and does not waste scarce resources that could be better used elsewhere. There are also ethical concerns to be considered in planning a research study, in collecting data, and in the use of research findings.

ETHICAL CONSIDERATIONS IN PLANNING A RESEARCH STUDY

In planning research studies, ethical considerations include making sure that the researcher's bias is clearly stated at the outset and then prevented from affecting the outcome of the study. Most researchers have some idea of what they expect or hope the findings of a research study will be. These expectations are reflected in the study's hypotheses. Researchers need to be careful to design their studies in such a way that their expectations do not bias the results of the study.

Another concern in planning a research study is protecting research subjects from harm. Generally speaking, most community health nursing interventions are not harmful, so there is little likelihood of harm arising from experimental treatments used in community health nursing research. The possibility of harm arises more often from withholding potentially beneficial interventions from groups used as controls in experimental research.[25] For example, if it is believed that improving family communication patterns will help prevent adolescent pregnancy, it may be harmful, and therefore unethical, to refrain from intervening in families at risk.

Withholding potentially beneficial interventions is a particular problem in community health nursing because of the profession's concern with the health of groups of people rather than individuals. Because this is the case, there is often a strong sense of urgency to use potentially beneficial interventions with all clients, not just a few. The community health nurse engaged in research can, however, ethically withhold an experimental intervention from a control group if the intervention has not yet been shown to be an effective one. Although the people in the control group might have benefitted from the intervention, their loss of this potential benefit is outweighed by the future benefit to others provided by empirical evidence of the intervention's effects.

If the community health nurse is still reluctant to deny interested subjects access to a particular intervention, he or she may use persons who voluntarily decline a particular service as a control group. This approach solves the ethical dilemma of denying an effective intervention to some subjects while giving it to others, but may create a subsequent problem of bias. Bias may occur because clients who agree to a service may differ substantially on critical factors from those who decline services.[3] For example, a nurse may be studying the effect of sex education on adolecents' use of contraceptives. The nurse might be reluctant to deny some adolescents access to information on sex while giving it to others, so he or she might use a group of adolescents who decided not to participate in the educational program as the control group. However, this approach might threaten the validity of study findings if the two groups are very different. If the group who chose to participate in the study were sexually active, while those who chose not to participate were not, any differences in their use of contraceptives would not be due to the education program, but to basic differences between the members of the two groups.

ETHICAL CONSIDERATIONS IN COLLECTING DATA

Ethical concerns in data collection include informed consent, voluntary participation, confidentiality, and the potential for harm to those who will collect the data. A further consideration particularly relevant to community health nursing is treatment for conditions uncovered in the course of the study. Most major educational institutions and health service agencies now have ***institutional review boards,*** which review prospective research in terms of ethical concerns prior to granting permission to conduct the study under the institution's auspices. The specific areas reviewed by the board include potential harm to subjects, provision for informed consent, protection of rights to refuse participation and to withdraw from participation, and provision for confidentiality and protection of subjects' privacy. Community health nurses may serve on institutional review boards or may be instrumental in establishing such review boards in their agencies.

Informed Consent

Informed consent, with respect to research participation, includes knowledge of the nature, duration, and purpose of the study, information on methods of data collection and how the data will be used, and an explanation of inconveniences, potential harm or discomfort, results, effects, and side effects of participation. Again, the question of actual harm arising from participation in a community health nursing research study is rare. However, there is the problem of how much information to give subjects when knowledge of the intent of the study might bias their responses. For example, if one is interested in identifying the beliefs of abusive and nonabusive parents about discipline, knowledge that they are participating in a study of this nature may cause the subjects to provide answers that do not truly reflect their beliefs, but reflect what they think they should say. The researcher must be careful to inform potential subjects of the intent of the study in such a way that the subjects can make informed decisions about participation, but not bias the results of the study.

Voluntary Participation

The right to refuse or withdraw from participation in a study must also be guaranteed to the subject. There must be neither overt nor covert coercion on the part of the researcher to motivate subject participation. This may be difficult to achieve in community health nursing situations because even when there is no coercion intended, the subject may perceive that he or she is being pressured to participate. Much of community health nursing research takes place in conjunction with organized health-care programs, and clients might feel that refusal to participate in the study will jeopardize their access to services. Community health nurse researchers must be sure to convey to clients that refusal to participate in a research study will not interfere with the provision of services. Participants must also clearly understand that they are free to withdraw from the study at any time.

Confidentiality

Consent to participate in a research study does not constitute waiver of subjects' rights to confidentiality. ***Confidentiality,*** or the assurance that subjects' responses will be kept private, is best protected when subjects are anonymous and not even the investigator can identify what information was derived from which subject. When anonymity is not possible because of the circumstances of the study, the investigator must assure subjects that their disclosures will not be publicly reported. The investigator must take whatever steps are necessary to prevent violation of subjects' rights of privacy.

Data Collection by Others

When agency staff or persons other than the researcher will be collecting data, they must be informed of the procedures and activities expected. If potential risks are involved in data collection, those collecting the data must be informed of those risks. There is also a need to inform staff at the time that they are hired that data collection for research purposes will be part of their job.[25]

Dealing with Other Conditions

Occasionally, other medical and health-related conditions are uncovered in the course of a research study. Thus, plans should be made to refer clients with serious illnesses for medical assistance.[14] More difficult decisions arise when referral for care may interfere with the results of the study. For example, the researcher might be reluctant to refer a research subject for care if the referral will mean that the subject is lost to the study. In such instances, the primary consideration should be the welfare of the client rather than the outcome of the study.

Ethical concerns may also surface when research leads to identification of illegal or dangerous behaviors. For example, a researcher who is studying family coping strategies may, in the course of the study, identify evidence of child abuse. In this case, the community health nurse has a clear responsibility to report suspected abuse to the proper authorities. The nurse has a legal and moral responsibility for the welfare of the child that transcends his or her responsibility to hold subjects' responses confidential. A situation of this kind can be addressed more easily if it has been anticipated and potential research subjects have been informed that evidence of abuse will result in a report to the authorities. Potential subjects then have the option of choosing not to participate in the study. This may create unavoidable bias in study findings if child abuse is one of the variables involved. In the case of other behaviors, where the safety of others is not jeopardized (for instance, illegal drug use by study subjects), the researcher may decide to refrain from notifying authorities.

ETHICAL CONSIDERATIONS IN THE USE OF RESEARCH FINDINGS

An ethical concern in nursing research that is seldom addressed is the issue of whether or not to publish the findings of a research study.[14] The question of publication of findings arises when there are methodological flaws in the research that may invalidate findings. The question then is whether one should publish the results, with a complete explanation of the flaws of the study, or refrain from publication altogether. When researchers are highly motivated by external pressure to publish, this question may be a very difficult one to resolve.[14]

The question of whether or not to publish research findings also arises when the study is well conducted and the researcher is confident that the results are valid. Publication of some research findings may be counter to the interests of the funding agency when the results are contrary to the agency's expectations. For example, should a researcher whose study was funded by a tobacco company publish results that confirm that smoking causes cancer? If researchers publish such findings, they will probably lose their source of research funds. On the other hand, the researcher who does not publish such findings has failed to warn the general public of potential hazards of smoking.

As noted earlier, there is some responsibility for researchers to acquaint the general public with the findings of their research when such information is in the public interest. When investigators go further than simply publishing in professional journals, however, it is important that such public dissemination of information not go beyond using data judged by one's peers as reliable and valid.[14] The same is true of the use of research findings to motivate social or political action. The researcher may not ethically make recommendations or take a position that is not supported by the actual data.

THE EPIDEMIOLOGIC PREVENTION PROCESS MODEL AND RESEARCH

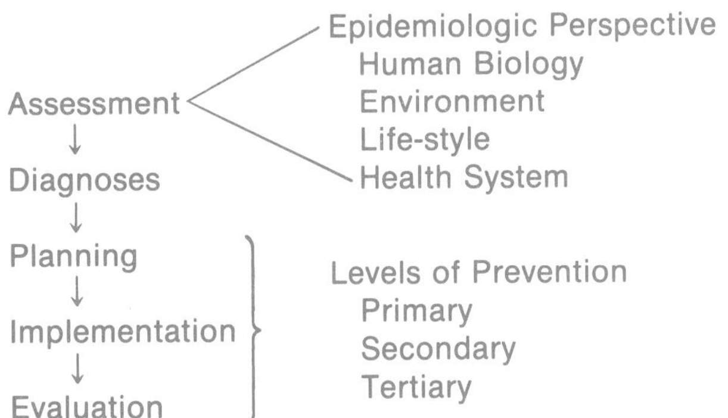

The epidemiologic prevention process model can be used to direct the activity of community health nurses in each of the four research roles discussed earlier. Aspects of Dever's epidemiologic perspective can assist in the identification of questions for community health nursing research, and the steps of the nursing process can be applied to the conduct of a nursing research study. For the sake of brevity, however, the discussion here will focus on the use of the epidemiologic prevention process model in the most common research role performed by community health nurses, that of the consumer of research.

ASSESSING RESEARCH RELATED TO COMMUNITY HEALTH NURSING

In the role of research consumer, the community health nurse assesses research related to community health nursing practice. Assessment in this context involves identifying relevant research, assessing the quality of the research, and assessing the readiness of research findings to be applied in practice.

IDENTIFYING RELEVANT RESEARCH

A wide variety of published research can be potentially applicable to community health nursing. However, it is neither possible nor appropriate for community health nurses to be conversant with all of this literature. This means that community health nurses must be selective and critical consumers of research. In their efforts to keep abreast of new knowledge in their field, community health nurses should scan the literature for articles relevant to their own areas of practice. For instance, if the nurse is dealing primarily with elderly clients in a home health situation, there is little need to delve deeply into the research literature related to the development of parenting skills or factors contributing to adolescent pregnancy. Articles of this type may be interesting but are not particularly relevant to the nurse's practice. Nurses, then, should be familiar with the literature in their field and should focus on journals that present research in those areas.

Even within one's own field of practice, there may be much literature that is not particularly significant, so nurses should spend their time reading studies that deal with significant questions. Information on the topic and its significance for an individual nurse's practice can be obtained by scanning the article or by reading an abstract if available. If in scanning, it does not appear that the article deals with a significant question relevant to one's practice, it should be set aside.

Research studies of interest to community health nurses might deal with factors in any of the four components of Dever's epidemiologic perspective. Research might indicate human biological, environmental, life-style, or health system factors that place certain groups of people at risk for specific health problems or might aid in identifying factors that promote health. Similarly, research might suggest nursing interventions that can modify or eliminate factors that contribute to health problems or that enhance factors that promote health.

ASSESSING THE QUALITY OF RESEARCH

Assessing the quality of the research conducted is the second aspect of assessing research related to community health nursing. Some of the questions to be addressed include the appropriateness of the research design for the problem studied, whether the sample was representative of the population studied, the reliability and validity of tools used to measure the variables, and the degree of control exercised over extraneous variables. A particularly important evaluative question is whether the conclusions drawn by the authors are consistent with the actual findings.

ASSESSING READINESS FOR APPLICATION

Another consideration in assessing the utility of research findings for community health nursing practice is whether the findings are ready for application. This means that there is sufficient evidence to suggest that findings are valid and reliable over time. This is not so much an evaluation of the credibility of one study as it is an examination of all the research in a particular area. Research findings that are ready to be used are consistent with prior research, maintain credibility when data are examined from other perspectives, meet criteria for statistical significance if applicable, and do not interpret unsupported or insignificant findings.[13] Generally speaking, the findings of a single study in any area are not ready to be applied in practice.

PLANNING TO USE RESEARCH FINDINGS

Planning for the application of research findings in community health nursing practice involves determining the applicability of findings to a specific population, communicating research findings to others, incorporating primary, secondary, or tertiary preventive measures supported by research in planning care for specific clients, and planning to evaluate the application of research findings.

DETERMINING THE APPLICABILITY OF RESEARCH FINDINGS

Even when research is conducted properly and findings are reliable and valid, the results may not apply to population groups with which the nurse is dealing. For example, a study indicating that a videotaped class on contraceptive use was effective in motivating white middle-class adolescents to use birth control does not mean that the same intervention will be equally effective with Latino adolescents. Community health nurses evaluating research must determine the degree to which findings are generalizable to the population groups with which they work.

COMMUNICATING RESEARCH FINDINGS TO OTHERS

Sometimes a particular community health nurse may not be able to apply research findings in practice because application would violate existing policies and procedures of the agency where the nurse is employed. In this instance, planning to incorporate research findings in practice will necessitate acquainting others in the agency with the findings and using the change and leadership processes described in Chapter 11, The Change, Leadership, and Group Processes, to bring about changes that facilitate application of research findings. One approach might be to apply the findings to the care of a specific group of clients as a pilot study to determine their utility in a particular setting.

INCORPORATING RESEARCH FINDINGS IN THE PLAN OF CARE

The community health nurse who wishes to apply research findings to practice will plan to incorporate primary, secondary, or tertiary preventive measures supported by research into care planning for specific clients. For example, if a certain approach to educating noncompliant clients about their hypertensive medications has been shown to improve compliance, the nurse would plan to use this approach in educating a noncompliant hypertensive client in his or her caseload. In this example, a secondary preventive measure, shown by research to be effective, is incorporated into the plan of care for a client with an existing problem of noncompliance. Research findings on the effects of a primary preventive measure like a group exercise program in increasing motivation to exercise might prompt a community health nurse to plan a group exercise program for employees of a bank. Or, if research indicates that education on contraceptive methods provided in the second trimester of pregnancy is more effective in preventing subsequent pregnancies than education provided in the first or third trimesters, the community health nurse might plan to incorporate education on contraceptives into the plan of care for an adolescent in the second trimester of pregnancy. In this instance, the intervention supported by research is at the tertiary level of prevention.

PLANNING TO EVALUATE THE APPLICATION OF RESEARCH

As in all aspects of community health nursing, planning to apply research findings in practice would include plans for evaluation. The community health nurse would plan to evaluate the outcome primary, secondary, or tertiary preventive measures suggested by research and used in the care of individuals, families, or groups of clients. For example, research might indicate that teaching parenting skills to unmarried, nonpregnant high school students reduces the incidence of child abuse. The community health nurse could teach parenting skills to a group of nonpregnant adolescents that the nurse encounters and plan to contact them several years later to determine the incidence of child abuse in the group. In this way the application of research findings leads to additional research that may support or refute the original findings.

IMPLEMENTING RESEARCH FINDINGS IN PRACTICE

The community health nurse would implement plans for incorporating research findings in the care of clients. Planned primary, secondary, or tertiary interventions supported by research findings would be carried out with specific clients. For example, a series of parenting classes would be presented to a group of nonpregnant adolescents. Or, the nurse might use a new technique for controlling incontinence in the elderly client, incorporating a secondary preventive measure supported by research. At the level of tertiary prevention, the community health nurse might suggest that a mother stop propping her baby's bottle, an intervention shown to lessen the frequency of middle ear infections.

EVALUATING THE APPLICATION OF RESEARCH FINDINGS

The community health nurse would then evaluate the effects of incorporating research findings in the plan of care using evaluative criteria developed in planning for the use of research findings. The use of primary preventive interventions suggested by research would be evaluated in terms of health-promotion and illness-prevention outcomes. Did the group exposed to the parenting education series have a lower incidence of child abuse than the general public or a comparable group that did not receive educational preparation for parenting? Did secondary preventive measures result in reduction or elimination of health problems? Or, were tertiary preventive measures successful in preventing the recurrence of a particular problem? As noted earlier, the evaluation of the utility of research findings in practice leads to new questions for research in community health nursing.

CHAPTER HIGHLIGHTS

- The steps of the research process are identifying a problem for study, reviewing related literature, identifying research variables, formulating hypotheses, selecting a research design, choosing a representative sample, collecting data, analyzing data, and communicating research findings.
- Research in community health nursing aids in development and testing of theory and provides evidence of the effectiveness of nursing interventions. Research guides practice and education for practice. Research can also be used to guide health policy formation.
- Societal needs, the level of theory development and prior research, the educational preparation of members to conduct research, and access to research funding are some of the factors that influence the type and extent of research conducted in a discipline.
- Community health nurses may perform any of four research-related roles including using research findings, identifying research questions, collecting data, and designing and conducting research studies. The last role is usually performed by nurses with advanced educational preparation.
- Research designs used in community health nursing research reflect the meld of nursing and public health sciences that comprise the specialty. Designs used may be descriptive or analytic in nature.
- Descriptive community health nursing research describes the nature of events of interest to community health nurses.
- Analytic research designs analyze patterns of relationships between variables, and include ecological and relational studies. Ecological studies compare the relationships between variables of interest in population groups, while relational studies examine relationships between variables within individuals.
- Relational studies can be observational or experimental. In observational studies, the researcher merely observes for the presence or absence of certain variables and identifies patterns of relationships. In experimental studies, nurse researchers control or manipulate independent variables and observe the effects on dependent variables.
- Observational studies can be retrospective, cross-sectional, or prospective in nature depending upon whether subjects have yet manifested the dependent variable.
- Experimental studies can be either prophylactic or therapeutic trials. Prophylactic trials study the effects of preventive measures and reflect primary or tertiary prevention. Therapeutic trials study the effects of interventions aimed at resolution of existing problems and reflect secondary prevention.
- Ethical concerns occur in all phases of a research study. Ethical considerations in planning research include selecting problems related to societal needs and protecting subjects from harm.
- Ethical concerns related to data collection address issues of informed consent, voluntary participation, confidentiality, protection of

(*continued*)

those who will collect data, and treatment of conditions identified during the study.

- Ethical considerations related to the use of research findings include issues of when and how to publish findings and their use in influencing the behavior of others.
- Prior to implementation in practice, research related to community health nursing must be assessed. Assessment consists of identifying relevant research, assessing the quality of the research, and assessing the readiness of findings to be applied in practice.
- Planning to use research findings in practice involves determining the applicability of findings to a specific client population, communicating the findings to others, planning to incorporate findings in client care plans, and planning to evaluate the application of research findings.
- Research findings that are ready for application and applicable to the selected client population are then implemented and their usefulness in practice evaluated, thus creating the opportunity for additional research.

Review Questions

1. Identify at least seven steps in the research process. Describe how each might be implemented in a research study related to community health nursing. (p. 180)
2. What are four factors that influence research in community health nursing? Give an example of the influence of each factor. (p. 181)
3. Describe at least three research roles for community health nurses. (p. 182)
4. Differentiate between experimental and observational studies. Give an example of each. (p. 184)
5. Describe the three types of observational studies. (p. 185)
6. Discuss at least four ethical concerns in community health nursing. Give an example of each concern. (p. 185)
7. Identify three aspects of assessment related to the role of the community health nurse as a research consumer. (p. 189)
8. Describe four considerations in planning for the use of research findings in community health nursing practice. Give an example of each. (p. 190)

APPLICATION AND SYNTHESIS

Mary Jones is a community health nurse working for the Clark County Health Department. Her responsibilities include home visits and work in child health, prenatal, family planning, sexually transmitted disease, and tuberculosis control clinics. Lately, she has received an increasing number of referrals for newborns who have positive urine screenings for drugs at birth. When she visits these babies and their mothers she notes that most of the mothers are teenagers and that they are very concerned because their babies cry a lot and cannot be comforted. Mary knows that irritability and inconsolability are common characteristics of drug-exposed infants. She has read that swaddling such infants and placing them in a darkened room may decrease their irritability, so she suggests these measures to the young mothers. Because of her concern about drug use during pregnancy, Mary also starts giving classes at the local high school on the effects of drugs.

1. What are some of the potential research problems that Mary might derive from her observations in practice?
2. What problems might relate to human biology? To environment? To life-style? To the health system?
3. What research questions come to mind in relation to primary, secondary, and tertiary prevention?
4. Choose one of the potential research questions you have identified. What research design would be most appropriate in answering that question? What are the variables involved? How might you go about collecting data for your study?
5. Once you have completed data collection and analyzed the results, where might you publish your findings? What specific journals might be interested in the outcome of your study?

REFERENCES

1. Lobiondo-Wood, G., & Haber, J. (1990). *Nursing research: Critical appraisal and utilization* (2nd ed.). St. Louis: C. V. Mosby.
2. Highriter, M. E. (1984). Public health nursing evaluation, education, and professional issues. In H. H. Werley & J. J. Fitzpatrick (Eds.), *Annual Review of Nursing Research* (Vol.2) (pp. 165–189). New York: Springer.
3. Oda, D. S., & Boyd, P. (1987). Documenting the effect and cost of public health nursing field services. *Public Health Nursing, 4,* 180–182.
4. Erickson, G. (1987). Public health nursing initiatives: Guideposts for the future. *Public Health Nursing, 4,* 202–211.
5. Green, J. L., & Driggers, B. (1989). All visiting nurses are not alike: Home health and community health nursing. *Journal of Community Health Nursing, 6*(2), 83–93.
6. Gulino, C., & LaMonica, G. (1986). Public health nursing: A study of role implementation. *Public Health Nursing, 3,* 80–91.
7. Jowett, S., & Armitage, S. (1988). Hospital and community liaison links in nursing: The role of the liaison nurse. *Journal of Advanced Nursing, 13,* 579–587.
8. Martin, K. (1988). Research in home care. *Nursing Clinics of North America, 23,* 373–385.
9. Barkauskas, V. H. (1983). Effectiveness of public health nursing home visits to primiparous mothers and their infants. *American Journal of Public Health, 73,* 573–580.
10. Combs-Orme, T., Reis, J., & Ward, L. D. (1985). Effectiveness of home visits by public health nurses in maternal and child health: An empirical review. *Public Health Reports, 100,* 490–499.
11. Norr, K. F., Nacion, K. W., & Abramson, R. (1989). Early discharge with home follow-up: Impacts on low-income mothers and infants. *JOGNN, 18*(2), 133–141.

12. Sereda, M. M. (1989). *Home health nursing survey.* Unpublished manuscript.
13. Hinshaw, A. S. (1988). Using research to shape health policy. *Nursing Outlook, 36,* 21–24.
14. Hessel, P. A., & Fourie, P. B. (1987). Ethical issues in epidemiological research. *SAMT, 72,* 863–865.
15. Highriter, M. E. (1977). The status of community health nursing research. *Nursing Research, 26,* 183–192.
16. American Nurses' Association Commision on Nursing Research. (1985). *Preparation of nurses for participation in research.* Kansas City, MO: American Nurses' Association.
17. Young-Graham, K. (1986). Research cuts breed new challenges for public health nursing. *Public Health Nursing, 3,* 69–70.
18. Keane, A., Larson, E., Naji, P., & Rom, M. (1986). Industry and nursing research: A compatible couple? *Nursing Economics, 4*(3), 128–130.
19. Ruffing-Rahal, M. A. (1985). Qualitative methods in community analysis. *Public Health Nursing, 2,* 130–137.
20. Valanis, B. (1986). *Epidemiology in nursing and health care.* Norwalk, CT: Appleton & Lange.
21. Lilienfeld, A. M., & Lilienfeld, D. E. (1980). *Foundations of epidemiology* (2nd ed.). New York: Oxford University Press.
22. Mausner, J. S., & Kramer, S. (1985). *Mausner and Bahn's epidemiology: An introductory text* (2nd ed.). Philadelphia: W.B. Saunders.
23. Vogt, T. M. (1983). *Making health decisions: An epidemiologic perspective on staying well.* Chicago: Nelson-Hall.
24. Friedman, G. (1980). *Primer of epidemiology.* New York: McGraw-Hill.
25. Jassak, P. F., & Ryan, M. P. (1989). Ethical issues in clinical research. *Seminars in Oncology Nursing, 5*(2), 102–108.

RECOMMENDED READINGS

Brink, P. J., & Wood, M. J. (1988). *Basic steps in planning nursing research: From question to proposal.* Boston: Jones and Bartlett.

Provides an introduction to the steps involved in planning a research study. Assists students through selection of a researchable problem to the writing of a research proposal.

Brooten, D., Gennaro, S., & Brown, L. P., *et al.* (1988). Anxiety, depression, and hostility in mothers of preterm infants. *Nursing Research, 37,* 213–216.

Describes the findings of a study of anxiety, depression, and hostility experienced by mothers of preterm infants at the time of infant discharge and at 9 months. Discusses changes in these measures over time.

Combs-Orme, T., Reis, J., & Ward, L. D. (1985). Effectiveness of home visits by public health nurses in maternal and child health: An empirical review. *Public Health Reports, 100,* 490–499.

Reviews findings of studies on the effects of community health nurse home visits to mothers and young infants.

DiIorio, C., & Riley, B. (1988). Predictors of loneliness in pregnant teenagers. *Public Health Nursing, 5,* 110–115.

Reports findings of a study of the relationship of self-concept and future orientation to loneliness among pregnant adolescents.

Duffy, M. E. (1988). Health promotion in the family: Current findings and directives for nursing research. *Journal of Advanced Nursing, 13,* 109–117.

Reviews research on health promotion in families and provides research questions for further study in this area.

Erickson, G. (1987). Public health nursing initiatives: Guideposts for the future. *Public Health Nursing, 4,* 202–211.

Describes results of a study to determine the roles performed by community health nurses in 15 official local health agencies in Connecticut. Also explores factors that affect community health nursing practice.

Jowett, S., & Armitage, S. (1988). Hospital and community liaison links in nursing: The role of the liaison nurse. *Journal of Advanced Nursing, 13,* 579–587.

Examines the findings of a descriptive study of the structure and process of the liaison or discharge planning role. Three models of linkage between hospital and community health services were identified and examined; the model that included community health nurses was found to be particularly effective.

Laffrey, S. C., Renwanz-Boyle, A., & Skagle, R., *et al.* (1990). Elderly clients' perceptions of public health nursing care. *Public Health Nursing, 7,* 111–117.

Presents findings of a study into the reasons why elderly clients seek care in a public health nursing program and their perceptions of the benefits received.

Lobiondo-Wood, G., & Haber, J. (1990). *Nursing research: Critical appraisal and utilization* (2nd ed.). St. Louis: C. V. Mosby.

Focuses on the application of research findings to clinical practice. Also provides an overview of the research process as used in nursing.

Norr, K. F., Nacion, K. W., & Abramson, R. (1988). Early discharge with home follow-up: Impacts on low-income mothers and infants. *JOGNN, 18*(2), 133–141.

Reports findings of a study on the effect of early discharge of mothers and babies with community health nurse follow-up shortly after discharge. Mothers and infants were compared with a group of mothers discharged at the usual time and mothers discharged early, but not accompanied by the baby.

Nuttall, P. (1988). Maternal responses to home apnea monitoring of infants. *Nursing Research, 37,* 354–357.

Details the findings on the types of upset experienced by mother of infants placed on apnea monitors at home. Identifies nine categories of upset described by mothers in the study.

Osofsky, J. D., Culp, A. M., & Ware, L. M. (1988). Intervention challenges with adolescent mothers and their infants. *Psychiatry, 51,* 236–241.

Examines the findings of a study into the effects of an intervention program for education and support of adolescent mothers on the development of their infants. Activities included home visitation by nonprofessional staff and a 24-hour support phone line.

Swanson, J. M., Forrest, K., & Ledbelter, C., *et al.* (1990). Readability of commercial and generic contraceptive instructions. *Image: Journal of Nursing Scholarship, 22*(2), 96–100.

Presents findings on the reading level of package inserts and generic instruction sheets dealing with contraceptives.

Tanner, C. A., & Lindeman, C. A. (1989). *Using nursing research.* New York: National League for Nursing.

Contains an overview of nursing research and its application to clinical practice in a variety of fields including community health nursing.

Tullman, L., Fawcett, J., Groblewski, L., & Silverman, L. (1990). Changes in functional status after childbirth. *Nursing Research, 39,* 70–75.

Reports findings of a study on factors affecting women's abilities and readiness to assume infant care responsibilities and resume normal activities within 6 months after delivery.

CHAPTER 11

The Change, Leadership, and Group Processes

KEY TERMS

changing
delegating
disconfirmation
driving forces
empirical-rational approach
force field theory
hygiene factors
motivators
normative-reeducative approach
participating
power-coercive approach
professional territoriality
refreezing
restraining forces
selling
telling
unfreezing

Reading of the accomplishments of early leaders in community health nursing like Lillian Wald and her compatriots, one may wonder how these women came to exercise such influence. The answer lies in their knowledge and use of the change, leadership, and group processes. They knew how to use their leadership abilities to influence individuals and groups of people to achieve desired changes in society and in the health-care system. Using these same processes, today's community health nurses can bring about changes in health care and in the health of those they serve.

The change, leadership, and group processes are interrelated. Community health nurses who seek to bring about change must exercise leadership, but leadership without systematic use of the change process may not achieve the desired outcome. Changes often occur as a result of the actions of a group of people rather than those of a single individual. Community health nurses exercise their leadership skills to direct group activity to accomplish desired changes. Knowledge of all three of these interrelated processes is essential to effective community health nursing practice.

(continued)

LEARNING OBJECTIVES

After reading this chapter you should be able to:

- Discuss the influence of driving forces and restraining forces in change.
- Describe four major considerations in planning for change.
- Identify three approaches to bringing about change.
- Describe the three stages of implementing change.
- Describe the relationship of follower maturity to leadership style.
- Identify three functions of the leader in implementing leadership.
- Describe two tasks in planning for group action.
- Describe two tasks in implementing the group process.
- Discuss two aspects of evaluation applicable to the change, leadership, and group processes.

THE EPIDEMIOLOGIC PREVENTION PROCESS MODEL AND CHANGE

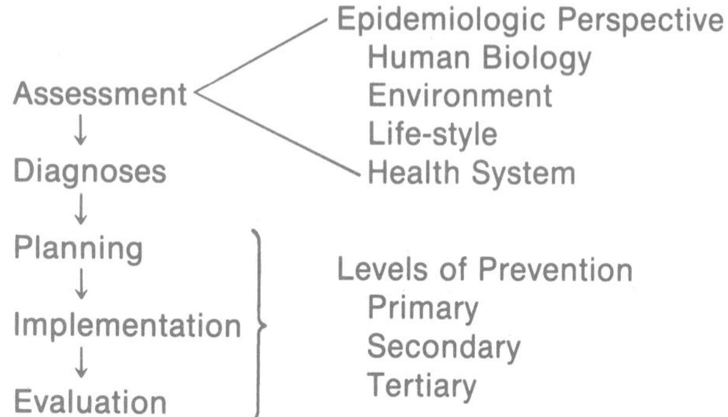

According to *force field theory,* there are always two types of forces that affect the likelihood of change in any situation—driving forces and restraining forces.[1] These two types of forces work in opposition, and it is the relative strength of each that determines whether change will occur.

Driving forces are those factors present in a situation that favor or facilitate change. ***Restraining forces,*** on the other hand, impede change. For example, staff frustration with cumbersome charting procedures may be a driving force that motivates a change to computerized record-keeping. In this situation, feelings of inadequacy regarding computer use and concern for depersonalization of clients may be restraining forces working against change.

Promoting change is a matter of manipulating the driving and restraining forces present in the situation. Community health nurses can increase driving forces, decrease restraining forces, or do both to bring about change. When driving forces are stronger than restraining forces, change will occur. In the change-agent role, the community health nurse can use the epidemiologic prevention process model to assess and modify driving and restraining forces that influence change in a given situation.

ASSESSING THE CHANGE SITUATION

To bring about change, the community health nurse must first identify a need for change. Factors related to human biology, environment, life-style, or the health system may give rise to a need for change. For example, a diagnosis of diabetes or heart disease will require a number of alterations in a client's life, while increases in the number of elderly persons in the population will necessitate changes for a community. Factors in the environment such as a flood or a rise in the unemployment rate also contribute to needs for change by individuals, families, and communities. Similarly, life-style factors, such as the number of people who drive while under the influence of alcohol or other drugs, give rise to the need for legal changes and other community activities to curb the problem. Finally, health system factors, like inequity in access to care or the emphasis on curative care at the expense of prevention, influence the need for change in the health-care delivery system itself.

HUMAN BIOLOGY

Human biological factors can serve as driving or restraining forces for change. Parents may wish that their small child would outgrow the need for diapers, but until the child develops the muscle control to be toilet-trained, the desired change will not occur. In this instance, the child's age and developmental level are restraining factors for change. For an adolescent son or daughter, however, developing an interest in the opposite sex—another maturational event—may lead to positive changes in hygiene practices the parents have been trying to encourage for years. In this case, age and developmental level are driving forces for change.

In a similar vein, physiologic status can either enhance or restrain the prospect of change. For example, a recent heart attack may motivate a person to quit smoking, while visual impairment may diminish a diabetic client's ability to change self-care patterns to include insulin injections.

ENVIRONMENT

Physical, psychological, or social environmental factors may also drive or restrain change in a given situation. For example, the community health nurse may encourage a client to make changes related to personal hygiene, but a lack of running water in the home may make it difficult for the client to perform the desired changes. In this instance, a physical environmental factor is acting as a restraining force for change. For another client, the psychological stresses of a recent divorce may hinder his or her ability to attend to the nurse's recommendations about dietary changes for the children. In both of these examples, environmental factors are functioning as restraining forces prohibiting change.

Social environmental factors might also act as driving or restraining forces for change. For example, low educational or income levels may prevent a client from making needed changes in housing arrangements for the family. On the other hand, support for a desired change from significant others serves as a driving force. Social factors in the form of legislation often bring about change. For example, increasing the tax on tobacco has significantly decreased smoking in Great Britain.

LIFE-STYLE

Driving and restraining forces may also be related to life-style. Substance abuse, for example, may be a restraining force in efforts to alter interaction patterns in violent families. On the other hand, substance abuse might be a driving force in a divorce.

Other consumption patterns may also create driving or restraining forces in a change situation. For example, adherence to a traditional cultural dietary pattern may make it difficult for a client to accept dietary changes necessitated by heart disease. Similarly, the busy executive may find it hard to change dietary patterns to accommodate the restrictions of diabetes.

HEALTH SYSTEM

Health system factors may also drive or restrain change. For example, active resistance by some health-care providers to health-care delivery reforms such as prospective payment and to national health insurance have impeded efforts to lower the cost of health care. On the other hand, political support by health-care providers has often resulted in legislative changes, such as mandatory seat belt laws, that protect the public.

DIAGNOSTIC REASONING AND CHANGE

Nursing diagnoses related to change can be performed at several levels. There may be a need for change in the behavior of an individual client or a family. Examples of diagnoses at these levels might be "need for change in dietary patterns due to pregnancy" or "need for change in family decision-making patterns due to increasing maturity of children."

Diagnoses of needed change might also be made in relation to groups or communities. For example, a community may have a high measles mortality rate in children under 1 year of age. Immunization for measles is usually given at 15 months of age. In this instance, however, there is a need to give the immunization at an earlier age to decrease both measles incidence and mortality. The community health nurse's diagnosis, in this case, might be a "need to change the routine immunization schedule due to increased measles mortality in infants."

Finally, the community health nurse may diagnose a need for change in the health-care delivery system itself. An example of such a diagnosis might be "need to provide low-cost health services due to high unemployment rates and low levels of health insurance." Another example of change needed in the health-care system may involve more effective recruitment and retention of qualified nurses, especially in community health nursing.

PLANNING FOR CHANGE

Change may occur with or without planning. In the absence of systematic planning, however, the change that occurs may not be desirable. As change agents, community health nurses approach change through "creative intentional intervention."[2] Planned change is a "conscious, deliberate, collaborative effort to improve the operations of a system."[3] Planning for change involves several tasks, including establishing goals and objectives, evaluating alternative approaches to change, delineating activities leading to change, and planning to evaluate the change.

ESTABLISHING GOALS AND OBJECTIVES

The first aspect of planning for change is determining what change should accomplish. This entails setting both broad goals and specific objectives. For example, the community health nurse might want to improve immunization levels among community residents. Increasing immunity in the population would be the broad goal, while immunizing 95 percent of children over 1 year of age against measles would be a specific objective. In this instance, the goal and objective reflect primary prevention, and primary preventive measures would be indicated to achieve them.

Goals and objectives for change may also reflect secondary or tertiary prevention. At the secondary prevention level, for example, change in an obese client's dietary patterns would be desirable. In this instance, the goal would be a balanced diet for the client. Specific objectives might include: (1) a decrease in caloric intake to 1800 calories per day, (2) inclusion of at least one iron-rich food in the diet daily, and (3) adequate intake of vitamins and minerals. Similarly, a change to more effective coping strategies by an abusive parent would be the goal of tertiary preventive measures planned in an abusive family situation. A related objective might be a decrease in the amount of alcohol consumed as a coping mechanism.

SELECTING AN APPROACH TO CHANGE

Generally speaking, there are three approaches that the community health nurse might take to bring about change. These are the empirical-rational approach, the normative-reeducative approach, and the power-coercive approach. Each of the three is appropriate in some change situations. The choice of a particular approach is dependent on the type of change to be achieved and the willingness and ability of those who require the change.[4]

The Empirical-Rational Approach

The ***empirical-rational approach*** to change assumes that people act reasonably and will follow the promptings of rational self-interest when the need for change is revealed to them.[5] In short, an awareness of a need for change will result in change. In this approach, change is accomplished by providing information about the need for change and how to bring it about. The community health nurse as change agent informs those who need to implement the change of an unfavorable condition and a desirable course of action, and those individuals carry out the change.

This approach to change is effective in situations when it is clear where one's self-interest lies, when there are few restraining forces operating, and the change does not pose a threat to those who must implement it. For example, school officials made aware of hazards posed by damaged playground equipment will probably take steps either to repair or remove the equipment. They can see the potential harm to the children and the possibility of lawsuits resulting from injuries, and they have no vested interest in retaining damaged equipment.

The Normative-Reeducative Approach

Unfortunately, human behavior is not always rational and is often heavily influenced by attitudes, values, and emotions. For example, a mother may know that her child needs immunizations but hesitates because she doesn't like to see her child hurt by the injection. Rather than trying to increase the mother's awareness of the need for immunization, the community health nurse as change agent could employ a ***normative-reeducative approach*** to change using educational strategies directed toward changing the mother's attitude. For example, the nurse might focus on how much greater the hurt would be if the child developed diphtheria or tetanus or one of the other diseases preventable by immunization.

As another example, teenagers often see unrestrained drinking as evidence of adulthood. By using a normative-reeducative approach the teens would be helped to see that refraining from drinking to excess is more characteristic of adult behavior than going on a Friday-night binge. The approach to behavioral change in this instance focuses on their attitudes to drinking.

The normative-reeducative approach would be used in situations in which those who need to make changes have a vested interest in maintaining the current situation or in which there are emotional and attitudinal restraining forces at work, but where attitudes are open and amenable to change.

The Power-Coercive Approach

Some people, however, cannot be brought to change behavior by rational argument or attempts to change attitudes. In these situations, the ***power-coercive approach*** to change may be effective. This approach uses the power to dispense reward and punishment to force change. As an example, children of parents who refuse to have them immunized are denied school entry unless there are religious or health reasons for nonimmunization. Using another example, empirical-rational strategies and normative-reeducative strategies have been somewhat effective in motivating people to use auto seat belts. Others, however, do not use seat belts. For these people, laws mandating seat belt use are a power-coercive strategy to force a change in behavior.

Information obtained by the community health nurse in assessing the change situation indicates the driving and restraining forces that are operating. When restraining forces are related to misconceptions and lack of knowledge about the need for change, the change itself, or its consequences, the nurse would select the empirical-rational approach to bring about the desired change. When restraining forces include attitudes unfavorable to the desired change but amenable to modification, the normative-reeducative approach may be chosen. When the assessment indicates strongly rooted attitudes and values that impede change or strong resistance to change, the power-coercive approach may be used. This approach is also appropriate in situations where the need for change is immediate and there is neither time for explanation nor for persuasion.

It should be remembered, however, that the power-coercive approach may result in temporary change and that those who are coerced may return to their previous behaviors as soon as coercive force is removed. For these reasons, the power-coercive method is the least desirable of the three approaches to change. This approach would not generally be used with clients, except in situations in which clients' behaviors are clearly dangerous to themselves or others as in the case of a client threatening suicide, child abuse, failure to obtain necessary medical care for a minor, or someone with a communicable disease who refuses to refrain from infecting others.

The power-coercive approach may be warranted, however, in advocacy situations and other similar occasions. For example, the community health nurse may find that the only way to motivate a landlord to comply with building safety codes is to threaten to report violations to the authorities. Or, health-care providers who discriminate against certain types of clients may be motivated to change their behavior if threatened with the loss of their jobs.

DELINEATING ACTIVITIES LEADING TO CHANGE

The next step in planning for change is to delineate specific activities required to meet the objectives for change. These activities may involve primary, secondary, or tertiary preventive measures. For example, if a change is needed in an infant's diet to accommodate the slowed rate of growth normal at the end of the first year of life, dietary education for the mother would be a primary preventive measure directed toward this change. Similarly, providing clean syringes and needles for intravenous drug users might motivate them to stop sharing needles and prevent exposure to hepatitis and human immunodeficiency virus (HIV).

Examples of secondary preventive strategies for change might include suggestions to minimize side effects of antituberculin drugs to resolve the problem of noncompliance, or assisting teenage alcoholics to explore their reasons for drinking. Educating a parent on the role of bottle propping in recurrent middle ear infections in an infant might be a tertiary preventive measure designed to produce behavior changes in the parent that prevent a recurrence of otitis media in the child.

PLANNING TO EVALUATE CHANGE

The last step in planning for change is to plan for evaluating the effects of the change and the process used to achieve it. Consequently, the community health nurse needs to determine how the change will be evaluated, what data will be collected, and what data-collection procedures will be used. In planning to evaluate change, criteria need to be developed that reflect the levels of prevention involved in the changes planned. If desired changes involve primary prevention, evaluative criteria will focus on the promotion of health and prevention of specific health problems. The emphasis in secondary prevention would be on criteria that reflect resolution of existing client problems, while evaluative criteria related to tertiary preventive measures would address prevention of complications or recurrence of problems. As an example, an objective for change at the level of

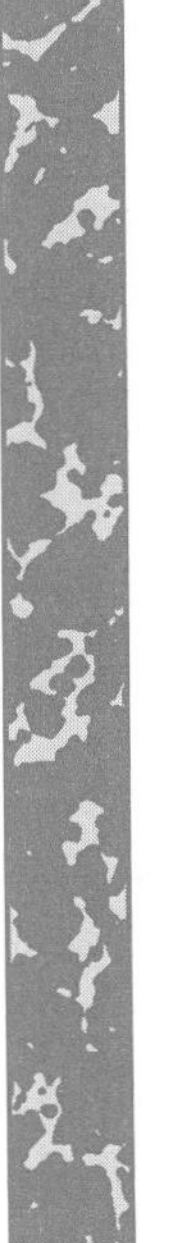

BOX 11–1

Considerations in Planning for Change

1. Evaluate and select an appropriate approach to change
   Empirical-rational approach: focuses on awareness of the need for change
   Normative-reeducative approach: focuses on attitudes to the change
   Power-coercive approach: uses power over rewards and punishments to enforce change
2. Delineate activities leading to change
3. Plan for evaluation of change

primary prevention might be increased use of condoms among male homosexuals to prevent HIV infection. Evaluative criteria for the achievement of change would focus on the proportion of homosexuals who use condoms consistently. Considerations in planning for change are summarized in Box 11–1.

IMPLEMENTING CHANGE

Whatever the approach to change selected in the planning stage, implementing it occurs in stages: unfreezing, changing, and refreezing.[6] All three stages apply to implementing changes of all kinds, including those related to individuals, families, and groups or communities as well as changes in nursing practice or in the health-care system.

UNFREEZING

Unfreezing is the process of creating an awareness of the need to change and developing motivation for the change. Unfreezing may be approached somewhat differently in each of the three approaches to change discussed earlier. For example, in the use of the empirical-rational strategy, the community health nurse as change agent may use a tactic known as disconfirmation to motivate others to change. ***Disconfirmation*** is an awareness that reality does not conform to the desired state of affairs. Creating disconfirmation involves presenting the client or target group with information to make them aware of differences between a desired state and reality. This awareness creates a feeling of discomfort with the current situation and fosters a willingness to change. For example, the community health nurse might present figures on the number of adolescent pregnancies occurring in a specific school to make parents aware of a need for sex education. The desired state is an absence of teenage pregnancies, but, as the community health nurse makes clear, this is definitely not the reality of the situation.

A second tactic used in unfreezing is introducing guilt. This tactic might be used in the normative-reeducative approach to change. When people are made to feel guilty about the current situation, they may be more likely to reexamine attitudes and institute change. For instance, the community health nurse might point out what poor role models smokers are for their children and what the effects of second-hand smoke might be on children's health. Guilt over possible damage to their own children's health might motivate some smokers to quit.

Providing a climate of psychological safety is another tactic used in unfreezing in the normative-reeducative approach to change. Again, using the change to computerized charting as an example, the community health nurse might assure the group that they will receive detailed instruction and demonstration of the system and will have opportunities to practice and receive feedback before the new system is implemented. These activities lessen fears of making mistakes and decrease restraining forces working against the change. In the power-coercive approach to change, unfreezing may be accomplished by presenting information on the need for change and the sanctions that will occur if the change does not take place.

CHANGING

Changing is the actual process of implementing or carrying out the planned change. Functions of the community health nurse as change agent during this stage include introducing new information needed to bring about the change; modeling and/or encouraging performance of the new behavior; allowing ample time to practice the behavior; and providing a supportive climate and opportunities to voice feelings of fear, anxiety, frustration, anger, and so on. Other functions include giving feedback on progress in implementing the change, acting as an energizer to maintain the momentum of the change, and decreasing resistance by continuing the activities of the unfreezing stage.[7]

Dividing the change into smaller segments and setting up effective communication channels can assist in the actual implementation of the change.[8] Delineation of activities needed for implementing the change during the planning stage of the change process may be done in such a way that segmental change is possible. For example, if community health nurses are asked to convert all existing client records to a computerized charting system, they may feel overwhelmed. However, if the change begins with newly opened records only, the change can be accomplished in manageable segments. As services to previously enrolled clients are terminated, there will be fewer and fewer records that have not been computerized.

Providing avenues for those involved in the change to communicate regarding problems experienced will also smooth the implementation process. Communication permits evaluation of the implementation of change on an ongoing basis and allows modification of the planned change or the activities required to implement it, thus resulting in a more effective change.

REFREEZING

Refreezing is the process of internalizing the change so it becomes part of the normal routine. In the com-

TABLE 11–1. STAGES IN IMPLEMENTING CHANGE AND FUNCTIONS OF THE NURSE AS CHANGE AGENT

Stage	Function of the Nurse as Change Agent
Unfreezing	• Create disconfirmation • Introduce guilt • Provide a climate of psychological safety
Changing	• Introduce new information required for change • Encourage performance of new behavior • Allow time to practice new behavior • Provide supportive climate for change • Provide opportunities to voice feelings about change • Give feedback on progress of change • Serve as an energizer • Continue activities of unfreezing stage
Refreezing	• Continue energizing activities • Continue to direct new behavior • Delegate greater responsibility for change to client or target group

puterization example, refreezing has occurred when the change to computerized charting has become internalized to the point that staff members wonder how they ever managed to chart the old way. Functions of the change agent at this stage include providing continuing motivation, directing the new behavior, and delegating greater responsibility for the change to others.[7] Stages in implementing change and the functions of the community health nurse as change agent are presented in Table 11–1.

EVALUATING CHANGE

Evaluating change involves assessing the change itself and the process used in achieving it. In evaluating change itself, the first question is whether the desired change was achieved. Has the individual client, family, or target group made the expected change in health-related behaviors? Are they now, for example, engaging in more effective communication patterns or eating a more appropriate diet? Is charting now done on computer?

The second consideration in evaluating change is its effects. It may be that, even though the change has been achieved, it has not had the desired effect. For example, the client may have changed his or her dietary patterns and still not be losing weight. Or, more immunization clinics may have been established without appreciably raising immunization levels.

In addition, change may have unanticipated effects that may or may not be desirable. For instance, the change to computerized charting may provide avenues for violation of client confidentiality because the computer increases access to client records. Or, the nurses may spend more time correcting computer errors than they spent in handwritten charting.

Another aspect of evaluating change is the evaluation of the process used to achieve the change. Were the need for change and the driving and restraining forces accurately identified? Was the change well planned? Was the appropriate approach to change selected given the factors involved? Was resistance adequately addressed? What activities were involved in unfreezing, changing, and refreezing? Were these activities appropriate to the situation? Answers to these questions will provide direction for action if the desired change has not yet been achieved and further attempts are warranted. They will also

BOX 11–2

Components of the Change Process

1. Assess the change situation in terms of:

   Factors giving rise to the need for change
   Driving forces for change
   Restraining forces for change

2. Diagnose the need for change
3. Plan for change

   Establish goals and objectives for change
   Evaluate approaches to change and select an appropriate one
   Delineate activities leading to change
   Plan for evaluation of change

4. Implement the change

   Facilitate unfreezing
   Facilitate the change itself
   Facilitate refreezing

5. Evaluate the change

   Evaluate the extent to which change has been accomplished
   Evaluate the effects of the change
   Evaluate the use of the change process

assist the community health nurse as change agent to use the change process more effectively in the future. Components of the change process are summarized in Box 11–2.

THE EPIDEMIOLOGIC PREVENTION PROCESS MODEL AND LEADERSHIP

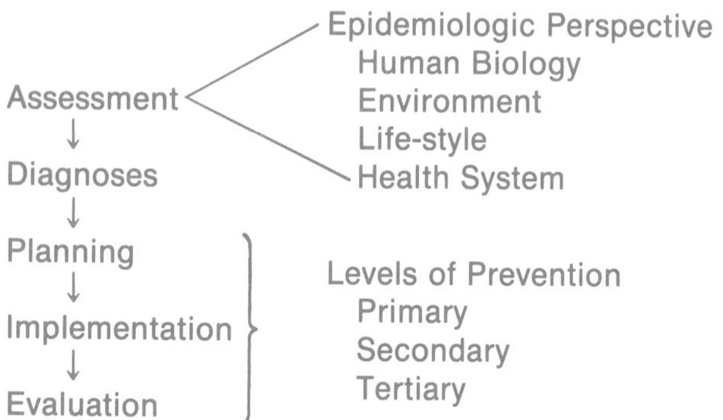

Initiating and directing change requires leadership on the part of the nurse. The 1988 Institute of Medicine report, *The Future of Public Health,*[9] cited a lack of leadership in public health. For this reason, community health nurses should prepare to provide leadership in the process of designing a health-care system that will meet the health needs of the public.[10,11] In this age of rising costs and diminishing resources, there is a particular need for leadership to assure that health resources are adequate to meet those needs.[12]

Community health nurse leaders may make use of a variety of theories—including trait theories, behavioral theories, motivational, and interactional theories—designed to explain the phenomenon of leadership. Because of the diversity of people who may be led by community health nurses, nurses need to have a repertoire of leadership styles and skills available to them. For this reason, we will focus on interactional theory in our discussion of leadership in the context of the epidemiologic prevention process model. Interactional theory describes the influence of the leader, the followers, and the situation on the outcome of any leadership effort.[7] Readers interested in other approaches to leadership can find information in a variety of nursing leadership textbooks.[7,13]

ASSESSING THE LEADERSHIP SITUATION

As the first step of the epidemiologic prevention process model applied to leadership, the community health nurse assesses the need for leadership as well as factors in the situation that will affect leadership and task accomplishment. The nurse as leader assesses factors related to oneself, one's followers, and the task to be accomplished in terms of Dever's epidemiologic perspective. The resulting information will direct the selection of a leadership style appropriate to the situation.

HUMAN BIOLOGY

One major consideration in leadership is the maturity of one's followers with respect to the task at hand. Maturity is a combination of expertise related to the task and motivation to perform the task.[4]

Age and developmental level can influence both leader and follower maturity. Children will usually have less expertise related to many tasks than will adults, although this is not always true. For example, a school-age child may have had more exposure to computers than many adults. If the task to be accomplished requires computer skills, the youngster may be more mature relative to the task than the inexperienced adult.

Physiologic function can also influence followers' abilities to complete necessary tasks. If, for example, one is trying to provide leadership in a disaster situation and all of one's followers are injured, their ability to perform required tasks will be influenced by the type and extent of their injuries. Biological factors can also influence the effectiveness of the leader. For example, an ill or injured leader might inspire less confidence on the part of followers than a strong and forceful one.

ENVIRONMENT

Aspects of the physical, psychological, and social environments can influence the leader, followers, and/or the leadership situation.

Physical Environment

The physical environment can give rise to the need for leadership or factors that influence that need. Potential for a flood, for example, might require leadership in the evacuation of local residents.

If followers are physically distant from the leader, this distance may influence how leadership is exercised. For example, if a community health nursing student is making a home visit without his or her instructor and encounters difficulties, the instructor may need to provide leadership and direction by phone rather than in person, and the approach taken to leadership in this situation might be different from the approach that might be used on-site. If there are other incoming telephone calls, for instance, the instructor might just tell the student to take specific action rather than assist the student with problem solving.

In addition, the physical environment may or may not contain the materials needed for task accomplishment. This lack of necessary materials might hamper the effectiveness of the leader in getting a given task accomplished. Suppose that the task to be accomplished is feeding a group of disaster victims. If there is no food available because transportation has been curtailed, it will be difficult to accomplish this task no matter how experienced the leader and followers are.

Psychological Environment

The psychological environment affects both leader and followers. Followers' motivation to act is a function of their psychological environment. For example, followers may be unwilling or unable to act in the manner desired by the leader if incapacitated by emotions such as fear, anxiety, or grief. In assessing the leadership situation, the nurse as leader will need to identify psychological factors motivating current behavior and those that might motivate followers to desired behaviors.

The resulting knowledge will allow the nurse to provide the types of motivation needed to promote desired behavior and task accomplishment by followers. For example, if followers are motivated by monetary considerations, monetary rewards might bring about the desired behavior. For other followers, presentation of a challenge might be a motivator.

The psychological environment can also influence the leader and his or her effectiveness. For example, lack of trust of the leader will detract from effectiveness in a leadership situation. Hesitancy on the part of the leader may also lessen follower confidence and willingness to act as directed. Lack of leader attention to the psychological needs of followers may likewise inhibit effectiveness.

Another aspect of the psychological environment is time and the resulting pressure for decision and action. Time constraints will influence the type of leadership style appropriate to the situation, as we shall see later in this chapter.

Social Environment

Social environmental factors also influence the leadership situation. Social factors such as low educational level or lack of exposure to similar situations can affect follower expertise and their ability to accomplish necessary tasks. In such cases, the followers are said to be "immature" with respect to the task to be accomplished.

Another aspect of the social environment is the position of the leader with respect to the followers. It is helpful, but not absolutely necessary, if the leader is in a position of authority vis-à-vis the followers. This position of authority gives the leader a certain amount of influence over followers. Followers' perceptions of the leader as being more knowledgeable than themselves regarding the task at hand also contribute to leader influence. Such perceptions might be attributable to the leader's educational level, social status, or other social environmental factors.

LIFE-STYLE

Life-style factors influence follower experience and expertise related to the task to be accomplished. Both occupation and leisure pursuits may provide followers with experiences relevant to a given leadership situation. For instance, a computer programmer or someone who uses computers for recreational purposes may have the skills needed for a computer-related task, while an experienced hiker may have tracking skills required to find a group of lost Scouts. These skills increase the task-related maturity of followers.

Similarly, life experiences might influence the leadership ability of the nurse leader. Functioning as a leader among co-workers should help prepare the nurse for leadership roles in other areas. For example, the community health nursing supervisor who applies leadership principles to direct the activity of staff members would use the same principles to assist abusive parents to form a self-help group.

HEALTH SYSTEM

Health system factors can also contribute to the effectiveness of the nurse leader. For example, the traditional hierarchical arrangement of the health-care team, which traditionally acknowledges physician leadership, may make it difficult for the nurse to assume a leadership role. This same traditional hierarchy may make it difficult for health-care consumers to act as leaders in health-related situations even when their leadership is warranted by the situation. In such circumstances, the nurse or consumer leader will need to pay particular attention to psychological factors motivating follower behavior.

Consumer perceptions of health-care providers and their intentions can also influence the ability of the nurse to lead in a situation in which health-care consumers are the followers. If health-care providers are perceived as intent on serving their own interests, their credibility and influence with followers will be minimal. If, on the other hand, providers are seen to be acting altruistically, they may have more influence on consumer behavior in a leadership situation.

DIAGNOSTIC REASONING AND LEADERSHIP

The community health nurse derives nursing diagnoses from data obtained in assessing the leadership situation. There are two aspects of nursing diagnosis related to leadership—diagnosing the need for action and leadership, and diagnosing follower maturity.

DIAGNOSING THE NEED FOR LEADERSHIP

The first type of nursing diagnosis involves identifying a need for action and for leadership to promote action. Very often, this is also a diagnosis of a need for change. For example, in assessing a community's health needs, the community health nurse may note a high incidence of pedestrian fatalities at a particular intersection. Action is needed in the form of a traffic signal to permit safe pedestrian crossing. However, local residents have no idea how to go about arranging for installation of a traffic signal. In this instance, the nurse has identified both a problem that requires action and a need for leadership to bring about that action. The nursing diagnosis derived might be a "need for leadership in preventing traffic fatalities due to community members' lack of experience with group action."

DIAGNOSING FOLLOWER MATURITY

The second aspect of nursing diagnosis in leadership is the diagnosis of follower maturity. Based on the assessment data obtained, the community health nurse should have an idea of both follower expertise and motivation regarding the action to be taken. Examples of possible diagnoses in this area might include "adequate follower expertise related to task but poor motivation due to anxiety," or "adequate motivation for action, but lack of expertise due to low educational level."

PLANNING FOR LEADERSHIP

Planning for leadership involves two considerations—selecting an appropriate leadership style and preparing followers for action. Other aspects of planning, such as delineating specific activities, and so on, are based on the general principles of planning discussed in Chapter 5, The Nursing Process, and Chapter 19, Care of the Community or Target Group.

SELECTING A LEADERSHIP STYLE

A successful leadership outcome is a function of the interaction among the characteristics of the community health nurse as leader, the followers, and the task or situation at hand. In planning for leadership, the community health nurse must select a style of leadership appropriate to all three of these components of the leadership situation.

One of four leadership styles that balance task-oriented and relationship-oriented behaviors by the leader may be appropriate to different leadership situations.[14] These four styles of leadership also reflect a continuum of follower maturity and range from "telling," which is used with the least mature followers, to "selling" and "participating," used when moderate levels of follower maturity are evident, to "delegating," which is used with mature followers. The community health nurse's expertise and comfort with each of the four styles will also influence the style selected in a given situation. Ideally, the nurse as leader will have developed the ability to use each of the four styles as needed in a given situation.

Telling

For a situation in which task accomplishment is a priority and relationship concerns are less important, or followers have limited expertise or motivation, ***telling*** may be an appropriate leadership style. In this style, the nurse as leader tells the follower what to do and how to do it. For example, if the community health nurse encounters a situation in which a client is in cardiac arrest, he or she would direct one family member to call for emergency assistance and order another to assist with CPR. There is no time to explain why certain things must be done or to worry about offending family members. Immediate action is required.

In another situation there may not be the sense of urgency involved in the previous example, but the followers may lack the experience required to determine what needs to be done or how to do it. In this instance, a "telling" or directive approach is also appropriate. For example, when people first begin to use computers, one focuses on telling them the exact steps to take to accomplish a task rather than on the principles behind computer operations. As they become more familiar with the use of computers, one might then change the approach to one that explains as well as tells what to do.

Selling

The second leadership style, ***selling,*** is used in situations in which both task accomplishment and interpersonal relationships are important. In this style, the leader works to persuade followers that a specific course of action should be taken. For example, the community health nurse might want to persuade school officials and parents that a school-based adolescent clinic is a good solution to identified health problems in this age group. The nurse as leader is not in a position to *tell* these people what to do, but must persuade them.

Participating

Participating is the third leadership style on the maturity continuum. A participative leadership style might be used by the community health nurse who is assisting parents of handicapped children to form a support group. In this instance, the nurse as leader would want to emphasize interpersonal relationships with less attention to the need to accomplish specific tasks. This leadership style is appropriate with a group of followers who are mature with respect to the group's goal, but need some guidance in reaching that goal.

Delegating

The fourth leadership style is ***delegating.*** In this style, followers are quite mature and can accomplish the group's goals with little or no direction from the leader. The nurse as a delegative leader places little emphasis on either task or relationship dimensions, but merely presents followers with a desired goal and leaves its accomplishment to them. For example, nursing faculty might delegate to the student organization the task of planning a graduation dinner expecting students to take care of all the details with minimal input from the faculty. The four leadership styles presented here are summarized in Table 11–2.

TABLE 11–2. LEADERSHIP STYLES AND CHARACTERISTIC FEATURES

Leadership Style	Characteristic Features
Telling	• Emphasis on task accomplishment rather than interpersonal relationships • Entails specific directions or orders given to followers without explanation • Appropriate in emergency situations • Appropriate when followers do not have expertise or motivation to act on their own
Selling	• High emphasis on both task accomplishment and interpersonal relationships • Entails persuasion of followers to take the desired course of action • Appropriate when followers have expertise but not the motivation to act on their own
Participating	• Emphasis on interpersonal relationships rather than task accomplishment • Entails allowing and encouraging follower input into decisions on action to be taken • Appropriate when followers have some expertise and are motivated to act but need some direction • Appropriate when time is not a factor
Delegating	• Low emphasis by leader on both task accomplishment and interpersonal relationships • Entails informing followers of task to be done and leaving them to accomplish it • Appropriate when followers are highly motivated and have the necessary expertise

PREPARING FOLLOWERS

The second aspect of planning for leadership is preparing followers for action. This can involve either enhancing their abilities to accomplish the task involved or improving their motivation to act.

Enhancing Followers' Abilities

Enhancing followers' abilities to perform a desired action might involve teaching new skills or providing opportunities to practice previously learned ones. For example, if the action required of followers involves use of interpersonal skills, the leader may plan to review principles of group dynamics and interpersonal communication with followers. Or, if the task involves use of computers, plans may need to be made to teach computer skills to followers or to broaden existing skills to encompass the desired action.

Improving Motivation

Because leadership is almost always directed to some type of action for change, improving followers' motivation to act may involve manipulation of the driving and restraining forces described in the earlier discussion of the change process. The community health nurse may need to plan to reduce restraining forces, enhance driving forces, or both. These forces may reflect the psychological motivators for behavior discussed earlier.

Two types of factors affect followers' motivation to act—hygiene factors and motivators.[15] ***Hygiene factors*** involve personal needs for comfort, safety, and security. In the absence of hygiene factors, followers may experience pain, insecurity, or fear regarding survival. Absence of hygiene factors leads to followers' dissatisfaction with a given situation. Identified hygiene factors include adequate salary, supervision, good interpersonal relationships, and a safe, tolerable environment.[7]

Motivators are factors that meet higher-order needs for personal growth and achievement. Their presence contributes to follower satisfaction. Specific motivators include meaningful activity, opportunity for achievement, appropriate responsibility, and recognition of ability and achievement.

People are motivated differentially by hygiene and motivation factors. For example, some followers may act to get a traffic signal installed at a dangerous intersection out of fear of injury to themselves or their loved ones. Others may be influenced to act by altruistic motives or because they like the challenge presented by a tussle with city hall.

Knowledge of what motivates a specific individual permits the use of motivators that will reduce restraining forces and enhance driving forces, increasing the potential for accomplishing the desired action. For example, if action is needed to improve the quality of nursing care provided, some followers may be motivated by threats of job loss, while others will be better motivated by recognition of a job well done. If the community health nurse has thoroughly assessed the leadership situation, this person will be able to plan for rewards and sanctions that motivate specific followers to action.

IMPLEMENTING THE LEADERSHIP PLAN

Two aspects of implementing a leadership plan include performance of designated activities by followers and performance of leadership functions by the leader. The first aspect is based on general principles of implementation discussed in Chapter 5, The Nursing Process, and will not be reiterated here. The second aspect of implementation is the performance of specific leadership functions by the nurse as leader. These functions include carrying out plans for follower preparation, coordinating and directing follower activity related to task accomplishment, and representing followers to outsiders.

Plans for preparing followers need to be executed. In this phase of implementation, the community health nurse provides whatever education is needed by followers to carry out the desired actions. The nurse also puts into operation planned rewards and sanctions designed to motivate followers.

In addition, the nurse coordinates group members' activities in planning and implementing the desired course of action. The amount of coordination required will depend upon the maturity of the group, their need for assistance, and the leadership style employed. For example, if the task was appropriately delegated to a mature group of followers, there will be little need for extensive coordination by the nurse as leader. If, on the other hand, the nurse selected the "telling" style of leadership, the leader might need to engage in quite a bit of coordination of follower activities.

Finally, the community health nurse as leader serves as the group's spokesperson. He or she supports group decisions and defends those decisions to outsiders when necessary. For instance, if the task remains unaccomplished because of a lack of necessary materials, the nurse as leader may need to explain difficulties in task completion to policymakers or supervisors.

EVALUATION AND LEADERSHIP

As was true in the change process, evaluation in a leadership situation addresses the outcome of leadership as well as the process used. Was the desired action or change brought about? Was the leadership style selected appropriate to the task and to the level

BOX 11–3

Components of the Leadership Process

1. Assess the leadership situation in terms of:

   Factors giving rise to the need for leadership
   Factors influencing the leadership situation

2. Diagnose the situation in terms of:

   The need for leadership
   Follower maturity

3. Plan for leadership

   Select an appropriate leadership style
   Plan to prepare followers for action
   Delineate actions to be taken

4. Implement the leadership process

   Enhance follower abilities
   Improve follower motivation
   Coordinate follower activities
   Represent group to outsiders

5. Evaluate leadership in terms of:

   Actions accomplished
   Use of the leadership process

of follower maturity? Were followers adequately prepared for action? These are a few of the questions that might be asked in evaluating leadership. Evaluation and other aspects of leadership in the context of the epidemiologic prevention process model are summarized in Box 11–3.

THE EPIDEMIOLOGIC PREVENTION PROCESS MODEL AND THE GROUP PROCESS

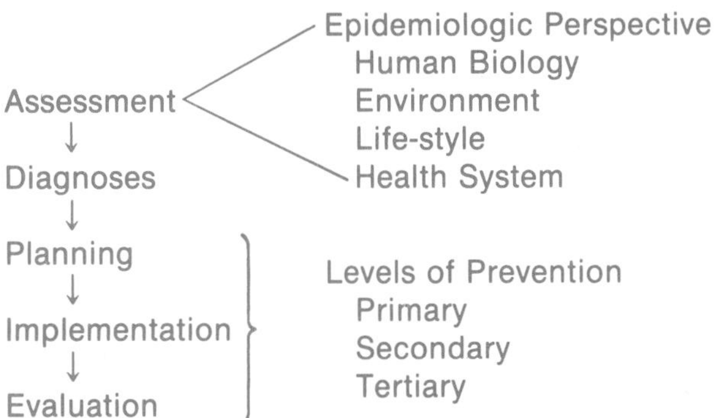

Change is often accomplished as a result of action by a group of people. This is particularly true of changes that occur in the health-care delivery system. Many of the problems that affect population groups cannot be solved by the action of one health-care provider, and cooperative activity by a group is required. Community health nurses are often called upon to initiate and direct group problem-solving activities; consequently, they must be conversant with the processes that govern the formation and operation of groups. Group-process skills are needed by community health nurses who are members, as well as leaders, or groups.

Group action has a number of advantages over actions taken by individuals. The greater range of knowledge and expertise of group members provides a broader base from which to derive solutions to health problems. For example, if community health nurses are concerned about drug abuse among elementary school children, to address the problem they might form a group that includes school officials, police, child psychologists, and parents. Each member of the group has expertise that can contribute to solving the problem. Police personnel have knowledge of means by which drugs are circulated, while school officials and parents can speak to factors in the school setting that contribute to drug traffic. The child psychologist can provide input into ways to motivate young people to refrain from using drugs. Working together, the group can generate a solution to the problem that is realistic and effective.

Another advantage to group activity is the increased efficiency realized by using each member's expertise and by eliminating duplication of effort. When people act cooperatively, those best suited to a particular function can perform that function. When one acts independently, one must carry out all the required functions despite one's level of expertise in those areas. In the drug-abuse example cited earlier, school officials and teachers can work on curriculum aspects of a drug-abuse prevention program while police concentrate on eliminating drug dealers from school grounds. Furthermore, group action also eliminates duplication of effort. For example, there is no point in the schools and the police department developing independent drug-education programs when drug education can be done more effectively and efficiently as a cooperative effort.

Finally, group action promotes communication among members of the group that may enhance problem resolution. Improved communication through group work can also lead to collaborative effort in other areas, which increases the resource network of each of the group's members.

The role of the community health nurse in group action to solve problems frequently involves initiating the group and directing its activity. In other instances, community health nurses are asked to serve on groups formed by others. In either case, knowledge of the group process will assist the nurse to make a greater contribution to the group effort.

In working with groups, community health nurses can use the epidemiologic prevention process model to direct group efforts. The model can be used both in group development and in the group's efforts to resolve health problems.

ASSESSMENT AND THE GROUP PROCESS

There are two aspects to assessment in group work. The first is assessment of the problem to be solved. This assessment is done from Dever's epidemiologic perspective with consideration of the human biological, environmental, life-style, and health system factors influencing the problem and its solution, as described in Chapter 6, The Epidemiologic Process.

The second aspect of assessment is assessing the group itself. Ideally, group members would be selected because they have characteristics that enable them to contribute to the group. Unfortunately, that is not always the case, and the community health nurse working with a group will need to assess group members to identify their strengths and weaknesses. One potential barrier to effective group action is lack of knowledge of the abilities and characteristics of group members that could enhance or undermine group effort. Careful assessment of group members by the community health nurse can help to eliminate this barrier. The assessment stage of the group process has been called the orientation phase of group development.[16]

HUMAN BIOLOGY

Some biological factors can often influence the group and its ability to function. Age and developmental level may determine the type of life experiences group members have had, and this, in turn, will affect their ability to generate solutions to problems. The physical health status of group members may also influence their ability to contribute. For example, if one group member is pregnant, the group will need to carry on in her absence if she goes into labor at a crucial time in the group's activity. For instance, a group of community health students who were organizing a health fair assigned the pregnant member tasks that could be completed prior to the fair (for example, publicizing the fair), just in case she went into labor early.

ENVIRONMENT

All three aspects of environment—physical, psychological, and social—can influence the activity of a group. If there are great distances separating group members, for example, much of the group's work may need to be done by mail or over the telephone. Similarly, if group members live in different parts of town, attention will need to be given to a centralized meeting place.

The psychological environment can pose several barriers to effective group work that arise out of the personal characteristics of group members. Members who are personally insecure or fiercely independent may feel threatened by the interdependence required in group work. Suspicion and lack of trust in other members may also hamper group effort. For example, in a community experiencing racial unrest, it may be difficult for members of different ethnic groups to work together.

Personal philosophies, values, and goals can also impede group effectiveness. It is important for the community health nurse to encourage group members to express their personal beliefs and attitudes both to the problem that needs resolution and to working as a group. It is vital for effective group function that all group members understand and accept the group's purpose and goals. For this reason, it is important that purposes and goals be developed jointly. When philosophical differences are identified early in the group's existence, those differences can be acknowledged and compromises achieved that would not be possible when such differences go unrecognized.

Paradoxically, another psychological barrier to effective group function arises out of commitment to the group on the part of its members.[17] This commitment entails group loyalty that may prohibit group members from acknowledging any weaknesses of the group, thus promoting a possible tendency to cover up any mistakes made.

The tendency of health-care providers to adopt a paternalistic attitude to health-care consumers is another psychological barrier to effective group work.[17] This can be a serious problem for community health nurses who frequently work in groups that include laypeople and consumers. In such situations, the community health nurse may need to function as an advocate for these individuals to ensure that their input is recognized by the group.

The interpersonal skills of each member will also influence the group's ability to work harmoniously. In groups whose members have good interpersonal skills, differences of opinion are dealt with more easily and the group can function more effectively. In groups whose members have poor interpersonal skills, the community health nurse may have to exercise his or her interpersonal skills to aid the group to work as a cohesive unit. The nurse may also need to foster interpersonal skills among group members.

The social environment can also give rise to barriers to effective group function. Some of the major barriers in this area relate to concepts of authority, power, status, and autonomy. For example, health-care policymakers may feel that their authority and power are threatened if health-care consumers are included in health planning groups. Or, group members of lower socioeconomic status may resent those from higher socioeconomic levels and have difficulty working with them. On the other hand, members from higher socioeconomic groups may have difficulty understanding the needs of those of lower status.

Culture is another social environmental factor that may affect the way a group functions. Cultures differ with respect to their ability to work in groups and commitment to group goals. They may also differ with respect to concepts of group leadership. For example, individuals from traditional Asian cultures may be very committed to working for group goals, but may be reluctant to advance ideas for problem resolution, expecting direction to come from the group leader. Members of various health disciplines also have unique cultures that might influence their ability to work in a group. For example, the use of medical and nursing jargon may be confusing to lay members of the group.

Differences in educational levels among group members can be barriers to effective group function. The community health nurse may find that group members need to be educated about both the problem and the group process. The need for education may be experienced by professional as well as lay members of the group. While professional members often have an understanding of the health implications of a problem and some idea of how to solve it, very few health professionals have been educated regarding the group process.

The final social environmental consideration in working with groups is the fact that a group is a social system, and whatever effects one part of the system will effect the entire system. For example, if a member who has assumed responsibility for gathering data needed by the group becomes ill or has a family emergency, the group will need to make other arrangements for gathering data. All group members must carry out assigned responsibilities adequately if the group is to function effectively. This means that group members must be concerned about the well-being of fellow team members and their ability to function. It also means that there must be a mechanism for integrating new members into the group in a way that their lack of familiarity with the group will cause the least possible disruption in group function.

LIFE-STYLE

Life-style factors affect group function in two ways. First, occupational and leisure aspects of life-style influence group members' areas of expertise. Health-care providers, for example, have certain expertise because of their occupations. Similarly, a lawyer or a nutritionist brings another area of expertise that might be needed by the group. Members' recreational activities may also give them specialized knowledge and skills that can be used by the group. For instance, a member who writes programs for computer games might help the group design a computer-assisted educational program on substance abuse for school-age children.

The second way in which life-style influences group function is the effect of people's schedules on group activity. For example, if members work and have several other responsibilities, it may be difficult for the group to schedule meeting times. This problem is particularly relevant in many groups with which community health nurses work. For instance, the nurse may be helping single parents form a support group. But because of group members' other responsibilities, the nurse as group leader may have to coordinate schedules so the group can meet. He or she may also need to coordinate group members' activities when assigned responsibilities are carried out independently.

HEALTH SYSTEM

Health system factors can also influence group function. Professional territoriality is one factor in this area that may hamper effective group function. ***Professional territoriality*** is the tendency of a discipline to regard certain activities as the sole province of their discipline and to resent others outside the discipline engaging in those activities. Because some health professions (and other disciplines) are not well defined, some health-care roles overlap, and group members may easily infringe on one another's sense of territory. One author aptly described the problem of role ambiguity in the following words: "Every profession is to some degree surrounded by a zone of ambiguity—The trouble with this zone of ambiguity is not that it is a no man's land, but that it seems to be everyman's land. And sometimes this leads to undeclared war between adjacent occupations."[18] Role ambiguity and professional territoriality may result in conflict that is detrimental to group effort.

Differences between health professionals and other disciplines in terms of their orientation to time, styles of interpersonal interaction, methods of organization, and value systems can also result in barriers to effective group action.[19] Health system factors that impair group function may also relate to concepts of authority and autonomy. Traditionally, physicians have been perceived as leaders in groups dealing with health.[20] In many instances, however, this may not be appropriate. It may be difficult for physicians and other health-care providers to see someone other than a physician as a legitimate leader in health-related groups.

Professional autonomy can also hamper group function. The joint effort required in group work decreases personal independence in favor of interdependence. Interdependence creates the potential for challenges or criticism of one member's beliefs or actions by other group members, a situation that may be threatening to the individual member. Again, use of good interpersonal skills by the community health nurse can create a climate in which group members do not feel threatened by interdependence.

DIAGNOSTIC REASONING AND THE GROUP PROCESS

Based on the assessment of group members, the community health nurse would diagnose group strengths and weaknesses. Diagnoses might also relate to group members' expertise and motivation relative to the problem to be solved. For example, the community health nurse working in a group might diagnose a "need for conflict resolution due to different perceptions of group goals by group members." Or, the nurse might derive a diagnosis of "effective group function due to successful accomplishment of tasks of group development." A third possible diagnosis might be a "need to educate members for group work due to inexperience with group dynamics."

PLANNING AND THE GROUP PROCESS

There are two aspects to planning in group work. One reflects the efforts of the group to resolve the problems in question. This aspect of planning uses the general planning principles discussed in Chapter 5, The Nursing Process, and Chapter 19, Care of the Community or Target Group. The second aspect of planning involves planning for the operation of the group itself and includes determining group modes of decision making, conflict resolution, communication, and role negotiation. These activities are carried out during what have been called the accommodation and negotiation stages of group formation.[16]

SELECTING A METHOD OF DECISION MAKING

Group action requires group decisions, and decisions must be made after careful consideration by group members. To facilitate decision making, group members should agree on the method by which decisions will be made. Because most people are not familiar with group processes or the deliberate need to select a decision-making strategy, the community health nurse may need to guide the group in this task.

Decisions can be made in one of six ways: by default, by the leader, by a subgroup, by majority vote, by consensus, or by unanimous consent. When decisions are made by default, they result from a lack of response by the group. For example, if a class of senior nursing students is invited by faculty to plan a graduation reception but fails to respond, they have, in fact, decided not to have a reception.

In the second method of decision making, decisions are made by the leader or person in authority. This method of decision making is appropriate in situations when a decision cannot wait on the slow-moving democratic process (for example, an emergency). The group may decide to give the group leader authority to make independent decisions in certain circumstances, but should decide in advance what circumstances warrant such independent decisions. In an effective group, this is not the method used for making most of the group's decisions.

In the third approach to group decision making, group decisions are made by a subgroup. This might involve "railroading," in which the subgroup uses its power and influence to force a decision on other group members. Or, the larger group may purposefully delegate the making of decisions to a subgroup. Many nursing organizations, for example, delegate authority to an executive board for decisions regarding everyday operation and only make major decisions as a total group.

Majority vote by group members is the fourth method of decision making. This is a frequently used method in many groups with which community health nurses work. The fifth method involves consensus or agreement by all group members despite reservations that individual members might have. Finally, decisions may be made by unanimous consent in which all group members agree without reservation. In both the consensus and unanimous-consent methods, the group may take a relatively long time to reach a decision because of the need for all members to agree. For the purposes of true collaboration in a group, majority vote, consensus, and unanimous consent are the most appropriate methods for group decision making.

DEVELOPING MECHANISMS FOR CONFLICT RESOLUTION

Breakdowns in the decision-making process are one source of conflict within the group. Other potential sources of conflict include incompatible goals, differences of opinion on the allocation of resources or rewards, and perceived threats to individual member's personal identity or rights. Conflict is a normal component of group effort and is to be expected. If the group has developed mechanisms for conflict resolution before conflicts arise, conflict can often be a positive experience for the group rather than a divisive one.

Recognition of conflict as a normal phenomenon is essential if the group is to plan ahead for conflict resolution. Again, many groups do not anticipate conflict, and when conflict occurs they are unprepared to deal with it. Strategies for resolving conflict constructively involve creating a climate conducive to discussion, identifying and eliminating sources of conflict, capitalizing on areas of agreement, and rational consideration of alternative solutions to conflict. The community health nurse can explore these approaches to conflict resolution with members of the group and assist members to select the most appropriate approach.

Creating a climate in which disagreement is acceptable can minimize or resolve conflict. Conflict resolution requires that all parties be fully able to express their perspectives through open communication.

Open communication cannot take place when there is pressure to conform and lack of acceptance of different opinions. Lack of communication contributes to conflict as well as hampering conflict resolution. As a group leader, the community health nurse may need to encourage group members to express thoughts and opinions that may not be congruent with those of other group members. Through the use of interpersonal skills, the nurse can assure that communications within the group are not accusatory, but deal with issues rather than personalities.

Recognizing the existence of conflict and identifying its sources and possible solutions are strategies for constructive use of conflict. A conflict that is ignored in the hope that it will resolve itself is likely to become worse. The community health nurse can encourage other group members to acknowledge that a conflict exists and help them explore the reasons for conflict. Again, the nurse should be alert to covert signs of conflict and bring them to the attention of the rest of the group. For example, a nurse working with a group trying to determine budget allocations among health-care programs within the county may notice that representatives of programs for the elderly are maintaining a stony silence during the discussion. The nurse may comment on the fact that they have not participated in the discussion and ask why. In the ensuing discussion, it may be learned that these group members feel that too much money is being allocated to maternal-child health programs and that the elderly are being shortchanged. Once this conflict has been exposed, the group can begin work to resolve it.

Another strategy for resolving conflict involves identifying small areas of trust and agreement between group members that can be expanded. For instance, although two group members may disagree on the "appropriate" approach to a problem, they can capitalize on their shared concern for clients' welfare. Finally, rational consideration of alternative solutions to a particular conflict using the group's decision-making process and the problem-solving process can result in conflict becoming a valuable learning experience in group problem solving. The community health nurse can assist the group to explore a variety of alternative solutions to a conflict and to select an approach that is agreeable to all members.

DEVELOPING COMMUNICATION STRATEGIES

Developing group communication strategies is another task in planning for group operation. The importance of an effective communication network cannot be overemphasized. The group must develop a common language that facilitates communication, and members should refrain from using jargon familiar only to members of their own discipline. When it is necessary to use terminology unfamiliar to others, efforts should be made to translate it into the common language. The nurse in this situation can either play the part of the translator or ask other members for clarification. For example, some members of a group may use acronyms unfamiliar to others, such as AFDC. The nurse should then explain to the group that this stands for Aid to Families with Dependent Children. If the nurse does not recognize the acronym, he or she would ask for an explanation of its meaning.

The group should also agree on the form that communication will take. For example, communications may be verbal, written, or a combination of both depending upon the situation. Perhaps the group will decide that communication with sponsoring institutions should take the form of formal written memoranda, while communications between group members should be more informal verbal messages.

Consideration should also be given to the fact that communication takes place outside of regular group sessions. The content of these informal encounters between group members should not undermine group function or provide a forum for airing grievances or denigrating other members. The community health nurse who encounters unproductive communication outside of group meetings can bring relevant issues to the attention of the entire group so open discussion can take place and conflict can be avoided or resolved.

Establishing a climate in which group members feel respected and in which differences are accepted will contribute to an effective communication network. This means that all group members should be encouraged to participate and should receive positive reinforcement for their contribution whether or not others agree with it. In the beginning of the group's operation, the nurse group leader may need to ask reluctant group members for their ideas and opinions. As their participation is received positively, they will begin to volunteer remarks.

NEGOTIATING ROLES

Another task to be accomplished in forming an effective group is role negotiation. As mentioned earlier, professional roles tend to overlap, and role negotiation is crucial to effective group function. When two or more group members possess similar skills, the group must decide who will be responsible for exercising those skills. These decisions may be made as a general rule of thumb, so that one member always has responsibility for certain activities, or may change with the needs of the situation. For instance, both teachers and nurses have educational skills. A group developing a health education program for the school system may decide that teachers will be responsible for general health education related to nutrition and hygiene, while the nurse deals with more complex health topics such as substance abuse and sexually transmitted diseases.

One particular group role that must be negotiated is the role of leader. This position incorporates functions related to group administration, liaison with outside groups, teaching, and coordination of group effort. The leadership role may be assigned to one member, may shift with the situation, or may reside with the group as a whole. In the latter instance, no one member acts as the leader, and leadership functions are performed by the group as a unit. In many instances, community health nurses fulfill the leadership role within the group, particularly in groups composed largely of nonprofessionals. In other cases, the nurse may need to help the group identify the person best suited to lead the group based on the needs of the situation.

IMPLEMENTATION AND THE GROUP PROCESS

Implementation in the group process involves actually assigning responsibilities for tasks required to achieve group goals and performing assigned tasks. Tasks are assigned on the basis of decisions made in the role-negotiation phase of planning. Actual implementation of tasks is based on the general principles of implementation discussed in Chapter 5, The Nursing Process.

Planned group operating procedures are also executed during the implementation stage. Decisions are made using the method of decision making selected and communication networks are established along lines determined by the group. If conflict should arise during group operation, the group will employ the conflict-resolution strategies selected during group formation.

EVALUATION AND THE GROUP PROCESS

Evaluation in the group process involves evaluating both the outcome of group activity and the process used to plan and execute group action. Tasks of this stage actually begin during planning and prior to implementation of group actions. The group identifies outcome criteria and plans mechanisms for evaluating the effects of group effort in terms of those criteria. Group members' responsibilities in evaluation should be negotiated in the same manner as other group roles and assigned on the basis of competency. For example, if the group has implemented a school nutrition program, teachers may evaluate students' knowledge of nutrition, while the community health nurse evaluates indicators of nutritional status such as height, weight, and hematocrit. The evaluation process itself is discussed in detail in Chapter 5, The Nursing Process, and Chapter 19, Care of the Community or Target Group.

The second aspect of evaluation involves evaluating the use of the group process. Concerns that might be addressed include the effectiveness of group decision making, conflict resolution, communication,

BOX 11–4

Components of the Group Process

1. Assess:

   The problem to be addressed by the group
   The members of the group in terms of factors influencing group function
   - Human biological factors
   - Physical, psychological, and social environmental factors
   - Life-style factors
   - Health system factors

2. Diagnose group strengths and weaknesses, expertise, and motivation

3. Plan for:

   Achievement of group goals
   Group operation in terms of:
   - Methods for group decision making
   - Mechanisms for conflict resolution
   - Methods of communication
   - Role negotiation

4. Implement:

   Activities designed to reach the group goal
   Group operating procedures

5. Evaluate:

   The outcome of group action
   The use of the group process

and role negotiation strategies. Were roles allocated in a way that facilitated group goal achievement? Was communication between group members effective? Were conflicts within the group adequately resolved? Answers to these and similar questions can assist the group to work together more effectively in the future and can prepare group members to function effectively in other groups.

The epidemiologic prevention process model can be used to facilitate group process in a variety of groups with whom community health nurses work. Community health nurses may use the model to assist a group of clients to achieve common goals. It can also be used with groups of health-care providers and policymakers to facilitate group process and achieve group goals. The components of the group process applied in the context of the epidemiologic prevention process model are summarized in Box 11–4.

CHAPTER HIGHLIGHTS

- The change, leadership, and group processes are closely interrelated and are frequently used in conjunction.
- The change process begins with an assessment of driving and restraining forces related to human biology, environment, life-style, and the health system that influence change in a given situation.
- Tasks in the planning stage of the change process include establishing goals and objectives for the change, evaluating and selecting an approach to change, delineating activities leading to change, and planning to evaluate the change.
- Three approaches to change are the empirical-rational, normative-reeducative, and power-coercive approaches. Each is useful in certain situations, but all have disadvantages as well.
- The three stages in implementing change are unfreezing, changing, and refreezing.
- In a leadership situation, the community health nurse as leader assesses factors related to human biology, environment, life-style, and the health system affecting the situation.
- Diagnosis in the leadership process includes diagnosing the need for leadership and diagnosing follower maturity with respect to the task to be accomplished.
- Planning for leadership includes selecting a leadership style appropriate to the situation, the leader, and the followers, and planning to prepare followers for action. Leadership styles that might be selected include telling, selling, participating, and delegating.
- The two aspects of preparing followers for action include enhancing their abilities to perform necessary tasks and improving followers' motivation to act.
- Three tasks of the leader in implementing the leadership process are preparing followers for action, coordinating follower activities, and representing followers to outsiders.
- The group process begins with an assessment of the situation and group members in terms of human biological, environmental, life-style, and health system factors that will influence group action.
- The two aspects of planning for group work are accommodating to group membership, and negotiation. Tasks of accommodation include selecting a method of decision making, developing mechanisms for conflict resolution, and formulating communication strategies. Negotiation of group members' roles is the other aspect of planning for group work.
- Two tasks in implementing group action are task assignment and performance of designated activities.
- Two aspects of evaluation are relevant to the change, leadership, and group processes—evaluation of the outcome of activity and evaluation of the process used.

Review Questions

1. Describe the influence of driving and restraining forces in a change situation. Give examples of each type of force. (p. 198)
2. What are the four major considerations in planning for change? Give an example of each. (p. 199)
3. What are the three approaches that may be taken to bring about change? Describe situations in which each approach might be appropriate. (p. 200)
4. Describe the three stages in implementing change. How might you facilitate movement through these stages? Give specific examples related to a change situation with which you are familiar. (p. 202)
5. Describe the relationship of follower maturity to leadership style. (p. 206)
6. What are the three functions of a leader in implementing leadership? Give an example of the performance of each function. (p. 208)
7. Describe two tasks in planning for group action. Give an example of the performance of each task. (p. 212)
8. Discuss two tasks in implementing the group process. Give an example of the performance of each. (p. 214)
9. What are the two aspects of evaluation applicable to the change, leadership, and group processes? Give examples of evaluative criteria for each aspect in each of the three processes. (pp. 203 and 214)

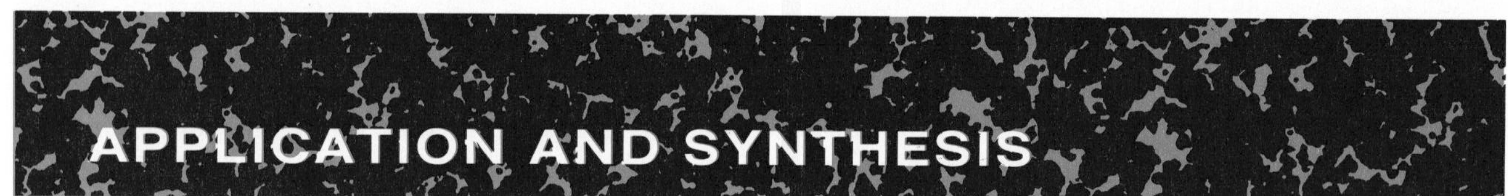

APPLICATION AND SYNTHESIS

In assessing the town of Clarkston, you, as community health nurse, note that there are high infant and maternal mortality rates. Part of the explanation for these high rates lies in a lack of prenatal care for large numbers of pregnant women. The local health department prenatal clinic is always full and clients may have a wait of 3 months or longer for an initial appointment. Because many of the pregnant women in the community don't seek care until their pregnancies are fairly far advanced, they may deliver before they can be seen. Seven private physicians in town provide obstetrical care, but their services are underutilized. This is primarily because most of the pregnant population come from low-income families and are on Medicaid, which these physicians do not want to accept. Because they are on the obstetrical staff of the local community hospital that accepts indigent clients, four of these physicians deliver many of these women, who have not had prenatal care. Two physicians have been sued as a result of complications experienced by these indigent women.

1. What changes or course of action might improve this situation?
2. What would be the objective of your change? Be specific.
3. What human biological, environmental, life-style, and health system factors are acting as driving and restraining forces in this situation?
4. As the leader in this change situation, who are your followers? How would you describe the maturity level of your followers?
5. What leadership style would be appropriate in this situation? Why?
6. How would you engage in unfreezing in this situation? What would you do to bring about the desired change? How would you promote refreezing?
7. How would you evaluate the outcome of the change and your leadership as a change agent?

REFERENCES

1. Lewin, K. (1951). *Field theory in social science: Selected theoretical papers.* New York: Harper & Row.
2. Flynn, J. M. (1988). Change theory. In J. M. Flynn & P. B. Heffron (Eds.), *Nursing: From concept to practice* (2nd ed.) (pp. 351–357). Norwalk, CT: Appleton & Lange.
3. Green, C. P. (1983). Teaching strategies for the process of planned change. *Journal of Continuing Education in Nursing, 14*(6), 16–23.
4. Haffer, A. (1986). Facilitating change: Choosing the appropriate strategy. *JONA, 16*(4), 18–22.
5. Chinn, R., & Benne, K. D. (1985). General strategies for effecting change in human systems. In W. B. Bennis, K. D. Benne, & R. Chinn (Eds.), *The planning of change* (2nd ed.) (pp. 22–45). New York: Holt, Rinehart, & Winston.
6. Schein, E. (1969). The mechanisms of change. In W. B. Bennis, K. D. Benne, & R. Chinn (Eds.), *The planning of change* (2nd ed.). New York: Holt, Rinehart, & Winston.
7. Tappen, R. M. (1989). *Nursing leadership and management: Concepts and practice* (2nd ed.). Philadelphia: F. A. Davis.
8. Rantz, M. J., & Miller, T. V. (1987). Change theory: A framework for implementing nursing diagnosis in a long-term care unit. *Nursing Clinics of North America, 22,* 887–897.
9. Institute of Medicine. (1988). *The future of public health.* New York: Academy Press.
10. McCreight, L. (1989). The future of public health. *Nursing Outlook, 37,* 219–225.
11. Salmon, M. E. (1989). Public health nursing: The neglected specialty. *Nursing Outlook, 37,* 226–229.
12. Josten, L. E. (1989). Wanted: Leaders for public health. *Nursing Outlook, 37,* 230–232.
13. Bernhard, L. A., & Walsh, M. (1990). *Leadership: The key to the professionalization of nursing.* St. Louis: C. V. Mosby.
14. Hersey, P., & Blanchard, K. H. (1988). *Management of organizational behavior: Utilizing human resources* (5th ed.). Englewood Cliffs, NJ: Prentice-Hall.
15. Herzberg, F. (1966). *Work and the nature of man.* Cleveland: World Publishing.
16. Brill, N. I. (1976). *Working together in human services.* New York: J. B. Lippincott.
17. Purtilo, R. B. (1988). Ethical issues in teamwork: The context of rehabilitation. *Archives of Physical Medicine and Rehabilitation, 69,* 318–322.
18. Merton, R. (1958). Issues in growth of a profession. In *Proceedings of the 41st Annual Convention of the American Nurses' Association* (pp. 295–306). Atlantic City, NJ: American Nurses' Association.
19. Mailick, M. D., & Jordan, P. (1977). A multimodel approach to collaborative practice in health settings. *Social Work in Health Care, 2,* 445–453.
20. Hutt, A. (1986). What exactly is the "team approach"? *Midwife, Health Visitor, Community Health Nurse, 22,* 340–342.

RECOMMENDED READINGS

Bennis, W. B. (1991). Learning some basic truisms about leadership. *National Forum, LXXI* (1), 12–15.

Describes the differences between leadership and management.

Bennis, W. B., & Nanus, B. (1985). *Leaders: The strategies for taking change.* New York: Harper & Row.

Presents the findings of studies of actual leaders and the strategies they employ. Also describes key skills of leaders.

Bernhard, L. A., & Walsh, M. (1990). *Leadership: The key to the professionalization of nursing.* St. Louis: C. V. Mosby.

Provides basic information on the leadership process as applied to nursing practice.

Desjardins, C., & Brown, C. O. (1991). A new look at leadership styles. *National Forum, LXXI* (1), 18–20.

Underscores the need for increased attention to relationship aspects of leadership.

Douglass, L. M. (1988). *The effective nurse: Leader and manager.* St. Louis: C. V. Mosby.

Offers an introduction to concepts of leadership and management by nurses.

Haffer, A. (1986). Facilitating change: Choosing the appropriate strategy. *JONA, 16*(4), 18–22.

Sets forth the three approaches to change and discusses the advantages, disadvantages, and applicability of each.

Lippitt, G. L., Langseth, P., & Mossop, J. (1985). *Implementing organizational change.* San Francisco: Jossey-Bass.

An overview of the change process and its implications for organizational change. Also addresses leadership styles in decision making and strategies for implementing change in organizations.

Rantz, M. J., & Miller, T. V. (1987). Change theory: A framework for implementing nursing diagnosis in a long-term setting. *Nursing Clinics of North America, 22,* 887–897.

Contains an overview of change theory and describes its application to change in a specific nursing unit.

Schorr, T., & Zimmerman, A. (1988). *Making choices: Nurse leaders tell their stories.* St. Louis: C. V. Mosby.

Describes the leadership approaches taken by many of nursing's current leaders.

Swansburg, R. C. (1990). *Management and leadership for nurse managers.* Boston: Jones and Bartlett.

Addresses the change and leadership processes and their implications for nursing management in organizational settings.

Tack, M. W. (1991). Future leaders in higher education. *National Forum, LXXI* (1), 29–32.

Enumerates the characteristics of effective leaders.

CHAPTER 12

The Political Process

Elizabeth Harper Smith

KEY TERMS

bill
campaigning
community organization
electioneering
health policy
laws
legislative proposals
lobbying
policy
policy-making
political process
power
power base
public-health policy
regulation

The change, leadership, and group interaction skills described in the last chapter are frequently used in the context of the political process, which many people equate with voting and legislation. The political process, however, encompasses more than these two activities. The ***political process*** is all of the activities that result in the formation of policies that guide societal behavior.

Policy guides and directs action in all spheres of social interaction including the provision of health-care services. For example, national defense policy determines the size of a standing army as well as the number and types of weapons that will be developed. Environmental policy guides decisions on the use of parklands, prohibition of offshore drilling, and disposal of hazardous wastes. In the same vein, health-care policy directs decisions and actions taken in the provision of health-care services. When nurses apply the change, leadership, and group processes to the development of health policy, they engage in the political process.

(continued)

LEARNING OBJECTIVES

After reading this chapter you should be able to:

- Identify at least three levels at which health-policy formation occurs.
- Describe at least five considerations in influencing health-policy formation.
- Identify four strategies for developing a power base for political influence.
- Describe at least four approaches to creating support for a proposed health policy.
- Outline the legislative process at the state and federal levels.
- Describe the regulatory process.
- Identify four criteria for evaluating a proposed health policy.

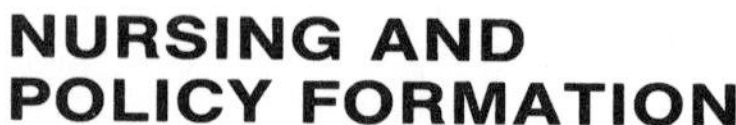

NURSING AND POLICY FORMATION

Early community health nurses were adept at the use of the political process in developing policies to promote the health of the population. These early leaders in community health nursing knew that the only way to make lasting changes in the social factors influencing health was to become involved in the formation of health policy at all levels. Nursing action to foster changes in sanitary conditions, to promote health legislation, and to change child labor laws are some examples of the early political activities by these nurses. They were active, as well, in many other social movements such as women's suffrage. They realized that the political process was a means of achieving their goal of improved health for all and that, because of its focus on the health of population groups, community health nursing is, by definition, political in nature.[1]

Over the years, many nurses became uncomfortable with the idea of political involvement, with the possible exception of exercising the right to vote. Politics had an unfavorable aura that was seen as incompatible with nursing's altruistic philosophy. More recently, nurses have begun to realize the need to influence health-policy decisions. Unfortunately, this activity has often been perceived as self-serving rather than being concerned with the health of clients.[2,3] For example, nurses have been encouraged to engage in political activity to ensure their "effectiveness in competing for scarce resources"[4] and to assure government funding for nursing research.[5]

There is a need for nursing input in health policy that affects not only the health of the population but also nursing practice. This need is apparent at all levels of government, but particularly at the federal level. The need for nursing influence at the federal level is underscored by the fact that, as of the fall of 1990, none of the 535 members of the U.S. Congress were nurses and only 11 members of their many staffs were nurses.[6] Despite their lack of expertise on health matters, these formulators of health-care policies for the nation rarely seek consultation from health-care providers.[2]

Political participation by nurses appears to be limited, although it is similar to that of women in other professional groups on measures of political participation. One study indicated that nurses were significantly less likely to vote than either female teachers or engineers; they were more likely than engineers to engage in protest activities and similarly unlikely to engage in campaign efforts and communal activities such as personal communications with policymakers, organizing and working with community groups, and writing letters to the editor. Nurses were also found to belong to significantly fewer professional organizations and to be less active than teachers or engineers in those organizations that might exert political influence.[7]

These findings suggest that nurses need to become more involved in influencing health policy at all levels. This is particularly true of community health nurses, whose responsibility is for the health of society at large.

HEALTH-CARE POLICY

Policy is the aggregate of principles directing the distribution of resources among the population,[8] while ***policy-making*** is the process of synthesizing those principles and the values, interests, and concerns that underlie them in response to an identified problem.[3] Policy is typically concerned with complex issues, and its formation involves the use of the political process. Policy is used by organizational systems, including governments, to determine goals, operating principles, and directions for action. In other words, policy is a value-based blueprint to guide subsequent action. ***Health policy*** is a defined set of principles used to guide activities to safeguard and promote the health of the public.

Public policy is a direction or course of action undertaken by a government or an official governmental agency. A public policy is a decision made by a society or its elected representatives that has material effects on members of the public other than those directly involved in the decision-making process.[9] Public policies determine the parameters for individual and collective social behavior in allocating and distributing resources.[10] A ***public health policy,*** then, is the way a society or its elected representatives allocate and distribute political and economic resources to meet the health needs of the populace.

The formation of health policy is not an end in itself. Health policy is a means to an end, ideally the improvement of the health status of the general public. Input by community health nurses into policy decisions may improve the potential for such favorable outcomes, but they are not assured.

LEVELS OF HEALTH POLICY

Policy can be made in any setting or organizational system where values are at issue, and policy formation takes place at many levels in society: family, community, institution, state, nation, even the international level.[3] Institutional goals and purpose shape policy decisions at the level of the health agency or institution. Examples of institutional policy related to community health would be decisions to create new programs or to expand or discontinue current ones. Decisions by local health departments to charge fees for previously free services such as immunizations are another example of institutional policy that affects the health of the public. Community health nurses need to be involved in the development of these and similar institutional policies to safeguard the interests of the public.

Health-policy decisions at the community level may be reflected in budget allocations for health-care programs, disaster preparation, housing codes, and so forth. At the state level, health-care policies focus on provision of health care and may include health programming decisions as well as policies related to licensure of health professionals, regulation of health-care institutions, and so on. At both the state and local levels, policies may also be formulated in legislation that regulates health-related behaviors by citizens. State laws and local ordinances that limit smoking in public places are examples of such policies.

National policy focuses on issues of concern to the society at large, and is exemplified by health-related legislation and regulations that are developed by federal agencies. While there are a number of health-related policies generated by the federal government, there is, at present, no single coherent health policy that directs provision of health care across the country.

The United States has allocated financial resources to create special programs that provide limited health-care services to selected populations of Americans. However, the provision of limited health-care services to small, select, underserved populations does not constitute a national health policy. Indeed, one of the major health-care issues facing the United States at this time is whether there should be such a national health policy.

The current lack of any comprehensive national policy related to health arises from a variety of factors. First, as noted in Chapter 3, The Health Care Context, there is no constitutionally mandated responsibility for health-care decision making at the national level. This lack of direct authority for health concerns has contributed greatly to the absence of a comprehensive and definitive national health policy. Up to now the health-care function has been viewed as a state responsibility, and the states have no authority to develop policies that apply to the nation as a whole.

Another factor in the absence of a definitive national health policy is the wide variety of health needs experienced by different segments of the population. It has been argued that a single national health policy generated at the federal level could not meet the health-care needs of the total population. It was this type of argument that led to the creation of regional health systems agencies, discussed below.

The lack of a definitive national health policy has resulted in the creation and demise of numerous health-oriented services and programs. Approaches and programs have changed as frequently as the members of the federal administrations that created them. Consequently, efforts to provide health-care services to targeted populations have been sporadic and poorly organized. Large gaps and costly overlaps in services have arisen from uncoordinated health-care programs. In addition, a pattern of inequitable distribution of resources and services has emerged. In some instances, one federal program has counteracted the effects of another.[11] An example of this is building large medical facilities in major metropolitan areas while simultaneously designing and implementing programs to attract health-care providers to rural areas. Excellent programs have often been well designed and instituted, but have not been provided with adequate funding for continued operation when a new administration shifted attention to other issues and concerns.

An example of federal programming intended to assist health policy development in all regions of the country was the Health Planning and Resources Development Act of 1974 (P.L. 93–641). Variations in health-care needs were to be addressed by regional health systems agencies (HSAs) that were created by the act. Each HSA was to assess area health needs, engage in systematic policy formation, and plan for the resources required to meet the specific health needs of the population served. The intent of the bill was to increase access to health care, increase the quality of health care, and decrease overall costs of health care.

During the operation of the HSAs, nursing was in a position to help achieve this policy agenda and to contribute to its own development as a profession. Nurse practitioner programs and clinical practice settings were developed. In addition, legislative changes occurred that supported reimbursement for nurse practitioner services. However, in some regions of the country there was little coordination with existing state planning agencies. In many of these regions, program overlap and competition occurred. Furthermore, the Health Planning and Resources Development Act provided no specific federal guidelines for the operation of HSAs, and individuals with expertise in systematic planning were not widely available to assist with HSA program development. Following changes in administration policies related to health, federal funds for HSA operations were eliminated. As a result, HSAs are no longer functioning as regional planning agencies directing health policy development and health-care delivery in their designated areas.

Health-oriented organizations such as the American Public Health Association (APHA) have long campaigned for a well-defined national health policy. The APHA's landmark call for a national health program was first made over 40 years ago. Since that time, the federal government has periodically made tentative efforts to develop a national health policy. Such efforts have not been sustained, and each tentative effort has been lost in the priority changes of successive administrations. Currently, a proposal for a national health program is being proposed by the major professional organizations in nursing.[12] This and similar plans for providing health care to the American population will be discussed in more detail in Chapter 13, Economic Influences on Community Health.

Business and industry, consumers, and lately Congress, have recognized that the United States is experiencing a health-care crisis that can no longer be tolerated. It is important for community health nurses and other health-care providers to work together to convince policymakers that a definitive national health policy is needed to provide a unified direction for the delivery of health-care services.

HEALTH POLICY VERSUS OTHER SOCIETAL ISSUES

Another issue related to health policy is the priority given to health concerns versus concerns for economic growth, international relations, national defense, energy resources, and so on. In a capitalistic economy such as that of the United States, economic concerns frequently override other social policy considerations. Rising costs for health care and other social programs coupled with the need for national defense and economic stability have generated much controversy in terms of national priorities.

Economic health is certainly vital to any society. Obviously, the economic health of the nation affects employment, and employment (or lack of it) will profoundly influence health status as well as access to health care. Less obvious is the fact that a significant portion of budgets such as that of the Department of Defense (DOD) is expended on health care, which affects the overall health of the nation. For example, a large share of the DOD budget is used to provide health services to active duty and retired members of the military and their dependents. The civilian sector is thereby relieved of the responsibility for providing services for this population under programs like Medicaid.

In addition, military health-care research also benefits the civilian population. For example, research conducted by the Army and the Air Force has contributed greatly to the available knowledge about AIDS. Similarly, the Army's occupational health program for civilian employees is the prototype for similar services in business and industry throughout the country.

Other endeavors that draw federal funding away from health programs may still contribute to improvements in health care. For example, health-related research undertaken as part of the space program has benefited the health of the general public.

Health-care providers need to be aware of the interplay of health-care issues and a variety of other national concerns in order to take responsible action in influencing policymakers on health-related issues. The community health professional should not focus exclusively on obtaining a "lion's share" of fiscal resources, but on the need to achieve a balanced distribution of finite resources.

It is particularly important that community health professionals, especially nurses, work toward policies that enhance coordination of health-care resources and services. Duplication of efforts is costly. Policies that promote a greater coordination between budgetary allocations—whether derived from the budgets of the National Institutes of Health, the Defense Department, or other programs—and coordination of services are greatly needed. The best method for accomplishing this coordination is for community health nurses to become well informed in all areas, not just with respect to health-care issues. Health and illness result from the interplay of multiple factors. Optimal health status and a definitive national health policy cannot be achieved by isolationist policies promoted by health-care providers.

AVENUES FOR FORMULATING AND IMPLEMENTING PUBLIC HEALTH-CARE POLICIES

Public health-care policy formation takes place via the political process. The two primary means of formulating and implementing health-care policies at state and national levels are legislation and regulation.

LEGISLATION

Laws are public-policy decisions generated by the legislative branch of government at the federal, state, or local level. Laws are created in a social system to express the collective values, interests, and beliefs of the society that generates them. As a society develops, so do its beliefs, values, and interests. Eventually, some laws enacted in earlier periods of a society's evolution will become obsolete. Sometimes laws will be created or revised to address new problems that have surfaced as the society changes. Modifications or changes in laws are legislative attempts to correct discrepancies that may have arisen between past and current social practices. Although this is a highly simplified description of the function of legislation, the point is that laws reflect societal needs and values and are subject to revision.

Policy formation via the legislative process is very similar at the federal and state levels. Figures 12–1 and 12–2 depict the typical progress of a bill through the state and federal legislative processes. The arrows in each of the figures indicate points in the process at which community health nurses might influence legislation.

Legislative proposals are statements of beliefs or interests that have been brought to the attention of a legislator. These interests may come to the legislator's attention through constituents or through his or her involvement on a legislative subcommittee dealing with specific issues. Community health nurses can influence the legislative process at this point by making lawmakers aware of the need to develop policy or to modify existing policies. After due consideration, constituents' beliefs or interests are drafted in a ***bill,*** which is a formally worded statement of the desired policy. Once a bill has been drafted, the sponsoring legislator submits it for identification, meaning that the bill will carry the legislator's name as sponsor. It is not unusual for a proposed bill to have multiple sponsors.

At the congressional level, the bill is assigned a number and listed by the House or Senate clerk and sent to a general committee for review. The committee may revise the language of the bill or amend it. In the normal course of events, the bill would then be sent on to the House or Senate floor for its "first reading." A first reading usually consists of a reference to the bill by number and title. The title may address the bill's content or the name(s) of its sponsor. The entire bill is not read at this time.

After its first reading, the bill might be referred to the appropriate subcommittee for hearings. At the congressional level there are six committees that deal with most health-related legislation. These include: (1) the Senate Finance Committee, which establishes policy related to the Medicare and Medicaid programs; (2) the House Ways and Means Committee, which oversees similar legislation for the House of Representatives; (3) the Senate Labor and Human Resources Committee; and (4) the House Energy and Commerce Committee, both of which address matters related to the programs administered by the Department of Health and Human Services; (5) the House Appropriations Committee; and (6) the Senate Appropriations Committee. The first four of these committees are enabling committees that deal with legislation establishing, modifying, or discontinuing health programs. The House Appropriations and Senate Appropriations committees are responsible for allocating the funds for the various federal programs. Similar committees exist at the state level.

Community health nurses can influence the legislative process at this point by contacting lawmakers and making their views known on legislation pending before them. Table 12–1 lists the addresses and telephone numbers of some of the significant congressional committees, as well as other agencies and organizations that may be of help to nurses in influencing health policy formation.

Committee members considering a particular piece of legislation can either review and modify a bill or decide not to report the bill out of committee, thus effectively killing it. Legislation can also bypass assignment to a committee and advance directly to a second reading on the House or Senate floor. The bill

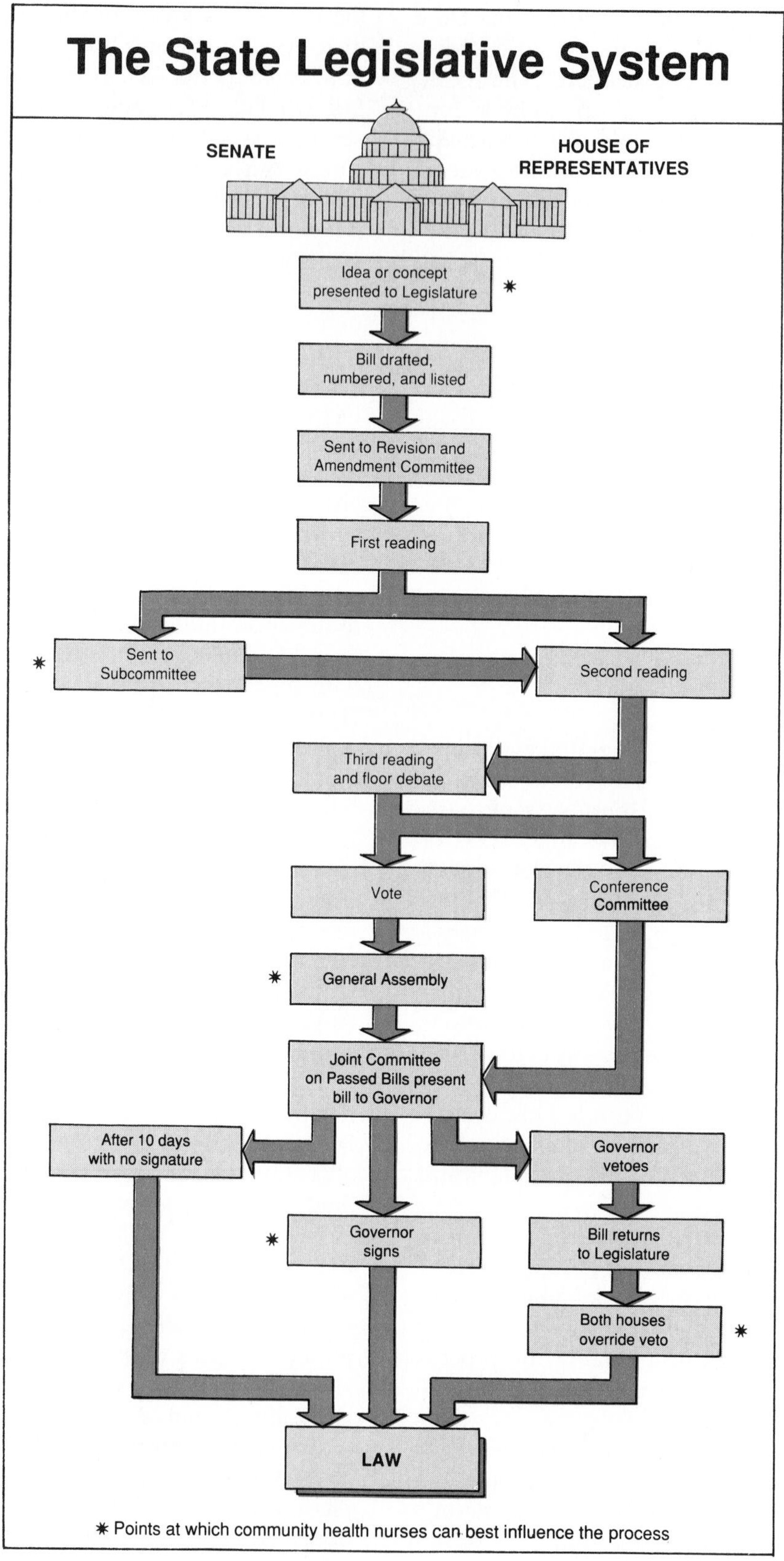

Figure 12–1. A typical state legislative process.

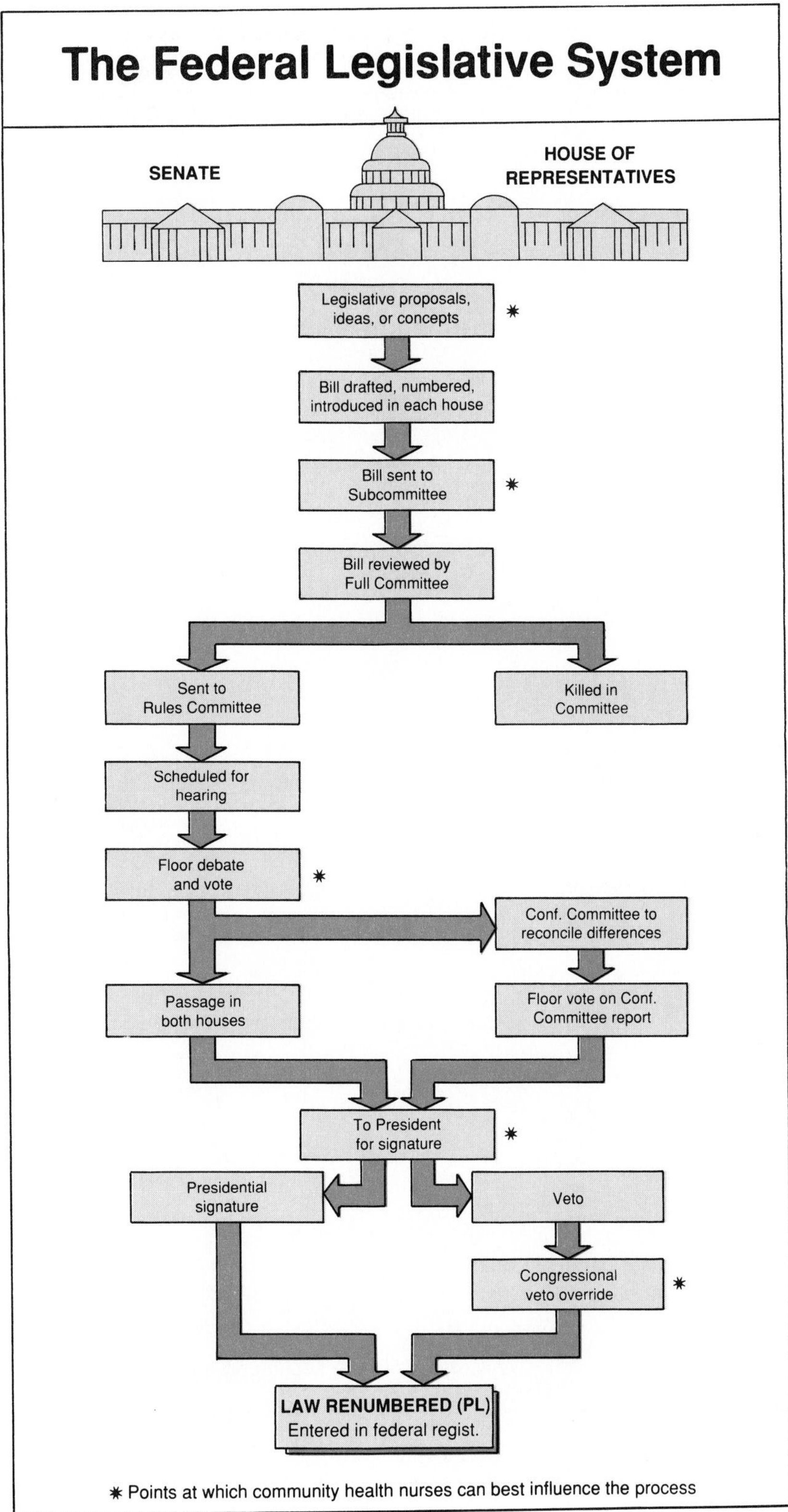

Figure 12–2. The federal legislative process.

TABLE 12–1. RESOURCES FOR NURSES CONCERNED WITH HEALTH-POLICY ISSUES

Agency or Organization	Mission
Center on Human Policy 724 Comstock Ave. Syracuse, NY 13244 (315) 423-3851	Information on law and policies related to disability, advocacy
Coalition for a National Health Service 116 Laburnam Cresent Rochester, NY 14620 (716) 442-1684	Education related to need for a national health service; advocacy on health system reform
Committee for National Health Insurance 1757 N Street, N.W. Washington, DC 20036 (202) 223-9685	Research, education on U.S. health-care system, advocacy, legislation
Health Policy Advisory Center 17 Murray Street New York, NY 10007	Information on occupational and environmental health policy
National Health Federation P.O. Box 688 Monrovia, CA 91016 (818) 357-2181	Advocacy for public rights to health care
U.S. Department of Health and Human Services Health Care Financing Administration 6401 Security Bldg. Baltimore, MD 21235 (202) 245-1319	Administers funds for health-care programs
U.S. Department of Health and Human Services Health Resources and Services Administration 5600 Fishers Lane Rockville, MD 20857 (301) 443-2216	Formulates health policy on services and facilities; funds program development; promotes education of health professionals
U.S. Department of Health and Human Services Social Security Administration 6401 Security Bldg. Baltimore, MD 21235 (301) 594-3120	Administers programs under Social Security Act
U.S. House of Representatives Committee on Ways and Means Subcommittee on Health 1114 Longworth House Office Bldg. Washington, DC 20515 (202) 226-3381	Health-policy formulation; deals with Social Security programs
U.S. House of Representatives Energy and Commerce Committee	Addresses general health-policy issues at the federal level
U.S. Senate Committee on Finance Subcommittee on Health SD-205 Dirksen Building Washington, DC 20510 (202) 224-4515	Health-policy formulation; deals with health programs; Medicare
U.S. Senate Labor and Human Resources Committee	Addresses general health-policy issues at the federal level

may then proceed to a third reading, be referred back to committee, or be sent to another committee for review and revision before advancing to the third and final reading. Following the third reading, the proposed legislation will be placed on the calendar for floor debate and, finally, voted upon. At this point in the legislative process, community health nurses can contact their own representatives and try to persuade them to support nursing's position on a particular bill.

If the legislation is passed in the chamber of Congress in which it originated, it will be sent to the other chamber for approval. In many cases, when a bill has advanced to this point, it will be passed by the second chamber without further modification. The bill can, however, be sent to another committee for review and modification. Once a bill has passed the second chamber, it will be returned to the house or chamber in which it originated for final approval. At the state level, a bill must be signed by the leaders of both houses of the legislature as well as the Secretary of State before it is forwarded for the governor's signature. After the governor signs the bill, it will be renumbered according to the appropriate lawbook code number, filed with the Secretary of State, and become law. A similar process occurs at the federal level after a bill is signed by the president.

In most states, if the two chambers of the legislature cannot agree on a similar version of a given bill, a special committee composed of members of both chambers will be formed. This committee is called a *joint conference committee.* The purpose of the joint committee is to develop a compromise bill. It is highly unusual for a joint committee recommendation not to be passed. Once the compromise bill has passed both houses of the legislature, it will be sent to the executive branch of the government (governor or president) for final approval.

The chief executive (governor or president) can either sign the bill or hamper its progress by not signing it or vetoing it. Lobbying may also be used at this point to influence the chief executive's disposition of a particular bill. If the executive vetoes a bill, it will be returned to the legislature. The legislature will then be required to meet a constitutionally prescribed majority vote (usually a two-thirds majority) to override the veto and enact the bill into law. Any bill that does not complete the legislative process during the legislative session in which it is introduced is dead, and it must be reintroduced in a subsequent session if it is ever to become law.

REGULATION

Policy decisions enacted as legislation are usually implemented by regulatory agencies charged with implementing specific types of legislation. For example, federal policies related to environmental issues are implemented by the Environmental Protection Agency (EPA), while state health-related policies are usually implemented by a state board of health or a comparable agency.

These agencies develop regulations that determine how legislation will be implemented. A ***regulation*** is a rule or order having the force of law that deals with procedures to be followed in implementing a piece of legislation. Regulations are intended to promote individual accountability for actions and to protect the public health and welfare. Regulations specify how policies are realized in actual behavior.

Regulatory agencies exert a great deal of control over health-related activities by both professionals and the general public. State agencies such as boards of nursing, for example, regulate who may practice nursing and how nursing licensure will be granted. These same agencies might also be responsible for determining which health-care providers can write prescriptions for medication in those states where such practices are authorized for personnel other than physicians.

When a piece of legislation authorizing an activity such as prescription-writing is passed, the legislature will usually designate an existing agency or create a new agency to implement the legislation. This agency develops the regulations that govern implementation of the law. In the case of prescription-writing privileges, the regulatory agency would determine who can write prescriptions and what additional qualifications might be required of those persons. For example, in California, nurses who are certified by the state as nurse practitioners may write prescriptions, but only if they have completed an approved course in pharmacology. Other regulations specify who is eligible for certification as a nurse practitioner in the state.

Another example of regulations that implement legislation is the procedures for handling hazardous substances in the workplace, which were developed by the Occupational Safety and Health Administration (OSHA). The enabling legislation mandated protection of employees from exposure to hazardous substances, but regulations developed by OSHA specify how certain substances should be handled. For example, certain types of ventilatory equipment are required in manufacturing processes using hazardous aerosols, so the risk of exposure to employees is minimized.

Regulations instituted by various agencies may dramatically influence the actual impact of a law.[3] For example, when prescription-writing by nurse practitioners was first instituted in Tennessee, one proposal was to restrict the privilege to nurse practitioners prepared at the master's level. Since this requirement would have excluded many nurse practitioners in rural counties where physicians were scarce, it would have undermined the intent of the enabling legislation—to provide greater access to health care for underserved populations.

Community health nurses can have input into regulations that affect their professional practice as well as into the legislation that shapes public-health policy. When a regulatory agency is in the process of formulating regulations, the public is informed that the process is being initiated. Generally, the agency formulates some preliminary regulations that are published for public review and comment. At the federal level, proposed regulations are published in the *Federal Register,* and similar registers exist in each state. Interested parties are then allowed to comment on the proposed regulations and suggest changes.

When regulations deal with particularly sensitive areas, the regulatory body involved may hold public hearings to solicit input from interested parties. Community health nurses may either comment on proposed regulations in written communications to the regulatory agency or provide testimony at public hearings. The regulatory agency can then use the input received to refine the regulations. Regulations are published in the appropriate state or federal publication and promulgated among individuals affected by them. For example, schools of nursing in California were informed in writing of changes requiring educational content on child abuse for public health nursing certification in the state.

INFLUENCING HEALTH-POLICY FORMATION AND IMPLEMENTATION

Community health nurses can influence health-related policies at all levels. To do so, however, they must be conversant with the political process and its use. Some of the considerations affecting the ability of community health nurses to influence policy formation are education, setting an agenda, defining and evaluating choices, obtaining data, developing a power base, and creating support for a particular policy or direction.

EDUCATION

It is important for community health nurses to understand the various processes involved in policy formation. Lack of educational preparation for political activity has been cited as one of the contributing factors in nursing's inability to influence health policy formation significantly,[3] and educational preparation in nursing has been found to be significantly related to political participation, with greater participation among better-educated nurses.[7]

It has been suggested that content on health policy be integrated into the overall curricula of baccalaureate, master's, and doctoral programs in nursing with separate courses in health policy as a potential elective for undergraduate students and as a requirement for graduate education. Content for health-policy education should address significant policy issues, the political process, analysis of health policies at several levels, strategies for presenting legislative proposals, and research related to health policy[4] as well as the significant legislative committees that review health-related legislation at the federal and state level.[2]

In addition to educating themselves for political activity, community health nurses can educate policymakers regarding the needs of the public. As noted earlier, policymakers rarely have backgrounds related to health and may be largely unaware of health issues or lack a sound understanding of their implications for the health of the public. It is the task of community health nurses and other health-care providers to educate policymakers in this regard. It is particularly important that these individuals be apprised of the findings of nursing research related to health-care delivery, since uninformed policymakers may profoundly influence the health-care delivery system.[13]

SETTING AN AGENDA

Community health nurses need to decide upon a policy agenda that they wish to support. There are many policy issues on which community health nurses may wish to have input, including issues related to the needs of the profession as well as those of the public. Choices among these issues must be made carefully to enhance the credibility of community health nurses with policymakers.

As noted earlier, health-care providers are often perceived by health-care policymakers as self-serving. For this reason, it is important for community health nurses to focus more on health-policy issues of concern to the public and less on issues of concern only to the nursing profession.[3] To influence health-policy decisions nurses need to approach policymakers regarding concerns related to important public issues such as AIDS, child and spouse abuse, substance abuse, and so on.[2] Other public concerns that should shape the nursing policy agenda include adolescent pregnancy, cost control, and care of the elderly. These concerns, rather than professional aspirations, should form the basis for use of the political process by community health nurses.[14]

DEFINING AND EVALUATING CHOICES

A third consideration in the efforts of community health nurses to influence health-policy decisions is defining and evaluating choices.[14] Many avenues can be taken in the development of health-care policies. Community health nurses have a responsibility to identify and evaluate alternative directions for health policy and to make policymakers aware of potential advantages and disadvantages of various alternatives. This means that community health nurses must keep abreast of issues and developments that affect the health of the public as well as potential approaches in dealing with health-related issues.

OBTAINING DATA

To be an effective influence on health policymakers, community health nurses must generate data that are relevant and persuasive. As noted in Chapter 10, The Research Process, community health nursing research can be geared to obtaining data needed to influence health-policy decisions. Factors that have hindered nurses' efforts in this area include the failure of nurses to replicate research and to develop cumulative findings that support specific policy directions, and failure to disseminate research findings beyond the professional community.[13] Research is also needed to define the role of community health nurses in health-care delivery and to support their inclusion in policy decisions.[14]

DEVELOPING A POWER BASE

Power generates influence, and community health nurses who wish to influence health-care policy need to develop a power base from which to do so. ***Power*** is the ability to influence the conduct of others without having one's own behavior modified. A ***power base*** is the resources that allow one person to influence another. Several strategies can be used to enhance one's power base. These include coalition building, bargaining, posturing, and increasing visibility.[15]

In coalition building, individuals or groups with common interests form a temporary alliance to work toward a common goal. The recent efforts of 18 major nursing organizations—including the American Nurses' Association, American Association of Colleges of Nursing, National League for Nursing, and others—to present a nursing proposal for a national health-care plan is an example of coalition building.

Bargaining, or trade-off, is another means of building a power base. In this strategy, individuals or groups relinquish something they want or provide something desired by another group, thus creating a mutual debt. For example, nursing might agree to support a policy direction favored by the American Medical Association in return for support of a nurse-sponsored initiative.

TABLE 12–2. STRATEGIES FOR DEVELOPING A POLITICAL POWER BASE

Strategy	Description of Strategy
Coalition building	Creating a temporary alliance among individuals or groups in order to work toward common goals
Bargaining	Trading or giving up something desired by another individual or group in return for support for one's own position
Posturing	Asking for more than one expects to get, with a subsequent retreat to a predetermined position
Increasing visibility	Purposefully engaging in activities that draw attention to an issue and to one's position on the issue

In posturing or bluffing, the individual or group who wishes to build a power base asks for more than one could really expect to get, and then falls back to a predetermined position beyond which the individual or group will not retreat. This is a tactic frequently employed in contract negotiations.

Increased visibility is achieved when individuals or groups purposefully engage in activities that place them in positions where they will be noticed for the right reasons. For example, when nurses choose to go on strike, reasons presented to the media usually deal with client-centered issues that gain public support and increase nursing's power and ability to influence policymakers. Strategies for developing a power base are summarized in Table 12–2.

CREATING SUPPORT

The last consideration in attempts to influence health-policy decisions is creating support for the policy alternatives supported by community health nurses. Several avenues are available for creating support in a policy situation. These include voting, community organization, campaigning, lobbying, presenting testimony, and holding office.

VOTING

Voting is perhaps the easiest means of influencing health-policy formation at governmental levels. Nurses can themselves vote and motivate others to vote to support policy directions that enhance public health. One vote alone may not seem important, but it may be a key factor in determining the outcome on an important issue. Because lawmakers in the United States are elected, they are susceptible to the power their constituents hold through the ballot box. Thus, voting is a vital component of the political process in which all nurses can participate.

In addition to voting, nurses can educate others regarding the need to vote. Legislative networks among nurses are intended to keep members informed of health-related issues and the need for support or lack of support of certain policy directions. Nurses can also educate the general public on legislative issues that come up for public vote. Finally, nurses can participate in voter registration programs that motivate the general public to exercise their franchise.

COMMUNITY ORGANIZATION

Another means of creating support for policy directions that may be employed by community health nurses is community organization. ***Community organization*** is a process of mobilizing community resources in support of planned change within the community. It consists of a systematic process of assessment, analysis, and planning, conducted within the context of the political process.[16] Steps in the community organization process include establishing legitimacy, defining the problem to be addressed, assessing and analyzing the problem, selecting goals, planning to obtain these goals, marketing, and evaluation.

Members of the community are involved in each step of the process and provide the motivating force behind the movement. The first step, however, is probably the most critical in creating support for health policy. Legitimizing the project requires development of authority to act. This may involve requesting officials to create a special task force to address a problem or including government officials in the planning body of the community organization structure.[16] Subsequent steps of the community organization process are similar to those of the nursing process and need not be reiterated here. It should be remembered, however, that the steps are carried out by members of the community rather than by the nurse.

Community organization can create a mechanism to influence policymakers in several of the ways discussed earlier in this chapter. Community groups can generate and evaluate policy alternatives and can collect data for presentation to policymakers. In addition, the organization provides avenues to educate voters and motivate their participation in policy decisions affected by voting.

CAMPAIGNING

Campaigning is a process designed to influence the public to vote in a particular way on an issue or a candidate. In campaigning, an issue or candidate is presented in a favorable light with the intent of influencing voters. Campaigning can be implemented via media presentations, group meetings or rallies, or in face-to-face contacts with the public.

Campaigning with respect to an issue involves presenting information related to the issue that persuades people to support nursing's position. Campaigning for a specific candidate can help ensure that policymakers who support nursing's position on important issues are elected. Campaigning for a candidate also creates a debt on the part of an elected official that may result in future support for a position promoted by community health nurses.

Much of the work of political action committees (PACs) is designed to support the candidacy of specific individuals. The American Nurses' Association Political Action Committee (ANA-PAC) was created in response to nursing's perceived lack of influence in the formulation of health policy. The purpose of ANA-PAC is to promote constructive national health-care legislation through the political "electioneering" process. ***Electioneering*** is the active process of endorsing candidates and contributing time and money to their campaigns. ANA-PAC and similar political action committees supported by nurses seek to enhance the political influence of nurses by supporting the election of candidates who back the profession and its position on significant health-related issues.

LOBBYING

Lobbying is a concerted effort to influence legislators to take certain positions on prospective bills, and it is another means of creating support for policies promoted by community health nurses. Individuals may engage in lobbying on their own initiative. Groups of people with common interests may also engage in organized lobbying efforts. For example, health-related organizations, such as the American Public Health Association, and professional organizations, like the American Nurses's Association, the American Medical Association, and others, employ paid lobbyists at both federal and state levels. The function of these lobbyists is to acquaint legislators with the position of the organization on a particular issue and to attempt to persuade them to back that position.

Individuals who engage in lobbying do so by contacting a legislator and making their position on an

TABLE 12-3. LOBBYING TECHNIQUES

Do	Don't
• Become familiar with the legislative process	• Make threats about loss of votes
• Become familiar with legislators	• Make promises that cannot be kept
• Know the issues	• Pretend to have influence
• Know your lobbying power	• Repeat the message too frequently
• Work through your own representatives	

issue known. It is not sufficient to acquaint a legislator with one's position, however. That position must be supported by data that will persuade the legislator to adopt a similar position. Whether lobbying is done by individuals acting on their own or at the instigation of organized groups, there are some strategies that can influence the effectiveness of lobbying. These strategies, as well as approaches to be avoided, are summarized in Table 12–3.

It is important for community health nurses who wish to influence legislators to know both the legislative process and the legislators involved. Legislators can be observed and their statements studied to provide information on their positions on issues influencing community health. Their voting records on significant issues can also be examined.

Once legislators' positions are known, they and their staff can be contacted to establish influential interpersonal relationships. Personal contacts through visits followed by telephone calls and follow-up letters or telegrams have been found to be effective means of influencing lawmakers. The point is made by some observers that one should not focus exclusively on legislators from one's own political party, but should contact members of both parties.[2] Legislators who support one's position can be encouraged in that support, while those who do not may be persuaded to change their position.

In addition to knowing a legislator's position on specific issues, nurses should be aware of which legislators serve on committees that deal with health-care issues. These legislators, along with one's own elected representatives, are appropriate targets for lobbying efforts. Knowledge of the legislative structure and committee assignments can assist nurses to target lobbying efforts in areas where they will be most effective.

Community health nurses also need to be conversant with the issues that they are addressing and with arguments on both sides of particular issues. Research related to health-policy issues can be presented to lawmakers and can be persuasive in promoting their support of a position. In discussing an issue, one should acknowledge the nature, source, and extent of possible opposition to one's position and should present the legislator with brief, factual, and documentable data related to the issue. It is usually preferable to provide legislators or their staff members with this data in written form and to include documentation. Some sources of information on policy issues of interest to community health nurses can be found in Table 12–1.

Generally speaking, individuals who lobby on their own should focus their efforts on legislators elected from their own districts. Legislators are usually more inclined to listen to constituents than to nonconstituents. Nurses can, however, network with each other so that several legislators are contacted by their own constituents regarding nursing's position on an issue.

Approaches to legislators that should be avoided when trying to exert influence include making threats regarding loss of voter support and making promises of support; pretending to have influence; repeating one's message too frequently; and demanding a commitment from a legislator before an issue has been completely explored. Such tactics can result in a loss of credibility and decrease one's ability to influence a legislator's behavior.

PRESENTING TESTIMONY

Policymakers sometimes hold public hearings or meetings to gather background information on an issue before attempting to draft legislative proposals or regulations. On occasion, such meetings are held by legislative subcommittees to explore the potential impact of a proposed piece of legislation. Writing and presenting testimony in a public hearing is another method community health nurses can use to influence policymakers.

Testimony presented by community health nurses should specifically address the issue in question and be brief, factual, and well documented. Legislative representatives are not health-care providers, so testimony given by a community health nurse needs to avoid medical jargon and be clearly understandable. A copy of the nurse's testimony should be given to the legislative representatives and staff either immediately preceding or at the time of the hearing. Documentation of sources of data permits later verification by the legislator or his or her staff.

HOLDING OFFICE

A final means of creating support for policy directions promoted by community health nurses is to become

BOX 12–1

Considerations Related to Influencing Health-Policy Formation

Education
- Educate community health nurses regarding the political process
- Educate policymakers regarding the health needs of the public

Setting an agenda
- Decide on a direction to be taken in health-policy formation

Defining and evaluating choices
- Identify alternative directions for health policy
- Evaluate advantages and disadvantages of health-policy alternatives

Obtaining data
- Conduct research related to policy formation
- Collect data related to specific policy issues

Developing a power base
- Create a power base from which to influence health-policy decisions

Creating support
- Develop and implement strategies to mobilize support for a proposed policy

a policymaker oneself. This may involve running for elective office or being appointed to a specific position. In either case, the community health nurse must first become politically active in some of the other ways described in this chapter to be sufficiently well known to be elected or appointed to a policy-making position.

One may also work in the background in policymaking by becoming a legislative staff person or a lobbyist for an organized group.[3] Again, such positions require familiarity with the political process and well-developed interpersonal relationships with legislators and other policymakers. Strategies for creating support for a policy position are summarized in Table 12–4, while considerations related to influencing health-policy formation and implementation are presented in Box 12–1.

TABLE 12–4. STRATEGIES FOR CREATING SUPPORT FOR A PROPOSED POLICY

Strategy	Description of Strategy
Voting	Exercising one's personal right to vote, encouraging others to vote, participating in voter registration drives
Community organization	Mobilizing community resources in favor of planned change or a proposed policy; establishing the legitimacy of the organization; defining the issue; assessing and analyzing the issue; selecting goals; planning to reach goals; marketing; evaluating effort
Campaigning	Providing endorsements or monetary support for specific policy proposals or candidates with the intent of influencing voters' responses
Lobbying	Engaging in personal communications with policymakers in an attempt to influence their actions in policy decisions
Presenting testimony	Providing information on an issue to policymakers at a public hearing
Holding office	Assuming a position as a policymaker by virtue of election or appointment to a specific office

THE EPIDEMIOLOGIC PREVENTION PROCESS MODEL AND THE POLITICAL PROCESS

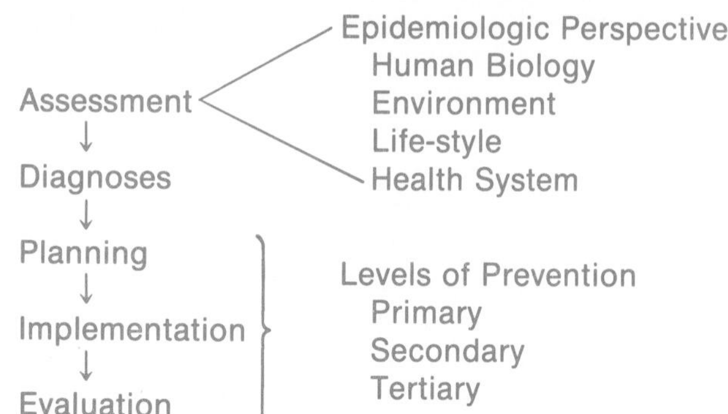

The epidemiologic prevention process model can be used to direct community health nurses' involvement in public-health-policy formation at all levels of society. Community health nurses working in specific organizations can assess the influence of institutional policies on the health of members of the organization.

They can also adapt strategies for policy formation to plan, implement, and evaluate programs that enhance rather than undermine health. In a similar fashion, community health nurses can use the epidemiologic prevention process model to assess and influence health-care policies at the local, state, and federal level.

ASSESSMENT IN HEALTH-POLICY FORMATION

Assessment of the health status of a community or population group may reveal the need for health policies. In addition, assessment may indicate areas in which existing policies impede achievement of the goals of public health.[17]

Once a need for health policy has been identified, the community health nurse can examine the situation in terms of the components of Dever's epidemiologic perspective for factors that influence the direction that policy should take. For example, recent human biological data indicate that a growing portion of the homeless population is comprised of young children, so policies dealing with the problem of homelessness will need to address the needs of this age group.

Other biological factors can also influence a given policy situation. If we use the homeless as our example, information on the types of health problems common in this population will influence the direction that policies should take. For instance, provision should be made for tuberculosis control and prevention of foot problems, two types of health problems frequently encountered among the homeless.[18,19]

Environmental factors can also affect policy formation. Again, using the homeless as our example, weather conditions in the Northeast make policies for this population a more critical issue than might be the case elsewhere, while the milder climate of the southwestern United States may encourage homeless individuals to migrate to these areas, thus compounding the problem of homelessness.

Factors in both the psychological and social environments also affect policy formation related to homeless populations. Because mental illness is prevalent among this group, issues of treatment must be addressed in any effective policy related to the homeless. Social factors such as unemployment and the lack of affordable housing will also need to be addressed if a policy for the homeless is to meet their needs on a long-term basis.

Life-style issues related to nutrition and sleep patterns as well as occupation and other consumption patterns affect policies designed to meet the needs of a homeless population. Policy development will have to consider avenues for feeding the hungry and for creating employment opportunities that permit the homeless person to afford housing.

Finally, health system factors influence the ability of homeless persons to receive necessary health care. Lack of access to care and appointment schedules that rely on possession of a timepiece are some of the factors that impede adequate health care for the homeless. Policy needs related specifically to the homeless population will be addressed in more detail in Chapter 24, Care of Homeless Clients.

DIAGNOSTIC REASONING IN HEALTH-POLICY FORMATION

Based on the outcome of his or her assessment, the community health nurse might arrive at diagnoses of the need for health-care policies to address issues raised. An example of such a diagnosis related to the homeless might be "need for a policy to address provision of health care for homeless individuals due to large numbers of the homeless and lack of present access to health care in this population." Another diagnosis might be a "need for special programs to house homeless women with children due to growing numbers in this population and their increased vulnerability to victimization."

PLANNING HEALTH POLICY

The community health nurse might then proceed to initiate or participate in plans to develop appropriate health policies. Planning policies to meet the needs of the homeless population might include primary, secondary, or tertiary preventive measures. For example, the local health department might suspend its fee policy for immunizations for homeless children in the state or the state Medicaid program might adopt a policy authorizing Medicaid benefits for homeless individuals without the proof of residence usually required for eligibility. Or, action might be taken to develop a policy creating jobs for homeless individuals within the local government and business community to enable them to become self-supporting and to prevent recurrent homelessness.

Whatever the level of prevention involved in planning health-care policies, the community health nurse will consider certain criteria that are characteristic of effective policies. These criteria include the adequacy of a proposed policy in meeting the health needs of the public, safeguards for the rights of individuals, equitable allocation of resources, and the capacity for implementation. The second and third criteria reflect ethical considerations that will be addressed in greater detail in Chapter 14, Ethical Influences on Community Health.

ADEQUACY FOR HEALTH NEEDS

Health policies must be developed that effectively address the health needs of the affected population. For example, a local government policy allowing homeless persons to sleep in city-owned buildings only addresses one small part of the plight of the homeless population. In this case, a more comprehensive policy that addresses both short-term and long-term solutions to the problems of homelessness is needed.

SAFEGUARDING INDIVIDUAL RIGHTS

Safeguarding individual rights is another criterion for sound health-care policy development. As an example, a policy that would require homeless individuals to surrender personal belongings to meet communal needs when admitted to a shelter would violate their property rights. There are circumstances, however, in which the good of society supersedes individual rights. For example, homeless persons may be prohibited from smoking in a shelter to prevent exposure of others to smoke or to prevent a fire. Whenever possible, though, health policies should be written in such a way that they do not violate the rights of individuals affected by them.

PROMOTING EQUITABLE ALLOCATION OF RESOURCES

Health policies should also promote equitable distribution of health-care resources. This means that policies should not discriminate against certain subgroups within the population. For example, open housing policies in homeless shelters may inadvertently discriminate against women and children who may be subjected to force to give way to adult males who desire shelter. Sex-segregated shelters that ensure access for both males and females provide for a more equitable allocation of resources.

CAPACITY FOR IMPLEMENTATION

For a specific health policy to be effective in promoting health or preventing illness, it must be capable of being implemented or enforced. For example, a local government might adopt a policy encouraging houses of worship to provide overnight shelter for homeless individuals. But, unless they are willing to cooperate, the policy cannot be implemented.

Community health nurses planning to influence health-policy formation should assess proposed policies or modifications of existing policies in light of these four criteria. Policies that do not meet the criteria should be redesigned, if possible, before they are presented to policymakers. If a proposed policy continues not to meet one or more criteria, its supporters should be prepared to justify the need for the policy. For example, nurses should be prepared to convince policymakers that a smoking ban in shelters for the homeless is warranted despite the violation of the individual's personal freedom of choice.

IMPLEMENTING HEALTH POLICY

Implementing planned policies often involves mobilization of support for the policy as well as actually putting the policy into operation. Community health nurses who desire to influence policy decisions should identify groups within the population who are likely to support the proposed policy. They should then develop specific strategies to elicit that support. These strategies may include educating the general public regarding the issues and proposed policy, or contacting health-related agencies and soliciting their support. Other community groups are also a source of support for policies that affect them directly or indirectly. In the case of programs related to care of the homeless, support might be derived from area churches, synagogues, etc., or business people on whose doorsteps homeless individuals are sleeping. Concerned health-care providers and educational institutions might also be sources of support for implementing health policies related to the homeless population.

EVALUATING HEALTH POLICY

In the evaluation phase of health-policy formation, the community health nurse might be actively involved in assessing the effects of health policies on meeting the needs of the particular target group, in this case, the homeless population. Community health nurses could assist in collecting data related to the outcomes of programs put into operation. For example, data might be gathered on the incidence of specific health problems among the homeless to evaluate the effects of policies designed to promote primary and secondary prevention. In addition, information could be collected regarding the number of persons who continue to be homeless despite assistance from established programs.

Finally, community health nurses would evaluate the effectiveness of the strategies used in policy development. For example, were insufficient funds allocated to implement established programs? Were nurses successful in motivating policymakers to address the problem of homelessness in a comprehensive fashion, or did the policies developed only deal with portions of the problem? The answers to these and similar questions can guide community health nurses' future efforts at influencing policy decisions not only on the issue of homelessness but the entire gamut of health-related issues.

CHAPTER HIGHLIGHTS

- Early community health nurses were adept at influencing health-related policy decisions. More recently, nurses, including community health nurses, have become less influential.
- The political process includes all of the activities that result in the formation of policy.
- Policy is the aggregate of principles directing the distribution of resources among the population, whereas policy-making is the process of synthesizing these principles and underlying values, interests, and concerns in response to identified problems.
- Health policy is a defined set of principles used to guide activities to safeguard and promote the health of the public. Public health policy is the way society allocates and distributes political and economic resources to meet the health needs of the public.
- Health policy is made at institutional or agency levels as well as at the level of local, state, and federal governments.
- Currently there is no single coherent health policy at the national level. The lack of a national health policy is, in part, due to lack of constitutional responsibility for health matters and to the diversity of health needs in different segments of the population. This lack of an overriding health policy has contributed to sporadic and poorly coordinated health-care efforts at the federal level.
- Health policy must be formed in light of other societal needs and cannot automatically supersede other needs for policy.
- Laws are public-policy decisions generated by the legislative branch of government. At the federal level the legislative process begins with the presentation of a need for policy, or a legislative proposal, to a lawmaker. This need is drafted into a policy statement, called a bill, which is sponsored by a legislator.
- After a general review, proposed legislation is sent to the House or Senate floor for its first "reading," which consists of a reference to the bill by number and title. The bill is usually then sent to the appropriate subcommittee for review, at which point it may be killed or sent for a second reading with or without modification.
- After its second reading, a bill may progress to the third and final reading, be referred back to the original committee, or be forwarded to another committee for review and potential revision. After the third reading, the bill is placed on the calendar for debate and vote. Bills that are passed are sent to the other chamber of the legislature for approval.
- Disagreement between the two chambers on proposed legislation is usually resolved in a joint conference committee. The revised bill is then returned for a vote in both chambers. After being signed by the leader of each legislative body, the bill is sent to the chief executive officer (governor or president) for signature. The bill may be signed or vetoed at this point.
- The legislature can decide to override an executive veto, usually by at least a two-thirds majority vote.
- Once a piece of legislation has been passed, it is forwarded to the appropriate agency for implementation. Implementation usually involves development of specific regulations. Community health nurses can have input into both the regulatory and the legislative process.
- Considerations in influencing health-policy formation include educating community health nurses for political activity and educating policymakers, setting a health-policy agenda, defining and evaluating policy choices, obtaining data, developing a power base, and creating support for a proposed policy.
- Strategies for developing a power base include coalition building, bargaining, posturing, and increasing visibility.
- Strategies for creating support for a proposed policy include voting, community organization, campaigning, lobbying, presenting testimony, and holding office.
- The epidemiologic prevention process model can be used to direct community health nurses' involvement in the political process. The nurse assesses the policy situation in terms of Dever's epidemiologic perspective, develops nursing diagnoses, and participates in planning, implementing, and evaluating health policies.
- Four criteria used in developing effective health-care policy are the adequacy of a policy for meeting the health needs of the targeted population, safeguarding individual rights, promoting equitable allocation of resources, and the policy's capacity for implementation.

Review Questions

1. Identify at least three levels at which health-policy formation takes place. (p. 221)
2. List and describe at least five considerations in influencing health-policy formation. Give an example of the influence of each on the participation of community health nurses in policy formation. (p. 228)
3. Identify four strategies for developing a power base for exercising political influence. Give an example of the use of each strategy. (p. 229)
4. Describe at least four approaches in creating support for a proposed health policy. (p. 229)
5. Outline the legislative process at the state and federal levels. Identify points at which community health nurses could influence the process. (p. 223)
6. Describe the regulatory process. How might community health nurses influence this process? (p. 227)
7. Identify four criteria for evaluating a proposed health policy. (p. 233)

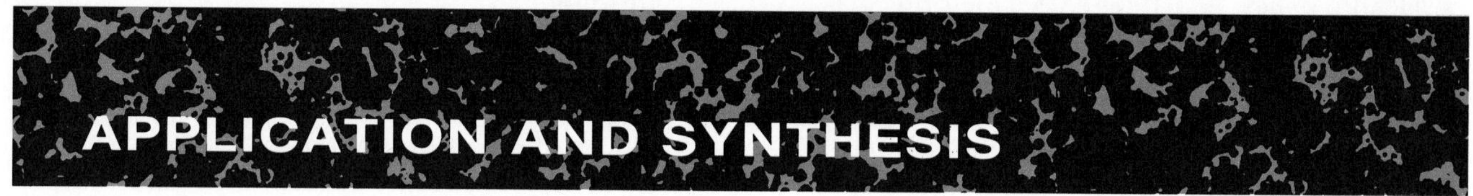

APPLICATION AND SYNTHESIS

Nurses in a southern state were concerned about the high incidence of motor vehicle fatalities in children under the age of 4. The state involved was largely rural with poorly maintained roads, and many accidents occurred in outlying regions or in crowded inner-city areas. Fatalities were particularly prevalent among low-income blacks in the cities, and among low-income whites and blacks in the rural areas. Few families had child-safety seats in their cars, and few adults used seat belts themselves. Many autos, especially in rural areas, were older models that did not even have seat belts. The state's population was about evenly divided between blacks and whites, and the educational levels in both groups were well below those of the rest of the nation.

The state nurses' association, in conjunction with the state Fraternal Order of Police, approached a newly elected state assemblyman who was willing to sponsor a bill requiring the use of approved car-seat restraints for all children under the age of 4. Both organizations mobilized their memberships in support of the bill. The state nurses' association represented approximately 10 percent of RNs licensed in the state, whereas the Fraternal Order of Police represented nearly 85 percent of the state's police officers. Neither of the two organizations approached members of the committees that would be reviewing the bill to enlist their support. Very little effort was made to educate the general public regarding the issue. Prior to their involvement in this cause, neither organization had been very active politically.

The bill was soundly defeated in the legislature. Some of the reasons given by various legislators for voting against the bill included beliefs that use of a child-safety seat is a parental, rather than a governmental, decision, beliefs that government already regulated too much of people's lives, concerns about the difficulties and costs of enforcing such legislation, and concerns about the cost of car seats for many poor families in the state.

1. What were the human biological, environmental, life-style, and health system factors operating in this situation?
2. What are some of the reasons why the nurses and police officers were ineffective in influencing policy formation in this situation?
3. In what ways did the proposed policy meet or fail to meet the criteria for effective health policy?
4. How might the nurses and police officers have developed a stronger power base to influence legislation?
5. What strategies could have been used to bring about a more positive outcome in this situation?

REFERENCES

1. White, M. S. (1982). Construct for public health nursing. *Nursing Outlook, 30,* 527–530.
2. Pearson, B. J. (1987). Judi Buckalew: Learning to play political hardball. *Nurse Practitioner, 12*(1), 49–54.
3. Stimpson, M., & Hanley, B. (1991). Nurse policy analyst: Advanced practice role. *Nursing & Health Care, 12*(1), 10–15.
4. Andreoli, K. G., Musser, L. A., & Otto, D. A. (1987). Health policy in nursing curricula. *Journal of Nursing Education, 26,* 239–243.
5. Hinshaw, A. S. (1988). Using research to shape health policy. *Nursing Outlook, 36,* 21–24.
6. Sharp, N., Biggs, S., & Wakefield, M. (1991). Public policy: New opportunity for nursing. *Nursing & Health Care, 12*(1), 16–23.
7. Hanley, B. (1987). Political participation: How do nurses compare with other professional women? *Nursing Economics, 5*(4), 179–188.
8. Miller, C. A. (1987). Child health. In S. Levine & A. M. Lilienfeld (Eds.), *Epidemiology and health policy* (pp. 15–54). New York: Tavistock.
9. Quade, E. S. (1982). *Analysis for public decisions* (2nd ed.). New York: North Hall.
10. Milio, N. (1981). *Promoting health through public policy.* Philadelphia: F. A. Davis.
11. Fein, R. (1980). Social and economic attitudes shaping American health policy. *Milbank Memorial Fund Quarterly/Health and Society, 58,* 349–385.
12. National League for Nursing. (1991, March). *Public Policy Bulletin.* New York: National League for Nursing.
13. Raudonis, B. M., & Griffith, H. (1991). Model for integrating health services research and health care policy formation. *Nursing & Health Care, 12*(1), 32–36.
14. Smith, G. R. (1989). Using the public agenda to shape PHN practice. *Nursing Outlook, 37,* 72–75.
15. Del Bueno, D. J. (1986). Power and politics in organizations. *Nursing Outlook, 34,* 124–128.
16. Courtney, R. (1987). Community practice: Nursing influence on policy formation. *Nursing Outlook, 35,* 170–173.
17. McCreight, L. (1989). The future of public health. *Nursing Outlook, 37,* 219–225.
18. Bowdler, J. E. (1989). Health problems of the homeless in America. *Nurse Practitioner, 14*(7), 44–51.
19. Wlodarczyk, D., & Prentice, R. (1988). Health issues of homeless persons. *Western Journal of Medicine, 148,* 717–719.

RECOMMENDED READINGS

Bagwell, M., & Clements, S. (1985). *A political handbook for health professionals.* Boston: Little, Brown.

Describes the political process in relation to health legislation and discusses strategies for influencing the process. Also addresses means to increase the political influence of health professionals.

Bradham, D. D. (1983). Health policy formation and analysis. *Nursing Economics, 1*(4), 47–50.

Discusses the processes of health policy formation and policy analysis.

Goldwater, M., & Zusy, M. L. (1990). *Prescription for nurses: Effective political action.* St. Louis: C. V. Mosby.

Provides guidelines for action by nurses who desire to influence the development of health-care policy.

Gorman, S., & Clark, N. (1986). Power and effective nursing practice. *Nursing Outlook, 34,* 129–134.

Presents the results of the Nursing Knowledge Project designed to evaluate the effect of specialized training on nurses' abilities to increase their power and influence in the clinical setting.

Williams, C. (1983). Making things happen: Community health nursing and the policy arena. *Nursing Outlook, 31,* 225–228.

Discusses the need for community health nursing involvement in health-policy formation.

UNIT THREE

Influences on Community Health

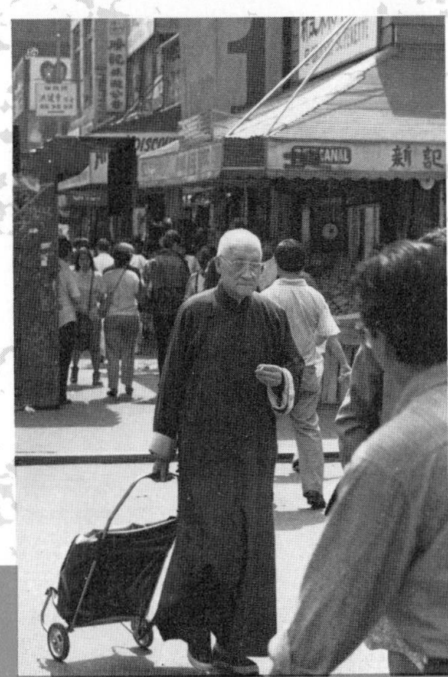

The health of the population is influenced both by societal factors and by individual behavior. Societal factors include economic, ethical, cultural, and physical environmental influences on health. Because community health nurses are concerned with any factor that may affect clients' health, the influences of these factors may need to be addressed through community health nursing interventions.

Economic factors influence the health of the public by affecting clients' access to the goods and services needed to promote, maintain, and restore health. Economic factors, for instance, may affect a family's ability to purchase nutritious food or adequate housing, or influence a community's ability to provide necessary services related to health, sanitation, and protection. Economic factors also influence the abilities of individuals, families, and communities to obtain needed health care.

Two current economic concerns for community health nurses are the high cost of health care and diminished access to care for some segments of the population. Chapter 13, Economic Influences on Community Health, examines these two concerns, explores mechanisms for financing health care, and discusses the role of the community health nurse in dealing with economic factors.

Ethical influences within society also influence the health of the population. These effects are felt by individuals and their families and by communities and other groups. For example, decisions may be needed about the care of a child with a life-threatening illness whose parents refuse medical assistance or about the use of technology to prolong life in a terminally ill elderly client. These and similar decisions at the individual and family level are made in all areas of nursing. In community health nursing, however, ethical decisions are also required at the group or aggregate level. Group decisions may be related to the allocation of scarce resources among primary, secondary, and tertiary preventive measures. Similar decisions might include whether mandatory seat belt use or prohibiting smoking in public places is ethical. Ethical decisions regarding the health of groups of people are the focus of Chapter 14, Ethical Influences on Community Health.

Culture guides and directs behavior, including health-related behaviors. Because community health nursing practice is directed toward promoting healthful behaviors among members of the population, community health nurses must understand the cultural basis for behavior. In Chapter 15, Cultural Influences on Community Health, readers are provided with an understanding of the basic premises of culture and are acquainted with the health-related effects of five subcultures found in the United States. The subcultures addressed are those of the Native American, Asian, black, Latino, and Appalachian populations. While there are many other cultural groups present in the United States, these subcultures have been selected because they are found throughout the country and are the groups most likely to be encountered by the majority of community health nurses.

Health is also influenced by the physical environment in which we live. In recent years there has been growing concern for the declining quality of the environment and for its adverse effects on health. Areas of particular concern are air and water pollution, exposure to radiation, noise pollution, and solid-waste disposal. Environmental conditions affect health both directly, as in the case of mercury poisoning through water pollution, and indirectly by decreasing the aesthetic quality of the environment and contributing to stress. Community health nurses can intervene to control the effects of environmental influences not only on individuals and families but also on groups of people. For example, a community health nurse may educate families on the appropriate disposal of hazardous wastes or on preventing lead poisoning in areas with high environmental concentrations of lead. At the aggregate level, political action and leadership in policymaking may reduce air and water pollution or prevent the effects of noise on health.

An understanding of economic, ethical, cultural, and environmental influences on health prepares community health nurses to intervene to meet clients' health needs by modifying factors contributing to those needs. This knowledge also enables community health nurses to identify and deal effectively with the health needs of the special target populations discussed in Unit Four, Care of Clients.

From the Community: A Nurse's Voice

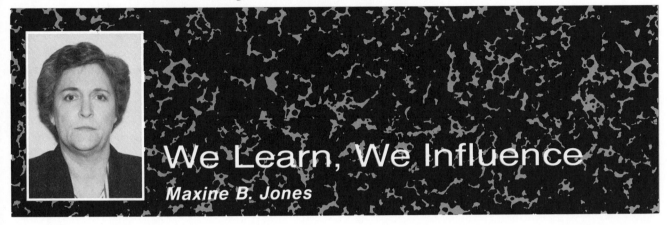

We Learn, We Influence

Maxine B. Jones

You might say that I entered community health nursing practice in an unusual manner; my educational preparation is adult health nursing. But I kept hearing my colleagues talking about how exciting, stimulating, and personally challenging community health nursing is, so I decided to investigate for myself. I liked what I found, and I engaged in postdoctoral study and clinical training for community health practice.

Because I am employed as a teacher in a collegiate school of nursing, I established a clinical rotation for my students in a local church that provides kitchen services for homeless persons. This community setting allows my students and me to work in a safe, structured environment with several at-risk population groups such as the homeless and the elderly, as well as with mentally ill and mentally retarded individuals who live in group homes within the surrounding neighborhood.

As a consequence, my students and I have learned a great deal about the needs and illnesses that are common among at-risk populations. But we've learned so much more! We've learned about human nature, about the value of maintaining supportive relationships with family and friends, about the pride and sensitivity of impoverished persons. Sometimes what we learned from clients was their gift to us, because their wisdom was the only thing they had to share. I was once cautioned, for instance, by two homeless brothers to carry a water bottle with me if I ever hitched a ride on a freight train so that I wouldn't hurt myself by jumping off the rapidly moving train to search for water.

Moreover, my students and I have learned how we as nurses can positively influence the health of the community we serve. We've learned to form coalitions with city agencies to provide systematic, effective health care to individuals who have almost no financial or health-care resources. We have seen the value of our health-care screening efforts in which hypertensive persons are identified and referred for early treatment, preventing cerebral vascular accidents and saving thousands of health-care dollars. We've helped mentally retarded people obtain early diagnosis and treatment for adult-onset diabetes. By persevering in devising ways to instruct these clients, despite their limited learning ability, we helped them to control their condition through diet alone.

Over time, my students and I have come to appreciate the truth of that old adage, "An ounce of prevention is worth a pound of cure." As community health nurses we learn from our clients, and in doing so we influence our community for the better.

CHAPTER 13

Economic Influences on Community Health

KEY TERMS

diagnosis-related groupings (DRGs)
economics
gross national product (GNP)
health maintenance organization (HMO)
preferred provider organization (PPO)
prospective reimbursement
retrospective reimbursement
utilization review

Economic factors influence the health of individuals, families, and groups, or communities. For individuals and their families, economic factors affect the ability to provide necessities like food and shelter. One's income also influences the ability to obtain health care. The general economic climate further influences health at the aggregate level, although this influence may be somewhat more indirect. For example, a declining economy contributes to high levels of unemployment. Unemployment, in turn, leads to reduced income for individuals and families and a reduced tax-base to finance government-supported health and welfare programs, both of which may result in inability to provide necessities, including health-care services. In addition, unemployment is usually accompanied by loss of employer-provided health insurance benefits, further reducing access to health care for certain segments of the population. Finally, economic factors that contribute to inflation affect the price of goods and services, including health services, further impairing the ability of the public to obtain necessities and health care. Some of the relationships between economic factors and health are depicted in Figure 13–1.

Relationships between economic factors and health are of concern to community health nurses because they influence the health of the individuals, families, and communities with which community health nurses work. While community health nurses cannot significantly influence the overall economic climate, they can modify the effects of that climate at both the individual/family level and the community level. At the level of individuals and their families, for example, the nurse can assist clients to budget their economic resources effectively or make referrals to financial assistance programs. At the community level, the community health nurse can use the change, leadership, and political processes discussed in previous chapters to influence policies related to economic issues, particularly those related to funding for health-care services. To do so, however, community health nurses must have some understanding of both current and proposed mechanisms for financing health-care services.

LEARNING OBJECTIVES

After reading this chapter you should be able to:

- Describe at least three relationships between economic conditions and health status.
- Identify two economic issues of particular concern to community health nurses.
- Differentiate between retrospective and prospective reimbursement.
- Identify three forms of publicly funded health insurance.
- Differentiate between per case and per capita prospective reimbursement.
- Identify at least four components of nursing's 1991 proposal for a national health-care plan.
- Describe at least three considerations in planning for a national health-care program.
- Describe at least three considerations in evaluating a national health-care plan.

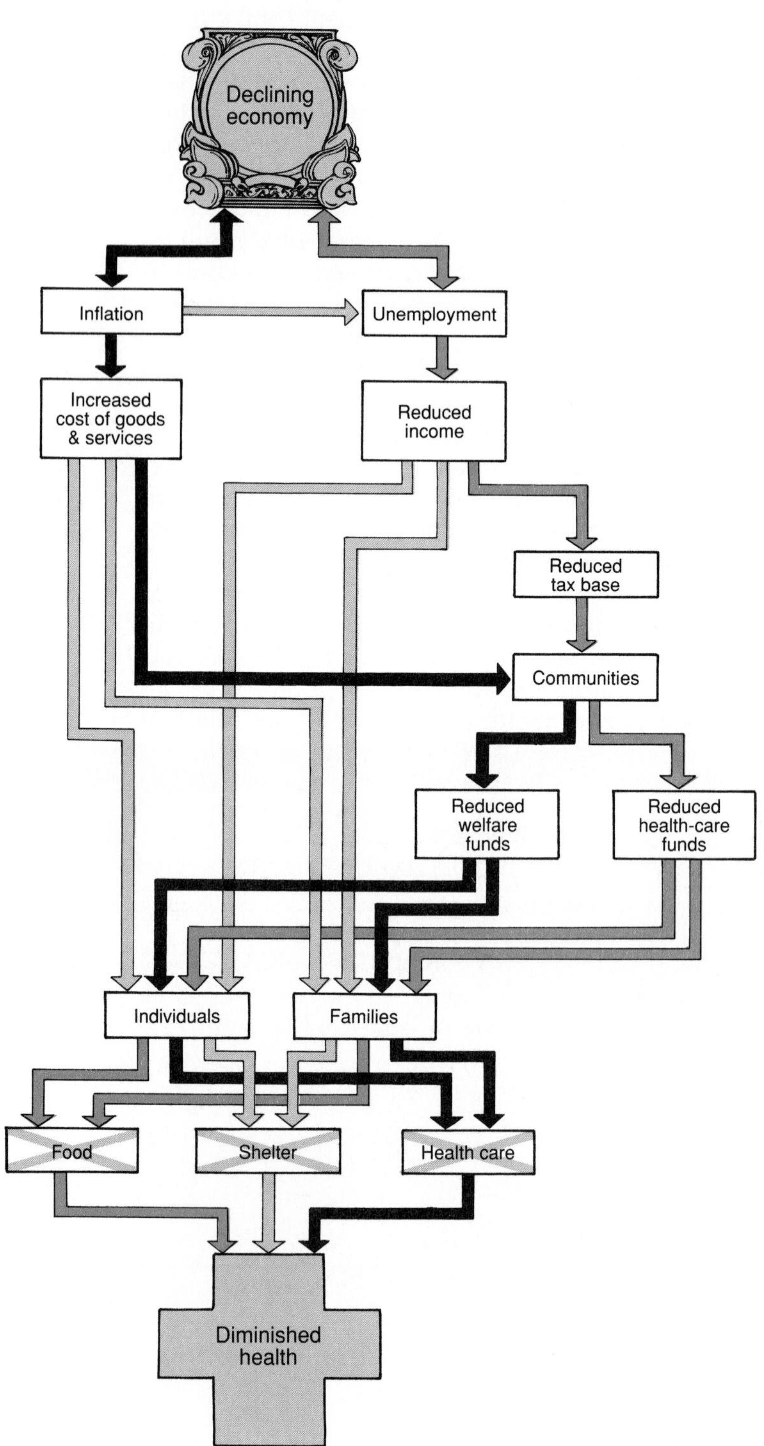

Figure 13–1. The relationship of selected economic factors to health.

ECONOMIC CONCERNS FOR COMMUNITY HEALTH NURSES

Economics is the science that addresses the production, distribution, and consumption of goods and services. A full discussion of economic principles is beyond the scope of this book, but within the area of economics as it relates to health are two major areas of concern for community health nurses. The first of these is the increasing cost of health care, while the second is decreased access to care brought about both by rising costs and by reduced income experienced by some segments of the population.

RISING HEALTH-CARE COSTS

Health-care costs increased by more than 300 percent in the 10 years from 1970 to 1980,[1] and costs continue to rise at an alarming rate. In 1985, for example, health care in the United States cost $425 billion and accounted for 10.7 percent of the gross national product (GNP).[2] The ***gross national product*** is the total monetary value of all goods and services produced by a nation during a specified period of time (usually a year).[3] In only 1 year, expenditures for health care had increased to $458 billion,[4] and by 1989, health-care costs had risen to $500 billion, or 11.1 percent of the GNP.[5] It is expected that the annual cost of health care in the United States will consume 13 percent of the GNP by 1995,[6] and will rise to $1.5 trillion (or 15 percent of the GNP) by the year 2000.[7] These projections translate to an increase in health-care spending from $1837 per person in 1986 to over $2000 in 1988[8] and $5500 per person by 2000.[4] At present, it is estimated that approximately $1 billion is spent each day on health care in the U.S.[9,10]

In spite of the tremendous amount of money spent on health care in the United States, the health status of the American public is not appreciably better, and in some cases is actually worse, than that of countries that spend far less.[7,9] For example, in 1986 Canada spent 8.5 percent of its GNP for health care and the United Kingdom spent 6.2 percent, while the United States expended 11.1 percent of GNP on health care. Both Canada and the United Kingdom have longevity and mortality rates comparable to those of the United States.[11] In terms of infant mortality, the United States ranks 18th, with higher infant mortality rates than those of such underdeveloped nations as Cuba, Greece, Singapore, and Hong Kong.[2]

Many reasons account for the high cost of health care in the United States. One reason, the use of advanced medical technology, has multiple effects that contribute to higher costs for health care. Advanced medical technology has saved many lives that might otherwise have been lost. These same technologies, however, have contributed to growing numbers of elderly and chronically ill people who require ongoing health-care services.

Both the advanced technology required to save them and the continued care needed by these groups of people increase health-care costs. In 1988, for example, 1647 heart transplants were performed at a cost of $150,000 to $200,000 each. Approximately 80 percent of those receiving heart transplants will survive, and each will require $12,000 in immunosuppressant drugs each year for the rest of their lives. In that same year, 1680 liver transplants were performed, each costing approximately $238,000. Only 65 percent of liver transplant recipients survive, but they will also require ongoing immunosuppression therapy. Kidney transplantation costs approximately $30,000 per person, the same amount required each year for dialysis, another high-tech procedure designed to prolong the lives of those who would otherwise die.[10]

Continued care for growing numbers of elderly people is also costly. For example, for those over age 75, health care accounts for 15 percent of total expenses versus 2.4 percent for those under age 25 and 5.5 percent for those age 55 to 64.[11]

In addition to its initial cost and the cost of maintaining lives saved, high-tech medical equipment tends to have the additional effect of being used more frequently to justify its cost. Consequently, more expensive diagnostic and treatment procedures may be chosen when less expensive ones might be equally effective. Health-care practitioners may also overuse expensive technology in an effort to prevent malpractice suits.[12] For example, obstetricians may be inclined to use cesarean section when a vaginal delivery would be perfectly safe because of the possibility of complications and subsequent lawsuits. Concern over malpractice suits has also contributed to the rise in malpractice insurance costs for health-care providers, further increasing the overall cost of health care.

Another factor in the high cost of health care in the United States is the increase in health insurance premiums, which rose 15–20 percent annually during the 1980s.[7] Health insurance benefits paid by U.S. employers in 1985 averaged 6.5 percent of payrolls.[7] Higher health insurance premiums not only boost the cost of health care but also the cost of business products and services. For example, it is estimated that the cost of employee health insurance benefits adds $300 to $500 to the cost of each auto produced by American car manufacturers.[2]

Increased coverage for medical care, whether by private health insurance companies or by publicly funded programs such as Medicaid and Medicare, has also contributed to escalating health-care costs by creating incentives for overuse. Health-care services have tended to be overused merely because they have become available at minimal cost to consumers and to the profit of health-care providers. In addition, because reimbursement under both public and private programs has often been tied to hospitalization, many clients were hospitalized for services that could have been provided as effectively, and less expensively, in clinics, offices, or clients' homes.

A further cost effect of both public and private health insurance programs has resulted from their focus on cure rather than health promotion or illness prevention. While the Medicaid program does provide some preventive and promotive services, particularly for children and pregnant women, most traditional health insurance plans cover only curative and restorative services. Because the cost of treating many health conditions exceeds the cost of preventing them, this emphasis on secondary prevention contributes to the overall rise in health-care costs. For example, it is estimated that every dollar spent on prenatal care saves over $3 on the care of low birth weight infants.[2] The relative costs of prevention and cure are exemplified in the fact that the amount of money spent by Humana Hospitals on the artificial heart equals the amount needed to completely eradicate smallpox around the world.[9]

Finally, publicly funded health insurance programs such as Medicare and Medicaid have the additional disadvantage of increased administrative costs. The paperwork needed for reimbursement under these programs not only increases the cost of care for the funding agency but also for the health-care provider who hires additional staff to handle the billing and bookkeeping tasks involved.

Another contributing factor in spiralling health-care costs has been recent advances made in salaries and benefits paid to nurses and other salaried health-care personnel. While few nurses would dispute the need for such advances, they have contributed to rapid escalation of health-care costs.

DIMINISHING ACCESS TO CARE

The second economic area of particular concern to community health nurses is decreased access to care among some segments of the population. Rising health-care costs, coupled with low income, have reduced access to care for many Americans.

The effects of escalating costs of health care have resulted in cutbacks in many services provided. In many areas, traditional community health programs that promote health and prevent illness have been reduced or eliminated completely. For example, decreased funds have been available to prevent sexually transmitted diseases such as syphilis because of the increased costs of AIDS prevention (Continuing increase in infectious syphilis, 1988).[13]

There has been an emphasis in community health, as in other areas of health care, on providing services that generate revenues. For example, in some parts of the country, local health departments give preference for well-child care to clients covered by Medicaid (a government program providing medical care for the poor) because the department can be reimbursed for its services by the Medicaid program. This policy effectively limits access to services for clients who are not covered and who cannot afford to seek health care from private providers.

The reverse may be true for clients with Medicaid who seek care for illness. Because of the cumbersome administrative structure of the Medicaid program, reimbursement of providers for services rendered takes some time, prompting some providers to refuse to see these clients. These clients are then forced to seek care in expensive settings such as emergency rooms or to go without care altogether.

Rising costs have also prompted some health departments to institute fees for formerly free services such as immunizations. While many departments set fees on a sliding scale based on clients' income, such fees continue to serve as a deterrent to clients who have no money to pay for health care and do not realize that a sliding scale exists.

Diminished access to care is also the result of lack of health insurance for many American families. From 1980 to 1985 the number of Americans without private health insurance increased by 45 percent; today approximately 37 million people in the United States are uninsured.[2] Of the 18 percent of the total U.S. population who are uninsured, roughly two-thirds have incomes above the poverty level[14] and more than half are employed full-time.[2]

As of 1987, over 13 percent of the U.S. population had incomes below the poverty level and more than 18 percent had incomes below 125 percent of the poverty level, yet only 6 percent of the total population received any form of public aid. In 1986, only 41 percent of those people with incomes below the poverty line were covered by Medicaid. In 1987, the Medicare program (a federal medical and hospital care program for the elderly) enrolled slightly more than 32.4 million Americans.[11] While some of these elderly people and those below the poverty line may be covered by private health insurance plans, there remain a large number of individuals who cannot afford health care and who have no form of health insurance.

For those who receive assistance under Medicare and Medicaid, services have been drastically curtailed in some areas. Eligibility requirements for programs such as Medicaid have been tightened so that fewer people are now eligible. For those individuals with Medicare, co-payments have risen 50 percent faster than their income. All of these facts point to decreased access to needed health care.

Thus it is obvious that current economic mechanisms for funding health care are not adequate to meet the needs of the American population. Community health nurses can be influential in bringing about changes in funding policies, but first they must have some understanding of current and proposed funding mechanisms.

MECHANISMS FOR FINANCING HEALTH CARE

Traditional means of funding health care have been retrospective in nature. ***Retrospective reimbursement*** is payment for services rendered based on the cost of those services. In a retrospective system, the cost of services is determined after the fact. In 1983, the federal government instituted prospective reimbursement for services provided under Medicare. ***Prospective reimbursement*** is payment at a predetermined, fixed rate for a specific health-care program or set of health-care services.

Prospective payment for services provided under the Medicare program is based on client's diagnoses, with set fees for care of clients who fall into specific diagnosis-related groupings (DRGs). ***Diagnosis-related groupings*** are categories of client diagnoses for which typical costs of care have been calculated, based on the cost of specific services required. In the DRG system, providers are paid a set fee based on clients' diagnoses and the typical costs of care for someone with that diagnosis. Prospective reimbursement systems are also a feature of some alternative modes of health-care delivery such as health maintenance organizations (HMOs) and preferred provider organizations (PPOs), both of which will be discussed later in this chapter.

Retrospective reimbursement has the disadvantage of encouraging health-care providers to give services that may not be necessary, merely because they are reimbursable. Under this type of system, the more care provided, the greater the economic gain for the provider. A provider who can be reimbursed for each office visit may be tempted to see a client three times for a particular condition, when two visits would suffice. Or, tests and treatments may be given that are not strictly necessary. For example, a surgeon might suggest a hysterectomy to a woman who has had minor problems with uterine bleeding when other less expensive measures would be equally effective.

Prospective reimbursement eliminates the incentive for overtreating clients. Because providers are paid at a fixed rate, extending the services provided to a client does not provide any additional revenue. In fact, continued service may be to the provider's disadvantage if the costs of service exceed the fixed rate paid for them. Providers, then, have an incentive to minimize the costs of care given.

Prospective payment systems also have disadvantages, however. They may promote prejudice against the very sick with health-care institutions attempting to avoid caring for them or providing inadequate care to minimize costs.[15] For example, under the DRG system, a hospital would be paid the same rate for a Medicare recipient hospitalized for diabetes, whether his or her hospital stay was 3 days or 30 days. Those who are very ill and who require more than the average stay for their diagnostic grouping may be discharged from services before they are actually ready for discharge. In the long run, such practices may lead to subsequent readmissions and to increased health-care costs.[15]

The DRG system has also been criticized as detrimental to provider-client relationships. Because providers may be pressured by hospitals and other institutions to minimize the cost of clients' care and maximize revenues, they may put the needs of the institution before those of the client and discharge clients before they are really ready for discharge. Or, physicians may mislabel clients' diagnoses to put them into groupings with higher reimbursement rates.[15]

CURRENT APPROACHES TO FINANCING HEALTH CARE

Current approaches to financing health care can be either retrospective or prospective in nature, and several different systems of reimbursement are to be found within the U.S. health-care system. Among these are the two-party and third-party reimbursement systems, per case prospective reimbursement, and per capita prospective reimbursement.

TWO-PARTY REIMBURSEMENT

In two-party reimbursement, the client pays the health-care provider directly. This is the traditional fee-for-service approach to the provision of health care, and, until this century, was the only way of paying for health-care services beyond charitable care.

The amount of direct payment by clients has steadily declined until the majority of health-care expenses are met by public or private third-party payments. In 1986, for example, only 28 percent of the total health-care expenditures in the United States were paid directly by consumers, while 30 percent was covered by private health insurance and nearly 40 percent by government-funded programs. Over 50 percent of out-of-pocket costs for health care were for the services of physicians and dentists and for medications, whereas only 14 percent of out-of-pocket expenditures were for hospitalization.[11]

Two-party reimbursement has the advantage of giving consumers some degree of control over the health care they receive. If one is unsatisfied with the care given, one can refuse to pay the bill for services, or one can seek care from another health-care provider. Consumers also have a wide choice among providers.

Both providers and consumers are conscious of cost factors in a two-party system. Consumers do not wish to pay too much for the services received, and providers do not want to drive clients away by charging higher fees than competing providers. Unfortunately, because of the high cost of health care, care for serious illness could bankrupt most individuals and families if they had to pay for everything themselves.

THIRD-PARTY REIMBURSEMENT

Third-party reimbursement mechanisms were designed to protect the average citizen from the financial devastation of serious illness and to supplement two-party payment. In a third-party reimbursement system, payment for health-care services is made by someone or some agency other than the individual receiving service, usually some form of public or private insurance.

Private Health Insurance

Third-party reimbursement can take place under either public or private auspices. The private component of the third-party reimbursement system consists of voluntary health insurance and includes the Blue Cross and Blue Shield nonprofit insurers and the commercial health insurance companies such as Aetna, Prudential, and so on. Blue Cross covers hospitalization costs, while Blue Shield covers the cost of physician's services. Commercial insurers operate on a for-profit basis and provide many different benefits packages with coverage for a variety of services.

In 1986, 180 million Americans were covered by some form of private health insurance. Nearly 82 percent of these individuals had coverage provided by an employer.[11] As noted earlier, the cost of health insurance has risen dramatically in the last several years. In 1970, for example, total expenditures for insurance premiums amounted to $16.8 billion compared to $140.7 billion in 1986.[11]

Employers, who pay the majority of the bill for health insurance, have begun to take several measures to decrease their costs. Some of the strategies used are reducing illness through preventive and health promotive efforts, shifting greater responsibility for payment to employees, using less costly health care services, negotiating for discounted prices on health care through preferred provider agreements, and self-funding insurance coverage for employees.[7,16] Use of preventive efforts, less costly services, and preferred provider arrangements will be discussed later in this chapter.

In an effort to make employees more conscious of health-care costs and to reduce their own expenditures, employers are shifting the cost of health insurance premiums to their employees through copayments and increased deductibles. In 1982, only 30 percent of employers required deductibles. By 1986, the number of employers requiring deductibles had risen to 63 percent.[7] Research has indicated that deductibles as high as $1000 reduce health-care expenditures by about 50 percent.[17] Unfortunately, such an approach discourages employees from seeking preventive health services and may, in the long run, increase the overall cost of health care by promoting a tendency to let health problems reach crisis proportions before care is sought.[7]

Many employers are also turning to self-insurance plans to reduce their health-related costs.[7,16,18] All fifty states have some form of legislation that mandates certain benefits when insurance is provided by private insurance companies. Because these laws do not apply to employers who self-insure their employees' health-care coverage, employers can provide basic coverage at a cost far less than they paid previously to purchase health insurance from private insurance carriers.[18] In addition, self-funded employer health insurance programs are exempt from state taxes that average 2–3 percent of the premium.[16]

More and more employers are taking this option to provide health-care coverage for their employees. In 1980, for example, only 25 percent of employers with 7500 to 10,000 employees self-funded their health-care plans compared to 75 percent in 1984.[7] Because employers are not required to offer mandated insurance benefits, the coverage provided is less than would be the case under private insurance and, again, health may suffer, resulting in higher societal costs for health care in the long-term.[18]

Publicly Funded Health Insurance Programs

Publicly funded health insurance programs are the second component of the third-party reimbursement system in the United States. Government funding accounts for a much lower portion of health-care financing in the United States than elsewhere in the world, just over 41 percent compared with 86 percent for the United Kingdom, 72 percent for Australia, 75 percent for Canada, and nearly 98 percent for Norway.[19] The public component of the third-party system consists of the Medicare and Medicaid programs and the Civilian Health and Medical Programs of the Uniformed Services.

Medicare. Medicare is part of the social insurance program arising from provisions of the Social Security Act. Under Medicare, people over 65 years of age who are eligible for Social Security benefits receive partial coverage of health services. Certain other individuals, such as the disabled, are eligible for Medicare coverage before age 65. In 1986, for example, there were more than 21 million individuals over the age of 65 and more than 2 million disabled people covered by the Medicare program.[11]

There are two components to Medicare coverage. Part A, the Hospital Insurance Program, covers inpatient services. Part B is a Supplemental Medical Insurance Program that covers services by a physician or a nurse or other health-care professional working under the direction of a physician. In the case of Rural Health Clinics, nursing services can be reimbursed with or without physician authorization.

Part A coverage is available to all participants in the Social Security program and is provided without additional premiums. Funding for Medicare Part A is derived from nonvoluntary Social Security taxes. Part B coverage is optional and entails payment of an additional premium similar to that paid for private health insurance, but much less costly. Under both components of the program, the client is responsible for a deductible and also pays a percentage of the cost of care (usually 20 percent) for services provided under Part B.

Part A covers hospitalization and related services including payment for a semiprivate room, laboratory and X-ray procedures, nursing care, meals, medications provided by the hospital, medical supplies and appliances, and the cost of operating room and recovery room services. Blood transfusions are also covered with an additional deductible. Care in a skilled-nursing facility may also be provided, but the client pays a co-insurance payment ($25.50 per day in 1990) for the first 8 days after which Medicare pays the total bill for a stay of up to 150 days. Beyond 150 days, Medicare pays nothing; thus long-term nursing home care is not covered.

Medicare Part A also covers home health services from nurses or physical and speech therapists for homebound clients on a physician's order. Coverage includes 80 percent of the cost of home equipment needs. Hospice care is also available for clients who are terminally ill. Finally, there is coverage for a total of 190 days of inpatient psychiatric care during a client's lifetime.[20]

Part B benefits include payment of 80 percent of allowable fees for physician care. Clients pay the additional 20 percent as well as any charges in excess of the allowable amount. Other benefits include outpatient clinic and emergency room services, physical and occupational therapy, outpatient psychiatric care, laboratory and ambulance services, and very limited coverage for medications.[20]

Medicare is administered at the federal level by the Social Security Administration. Information on benefits, eligibility requirements, deductibles, and copayments for Medicare Part A and Part B is summarized in Table 13–1.

As noted earlier, the Medicare program instituted a prospective payment system based on DRGs in 1983. At present the DRG system only applies to hospital costs covered under Medicare Part A. There is work going on at present, however, to extend the prospective payment system to cover the cost of physician services under Part B. A fee schedule based on a resource-based relative value scale (RBRVS) is expected to be implemented by January 1992. Under this system, physician fees will be determined for each of 33 medical specialty areas, and physicians will be paid for care provided on the basis of those fee schedules.[21]

Medicaid. Medicaid is jointly funded by federal and state revenues, although the distribution of costs varies from state to state, with the federal government paying for a larger share in states with limited resources. The Medicaid program provides health care to persons who are medically indigent. Services provided and eligibility vary somewhat from state to state, but all states must provide certain federally mandated services. These services include inpatient and outpatient hospital services; skilled nursing care; physician services; home health care; family planning services, and early and periodic screening, diagnosis, and treatment services (EPSDT) for eligible children under age 21. The EPSDT component of Medicaid is designed to provide periodic health screening for children and follow-up care for any abnormalities detected. Additional services, such as dental care, medications, and so on, may be provided in some states.

Certain groups are considered "categorically needy" and are automatically eligible for Medicaid. These groups include persons receiving Aid to Families with Dependent Children (AFDC) and those who receive Supplemental Security Income (SSI) due to low income and age, blindness, or disability. In 1987, approximately 4.3 million people received SSI payments and 3.7 million families received AFDC.[11]

The "medically needy" are also eligible for Medicaid. The medically needy are those individuals who meet income eligibility criteria for the program. Medicaid is funded by general tax revenues rather than through mandatory contributions as in the case of Social Security and Medicare.

While Medicaid meets the health-care needs of some Americans, there are many people in need who are not covered by the program. Because of cutbacks in funding, the number of individuals below the pov-

TABLE 13–1. MEDICARE BENEFITS, DEDUCTIBLES, CO-PAYMENTS, AND REQUIREMENTS, 1989

Benefit	Deductible	Co-payment	Requirements for Care
Part A			
Hospital services Semiprivate room Lab tests X-rays Nursing services Meals Drugs provided by hospital Medical supplies Appliances Operating room services Recovery room services	$560	None	Hospital admission
Blood transfusion	Additional	Cost of replacing first 3 pints	Need for more than 3 pints of blood
Skilled-nursing (150-day maximum)	None	$25.50 per day for the first 8 days	Provided in a Medicare-approved facility, need certified by physician, facility accepts client
Home health care	None	20% of allowable charge for medical equipment plus excess charges if any	Care provided by a Medicare-certified agency, client is homebound, client requires intermittent skilled nursing, physical or speech therapy, care is ordered and reviewed periodically by physician
Hospice care	None	$5 or 5% of cost of pain-relief drugs if needed	Physician certification of terminal illness
Inpatient psychiatric care	$560	None	Limited to 190 days in client's lifetime
Part B			
Physician's services	$75 for all Part B care	20% of allowable charges plus excess charges	Physician accepts client
Outpatient hospital services	No additional		
Emergency services	No additional		
Blood transfusion	No additional	20% of allowable charges plus cost of replacing first 3 pints of blood	None
Physical & occupational therapy	No additional	20% of allowable charges in Medicare-approved agency or costs over $400 for care by a private Medicare-certified therapist	Physician prescribed treatment plan with periodic physician review
Outpatient psychiatric services	No additional	38% of allowable charges & all costs over $1100	None
Laboratory fees	No additional	Excess charges only	Performance of tests in Medicare-certified labs
Ambulance services	No additional	20% of allowable charges plus excess charges	Medical need, ambulance meets Medicare standards, other forms of transport could endanger client's life
Drugs	No additional	20% of allowable charges plus any excess charges	Need for injections in physician's office or immunosuppressive therapy after organ transplant

(Source: Consumer Reports[20]*)*

erty line covered by Medicaid has declined in recent years. In 1984, for example, Medicaid covered 64 percent of those with incomes below the poverty level.[22] By 1990, the program covered only approximately half of those with incomes below the poverty threshold.[2]

CHAMPUS. CHAMPUS is a program that provides payment for medical services for the dependents of active duty or retired military personnel. CHAMPUS is usually used to pay for inpatient services not available through a uniformed services medical facility (for example, a naval hospital or an army medical center). CHAMPUS may also be used to finance outpatient services to dependents. While care provided through a uniformed services medical facility is free (except for a small daily fee for inpatient services), there is a deductible of $50 (or $100 per family) for outpatient services provided under CHAMPUS. In addition, CHAMPUS pays only 75–80 percent of the allowable costs for outpatient care, and the client or family must pay the balance of the cost of services received.[23] Funding for CHAMPUS is derived from and administered by the Department of Defense.

Per Case Prospective Reimbursement

Prospective reimbursement may be made on a per case or per capita basis. In the per case approach, health-care providers are paid on the basis of cases seen with specific diagnoses or problems. One form of per case reimbursement is the DRG system implemented by Medicare that was discussed earlier. Another type of per case prospective reimbursement is found in preferred provider organizations (PPOs).

Preferred provider organizations are negotiated associations between a funding source (usually an employer, although the source may also be an insurance company) and health-care providers, whereby providers give discounted services to a defined group of people (for example, employees). When employees use these "preferred" providers, the employer usually covers the bulk of charges. When someone chooses to use other providers, their out-of-pocket costs are higher than if they choose a preferred provider. For example, one company pays 90 percent of the costs of care when employees use preferred providers, but employees must pay 20 percent of costs when other providers are used. This arrangement resulted in health-care cost savings of 20 percent for the company involved.[24] In other instances, PPOs have demonstrated a 15 percent savings in health-care costs.[7]

For providers to remain on the preferred list, they must provide quality services at a reasonable cost, thus encouraging efficiency, but not at the risk of quality. In a PPO, providers are paid for specific services on a per case basis at a predetermined fee, and providers are independent of the reimbursement system. PPOs decrease the per visit cost of health care, but, if the number of visits increases, may not reduce the overall cost of health care to the employer or to society. Utilization review programs, however, can help to minimize overall costs in a PPO arrangement.

Utilization review involves a review of cases to determine appropriate use of resources and may include several approaches such as preadmission review for nonemergency conditions, continued stay reviews, second opinions prior to surgery, and bill auditing. In one survey of 100 large companies, 95 percent engaged in preadmission reviews and continued stay reviews, 94 percent required a second opinion prior to elective surgery (as opposed to emergency surgery), and 68 percent audited bills for services provided.[7] There is some question whether or not a second opinion related to surgery is a cost-effective review strategy, since the second opinion adds an additional cost factor.[16] There is evidence, on the other hand, to suggest that bill auditing is warranted. In one study, over 97 percent of hospital bills had errors.[25]

In 1986, there were over 300 PPOs throughout the country and approximately 10 percent of hospitals were involved in some form of PPO arrangement.[26] In addition to PPO arrangements made with employers, many health-care providers have become preferred providers for both profit and nonprofit insurance companies.[24]

Per Capita Prospective Reimbursement

In a per capita prospective system, health-care providers receive an annual lump sum for each client enrolled in the program. The net effect is a fixed budget for the program. The health-care provider agrees to provide all covered services needed by enrollees. Health maintenance organizations (HMOs) operate on a per capita prospective reimbursement basis.

A ***health maintenance organization*** is an organized health-care delivery system providing a wide range of health services to a voluntarily enrolled population for a fixed prepaid fee. Under the Health Maintenance Organization Act of 1973, federally designated HMOs must exhibit four characteristics: (1) an organized system to provide health care in a particular geographic area, (2) an agreed-upon set of services for health maintenance and treatment, (3) a voluntarily enrolled membership, and (4) rates based on those for similar services in the surrounding community.[11]

The number of HMOs throughout the country

has increased dramatically, as has enrollment. In 1976, for example, there were only 175 HMOs operating with a total enrollment of slightly more than 6 million people. By 1987, the number of HMOs had increased to 662, and more than 28.5 million people received health-care services from an HMO.[11]

An HMO provides most of the preventive, curative, and rehabilitative health services needed by its members for a set fee. It is similar to private health insurance in that yearly premiums are paid. The emphasis in an HMO is on ambulatory care, preventive services, and efficiency. Because the HMO has a fixed income based on the number of members enrolled, it is important that the cost of care be minimized. Generally speaking, it costs less to prevent a health problem than to cure it. Ambulatory care costs less than hospital care, and efficient service is less costly than inefficient service. The healthier the membership remains, the fewer the dollars expended in providing service and the lower the premiums.

The HMOs can be either public or private agencies and all are regulated under the HMO Act of 1973. This act specified the minimum types of service to be provided, the manner in which the HMO is to be organized, and a mechanism of initial federal support for development. It also specified that industries that subscribe to an HMO must offer employees the option to choose either membership in the HMO or more traditional health insurance coverage. Also according to this act, one-third of the governing board of an HMO must be health-care consumers.

The HMOs incorporate the concept of per capita prospective payment in that the enrolled population pays a lump sum annual premium that assures access to all needed services covered by the program. As noted earlier, the fixed budget of an HMO leads to cost-consciousness on the part of health-care providers and contributes to more efficient use of resources and lower overall costs. In fact, HMOs have been demonstrated to reduce overall health-care costs by 25 percent, largely because of lower rates of hospitalization.[7]

Because their fees are based on a per capita prospective payment system, an HMO will lose money if its enrolled members require a great deal of care. This fact leads to the potential for discrimination against the elderly or those with chronic illnesses that require frequent and/or extended periods of care.[15] Such people may be prohibited from enrolling in an HMO, although such practices are prohibited by law in HMOs receiving federal funding.

In other attempts to contain costs, an HMO may place restrictions on the types of diagnostic and therapeutic procedures that providers can employ or on the number of visits that are covered. Such activities may reduce the quality of care that can be provided and may jeopardize the health of enrolled members.[15]

A NATIONAL HEALTH PROGRAM

As noted earlier in this chapter, current mechanisms for financing health-care services leave 37 million Americans without access to health care. In spite of massive expenditures for health care, the health status of the American people is no better, and in some respects is worse, than that of nations that spend far less. For this reason, many people have called for a new approach to providing health-care services—a national health program.

The issue of a national health program, or national health insurance, has been debated for over 75 years.[22] During that time, a number of proposals have been advanced and defeated in Congress. Various proposals for national health insurance have been put forward and tend to fall into two categories, those in which the government pays for care by other providers as a third-party payer and those in which health-care providers are salaried government employees. The first type of plan is exemplified by the Canadian health-care system, while the British system is an example of the second type. Both of these national plans were discussed in Chapter 3, The Health-Care Context. Both the government-as-third-party-payer approach and the government-as-provider approach have two subcategories, plans that provide narrow coverage and those providing wide coverage.

NARROW COVERAGE PLANS

Proposals for narrow coverage usually include coverage of the entire population but within very narrow limitations; for example, catastrophic illness. Catastrophic illness is a serious condition that, because of its severity and the cost of care needed, could exhaust the financial resources of clients if they were required to pay the costs themselves. Plans designed to cover catastrophic illness generally focus on health-care funding for secondary prevention, or treatment of existing illness.

Several plans for catastrophic illness coverage have been introduced at the federal level. Some of these are designed to provide coverage for catastrophic illnesses for all members of society. Others are geared toward selected groups of people. One such plan was enacted in 1989 for coverage of the elderly under Medicare. This legislation was subsequently repealed as a result of active lobbying by those opposed to the increased Medicare premiums required.[7]

Some states have also moved to create catastrophic insurance plans. One approach taken by some states to catastrophic coverage is direct financing of catastrophic medical expenses from the general revenues of the state. Five states currently have such programs in operation. This type of approach meets the needs of the poor and those on fixed incomes such as the elderly. Another approach along this line taken by some states is the expansion of Medicaid eligibility requirements to cover a larger proportion of those who have no insurance.[27]

WIDE COVERAGE PLANS

Health-plan proposals of the wide coverage type can also be divided into several subcategories. One of these is mandatory enrollment by self-supporting people in existing insurance programs with a separate program for the indigent or insurance premiums paid by the government. A variation of this type of program would require all employers to provide health insurance coverage to their employees.[28]

A second type of wide coverage plan calls for voluntary enrollment in existing private insurance programs, again with government subsidy for the indigent. A third approach to wide coverage calls for universal coverage with a comprehensive range of benefits and limits set on provider and hospital costs. The most sweeping type of wide coverage proposal would result in changes in the entire U.S. health-care system with the government providing all health care in a system similar to those of many European countries (see Chapter 3, The Health-Care Context).

National health-care proposals have recently been advanced by several groups of health-care professionals including a coalition of nursing organizations and the Physicians for a National Health Program. The latter group, which consists of 2500 doctors across the country, has developed a proposal based on the Canadian health-care system.[29] Under this proposal the federal government would fund a basic program of health-care services for all citizens. In this program, physicians would negotiate fees with state agencies for covered services, and hospitals would be paid a lump sum each year for covered hospitalization benefits.[30] Other features of this plan are summarized in Box 13–1.

In February 1991, a coalition of nursing organizations, including the American Nurses' Association, the American Association of Colleges of Nursing, the National League for Nursing, the Association of Community Health Nurse Educators, the National Association of School Nurses, and others, put forth a proposal for a national health program believed to meet the health-care needs of the American public. Components of the plan included (1) a defined standard package of health-care services, including primary

BOX 13–1

Features of the Physicians for a National Health Program Proposal

- Universal coverage of all medically necessary services
- Covered services to be determined by boards of experts and community representatives
- Elimination of deductibles and co-payments
- Lump-sum annual payments to hospitals for covered services
- Prohibition of use of hospital funds for expansion, profit, or major capital purchases or leases
- Fee-for-service or salaried positions in hospitals or group practice options for health-care providers
- Physician billing of individual clients only for uncovered services
- Optional lump sum payments to institutions providing outpatient, home health, health education, preventive, and physician services
- Optional per capita payment to HMOs, PPOs and similar institutions
- Separate planning for coverage for long-term care (in process)
- Funding for facility construction or renovation distributed by regional health-planning boards of experts and community representatives
- Coverage of necessary and useful drugs and outpatient equipment
- Disbursement of all funds by a national health program
- Funding based on income or other progressive tax, employer contributions, and current Medicare and Medicaid allocations
- Elimination of private insurance plans duplicating covered services

(Source: Himmelstein[30])

BOX 13–2

Features of Nursing's Proposal for a National Health Plan

Provision of a defined standard package of services
Universal access to health care for all people
Control of health-care costs through case management
Incremental implementation with priority given to pregnant women, infants, and children
Financing through government and private funds from taxes, employer contributions, and individual contributions
Continued operation of private insurance companies, with mandated minimum benefits packages
Options for purchase of additional services by employers or individuals if desired
Mandatory employer-provided insurance coverage of employees either through the public plan or through private insurance
Controlled health system growth through planning and resource allocation
Consumer and provider incentives for cost-effectiveness
Linking of reimbursement to outcomes of care demonstrated by research
Control of administrative costs
Consumer choice among a range of health-care providers

(Source: American Association of Colleges of Nursing[32]; National League for Nursing[31])

care and preventive services, for all residents; (2) improved consumer access to care; (3) control of health-care costs through case management; and (4) incremental implementation of the plan with priority given to pregnant women, infants, and children.[31]

Financing for the program would be accomplished through a combination of public and private funding sources. As envisioned, the public portion of the program will provide standardized services for the poor and will also be available for purchase by employers and individuals. Private insurance programs would continue to operate, but would be required to provide the minimum standardized benefits. Both employers and individuals could purchase additional services as desired. Employers must offer employees either private insurance coverage or buy into the public plan.[32]

The nursing proposal also includes strategies to reduce health-care costs. Some of these strategies include managed care; controlled health-care system growth through planning and resource allocation; consumer and provider incentives for cost-effectiveness; tying reimbursement to care outcomes demonstrated by research; controlling administrative expenses; and promoting consumer choice of providers.[32] This last can be accomplished by promoting the use of nurse practitioners who are cost-effective providers of primary-care services. In fact, in those industries that offer on-site primary care, the use of nurse practitioners has resulted in cost savings.[33–35] Features of the national health program proposed by nursing are summarized in Box 13–2.

The proposals discussed here are only two of many advanced in the recent past. During the 101st Congress alone, more than 11 major bills were introduced, all dealing with some form of national health insurance plan. Some of these proposals dealt with selected target groups, while others addressed the health-care needs of the entire population.[36] In addition, 15 health-related agencies and organizations have developed proposals or statements on health-care funding.[37] One can conclude from the extent of activity directed toward development of a new system of funding health-care delivery that such a system will not be long in coming.

THE EPIDEMIOLOGIC PREVENTION PROCESS MODEL AND A NATIONAL HEALTH-CARE PLAN

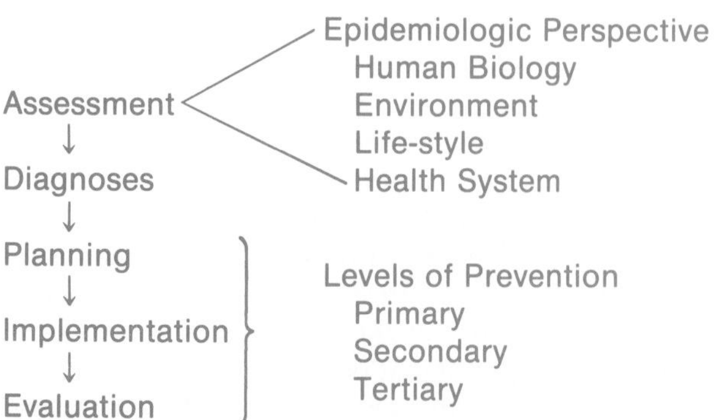

At present, tremendous potential exists for shaping economic influences on health care, particularly for influencing mechanisms of health-care financing. Because community health nurses are concerned for the health of the total population, they should be intimately involved in the development of funding mechanisms that best meet the health-care needs of the public. In the following discussion the epidemiologic prevention process model is applied to the development of a national health program that meets those needs.

ASSESSING THE NEED FOR A NATIONAL HEALTH PLAN

Assessment in the development of a national health-care plan should focus primarily on identifying the groups of people to be addressed by the plan and the types of services that need to be covered. Information related to human biology, environment, life-style, and the current health system can provide answers to these questions of coverage.

HUMAN BIOLOGY

Considerations of maturation and aging suggest that certain subgroups within the population should receive priority, even in a national health program that will eventually address all members of the population. As noted earlier, the nursing proposal for a national health plan targets pregnant women, infants, and children as care recipients in early phases of plan implementation. Access for health care for young children is a serious concern in the United States. Failure to promote health and prevent illness in the young contributes to chronic health problems and escalating health-care costs in later life.

In 1985, more than 15 percent of children under 16 years of age had no form of health insurance. The number of children growing up in poverty and with reduced access to health care is increasing. In 1970, just under 15 percent of children lived in families with incomes below the poverty level. By 1987, 20 percent of children were part of families with incomes below this level.[11] Forty percent of all children under 4 years of age and 80 percent of minority children have not completed an initial immunization series, in part due to the cost of health care. Prenatal care, which can give a newborn a healthier start on life, is received by fewer pregnant women than ever before.[2]

The elderly are another population group that need access to health-care services often denied in the present system. As noted earlier, the elderly expend a greater percentage of their income on health-care services than do other age groups. Despite advances in incomes for the elderly due to Social Security, more than 12 percent of those over the age of 65 remained below the poverty level in 1987.[11]

The size of the elderly population is expected to continue to expand, placing additional strain on available health-care resources. In 1985, the elderly constituted 11 percent of the U.S. population, but accounted for 29 percent of health-care costs. Given current projections, by the year 2050 the population over 65 years of age will comprise 69 million people, 15 million of whom will be over 85. Between 1980 and the year 2000, the elderly population is expected to increase by 18 percent, but the functionally dependent will increase by 38 percent to 15 million people.[10]

The growing number of retirees in the population has increased the health-care cost burden for business and industry. For instance, in 1985, industry spent more than $4.5 billion on health care for retirees. Many employers are responding to this financial drain by reducing health-care benefits for retirees and increasing retiree responsibility for a greater portion of the health-care services they receive.[7]

Funding for long-term care for the elderly and chronically ill is another area of concern related to both biological aging and physiologic function. Medicare does not cover long-term nursing home care, and Medicaid coverage begins only after clients have exhausted all personal resources. In one study, half of single people over 75 years of age admitted to a nursing home exhausted their savings within 3 months, and 83 percent were impoverished within a year.[38]

The relationship between physiologic function and health care is a dual one. Those who have physiologic abnormalities require more health services than those who do not. Conversely, lack of access to illness-preventive and health-promotive care contributes to more illness. Health-care costs related to disability in 1981 amounted to $114 billion.[7]

A special area of concern in terms of physiologic function is the cost of care for persons with AIDS (PWAs). Currently, 25–40 percent of states' Medicaid budgets are spent on care for those with AIDS. In 1986, this amounted to $2.3 billion. Projected Medicaid expenditures for PWAs in 1991 are $47 billion. Attention is also needed with respect to a variety of other communicable and chronic conditions.

ENVIRONMENT

Elements of the social and psychological environments will influence health-care financing reforms. The effects of poverty and unemployment on health and one's access to health care have already been addressed, but these are the types of social environmental factors that community health nurses would need to consider in influencing the direction to be taken by a national health program. Any such program would need to include mechanisms for providing health care to the poor and those who are not covered by any form of health insurance.

A generally depressed economic climate, another social environmental factor, suggests that a health program based exclusively on employer contributions would not meet the health needs of the population. Business and industry are adversely affected by a declining economy and could not bear the added burden of completely funding a national health-care system. In addition, as already noted, only about half of those people without health insurance coverage are employed. These individuals would be left out of any plan that relies exclusively on employer contributions.

A psychological environmental factor that would influence the development of a national health program is the prevalence of mental health problems. At present, approximately 7–10 percent of insurance payments are for treatment for mental and nervous disorders including substance abuse. The majority of these expenses (80 percent) are for inpatient treatment. It is estimated that over 29 million Americans suffer from some form of mental disorder and that more than 20 percent of them, including 2 million seriously disturbed children, receive no care for their illness.[7] Clearly, an effective national health plan will need to address problems of mental illness.

LIFE-STYLE

Life-style factors contribute to a variety of illnesses in today's society, thereby adding to the overall costs of health care. Many life-style factors can be modified through primary prevention programs related to diet, exercise, smoking, and other behaviors that affect health.

Substance abuse is a life-style factor that significantly influences health-care expenditures. In terms of related health-care costs, it is estimated that alcohol abusers use eight times as much medical care as do nonabusers, are absent from work 2.5 times as often, and have 3.6 times as many accidents as do nonabusers.[7] Factors contributing to substance abuse and its control are addressed in Chapter 34, Substance Abuse.

HEALTH SYSTEM

The potential effects of a national health-care plan on the health system and the quality of care provided should also be considered. As noted earlier, many health-related groups are actively supporting some form of health-care program. Others are resistant to changes in health-care financing that could affect their practice. Because of the long-standing independence of health-care providers in the United States, a system in which all providers were salaried employees of governmental agencies would probably be unpalatable. For this reason, a viable national health-care program would probably have to incorporate both salaried and independent modes of practice by health-care providers.

DIAGNOSTIC REASONING AND A NATIONAL HEALTH-CARE PLAN

Based on the assessment of factors influencing health-care funding and health-care needs within the population, the community health nurse would develop nursing diagnoses to guide the development of a national health plan. Diagnoses would reflect the population to be covered by the plan as well as the types of services to be provided. For example, the nurse might diagnose a "need for a national health-care program to provide a basic set of standardized services to all Americans due to lack of access to care among some segments of the population." A related diagnosis would be a "need for attention to the health-care needs of special target groups such as the very young and the very old due to their increased vulnerability to health problems." In a similar vein, the nurse might diagnose a "need for special funding programs to meet the needs of the poor, the uninsured, and the uninsurable due to their increased risk of disease and decreased access to health care."

Nursing diagnoses might also reflect the directions to be taken by a national health-care plan in the types of services provided. For example, the community health nurse would identify a "need for coverage of primary preventive activities for chronic and communicable diseases and for mental illness due to the high incidence, cost, and preventable nature of many of these conditions." Such a diagnosis suggests that primary preventive services should be covered by the plan as well as curative and restorative services. Additional diagnoses would include the "need for secondary and tertiary preventive services due to the incidence of existing health problems and the cost to society of problems left untreated."

PLANNING A NATIONAL HEALTH-CARE PROGRAM

Planning a national health program should involve input from community health nurses who are conversant with the health-care needs of the general public. Community health nurses should communicate the needs of the public to policymakers and influence the development of health-care financing policy through the change and leadership processes discussed in Chapter 11, The Change, Leadership, and Group Processes, and the political processes discussed in Chapter 12, The Political Process.

Areas to be considered in planning a national health program would include basic services to be covered, mechanisms for paying for care, who will provide care, where care will be provided, and relationships among providers, the health-care system, and funding agencies. As noted earlier, an effective national health program needs to address plans for services at all three levels of prevention with an emphasis on primary prevention designed to minimize the occurrence of health-care problems and, thereby, reduce the overall cost of care. Primary preventive measures covered would include illness-preventive services such as immunizations and education on risk factors for specific illnesses, as well as general health-promotive interventions such as counseling on basic nutrition, exercise, and coping strategies.

Secondary preventive activities covered by the plan would emphasize early detection and treatment of existing physical and emotional problems to prevent exacerbation and higher costs later on. Routine screening services as recommended by the U.S. Preventive Services Task Force[39] would be incorporated into the basic services provided under the plan (see Chapter 32, Chronic Physical Health Problems, for a discussion of recommended screening procedures). The national plan would also emphasize treatment in the least expensive setting, and treatment facilities would be made easily available to members of the population.

Provision would also be made for tertiary prevention, but with less emphasis than primary and secondary prevention. If primary and secondary preventive efforts are successful, there is less need for tertiary prevention.

Another area to be addressed in a national health program is funding of health care. As noted, a variety of proposals have been made that incorporate funding from employer contributions, individual contributions, tax revenues, and so on. In the United States, a combination of all of these sources of funding would probably be most effective, but the plan would need to spell out how each aspect of funding would be handled and should make provision for strategies to control administrative costs.

Questions of who should provide care and in what settings should be resolved by a broad range of consumer choice of providers and settings. Any plan proposed should include incentives to use cost-effective providers (for example, nurse practitioners rather than physicians for routine primary care) and to seek care in the least expensive setting possible. Community health nurses can contribute in this area through research on cost-effective modes of health-care delivery.

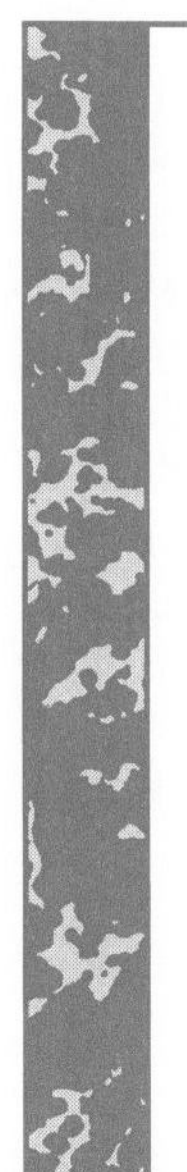

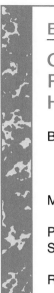

BOX 13–3

Considerations in Planning a National Health-Care Program

Basic services covered under the plan
- Primary preventive services
- Secondary preventive services
- Tertiary preventive services

Mechanisms for financing health-care services

Providers of health-care services

Settings in which health-care services will be provided

Relationships between health-care providers and funding agencies

A final consideration is that of the relationship of providers to the funding source and to the health-care system in general. Should providers be independent practitioners, members of practice associations, or salaried employees? As noted earlier, given the independent tradition of health-care practitioners in the United States, a combination of arrangements would probably be most appropriate in meeting the needs of the citizenry. Community health nurses influencing the planning of a national health-care program can acquaint policymakers with various options for provider-funding source relationships and the utility of independent practice by nurses. Considerations to be addressed in planning a national health-care program are summarized in Box 13–3.

IMPLEMENTING A NATIONAL HEALTH-CARE PLAN

Implementing a national health-care program includes developing sufficient support in Congress to pass the required legislation, educating both health-care providers and consumers about the plan, and planning for incremental implementation of the plan. As noted earlier, certain vulnerable populations such as young children, pregnant women, the elderly, and the poor should receive priority for plan implementation.

Several strategies have been suggested for nursing to exercise its influence in plans for a national health-care program. Among them are the need to unify nursing support for such a program, increasing visibility in campaigns for good health, marketing nursing services in health promotion, identifying the types and numbers of nurses that will be needed to implement the plan, and educating nurses, other health-care providers, and policymakers about nursing's proposed plan. Nurses can also seek positions as policymakers and use political strategies discussed in Chapter 12, The Political Process, to develop a power base to influence legislators toward a national health-care program.[2]

EVALUATING A NATIONAL HEALTH-CARE PLAN

Evaluation of a national health-care plan would be undertaken from a variety of perspectives. One evaluative criterion would be the extent to which the plan assures access to necessary services for the entire population. Are people, particularly those who have been underserved in the past, able to receive the health-promotive, illness-preventive, curative, and restorative services needed to achieve optimal health?

A second area for evaluation would be the effects of the plan on the overall cost of health care. Has the plan reduced expenditures or merely shifted them to other areas? Have expenditures actually increased because of the plan? If so, is this a temporary phenomenon to be replaced by long-term gains, or will health-care costs continue to rise?

A third general area for evaluation would be the effects of the plan on the quality of care provided. Have cost considerations lowered the quality of care provided? If so, what effect has this had on the health status of the American public? In addition, one would look at consumer satisfaction with the care received under any national program.

Finally, one would evaluate the outcomes of the program for those served. Here, emphasis would be placed on the effectiveness of primary, secondary, and tertiary preventive components of the program in improving the overall health of the population. Have primary preventive efforts decreased the incidence of illness? Have health-promotive efforts enhanced the health status of the population? In the area of secondary prevention, one would examine the effects of the program on mortality rates and disability due to existing health problems. Are secondary preventive services provided under the plan contributing to reduced mortality from cardiovascular disease, greater longevity for persons with AIDS, and so on? Are those with existing chronic diseases better able to function adequately with less disability because of services provided? With respect to tertiary prevention, one would examine the extent to which services offered under the national health plan have prevented recurrent health problems and minimized complications of existing problems.

Community health nurses could be actively involved in all of these areas of evaluation. They could participate in identifying evaluative criteria, gathering evaluative data, and interpreting findings through research in these areas. Nurses should also be involved in using evaluative findings to revise or modify the plan as needed through their use of the change, leadership, group, and political processes. Considerations in evaluating a national health program are summarized in Box 13–4.

BOX 13–4

Considerations in Evaluating a National Health-Care Plan

- The extent to which the plan provides access to care for all people
- The effect of the plan on the overall cost of health-care services
- The effect of the plan on the quality of care provided and consumer satisfaction with care
- The effect of the plan on the health status of the population in the areas of:
  - Primary prevention
  - Secondary prevention
  - Tertiary prevention

CHAPTER HIGHLIGHTS

- Economic factors influence the health of individuals, families, and groups or communities. Economic factors affect the abilities of individuals and families to obtain basic necessities and access to health-care services. Economic factors also influence a community's ability to provide citizens with basic necessities and with health-care services.
- Because of their impact on health, two economic factors of particular concern to community health nurses are the rising cost of health care and diminishing access to care for some segments of the population.
- Reasons for the high cost of health care include the use of expensive technology; the need for continuing care for many elderly and disabled individuals; ever-higher health insurance premiums; overuse of health-care services due to availability; high administrative costs for publicly funded health-care programs; and recent advances in salary and benefits by nurses and other providers.
- Diminishing access to care is the result of rising costs for health-care services, decreased income due to unemployment, lack of health insurance for many people, and the reluctance of some providers to accept certain forms of reimbursement.
- Health-care financing mechanisms can be retrospective or prospective in nature. In retrospective reimbursement, the cost of services is determined after services are provided and is based on the cost of the care given. In prospective reimbursement, payment is based on a predetermined fee for specific types of care or specific diagnoses.
- Retrospective reimbursement systems have the disadvantage of providing incentives to give unnecessary care because it is reimbursable. Prospective systems provide incentives to minimize the cost of care, but may, thereby, reduce the quality of care given.
- Current modes of health-care financing in the United States may involve two-party or third-party reimbursement. In two-party reimbursement, the client pays the health-care provider directly for services rendered. In a third-party system, providers are reimbursed by a third party, usually via some form of health insurance.
- Third-party reimbursement can involve either private or publicly funded health insurance or per case or per capita prospective reimbursement. Public health insurance programs include Medicare, Medicaid, and CHAMPUS.
- Medicare provides health care for elderly and disabled people who are eligible for Social Security benefits. It consists of two parts: Part A pays for hospitalization costs, and Part B requires an additional premium and covers physicians' costs and other services. Medicare is administered by the federal government.
- Medicaid provides coverage for the categorically needy and the medically needy. Medicaid is administered by each state and benefits may vary somewhat from state to state beyond federally mandated minimum benefits.
- CHAMPUS provides care for dependents of active duty and retired military personnel that is not provided by military health units under the Department of Defense.
- In per case prospective reimbursement, fees for health-care services are predetermined, and payment is made on the basis of cases seen. PPOs operate on a per case prospective reimbursement system. In a PPO, providers give discounted services to funders, who encourage members to use the preferred providers.
- HMOs are examples of per capita prospective reimbursement mechanisms. In an HMO, health-care providers receive a lump sum payment based on the number of participants enrolled in the program. They then provide all agreed-upon health services required by enrolled members.
- There is growing support for some type of national health-care program, and several proposals have been introduced in Congress. Proposals can be either wide or narrow in terms of the population and services covered. They also differ in terms of their approach to financing health care.
- Two proposals for a national health-care system introduced in recent years are that of the Physicians for a National Health Program and the proposal put forth by organized nursing in 1991.

(continued)

- The epidemiologic prevention process model can guide nurses in the design of a workable national health-care plan. Assessment would identify services to be offered and populations to be targeted by the plan.
- Planning for a national health-care program would need to address such considerations as benefits, funding mechanisms, who will provide care, where care will be provided, and relationships between providers and funding sources.
- Implementing a national health-care program will require use of the change, leadership, group, and political processes in influencing policymakers and the general public.
- Considerations in evaluating a national health plan would include the effects of the plan on access to health care for all Americans; on the overall cost of care; and on the quality of care provided; outcomes of the plan in terms of primary, secondary, and tertiary prevention would also have to be assessed.

Review Questions

1. Describe at least three ways in which economic conditions may influence the health status of the population. (p. 241)
2. What two economic issues are of particular concern to community health nurses? (p. 244)
3. What is retrospective reimbursement? How does it differ from prospective reimbursement? (p. 247)
4. Identify three forms of publicly funded health insurance. Describe the beneficiaries of each. (p. 248)
5. How does per case prospective reimbursement differ from per capita prospective reimbursement? Give an example of an approach to health-care delivery that involves each type of reimbursement. (p. 251)
6. Identify at least four components of the national health-care plan proposed by nursing in 1991. (p. 254)
7. Describe at least three considerations in planning for a national health-care program. (p. 257)
8. Describe at least three considerations in evaluating a national health-care plan. (p. 258)

APPLICATION AND SYNTHESIS

You have been appointed to the mayor's task force on health care in the midsize community in which you work as a community health nurse. The assessment of community health and economic status conducted by the task force indicates that the bulk of the population's health-care needs are adequately met at all three levels of prevention. The exception to this, however, is the population of the migrant farm camp at the edge of town.

This group is comprised primarily of male Mexican workers who have entered the United States on legal work visas. Very few of the workers have brought their families with them. Most of this population receive no health care except for treatment in the emergency room of the community hospital. Usually this care is provided for work-related injuries or serious illness. Members of this group receive no primary preventive care and do not seek care for minor illnesses because of their inability to pay.

Because most of these people are in the United States legally, they would be eligible for Medicaid. However, very few have applied for this program because of language barriers, lack of transportation to the social services office, and inability to afford to take the time off work to submit an application. Even if they did receive Medicaid assistance, they would be unlikely to find a regular health-care provider who accepts Medicaid reimbursement. Only one community clinic and one independent nurse practitioner, in addition to the community hospital, accept Medicaid. Local physicians receive adequate income from private paying clients and those with private health insurance. Because of the extended time between provision of services and receipt of Medicaid reimbursement, these physicians no longer accept Medicaid clients.

The rest of the population is well-off compared to state and national average incomes. With the exception of the migrant workers, most residents are employed by three large industries and receive salaries that are quite adequate to meet the cost of living. Because of the industry present in the community, the local tax base is more than adequate. The community does not budget any public funds for health care as the majority of the population are adequately served by private providers. There is no local health department, but the county offers public health services in a town 50 miles away.

1. What human biological, environmental, life-style, and health system factors are influencing the health status of the migrant group?
2. How would you go about arranging to finance health care for this population group?
3. What kind of funding mechanisms might be most appropriate for providing care to the migrant population? Why?

REFERENCES

1. Simmons, H. E. (1981). Medicare in the '80s. *Journal of the Tennessee Medical Association, 74*, 575–582.
2. Johnson, P. A. (1990). A national health insurance program: A nursing perspective. *Nursing & Health Care, 11*, 416–418, 427–429.
3. Wilson, W. H. (1972). *Life on paradise island*. New York: Lothrop, Lee, & Shepard.
4. Division of National Cost Estimates, Health Care Financing Administration. (1990). National health expenditures. In P. R. Lee & C. L. Estes (Eds.), *The nation's health* (3rd ed.) (pp. 207–221). Boston: Jones and Bartlett.
5. American Public Health Association. (1989). *Action alert*. Washington, DC: American Public Health Association.
6. Solovy, A. (1989). Health care in the 1990s: Forecasts by top analysts. *Hospitals, 63*(14), 34–46.

7. Rooney, E. (1990). Corporate attitudes and responses to rising health care costs. *AAOHN Journal, 38,* 304–311.
8. Levit, K. R., Freeland, M. S., & Waldo, D. R. (1990). National health care spending trends: 1988. *Health Affairs, 9*(2), 171–185.
9. Lamm, R. D. (1990). The 10 commandments of health care. In P. R. Lee & C. L. Estes (Eds.), *The nation's health* (3rd ed.) (pp. 124–133). Boston: Jones and Bartlett.
10. Starck, P. L. (1991). Health care under seige: Challenge for change. *Nursing & Health Care, 12,* 26–30.
11. United States Department of Commerce. (1990). *Statistical Abstract of the United States, 1989* (109th ed.). Washington, DC: Government Printing Office.
12. Relman, A. S. (1989). The National Leadership Commission's Health Care Plan. *The New England Journal of Medicine, 320,* 314–315.
13. Continuing increase in infectious syphilis—United States. (1988). *MMWR, 37,* 35–47.
14. Rubin, R. J., Moran, D. W., Jones, K. S., & Hockbarth, M. A. (1988). *Critical condition: America's health care in jeopardy.* Washington, DC: Lewin/ICF.
15. Dougherty, C. J. (1988). *American health care: Realities, rights, and reforms.* New York: Oxford Press.
16. Williamson, W. H., & Moore, P. V. (1987). Health care cost containment: Current societal forces and health care trends. *AAOHN Journal, 35,* 444–448.
17. Herzlinger, R. (1985). Corporate America's "mission impossible": Containing health-care costs. *Technology Review, 88*(8), 41–44, 46–51.
18. Rublee, D. A. (1986). Self-funded health benefit plans: Trends, legal environment, and policy issues. *JAMA, 225,* 787–789.
19. Schieber, G. J., & Poullier, J. (1989). International health care expenditure trends: 1987. *Health Affairs, 8*(3), 169–178.
20. Beyond Medicare. (1989). *Consumer Reports, 54,* 375.
21. Fee Schedule for physicians moving toward implementation. (1991, January). *The Nation's Health,* p. 5,
22. Harrington, C. A. (1988). A national health care program: Has its time come? *Nursing Outlook, 36,* 214–255.
23. CHAMPUS Public Affairs Branch. (1990). *CHAMPUS handbook.* Aurora, CO: CHAMPUS Public Affairs Branch.
24. Froh, R. (1986). Changing patterns in health benefits design. *Nursing Economics, 4,* 117–121.
25. Kimbrough, A. W. (1985). Auditors found errors in 97 percent of hospital bills. *Atlanta Journal,* p. 10.
26. Scheier, R. L. (1986, February 21). Market-place is the new frontier, analysts warn. *AMA News,* pp. 32–34.
27. Merritt, R. (1987, May–June). Legislatures expand medicaid eligibility. *The Nation's Health,* p. 11.
28. Sorian, R. (1987, July). Kennedy proposes mandatory insurance. *The Nation's Health,* p. 4.
29. Frisof, K. B. (1990). The case for universal health insurance. *The Journal of Family Practice, 30,* 465–467.
30. Himmelstein, D. U., Woolhandler, S., & the Writing Committee of the Working Group on Program Design. (1989). A National Health Program for the United States: A physicians' proposal. *The New England Journal of Medicine, 320,* 102–108.
31. National League for Nursing. (1991, March). *Public Policy Bulletin.* New York: National League for Nursing.
32. American Association of Colleges of Nursing. (1991, January 25). *Nursing's agenda for health care reform: Executive summary.* Washington, DC: American Association of Colleges of Nursing.
33. Yeater, D. C. (1985). 1985 health care cost management update. *Occupational Health Nurse, 33,* 594–599.
34. Lawler, T. G., & Bernhardt, J. H. (1986). Nurse practitioners and HMOs in occupational health. *AAOHN Journal, 34,* 333–336.
35. Dellinger, C. J., Zentner, J. P., McDowell, P. H., & Annas, A. W. (1986). The family nurse practitioner in industry. *AAOHN Journal, 34,* 323–325.
36. American Nurses' Association. (1990a). Capitol Update, *8*(7), 1–8.
37. American Nurses' Association. (1990b). *Overview of statements on health policy by public and private organizations.* Kansas City, MO: American Nurses' Association.
38. Newald, J. (1987). Long-term care financing: Will it bury tax reform? *Hospitals, 61*(5), 42–47.
39. United States Preventive Services Task Force. (1989). *Guide to clinical preventive services.* Baltimore: Williams & Wilkins.

RECOMMENDED READINGS

American Nurses' Association. (1990). *Overview of statements on health policy by public and private organizations.* Kansas City, MO: American Nurses' Association.

Provides a summary of the components of statements on health financing reform of 15 health-related agencies and organizations.

Enthoven, A. C. (1990). Health care costs: Why regulation fails, why competition works. How to get from here to there. In P. R. Lee & C. L. Estes (Eds.), *The nation's health* (3rd ed.) (pp. 286–293). Boston: Jones and Bartlett.

Discusses a health-care system based on fair competition and the principles under which such a system would operate. Presents arguments for competition among health-care providers as the primary approach to cost containment.

Ginzberg, E. (1990). A hard look at cost containment. In P. R. Lee & C. L. Estes (Eds.), *The nation's health* (3rd ed.) (pp. 246–252). Boston: Jones and Bartlett.

Examines successes to date in health-care cost-containment as well as future directions for cost-containment efforts and projected outcomes.

Maxwell, R. J. (1988). Financing health care: Lessons from abroad. *British Medical Journal, 296,* 1423–1426.

Presents a British perspective on the percentage of national income that should be spent on health-care services for the general population.

Rice, D. P. (1990). The medical care system: Past trends and future projections. In P. R. Lee & C. L. Estes (Eds.), *The nation's health* (3rd ed.) (pp. 72–93). Boston: Jones and Bartlett.

Describes past and current trends in health-care delivery and health status and factors influencing both. Also reviews policy issues related to reimbursement, access, long-term care, and corporate medicine.

Scott, C. L., & Harrison, O. A. (1990). Direct reimbursement of nurse practitioners in health insurance plans of research universities. *Journal of Professional Nursing, 6*(1), 21–32.

Reports the findings of a study on the extent to which nurse practitioner services are reimbursed under the health insurance benefits plans of major health-care research and educational institutions.

Vladeck, B. C. (1990). The market vs regulation. In P. R. Lee & C. L. Estes (Eds.), *The nation's health* (3rd ed.) (pp. 277–285). Boston: Jones and Bartlett.

Presents arguments for government regulation of health care as the primary approach to cost control.

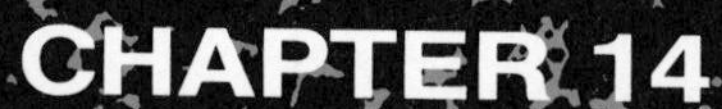

CHAPTER 14

Ethical Influences on Community Health

KEY TERMS

act utilitarianism
autonomy
beneficence
consequentialist theories
contractarianism
deontology
durable power of attorney
egalitarian perspective
egoism
ethical dilemma
ethics
euthanasia
justice
libertarianism
living will
macroallocation
microallocation
nonconsequentialist theories
private consumption goods
restorative justice
rule utilitarianism
social good
utilitarianism

The goal of community health nurses is to enhance the health of the public. But what happens when enhancing the health of one segment of the population results in harm to others? Or, when enhancing the health of a single individual harms that individual in some other way? These are some of the ethical questions faced by community health nurses.

Ethics are the values or standards that govern the behavior of a group and determine the rightness or wrongness of action. Community health nurses have to be concerned with both medical ethics and community health ethics. Medical ethics deals with values, choices, and personal moral behavior as they pertain to interactions with individual clients, whereas community health ethics relates to those same types of values and choices and social morality as applied to the health of population groups.[1] Although both types of ethics are important to community health nurses, the ethics of providing health care for individuals and their families are addressed in other books.[2,3] For this reason, this chapter will focus on the ethics of providing health care to population groups.

(continued)

LEARNING OBJECTIVES

After reading this chapter you should be able to:

- Identify three basic principles of ethics.
- Distinguish between consequentialist and nonconsequentialist ethical theories.
- Describe at least three theories of ethical decision making.
- Identify at least two sources of ethical dilemmas in health care.
- Describe at least four ethical dilemmas encountered in community health practice.
- Identify two levels of nursing diagnosis related to an ethical dilemma.
- Describe two tasks in planning to resolve an ethical dilemma.

BASIC PRINCIPLES OF ETHICS

Although there is disagreement on the length of the list and the labels given to the concepts, many ethicists would agree that ethical behavior is based on the exercise of several basic principles. The principles most often encountered in the ethical literature are beneficence, autonomy or self-determination, and justice or equity.[4–6]

BENEFICENCE

Beneficence involves benefitting or promoting the good of clients.[7,8] The principle of beneficence requires that the community health nurse or other health-care provider take positive steps to help the client.[4] These steps may involve preventing harm to the client (sometimes referred to as nonmaleficence),[8] removing harm, or actively promoting the client's good.[9] For example, community health nurses advocating legislation that mandates helmet use by motorcyclists would be taking steps to prevent harm. Political campaigns to clean up toxic waste sites work to remove harm, while legislation that mandates specified physical education requirements for school children would promote health.

AUTONOMY

Autonomy is a form of personal liberty in which the individual chooses his or her own course of action.[4] The principle of autonomy is also known as "self-determination."[5] This principle is sometimes subsumed under the broader heading of "respect for person," which also includes principles of privacy and confidentiality, truth-telling or veracity, and the right to refuse treatment.[9,10] Support for a living will or the right to refuse, in advance, extraordinary life-saving measures is based on the principle of autonomy, or the client's right to determine his or her own course of action. Opposition to motorcycle helmet laws is also based on the principle of autonomy.

JUSTICE

The principle of ***justice*** or equity involves the fair distribution of benefits and burdens among members of society.[4,5] Under the principle of justice, all things being equal, all groups of people should be treated equally. Ethical decisions based on the principle of justice are grounded in the belief that society's resources should be equitably distributed. There are several perspectives on justice. The first of these, the ***egalitarian perspective***—that all individuals are entitled to the same amount of available goods and services, is based on a belief in the fundamental equality and worth of all persons. According to this perspective, each person should receive the same amount of goods and services regardless of one's needs. The argument is usually made, however, that everyone should receive a "decent minimum" of the goods and services available. The problem then becomes one of determining what constitutes the decent minimum to which everyone is entitled.

The second perspective on distributive justice is that goods and services should first be provided to those most in need of them.[11] From this perspective, distribution of goods and services should benefit those who are the least advantaged in the society. This is the principle on which assistance programs with income eligibility criteria are based. Such programs are designed to meet the needs of the most disadvantaged segments of society, even though other segments might benefit as much or more from such programs.

Finally, decisions regarding distribution of goods and services might involve a ***restorative justice*** perspective in which primary emphasis is placed on meeting the needs of those persons whose conditions

TABLE 14–1. BASIC ETHICAL PRINCIPLES

Ethical Principle	Description of Principle
Beneficence	Ethical action benefits the client through preventing harm, removing harm, or promoting the client's welfare.
Autonomy	Ethical action promotes the client's right to decide the course of action to be taken.
Justice	Ethical action promotes fairness or equity in the allocation of goods and services among the members of a society. Allocation decisions can be based on equal distribution to all, distribution to those most in need, or distribution to those who have been victims of past injustice.

arise out of prior injustice. From this perspective, it could be argued that society has a responsibility to care for the victims of criminal acts because their needs for care are the result of injustice. In the same vein, victims of racial discrimination in employment have a greater right to scarce jobs or assistance than those who have not been subjected to discrimination. Basic ethical principles are summarized in Table 14–1.

APPROACHES TO ETHICAL DECISION MAKING

Ethical dilemmas require choices between alternative actions (one of which may be not to take any action). To make appropriate choices, community health nurses and other health policymakers need to use a systematic approach to ethical decision making. Doing so helps to produce decisions that are based on consideration of the factors involved,[8] and to avoid decisions based on emotional responses that may not truly be in clients' best interests. Systematic approaches to ethical decision making can be based on any of several ethical theories. The ethical theories addressed in this chapter can be divided into two categories—consequentialist theories and nonconsequentialist theories.

CONSEQUENTIALIST THEORIES

Consequentialist theories are those in which ethical decisions are based on the consequences of an action rather than on the action itself.[10] Other terms for consequential ethics are situational or teleological ethics.[5] From the consequential perspective, the morality of a particular act is judged on whether it results in a good outcome. Consequential theories to be addressed include egoism, utilitarianism, and libertarianism.

EGOISM

Egoism is an ethical perspective in which ethical decisions are based on what is best for the decision-maker.[9] The community health nurse, or other health policymaker, who acts from an egoist perspective makes decisions based on self-interest.[12] For example, a community health nursing agency may decide to curtail home nursing services to clients who are not covered by Medicare or private insurance to assure the financial solvency of the agency. In this instance, policymakers are acting on the basis of what is best for the agency rather than what is best for individual clients.[13]

Community health nurses might also act from an egoist perspective in dealing with individual clients. For example, a nurse who puts off visiting a terminally ill client because the nurse is made uncomfortable by impending death is operating ethically as an egoist. In one study of hospital nurses' reasons for certain decisions in hypothetical ethical situations, self-protection or egoism was a consistent reason given for resuscitation decisions with clients with poor prognoses.[14] It is to be supposed that community health nurses, being human, would also act from an egoist perspective on occasion.

UTILITARIANISM

Utilitarianism is an ethical approach in which ethical decisions are based on perceptions of the greatest good or happiness (or the least harm) for the greatest number of people.[13,15] In this perspective, one looks at the consequences of an act for general human welfare to determine the rightness or wrongness of an act.[16] The overriding ethical principle in utilitarian theory is beneficence, the doing of good for the client.

Two approaches can be used in the utilitarian perspective to make decisions about the consequences of an action. The first is called ***rule utilitarianism.***[17] Using this approach, decisions are made on the basis of a general rule of thumb that, in most similar situations, the greatest good is achieved by taking a specific action. Following this approach to ethical reasoning, health-care policymakers could decide to withhold expensive treatment for multiple congenital anomalies on the grounds that the money could be better spent on prenatal care that would prevent congenital defects in a large number of babies. Rule utilitarianism usually is used with respect to questions of ***macroallocation,*** decisions about the distribution of health-care resources to groups of people.

The second approach to utilitarian decision making is ***act utilitarianism.***[17] Here the emphasis is on the consequences of a specific act in a given situation rather than on a general rule. Such an approach usually is applied to ***microallocation*** decisions—namely what health-care resources should be provided to a particular client. For example, owing to the needs of other clients, a community health nurse might decide to discontinue services to a client who is not benefitting from them. In this instance, greater good for society can be achieved by serving those who will benefit from services rather than continuing to serve those who will not.

LIBERTARIANISM

Libertarianism is an ethical framework in which actions are judged favorably to the extent that they protect individual liberties. From the libertarian perspective the ethical principle that supersedes all others is autonomy, or self-determination, the right to choose for oneself. This means that people have a right to choose behaviors that may be detrimental to their own health. Libertarian arguments have been advanced against legislation mandating the use of helmets by motorcyclists, seat belt use by adults, and so on. Problems arise, however, when an individual's right to choose conflicts with the rights of another. For example, the right of a person to choose a smoke-free environment may conflict with the right of someone to smoke. The libertarian approach also endorses the position that people are entitled only to the amount of health care for which they are able to pay.[18]

NONCONSEQUENTIALIST THEORIES

Nonconsequentialist theories are those in which ethical decisions are based not on the outcome of an action but on the rightness or wrongness of the action itself.[10] According to these theories, there are certain rules or duties that are unchanging and that apply to all situations. Codes of ethics, such as the one developed by the American Nurses' Association, are based on notions of duty and are derived from nonconsequentialist theories.[9] Nonconsequentialist theories to be addressed here include deontology and contractarianism.

DEONTOLOGY

Deontology is an ethical perspective in which decisions are based on formal rules or obligations.[16] A community health nurse operating from a deontologic perspective would behave according to a set of rules arising from underlying beliefs about one's duties in relationship to others. The rules underlying this perspective stem from an awareness of the fundamental value of each human being[15] and are held to be immutable. Behavior is based on the merits of the action proposed and the principles or rules involved. Under the deontologic perspective, it would be considered wrong to steal even if one was starving. Also, in this perspective, there are certain actions or duties to which one is obligated regardless of the circumstances. These include the duty to prevent harm (the principle of nonmaleficence), the duty to promote good (beneficence), the duty to be fair (justice), the duty to keep promises (fidelity), and the duty to respect others (autonomy).

The "virtue-based" medical ethic or standard advocated by some authors is based on deontologic theory. Under this ethic, health-care providers recognize their obligation based on their assumption of a provider role. This approach is the basis for arguments that health-care providers, by virtue of having voluntarily selected their professions, have a duty to care for persons with AIDS despite the potential for personal harm.[19]

CONTRACTARIANISM

Contractarianism is an ethical perspective in which ethical decisions are based on the duties that arise from an implicit or explicit contract between individuals or groups of people. The contractarian approach to ethical decisions acknowledges the social nature of human beings and the existence of an implied contract between the individual and society. This contract presumes individual behavior that will support the continued existence of society, while charging society with the obligation of providing for the needs of individuals and of safeguarding their rights. Under such a contract, individuals could expect society to assure them equal measures of liberty, opportunity, wealth, and so on, unless differences in these attributes would be to the advantage of the society at large. For example, it was appropriate in primitive societies for the men to have the greatest share of food supplies in times of shortage, because they were the hunters who supplied food for the entire group.

The contractarian approach has frequently been used to justify some health-care providers' refusal to care for some persons. Private providers have refused care to those who could not pay their fees; more recently, some private physicians have refused to care for AIDS patients for fear of personal exposure. The argument made in these cases is that the physician is free to choose not to enter into a contractual arrangement to provide care. The same argument could be used to deny home health nursing services to those

TABLE 14–2. SELECTED ETHICAL DECISION-MAKING THEORIES

Ethical Theory	Basis for Ethical Decision Making
Egoism	The needs, wants, or desires of the decision-maker
Utilitarianism	The greatest good (or least harm) for the greatest number
Libertarianism	Protection of personal liberty
Deontology	Duties or obligations arising from universal rules or principles
Contractarianism	Duties or obligations arising from an implicit or explicit contract between individuals or groups

with AIDS. This type of approach is in direct opposition to the virtue aspect of the deontologic perspective. Theories of ethical decision making presented here are summarized in Table 14–2.

ETHICS IN HEALTH CARE

Health-care ethics guide health-care providers in determining the morally right action in a given situation. Often the action to be taken is obvious. The provider should do whatever is going to be of greatest benefit to the client. Sometimes, however, it is not clear what course of action will be of greatest benefit (or least harm). When this occurs, one is faced with an ethical dilemma. An ***ethical dilemma*** exists when there is a conflict over the morally right action to be taken,[7] or between two courses of action that are equally desirable or undesirable.[4,10]

SOURCES OF ETHICAL DILEMMAS IN HEALTH CARE

Ethical dilemmas in health care arise from societal factors that place values in conflict. One source of ethical dilemmas in health care is society's choice of some goals over others. When society chooses to work toward certain goals, values implicit in those goals are emphasized, while the values implicit in other goals are minimized. For example, because the American health-care system emphasizes curative care, the value of preventive care is minimized. Conversely, a focus on prevention would minimize the values inherent in the care of people with existing health problems. In a society that does not have the resources to provide the needed level of care in both areas, the need to choose one focus over the other creates an ethical dilemma.

Another source of ethical dilemmas in health care is the choice of target groups that will benefit from health-care programs. The choice of one segment of the population as beneficiaries discriminates against other groups constrained by limited resources. For instance, health-care programs, such as Medicaid, that assist the poor discriminate against those with moderate incomes who are not eligible for services, but who must pay for them through taxes.

A third source of ethical dilemmas is the means chosen to achieve some common public health-care goal. Approaches that seem to benefit the majority of the population might infringe on the rights of certain other individuals. Prohibiting smoking in public buildings, for example, infringes on the rights of smokers.

Finally, ethical dilemmas in health care can arise as consequences of social change. For example, a declining economy and reduced tax base might force policymakers to curtail some health-care services. The choice of what services to curtail could constitute an ethical dilemma because any reduction in services will affect some group of consumers adversely.

ETHICAL DILEMMAS IN COMMUNITY HEALTH

Health-care providers, including community health nurses, are faced with a variety of ethical dilemmas that affect the health status of population groups. These include determining whether responsibility for health lies with the individual or with the society; decisions on the preeminence of individual or societal good; allocating scarce resources; and dealing with issues related to death and dying.

PERSONAL OR SOCIETAL RESPONSIBILITY FOR HEALTH

Ethical questions related to responsibility for health can be of two types. The first deals with a person's right to make health-related decisions; the second deals with the extent to which society is responsible for providing health care for its citizens.

Personal freedom is one of the hallmarks of American society. But freedom can have its limits. Should one be free to make one's own decisions regarding health matters, or is this an area in which government regulation is appropriate?

The ethical dilemma here often takes the form of controversies over whether individuals should be compelled to engage in behaviors that are for their own good. Examples of dilemmas of this sort include controversies over compulsory helmet laws for motorcyclists, or compulsory tests of thyroid function for all newborns. For cases in which the activity of one person is obviously harmful to another, it is easier to decide that the freedom of one individual should not be construed as liberty to harm others. However, when it can be argued that one's behavior (for example, hang gliding or riding a motorcycle without a helmet) does not directly harm others, should one be allowed to make one's own decisions? An affirmative answer to this question would be based on the principle of autonomy, while arguments that people need to be prevented from engaging in unhealthful behaviors would be based on the principle of beneficence.[4]

A related question is: Should one who chooses to act in an unhealthful manner be held responsible for the consequences of that choice, or does society have a responsibility for the health of these people? Should the smoker who develops lung cancer, for example, be held responsible for the costs of expensive therapy needed to treat his or her disease? Or does society have some responsibility to assist the individual to deal with the consequences of his or her actions?

Questions of individual versus societal responsibility arise again and again in health care. Who should pay for the lifetime expenses of the quadriplegic injured in a motorcycle accident? Should the person injured pay the costs for care if he or she was not wearing a helmet? Should society assume these costs if the motorcyclist took appropriate precautions, but injury occurred anyway? Some authors[20,21] point out that assigning responsibility for one's behavior assumes that the specific consequences of that behavior for health are known (for example, supported by research findings) and understood by the individual involved. They caution that this perspective may result in *blaming the victim* or assigning total responsibility for health to the actions of the individual without acknowledging the influence of social and environmental factors.[20]

The second aspect of the question of personal versus societal responsibility for health is the extent of society's responsibility to provide health-care services. The answer lies in the way in which society defines health.[22] If health is defined as a ***social good***—one that benefits all of society—health care should be financed by the society at large. If health and health care are perceived as ***private consumption goods***—goods that benefit the individual and can be obtained if one can afford them, like a car or a swimming pool—health care should be financed by the individual recipient. Unfortunately, this is a question that has not yet been adequately resolved in American society.

INDIVIDUAL VERSUS SOCIETAL GOOD

An ethical dilemma closely related to the previous discussion is the relative merit of individual rights or good versus those of the society at large, when the two are in conflict. Does a person with a communicable disease, for instance, have a right to refuse treatment if he or she is likely to infect others? Or does society have a right to impose some restrictions on individual freedoms to protect the health of the majority?

Perhaps the most compelling ethical conflict of this sort today is the need to protect the identity of individuals who test positive for human immunodeficiency virus (HIV), the virus that causes AIDS, versus the need to protect others from becoming infected. Control of AIDS is hampered in many jurisdictions because of privacy laws that expressly prohibit notifying contacts that they have been exposed to HIV. In this instance, the right of the individual to privacy has been given primacy over the rights of others to know of possible infection and over the rights of still others to be protected from exposure to a fatal disease. In view of concerns for both confidentiality and protection from harm, several criteria have been proposed for determining the appropriateness of mandatory screening and reporting of HIV test results.[23] These criteria include expectations that:

1. the target population has an identified reservoir of infection;
2. the environment of the population poses a significant risk of spreading the disease;
3. knowledge of test results would enable authorities to take preventive measures;
4. the consequences of testing would not outweigh the benefits, and;
5. there are no other alternatives that would be as effective in meeting health objectives.

Relaxation of confidentiality statutes to allow notification of contacts to persons with HIV-positive tests have been proposed. Contacts can then engage in measures to prevent the spread of the disease to others. In a recent California decision, the court ruled that health-care providers have an obligation to protect third parties from harm even if doing so means violating client confidentiality.[24] Although the legal status of the issue may have been addressed, the ethical question remains whether the individual right to confidentiality outweighs the right of others to know of their possible exposure.

Some authors[25] have asserted that any situation in which societal rights clearly take precedence must be necessarily related to the common good. In many instances, however, it is difficult to make that distinction, and health-care providers must use their own ethical principles to resolve the ethical dilemma.

Other providers[26] have made the point that an emphasis on population-wide benefits may distort decisions with respect to individual clients. It may be that, in the interests of enhancing the overall health status of society, individuals are being subtly coerced to more healthful behaviors. A case in point is the tremendous pressure brought to bear on people to quit smoking. The ethical conflict lies in the individual's freedom to determine his or her own behavior versus society's right to decrease the societal costs of such conditions as heart disease and cancer.

RESOURCE ALLOCATION

Another ethical dilemma that faces today's public health policymakers is the allocation of scarce health-care resources.[27] Modern medical technology makes possible many previously undreamed of health benefits. Unfortunately, because of limited economic resources, not all of this medical technology can be made available to everyone. Two questions then arise. First, who should benefit from medical technology? The answer varies depending on the approach to ethical decision making taken. Should those in greatest need receive help first (a justice approach)? Or should those most likely to contribute to society in the future, or those who have contributed to society in the past, be aided?

The second question is whether society should use health-care resources to cure existing illness.[28] Should society use advanced technology to provide heart transplants, for example, or should society instead use available resources to prevent heart disease in persons who are presently healthy? From the utilitarian perspective, the greatest good comes from preventing heart disease in many people rather than in performing heart transplants in the few. Different answers to the question of appropriate resource allocation would be derived from other perspectives.

DILEMMAS RELATED TO DEATH AND DYING

Ethical dilemmas related to death and dying abound in today's society. These dilemmas include whether a person has a right to refuse extraordinary treatment to prolong life, the corollary issue of whether someone has a right voluntarily to terminate his or her life, and the manner in which one dies when death is inevitable. Some of the approaches taken to resolve these dilemmas will be examined here.

The Living Will

A ***living will*** is a document drawn up by an individual while in a state of relative health. The living will states that the signer chooses not to be subjected to extraordinary life-saving measures should the time arise when he or she is unable to make choices regarding care. Living wills are recognized as legal documents in 41 states.[29] Most living-will legislation includes four provisions: (1) a definition of terminal illness as a condition that would result in death despite any intervention employed; (2) execution of a written document expressing the wish that extraordinary measures be withheld or withdrawn; (3) agreement of two or more physicians as to the hopelessness of the situation; and (4) relief of the physician and the institution of liability from the decision.[30]

A suggested alternative to the living will is the durable power of attorney. A ***durable power of attorney*** is a legal document by which someone gives another person the authority to make decisions regarding extraordinary life-saving measures should that person be unable to make these decisions on one's own. A durable power of attorney has the advantage of allowing decisions to be made on the basis of factors involved in a particular situation rather than as a one-time decision that may not reflect the individual's wishes at the time.[31] For example, if one signs a living will, then changes one's mind but fails to destroy the living will, extraordinary measures may not be taken even though that would be the client's true desire. The durable power of attorney would allow for changes of mind or special circumstances that would alter the client's decision if he or she could make one. The person designated as the one to make decisions would most likely be aware of the client's wishes in a specific situation.

There are a number of potential drawbacks to resolving ethical dilemmas related to extraordinary measures. The power of attorney may be interpreted to cover more than what was intended (for example, as giving someone else control over one's finances). The other problem is that power of attorney is granted to a specific person, who may or may not be available to make decisions regarding treatment at the point when the client is incapacitated. For example, the person designated may die before the client even becomes ill.

Living wills and durable powers of attorney may pose problems for providers who specialize in curative care. To allow a client to die when measures are available to prolong life could cause feelings of guilt in those whose aim is to prevent death. For this reason, living wills are sometimes disregarded by health professionals. Providers also may be inclined to disregard living wills because of fear of litigation by family members if the client's will is honored. However, designation of a living will as a legally binding document in many states has helped to alleviate some of this fear. More information on the living will can be obtained from The Society for the Right to Die, 250

West 57th Street, New York, NY 10107.

The living will does not address the right of a parent or guardian to refuse extraordinary medical treatment when the client is a minor or other individual whose care decisions are made by others. The so-called Baby Doe regulations issued by the federal government in 1984 are an attempt to deal with this question. These regulations allow denying medical treatment for an infant when the infant is irreversibly comatose or when providing treatment would merely prolong death or would be futile in terms of the child's survival and would be inhumane.[32] While the courts have seemingly resolved the question on a legal basis with respect to infants, the ethical question of when it is or is not appropriate to withhold extraordinary measures still remains.

Hospice

The hospice movement is related to the issue of how one decides to face death. Hospice can be a *place* or an *attitude* toward death. The term "hospice" derives from the medieval word for a resting place for travelers on a pilgrimage to the Holy Land. It is used in its current sense to connote the Christian belief that death is a part of the journey to new life.[33] The hospice movement was initiated to provide terminally ill patients with an option to die with dignity in a caring atmosphere and with loved ones close by. As stated by proponents of this movement, "What people need most when they are dying is relief from the distressing symptoms of their disease, the security of a caring environment, sustained expert care, and the assurance that they and their families won't be abandoned."[34] That there is a need for this type of care is evident in the growth of the hospice movement in the last few years and in the endorsement of the hospice concept by the American Hospital Association Board of Trustees in 1979.[35] In Kentucky, for example, increases in admissions to hospices between 1982 and 1985 were so substantial that in some counties as many as 40 percent of terminally ill cancer patients were served by hospices.[36]

Euthanasia

The living will and the hospice movement are responses to the issue of withholding extraordinary measures to prolong life. A related issue that is not addressed by these responses is that of euthanasia. ***Euthanasia*** is the practice of providing a merciful death for those who are hopelessly sick or injured. Euthanasia can be voluntary or involuntary, active or passive. In voluntary euthanasia, termination of life is performed with the consent of the person involved. In involuntary euthanasia, the person's consent has not been obtained. Legally, this form of euthanasia is equivalent to murder. Passive euthanasia involves failure to use measures that would prolong life and is addressed by the living will, the durable power of attorney, and the hospice movement.

Active euthanasia involves the use of interventions that will bring death about sooner than would otherwise be the case.[37] Active euthanasia or "mercy killing" is currently illegal in all states. Legislative efforts to legalize the practice are aimed at eliminating criminal prosecution for health-care providers and/or loved ones who assist terminally ill individuals to commit suicide.

Arguments supporting legislation permitting active voluntary euthanasia often advance the claim that current laws force physicians to keep clients alive in violation of clients' wishes, force clients to endure pain and loss of dignity, and abrogate clients' absolute rights to control their own health-care decisions. Opponents of such legislation argue that individuals can choose to refuse treatment and die in the normal course of events. Further, it is argued that, although terminally ill patients may suffer pain and other consequences of disease, termination of life is an inappropriate approach to symptom control.[38] Rather, efforts should be directed at providing symptom relief and restoring the dignity of the terminally ill.

Finally, opponents of legislation permitting active voluntary euthanasia argue that the right to self-determination may not be exercised to the harm of others. Such legislation might be interpreted as a mandate requiring health-care providers to assist clients in active euthanasia, possibly forcing providers to violate their own ethical principles. Harm might also occur to clients and society if such legislation is interpreted as condoning involuntary euthanasia, as has occurred in the Netherlands.[39] In such an event, persons felt to be a drain on society might be eliminated with or without their consent. To prevent the potential for such harm to individuals, to health-care providers, and to society, many ethicists believe continued prohibition of active euthanasia is warranted.[40]

DENIAL OF SERVICE

At what point and for what reasons is refusing to care for a client justifiable? Denial of services is an ethical issue closely related to those of resource allocation and the use of extraordinary measures to prolong life.

In some instances, hospitals and other health-care institutions are turning away people who have no apparent means of paying for the care received. Is this justifiable? Even if one argues that everyone has a right to life-sustaining health care, many questions still arise. Who, for example, has the responsibility to pay for life-sustaining care when the client cannot? If a society with limited resources has the responsibility for providing such care, who decides what other services will be curtailed? Is it ethical to curtail community health nursing services to individuals who cannot pay for them, or should this be considered "abandonment"?[41]

Another issue that has surfaced in the last few years with respect to the denial of service is the refusal to care for individuals when providing care might jeopardize the safety of the provider.[42] For example, can a community health nurse working in home health ethically refuse to start intravenous therapy for a client with AIDS because of the potential for exposure to HIV? Or, can a community health nurse refuse to accept as part of his or her caseload a psychiatric client with a potential for violence? Arguments in the medical community for and against the right to refuse care tend to be based on contractarian models; on the belief in the right to health care upheld by the principle of justice; on the libertarian model; or on the deontologic model.[19] In the contractarian model, it is argued that providers and clients voluntarily enter into a contract for health-care services. Because the contract is perceived as voluntary on both sides, providers may refuse to enter a contract with certain persons.

When the principle of justice is applied, it is assumed that all people, regardless of the nature of their disease or other circumstances, have a right to health care. If this right is acknowledged, society has a concommitant responsibility to provide health care, including care for persons with AIDS. The health-care provider operating from a libertarian model would contend that the primary guiding principle is his or her right to decide on a personal course of action. This provider could then refuse services to selected clients and remain within the libertarian ethical framework.

In the deontologic model, health-care providers are believed to have a duty to provide health care to members of society whatever their circumstances. This belief is based on the assumption that people who voluntarily enter a profession assume the duties assigned by society to that profession despite the personal risks involved.

Nursing has attempted to address the question of refusal to care for a client based on potential for harm to the nurse. According to the American Nurses' Association Committee on Ethics, nurses must care for clients except when the risk to the nurse outweighs the benefit to the client.[43] In light of current information, for example, it appears that the risk of HIV infection for nurses caring for clients with AIDS is minimal when adequate precautions are taken. Given this information, it is reasonable to assume that nurses are obligated to care for people with AIDS as well as for those with other communicable conditions.

THE EPIDEMIOLOGIC PREVENTION PROCESS MODEL AND ETHICAL DILEMMAS

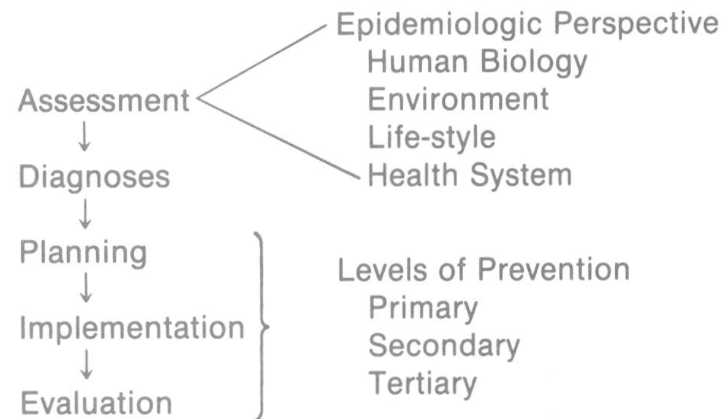

The ethical dilemmas discussed here have implications for the behavior of community health nurses at both individual and aggregate client levels. At the individual level, the community health nurse would function as a client advocate, ensuring that the health care provided to clients and their families is based on sound ethical principles. Community health nurses do not usually make unilateral ethical decisions at the aggregate level, but they have a responsibility to ensure that health policy is consistent with ethical principles.

To promote ethical action at both the individual and aggregate client levels, community health nurses must examine their own ethical values and use an approach to ethical decision making consistent with those values. Ethical decision making should be a deliberative process engaged in by nurses and others involved in an ethical dilemma. Deliberation in an ethical dilemma can be guided by the use of the epidemiologic prevention process model. Using the model in an ethical dilemma, the community health nurse would not only facilitate assessment and diagnosis of the ethical situation but also plan, implement, and evaluate actions to be taken to resolve the dilemma.

ASSESSING THE ETHICAL DILEMMA

The community health nurse and others involved in ethical decision making assess both factors that contribute to an ethical dilemma and those that influence decisions on an appropriate course of action. This assessment can be conducted in terms of Dever's epidemiologic model.

HUMAN BIOLOGY

Human biological factors can influence both an ethical dilemma and decisions regarding its resolution. For example, the ages of persons involved might be an influencing factor. The decision to perform a hysterectomy on a woman past child-bearing age would be easier to make than in the case of a younger woman who wants to have children. On the one hand, a younger woman may want to be cured of her uterine cancer. On the other hand, she may also desire to have a child. The decision becomes even more complicated if the physiologic factor of pregnancy is added. Should the woman have the hysterectomy, or should she carry the pregnancy to term?

Another example of age as an influencing factor might arise in resource allocation decisions related to the use of expensive medical technology. If the recipients of organ transplants are primarily young children, policymakers may decide that this is a more worthwhile expenditure of available health-care funds than if most recipients are elderly. The reasoning here is that children who are saved through transplants have their entire lives ahead of them and can become productive members of society, whereas older persons have already lived most of their lives and would have a limited number of productive years left even with the transplant.

As noted earlier with respect to pregnancy, physiologic factors may also affect ethical dilemmas and decisions related to them. For example, in a situation of limited resources, policymakers might choose to provide care to those who are in relatively good health, judging that their chances of survival are greater than, say, someone who has other debilitating life-threatening conditions.

ENVIRONMENT

Environmental factors, particularly those in the psychological and social environments, can influence ethical dilemmas. Ethical issues are usually emotionally charged, and the psychological environment can greatly influence decisions. For example, the fear of contracting AIDS has led some health-care providers to refuse care to people with AIDS. Similarly, feelings about crime and criminals influence decisions about the provision of health care in correctional settings.

Social environmental factors can also influence ethical dilemmas. Fears of malpractice suits may influence providers in decisions to terminate life-support services. The cost of health care and lack of access to care also contribute to ethical dilemmas. For example, should parents be held responsible for their child's death from pertussis because they failed to obtain immunizations they could not afford?

Cultural beliefs about human dignity, self-determination, and the worth of human life also contribute to ethical dilemmas. In the United States, for example, where personal liberty is a predominant value, health-care policies that curtail individual freedom in favor of the common good are frequently resisted. In making such decisions, policymakers have to take into account the relative merits of personal liberty versus the benefit to society of curtailing certain liberties.

Similarly, beliefs about the worth of individuals often influence situations in which policymakers must decide between allocating resources to care for those with existing illness or preventing illness in the larger population. With a cultural value of individual worth, it is difficult to decide that society will not pay for a liver transplant for a sick child because the money is needed to keep other children healthy. Beliefs about human dignity and the value of life can also influence policy decisions related to living wills, hospice care, and euthanasia.

LIFE-STYLE

Life-style factors also play a part in the development or resolution of ethical dilemmas. Sometimes the dilemma itself arises out of behaviors related to one's life-style. For example, should society accept the burden of care for someone who is injured while hang gliding? Should the motorcyclist who refuses to wear a helmet or the person who drinks and drives be eligible for public assistance in overcoming the effects of a serious accident?

Other ethical dilemmas arise out of the dominant American life-style of personal freedom and independence. To what extent should society be allowed to compel healthful behaviors such as the use of seat belts or the avoidance of smoking? In what circumstances does the protection of society supersede individual rights?

HEALTH SYSTEM

Health system factors give rise to ethical dilemmas when the rights and needs of health-care providers conflict with other societal values. For example, do providers have a right to charge fees that afford them a reasonable income despite the inability of some clients to pay those fees? Should providers be expected to be on call 24 hours a day, 7 days a week? Should government have the right to dictate how health-care providers practice their professions? What happens when the moral beliefs and values of a provider conflict with the desires of clients, or the policies of an employer or society at large? Must providers jeopardize their own safety in the care of clients who are potentially communicable or who are violent? Should employers be required to protect health-care personnel from hazardous conditions? Should they, for example, be required to provide expensive immunizations against hepatitis B?

DIAGNOSTIC REASONING AND ETHICAL DILEMMAS

Based on factors identified in assessing the ethical dilemma, the community health nurse would derive nursing diagnoses at two levels. The first level relates to the existence of an ethical dilemma, whereas second-level diagnoses address the values and value conflicts involved in the dilemma.

DIAGNOSING THE EXISTENCE OF AN ETHICAL DILEMMA

The first level of nursing diagnosis involves confirming that an ethical dilemma does, in fact, exist. The nurse would support this diagnosis with a description of both the problem and the disadvantages posed by all of the potential alternatives to its solution that constitute an ethical dilemma. When there is an alternative without ethical disadvantages, there is no ethical dilemma to be solved. An example of a nursing diagnosis at this level might be the community's "need for an ethical decision on what programs will be eliminated due to reduced funds."

DIAGNOSING CONFLICTING VALUES

The second level of nursing diagnosis involves identifying the values and value conflicts inherent in the ethical situation. The community health nurse would specify the values operating in the situation and identify the individuals holding those values. For example, in the case of mandatory use of motorcycle helmets, cyclists may value freedom of choice, convenience, and lack of constraints on vision entailed in helmet use. Health-care providers supporting legislation for mandatory helmet use value protection of life and health, while lawmakers may value personal freedom, protection of life and health, and protection of society from the economic burden of caring for individuals injured because of failure to use helmets. A nursing diagnosis in this situation might be "conflict between the values of personal freedom and protection of life and health." Another nursing diagnosis might reflect the conflict between the values of personal freedom and protection of society from the costs of accidental injuries.

PLANNING TO RESOLVE AN ETHICAL DILEMMA

Using the epidemiologic prevention process model, planning to resolve an ethical dilemma involves three tasks. The first task is to give priority to the values involved in the dilemma, whereas the second involves evaluating alternative courses of action. The third task is to select the alternative that best fits the paramount values operating in the situation.

GIVING PRIORITY TO VALUES INVOLVED IN THE DILEMMA

The first consideration in planning to resolve ethical dilemmas is assessing the priority of the values involved. Values would be given priority on the basis of the ethical theory selected by community health nurses as most in keeping with their personal and professional values. Suppose, for example, a group of community health nurses are trying to decide whether to support proposed legislation for mandatory helmet use by motorcyclists.

An egoistic perspective on the part of the nurses might result in no action being taken by the group in regard to the proposed legislation. If the nurses perceive that they will neither gain nor lose as a result of the decision, they may ignore the issue altogether. If, however, the nurses perceive the costs of medical care for motorcycle injuries as the cause of increases in their taxes, they will probably decide to support the legislation. If, on the other hand, the costs of enforcing the legislation were perceived as likely to increase their taxes, they would probably take collective action to oppose the legislation.

If deontologic theory is being used by the nurses, top priority will be given to values that conform to notions of duty and obligation. For example, the nurses might believe that individuals have a duty to protect their own health and that the legislature has a duty to protect society. In this situation, the nurses would give protection of health and protection of society greater priority than personal freedom, and would support mandatory helmet use.

Viewing the dilemma from a utilitarian perspective, the nurses would see the good of society as the primary deciding factor. For this reason, they would probably assign first priority to the value of protecting society from economic burdens and again support the legislation.

Using the contractarian approach, the community health nurses might assess values differently based on their view of their relationship to society. If they see their role as community health nurses in the light of a contract with society to protect it from the burden of health-care costs engendered by motorcycle accidents, they will support the legislation.

The libertarian perspective used in this situation would result in personal freedom being considered the most important value. For nurses using this perspective, the right to choose for oneself always supersedes all other rights and values. Given the priority of this value over the values of protecting individuals and society from harm, the nurses would decide not to support the legislation.

SELECTING A COURSE OF ACTION

Once the values operating in a given ethical situation have been assigned priority, it is possible to evaluate alternative courses of action in terms of their conformity to the values given highest priority. Then the course of action that best supports those values would be selected. Using the previous example, if the highest priority is protection of society, legislation mandating helmet use would be supported. If the value of personal freedom is given greater priority, nurses would vigorously oppose proposed legislation.

IMPLEMENTING AN ETHICAL DECISION

Once a course of action in keeping with the ethical principles of the decisions-makers has been selected, steps are taken to implement the decision. In the example above, if the community health nurses have decided to support the proposed legislation for mandatory helmet use, they will engage in some of the political strategies described in Chapter 12, The Political Process, to influence legislators to support their position. They would use these same strategies to implement the decision to oppose the legislation.

EVALUATING AN ETHICAL DECISION

Two aspects are involved in evaluating ethical dilemmas. The first is evaluating the outcome of actions taken. Did the selected course of action result in an outcome consistent with important values? In the case of laws mandating helmet use, for example, one might evaluate whether helmet laws decreased the severity of motorcycle injuries and thereby reduced the economic burden on society.

The second aspect of evaluation deals with the decision-making process used. Were the nurses involved in the ethical decision unsure of the ethical theory to which they subscribed? Were they unclear on what values were really most important to them? If the answer to these and similar questions is yes, there is a need for individual or group clarification of the moral principles and values that are espoused before dealing with another ethical dilemma.

CHAPTER HIGHLIGHTS

- Ethics are the values and standards that govern the behavior of a group and determine the rightness or wrongness of action.
- The three basic principles of ethics are beneficence, autonomy, and justice.
- Approaches to ethical decision making can be categorized as consequentialist or nonconsequentialist theories. In consequentialist theories, decisions are based on the outcomes of action. In nonconsequentialist theories, decisions are based on the morality of the act itself.
- Consequentialist theories include egoism, utilitarianism, and libertarianism. In egoism, the decision-maker bases an ethical decision on the outcome for oneself.
- Ethical decisions made from a utilitarian perspective are based on the action that will achieve the most good (or the least harm) for the most people. Rule utilitarianism is based on generalizations regarding outcomes in similar situations, whereas in act utilitarianism, decisions are grounded on the anticipated consequences of a specific action in a given situation.
- In libertarianism, the overriding principle is that of personal liberty, and ethical decisions are made to protect the right of the individual to self-determination.
- Nonconsequentialist ethical theories include deontology and contractarianism. In both, decisions are based on notions of duty and responsibility.
- In the deontologic perspective, ethical decisions are based on formal rules or obligations.
- In the contractarian approach, ethical decisions are based on duties arising from explicit or implicit contracts between individuals or groups of people.
- Ethical dilemmas in health care arise as a result of society's choice of some goals over others, the choice of target groups to benefit from health-care services, the means chosen to achieve common health-care goals, or as consequences of changes in social factors.
- Ethical dilemmas facing community health

practitioners today include questions of personal or societal responsibility for health, individual versus societal good, resource allocation, dilemmas related to death and dying, and denial of services.

- Nursing diagnoses related to ethical dilemmas occur at two levels. At the first level, the community health nurse diagnoses the existence of an ethical dilemma. At the second level, diagnoses of underlying value conflicts are made.
- Two tasks involved in planning to resolve an ethical dilemma are giving priority to the values involved in the dilemma and selecting a course of action.
- In evaluating an ethical decision, the community health nurse would focus on the effects of the decision in supporting the important values in the ethical dilemma and the use of the ethical decision-making process.

Review Questions

1. What are the three basic principles of ethics? Give an example of each principle related to community health nursing. (p. 266)
2. Distinguish between consequentialist and nonconsequentialist theories of ethical decision making. (pp. 267–268)
3. Describe the basis for ethical decisions in each of four theories of ethical decision making. (pp. 267–269)
4. Identify at least two sources of ethical dilemmas. Give an example of an ethical dilemma related to community health that might arise from each. (p. 269)
5. Describe at least four ethical dilemmas encountered in community health practice. (pp. 269–273)
6. What are the two levels at which nursing diagnoses are made in an ethical dilemma? (p. 274)
7. What are the two tasks in planning to resolve an ethical dilemma. (p. 275)

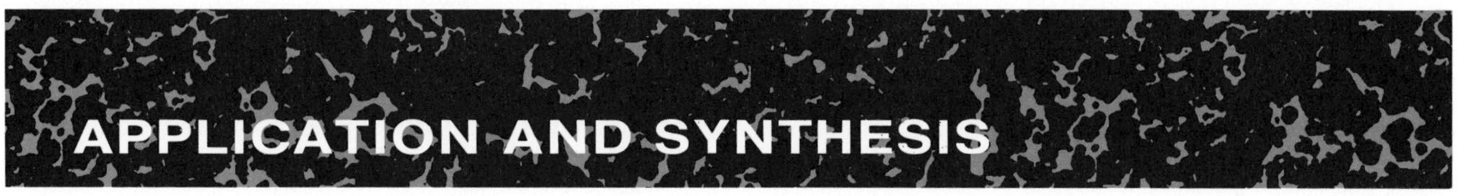

APPLICATION AND SYNTHESIS

A community health nurse is helping with casualties resulting from her apartment building collapsing after a major earthquake. There are many severely injured persons who need immediate care. At present, the nurse is the only health-care provider available, and decisions must be made as to who should receive care first. One of the victims who will probably not survive unless she receives immediate attention is the 88-year-old mother of the community health nurse. This older woman has had a heart attack. Other victims include an 8-year-old who has a head injury and a woman with a sprained wrist who is hysterical because her toddler is trapped in the building. A neighbor who was trying to help others trapped in the rubble has suffered a severe laceration on his thigh and needs to have the wound cleaned and dressed.

1. What human biological, environmental, life-style, and health system factors will influence the community health nurse's decision?
2. What are the values operating in this situation?
3. How would the egoist resolve this situation? The deontologist? The utilitarian? The contractarian? The libertarian?
4. How would you resolve the dilemma? Why would you take this approach?

REFERENCES

1. Roemer, R. (1987, May/June). Public health ethics and the law. *The Nation's Health,* p. 2.
2. Bandman, E. L., & Bandman, B. (1985). *Nursing ethics in the life span.* Norwalk, CT: Appleton-Century-Crofts.
3. Fowler, M. (1990). *Nursing ethics.* Philadelphia: J. B. Lippincott.
4. Rogers, B. (1988). Ethical dilemmas in occupational health nursing. *AAOHN Journal, 36,* 100–104.
5. Starck, P. L. (1991). Health care under siege: Challenge for change. *Nursing & Health Care, 12,* 26–30.
6. Thompson, I. E. (1987). Fundamental ethical principles in health care. *British Medical Journal, 295,* 1461–1465.
7. Aroskar, M. A. (1989). Community health nurses: Their most difficult ethical decision-making problems. *Nursing Clinics of North America, 24,* 967–975.
8. Jenkins, H. M. (1989). Ethical dimensions of leadership in community health nursing. *Journal of Community Health Nursing, 6,* 103–112.
9. Lanik, G., & Webb, A. A. (1989). Ethical decision making for community health nurses. *Journal of Community Health Nursing, 6,* 95–102.
10. Bunting, S. E., & Webb, A. A. (1988). An ethical model for decision-making. *Nurse Practitioner, 13*(12), 30–34.
11. Churchill, L. R. (1987). *Rationing health care in America.* Notre Dame, IN: University of Notre Dame Press.
12. Bandman, E. L., & Bandman, B. (1988). Ethical aspects of nursing. In J. M. Flynn & P. B. Heffron (Eds.), *Nursing: From concept to practice* (2nd ed.) (pp. 261–276). Norwalk, CT: Appleton & Lange.
13. Schultz, P. R. (1987). Clarifying the concept of "client" for health care policy formation: Ethical implications. *Family and Community Health, 10*(1), 73–82.
14. Lawrence, J. A., & Helm, A. (1987). Consistencies and inconsistencies in nurses' ethical reasoning. *Journal of Moral Education, 16*(3), 167–175.
15. DeWolf, M. S. (1989). Ethical decision-making. *Seminars in Oncology Nursing, 5*(2), 77–81.
16. Schultz, R. C. (1987). Ethics and community health: Philosophical traditions and recent turnings. *Family and Community Health, 10*(1), 1–7.
17. Dougherty, C. J. (1988). *American health care: Realities, rights, and reforms.* New York: Oxford University Press.
18. Brody, B. A. (1988). Justice in the allocation of public resources to disabled citizens. *Archives of Physical Medicine and Rehabilitation, 69,* 333–336.
19. Zuger, A., & Miles, S. H. (1987). Physicians, AIDS, and occupational risk. *JAMA, 258,* 1924–1928.
20. McLeroy, K. R., Gottlieb, N. H., & Burdine, J. H. (1987). The business of health promotion: Ethical issues and professional responsibilities. *Health Education Quarterly, 14*(1), 91–109.
21. Wikler, D. (1987). Who should be blamed for being sick? *Health Education Quarterly, 14*(1), 11–25.
22. Reinhardt, U. E. (1990). Rationing the health-care surplus: An American tragedy. In P. R. Lee & C. L. Estes (Eds.), *The nation's health* (3rd ed.) (pp. 104–111). Boston: Jones and Bartlett.
23. Gostin, L., & Curran, W. J. (1987). AIDS screening, confidentiality, and the duty to warn. *American Journal of Public Health, 77,* 361–366.
24. Kleinman, I. (1987). Transmission of human immunodeficiency virus: Ethical considerations and practical recommendations. *Canadian Medical Association Journal, 137,* 597–599.
25. Fleisher, S. M. (1980). The law and basic public health activities. In M. Roemer & McKray (Eds.), *Law and health policy: Issues and trends.* Westport, CT: Greenwood Press.
26. Forrow, L., Wartman, S. A., & Brock, D. W. (1988). Science, ethics, and the making of clinical decisions: Implications for risk factor intervention. *JAMA, 259,* 3161–3167.
27. La Puma, J., Cassel, C. K., & Humphrey, H. (1988). Ethics, economics, and endocarditis. *Archives of Internal Medicine, 148,* 1809–1811.
28. Weil, M. H., Weil, C. J., & Rackow, E. C. (1988). Guide to ethical decision-making for the critically ill: The 3 R's and Q.C. *Critical Care Medicine, 16,* 636–640.
29. Is a living will the way to go? (1987). *U.S. News & World Report, 103*(8), 65.
30. Rizzolo, P. J. (1978). The living will. *Journal of Family Practice, 6,* 881–885.
31. Johnson, A. (1983). A concord in medical ethics. *Annals of Internal Medicine, 49,* 263–264.
32. York, G. Y., Gallarno, R. M., & York, R. O. (1990). Baby Doe regulations and medical judgment. *Social Science and Medicine, 30,* 657–664.
33. Lamerton, R. C. (1973, January 23). The need for hospices. *Nursing Times,* 155–157.
34. Craven, J., & Wald, F. S. (1975). Hospice care for dying patients. *American Journal of Nursing, 75,* 1816–1822.
35. Experts probe issues around hospice care. (1980). *Hospitals, 54,* 63–67.
36. Bonham, G. S., Gochman, D. S., & Burgess, L. (1987). Hospice in transition: Kentucky 1982–85. *American Journal of Public Health, 77,* 1535–1536.
37. Musgrave, C. F. (1987). The ethical implications of hospice care. *Cancer Nursing, 10*(4), 183–189.
38. Fowler, M. D. M. (1988b). Legislation to legalize active euthanasia. *Heart & Lung, 17,* 458–459.
39. Fowler, M. D. M. (1988a). Ethical guidelines. *Heart & Lung, 17,* 103–104.
40. President's Commission for the Study of Ethical Problems in Medicine. (1983). *Deciding to forego life-sustaining treatment.* Washington, DC: Government Printing Office.
41. Reckling, J. A. B. (1989). Abandonment of patients by home health nursing agencies: An ethical analysis of the dilemma. *Advances in Nursing Science, 11*(3), 70–81.
42. Walters, L. (1988). Ethical issues in the prevention and treatment of HIV infection and AIDS. *Science, 239,* 597–603.
43. Freedman, B. (1988, April/May). Health professions, codes, and the right to refuse to treat HIV-infectious patients. *Hastings Center Report,* 20–25.

RECOMMENDED READINGS

Cunningham, N., & Hutchinson, S. (1990). Myths in health care ethics. *Image: Journal of Nursing Scholarship, 22*, 235–238.

Explores several misconceptions regarding ethical behavior in health care including the relationship of ethics to science, the predominance of values, and the consistency in ethical thinking.

Huggins, E. A., & Scalzi, C. C. (1988). Limitations and alternatives: Ethical practice theory in nursing. *Advances in Nursing Science, 10*(4), 43–47.

Discusses the limitations of various theories of moral development as frameworks for studying ethical decision making in nursing.

Reckling, J. A. B. (1989). Abandonment of patients by home health nursing agencies: An ethical analysis of the dilemma. *Advances in Nursing Science, 11*(3), 70–80.

Examines the ethical dilemma of discontinuing home nursing services to clients who can no longer pay for them. Addresses the responsibility of nurses in such situations.

Reinhardt, U. E. (1990). Rationing the health-care surplus: An American tragedy. In P. R. Lee & C. L. Estes (Eds.), *The nation's health.* (3rd ed.) (pp. 104–111). Boston: Jones and Bartlett.

Addresses the ethical implications of rationing health-care services in a time of scarce resources. Describes notions of a right to health care and sources of resistance to that position.

Sciegaj, M., Wade, T. E., Dever, G. E. A., & Alley, J. W. (1987). A framework for applying ethical theory to public health practice. *Family and Community Health, 10*(1), 15–23.

Describes an ethical model used to make resource allocation decisions for the State of Georgia. Addresses the ethical implications of resource allocation.

Thomasma, D. C. (1989). Ethics and professional practice in oncology. *Seminars in Oncology Nursing, 5*(2), 89–94.

Identifies ethical issues related to care of clients with cancer and presents the nursing implications of each issue.

Thompson, I. E. (1987). Fundamental ethical principles in health care. *British Medical Journal, 295*, 1461–1465.

Discusses the grounds for justifying a set of fundamental ethical principles that apply to all areas of health care, rather than discrete branches of ethics related to medicine, nursing, and so on.

Weil, M. H., Weil, C. J., & Rackow, E. C. (1988). Guide to ethical decision-making for the critically ill: The three R's and Q.C. *Critical Care Medicine, 16*, 636–640.

Presents a model to guide decisions on the use of medical technology for critically ill clients. Components of the model address questions of whether proposed measures are rational, redeeming, and respectful as well as concepts of quality of life and cost-effectiveness.

Wikler, D. (1987). Who should be blamed for being sick? *Health Education Quarterly, 14*(1), 11–25.

Sets forth the ethical implications of assigning personal responsibility for health to the individual client and the tendency to "blame the victim" when social and environmental factors may be the underlying causes of poor health.

CHAPTER 15

Cultural Influences on Community Health

KEY TERMS

cultural accommodation
cultural blindness
cultural conflict
cultural imposition
cultural pluralism
cultural sensitivity
cultural shock
culture
ethnicity
ethnocentrism
expressive functions
instrumental functions
race
stereotyping

The health status of individuals, families, and communities is the product of interaction between the client and the environment. One significant component of the environment that has considerable influence on clients' health is culture. Culture is a pervasive social phenomenon that colors attitudes, values, and beliefs about the world, and guides interactions with that world. Culture directs most human behavior, including health-related behavior. For this reason, it is particularly important for community health nurses to consider their clients' cultural backgrounds in formulating care to meet health needs.

Unfortunately, community health nurses may not always feel adequately prepared to deal with the health needs of clients from other cultures. One study indicated that many community health nurses do not feel confident of their abilities to care for a culturally diverse clientele.[1] The nurses surveyed felt least confident in providing care for Southeast Asians and most confident in caring for blacks. Levels of confidence in caring for Latinos of Puerto Rican origin were found to be in the intermediate range. These community health nurses were most knowledgeable about the appropriate use of an interpreter and less knowledgeable about beliefs related to respect, authority, and modesty and about health beliefs and practices of clients from other cultures. These findings suggest the need for cross-cultural content in basic nursing education and for the inclusion of this content in community health nursing education.

(*continued*)

LEARNING OBJECTIVES

After reading this chapter you should be able to:

- Differentiate among culture, race, and ethnicity.
- Identify six characteristics common to all cultures.
- Describe at least four potential negative responses of nurses to people from other cultures.
- Identify six characteristics common to all cultures.
- Describe four principles of cultural assessment.
- Identify three considerations in assessing the human biological component of a culture.
- Identify at least five aspects of the environment to be considered in a cultural assessment.
- Describe at least three life events to be considered in a cultural assessment.
- Describe at least three similarities and four differences between folk and scientific health-care systems.
- Describe at least four considerations in assessing the influence of folk health-care systems.

RACE, CULTURE, AND ETHNICITY

Three terms that are frequently, and inaccurately, used synonymously in discussions of client groups are "race," "culture," and "ethnicity." ***Race*** is an attribute that allows classification of human beings on the basis of certain biological characteristics such as the color of skin, eyes, or hair or features such as hair texture or the shape of the eyes, nose, lips, and so on. Such distinctions, however, are unreliable as scientific classifications.[2] A case in point is the racial admixture found among Latinos, whose forebears may have included Caucasians, Indians, blacks, and Asians. Racial distinctions are useful primarily for political and socioeconomic categorization.

Culture, according to one observer, is the shared values, beliefs and practices that guide thinking and action among a particular group of people.[3] Or, according to another, cultures are "systems of shared beliefs and orientations unique to groups."[4] For the purposes of this chapter, ***culture*** is the collection of beliefs, values, and behaviors that permit a group of people to interact effectively with their environment.

A group's culture is unique. The beliefs and behaviors that constitute a particular culture arise from the unique constraints faced by a given group of people in dealing with problems common to all humankind. These unique situational constraints are the source of cultural variation among groups of people. For example, exposure to periodic drought and famine in India may have resulted in the Hindu prohibition on killing cattle.[5] Because the cow was a source of milk and assistance in plowing the farmer's fields, killing and eating the family's only cow in a time of deprivation would decrease the family's chances of long-term survival and also jeopardize the survival of the society. Reinforcing this supposition is the observation that, in areas where droughts and mine were not experienced on a regular basis, the need to protect cattle did not arise. In this instance, the environmental constraints imposed on Hindu society led to the development of a specific cultural practice that ensured society's survival in times of drought or famine.

Ethnicity is the designation by self or others as a member of a distinct population group on the basis of specific national and/or biological characteristics.[2] Members of an ethnic group may or may not share elements of a common culture. For example, many blacks do not adhere to the norms of traditional black culture derived from an African heritage, yet they are considered part of the black ethnic group based on their skin color. Questions of ethnicity arise only when one group of people is identified as different from another group, and "the essence of the concept is one of contrast between two or more groups, not the objective cultural content possessed by one of the groups in and of itself."[2] In other words, culture may contribute to ethnic distinctions among groups, but it is not equivalent to ethnicity.

In this chapter we will explore some of the cultural differences that contribute to ethnic diversity and influence the health status of specific population groups in the United States. In addition to identifying cultural differences, we will investigate their implications for planning, implementing, and evaluating health-care activities in the community health setting.

CHARACTERISTICS OF CULTURE

Although cultures vary among groups, certain identifiable characteristics are common to all cultures. Culture is a universal experience. All people engage in culturally prescribed behavior patterns. Curiously, though, the influence of culture is largely unconscious. Culture encompasses and directs most aspects of life. However, the influence of culture is rarely consciously noted, unless one purposefully undertakes a study of one's one culturally determined behavior. What is more, the culture of any particular group is unique. While several cultures may exhibit certain commonalities, no two cultures, like no two individuals, are exactly alike.

Another characteristic of culture is its stability. Cultural characteristics tend to endure across generations. Culture, however, is neither static nor immutably fixed; it is subject to change. Although the superficial aspects of cultural can change relatively easily, basic cultural values and beliefs change slowly and may provide the basis for strong resistance to change.

Finally, the degree to which an individual adheres to cultural beliefs, values, and customs is affected by many factors. Among these are an individual's educational level, social status, facility with the dominant language, length of exposure to the culture of the larger society, and whether the individual resided in an urban or rural setting in the country of origin.[6] Generally speaking, the higher the individual's educational level and social status and the greater the use of the dominant language, the greater the identification with the culture of the larger society and the less the adherence to subcultural norms. General characteristics of culture are summarized in Box 15–1.

BOX 15–1

Characteristics of Culture

Universality: Culture is a pervasive phenomenon that involves all human populations.

Uniqueness: All cultures are unique and, while there may be similarities between cultural groups, no two cultures are exactly alike.

Stability: Culture is lasting and endures through generations.

Changeability: Culture changes over time. Superficial aspects of culture change more readily than deeply held beliefs and values.

Unconsciousness: Culture directs behavior, but its influence is largely unnoticed.

Variability: The degree of adherence to cultural beliefs, values, and behaviors varies with individual members of the culture and depends upon a variety of factors.

NURSING RESPONSES TO CLIENTS FROM OTHER CULTURES

Community health nurses frequently encounter clients whose cultures differ from their own. The response of nurses to these differences may be either positive or negative. Potentially negative reactions include ethnocentrism, cultural blindness, cultural shock, cultural conflict, cultural imposition, and stereotyping. A positive response on the part of the nurse involves cultural sensitivity.

NEGATIVE RESPONSES

Ethnocentrism is a common response to cultural differences. ***Ethnocentrism*** is a conviction that one's own way of life, values, beliefs, and customs are superior to those of others.[7] Ethnocentric convictions may lead a nurse to ridicule or denigrate the beliefs and behaviors of others, thus impairing his or her ability to accept and work with clients as unique individuals. The community health nurse who ridicules the use of amulets and other objects to ward off evil without attempting to understand the basis for the practice is engaging in ethnocentrism.

Cultural blindness involves ignoring cultural differences between nurse and client.[8] The nurse who is culturally blind behaves as though these differences did not exist. Cultural blindness occurs, for example, when community health nurses engaged in nutrition counseling ignore clients' cultural food preferrences.

Cultural shock occurs when a nurse is only too aware of the cultural differences between his or her background and those of clients.[8] The nurse may be stunned by the differences perceived and, in effect, immobilized until he or she can come to terms with the "shocking" aspects of the alien culture. Cultural shock is frequently experienced by students new to community health nursing who have difficulty overcoming their feelings about homes they consider "dirty." They may be so caught up in their reactions to the dirt that they have difficulty achieving a therapeutic relationship with the client.

Cultural shock is most likely to occur in response

to behaviors approved in one culture that are disapproved in the nurse's own culture. The stronger the taboos against the behavior in the nurse's culture, the greater the shock when that behavior is an accepted practice in another. Cultural shock can also arise from communication difficulties. The nurse may become perplexed and frustrated when familiar words and gestures suddenly acquire unfamiliar meanings.

Cultural shock is a phenomenon that may be experienced by nurses caring for clients from cultures other than their own. But cultural shock can also affect clients who have suddenly found themselves immersed in an unfamiliar setting. Nurses take action when they encounter clients experiencing physiologic shock; the same should be true of nurses who deal with clients experiencing cultural shock. This is difficult, though, when the nurse is in cultural shock as well.

Cultural conflict can also impede a nurse's ability to respond adequately to the needs of clients from other cultures. In ***cultural conflict,*** a nurse is aware of differences between his or her culture and that of the client, and feels threatened by these differences.[8] The nurse may respond by ridiculing the client's beliefs and customs to bolster his or her own personal cultural values. This behavior contrasts with that of the ethnocentric who is truly convinced that his or her cultural beliefs and practices are superior. The nurse experiencing cultural conflict does so precisely because the recognition of cultural differences causes him or her to doubt the validity of personal beliefs and behaviors, doubt that may, in turn, threaten the nurse's self-esteem.

Cultural conflict can be illustrated by the case of an American nurse serving with the Peace Corps in India. Many of the villagers found it hard to accept that the nurse did much of her own housework when they knew she could afford servants. In an extremely class-conscious society whose upper-class members do not engage in menial labor, the idea of doing one's own housework was perceived as a threat to the established order. The villagers were unable to comprehend that most American women do not have servants. They finally reconciled themselves to the nurse's behavior by labeling it "another crazy American habit." Denigration of the nurse's culturally prescribed behavior preserved the villagers' belief in their own behaviors as "correct."

Cultural imposition refers to a nurse's expectation that everyone should conform to his or her own cultural practices, whatever their personal beliefs.[8] This response to cultural differences is an extension of ethnocentrism in that the nurse not only ridicules other practices but also expects them to be abandoned and those of the nurse's culture assumed. The expectation of some community health nurses that everyone who lives in the United States should speak English is an example of cultural imposition.

Stereotyping is the belief that members of a particular cultural group will conform to some cultural pattern associated with that group. Stereotypes may have their basis in fact or fiction. But, even when the stereotypical notion conforms to an actual cultural norm, expectations that all members of a group will conform to that norm can be as detrimental to nurse/client interactions as ignoring cultural differences. Stereotypes are the means people use to avoid dealing with each other as individuals.[9] Nursing, as a profession, maintains a belief in the uniqueness of the individual. Nurses who engage in stereotyping are not viewing clients as individuals but as "copies" of the typical member of a cultural group.

Stereotyping arises from three common behaviors.[10] The first of these is hasty generalization based on limited observation and understanding. For example, the community health nurse who assumes that all Mexican Americans engage in the same behaviors that his or her Mexican American friends do is generalizing inappropriately. The nurse's exposure to Mexican American culture has been too limited to make such a broad generalization.

The second source of stereotypes is generalization from nontypical subgroups to the whole culture. For example, many people base their concept of Asian Indian culture on the beliefs and behaviors exhibited by students who come to the United States to study. These students usually come from upper-class Indian families living in large cities. Their behavior, in many respects, is not typical of Indian culture as a whole, although they retain much of their cultural heritage.

Finally, stereotyping may result from failure to concede the possibility of variation and change within a particular culture. As noted earlier, not every member of a group will display the same behaviors. Also, culture is stable, not static. Cultures change, albeit slowly, and any member of a cultural group is apt to display variations in values, beliefs, and behaviors based on his or her position relative to those changes. Generally speaking, younger members of a group and those experiencing the most contact with the culture of the larger society will most likely exhibit changes from traditional beliefs and behaviors.

Nurses need to be familiar with the various dimensions of their clients' cultures and the influence of culture on health. However, they must also consider the unique qualities of each individual, family, or group. The nurse who ascertains the degree to which a client engages in typical cultural behaviors will tend to avoid the pitfall of stereotyping.

CULTURAL SENSITIVITY

The negative responses to people of other cultures described above are normal responses when one is faced with a culture different from one's own. These responses, however, interfere with a community health nurse's ability to promote the health of people from other cultural groups. Most nurses learn to overcome negative responses to clients of different cultural backgrounds. Eventually, most nurses recognize the existence of cultural diversity among clients and use their knowledge of these differences to develop culturally sensitive interventions designed to meet their client's health needs. ***Cultural sensitivity*** is an awareness on the part of care-givers of the significance of cultural factors in health and illness. Cultural sensitivity is a prerequisite for individualized, holistic health care. The culturally sensitive community health nurse recognizes and accepts the variety of cultural behavior patterns displayed by clients. He or she responds to this variation through ***cultural accommodation,*** the modification of health-care delivery in keeping with the client's cultural background.[8]

Several arguments have been advanced in favor of culturally sensitive nursing practice. If the goal of nursing is service to society, then nurses must understand the characteristics of the society in which they live and work. Extending this argument, some nursing writers have contended that it is the nurse's responsibility to create a health-care environment as similar as possible to the client's living environment.[11] To do so, the community health nurse must understand the client's culture as part of that environment. Finally, cultural differences are least detrimental to achieving health-care goals when they are understood. Community health nurses will make greater headway in promoting clients' health if their interventions are based on an understanding of clients' cultural backgrounds. Culturally consonant health care may serve to enhance client participation in behaviors designed to foster health.

Cultural sensitivity is characterized by several identifiable features.[12] The first of these is respect for people as unique individuals and respect for their culture as one factor contributing to their uniqueness. The culturally sensitive nurse does not expect all persons to conform to the majority culture. Nor does the nurse expect all members of one cultural group to behave in exactly the same way. He or she avoids stereotyping by gathering information relative to the specific culture and then assessing the individual client's degree of conformity to cultural beliefs and practices.

The second aspect of cultural sensitivity is an awareness that ethnic or cultural groups have culturally prescribed beliefs and practices related to health. Health and illness are defined culturally, as are practices that promote health and prevent or cure illness. Cultures also vary in their attitude toward and priority placed on health. The community health nurse who is sensitive to the implications of cultural health beliefs and attitudes will realize that health may not be viewed as a high priority in some situations.

A third feature of cultural sensitivity involves modification of nursing care to incorporate folk health practices whenever possible. Finally, cultural sensitivity is characterized by an ability on the part of the nurse to act as an advocate for persons of other cultural groups who are denied adequate care.

As noted earlier, community health nurses may respond positively or negatively to clients from cultures that differ from their own. Negative responses impair the nurse's ability to interact effectively with clients, whereas the positive response of cultural sensitivity enhances the nurse's ability to intervene effectively to meet client needs. Potential responses to clients from other cultures are summarized in Box 15–2.

RELATIONSHIPS BETWEEN CULTURE AND HEALTH

Culture has both direct and indirect effects on a client's health. Direct effects stem from specific culturally prescribed practices related to diet and food or to health and illness. For example, all cultures have prescribed practices intended to promote health and prevent illness or to restore health when illness occurs. Similarly, all cultures have particular dietary practices that contribute to the nutritional status and, thereby, to the health status of their members.

Culture also affects health indirectly. These indirect effects result from cultural definitions of health and illness, acceptability of health-care programs and professionals, and cultural influences on compliance with suggested health or illness regimens. Cultural definitions of health and illness determine what kinds of health problems are considered worthy of attention and what conditions are likely to be disregarded. If, for example, certain behaviors that are perceived as evidence of mental illness by the larger society are considered normal in the client's culture, then the client is unlikely to take any action to deal with the problem. Similarly, minor illnesses may be ignored if health is defined in terms of one's ability to work or to perform other social roles. In general, people are likely to disregard any type of condition that is not

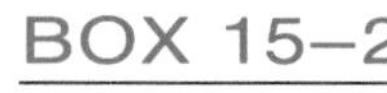

BOX 15–2

Positive and Negative Responses to Clients from Other Cultures

POSITIVE RESPONSE

Cultural sensitivity: recognition of the significance of cultural factors in health and illness, characterized by:

- Respect for people as unique individuals and for cultural variables as one measure of uniqueness
- Recognition and acceptance of a variety of cultural beliefs and behaviors and their implications for health
- Modification of health-care delivery in light of cultural factors
- Advocacy for clients from other cultural groups

NEGATIVE RESPONSES

Ethnocentrism: belief that one's own culture is superior to that of others

Cultural blindness: failure to recognize cultural differences

Cultural shock: immobilization due to perceptions of overwhelming cultural differences

Cultural conflict: ridicule of cultural beliefs and practices of others because of perceived threat to one's own beliefs

Cultural imposition: belief that everyone should conform to the dominant culture

Stereotyping: belief that all members of a cultural group will conform to a typical set of real or perceived beliefs and behaviors

defined as illness in their own culture. This cultural propensity can lead to serious health consequences.

Cultural factors may also determine the acceptability of both health programs and health providers. For example, cultures that eschew scientific medicine in favor of healing based on faith in God may view immunization programs as inimical to their beliefs. In other cultures, health-care providers may be considered lower-class persons not to be associated with, effectively preventing people from taking advantage of many health opportunities. For example, nursing is considered a lower-class occupation in India, and nurses have little opportunity to influence the health of their clients for the better because of their low social status.

Finally, cultural factors often determine whether clients will comply with recommendations when they do seek professional help. If the recommendations of health-care providers are too far removed from normal cultural practices in a given situation, the client is unlikely to comply with those recommendations. For example, a community health nurse may suggest reducing the caloric intake of an infant who is overweight. If the mother's culturally derived perception is that a fat baby is a healthy baby, she is unlikely to follow the nurse's suggestions.

SELECTED CULTURAL GROUPS IN THE UNITED STATES

American society is distinguished by its ***cultural pluralism,*** the simultaneous existence of many cultures within the larger society. The American subcultural groups to be examined here include Native Americans, Asian Americans, Black Americans, American Latinos, and Appalachian Americans.

NATIVE AMERICANS

According to the 1980 census, approximately 1.5 million people were listed as American Indian, Eskimo, or Aleut, comprising the group designated as Native Americans.[13] This figure represents a substantial increase from just over 333,000 persons of Native American descent in 1940.[14] American Indian tribes are further classified by the region of the country in which they originated (Plains, Southwestern, etc.) or by their traditional staple food (buffalo, carribou, etc.).[15]

Over half of the Native American population is located in the Pacific and Mountain regions of the western United States. However, there is no state in which persons of Native American origin are not found.[16] Today, approximately 70 percent of Native Americans are found in urban areas, compared to only 8 percent in 1940.[14]

It is difficult to generalize regarding the Native American cultural group. Each of the approximately 400 tribes in the United States has its own unique culture, and health beliefs and practices vary widely from tribe to tribe.[17] Members of each tribe consider themselves a people distinct from those of other tribes, and the designation "Native American" is assigned by the larger culture to those individuals descended from the peoples inhabiting the American continents when European settlers first arrived. There are, however, certain commonalities among these subcultural groups. Some of these commonalities, as well as some distinct differences, will be addressed later in this chapter.

ASIAN AMERICANS

Persons of Asian or Pacific Island descent comprised 1.5 percent of the total U.S. population at the time of the 1980 census. This figure amounts to 3.7 million people.[13] By 2010, this group is expected to comprise more than 12 percent of the population.[2] Like Native Americans, Asians are dispersed among all 50 states and the District of Columbia. Approximately two-thirds, however, reside in the West.[16]

Nurses working with Asian clients will confront a wide diversity of cultures. While there are some commonalities, each nationality has its own unique culture. The classification "Asian" includes such diverse peoples as Chinese, Japanese, Filipinos, Laotians, Vietnamese, and Koreans. Within each group there are three subgroups exhibiting cultural differences.[7] The first group consists of persons born in Asia who migrated to the United States several years ago. Members of the second group include relatively new arrivals, while the third group is composed of first- and second-generation Asian-Americans born in the United States. Many of the second group came from parts of Asia in which there has been some exposure to Western medicine (more in some countries than others). The third group tends to be oriented to Western health care but may engage in a variety of folk health practices as well.

In reflecting on these categories of Asian immigrants, however, one must keep in mind the change in Asian arrivals in recent years. Previous arrivals who now have American-born children usually emigrated voluntarily. They came to the United States with certain goals and expectations. More recent arrivals, particularly from Southeast Asia, tend to be refugees, not immigrants.[18] Rather than *coming* to this country by choice, many of them are *fleeing from* their homeland out of necessity. This fact may profoundly affect their health, and most particularly their mental health.

The ability of these new arrivals to adapt to a new way of life is further hampered by loss of worldly possessions and, in many cases, by loss of family members and friends. These individuals may have lived for protracted periods of time in a state of uncertainty regarding their very survival. The behavior resulting from this uncertainty has been labeled "survival syndrome," and is characterized by a wait-and-see attitude and by an unwillingness to make decisions.[18] All of these factors complicate the multiple health problems a community health nurse may encounter working with these new immigrants.

By September 1986, over 800,000 refugees from Southeast Asia had entered the United States. Not quite two-thirds of these refugees are Vietnamese, while Laotians and Cambodians constitute 17 percent and 20 percent of the refugee group respectively.[19] While the total Asian population is more widely distributed throughout the United States, almost half of the Southeast Asian refugee group is concentrated in 13 western states.[20] Like the Native American population, the majority of Asians in the United States are found in urban areas.

BLACK AMERICANS

Approximately 12 percent of the American population is black; this amounts to almost 29 million people spread across the United States.[13] The percentage of black Americans in the population is expected to increase to nearly 15 percent by the year 2010.[2] The states with the highest black populations include New York and California, and 16 states have a black population of a million or more. In the South, black Americans are a large percentage of the population (36 percent in Mississippi, 31 percent in South Carolina, and 30 percent in Louisiana). The majority of black Americans (more than 80 percent) live in metropolitan areas, particularly New York, Chicago, Los Angeles, and Philadelphia.

Black Americans no more subscribe to one set of cultural beliefs and practices than do Native Americans or Asians. Within the black population, subcultural groups include descendants of former slaves brought from Africa as well as Black Muslims and persons of cultural heritages from Trinidad, Jamaica, and other parts of the world.

AMERICAN LATINOS

As of 1987, the Latino population in the United States included 18.7 million persons.[13] By the year 2000, Latinos are expected to represent the largest minority group in the United States.[21] About half of the Latino population resides in the West. One-third lives in California, with large numbers of Latinos also found in Texas, New York, and Florida.[22]

People of Spanish origin are a culturally diverse group who usually refer to themselves as "Latino" rather than "Hispanic." The Latino population consists of persons whose families have come from Mexico, Cuba, Puerto Rico, Chile, El Salvador, Guatemala, Nicaragua, and the Dominican Republic.[23] Two characteristics shared by members of these culturally diverse groups are a heritage of Spanish conquest and use of Spanish as the primary language. Even these features, however, are not uniform because Spanish language and culture have been blended with aspects of native languages and cultures found among each conquered people.

APPALACHIAN AMERICANS

Census figures do not delineate members of the Appalachian cultural group. Because of their lack of visibility as an identifiable ethnic group, Appalachians have been neglected as a minority culture.[24] As defined by the federal government in the Appalachian Regional Act of 1965, Appalachia consists of 195,000 square miles of territory in 397 counties, within 13 states: Alabama, Georgia, Kentucky, Maryland, Mississippi, New York, North and South Carolina, Ohio, Pennsylvania, Tennessee, Virginia, and all of West Virginia. There are 24 million people in Appalachia, including 6 million in the 80,000 square miles of the poorer Southern Appalachian Region comprised of 190 counties in Alabama, Georgia, Kentucky, North Carolina, Tennessee, Virginia, and West Virginia.[25] Appalachians, as a cultural group, are the people from this region of the country who adhere to a cultural blend derived from the American Indian tribes and the original Scots-Presbyterian settlers of the area.

Obviously nurses working in Appalachia should be familiar with the local culture. However, nurses are not the only ones for whom a study of Appalachian culture is appropriate. Because of the lack of economic opportunity, particularly in Southern Appalachia, many Appalachians are relocating in areas where jobs are available. Between 1950 and 1977, 3.5 million Appalachians migrated to major urban areas such as Cleveland, Detroit, Cincinnati, Pittsburgh, and Chicago.[24]

THE EPIDEMIOLOGIC PREVENTION PROCESS MODEL AND CULTURAL INFLUENCES ON HEALTH

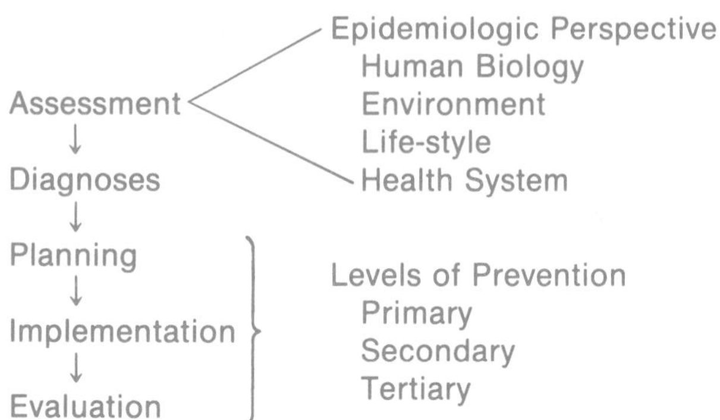

The epidemiologic prevention process model can be used as a framework for exploring other cultures as well as for organizing care for clients from specific cultural groups. Using the model, the community health nurse examines racial, ethnic, and cultural factors that influence clients' health. The nurse then uses the model to design culturally sensitive interventions to meet the needs of specific clients.

ASSESSING RACIAL, CULTURAL, AND ETHNIC FACTORS INFLUENCING HEALTH

The first task in working with clients from other cultures is obtaining information about the client. Community health nurses can use Dever's epidemiologic perspective to collect, organize, and analyze information about cultures frequently encountered in their practice. Prior to examining some of the human biological, environmental, life-style, and health system factors influencing the five cultural groups discussed in this chapter, several general principles involved in the study of another culture will be explored.

PRINCIPLES OF CULTURAL ASSESSMENT

Four basic principles should guide nurses engaged in the study of other cultures. First, view all cultures in the context in which they developed. As noted earlier, cultural practices arise out of a need to meet common human problems in a particular human setting. That setting must be considered in exploring other cultures.

Second, examine the underlying premise of culturally determined behavior. What was the intended purpose for the behavior when it originated? Does the behavior still fulfill this purpose? When one knows the underlying reason for behaviors that seem strange to an outsider, such behaviors may not seem quite so strange after all. The nurse should also examine the meaning of the behavior in the cultural context. The meaning of certain behaviors from the perspective of the nurse's culture may be very different from the behavior's meaning in the context of the client's culture. For example, resistance to having one's head shaved for a cranial surgical procedure may be interpreted as vanity from the nurse's perspective. However, when the nurse understands that some clients view the head as the home of the soul, such resistance is more understandable.

Finally, recognize the existence of intracultural variation. Not every member of any given cultural group will display all of the typical cultural behaviors. There may be several subgroups within one cultural group with different behavior patterns. Or, individual clients may be more or less acculturated to the larger society. When the nurse expects to find intracultural variation, he or she will tend to avoid stereotyping and responding to clients as if they were typical representatives of their cultural group. Principles of cultural assessment are summarized in Box 15–3.

OBTAINING INFORMATION ABOUT OTHER CULTURES

How does one become knowledgeable of other cultures? Perhaps the easiest way to begin a study of another culture is to read literature related to that culture. In reading, the community health nurse should examine the qualifications of the authors writing about cultural minorities. He or she should determine whether the book or article is based on empirical data derived from research, on personal experience with a particular culture, or on stereotypes.

A second means of acquainting oneself with another culture is to interview colleagues who are members of that culture. Explore with them their concepts of health, illness, and attitudes and practices affecting health. Discover how these may differ from those held by previous generations or other members of their family. The health professional, by virtue of his or her knowledge of health matters, is likely to have achieved a greater degree of acculturation and conformity with the culture of the larger society with respect to health practices than nonprofessionals from the same group. However, these individuals remain a valid source of information regarding cultural health beliefs and practices.

One of the best ways to become familiar with a particular culture is to spend time living within it. This approach is not always feasible, however. Alternatives include home visits to families within the group to observe daily living in the cultural context or questioning clients and families regarding health-related beliefs and practices. Another possible approach is observation of activities and interactions at health facilities and community or religious functions.

When assessing a culture directly, the community health nurse should follow a few useful guidelines.[26] First, look and listen before asking questions or taking action. Observation aids in asking pertinent and timely questions and forestalls actions that may be inappropriate. Second, explore how the group feels about being studied. Explain that your reasons for studying the culture are practical and do not arise out of idle curiosity. Third, discover any special protocols. Should one speak to a local leader before beginning to observe a group? Is there a council or leadership group who should grant permission for participation in group activities? Fourth, foster human relations, putting them before the need to obtain information. Information will not assist the nurse to provide care if he or she alienates members of the group. Social amenities are very important in many cultures and should be attended to before the "business" of information gathering begins in earnest. In fact, information about social amenities is part of the data needed by the nurse.

Many people, in exploring another culture, look for differences from the culture of the larger society. However, the nurse should also look for cultural similarities that can be used as a foundation in aiding clients to accept and use health-care services. In addition to recognizing cultural similarities and differences, the nurse should accept cultural differences as normal rather than bizarre or strange.

BOX 15–3

Principles of Cultural Assessment

- View all cultures in the context in which they developed.
- Examine underlying premises for culturally determined beliefs and behaviors.
- Interpret the meaning and purpose of behavior in the context of the specific culture.
- Recognize the potential for intracultural variation.

Locate reliable informants who are conversant with the culture. Some suggested informants are group leaders and respected residents, those considered wise, "ordinary" group members, and clients. Critics of the traditional aspects of the culture may also be interviewed to provide a balanced picture.

Participate as well as observe. The nurse must assess each situation as it occurs to determine whether participation or observation is the more appropriate activity. Participation conveys an openness to cultural differences and a willingness to engage in culturally prescribed activities rather than ridicule them. However, there may be some activities that are closed to outsiders in which the community health nurse's participation would not be welcomed.

When exploring another culture, the nurse should also consider the feelings of group members about questions asked. The nurse should ascertain what types of questions are acceptable or offensive in a particular culture. For example, Americans in India find it difficult to adjust to frequent questions about their salary, how much their clothes cost, and so on. Such questions are perfectly acceptable in India, but considered impolite or "nosy" in the United States.

A little forethought as to the phrasing and timing of questions can prevent a serious faux pas. Ask questions positively without implying value judgments. For example, saying "I notice you put garlic on a string around the baby's neck; can you tell me what it's used for?" is far more acceptable than saying, "Why in the world do you hang that smelly garlic around the baby's neck?"

Nurses might ask the same questions of themselves and gauge their own emotional reaction to the questions.[26] A nurse can also try out questions on colleagues who are members of the culture being explored. Suggestions for modes of cultural exploration discussed here are summarized in Box 15–4.

BOX 15–4

Modes of Cultural Exploration

- Review the existing literature on beliefs, values, and behaviors of specific cultural groups.
- Interview colleagues who are members of the cultural group in question.
- Immerse oneself in the culture to be studied.
- Observe members of specific cultural groups.
- Interview members of cultural groups studied, particularly group leaders.
- Interview other informants conversant with the culture.

COMPONENTS OF CULTURAL ASSESSMENT

To gain knowledge of those aspects of culture most relevant to health and health care, nurses need to organize the collection of data. The epidemiologic prevention process model provides a framework for organizing data collection related to the human biological, environmental, life-style, and health system aspects of culture.

HUMAN BIOLOGY

It is important to keep in mind that a thorough assessment of persons from other ethnic and cultural groups should not focus exclusively on social factors or culturally determined behaviors. Differences related to genetic inheritance and physiologic function must be considered as well.

GENETIC INHERITANCE

Among the five cultural groups presented in this chapter, some physical differences deriving from genetic inheritance have implications for nursing.[27] For example, black youngsters tend to exceed standard heights and weights at all ages, whereas Asians are usually smaller. Groups also differ in rates of maturation, with blacks and Asians reaching puberty earlier than Caucasians. The dry ear wax normal in Asian or Native American clients is best dealt with using irrigation techniques while the wet wax common in blacks and Caucasians is more appropriately removed with a curette.

Epicanthic folds are commonly seen among Asians, while lumbar lordosis is a common normal finding in black children. The size, number, and shape of teeth also differ among ethnic groups. Differences in skin pigmentation of some groups can hinder assessment of changes in skin coloration unless one recognizes variations in normal coloration for a particular group. Hair texture differences, food intolerance, and differences in drug metabolism may necessitate changes in approaches to physical care and require knowledge of such variations on the part of the nurse. For example, milk is not always considered a suitable source of protein for blacks and some Asians owing to the relatively high incidence of lactose intolerance in these groups.[7,28] Community health nurses working with these clients would suggest other sources of protein in place of milk. Differences exist in normal lab values among different cultural groups. For example, normal hematocrit levels are slightly lower for black clients than for Caucasians.

Genetic inheritance may also play a part in the types of health problems commonly seen in members of some ethnic and cultural groups. For example, diabetes is a common problem in many Native American tribes, whereas sickle cell disease is a genetically transmitted disease particularly prevalent among African Americans.

PHYSIOLOGIC FUNCTION

Physiologic function is the second aspect of human biology considered in the study of another culture. Three categories of physiologic considerations need to be addressed. These include attitudes toward body parts and physiologic functions as well as folk and scientific designations of physical illness commonly encountered in the particular group.

Attitudes to Body Parts and Physiologic Functions

The physical differences described previously may lead to different cultural attitudes and approaches to physiologic function in different cultures. Care of one's body and attention to basic physiologic functions will differ from one group to another. One area that the nurse will want to explore includes approaches to hygiene. Questions that might be asked include how and when group members bathe and ways in which hair, skin, and teeth are cared for.

Special significance may be attached to certain body parts in a particular culture. For instance, in some cultures, the head is considered sacred and is to be treated with respect. In these cultures, bumping someone's head is considered an insult. Among many Vietnamese, for example, touching the head is thought to cause loss of the soul.[29]

In many cultures, certain body parts are believed to be responsible for functions and conditions that are not in accordance with scientific knowledge of physiology. In many Asian folk medicine systems, for example, the heart is thought to be responsible for insomnia, dreams, forgetfulness, insanity, and delirium. The kidneys, on the other hand, are believed to control water, birth, development, reproduction, and maturation.[30] Beliefs and attitudes to body parts and physiologic function may influence acceptance of such scientific medical procedures as transfusions, venipuncture, transplantation, and autopsy.[31]

Of course, exposure of certain body parts is appropriate in some cultures and not in others. In some regions of the world, neither men nor women cover their breasts, yet for the U.S. female, exposing the breasts is generally unacceptable. In India, uncovering the shoulders and upper arms is considered indecent.

Differences also exist between cultures in terms of what body parts may appropriately be touched and who may touch them. For example, among the Zuni of New Mexico it is inappropriate to view or touch the genitals at certain times, even for health-care purposes.[32] There may be restrictions on touching between members of the opposite sex or members of the same sex. For instance, it would be unusual for adult members of the same sex to hold hands or to kiss in public in the United States. In other cultures, same-sex touching or kissing may be perfectly acceptable, while similar behavior by members of the opposite sex are thought to be inappropriate.[33]

Another consideration to be addressed relative to physiologic function is that of privacy. Cultures differ in terms of what physiologic functions may be performed in public and those for which privacy is required. For example, American tourists are frequently shocked by urination or defecation in public that is sometimes commonplace in many undeveloped countries. Latinos, also, exhibit a great deal of modesty regarding urination and defecation as well as bathing and dressing.[31] Similarly, people from other cultural groups may have difficulty accepting the presence of the husband or father during delivery. In some cultures, children are allowed or even encouraged to observe a delivery, while in others, birth is not an appropriate event for them to witness.

In exploring cultural attitudes to physiologic function, the nurse may also need to determine whether there are periods of time during which individuals are considered ritually unclean. In many cultures, for example, postpartum or menstruating women are considered unclean, and their activities and interactions with others are restricted.

Recognized Folk Illnesses

Health is an area of concern to most people, and there are few cultural groups that do not have some systematized way of dealing with illness. Many folk cultures have a unique method of classifying illnesses that aids in their identification and their treatment within the culture. Of the cultural groups presented in this chapter, Appalachians, blacks, and Latinos have such systems that include specific recognized folk illnesses.

Black and Appalachian folk medicine systems recognize a number of similar conditions related to the character of the blood. Among these are high blood, low blood, thin blood, bad blood, and poison blood. "High blood" refers to an "excess" of blood in the body, and is not related to a medical diagnosis of high blood pressure. High blood is thought to result from the ingestion of rich food, particularly red meat. Treatment includes ingesting lemon juice, vinegar, Epsom salts, or other "astringents" that are thought to open the pores and allow excess blood to be "sweated" out.[29,34]

"Low blood" is believed to be a condition of "too little" blood in the body and is comparable to anemia. Its perceived cause may include too vigorous treatment for "high blood," too many astringent foods, or prolonged use of medications for hypertension. Treatment usually includes decreasing astringents and increasing the intake of red meat. Other forms of treatment for low blood involve the principle of imitative magic (for example, ingesting something the color of blood such as beets, wine, grape juice, liver, blood sausage, blood from a freshly slaughtered animal, or water in which a nail has rusted).[34]

"Thin blood" describes a supposed increased susceptibility to illness. It is believed that thin blood can be prevented by the use of warm clothing and by staying indoors during cold weather. "Bad blood" refers to sexually transmitted disease and is believed to be acquired through sexual promiscuity. This belief may be totally unrelated to scientific concepts of bacteriologic infection. In some places, for example, it is thought that a woman who has intercourse with seven men will acquire bad blood whether or not her partners are infected.[34]

The term "poison blood" may refer to septicemia, but may also indicate illness due to witchcraft. Rashes are thought to be indicative of impurities in the blood rising to the surface. Among both Appalachian and black clients, catnip tea is given to newborns to drive out impurities acquired in utero. Impurities of the blood may also be treated by purging with sulfur and molasses, castor oil, or any number of other purgatives and cathartics. Spring is a time when purging commonly is recommended, as impurities that have lain dormant throughout the winter are thought to rise with the coming of spring.[34]

Members of Latino cultures also recognize a number of specific conditions unknown to science. These include *susto, empacho, caida de mollera, mal de ojo* (or *mal ojo*), *mal puesta, serena, coraje, espanto, pujos,* and *ataque*.

Susto is a condition believed to be caused by magical fright and loss of the soul. It may be due to an inability to cope with a situation, a sudden surprise, danger, or terror. Symptoms include nervousness, sleeplessness, and loss of appetite.[35] Prevention involves avoiding excitement, alertness for danger, and drinking water. Diagnosis and treatment occur in four stages.[36] In the first stage, the client describes his or her symptoms, after which bedrest is recommended. A more detailed description of the event causing the condition is obtained as the second stage is entered. The third stage focuses on draining away the illness and returning the soul. This stage may involve calling the person's name and begging the soul to return, reciting the Apostles' Creed, confessing sin or discussing the victim's life, or sweeping the recumbent body of the victim with the branches of a sweet pepper tree. The final stage of intervention is the gradual return of the client to his or her usual social role. Because of their believed innate weakness, women and children are thought to be highly susceptible to *susto*.

Empacho is believed to be caused by a bolus of undigested food adhering to the walls of the stomach or intestine. It may result if one is forced to eat when one does not want to or when one is upset or from eating too much rice, potatoes, or banana. Common symptoms include stomach pain, diarrhea, vomiting, and anorexia. Additional symptoms include thirst and abdominal swelling.[35] Treatment can include massaging the abdomen or back, or administering a laxative.[37] Other treatments include increasing fluid intake, slapping the skin in the costovertebral angle, or ingesting a "cold metal" (for example, quicksilver) followed by a "hot" laxative such as castor oil. Prevention is accomplished by means of a periodic purge of the gastrointestinal system.[38]

Caida de mollera or "fallen fontanel" is a condition of young infants believed to result from being bounced too vigorously, from head trauma, or from rapid or rough removal of a nipple from the baby's mouth. This condition is characterized by a depressed fontanel, vomiting, diarrhea, irritability, and an inability to suck. It may be treated by exerting pressure on the infant's palate to push the fontanel back in place, by herb teas, by application of a poultice of egg white, rue, and other herbs to the fontanel, or by holding the infant by the ankles and immersing the fontanel three times in a pan of water.[35]

Mal de ojo or "evil eye" is believed to be caused when one either admires a child or envies its parents and does not touch the child. Generally, the result of *mal de ojo* is unintended. *Mal de ojo* is characterized by constant crying, fever, diarrhea, vomiting, and irritability. Prevention by means of touching a child one admires is encouraged. Treatment involves passing a whole egg over the child's body or rubbing the egg on the body while reciting prayers. The egg is then broken and left in a bowl under the head of the child's bed all night to draw out the fever. Another approach is the use of prayer and oil massage.[35]

Mal puesto refers to conditions caused and cured by magic. The usual precursor to a case of *mal puesto* is believed to be a problem in one of three types of social relationships: a lovers' quarrel, unrequited love, or envy of one's good fortune by another.[38] *Mal puesto* may be characterized by unusual patterns of behavior, emotional lability, or convulsions. Treatment consists of magical intervention by a *brujo* (witch) or *curandero* (healer), and varies with the type of hex involved.[37]

Serena or "draft" is a condition in which dampness or evil spirits cause symptoms of an upper respiratory infection.[39] *Coraje* or "rage" is characterized by psychomotor hyperactivity, screaming, crying, and yelling believed to result from an emotional response to a particular situation, while *espanto* is severe fright after witnessing supernatural beings or events.[40]

Pujos is characterized by grunting and umbilical protrusion in an infant, and is believed to occur as a result of contact between the infant and a menstruating woman. Treatment involves tying a piece of fabric from the woman's clothing around the infant's waist for three days.[35]

Ataque is a condition recognized by Latinos of Puerto Rican descent. It is characterized by hyperkinetic seizures, aggression, or stupor. *Ataque* may result in response to tension and stress[17] or may be an expression of grief at the death of a loved one.[41]

Common Scientific Medical Diagnoses

In addition to the folk illnesses recognized by some ethnic and cultural groups, the cultural groups explored in this chapter experience a number of health problems diagnosed by the scientific health-care community.

Native Americans. With the coming of white settlers, the health status of Native Americans began to deteriorate because of exposure to new pathogens and to changes in diet and life-style.[42] Although health conditions have improved in recent years, Native Americans are still afflicted by unusually high rates for some health problems. The life-expectancy of the Native American at birth is only 44 years compared to 70 years for the average American.[17] A high unemployment rate, low income, high birth rate, and inadequate housing are some of the factors that contribute to a multitude of health problems.

To a large extent, acculturation to the larger society has been detrimental to Native Americans' health status. A sedentary life-style and a diet high in fat and carbohydrate consisting of foods supplied by government agencies have contributed to increased incidence of obesity, hypertension, heart disease, and diabetes.[43] Heart disease is the leading cause of death among Native Americans.

The overall infant mortality rate among Native Americans is now comparable to that of the general population. Rates for birth trauma and asphyxia, however, are more than double those for the United States, and the rate of fetal alcohol syndrome is six times that of the nation.

Chronic diseases are also prevalent. Fifteen percent of the Native American population over 45 is affected by diabetes, and diabetic death rates are twice those for the general population. End-stage renal disease is encountered nearly three times as often among Native Americans as in the general population. More than half of the end-stage renal disease in Native Americans is due to diabetes, compared to only 27 percent of cases of renal disease in Caucasian clients.[44] These figures suggest that efforts to control diabetes are less than effective in the Native American population. Other frequently encountered chronic diseases include arthritis, diseases of the spine and connective tissue, and chronic obstructive pulmonary disease (COPD).

Mortality from infectious diseases among Native Americans is still twice that of the general population. Meningitis, hepatitis, and sexually transmitted diseases are significant problems.[45] Tuberculosis mortality has been from 2 to 10 times higher for Native Americans in some parts of the country than for Caucasians, blacks, and Latinos. Native American mortality from other infectious respiratory diseases has decreased dramatically (82 percent since 1955), but remains 31 percent higher than national rates.[45] Other infectious diseases causing increased mortality in this group include parasitic infections, pneumonia, and kidney infection.[46] Deaths due to infections, respiratory diseases, neoplasms, and cerebrovascular hemorrhage are of particular concern among Alaskan Natives.[47]

Death is not the only measure of illness in this population, however. The incidence of tuberculosis (TB) is more than four times that of the Caucasian population. Thirty-five percent of those with TB are under 35 years of age. This is an age group for whom preventive chemotherapy is routinely recommended on exposure.[48] The large number of cases affecting those under age 35 indicates that contacts to active cases of tuberculosis are not being adequately followed and that preventive therapy is not being instituted when contacts are identified.

Mental health problems are also prevalent, particularly those related to substance abuse. Alcohol-related mortality is four times that of the nation as a whole, and Native Americans exhibit the greatest prevalence of alcohol-related problems of any ethnic group. Traumatic injury related to alcohol and substance abuse, accidents, and interpersonal violence is a leading cause of death in this population. In fact, trauma accounts for 71 percent of premature mortality among Native Americans in states such as New Mexico. In 1987, the New Mexico motor vehicle fatality rate for young Native American males was nearly four times that of 15- to 24-year-old Caucasians across the nation.[49]

Asian Americans. Health problems are common among Asian Americans as well, and they are complicated by language and cultural barriers. Health problems frequently encountered include tuberculosis, mental illness, malnutrition, and chronic diseases associated with aging. Suicide rates are high among both Southeast Asian refugees[50] and Chinese Americans.

In 1970, the TB rate for Chinese in San Francisco was four times that of the city's general population.[51] Tuberculosis continues to be a serious problem, particularly among Southeast Asians. The incidence of TB among Southeast Asian refugees is 8.7 times higher than for the Caucasian population of the United States. As is true among Native Americans, over half of those with TB among this group are under 35 years of age, suggesting that routine chemoprophylaxis is particularly warranted.[52]

Other common problems include various respiratory infections, communicable diseases, and cancer, as well as parasitic infestations, hepatitis, dental problems, arthritis, and hearing and vision problems. Screening tests for TB and type B hepatitis were positive in 62 percent and 26 percent, respectively, of Asian refugees screened in one clinic.[53]

Some progress has been made in meeting the health-care needs of Southeast Asian immigrants. Research has indicated that U.S. residence had resulted in a decrease in low birth weight babies in this population. There has been a decline in low birth weight from 7 percent of infants born in 1980–1981 to 5.4 percent of those born to Southeast Asian refugees in 1986.[54] These figures remain relatively high compared to the general population, however, and additional efforts are needed to improve pregnancy outcomes for Asian clients.

Black Americans. Black clients experience increased incidence and prevalence rates for many of the same health problems as members of other cultural groups. These problems include higher overall death rates and increased incidence rates for TB, cancer, and hypertension. Other major health problems experienced by the black population include heart disease, stroke, malnutrition, and alcoholism. In one study comparing blacks and whites in Washington D.C., the age-adjusted mortality rate for blacks exceeded that of the Caucasian population by 37 percent. Higher mortality rates for black males were found for SIDS, suicide, homicide, prematurity, chronic liver disease and cirrhosis, and accidental injuries. Black women exhibited higher death rates for diabetes, pneumonia, and influenza.[55] Black women also have been found to have a higher prevalence of obesity than do white women (35 percent vs. 20 percent). In addition, black females are twice as likely as whites to have low birth weight babies.[56]

Blacks are also less likely to seek attention for chest pain than their Caucasian counterparts. In one study, nearly half of black clients with recurrent chest pain had never sought medical care compared to 27 percent of whites. These differences were explained, in part, by different perceptions blacks have of the seriousness of cardiac symptoms and by prior unsatisfactory health-care experiences.[57] Like some other cultural groups, blacks generally have poor access to health care. The physician-to-patient ratio in the white community is approximately 1:538, while that for blacks is 1:4100. In 1970 only 2 percent of physicians in the United States were black[58] and that number has not grown appreciably in the last decade.

American Latinos. Particular problems in the Latino population include a higher incidence of complications of pregnancy for Puerto Rican women[59] and tuberculosis. Tuberculosis rates are four times those of the non-Latino population. Again, a large portion of these cases are under 35 years of age.[22]

Additional problems are the high incidence of AIDS among Latino women in some parts of the country and increased mortality from infectious diseases. Latino women in New York City have an incidence rate for AIDS more than 11 times that of the Caucasian population and account for 13 percent of all Latino AIDS deaths since 1980.[60] These figures are most probably the result of the high incidence of intravenous drug use in the Latino population of New York.

Latinos also experience higher rates of death than the non-Latino Caucasian population from infectious causes such as pneumonia[46] and traumatic injury related to alcohol, drug abuse, accidents, and violence.[49] Special problems found among Latino refugees from Central and South America include gastroenteritis and parasitic infestations, as well as the physical and emotional after-effects of torture.[23]

Appalachian Americans. Major health problems among Appalachians include chronic lung diseases, infections, and diseases of bones and joints. Depression, arthritis, allergies, heart problems, and serious lung conditions are among the maladies identified by Appalachians themselves. Other problems include difficulties with vision and hearing, dental problems, and severe emotional disorders.[61]

The typical Appalachian has limited access to health care because of a dearth of health professionals. According to some estimates, there are 34 percent fewer physicians and 20 percent fewer dentists in Appalachia than in the nation at large.[24] Because the number of nurses in Appalachia is only 5 percent below the national average, nurses have become the primary providers of care in many areas. Despite the efforts of these nurses, the insufficient number of health-care professionals in Appalachia has resulted in crisis-oriented health care.

ENVIRONMENT

Aspects of the physical, psychological, and social environments influence culture and its effects on the health status of population groups.

PHYSICAL ENVIRONMENT

The geographic isolation created by some physical environments may contribute to the development and continuation of cultural variations. For example, the isolation of many Appalachian mountain communities led to the development of a unique culture that has withstood many incursions by the larger society. The insularity created by geographic or social isolation also contributes to lack of change within a culture over time.[28,61]

Cultural groups differ in their view of the relationship between human beings and their environment. These differences can be referred to as the "man-nature" orientation of a culture.[62] This orientation may reflect a view of people as subject to, in harmony with, or having mastery over the environment. Black, Latino, and Appalachian clients tend to perceive human beings as subject to the environment and as having little control over their own destiny. Asian and many Native American cultures tend more toward the view of people acting in harmony with nature, while the dominant American culture emphasizes society's mastery of nature.

The type of man-nature orientation typically exhibited by members of a cultural group has implications for health-related action. For example, people who see themselves as subject to the environment may see little use in attempts to change environmental factors impinging on their health.

PSYCHOLOGICAL ENVIRONMENT

Areas to be considered in assessing the psychological environment include attitudes and beliefs regarding mental illness, the importance of individual versus group goals, modes of authority and decision making, attitudes to change, and the character of relationships with the larger society.

Attitudes to Mental Illness

Many cultures fail to make a distinction between mental and physical illness. Emotional distress may be somatized and experienced as physical symptoms or an inability to perform one's usual social roles.[7] Several of the cultural groups addressed here, however, do have some concept of disease caused by psychological factors. Blacks, for instance, view stress as a source of illness. Stress is believed to arise from negative emotions such as envy, guilt, and ineffective interpersonal relationships.[63] Similarly, Laotians may believe that worry results in illness.[64]

Many Latinos also distinguish between physical and emotional illness and further subdivide the category of emotional illness into mental and moral conditions.[65] The client with a mental illness is seen as a victim of circumstances with no responsibility for his or her condition. The client's condition may be the result of a blow to the head, fright, or anxiety, or may be due to the malign effects of witchcraft. Moral illness, on the other hand, is the result of moral weakness on the part of the client and might be manifested as excessive emotion, as in the case of *coraje,* weakness of character, as in alcoholism, or a propensity for engaging in vice, such as drug abuse.

A diagnosis of mental illness may be perceived by members of many cultural groups as shameful. Chinese clients, for example, might try to hide mental illness in a family member, keeping the person at home as long as possible. Typical Western approaches to psychotherapy are frequently ineffective with members of other cultures because assertiveness and independence, expression of feelings, and confrontation are culturally prohibited behaviors frequently encouraged in psychotherapy.[7,33]

Individual Versus Group Goals

The nurse exploring the norms of another culture would assess the relative importance of individual versus group goals. Western medicine (and nursing in particular) emphasizes the worth of each individual. It sometimes comes as a great shock to community health nurses to realize that this is not true in all cultures. For example, an American community health nurse working with the Peace Corps was serving in India where a young woman developed tetanus. Therapy was available at the missionary hospital 2 hours away. However, the family determined that the cost of transporting the woman to the hospital was too high and decided to let her die rather than spend what little money they had. While the family's decision may seem callous, it was made on the basis of what was best for the entire family rather than on the needs of an individual member. Money that could have been used to transport the woman to the hospital was needed to feed many other mouths. In this instance, the welfare and continued survival of many took precedence over the life of one. Nurses in a relatively affluent country, such as the United States, are seldom forced to make decisions of this sort, and may find it exceedingly difficult to accept such a philosophy on the part of clients with different cultural backgrounds.

In Native American culture, the individual is considered an independent agent. This orientation is particularly true of the Navajo, among whom even small children are encouraged to voice their opinion. It is believed that no one has the right to speak or make decisions for another. It is sometimes surprising to the nurse that young children are allowed to determine for themselves whether they will take a prescribed medication.[11,66]

There is also a strong commitment to family and to tribe among Native Americans. This commitment does not, however, take precedence over individual development or freedom of choice. In such cultures where individual autonomy is valued, the nurse will need to address the motivation of the individual client to carry out desired health-care practices.

The typical Appalachian client is ruggedly individualistic from the point of view of outsiders. There is little sense of community, and values such as self-reliance and independence are highly regarded.[67] Personal independence and individual growth and development, however, are subordinated to the needs of family or kin.[68] Pride and reliance on self and family to meet one's needs have been major deterrents to the use of governmental health and service programs.

In contrast to the Appalachian client who subordinates personal independence and individuality to group needs only when necessary, the Asian client's individuality is subordinated to the family.[7,67] In traditional Chinese society, for example, the family or clan and some other community associations fulfilled the social needs of the individual. As families were separated after coming to America, the newly arrived family groups and benevolent associations took on the responsibility of meeting the social welfare needs of immigrant Chinese.[51] The relationship of the individual Chinese to the group remains very strong, and the individual is expected to direct his or her energies to the benefit of the group. For example, the careers of children might be planned, not on the basis of interest, but in terms of the accomplishment of family goals. Group ties are similarly strong in the traditional Japanese culture.

As well as being family and group-oriented, many Asians are also class conscious. This is particularly true of the Southeast Asian refugee group.[50] This may present problems when members of the same culture, but different social classes, act as providers of health care or as interpreters.

Like the Asian client, many persons of Latino origin place greater emphasis on the group than on the individual. This is particularly true with the family. Individual needs tend to be subordinated to family needs.[69]

Authority and Decision Making

Cultural patterns of authority and decision making frequently correspond to individual versus group goal orientations. Groups that emphasize family or community goals frequently vest authority and decision-making power in elders rather than in individuals.

Respect for authority is another feature of culture that influences the psychological environment and its effects on health. Seeming agreement and compliance on the part of some clients may only reflect an attitude of respect for the health-care provider rather than genuine motivation toward healthy behavior. Respect for authority can enhance or detract from a therapeutic regimen. When a client's respect for authority leads to compliance with medication orders and other recommendations, for example, it enhances the therapeutic effect of health care. A client's respect for authority can also hinder health-care providers' efforts. For example, a client's respect for authority may detract from the effectiveness of a community health nurse's efforts to enhance the client's reliance on his or her own abilities to resolve health problems.

Decision-making processes within a cultural group are indicative of its attitude to authority. The community health nurse should assess how decisions are made. Are they arrived at in a democratic fashion where all concerned have equal input? Or, are they made by a central authority figure or group? The traditional Latino family identifies the husband/father as the primary decision-maker. More recent research indicates that many decisions are made jointly by husband and wife, particularly in those families where the woman is employed.[4] In some Native American tribes, on the other hand, all family members (including children) help make decisions.[11] In other tribes, decisions are made by the female head of the family.

Attitudes Toward Change

Group attitudes toward change also influence the psychological environment and health care for group members. In assessing a particular cultural group, the nurse will want to explore what changes are taking place within the culture itself as well as how open or resistant to change the group is. Resistance to change among farmers in India, for example, hampered efforts of Peace Corps volunteers to introduce new agricultural practices. On the other hand, openness to change on the part of small businessmen in India made business-related Peace Corps programs much more effective.

Closely allied to group attitudes toward change are culturally based attitudes of resignation and acceptance. In many areas of the world, notably underdeveloped countries, people have little access to the means to change the circumstances of their lives. Over many generations, people in such cultures often become resigned to their condition. Widespread resignation within a cultural group can frustrate health professionals who see ways in which people could better their situation if they were only motivated to act. In fact, an attitude of resignation is often misinterpreted as a lack of motivation on the part of clients from other cultures.

Relations with the Larger Society

The last cultural feature that may significantly influence the effects of the psychological environment on health is the quality of a cultural group's relationships with the larger society. Relationships between subcultures and the larger cultural group can be complementary, "colonial," competitive, or conflictive in nature.[2] Complementary relationships exist when interaction between groups is mutually supportive. To a large extent, complementary relationships exist between Americans and Canadians. Colonial relationships occur when one group is exploited by another. This type of relationship is frequently seen in the United States in interactions between Latino migrant farm workers and the larger society and occurred historically with the Chinese brought to the United States to build the railroads and the black Africans brought as slaves to the southern states.

Competitive relationships occur when cultural groups compete for the same resources on an essentially equal basis. This type of interaction was typical between Irish and Italian immigrants during the industrial development of the northeastern United States. Finally, a conflictive relationship exists when one cultural group attempts to dominate the other and the second group resists attempts at domination. Attempts by Caucasians to continue to dominate African Americans have been actively resisted since the advent of the civil rights movement in the United States, creating conflictive relationships in many parts of the country.

In assessing a subculture's relationships with the larger society, the community health nurse would consider how the subculture views itself with respect to the larger society. Do group members tend to assume a subservient posture or one of superiority in their interactions with the larger group? Do they view themselves as the equals of other members of the society? How do members of the larger society view the subculture? Are the views of members of the subculture respected by the larger society? Is their participation in society sought or rejected?

SOCIAL ENVIRONMENT

The social environment within a specific culture also influences health and health practices. Each culture has norms that govern the social interaction of its members. Areas for consideration in assessment include interpersonal relationships, communication, beliefs and values, and the place of religion and magic in the culture. The nurse would also explore the effects of the larger society on the subculture.

Interpersonal Relationships

The types of interpersonal relationships that are important in a particular culture and the rules governing those relationships can profoundly influence the health of members of the cultural group and their relationships with health-care providers.

Family Relationships. One of the primary concerns in cultural assessment is determining the place of the family within the culture and the role of the family with respect to health and illness. The community health nurse should be aware of the influence that the family exerts on its members in a particular culture. To what extent do family beliefs and values influence individuals' behavior?

The structure of family life also merits exploration, including the family's typical organizational structure and patterns of residence. Do families tend to be nuclear or extended in structure? Who lives with whom? Is descent determined matrilineally (through the mother, as in the case of some Native American tribes) or patrilineally (through the father)?

Another consideration is that of family roles. What tasks do family members typically assume? Are these tasks interchangeable? Who assigns tasks? Are family tasks gender-specific, with males taking on certain functions and females responsible for others? The development of gender roles in ethnic groups is influenced by several conditions in the larger society.[4] These conditions include the position of the cultural group vis-à-vis other groups in the larger society, the presence of an identifiable ethnic community, and the degree to which group members self-identify with the cultural group. The greater the identification with the group, the greater the identifiability of an ethnic community; the less the interaction with the larger society, the more likely it is that gender roles follow traditional cultural patterns. In exploring any particular cultural group, the community health nurse would identify typical gender roles and patterns and how they are exhibited within families.

The role and status of individual family members is a major consideration with implications for health care. In some cultures, children are central figures in the family. In others, life centers around the older members. Who in the family makes decisions regarding health and illness? In some instances, individuals decide for themselves when and where to seek health care. In others, those decisions are made by the authority figures within the family.

Another question is: What roles are assumed by family members with respect to illness? There may be specific family members whose task it is to care for the sick. Or, the entire family may expect to participate in the care of ill members.[70]

Family ties are of great importance in each of the five cultural groups presented in this chapter. Family roles differ, but there are specific expectations of family members. These expectations extend into the realm of health behaviors as well as other aspects of family life.

Native Americans: In most Native American cultures, the family is very important, particularly in the care of the sick. Recovery from illness is believed to require the aid of family members.[66] The importance of the extended family is widely recognized in these groups. Native American families provide care for their elderly and orphaned children as respected members of the family.[11] The elderly are revered for their wisdom and experience.

Children are welcomed in the family, and child-rearing practices are lenient by the standards of the larger society. Native American children are not forbidden to engage in an activity, but are told the possible consequences and allowed to make their own decisions. There is little physical punishment, because positive rather than negative reinforcement of behavior is emphasized.[66,71]

Descent in many Native American families is matrilineal, and the woman has a great deal of power within the family, particularly among the Navajo.[72] In some tribes, it is the maternal grandmother who must grant permission for health care for family members. Family roles tend to be interchangeable, and decision making is shared.[17] An Indian child may have several "mothers" responsible for his or her well-being, while the grandmother may take primary responsibility for health.[31]

The presence of family during illness is very important to the Native American client. Families participate in healing rituals and the client becomes the center of interest.[73] Family members are expected to be present in the case of illness, particularly if death is imminent. Visits by family members are comforting to hospitalized clients. Specific family members have designated roles in the care of the sick and should be allowed and encouraged to participate in the care of the client.

Asian Americans: In the traditional Asian family, the father is the undisputed head of the household.[7,74] There is more emphasis on the extended than the nuclear family. The extended family may include deceased ancestors as well as living members.[6] The oldest living male member is the head of the family. At his death, he is succeeded in this position by the eldest son.

Dominance and deference are the roles ascribed to parent and child, respectively.[17] The traditional Asian family has been patriarchal with the wife assuming a subordinate role. The woman is largely uneducated, and the husband functions as the family spokesman. The woman acquires power through her sons and, in later life, could assume a matriarchal role. In Korean society, the woman who dies before marriage is thought to be of no value and is not included in ancestor rituals. The female role in this and similar Asian cultures is defined by the duty to produce an heir.[74] Respect for elders is ingrained in Asian children.

Large families have traditionally been desirable by reason of high mortality and the need for family manpower. Because the family is close-knit, members may tend to avoid contact with outsiders unless necessary.[18] Care of the sick is very much a family function, and families expect to be able to participate in the care of a hospitalized member.

It is the responsibility of the traditional Asian male to support the family financially, while the woman cares for the home and children. In the United States, the frequent need for both parents to work conflicts with traditional roles and may contribute to feelings of shame and guilt on the part of the male.[18] The nurse working with either the Appalachian or Asian client should include the husband as decision-maker in planning for health care for family members.

Asian children are actively involved in family life.

They are taught early in life about their cultural heritage. Asian parents often discipline by invoking feelings of shame and guilt.[7]

Many Asian families have sharply defined member roles related to health care. For example, in Korean families, mothers-in-law have a specific responsibility for the care of the pregnant woman from the beginning of the birth process through the postpartum period.[74] Among the Hmong of Laos, the family group must approve bedrest for an ill member, and family members often stay with an ill member until the time of recovery or death.[64]

Black Americans: Black families were traditionally stereotyped as matriarchal households.[9] Research has indicated, however, that this is not usually the case. In 1987, for example, more than half of all black families consisted of both husband and wife, while less than a third were composed of single women with children.[13]

Female roles in the black family include providing child care, housekeeping, and financial support, although these roles are shared by the male.[75] Unlike traditional Asian families, decision making is shared between husband and wife in the black family. Family roles are flexible rather than rigid. Both instrumental and expressive family functions are shared by husband and wife.[33] ***Instrumental functions*** are those dealing with the material welfare of the family such as economic support. ***Expressive functions*** deal with interpersonal relationships involved in child care and so on. This role adaptibility allows the black family to function even when key members are absent.

Family role adaptability is only one of five strengths that characterize black families. Others include strong kinship bonds, strong work orientation, strong achievement orientation, and strong religious orientation.[76] Family ties are strong within both nuclear and extended black families. Parent-child relationships are close and the father-child relationship may be as significant as the bond between mother and child.[77]

Children are highly valued in the black family. Adult roles are assumed somewhat earlier than is the case in the larger society, and adolescents and preteens frequently have more family responsibilities than would be the case with their Caucasian counterparts.[77]

Care of children, the elderly, and the sick remain strong family functions. Often, other persons without blood ties are "adopted" into the family because they have no other resource. Care of the sick takes place within the family whenever possible. It is frequently a female relative with knowledge of a variety of home remedies who assumes this responsibility.[33]

American Latinos: Like Asian families, the traditional Latino family is essentially patriarchal in nature, and family roles are clearly defined. Traditional Latinos typically have a firm belief in male superiority but perceive women as the life force that keeps the family together.[69] In traditional Latino cultures, the father is the decision-maker and provider.[21] Women decide when illness exists, but men decide how it will be dealt with. Once this decision has been made, mother or grandmother is responsible for implementing the decision and providing the actual care of the sick.[65,78,79] As noted earlier, this traditional role structure has been replaced by a more egalitarian approach in many families in which husband and wife share decision-making authority.

Children are welcomed and highly valued in traditional Latino cultures.[69] They are expected to obey and respect their elders, work toward the good of the family, and maintain family honor.[80] Latino parents may be seen by the larger society as overprotective and may use guilt as a form of discipline to encourage appropriate socialization.[21]

The extended family is important in Latino cultures, although the basic family unit remains the nuclear family. The Latino extended family might also include additional persons called *compadres,* which means "co-parents." A *compadre* is a close friend, unrelated by blood, who assumes parental functions within the family similar to those of a godparent in some other cultures.

Care of the sick is very definitely a family matter in traditional Latino cultures. Only when the family cannot cope with illness through traditional remedies is help sought from outsiders. Folk health practices incorporate a great deal of family participation, and family members frequently accompany the client to the physician's office, clinic, or hospital.

Appalachian Americans: The family centeredness exhibited by Appalachians provides a shared source of resources that enables them to provide for many of their needs without outside assistance.[81] The basic family unit in Appalachia is the nuclear family, headed by a strong authoritarian father, with close ties to the extended family of both mother and father.[82]

Family roles are well defined in traditional Appalachian culture. The husband/father is head of the family and the decision-maker. He is responsible for providing transportation for family members to go anywhere, including trips for health care. The husband is the family spokesman, while the wife is expected to stay at home. The wife is responsible for the care of the home and children, while her husband works outside the home.[83]

A large family is favored in Appalachian culture because childbearing and child rearing are considered one of a woman's main functions. A woman's role also includes care of the sick, and it is primarily Appalachian women who have perpetuated the folk health practices typical of this culture.[10] Some of these practices will be examined later in this chapter.

Kinship ties are of primary importance to the Appalachian client. One's importance in society is judged not so much by what one does as whose son or daughter one is. Outsiders must be accepted within the kinship network before they can hope to accomplish any change in the system. The extended family system is held together by ties of obligation rather than affection, but a strong maternal-child relationship exists that results in the capability for trusting relationships with others.[84] The Appalachian client turns to the family for help in coping with the fear and anxiety engendered by illness.

Socialization of children in Appalachia is primarily a family function. Schools have tended to be distrusted, as they drain the manpower necessary to maintain the family economy.[82]

Appropriate Demeanor in Interpersonal Relationships. Another aspect of interpersonal relationships within a specific culture that is of particular concern to community health nurses is the demeanor or behavior expected in one's interactions with others. In every culture there are certain behaviors that are acceptable and others that are not. If community health nurses are to work effectively with clients from other cultures, they must engage in acceptable behaviors and avoid behaviors that might give offense.

Behaviors acceptable in one culture are not necessarily acceptable in another. For example, it is not unusual in some cultures for men to embrace or for women to hold hands while walking down the street.[85] In the United States, however, such behavior might be interpreted as homosexuality. By the same token, members of the opposite sex holding hands in public is acceptable in the United States and unacceptable in other parts of the world.

It is beyond the scope of this book to list all of the possible behaviors considered acceptable and unacceptable in the five cultural groups presented here. However, Table 15–1 presents several examples of acceptable and unacceptable behaviors for each cultural group. Several other acceptable and unacceptable behaviors are discussed in other sections of the chapter.

Communication

Communication is another important consideration in assessing the social environmental aspects of cul-

TABLE 15–1. SELECTED EXAMPLES OF CULTURALLY UNACCEPTABLE BEHAVIOR

Unacceptable Behavior	Recommended Approach
Disrespect for elders and other authority figures	Show respect for elders and those in authority
Using informal forms of address inappropriately	Use appropriate forms of address (for example, using formal mode of speech with older persons)
Direct eye contact (Native American, Latino)	Look at the ground or to the side when speaking to another
Assuming authority over others (Appalachian)	Avoid conflict
Arguing with authority figures (Asian, Latino)	
Competing with others (Appalachian, Native American)	Cooperate with others
Causing others to "lose face" (Asian)	Prevent others from losing face
Strong hand clasp (Native American)	Display modesty and respect for privacy
Writing a "life-story" (Native American)	
Self-disclosure (Native American, Asian, Appalachian, Latino)	
Overt discussion of sexuality (Asian, Latino)	
Aggressiveness or self-assertion (Native American, Latino, Asian)	Display humility and self-effacement
Drawing attention to oneself (Native American, Asian)	
Expressing personal opinions (Asian)	
Ridiculing others (Asian)	Direct humor at self (especially with Appalachian clients)
Dependence on others (Appalachian)	Display self-reliance and stoicism (Appalachian, Asian)
Complaining (Asian)	
Displaying emotion (Asian, Native American)	Control emotions (Asian, Native American, Appalachian)
Getting right down to business (Asian, Native American, Latino, Appalachian)	Observe social amenities before conducting business
Saying no to a request (Asian)	
Refusing hospitality (Asian, Appalachian)	Graciously accept hospitality

ture. Both verbal and nonverbal forms of communication should be explored.

Language is the major means of transmitting culture. As such, it is an important consideration in cultural assessment. The community nurse should determine the language with which the client is most comfortable. Whenever possible, employ the client's native language (and dialect, if relevant).[12] This is particularly important when there is a need to discuss intimate topics. Such areas are even more difficult to discuss in a second language than in one's mother tongue.[21]

As far as possible, the community health nurse should strive to become familiar with the spoken language of a cultural group. Some languages include both formal and informal modes of address, and the nurse should become familiar with the circumstances in which each mode of address is used. For example, one would usually use an informal mode when speaking to a family member, a close friend, or a child. Formal modes of address are usually used when conversing with strangers and casual acquaintances, people in positions of authority, and older persons. In Korean culture, for example, it is considered disrespectful to address elders in the informal mode, and only children are addressed by name.[74]

It is wise to remember that the nurse with a poor command of a foreign language is at the same disadvantage as a client with little facility in English. In this situation, an interpreter is in order, preferably one with a cultural background similar to that of the client and conversant with the larger society as well. An interpreter who is not familiar with the larger culture may not be able to translate a concept that he or she doesn't understand. For example, the interpreter may not be able to translate a question about the use of contraceptives unless that individual understands the meaning of contraception.

Knowledge of a client's language will also allow community health nurses to obtain or create health-related literature in the client's native tongue for clients who are literate. Unfortunately, many foreign-language materials related to health are literal translations of materials written in English and may not be comprehensible to the client. Translated educational materials should make use of native idioms whenever possible.

The words used are only one aspect of communication. Another aspect is the context in which the message is conveyed.[86] In a "low context" culture such as that of the United States, the essence of a message is conveyed in the *words* used. In a "high context" culture, on the other hand, much of the message is communicated by the *context* in which the message is relayed rather than in the words used. Suppose, for example, that the nurse asks a mother when she plans to follow up on an immunization referral. In some cultures, it is polite to respond with the answer that one believes is expected, and the client might reply that she plans to get the immunizations that week. When the nurse visits the following week and finds that the mother has not yet had the child immunized, the nurse may interpret the client's previous statement as a lie. Yet, in the context of the client's culture, she was giving the appropriate response. If the nurse is aware of this cultural context, he or she is more likely to interpret correctly the mother's response as meaning that she will get the immunizations in the not too distant future.

Conflict can occur between individuals from high-context and low-context cultures primarily as a result of misinterpretation of communications. Those from the high-context culture may be reading into the message contextual considerations that might not exist. At the same time, the low-context person may be missing a large portion of the content of the message through neglect of contextual considerations.

Contextual considerations might include the need to observe certain social amenities before directing the conversation to the area of interest. For example, Puerto Ricans, as well as members of other cultures, might expect to learn something about the nurse as a person before getting down to the business at hand.[17]

Culturally prescribed reticence, courtesy titles, epithets, and gestures are other culturally determined aspects of communication. Culturally prescribed reticence refers to the relative openness about personal matters expected in casual encounters with others. Orientals, for example, display a high degree of reticence. They traditionally consider it impolite to ask personal questions and are uncomfortable discussing personal matters with casual acquaintances, including health professionals.[31] Native Americans are also socialized to little self-disclosure,[85] and the Western Appache may remain silent rather than speak in ambiguous or unpredictable situations.[31]

Latinos are also frequently reluctant to discuss personal matters with relative strangers.[69] In a similar vein, Latinos tend to provide responses that they believe are expected by health professionals and often keep their true feelings to themselves.[21]

Appalachians also tend to be very private persons and may resent intrusion by strangers. This cultural reticence is compounded by a mistrust of outsiders that is a historical product of the exploitation of Appalachia and its resources by others.[87]

Gestures are another important contextual factor. Gestures, like words, can convey totally different meanings in different cultures. In the larger American society, for example, one apologizes for accidentally bumping into someone else, but thinks nothing of pointing the sole of one's shoe at another. Clients from India would be highly insulted to have the soles of one's shoes directed toward them or, worse yet, to be touched by someone's shoe. Footwear is considered dirty and contaminated in India, and the implications of intentionally touching someone with your shoe would be comparable to spitting in someone's face in the United States.

Other gestures, even if not insulting, may convey different meanings in different cultures. For example, in the dominant American culture, one indicates agreement by nodding the head, whereas in India one says yes by tilting the head toward the shoulder. Peace Corps volunteers who developed this habit were sometimes thought to have a nervous tic on their return to the United States.

Cultures also differ with respect to their use of first or last names and courtesy titles. As with any client, it is wise to ask how a client from another culture wishes to be addressed. Often the use of a first name is restricted to close friends or children. Adults may be referred to by last name with or without the appropriate title (for example, "Gordon" vs. "Mrs. Gordon"). In Korean culture, family members are addressed in terms of their relationship to the youngest child in the family (for example, "Sung's grandmother"). As other children are born into the family constellation, the individual's relationship changes and forms of address change. For this reason, many elderly Koreans may not remember their given name after being addressed in terms of multiple relationships for years.[74]

Some epithets are considered insulting in different cultures. An epithet is a word or phrase used in place of the correct designation and may or may not be derogatory in nature. When cultural differences intervene, generally innocent words may take on the character of insults. Most nurses are sensitive enough to refrain from calling a black male "boy." Mexican-Americans may or may not be offended by being referred to as *chicano* depending upon the degree of their involvement with the cultural movement *La Raza.* Again, ask the individual client the preferred form of address.

Beliefs and Values

Cultural beliefs and values also influence health-related behavior. A culture's value orientations should be investigated as part of cultural assessment as well as the values attached to material goods, success, and competition.

All cultures develop value orientations related to questions common to all groups of people.[62] These value orientations address the character of human nature (the human nature orientation), the relation of human beings to their natural environment (the man-nature orientation), the temporal focus of life (time orientation), the modality of human activity (the activity orientation), and the relation of human beings to each other (the relational orientation).

Variations in these five value orientations are believed by some researchers to result in the major differences that occur between cultures.[62] Each of the five cultural groups presented in this chapter differs markedly from the value orientations typical of American culture. Understanding these variations in value orientations will help the community health nurse understand differences in behaviors that arise out of beliefs and values. Such an understanding will also aid the nurse in planning culturally consonant interventions.

Earlier in this chapter, the man-nature orientation was described as the way in which members of a specific cultural group view their interaction with the physical environment. The human nature orientation refers to the cultural view of human beings as inherently evil, inherently good, or any of several combinations of good and evil. Native American and Asian cultural groups tend to see humanity as fairly neutral, neither good nor evil. Traditional Appalachian, black, and Latino cultures, on the other hand, view human beings as sinful, but redeemable.

All cultures deal, to some extent, with the three aspects of time orientation: past, present, and future. Differences between cultures lie in the emphasis placed on each aspect. For example, Native Americans, blacks, Latinos, and Appalachians tend to be oriented to the present[17,33] whereas Asian clients may be oriented to the past and to tradition. American society in general is oriented to the future.

Another aspect of time orientation is that of scheduling. Members of Western cultures tend to order much of their lives in relation to the clock. Cross-cultural conflicts can arise as a result of different orientations to time. For example, Puerto Rican clients are oriented in the present and value completing a current activity rather than interrupting it to keep an appointment elsewhere. Clients from other cultural groups are also less concerned with specific schedules than health professionals are likely to be.

Another consideration in cultural orientations to time relates to the timing of home visits. As noted in Chapter 8, The Home Visit Process, community health nurses should cultivate knowledge of the daily habits of all clients and plan home visits (or clinic appointments) at times that are least disruptive to family life. A home visit at an inappropriate time is likely to be unproductive and may even be destructive of the rapport between client and nurse. As a general rule, times to be avoided include rest periods, periods when intensive work is performed, times of religious ceremonies and rituals, and bathing times. Mealtimes should also be avoided unless the nurse has a specific purpose in visiting at that time. For instance, visiting during lunch is one way of validating a client's compliance with a special diet. Because the times at which certain activities are routinely performed may vary from culture to culture, the community health nurse should become familiar with daily patterns typical of specific cultural groups.

One of the most frustrating manifestations of different cultural orientations to time for health-care providers involves late or broken appointments. Because some cultural groups are not as time conscious as the typical American, clients may tend to arrive at a time convenient to them, and not at their appointed time. Latino clients, for example, do not adhere rigidly to schedules, while in some Asian cultures it is considered polite to arrive an hour late for an appointment.[53] Appalachians as well have a different orientation to time, which may give rise to difficulties with formal work schedules and in keeping appointments.[82]

A variety of approaches can be employed to deal with the problem of differing cultural orientations to time. Appointments can be made for a specific day rather than a specific hour, with clients seen on a first-come, first-served basis. Another possibility is to schedule several clients at the same hour in the hope that at least one will be there on time. A third approach is to do away with scheduling altogether or schedule people 2 to 3 hours before you actually expect them to appear. Clinics can also be scheduled at more convenient times (for example, evenings or weekends, or during slow periods for seasonal workers). None of these approaches may prove successful, however, and community health nurses might need to learn to cultivate patience to cope with their own feelings of frustration.

The activity orientation refers to the purpose of human activity. "Being" is emphasized in Latino, black, and Native American cultures. In these cultures the emphasis is on spontaneous self-expression. In the "being-in-becoming orientation," the purpose of human activity is developing all aspects of the self as an integrated whole. This is the typical emphasis among Asian cultures. A "doing orientation," on the other hand, characterizes American society and emphasizes activities that lead to visible accomplishments such as career success, wealth, and so on.

A culture's relationship orientation describes the value that members of the group place on specific categories of relationships. In some cultures the most important relationships are those that occur between generations within the family. This is typical of Asian clients, who function within a group identified primarily by direct lineal descent from father to son.

Collaterally oriented cultures place more emphasis on relationships with others on one's own level (for example, among one's siblings and cousins). The extended families of blacks and Native Americans are examples of this type of relationship. Appalachian and Latino cultures, however, tend to emphasize both lineal and collateral relationships. In contrast, American society as a whole tends to place greater emphasis on individualistic relationships in which relationships with those outside the family are often more highly valued than those with family members. Individualistic relationships are characterized by impersonality, while more intimate personal relationships are characteristic of lineal and collateral orientations.

Cultural values related to material goods, success, and competition are also explored in relation to the particular culture studied. Do members of the cultural group value economic success as measured by material goods and wealth? Is career success valued? Formal education, work, and achievement are valued in black, Asian, and Latino cultures, but attitudes toward material measures of success are viewed somewhat differently from what is typically the case in American society. For example, achievement is valued by the Asian client because it reflects on family honor and status.[7] Among many Native Americans, formal education is valued because it enhances prosperity.[66] Although prosperity is valued, generosity commands the respect of others, and acquisition of material goods can lead to social ostracism.[17]

Another important value involves the emphasis placed on competition. In American culture, competition is highly valued. It is less valued, or even considered impolite, in some other cultures. For example, Native American children may do less well in school than other youngsters. This is not due to an innate lack of ability, but to a cultural attitude. In many Native American tribes, as well as Asian and Appalachian cultures, it is considered impolite to compete with others. Cooperation is the valued behavior rather than competition.[17]

Religion and Magic

Religion and magic are other important considerations in cultural exploration. Religion is an organized system of beliefs regarding the origin, nature, and purpose of the universe. Individual and group experiences related to religion differ along five dimensions: the experiential, ritualistic, ideologic, intellectual, and consequential dimensions.[41] The experiential dimension reflects the emotional aspects of religion. For example, religious beliefs and practices may bring feelings of comfort, joy and elation, remorse, and so on for different people or different groups. Religions also have a ritualistic dimension. Members of most religious groups are expected to engage in certain prescribed behaviors or practices. These can include lighting candles, chanting specific prayers, participating in special ceremonies like a Mass or worship service, handling snakes, or using hallucinogenic substances. The ideologic dimension of religion consists of the spiritual beliefs held by members of the religious group. For example, Christians believe that Christ is the Son of God sent to save the world. For members of other religious groups, Christ is one of several prophets. The intellectual dimension of religion reflects members' knowledge of these beliefs and their familiarity with the sacred writings of the group. Finally, the consequential dimension of religion consists of the standards of conduct expected of group members.[41] The five dimensions of religion are summarized in Box 15–5.

Religion can be a contributing factor in the phenomenon of resignation noted earlier.[21] "Who can challenge the will of God?" may be the fatalistic response to efforts toward change in Appalachian, Asian, and Latino cultures. Black culture is more amenable to change.[77]

BOX 15–5

Dimensions of Religion

Experiential dimension: emotional effects of participation in religion and religious observances

Ritualistic dimension: expectations regarding participation by group members in specific rituals and practices

Ideologic dimension: beliefs held by the members of the group

Intellectual dimension: knowledge of religious beliefs and sacred writings and how these are conveyed to group members

Consequential dimension: Expectations regarding standards of conduct based on religious beliefs

Religion can affect health in ways other than contributing to fatalistic attitudes. The nurse exploring another culture may encounter religious practices that enhance or detract from health. Most people are familiar with the prohibition against blood transfusions among some religious sects and the stand of the Roman Catholic Church against artificial forms of birth control. Either of these practices can be detrimental to health in situations where a transfusion is indicated or where pregnancy is medically contraindicated. On the other hand, the Jewish proscription against pork probably originated as a measure designed to promote health by preventing infestation with trichinosis.[5]

A community health nurse needs to assess several features of a culture's relationships to religion to determine the importance of religions in the health of a community.[10] First, one would explore the extent to which religion is involved in health care. Are there specific religious beliefs regarding the cause of illness or appropriate treatments? Do members of religious groups play a role in the diagnosis and treatment of illness? For example, belief in faith healing is strong in Appalachia. Here, religion takes on a direct curative aspect in the treatment of illness. The healer is believed to have been "called by God" and exercises healing powers through divine intervention.

Second, one should explore the influences of religion on the health of a cultural group's members and on the health-care system. Are certain religious practices detrimental to health? Examples of potentially dangerous religious practices are snake handling in some parts of Appalachia and the use of peyote and other hallucinogens in some Native American religious ceremonies. Another related area of inquiry is determining the degree to which religious and health-care systems either conflict with or complement each other.

A third aspect of the impact of religion on health is the effect of religious sponsorship on the use of health services. Does this sponsorship enhance or detract from the acceptability of health programs? For example, if the only hospital in the community is a Roman Catholic hospital, are protestant Appalachian clients reluctant to obtain services there? The fourth consideration is the relationship between religious leaders and healers with health-care personnel. Is this a cooperative relationship? Or are they in competition with each other?

Religion and magic are closely intertwined in many cultures. Distinctions between the two are based on the agent of action. Religion is viewed as supplicative; the person typically conciliates personified supernatural powers, requesting specific action on their part. For example, a particular client may make an offering to gods or spirits or pray for a cure for his or her illness or relief from suffering. Magic on the other hand is considered manipulative. In using magic, an individual manipulates impersonal powers to achieve a desired result.[88] Magic is based on the principle of sympathy. Sympathetic magic arises from an assumed connection between everything in the universe and the belief that an understanding of the connection provides the power of manipulation.[63]

Magical practices are divided into two categories—contagious magic and imitative magic. Contagious magic is based on the assumption that things that have been connected remain connected even though physically separated from each other. Whatever one does to the part influences the whole. This is why fingernail parings or a lock of hair are frequent ingredients of magical rituals. It is believed that damage done to these things formerly connected to an individual will cause damage to the individual.

In imitative magic, the operating principle is "like follows like" in which similar objects have similar properties and react in similar ways. Pins inserted into a doll made to look like an enemy, for example, will cause the enemy pain and injury. By the same token, a knife placed under the bed of a woman in labor is believed to "cut the pain" of contractions. In some Mexican Indian groups, imitative magic makes use of intricate paper figures believed to represent an individual's soul force or *zaki*.[89]

Native Americans. Religion, medicine, and magic are inextricably bound in most Native American cultures. The Indian concept of medicine embraces forces beyond treatment of illness and healing of wounds.[90] Death is viewed as a part of the life cycle, and is an essential component of the natural harmony that is health.[73] Therefore, Indian medicine is not always directed toward a cure for illness.

Magic can be either a causative or curative force in the Native American concept of illness. Sorcery and witchcraft, as well as taboo violation, are some of the recognized causes of illness.[42,89] The medicine man is skilled in magical as well as physical aspects of healing. The medicine man would seem to be the practitioner of choice for illnesses that the larger society would consider "psychological" in origin. However, Native Americans consider all diseases within the province of folk medicine.[73]

Asian Americans. Religion also plays an important part in the health practices of certain Asian cultures. For example, illness is attributed by Filipinos to the will of God. Filipinos tend to deal with illness through prayer and the hope that God's will includes recovery.[91] Religion also influences the response of other Asian clients to illness and pain. Buddhism promotes acceptance of life and discourages display of strong emotions. This tends to foster a stoic, uncomplaining response to pain and illness.[33]

Like Native American clients, Asian clients may hold a belief in evil spirits. Vietnamese parents, for example, dress their newborns in old clothes and avoid praising them for fear that jealous spirits will steal them away.[6] A related belief is that blood is an irreplaceable source of the body's strength, so Asian clients may vigorously resist the taking of blood samples.[92]

For Southeast Asian clients, the head is the dwelling place of the spirit. Thus, one should not touch someone else's head without permission for fear of possible damage to the spirit.[50] Charms of gold or silver or strings around the waist, wrist, or neck of an infant are used to ward off evil spirits. They are thought to bring good luck and health and should not be removed.

Other Asian cultural groups also engage in preventive measures related to supernatural agents. Cambodian women have hot coals placed beneath their bed during labor to drive away evil spirits. Parents also verbally claim their baby after delivery, giving notice to spirits that the child belongs to them.[6]

Black Americans. Religion in black culture provides a means of reducing tension. Religious practices and rituals are very expressive and emotion-laden and blacks usually have a strong religious orientation.[31] Religion is also a stabilizing force for the black family, providing support in times of adversity. Religion assists many black clients in understanding their place in life, understanding death, and developing identity and inner strength.[93] For many blacks, religion also provides a basis for developing values related to life and health. Good living is viewed as a means of promoting physical and mental health. When illness occurs, God is perceived as the ultimate source of healing, whether the cure is achieved by folk remedies, a faith healer, or scientific medicine. All forms of therapy are believed to be enhanced by faith and prayer.

Black religious groups often engage in community-oriented activities and provide excellent resources for promoting and implementing health programs. Black churches also serve as sources of social change, and the minister is usually a strong and influential individual.[77]

In black culture, *maleficia* is the term given to occurrences attributable to evil influences.[94] Witchcraft is suspected whenever an illness proves not to be amenable to treatment by a physician or when an individual consistently acts in an antisocial manner or differs significantly from his or her usual behavior. This last action is also true of Asian cultures. For example, witchcraft may be seen as the cause of an Asian son's unfilial behavior in arguing with his father. No normal son would do such a thing. Therefore, he must be bewitched.

Any of a variety of methods can be employed in casting a spell. Those frequently used in black witchcraft practices include causing the victim to ingest some evil substance (for example, powdered snake skin), placing a "conjure" where the victim will step over or be in close proximity to it, or manipulating occult materials.[94] The phenomenon of the evil eye is also recognized in black folklore.

In black culture, witchcraft is employed with care as a means of settling differences with an enemy. Belief in the homing tendency of spells is the reason for such care. It is believed that a spell is indestructable. If removed from the intended victim, a spell rebounds on the individual who requested it rather than on the practitioner of magic.[94]

Voodoo involves magical practices that may be either good or evil in intent. The term "voodoo" derives from Vodu, the God of snake worshippers who came as slaves to the West Indies.[95] Voodoo can involve white magic, which is beneficial, or black magic, which is very dangerous.

Magical practices involved in voodoo employ a variety of symbols. *Gris-gris* is the term given to one such category of symbols. Gris-gris can be used to prevent or cause illness and can therefore be either good or bad. Good gris-gris can include pleasantly scented powders and oils, whereas foul-scented ones are used as bad gris-gris. Candles of various colors are also widely used, with the color symbolic of the intent of the spell. Black, for example, is symbolic of evil.[95]

American Latinos. For the person of Latino origin, an attitude of submission to the will of God strongly influences health behavior.[21] Illness may be the result of *castigo* (punishment for sins) or suffering, which is part of humankind's lot in life. The Latino client often looks forward to reward in the afterlife. Attempts to interfere with the will of God may result in further punishment, so acceptance and compliance are the primary responses to illness. Religion is also influential in terms of the treatment of illness in Latino cultures, and many religious rituals are employed in healing.

Belief in witchcraft and supernatural forces that result in illness is relatively common in Latino cultures. The evil eye or *mal ojo* has already been discussed. A second category of unnatural illness recognized by Latinos occurs as a result of *brujeria*, or witchcraft.[65] As in any other folk belief system, illnesses caused either by *mal ojo* or *brujeria* are not amenable to intervention by health professionals, at least according to believers.

Appalachian Americans. Appalachians are a strongly religious group. This religiosity is derived from their Scots-Presbyterian ancestry.[96] The predominant churches in Appalachia are Christian fundamentalist, emphasizing the literal interpretation of Scripture. Religion provides an outlet for frustrations engendered by a hard life, with the promise of afterlife providing some compensation for suffering in this one. Appalachian culture fosters a strict moral code prohibiting such activities as dancing, drinking alcohol, gambling, infidelity, and fighting.[82] Religion in Appalachia influences health in terms of its importance in curing disease. A study of Appalachian migrants to Detroit reported that all of the subjects considered faith an important factor in curing disease and that more than 75 percent of them believed in faith healing.

Appalachian witchcraft beliefs stem from black, pioneer, and European folklore.[97] The evil eye is one supernatural cause of illness and misfortune subscribed to by the Appalachian. The evil eye results when someone who has the power looks upon the victim and illness results. This can be an intended or unintentional occurrence and may even occur as a result of merely envying the good fortune of another. As in most other magically caused illnesses, the evil eye cannot be cured by a physician, according to believers. Intervention can only be done by the person who cast the evil eye or by a mediator who is assisted by supernatural powers.

Knowledge of beliefs regarding the influence of magic on health and health practices is useful to community health nurses. If a nurse determines that the client or family attributes illness to witchcraft, he or she can encourage consultation with a practitioner of folk medicine *in addition* to compliance with a medically prescribed regimen. An understanding and acceptance of such beliefs will also enable the nurse to contribute to the client's emotional health by promoting expression of fears and anxieties.

Economic Status

Assessment of a cultural group also includes consideration of the economic status of group members relative to the larger society. Members of the subcultures discussed in this chapter tend to be economically and educationally disadvantaged as a result of a number of factors, including language barriers and limited job opportunities. Community health nurses should assess the economic and educational status of members of the cultural group and the effects of these factors upon the health of group members.

Native Americans typically have low levels of income and education compared to the larger society. According to 1980 census figures, almost 24 percent of Native American families had incomes below the poverty level. Unemployment among Native Americans in 1980 was twice as high (13 percent) as the general population (6.5 percent).[13] Over 40 percent of Indian males and 16 percent of females are 2 years or more behind in school compared to others of comparable ages.[14] Among Native Americans 25 years of age or older, over 8000 have less than a fifth-grade education, and only 1 percent have four or more years of college.[13]

Asian Americans as a total group fare somewhat better than their Native American counterparts. In 1980, less than 11 percent of Asian families had incomes below the poverty level, and less than 5 percent of this group were unemployed. Thirty-four percent of Asian Americans had completed 4 or more years of college, while only 6 percent of the population had less than 5 years of education.[13]

Income figures for American blacks indicate that in 1987, over 31 percent of black families had incomes below the poverty level, and the rate of unemployment for this group was more than twice as high as that of the general population (13 percent vs. 6.5 percent). In 1987, more than 18 percent of blacks had less than an eighth-grade education compared to less than 13 percent of the total population. Only 10 percent had 4 or more years of college compared to more than 20 percent of Caucasian Americans.[13]

Approximately 27 percent of Latino families had incomes below the poverty level in 1987, whereas the unemployment rate for this group was almost 9 percent. Slightly over 35 percent of American Latinos in 1987 had less than an eighth-grade education, and less than 9 percent of this population had 4 or more years of college education compared to nearly 20 percent of the total U.S. population.[13] Because of their lack of status as an easily identified population group, economic and educational statistics for members of the Appalachian subculture are not available.

LIFE-STYLE

The life-style typical of a particular cultural group can also have significant effects on the health status of its members. Aspects of life-style to be assessed by the community health nurse include dietary practices and other consumption patterns as well as practices related to specific life events.

DIETARY PRACTICES

Dietary practices include preferences for specific foods, typical modes of food preparation, and food consumption patterns. Community health nurses should also explore the therapeutic uses of food and the social and religious symbolism of certain foods.

Food preferences are defined culturally, and what is considered food in one culture may not be considered as such in another. The practice among southern blacks of eating animal viscera or "chitlins" originated from the practice of white masters leaving the offal from slaughtered livestock for their slaves. Dog, rats, rattlesnakes, and snails are considered food in some cultures. Latinos may not always perceive green vegetables as food, whereas Vietnamese clients may use both shells and bones as food items.[29]

Because nutrition is such an integral part of health, nurses must be aware of the food practices of their clients. This awareness enables the nurse to incorporate these practices, as well as specific food preferences, into the plan of care whenever possible. The nurse must consider not only the type of food preferred but also the preferred means of preparation.

Methods of preparation can affect the nutritional status of many foods. For example, the rapid cooking of vegetables by Asians helps to retain the vegetables' vitamin content,[29] while overcooking by other groups causes loss of nutrients. Frying foods in animal fats, a common practice among many southern blacks, increases their cholesterol consumption and dietary fat content.

Other areas for consideration in nutritional assessment include the frequency of meals eaten away from home and the degree of regularity of consumption patterns.[98] For example, blacks tend to eat larger, more elaborate meals on weekends than during the week. For this reason, a 3-day diet history, a frequent method of assessing dietary patterns, may not provide an accurate picture of a black client's nutrition or food consumption patterns. Even the times at which specific meals are eaten can vary among cultural groups. For example, in warmer climates, the evening meal is often eaten quite late to provide a cooler, more relaxed atmosphere in which to dine.

A great deal of symbolism is attached to food in every culture. Food can function as a focus of emotional association, a channel for interpersonal relationships, or as a means of communicating love, disapproval, discrimination, and so on. What parent has not shown love of a child by providing a favorite food or indicated disapproval by sending a child to bed without dessert?

In most cultures, the sharing of food indicates acceptance and intimacy. When new neighbors move in, for example, one might invite them over for coffee to get acquainted. Food practices also convey many associations with family sentiment. In many households, it is not Christmas without a special cookie, dessert, or meal. Many cultural traditions revolve around food. For many generations, eating fish on Fridays symbolized sacrifice on the part of Roman Catholics. Fasting still has this connotation in many cultures.

Within everyday family life, certain meals have more or less symbolism than others. In many cultures, the evening meal is the specific gathering time of the family. Morning and noon meals have less significance in these cultures. In rural America, however, the noon meal was the more important meal of the day.

Food items can also be used for preventive and therapeutic purposes by members of cultural groups. For example, many cultures uses a variety of herbal teas to prevent or cure illness. Some of the therapeutic uses of specific foods will be presented later in this chapter.

As is the case with other culturally determined behavior, dietary practices vary with the extent to which an individual client has adopted the culture of the larger society. Pressures to change food practices arise from two sources—the environment and demands for acculturation.[98] The environment causes changes in dietary practices when usual food sources or ingredients are not available or when changes in one's living environment make certain foods or practices inappropriate. For example, movement from a nomadic-hunter society to a sedentary existence has caused the high fat consumption of the Pima Indians to become inappropriate and has resulted in widespread obesity.[43]

Demands for acculturation, or a desire not to be "different," can lead to either positive or negative changes in eating habits. For instance, the desire to fit Western cultural norms has led to decreased breast feeding among Southeast Asian women, a negative result of acculturation.[99]

Native Americans

Food has social as well as nutritive value among cultural groups. For Native Americans, some foods, particularly corn, have sacred symbolism and are used in tribal ceremonies.[100] These ceremonies might take place in the health-care setting. Nurses should make an effort to understand the ritual significance of certain foods and act accordingly. For example, rather than objecting to the diabetic client eating certain foods, nurses can help the client adjust the day's diet by figuring the appropriate exchanges.

Most Native Americans, in past years, ate a relatively balanced diet, although they had no knowledge of nutrition.[42] Common staples included meat and a variety of vegetables.[101] As a result of changes in lifestyle, many families no longer farm or raise livestock. Forced to buy meat and vegetables at today's inflationary prices with limited income, their access to adequate nutrition has been limited.[72]

A study of the traditional foods of North Dakota Indians indicated that the nutrient content of the Native American diet of the past was quite high. Of seven traditional foods examined, only two (corn bread and Indian fried bread) were not considered nutritious. Unfortunately, fried bread is the only one of these traditional foods regularly eaten today. Study results indicate that reversion to more traditional foods would preserve cultural heritage as well as improve nutritional status among many Native Americans.[101]

The typical diet among many Native Americans today includes indigenous and processed foods and few fresh fruits and vegetables, especially in urban areas. Among some groups, such as the Navajo, meat and blue cornmeal are believed to give strength, while milk is considered a weak food. As noted earlier, corn has a special mystical significance and is considered a sacred food in many tribes.[29]

Asian Americans

The typical Asian diet is high in sodium because of widespread use of soy sauce and, in the case of Filipinos, salt. A balanced meal in Asian cultures is thought to incorporate both "hot" and "cold" foods. Hot and cold do not refer to the temperature of the food, but to its relationship to the forces of Yin (cold) and Yang (hot). Yin and Yang are the two opposing forces of the universe that regulate the normal flow of energy.[30] An imbalance in these forces is thought to result in illness. Typical foods eaten by Asian clients include a wide variety of vegetables, eggs, rice, wheat, pork, and chicken.[29]

Particular foods might be used in the treatment of specific conditions because of their "hot" or "cold" properties. When Yin is in excess, "hot" foods such as chicken broth and ginger are given and "cold" foods such as fruits and vegetables are avoided.[29] Other "hot" foods include rice, pork, chicken, eggs, vinegar, and peanuts.

Special foods and herbs are used at certain times. Ginseng is frequently given to pregnant women. "Hot" foods are used during the postpartum period by clients of both Korean and Chinese ancestry. Iron is believed by some Asians to "harden the bones" resulting in a difficult delivery. For this reason, some Asian clients may refuse prenatal vitamin and mineral supplements that contain iron.[102]

Asian clients may refuse ice water in the belief

that it "shocks the heart." Vegetables and beef are preferred well cooked, while milk and milk products are frequently disliked by Chinese clients.[51] Many Southeast Asian clients display an actual intolerance to lactose and have vomiting and diarrhea with the ingestion of milk products.[7,50]

Black Americans

As noted earlier, many food preferrences among blacks are the result of the availability of such foods to slaves. In addition, fried foods and starches are favored, as are many "junk" foods. Foods typically eaten include corn, pork, lard, legumes, greens, and hot breads. The diets of southern blacks are frequently deficient in sodium, calcium, iron, niacin, and calories.[29]

Certain foods are perceived by some blacks as providing strength. These foods include milk, meat, and vegetables.[29] Some combinations of foods, such as watermelon and whiskey or milk and fish, are thought to result in illness or death.[103] Many black people also subscribe to the idea of "hot" and "cold" foods and use certain foods in dealing with specific conditions. For example, pregnancy is thought to be a "hot" condition, so meat is avoided and additional sodium consumed.[29] Such practices may increase the potential for both anemia and eclampsia during pregnancy.

American Latinos

Latino clients share the Asian classification of foods into "hot" and "cold" categories. They also believe that "cold" foods should be consumed during "hot" illness and vice versa. Chili peppers, garlic, onions, fish, turkey, and most starches are considered "hot" foods. Most other vegetables, beef, lamb, cow's milk, rabbit, chicken, legumes, corn tortillas, and human milk are considered "cold."[104] Clients from Mexico employ a number of condiments, particularly red and green chili peppers, that make their food quite spicy. Puerto Rican food, on the other hand, is much more bland. Typical foods eaten by Latinos include beans, flour and corn tortillas, eggs, chicken, several vegetables, sweetened packaged cereals, milk in hot drinks, canned fruit, ice cream, and gelatin. The typical Latino diet is apt to be deficient in vitamin A, iron, and calcium intake.[29]

Appalachian Americans

Soup beans, corn bread, greens, fried meats, biscuits, and gravy are some of the staple foods of the typical Appalachian client. Some Appalachians believe that tomatoes are harmful and may cause cancer. Avoidance of other foods such as pork, cabbage, instant coffee, "store tea," fish without scales, web-footed fowl, oysters, grapefruit and several other fruits, as well as salt and artificial sweetners, is recommended by one modern-day folk healer.[105]

LIFE EVENTS

A great deal of variation exists among cultural groups in the attitudes and behaviors expected in relation to certain life events such as conception, birth, and death.

Conception and Contraception

Beliefs and practices related to conception and contraception vary from culture to culture. In many traditional Latino families, the wife expects to become pregnant shortly after marriage. Should conception not occur, certain herbs may be used to "heat the womb" and promote conception.[106] Korean women traditionally define their self-identity in terms of the mother role and their duty to produce an heir, so conception shortly after marriage is valued.[74] Family-planning information is likely to be unwanted by women who adhere to such traditional beliefs about childbearing.

Blacks and Native Americans tend to view contraception as an individual decision or one made for the good of the family. Latinos, on the other hand, may not be open to artificial forms of contraception such as birth control pills, IUDs, and so on, because of religious doctrines of the Roman Catholic Church, the primary religion of 85 percent of Latinos.[21] Filipinos often resist contraception on similar religious grounds. Asian women might be reluctant to seek family-planning services if they believe that they will be examined by male health-care providers; feminine modesty is highly valued in Asian culture.

While illness-preventive behaviors are not widely accepted by Appalachians, contraception is a widely practiced preventive behavior. In one study, approximately 83 percent of married women in rural Appalachia were using some form of contraception, and 87 percent of those women were using reliable methods such as sterilization, oral contraceptives, or an IUD.[107]

Birth

Birth is a life event surrounded by many cultural beliefs and practices. Many folk health beliefs and practices are related to conception, pregnancy, labor and delivery, and postpartum care.

Among Asians, childbirth is not considered an illness, but is a period of danger for both mother and infant. Special foods and herbs such as ginseng are used to safeguard the pregnant woman. Iron in the prenatal period is thought to harden the bones and make delivery more difficult.[102] Therefore, many

Asian women will resist taking vitamin preparations containing iron.

Many Asians, including Vietnamese[6] and Chinese,[102] believe that body heat is lost during labor and delivery. The Vietnamese use hot coals beneath the bed to counteract this, and both Vietnamese and Chinese use "hot" foods to replenish body heat. Hot foods include rice, chicken soup, peanuts, vinegar, and ginger. Cold foods such as most fruits and vegetables are avoided. Koreans use a seaweed soup with rice during the postpartum period to cleanse the blood and increase milk production.[102]

Practices related to birth itself vary from one group to another. Among the Hmong, for example, the placenta is buried after delivery with the place of burial specifically defined for male and female infants. The placenta is to be buried near the center pole of the house after the birth of a male child and under the parents' bed for a girl. It is believed that the place where the placenta is buried is the person's "true home" and burial in the wrong place will lead to misfortune.[108]

After delivery, Asian clients are exhorted to avoid "cold" and exposure to unclean things. Showers and baths, except sponge baths, are contraindicated. Water applied to the body is thought to cause loss of nutrients through the skin. Women remain at home for some time after delivery[102] and avoid early ambulation and strenuous activity to protect internal organs.[6] Abstinence from intercourse lasts from 2 to 3 months after delivery, and the use of contraceptives is discouraged.

For the pregnant Latino, especially the primipara, pregnancy is a time of many controls on activity, food, and so forth. Fewer restrictions are placed on the woman who has had several previous pregnancies.[106] Bathing is encouraged and cravings satisfied or the child will have a defect related to the food craved by the woman.[69,106] The pregnant woman is encouraged to keep active and to sleep on her back. Special massage may be used to "fix" the baby in an appropriate position for delivery. Milk might be avoided in the diet in the belief that it will result in a larger baby and a more difficult delivery.[106]

In some Latino cultures, pregnant women are believed to be particularly susceptible to *coraje,* or rage, which may result in spontaneous abortion, premature delivery, or knots in the umbilical cord. For this reason, the pregnant woman is encouraged to cultivate serenity and remain calm. She should also refrain from hanging laundry or reaching up, sitting tailor fashion, or crossing the legs as these behaviors may lead to a knotted umbilical cord. Sexual intercourse is continued throughout the pregnancy to ensure adequate lubrication of the birth canal to facilitate delivery, but baby showers are not held until close to the time of delivery to avoid envy and the evil eye.[106]

The Appalachian client might display numerous beliefs and practices related to childbearing. These range from explanations of when fertility is greatest, to beliefs as to how the sex of the child is determined, to means for speeding up labor and preventing complications. In traditional Appalachian culture, prenatal care, delivery, and postpartum care are the responsibility of the older, experienced female members of the family. The prenatal and postpartum examinations performed by most physicians are considered unnecessary and humiliating. However, the Appalachian client is more amenable to seeking professional care for a simple, natural condition such as pregnancy than for many illnesses.[83]

In Appalachian culture, specific health practices are to be observed in the prenatal, labor and delivery, and postpartum periods. The pregnant woman should eat a balanced diet and avoid strong emotion.[34,109] Strong cravings, fright, or surprise can cause the infant to have a birthmark. Abortion can result from jumping from a height such as a barn roof, stepping over a rail fence,[88] or drinking ginger root tea.[105]

Labor pains may be eased by placing a sharp implement such as a knife, scissors, or razor on or under the bed to "cut" the pain. Labor can be speeded up by wrapping the mother's ankles in warm cloths[34] or by the physical presence of the father or an article of his clothing in the labor room. This last practice is an instance of the principle of contagious magic, as the presence of the father or his clothing is believed to impart male strength to the woman, increasing the force of contractions.[88]

Practices used in the postpartum period include bed rest, a dose of castor oil or paregoric to purge impurities from the mother, and avoidance of fresh fruit.[109] In both Appalachian and black cultures, catnip tea is given to the newborn to cleanse the liver and bring out impurities in the form of hives.[34] Postpartum hemorrhage may be stopped by recitation of certain biblical verses, particularly Ezekiel 16:6. Postpartum pains may be alleviated by a strong drink of whiskey or, again, by imparting strength by hanging the husband's pants on the bedpost.[88] Beliefs and behaviors related to childbearing in the cultural groups presented here are summarized in Table 15–2.

Death and Dying

The last life event to be considered in a cultural assessment is death. All cultural groups have beliefs and practices related to death and dying, and culture influences death and dying in a number of ways.[31]

TABLE 15–2. SELECTED CULTURAL BELIEFS AND BEHAVIORS REGARDING CHILDBEARING

Focus	Belief or Behavior
General	• Menstrual cramping can be alleviated by avoiding spicy food. (Appalachian, Latino) • Menstruation is a "hot" condition, so "cold" foods should be eaten. (Appalachian) • Childbirth is a natural event. (Appalachian)* • A pregnant women is considered ill. (Latino) • Pregnancy is a time of danger for mother and child, but is not an illness. (Asian)
Contraception	• Herbal preparations can be used to prevent pregnancy. They may be given as teas, suppositories, douches, applied topically, or inhaled. (Latino) • Pregnancy should be prevented through abstinence. (Asian) • Oral contraceptives cause birth defects and ill health for the mother. (Appalachian) • Abortion can be caused by drinking ginger root tea, jumping from a height, or stepping over a rail fence. (Appalachian)
Conception	• Herbs can be used to "heat" the womb to promote conception. (Latino) • The fertile period for a woman is a few hours of a "heat cycle" midway between menstrual periods. (Appalachian)* • The child's sex is determined by the side the mother turns to after intercourse. (Appalachian) • The right ovary produces "girl seeds," the left produces "boy seeds." (Appalachian)
Pregnancy	• Pregnant women should eat a balanced diet and avoid sweets and snacks. (Appalachian)* • Pregnancy is a "hot" condition so meat should be avoided and sodium intake increased. (Black)† • Red meat should be avoided during pregnancy to prevent "high blood." (Black, Appalachian)† • Iron in the prenatal diet causes hardening of the bones and a difficult delivery. (Asian)† • Milk during pregnancy may result in a large baby and a hard labor. (Latino)† • Soy sauce and shellfish should be avoided during pregnancy. (Asian) • Unclean foods should be avoided during pregnancy. (Asian) • Cravings should be satisfied to prevent a defect related to the food craved. (Latino, Appalachian) • Ginseng tea will strengthen the pregnant woman. (Asian) • Strong emotions during pregnancy will leave a mark on the baby. (Appalachian, Latino) • Fright or surprise during pregnancy can injure the baby. (Latino, Appalachian) • Pregnant women should avoid raising their arms or hanging laundry to prevent knots in the umbilical cord. (Latino) • Sitting cross-legged fashion will cause knots in the umbilical cord. (Latino) • Bathing should be encouraged during pregnancy. (Latino)* • Pregnant women should sleep on their backs. (Latino) • Pregnant women should keep active. (Latino)* • Nausea and vomiting can be treated with a mixture of flour and water, lemon and water, or chamomile tea. (Latino) • Violent purging herbs can be used for constipation in pregnancy. (Latino)† • Prenatal care and delivery by an older woman is preferred. (Appalachian, Asian) • Pregnant women should be accompanied to the doctor by husbands or female family members. (Latino) • Periodic massage during pregnancy can help fix the fetus in the correct position for delivery. (Latino) • Baby showers should be held close to the time of delivery to prevent envy and the "evil eye." (Latino) • Sexual activity should be continued throughout pregnancy to keep the birth canal lubricated. (Latino)
Delivery	• There is a correlation between the hour of conception and the time of delivery. (Appalachian) • Labor can be stimulated by the use of various herbal preparations. (Latino) • Wrapping warm clothes around the mother's ankles will speed labor. (Appalachian) • The presence of the father or an article of his clothing will speed delivery. (Appalachian) • The father or one of his relatives should deliver the child. (Hmong) • Husbands should not be present during labor and delivery. (other Asian) • It is inappropriate to exhibit pain during labor. (Asian) • Labor pains can be "cut" by placing a sharp implement under the bed. (Appalachian) • Aspirin given for pain will thin the blood and cause increased bleeding. (Appalachian)* • Recitation of certain biblical passages will stop hemorrhage. (Appalachian) • Delivery should take place in a squatting position. (Asian) • Delivery causes a loss of body heat that must be replaced. (Asian)

(*continued*)

TABLE 15–2. (*Continued*)

Focus	Belief or Behavior
Postpartum	• Castor oil or a paregoric should be given to the woman after delivery. (Appalachian)†
	• Fresh fruit and other "cold" foods should not be eaten after delivery. (Appalachian, Asian)
	• Salads and sour foods cause postpartum incontinence. (Asian)
	• Postpartum fluid intake should be decreased to prevent stretching the stomach. (Asian)†
	• Beef and seafoods cause itching at episiotomy site. (Asian)
	• Alcohol in rice wine causes bleeding. (Asian)
	• Prolonged bedrest and avoidance of strenuous activity prevent complications after delivery. (Appalachian, Asian)†
	• Outside visitors should be discouraged after delivery. (Korean)
	• Strangers in the home after delivery may steal the mother's milk. (Hmong)
	• Postpartum pain can be relieved by whiskey, or by hanging the husband's pants over the bedpost. (Appalachian)
	• Herbal preparations can relieve afterpains. (Latino)
	• Burning or burying the placenta will prevent harm to mother and child. (Appalachian, Hmong)
	• Drinking cold water should be avoided after delivery. (Asian)
	• Intercourse should be avoided 2 to 3 months after delivery to prevent disease. (Asian)
Infant	• A raisin on the umbilical stump will prevent air entering the infant's body. (Latino)†
	• Castor oil will seal the umbilical stump. (Appalachian)†
	• A belly band on the infant will prevent umbilical hernia. (Appalachian)
	• A silver coin taped over the umbilicus will prevent umbilical hernia. (Latino)
	• Infants should be given a purge or tonic (may contain lead). (Asian, Black)†
	• A second stillbirth can be prevented by placing a dead infant face down in the coffin. (Appalachian)
	• Exposure to a menstruating woman may cause an umbilical hernia. (Black, Latino)

* Beliefs or practices consistent with scientific health care.
† Potentially harmful beliefs or practices.

One area of influence is the need for comfort experienced by the dying client. In those cultures where death is seen as a normal part of life, there may be less need to comfort the dying and his or her family; conversely, in cultures where death is feared, comfort may be needed and appreciated.

The community health nurse should assess whether those she is dealing with have a cultural belief in an afterlife. Some non-Western religions, including Hinduism, believe in reincarnation until the soul has achieved perfection and passes to Nirvana. Do religious beliefs regarding death and afterlife offer a source of comfort to clients and families or do they engender fear and anxiety?

Attitudes toward death within a cultural group can also vary depending on the nature of the death. Violent deaths may be more difficult to accept as a normal part of life. Among blacks, violent deaths provoke more emotional outbursts, anger, and rage than do natural deaths,[31] while the Lao people see violent death as punishment for misdeeds.[64] For the Cheyenne, violent death is believed to lead to a disturbance in spiritual balance and eternal wandering of the departed soul.

Cultural responses to suicide differ from cultural responses to death from natural causes. For example, Latinos are more likely to conceal a suicide than members of other groups. This may be a result of past refusal by the Catholic Church to bury suicide victims in hallowed ground.[110] Among Filipinos, suicide is considered shameful.[31]

Culture also influences the selection and perception of health-care providers when death is imminent. Some cultures believe that one should die at home and are, therefore, unlikely to seek medical care for the dying client for fear that he or she will be removed from the home and placed in a hospital to die. The Hmong, for example, believe that death should take place in the home.[64] For many people, going to the hospital is seen as evidence that death is inevitable. For example, Asian, Native American, and black clients may equate hospitalization with imminent death.[7,31]

Care of the body following death, and funeral and burial practices, are also influenced by culture, as are expectations regarding grief and mourning and practices to be observed during this period. Mourning is "the culturally defined patterned behavioral response to a death,"[31] and practices related to mourning will vary from one group to another.

Finally, culture influences communication regarding death, particularly with respect to children and their knowledge of and participation in the rites that accompany a death. For example, Appalachians are usually quite open in their communication about death, and Native American and Latino children help with the care of the dying family member and participate in funeral and grieving practices. Despite this participation, one study of Latinos indicated a widespread belief that the dying person should not be informed of his or her prognosis.[110]

Other questions relate to who should attend the dying client. The eldest son of a Chinese client should be present with his dying parent, whereas in some Native American tribes, the maternal aunt is the more important figure.[70] Members of other tribes believe that the spirit cannot leave the body until family members are present.[31]

Among Native Americans, death is considered a part of life, and funerals are accompanied by feasting and gift giving.[90] Many tribes, including the Navajo and the Tlingit, prefer not to touch a dead body.[31] This may be a measure designed to prevent intrusion by the dead person's ghost. Among the Sioux, on the other hand, family members are expected to prepare the body for funeral rites. Nurses should be familiar with the death rites of specific tribes so they can assist the family through their time of grief. Should the nurse wash and prepare the body or is a family member responsible for this? Should personal belongings be left with the body or given to the family? The nurse should learn the answers to such questions when working with clients from these cultures.

Generally speaking, there is no belief in an afterlife among traditional Native American tribes. Nurses who use this approach to comfort clients with terminal disease will find it ineffective. They may be confused and frustrated by this lack of response unless an understanding of the cultural beliefs involved has been achieved.

Members of many Native American tribes see the body as a "seed to be planted" and believe that the body must be disposed of in its entirety. Thus, family members may request amputated limbs to be kept until death and disposal of the body. They may also resist having an autopsy performed.[31] Disposal of the body can vary among tribes. For example, cremation is traditionally practiced by the Tlingit and Quechan tribes, whereas the Sioux place the dead on elevated platforms, and members of Pueblo tribes bury their dead. Among many tribes, such as the Navajo, the body is dressed in fine clothes and jewelry and wrapped in new blankets. As noted earlier, the Tlingit fear to touch a dead body, so the client may be dressed in funeral clothes several days before death.[31]

Mourning can be very emotional in some Native American tribes, but it usually lasts a very short time. For instance, following 4 days of mourning, the Cheyenne and Quechan cease grieving, as do members of some other tribes. In some tribes, the name of the deceased is never spoken again and memory of the deceased is actively suppressed.[31]

Approaches to death and dying also differ between Eastern and Western cultures. Veneration of one's ancestors is common in the East. Vietnamese believe, for instance, that the dead continue to remain close to living family members. Thus it is very important for the Vietnamese client to die at home.

Clothing assumes special meanings when it comes to dying. The clothing of a deceased Chinese is believed to contain evil spirits. Family members of hospitalized clients should be encouraged to take clothing home until the client is discharged. If the client should die, the family may be reluctant to accept the deceased's personal effects.[51] Clothing is also used to symbolize mourning, and mourning garments are worn for varying lengths of time in different cultures.[18] The color of mourning can also vary. For example, black is the color of mourning for many cultures, but white signifies mourning among the Hmong, while black is worn for weddings and other celebrations.[108]

In traditional black culture, death is perceived as a passage from one realm of life to another. Funerals are generally occasions for celebration despite the grief of family members left behind. Some blacks also have the practice of passing a child over the dead body to carry away any illness the child may have.[95] As is true in the larger society, funerals and wakes are seen as a psychosocial mechanism that facilitates grieving.[31] It has been suggested by some authors that blacks may be less accepting of death than other cultural groups because of demonstrated expectations and desires for long life, despite figures indicating reduced longevity in this group.[110]

Funerals among Latinos are evidence of their deep religious belief in an afterlife. Death is perceived as the will of God. After death, the body is prepared by a commercial mortuary and placed on display during the Rosary ceremony that takes place prior to the funeral. The Rosary is an occasion for friends to join the family in saying the specified prayers of the Rosary and to offer condolences. Following the Rosary, the funeral mass is held and the body laid to rest. *Novenarios,* or nine days of evening prayer services, begins on the Monday following the death. Services are held in the home of the deceased or his or her family. In the traditional Latino family, mourning is observed for 6 months, during which survivors wear black and restrict their social activities.[65]

As we have seen, beliefs and behaviors regarding death and dying vary among different cultures. Table

TABLE 15–3. SELECTED CULTURAL BELIEFS AND BEHAVIORS REGARDING DEATH AND DYING

Focus	Belief or Behavior
General	• Death is a normal part of life. (Native American, Asian) • Death is passage from one realm of life to a better one. (Black) • Death is passage into the next life. (Asian) • No belief in afterlife. (Native American)
Violent death	• Violent death provokes stronger emotional outbursts than does a normal death. (Black) • Violent death is punishment for misdeeds. (Lao) • Violent death creates a ghost to wander forever. (Navajo, Cheyenne)
Suicide	• Suicide should be concealed because of shameful nature. (Latino, Filipino) • Suicide may be used to save family honor. (other Asian)
Place of death	• Hospitalization means death is imminent. (Black, Asian, Native American) • Death should occur at home. (Hmong, Vietnamese)
Preparation and disposal of body	• Touching a dead body may bring misfortune. (Navajo, Tlingit) • Passing a child over a dead body may cure illness. (Black) • Entire body must be disposed of together. Autopsy may be resisted. (Native American) • Bodies should be cremated. (Tlingit, Quechan) • Bodies should be buried. (Pueblo tribes) • Bodies should be exposed to air on funeral platform. (Sioux) • The dying person should be dressed in funeral clothes before death. (Tlingit) • Family members should prepare the body for burial. (Sioux) • Bodies are prepared for burial by commercial mortuary. (Latino) • Bodies should be richly dressed and wrapped in new blankets. (Navajo) • Clothing of a dead person may contain evil spirits. (Chinese)
Grief and mourning	• Emotional grieving lasts for 4 days after which the name of the dead is never spoken. (Cheyenne, Quechan, Navajo) • White should be worn during the mourning period. (Hmong) • Black should be worn during the mourning period. (Latino) • Social activities should be restricted during the mourning period. (Latino) • The dead should be included in rituals commemorating ancestors. (Vietnamese) • The funeral and wake are a time to rejoice for the dead and comfort the living. (Black) • Funeral Mass is preceded by saying the Rosary. (Latino) • The first Monday after death begins 9 days of evening prayer for the dead. (Latino)
Participation and knowledge	• Dying clients should be protected from knowledge of impending death. (Latino) • Children should participate in the care of dying family members, funerals, and mourning. (Native American, Latino) • The eldest son should be present at the death of a parent. (Chinese) • Family members must be present for the spirit to leave the body. (Native American)

15–3 summarizes selected behaviors related to death and dying for the cultural groups presented here.

OTHER CONSUMPTION PATTERNS

A final consideration in investigating life-style factors in another culture is that of consumption patterns other than dietary practices. These include the use of tobacco, alcohol, and other abused substances. Alcoholism is a serious problem among Native Americans and has contributed to rising mortality rates due to alcohol-related motor vehicle accidents.[49] Peyote and other hallucinogens may be used in religious ceremonies by members of the Native American Church.

The use of alcohol is disapproved by many Appalachian families, although brewing alcoholic beverages for sale to outsiders is a lucrative enterprise in some parts of Appalachia. Asians have a relatively low incidence of alcoholism, which many believe is due to early introduction of children to moderate use of alcoholic beverages such as fruit wines and saki. Among blacks and Latinos, use of alcohol is considered part of the male adult image. Alcoholism and substance abuse are prevalent among many minority groups including blacks, Native Americans, and Latinos, not so much because of cultural practices related to alcohol but because of the stress of life for minority group members.

Tobacco use is high among all of the minority groups presented here. As is the case among Americans at large, smoking tends to decline as educational levels increase. A recent study of smoking among Latinos in San Francisco indicated that fewer acculturated males and more females smoked than among their less acculturated counterparts. For those who did smoke, however, the more acculturated smoked more cigarettes per day.[111] These findings suggest that educational messages regarding smoking should be targeted differentially among various cultural groups.

HEALTH SYSTEM

Areas of cultural assessment related to the health system include the folk health system within the culture, as well as group members' use of the scientific system. Components of the folk health system to be addressed include cultural perceptions of health and illness and disease causation, folk health practitioners, and culturally prescribed health practices.

PERCEPTIONS OF HEALTH AND ILLNESS AND DISEASE CAUSATION

All cultures have concepts of health and illness and theories of disease causation, although these may differ widely from group to group. It has been suggested that each culture has an "explanatory model" of illness that defines the nature of illness, its treatment, and the type of relationships that should occur between client and health-care provider.[112] Nurses who wish to understand clients' conceptions of health and illness must investigate the explanatory models found in each client's culture.

Native Americans

Among Native Americans, cultural concepts of health and illness are fairly consistent across tribes. The health beliefs of the Navajo are relatively typical of those of Native Americans in general. According to a Navajo nurse, "The Navajo believes everything is in harmony and all of nature works with itself rather than against itself. When illness occurs, a Navajo has violated this law."[72] Health is viewed in terms of the life cycle, which encompasses birth, life, and death. Health is the result of harmony between man and universe, as well as an ability to survive in difficult circumstances and not be vulnerable to threatening situations.[66] Human beings are not viewed as the dominant force in nature but as interdependent with other beings and forces. Illness results from disharmony with the environment. This disharmony may result from human violation of a natural law or from such natural phenomena as storms, lightning, and so on.[73]

Other potential causes of illness are witchcraft, spirits, and animal contamination. Disease is thought to be caused by object intrusion, spirit intrusion, soul loss, or insults to nature. Object intrusion occurs when one's body is invaded by a worm, snake, insect, or small animal and occurs as a result of sorcery.[89] Spirit intrusion involves possession by ghosts, either animal or human. Some hunting rituals involve appeasement of the ghosts of animals killed.[42] Soul loss occurs during dreams when the soul wanders from the body.

Among the Otomi Indians of Mexico, distinctions are made between "bad illness" caused by evil people or beings and "good illness" that is amenable to scientific medicine. "Airs" or wandering ghosts of those who met a violent end may also cause disease.[89] The Zuni also attribute disease to both natural and unnatural causes. Natural illnesses may result from injury, insect bite, and so on. Unnatural conditions may result from sorcery, object intrusion, and breach of taboo.[100]

Asian Americans

The emphasis in Asian folk medicine is primarily preventive, whereas that of Western medicine is oriented to "crisis intervention."[113] Most Asian medicine is based on Chinese medicine adapted as the Chinese moved throughout Asia.[30] The Asian concept of health involves achieving a state of *Qi* (pronounced "chee"), which is a balance of Yin and Yang.[17] An imbalance between Yin and Yang results in disharmony or illness.

Most Asian cultures believe that all components of the universe, including humans, are composed of a Yin and a Yang. The Yin is the negative female force, characterized by darkness, cold, and emptiness. The Yang is the positive male force producing light, warmth, and fullness. The Yin and Yang may be likened to the actions of the sympathetic and parasympathetic nervous systems. The Yang is comparable to the defensive action of the sympathetic system in that it protects the body from external invasion. The Yin, like the parasympathetic nervous system, is concerned with restoring and conserving bodily energy. An overabundance of either Yin or Yang is thought to trigger illness. For example, an excess of Yin may result in frequent colds, nervousness, and gastric problems. Too much Yang may cause fever, dehydration, irritability, and tenseness.[51]

Similar concepts to the Yin and Yang of Chinese medicine are found among the Vietnamese. A balance between Am and Dong is required for health, and that balance is maintained through judicious use of "hot" and "cold" substances. Imbalance results in disease.[99] Illnesses that result from an excess of Yin include diarrhea, dizziness, and blurred vision, whereas Yang conditions include pimples, pustules, and constipation.[114]

For the Khmer of Cambodia, health is a reflection of previous behavior and moral action. Misfortune and illness are the result of violations of moral and ethical codes. Illness may also be due to invasion by evil spirits or an imbalance of Yin and Yang.

Among Lao and Hmong clients, illness is believed to be due to the absence of one or more of a defined number of souls that comprise one's life force. The number of souls that should be present ranges from 8 to 32 depending upon the cultural group. Conversely, health is the presence of all the requisite souls. Soul loss may be caused by the influence of the spirits of dead ancestors. Hmong clients may also believe that illness is the result of bad blood.[64] Other causes of disease found among Southeast Asian clients include inharmonious or inappropriate behavior by the client, his or her relatives, or neighbors. While Thai clients may believe that disease is caused by germs, they may also believe that these germs must be activated by sorcery to cause disease.[115]

Health is viewed by most Asian cultures as an exclusively physical matter.[30] Mental illness is taboo and carries a definite stigma. Families in which an emotional illness occurs are shamed and may try to hide the problem as long as possible. Mental illness is thought to be the result of punishment for the sins of the entire family.

Black Americans

Blacks frequently attribute illness to punishment for wrongdoing, to magic, diet, life-style, impurities in air, food or water, poor hygiene, and irregular bowel movements.[63] Blacks tend to classify illnesses as natural or unnatural,[34] and they place them in three etiologic categories:[28] environmental hazards, divine punishment, and impaired social relationships that may result in worry or the incursion of spells and witchcraft.

In traditional black culture, all illnesses are thought to be curable, and the concept of chronic disease is difficult to accept. The belief in a cure for every illness is derived from the principle that for everything, including disease, there exists its opposite.[34] Blacks tend not to separate mental and physical illness.[28]

American Latinos

In Latino cultures, as well, illness is viewed as more than a mere biological occurrence and is seen in terms of its spiritual and social ramifications. Latino clients also differentiate between natural and unnatural illnesses. Natural illnesses are thought to occur as the result of a personal violation of the balance among human beings, nature, and God.[36] Unnatural or supernatural illness is secondary to satanic forces.[80]

Many Latinos have a complex classification system for diseases that includes both physical and emotional illness.[65,78] Physical illness can be temporary (no treatment needed), mild (able to be treated at home), or grave. Grave or serious illnesses are further categorized as painful or chronic. Emotional illness can be of a mental or moral nature. Mental illness includes derangement due to head trauma, fright, or worry, as well as hex illnesses due to *mal ojo* or witchcraft, and hereditary diseases such as mental retardation and epilepsy. Clients with mental illness are perceived as victims with no responsibility for their condition. Moral illness, however, is the fault of the person affected. Moral illness may include excessive exhibition of emotions such as rage and jealousy, character weakness such as alcoholism or kleptomania, or a tendency toward vice exemplified by marijuana or drug use.[65] Illness can also be a result of imbalance in "hot" and "cold" humors, concepts similar to the hot-and-cold balance seen in Asian cultures.[78]

Other conceptualizations of disease also exist among members of Latino cultures.[38] First, illness may be used as a rationalization for inappropriate behavior, thereby absolving the miscreant and family of responsibility for his or her actions. For example, a daughter who defies her parents to marry an "outsider" may be thought to be the victim of an illness caused by witchcraft.

Second, illness following interpersonal problems may be a precursor to their solution. For example, the daughter who falls ill when her father will not allow her to marry the man she loves may convince her father to change his mind rather than see her suffer. Finally, illness may be the expected result of violating a traditional value. For instance, loss of a first child may be perceived as retribution for lack of filial behavior on the part of the girl who marries against her parents' wishes.

In Latino cultures, chronic illness is seen as punishment for evil. The Latino attitude toward health and illness is fatalistic. It is believed that health is a matter of chance and little can be done to maintain or enhance it. Health is perceived as a gift from God and is defined in terms of three criteria: freedom from pain, a well-fleshed body, and a high level of physical activity. Health is equated with strength, and illness equated with weakness.

Appalachian Americans

In Appalachia illness is regarded as a state of disequilibrium, while health is equated with harmony with one's environment. A study of older Appalachians found that most subjects defined health as being able to work, to take care of themselves, and to do the things that one likes to do.[116] Physical symptoms or limitations related to activities of daily living

TABLE 15–4. SELECTED CULTURAL BELIEFS REGARDING DISEASE CAUSATION

Focus	Belief
General	• Illness can result from either natural or supernatural causes. (Native American, Asian, Appalachian, Black, Latino)
Natural illness	• Illness can result from violation of a natural law. (Native American) • Natural phenomena such as storms, lightning, and other disturbances may cause disease. (Native American) • Germs may cause disease. (Appalachian) • Environmental hazards (e.g., bad air, water) may result in illness. (Black) • Imbalance among man, nature, and God may cause illness. (Latino) • Imbalance between "hot" and "cold" forces may cause illness. (Latino, Asian, Appalachian) • Natural illnesses may result from insect bites, bruises, or injuries that cause fractures. (Zuni) • Bad blood may cause disease. (Hmong) • Illness may be due to inharmonious relationships or inappropriate behavior by client, relatives, and/or neighbors. (Southeast Asian) • Natural diseases result when one confronts the forces of nature without adequate protection. (Black) • Poor health habits and bad hygiene may cause disease. (Black) • Irregular bowel habits might bring on illness. (Black, Appalachian)
Supernatural	• "Bad" illnesses are caused by the evil action of people or spirits. (Otomi) • "Airs" or wandering ghosts of those who met violent ends may cause illness. (Otomi) • Disease may result from spirit intrusion or object intrusion. (Otomi, Zuni, other Native American) • Breach of taboo may result in disease. (Zuni) • Germs must be activated by a sorcerer before they can cause disease. (Thai) • Evil spirits cause disease. (Hmong, Latino, Black) • Illness may be a punishment for sins or a test of faith. (Black, Appalachian, Latino) • Soul loss may cause disease. (Lao, Hmong, Native American) • Illness may be due to magic. (Black, Latino, Asian, Appalachian)

were seen as the opposite of good health. The Appalachian client acknowledges several sources of illness including germs, magical causes[117] and punishment for sins.[37]

Illness in Appalachia is defined in terms of the subjective feelings of the client. One is not ill unless one feels ill.[24] This definition of illness makes compliance with a medical regimen uncertain in illnesses such as TB in which the client usualy does not feel ill. Symptomatic physical illness may engender strong fears and anxieties on the part of the client, particularly if hospitalization is required.[84] Emotional illness is viewed as weakness to be dealt with privately rather than through outside assistance.[118] Beliefs regarding the cause of disease among the cultural groups presented here are summarized in Table 15–4.

FOLK HEALTH PRACTITIONERS

Every culture has its own folk health practitioners. The most important attributes of folk practitioners were well captured in this description:

> The folk practitioner uses a combination of rational, irrational, and psychological techniques in curing; his diagnosis is minimal; he has folk medical theories based on such things as a simplified notion of the body, religion, astrology, and plant lore; he treats more commonplace or chronic conditions than he does acute ailments or infectious diseases; he is charismatic and a good showman; and he reinforces the value system of his clients.[105]

In assessing any cultural group, the nurse will want to explore several areas related to folk health practitioners. Among these are the types of practitioners recognized by the group, the health-related services provided, and the methods employed. Other questions to be asked include: Who and where are the practitioners? Is there a recognized hierarchy among practitioners? Does referral or cooperation exist between folk and professional practitioners? Who uses the folk practitioner and what is the prevailing attitude of community members toward folk practitioners? Finally, the nurse will explore the expectations involved in the client-practitioner relationship.

Native Americans

Native American tribal medicine has been described as a combination of rational and religious practices. The Native American seeks care from someone who can restore harmony with his or her surroundings. Several sources of health care, in addition to health professionals, are available to Native American clients. Generally, the client first seeks assistance from a family member who is responsible for care of illness. If this route proves unsuccessful, he or she may see a community specialist who has knowledge of healing but does not have the religious affiliation of the medicine man.[119]

The central healing figure, however, is the medicine man. Medicine men often fall into specific classes within a tribe. These include practitioners of medical magic who can deal with supernatural causes of illness,[119] herbalists, and seers or prophets. Herbalists have knowledge of the use of herbs in healing, while prophets or seers can assist one to avoid harmful situations or determine one's prognosis.[42] Interestingly enough, physicians are considered herbalists, because they are knowledgeable about the use of medications but cannot restore harmony with nature.[11]

Folk health practitioners vary from tribe to tribe among Native Americans. Among the Zuni, for example, there are three broad classifications of healers.[32] Medicine men employ meditation, chanting, massage, and herbs to draw out evil forces causing disease. Bone pressers realign and reset bones and deal with skeletal injuries and arthritis using a form of physical therapy. Belly rubbers, who are usually women, are persons who have been struck by lightning, thereby acquiring the ability to deal with gastrointestinal and liver complaints by rubbing the abdomen.[32]

The primary healer among the Lakota-Ogalala people is the Yuwipi man. This person usually had a mystical experience as a child and experienced a misfortune in middle age that was associated with illness or injury and communication with ghosts. This experience is followed by consultation with an established Yuwipi man and an apprenticeship. Following apprenticeship, the person practices on his own until the occurrence of another misfortune, at which time his healing powers seem to disappear. The Yuwipi healing ritual involves a trance during which the healer calls on spirits who tell him how to cure the client's illness. Services of the Yuwipi man are usually sought for supernatural illness.[120]

Navajo healers frequently engage in a healing ritual called the Blessingway, or Beautyway. This ritual consists of chants and other practices aimed at restoring harmony and health.[66]

Asian Americans

Chinese medical practitioners can be classified as acupuncturists, herb pharmacists, or herbalists.[51] The herbalist diagnoses illness and prescribes an herbal remedy, which may be prepared by the herbalist or by the herb pharmacist. Clients may also go directly to the herb pharmacist, who will provide a remedy based on the client's description of symptoms. The herbalist is more of a diagnostician than is the herb pharmacist. The herbalist obtains a history, observes the client's tongue, color, and perspiration, listens to body sounds, and takes the pulse to diagnose illness.

The acupuncturist employs the same diagnostic techniques but uses acupuncture rather than herbs as therapy. In the acupuncture technique, the practitioner inserts fine needles into any of 361 meridians, or channels, influencing the area affected. Meridians selected are those that serve the body part affected by disease, those known to have specific therapeutic properties related to certain kinds of disease, or those in close proximity to the area involved. Acupuncture has achieved a certain degree of recognition as a treatment modality in the scientific health-care system, and acupuncturists are licensed as independent practitioners in 16 states and can practice under the supervision of a physician in 10 others.[30]

Among the Lao, *maw*, or healers, are classified by their specialty area and include the spirit expert, the magic expert, the medicine expert, and others who provide technical services such as midwives, herb merchants, and injectionists. Spirit and magic experts deal with illnesses believed to be caused by evil spirits or magic, respectively. The medicine expert uses herbal medicines to treat illness, while the herb pharmacist dispenses the herbs required for recommended treatments, and the injectionist gives injections prescribed by other practitioners including Western physicians.[64]

Hmong clients may seek the services of a medicine healer for externally visible symptoms. The medicine healer employs diet, massage, and herbal remedies to deal with illness. For invisible sources of pain or disability, clients may see a shaman, or *neeb*, who will enter a trance to determine which of the client's souls are missing and where they have gone. During the trance, the shaman will attempt to cajole the souls to return to the client or may have to fight evil spirits that are preventing the return of the souls.[64]

Black Americans

Among many blacks, the ability to heal is perceived as a divine gift. Practitioners can be classified into three groups based on the means by which this power was acquired.[28,63] The first and lowest rank consists of those who learned their craft from others. This category includes the housewife as well as the medical doctor. These individuals are believed to be capable of dealing only with simple conditions attributable to natural causes.

The second category of healer includes those who acquired their healing power during a religious experience in later life. The spiritualist is an example of this type of healer and is capable of dealing with problems of a financial, personal, spiritual, or physical nature.[37]

The most gifted individual is the one born with healing abilities. This person is identifiable at birth or even during gestation. Birth order may be an indication of healing powers. For example, a seventh son or daughter or a child born after twins is thought to have special powers. Children born with the amniotic sac covering the face are thought to have innate healing abilities. Occasionally, a fetus in utero may demonstrate healing capabilities even before birth. It is the person born with the skill of healing who is capable of curing all illnesses, even those of magical origin.[34]

An additional type of healer recognized in black cultures is the voodoo priest or priestess or conjurer. Other terms for this type of practitioner are "root doctor," "herb man," or "herb doctor" (not to be confused with the herbalist of other cultures), "underworld man," "conjure man," or "goofuhdus man."[28] The conjurer may be trained by another or inherit the ability from his or her father or mother. The skills of the conjurer are believed to be effective against all forms of magically wrought illness.

American Latinos

Latino folk medicine also recognizes a variety of healers. Assistance with health matters is usually first sought from *el (la) que sabe,* a family member conversant with folk remedies. This person deals with common minor ailments.[80] The *yerbero* is knowledgeable in the use of herbal remedies. Herbs are employed in both preventive and curative practices and the activities of the Latino *yerbero* are similar to those of the Asian and Appalachian herbalist.[37]

Curanderismo is a healing tradition prevalent in Mexico that derives from both Indian and Roman Catholic tradition. Major elements of *curanderismo* are the belief that God heals all illnesses, a compendium of folk illnesses that respond to treatment by the *curandero,* and belief in mystical diseases such as *susto.*[121] The treatment practices of this healing tradition commonly include herbal remedies, prayer, healing trances and rituals, suggestion, massage, advice, dietary intervention, magic, and discussion of the problem that is causing the disease.[36] These practices are used in the treatment of such conditions as *mal de ojo, empacho, caida de mollera,* and *mal puesto.*

The *curandero* usually receives the gift of healing through divine intervention, but may also be trained in healing arts by another *curandero.* One may become a *curandero* as a result of dreams, visions, or by experiencing a feeling of oneness with some force beyond the individual. The principal characteristic of the *curandero* is religious faith. The failure of a cure is attributed to the will of God rather than the ineptness of the practitioner. Other attributes seen among *curanderos* include seizures, fainting spells, episodes of sleepwalking or talking during sleep, or trances.[38]

Espiritismo or spiritualism is another traditional system of healing that is common among Puerto Ricans.[36] Its origins lie in African and French traditions combined with elements of Roman Catholicism.[36,122] Adherents of this tradition believe there is an invisible world of spirits of the deceased who attach themselves to the living for either good or ill. One's body is believed to have an aura that reflects one's health status, a second aura that reflects emotional state, and two surrounding envelopes separated by black space. Each envelope consists of electrical particles that circulate either clockwise (the inner envelope) or counterclockwise (the outer envelope).

The spiritualist employs healing passes ("magnetic" discharges from his or her fingers), counseling, and the use of homeopathic remedies (substances that are thought to be like the condition or its cure) to restore health.[122] The spiritualist or medium also attempts to commune with the spirit world to induce good spirits to ward off bad spirits that may be causing disease.[36] Requirements to become a spiritualist include a desire to cure, the ability to receive the curing spirit, purity of heart and body, and faith in God.[122]

According to Finkler,[123] healer-client interaction in the spiritualist tradition occurs in four phases. The first phase is one of dislodgement, in which a *limpia,* or cleansing ceremony, is used to cleanse the client. In the second stage, the client describes his or her symptoms. The third stage consists of the healer's statement of the treatment needed; the fourth stage is a recapitulation of the required treatment. In addition to the healing phases, the healer may use a combination of herbal teas, baths, massage, and patent medicines.[123]

Like *espiritismo, santeria* is a folk healing approach derived from Roman Catholic ritual and African tribal beliefs. It is particularly prevalent among Cubans.[36] While the *espiritualista* works primarily through the power of spirits and deals with solving existing problems, the *santero* emphasizes health promotion. The *santero* deals with illnesses arising from object intrusion, imitative or contagious magic, soul loss, spirit intrusion, and diseases caused by the anger of the gods. Treatment by a *santero* usually consists of a prolonged ritual involving cleansing of evil spirits, rebirth, and protection from future evil. Such rituals commonly involve a special bath, drinking the blood of sacrificed animals, eating farina, and chanting.[36]

The *sabador* uses massage and manipulation to treat both traditional and nontraditional illnesses affecting the musculoskeletal system. The *sabador* may also deal with conditions such as *caida de mollera* and *empacho.*[65] The final category of practitioner found in Latino cultures is the *brujo,* or witch, who uses magic to inflict, prevent, or cure illness.[65] The *brujo* is comparable to the conjurer found in black cultures.

Appalachian Americans

Four categories of traditional folk practitioners exist in Appalachia: herbalists, faith healers, psychic healers, and midwives.[117] Much of the Appalachians' knowledge of herbal remedies was acquired from their Indian neighbors, particularly the Cherokee.[105] Herbalists possess several qualifications for their craft. First among these is a belief in the healing power of plants. Second, the herbalist must have skill in identifying, collecting, preparing, and using herbs. A third requisite is belief in the assistance of God. Religion and healing are closely intertwined in Appalachia, and a cure cannot be achieved without divine intervention. The final requisite for the herbalist is experience, which is frequently a part of the natural socialization process for young girls in Appalachia. If a family member is skilled in the use of herbal remedies, the girl will serve an apprenticeship learning this skill.[124]

A strong interpersonal relationship between client and healer is required in all types of healing, but is particularly necessary with faith healers. Faith healers exercise their skill by means of the laying on of hands, assisted by the divine presence. Timing and belief are important components in faith healing. The faith healer generally employs words of power that are closely guarded secrets. One powerful phrase used is "Three ladies come from the east, one with fire, two with frost, out with fire, in with frost."[124]

Psychic healers are believed to use special powers to project healing forces into the sick person. A psychic healer is thought to possess healing energy that can be transmitted to others usually by some form of touch. Untrained midwives are usually mature women who assist with childbirth. They may provide advice, herbal tonics, and other remedies during pregnancy.

Generally speaking, healing is the province of Appalachian women. Men, however, may also participate in healing responsibilities. Healing functions related to childbirth, aches and pains, wounds, burns, fits, and spells are the responsibility of women, whereas men deal with warts, chills, and fevers.

FOLK HEALTH PRACTICES

Members of all cultural groups engage in certain culturally prescribed health practices. It is wise for the community health nurse exploring the health practices employed by a cultural group to recognize that these practices are designed to meet specific needs and have meaning and importance to group members.

Traditional health practices can be categorized into those related to primary and secondary prevention. Childbirth practices, a special category of primary preventive measures, were discussed earlier in this chapter.

Primary Preventive Practices

Health promotion and illness prevention also are important aspects of a folk health system. Table 15–5 presents some common cultural beliefs and behaviors related to health promotion and illness prevention for each of the five cultural groups presented in this chapter.

Native Americans. Native American folk medicine uses both preventive and curative health practices. Some of the preventive measures include herbal teas and charms and fetishes to ward off evil spirits that cause disease.[119] Another preventive measure is the cultural taboo against cutting one's hair. Long hair is a sign of health and strength. Cutting the client's hair is thought to weaken the person and may bring about, prolong, or prevent recovery from illness.[90] Among the Otomi, the *limpia,* or cleansing ceremony, might be used on a regular basis as both a preventive and curative measure in the case of illness.[89]

In some tribes, the "writing of one's story" is thought to cause loss of some spirit life.[11] The nurse should ascertain if this belief is held by a client before obtaining a health history or making other notations on the client's record. It may be necessary to go into less detail in a health history than would otherwise be the case.

Native Americans have also developed a number of precautions related to communicable diseases without benefit of knowledge of pathogenic organisms. Isolation is a common practice for illnesses known to be contagious or considered unclean. Items in contact with the infected person are burned and clothing washed. Refuse is also burned as a sanitation measure. In some tribes, men wounded in battle were placed in individual huts, away from the rest of the village, during their convalescence. This practice is comparable to the modern concept of reverse isolation.[42]

TABLE 15–5. SELECTED CULTURAL BELIEFS AND BEHAVIORS RELATED TO HEALTH PROMOTION AND ILLNESS PREVENTION

Focus	Belief or Behavior
General	• Carrying a printed prayer on one's person will prevent mishap. (Appalachian, Black) • A variety of herbal preparations can be used to promote health and prevent illness. (Asian, Black, Appalachian, Latino, Native American, Southeast Asian) • Periodic purges keep the system open and prevent disease. (Black) • Silver or copper bracelets worn by young girls warn of impending illness by turning the surrounding skin black. (Black) • A *limpia* or cleansing ceremony may be used as a general preventive measure. (Otomi)
Diet	• Children, pregnant women, convalescents, and the elderly should avoid red meat to prevent "high blood." (Black, Appalachian) • Pork, cabbage, instant coffee, "store tea," fish with scales, round-hoofed animals, oysters, potatoes, plums, grapefruit, cherries, cranberries, graham crackers, salt, and saccharin lead to waste buildup and illness, and should be avoided. (Appalachian) • A balance of hot and cold foods should be eaten. (Asian, Latino, Appalachian)
Life-style	• Excess in food, drink, and activity should be avoided. (Black) • Keeping the body clean inside and out will prevent illness. (Black)
Magic	• Charms worn around the neck ward off evil and prevent illness. (Appalachian, Black) • Asafetida, or rotten flesh, worn in a bag around the neck prevents communicable disease. (Black) • Charms made of the fat of a person who died a violent death can scare away evil spirits. (Lao) • Amulets, chains, and tattoos prevent spirit invasion. (Khmer) • A string on the wrist or neck protects the infant from evil spirits. (Hmong) • Prayer and veneration of the relics of saints can prevent illness. (Latino) • Charms and fetishes will ward off evil. (Native American)
Specific prevention	• Eating onions or baking soda will prevent "flu." (Appalachian) • Avoiding tomatoes will prevent cancer. (Appalachian) • Avoid cutting infants' fingernails to prevent heart disease. (Asian) • Nosebleeds can be prevented by not becoming overheated. (Latino) • Prevent chills by not eating or drinking cold things when hot. (Latino) • Not cutting one's hair will prevent loss of strength. (Native American) • Avoid writing one's story to prevent loss of life spirit. (Native American) • Isolation will prevent the spread of communicable disease. (Native American)* • Isolating ill persons will prevent them from becoming worse. (Native American)* • Burning refuse will prevent disease. (Native American)* • A gold ring on a red ribbon around the neck will prevent anxiety. (Latino) • Wearing coral around the neck or wrist will prevent depression and "evil eye." (Latino) • Not going barefoot will prevent tonsillitis. (Latino)

* Beliefs or practices consistent with scientific health care.

Asian Americans. All of the many Asian cultural groups engage in a variety of unique practices. There are, however, some common preventive and therapeutic behaviors among them. Some common health practices include massage, use of herbs, and meditation.

Herbal teas are widely used to prevent a variety of illnesses, especially among Southeast Asian groups.[125] Some Asians also avoid cutting an infant's fingernails to prevent heart disease.[6] The Khmer may use amulets, chains, and tattoos to prevent spirit invasion,[114] while the Lao and Hmong also use charms against sorcery. A most powerful charm used by the Lao is made from the fat of a person who has met a violent death. Among the Hmong, a charcoal cross on the forehead is thought to provide protection against evil spirits.[64] Finally, ginseng preparations, as well as other special foods, are given during pregnancy to provide strength and prevent complications.

Black Americans. Many of the preventive measures used by blacks are similar to those of Appalachian clients. Practices that the two groups have in common include prevention of "high blood" by avoiding red meat, the use of charms, and carrying a printed prayer. Many blacks also believe, in common with Latinos, that the touch of a menstruating woman may be harmful to the newborn infant. Keeping the body clean inside and out is another measure used to prevent illness. This may lead to excessive use of laxatives to purge the body of impurities.[63] One scientifically sound preventive measure is avoidance of late nights and excessive consumption of food and drink. Other preventive measures were described earlier in conjunction with the traditional folk illnesses for which they are used.

American Latinos. Prevention in Latino cultures involves a number of dietary measures as well as activities and charms and relics thought to possess supernatural powers. *Mal aire* or "bad air" causes several conditions that can be prevented by avoiding drafts, covering one's head while outdoors, and keeping the windows closed at night. Herbs and spices are used in various teas to prevent and cure illness. Charms such as a gold ring on a red ribbon or coral worn around the neck or wrist may also be used to prevent anxiety, depression, and *mal ojo*.[78] Red clothing may also be used to protect infants from *mal ojo*.[69]

Latinos believe that their diet should include a balance of "hot" and "cold" foods. Excess consumption of rice, bananas, apples, fried foods, coffee, and tamales should be avoided. Eating or drinking cold foods when overheated or sitting in a draft can cause chills.[80] Overheating oneself through strenuous exercise can also bring on nosebleeds, so such activities should be avoided.[34] Several other Latino preventive measures were discussed earlier in this chapter in conjunction with the folk illnesses for which they are used.

Appalachian Americans. Appalachian folk health practices include a variety of preventive measures. Many of these include dietary practices involving consumption or avoidance of specific foods. For example, eating raw onions or taking baking soda are thought to prevent influenza. Foods to be avoided include tomatoes, meat from round-hoofed animals, fish without scales, several fruits, and commercial preparations such as instant coffee and teas purchased at the store rather than brewed from wild herbs.[105] Persons who are considered weak and susceptible to illness, such as pregnant women, children, the elderly, and convalescents, should also refrain from eating red meats to prevent "high blood."

Magical interventions include carrying a printed prayer on one's person to prevent a variety of mishaps including drowning and various illnesses and other accidents.[34] Wearing charms is also thought to ward off evil and prevent conditions like rheumatism, cramps, leg pains, nightmares, and illnesses caused by witches.[124]

Secondary Preventive Practices

When illness occurs, members of a cultural group turn to practices designed to diagnose and treat illness. Many similarities exist between cultures in such practices.[37] Some common therapies include diet, herbs, application of heat and cold, massage, bone setting, exercise, and rest. Table 15–6 includes selected cultural beliefs and practices related to diagnosis and treatment of illness.

Native Americans. Some Native American tribes use dreams as a diagnostic tool.[42] In areas where this is the case, nurses should inquire about the client's dreams as a means of establishing credibility and to gain a clearer picture of the client's state of health and related cultural beliefs. Seers or prophets within the tribe may be responsible for interpreting dreams and should be incorporated into the plan of care if necessary. Another type of diagnostician is the "hand trembler" who identifies the locale and cause of disease.[73]

While healing rituals may vary among tribes, there are some universal treatment techniques used. One common principle is that "like cures like." In addition, many common remedies incorporate the administration of herbal medicines that may be ingested or applied to affected areas of the body. Many herbs are thought to derive their healing power from ritual ceremonies. Certain herbs are considered useful because they are distasteful to evil spirits[42] and cause them to depart the client's body.

Among many preparations used for their healing properties by the Otomi of northern Mexico are green vegetables and onions for respiratory disease, herb poultices, and teas for pain or to draw out evil illnesses. Herbs are used in sweat baths to draw out evil. Cooked onions are used to gain weight, while raw onions are used to lose weight. Heavy or prolonged menstrual bleeding may be treated with boiled banana peels or stems, and purgatives are frequently used in poisoning cases.[89]

The Zuni use sap from pinon trees to treat leg ulcers and its gum as an antiseptic. Poultices made of juniper ash are used to reduce edema due to injury, and goldenrod or "Zuni tea" is given for colds, sore throat, and cough. For fever, and for gastrointestinal or genitourinary problems, a concoction made of thistles is used, while sage and mustard are used to treat burns and headache, respectively.[32]

Another major healing ceremony is the "sing." This is a ritual performed by a medicine man or a singer consisting of "ritual, prayers, and chants which must be performed in precisely the right manner to be effective."[73] A sing is a community affair that involves the client, the singer, and associates, family, and friends. A sing can last as long as 9 days, but most are considerably shorter.[73] Sings are also used to confer or increase the power of herbs and other implements of healing or to renew that power.[42]

TABLE 15–6. SELECTED CULTURAL BELIEFS AND PRACTICES RELATED TO DIAGNOSIS AND TREATMENT OF ILLNESS

Focus	Belief or Behavior
Diagnosis	• Diagnosis made by means of dreams or by a "hand trembler." (Native American) • Diagnosis made using techniques of inspection, listening, questioning, and palpation. (Chinese, other Asian) • Diagnosis made by iridology—the condition of the iris. (Asian)
General treatment	• Exercise may be suggested as a remedy for illness. (Asian) • Herbal preparations are frequently used to treat illness. (Native American, Asian, Appalachian, Black, Latino) • Sweat baths may be used to treat illness. (Native American, Lao, Khmer) • Massage may be used to treat illness. (Otomi, Zuni, Lao, Hmong, Chinese) • Onions placed on the wall of a sickroom will absorb illness. (Appalachian) • Signs of the zodiac indicate susceptibility to specific diseases. (Appalachian) • Signs of the zodiac should be consulted when planning surgery. (Black) • Prayer may bring about cure of illness. (Latino, Native American) • Pressure on specific points on the foot (reflexology) may relieve illness. (Japanese) • Medication should be discontinued when symptoms disappear. (Lao, other Asian, Black)* • Wounds should be covered to keep them clean. (Lao) • Medicines are usually prepared by boiling herbs in a prescribed amount of water and taking all of the preparation. (Chinese, other Asian)* • Scientific medicines are considered "hot" and may not be taken if the illness is considered "cold." (Otomi, Asian)*
Diet	• "Hot" foods should be taken to treat "cold" illnesses and "cold" foods to treat "hot" illnesses. (Asian, Appalachian, Latino)
Magic	• Gather bark from the east side of a tree to appease the gods (Native American) or for greater potency. (Appalachian) • Like cures like. (Appalachian, Black) • Use invocations to spirits accompanied by rattle or drum in healing rituals. (Native American) • Songs or chants amplify the forces of good in their battle with evil. (Otomi, other Native American) • Garlic on one's person or in a room will ward off evil spirits. (Black) • A *limpia*, or cleansing, may be accomplished by passing an object over the body to pick up evil. (Otomi) • Recital of the Twenty-third Psalm, reading Scripture, prayer, and positive reminiscences may cure illness caused by a hex. (Black) • A *baci* ceremony may be used to placate spirits causing illness. (Lao)
Treatment for specific conditions	• Coining is used to treat pain, colds, vomiting, and headache (Khmer), heat stroke, indigestion, and colic. (Chinese) • Cupping is used to treat headache and bodyache by removing noxious elements (Khmer). Cupping may also be used to treat arthritis, abdominal pain, abscess, and stroke paralysis. (Chinese) • Moxibustion is used to treat mumps, convulsions, and nosebleed. (Chinese) • Treat pain with acupuncture, acupressure, blowing in the ear, painting with a purple spot, pinching, cupping, or coining. (Asian) • Sweat baths are useful treatments for childbirth, opium withdrawal, mental disorder, and psychosomatic illnesses. (Lao) • Warts can be removed with water from the rotted stump of a chestnut tree. (Appalachian) • Herbal teas may be used for fatigue, cold, sore throat, cough, chest ailments, and other conditions. (Appalachian) • Sassafras is used for agues, lung fever, ulcers, stomach problems, skin conditions, sore eyes, catarrh, gout, dropsy, syphilis, and anemia. (Appalachian) • Use goldenseal (herb) for weak stomach, liver, or intestinal problems, hemorrhages, poor circulation, and "nerves." (Appalachian) • Use ginseng for stomach and female problems, aging, sore eyes, asthma, poor appetite, rheumatism, longevity, and luck. (Appalachian) • Any plant root or plant with a yellow cast can be used to treat jaundice. (Appalachian) • Use yellow root tea for sore throat, stomach upset, high blood pressure, canker sores, or tonic. (Appalachian) • Use boiled green persimmons for diarrhea. (Appalachian) • Smoke jimson weed for asthma (Appalachian) • Use ginger to strengthen the heart and treat nausea and dyspepsia. (Asian) • Treat object intrusion by massage to draw the object up, then sucking over the area. (Otomi) • Use green vegetables and onions to treat respiratory disease. (Otomi)

(*continued*)

TABLE 15–6. (*Continued*)

Focus	Belief or Behavior
Treatment for specific conditions (*continued*)	• Use cooked onions to gain weight, raw onions to lose weight. (Otomi) • Dissolve certain tree insects in the mouth to treat sores or drink the juice of the insect. (Otomi) • Grind up guava and put in the mouth to treat sores. (Otomi) • Poultices may be used to treat heart pain. (Otomi) • Boiled banana peel or stems will stop heavy or prolonged menstrual bleeding. (Otomi) • A tamarind bath can be used for the chronically fatigued child. (Otomi) • Purgatives should be used for "poison." (Otomi)* • Drink sugar and turpentine for worms, rub it for backache. (Black)* • Use "bluestone" powder in open wounds. (Black) • Use stale bread or sour milk on lacerations. (Black) • Use lemon and honey for colds or camphor and oil rub for cough. (Black) • Onions applied to the feet and use of several blankets will cure fever. (Black) • Fluid intake should be decreased with fever. (Khmer)* • Pinon sap is used to treat leg ulcers. (Zuni) • Goldenrod tea is used for cold, sore throat, and cough. (Zuni) • Pinon gum may be used as an antiseptic. (Zuni) • Thistle concoctions can be used for fever, gastrointestinal problems, or genitourinary infections. (Zuni) • Mustard plant can be used to treat headache or sunburn. (Zuni) • Sage can be used to treat burns. (Zuni) • Anemia may be treated with blood pudding. (Latino) • Raw potato soaked in vinegar may be placed on the forehead to treat headache. (Latino) • Skin conditions may be treated with grated potato or tomato. (Latino) • Oregano tea may be used for cough. (Latino) • Earache is treated with a preparation of rue on cotton placed in the ear. (Latino) • Hot tea or a dock (weedy plant) or saline gargle can be used to treat sore throat. (Latino) • Fever may be treated with an enema of "malva leaves." (Latino) • Tape treated with camphor balm can be placed over the temples to treat headache. (Lao) • Greta or azarcon may be used to treat *empacho* (both have high lead content). (Latino)* • Chamomile tea is good for high blood pressure. (Latino) • High blood pressure may also be treated by eating pears, being tranquil, and eating garlic (to prevent stoke). (Latino) • Rattlesnake capsules may be used to treat a variety of chronic conditions. (Latino)*

* Potentially harmful practice.

Songs are also used in Otomi healing rituals and are believed to amplify the forces of good in their battle with evil forces causing disease.[89]

Sleight of hand is sometimes performed to symbolize the extraction of foreign objects placed in the client's body to cause illness. In some tribes such practices are not acknowledged,[89] whereas in others the sleight of hand is recognized but believed to be symbolic of the healing action of the gods.[100]

Asian Americans. Asian folk medicine employs four diagnostic techniques: visual inspection, listening, questioning, and palpation.[126] Visual inspection includes assessing the client's nutritional condition and skeletal development; the color and condition of the skin; the condition of five "rooted" organs (eyes, tongue, lips and mouth, nose, and ears), each of which is believed to reflect the condition of other body parts; the condition of the nails and hair; and the character and color of excreta.

In the technique of listening, the Asian practitioner assesses the quality of the speaking voice, respiratory sounds, the presence or absence of cough, yawning, or sneezing; the character of abdominal sounds, and the presence of delirium. Questioning involves obtaining information related to five tastes (salty, bitter, sweet, sour, and hot or spicy), five fluids (sweat, tears from crying, dribbling saliva, tears from weeping, and spitting saliva), five states of mind (anger, happiness, worry, sadness, and fear); fever, sweating, appetite and diet, excretory functions, dry mouth, vomiting, coughing or respiratory abnormality, hemorrhage and menstruation, and pain. Other questions focus on dizziness, tightness of the shoulders, insomnia or sleepiness, palpitation or other cardiovascular abnormality, coldness of the extremities or feeling hot, unusual movement of the extremities, or one's sexual life.[126] As one can see from this list, the Asian practitioner examines many of the same areas covered in a thorough health history obtained by Western medical professionals.

Using the technique of palpation, the practitioner examines several pulses, the abdomen and chest, the back, and the meridians that carry the *Qi* or life force.[126] One other diagnostic approach that may be used by some practitioners is that of iridology, or examination of various parts of the iris. Practitioners of this form of diagnosis believe that the condition of certain portions of the iris reflect the condition of specific body parts.[127]

Southeast Asian clients employ four major forms of self-care for illness.[20] These include offerings to spirits, dermabrasion, maintenance of hot-cold balance, and use of herbal medicines. Illness in children may be interpreted as an attempt by spiritual parents to take them back and is treated by offerings of chicken to placate the spirits.

Several treatment modalities are used by Asian cultural groups.[7,114,128,129] These include cupping, pinching, coining, steaming, the use of herbal preparations, massage, moxibustion, burning, acupuncture, acupressure, and reflexology. Cupping consists of burning an alcohol swab in a cup and placing the heated cup over the painful area to draw out noxious elements. Cupping leaves a circular bruised area. This procedure is commonly used to treat headache and body aches, arthritis, abdominal pain, abscesses, and paralysis due to stroke.[7,114]

Pinching, believed to bring out wind, produces welts or bruises. Pinching is commonly done on the neck and over the bridge of the nose. It leaves severe asymmetric ecchymoses in the area pinched. Coining or rubbing is performed on lubricated skin with a spoon or coin. It is used to treat pain, colds, vomiting, headache, stroke, deafness, facial paralysis and epilepsy.[7,114] Coining results in circular excoriations that resemble cigarette burns.

Steaming is used to improve the complexion of postpartum women and for respiratory difficulties in children. Hot water with herbs is poured over a hot rock and the steam inhaled. Remedies including tiger balm and ginger root are also frequently used for various illnesses.[114] Eight categories of action of herbal remedies in Chinese medicine have been described.[7] These include emetics, purgatives, herbs that induce perspiration, heat inducers, tonics, diuretics, detoxins, and neutralizers.

Massage is used to improve the circulation of energy and blood, to increase movement of stiff joints, and to increase resistance to disease. Two types of massage employed are a pushing and grasping technique, used for neurasthenia, ulcers, and chronic hepatitis, and a technique of palpating and massage used to bring about the other effects listed above.[7]

Moxibustion consists of the application of pulverized and heated wormwood or moxa plant over specific meridians or areas that indicate points of entry to channels leading into the body. It is commonly used to treat conditions such as mumps, nosebleed, and convulsions.[7]

Burning is used by some Asian groups to compensate for heat loss due to diarrhea. Burning consists of touching a lighted cigarette or burning cotton to the skin, usually on the abdomen.[20] Because burning and dermabrasive techniques such as coining, cupping, and pinching leave unusual bruises or lesions, they may be interpreted as signs of child abuse; thus great care should be taken in the presence of such findings to elicit an accurate history of their occurrence. These practices are not usually physically dangerous and may even contribute to the client's sense of well-being, so they should be permitted or, at times, even encouraged.[20]

As noted, herbal medicines are frequently used in both Asian and other cultures. For the most part, the use of these remedies can be encouraged. However, the community health nurse should try to determine the actual ingredients of these remedies whenever possible as some have been shown to contain high levels of lead, arsenic, and mercury.[130]

As in the case of dietary therapeutics in Asian cultures, "hot" treatments are used for "cold" illnesses and vice versa. Acupuncture is a "cold" treatment and is used in conditions caused by an excess of Yang. Moxibustion, on the other hand, is "hot" and is used to treat an excess of Yin.[95] Shiatsu acupressure, a Japanese technique related to acupuncture, makes use of pressure, rather than the insertion of needles over acupoints or valves that control the flow of *Qi* along the body's meridians.[128,129] Another related technique is that of reflexology in which certain points on the foot are stimulated with pressure so as to achieve specific therapeutic effects in related parts of the body.[128]

Among the Lao, common remedies include the use of moxibustion, massage, bandages, compresses and splints. Tape treated with camphor balm is placed over the temples for headache, while sweat baths are commonly used for childbirth, opium withdrawal, mental disorders, and psychosomatic illnesses. The Lao use a *baci* ceremony to placate spirits. Medicines can be of animal, vegetable, or mineral origin.[64] One folk remedy for fever called *pay-loo-a* contains high levels of lead and may result in lead poisoning.[127] The Hmong use similar types of medicine and massage. Cupping is also performed, but a cow horn is used rather than a cup.[64]

Many Asian clients have a different orientation to treatment than do Westerners. This is particularly true with respect to medications. The Chinese, for example, believe that one dose of an herbal preparation should cure the condition and are confused by multiple-dose therapies. Also, medication is usually taken in liquid form with very specific instructions as to its use. Western medications tend to be dispensed in pill form with few directions, which further confuses clients.[51] The Lao client, rather than relying on a single dose for cure, may take several doses in the belief that, if one is good, more is better.[64] On the other hand, members of Lao, Khmer, and other Asian cultures may reduce the prescribed dose or discontinue medication use because of side effects.[64,114]

Black Americans. Many black cultural practices involved in healing have already been discussed in relation to the folk illnesses for which they are used. One additional behavior that warrants mention is the practice of consulting the zodiac prior to scheduling any surgical procedure. It is believed that blood is more plentiful in certain areas of the body during the influence of certain astrological signs. Levels of blood present in each region of the body fluctuate with changes in the zodiac, much like tides are influenced by the moon. Therefore, to prevent hemorrhage, a surgical procedure should only be scheduled when the amount of blood at the operative site is expected to be at a minimum.[34] Specific remedies used for illnesses caused by evil spells include reading Scripture, recitation of the Twenty-third Psalm, prayer, and positive reminiscences.[63]

American Latinos. Latinos typically treat illness in one of three ways depending upon its perceived severity. Criteria used to determine severity include the extent of pain and the presence of bleeding.[78] Minor illnesses are dealt with at home using a variety of herbs and kitchen vegetables. When these remedies fail, over-the-counter medications may be tried. For serious illness, outside help is sought in the form of medical prescription[65] or through the traditional folk healers discussed earlier. Some traditional remedies include blood pudding to treat anemia, application of raw potato slices soaked in vinegar to the forehead for fever and headache, and the use of grated potato or tomato for skin conditions.[78] High blood pressure is treated with chamomile tea, pears, cultivating tranquility, and eating garlic to prevent stroke.[131] Oregano tea or steam inhalation is used for cough, while rue on cotton is often placed in the ear for earache. Sore throat is treated with hot tea or gargles of dock (a weedy plant) or saline. Treatment for fever might include an enema with a solution made from "malva" leaves.[65] Cooked prickly pear cactus is used for diabetes. This preparation is known to have a mild lowering effect on blood glucose[69] and may precipitate a hypoglycemic reaction in diabetic clients taking hypoglycemics.

Two folk remedies that have been widely used for treating *empacho* are *greta* and *azarcon*. Both have extremely high levels of lead (as much as 90 percent) and can be quite toxic.[127] Both were widely used in many Mexican-American communities until widespread public education campaigns limited their use. They remain a danger, though, for recent arrivals to the United States from Mexico, those who may not have been reached by the educational campaign.[121]

Another Latino folk health practice that has potentially harmful effects is that of ingesting rattlesnake capsules. Rattlesnake capsules are an old Mexican folk remedy used for a variety of chronic illnesses. The capsules, made of pulverized rattlesnake, frequently contain *Salmonella arizona*, a pathogenic bacteria that causes diarrheal disease. Their pathogenic effects are particularly severe for those who are immunocompromised.[132]

Appalachian Americans. One Appalachian healer described a common practice of consulting the signs of the zodiac to determine one's susceptibility to certain "two-way viruses." Each sign of the zodiac is associated with a particular part of the body. Aries is the "head" sign, so persons under this sign are susceptible to head colds. Those whose sign is Saggitarius, a "thigh" sign, are thought to be susceptible to problems in the loins, evidenced by cramps, aching, and so on.[105]

Treatment of illness among Appalachian clients tends to involve two stages.[24] In the first stage, clients try a variety of home remedies. In the second stage, they may seek the assistance of a "granny midwife," an herbalist, or a faith healer. Only in an emergency will the traditional Appalachian usually consult a physician.

Herbal preparations are used to cure as well as prevent illness in Appalachia. Some herbs are used singly, while others are strengthened when used in combination. For example, "white lightning" (homemade whiskey) added to snake oil makes a more effective rub for sore muscles than snake oil alone.[105]

FOLK VERSUS PROFESSIONAL HEALTH CARE

When the health practices followed by individual members of a culture are not successful and illness results, there is a need to seek assistance from a health-care provider. Given the relative inaccessability of professional health care, coupled with a distrust of professional providers in some groups, it is not surprising that members of many cultures turn to folk healers for assistance.

In many cultures, illnesses tend to be divided into two major categories: those amenable to folk medicine and those amenable to scientific medicine. Illnesses considered amenable to folk medicine tend to be chronic, nonincapacitating maladies and those believed to be caused by supernatural agents. Critical, incapacitating conditions, on the other hand, tend to require scientific medicine.

Several similarities can be observed in both folk and scientific health-care systems.[36] Both employ similar diagnostic skills such as listening and observation and both make use of verbal and nonverbal communication skills. Both systems engage in psychological and somatic techniques of naming illnesses, creating positive expectations, suggestion, interpretation, emotional support, and manipulating the environment. In addition, both systems use medicinal substances and engage in some forms of laying on of hands or massage. Finally, both the folk and scientific systems are based on an unequal relationship in which one party is an expert and one is a layperson.

Additional similarities between folk and scientific health systems include provision of a rationale for treatment, an explanation of illness, and a rationale for social and moral norms.[17] For example, both traditional black culture and the scientific health-care system explain the cause of AIDS in terms of life-style behaviors related to sexual behavior and drug use. They also provide rationale for selective sexual activity and refraining from drug abuse as a means of preventing AIDS.[63] However, the reasoning process used to reach these conclusions is different in each system.

Differences between the two systems are also evident.[36] Traditional folk medicine takes into account the religious and moral implications of disease, while the scientific system does not. Scientific medicine makes a definite distinction between mental and physical illness, while many folk health systems do not. Folk medicine is community-oriented, whereas scientific medicine is more oriented to the individual client. Folk medicine also tends to take place in familiar surroundings, whereas care in the scientific system is frequently provided in a distinctly foreign environment.[36]

Other differences have also been noted between folk and professional health-care systems.[133] Folk health care is primarily humanistic in nature, whereas scientific care is impersonal. Emphasis is placed on familiar, practical, and concrete facts in the folk system and on unfamiliar and more abstract concepts in the scientific system. The folk system is holistic in its orientation; the scientific system tends to be more fragmented. The focus is on *caring* in the folk system and on *curing* in the scientific system. The folk system stresses prevention of illness; the scientific system emphasizes diagnosis and treatment.

Cost of services is another significant difference between the two systems, with moderate costs for folk health care and high costs for scientific care. There is also less emphasis on cultural support systems in the scientific system than in the folk system. Similarities and differences between folk and scientific health-care systems are summarized in Box 15–6.

The choice of one system over the other is influenced by a variety of factors. Reasons for choosing folk health practices over scientific medicine include:

1. underestimating the severity of disease
2. inability to afford scientific medicine
3. religious beliefs and practices
4. inability to communicate because of language barriers
5. distrust of health professionals owing to impersonality of service, long waits, etc.
6. pride and modesty
7. fear of unfamiliar practices, hospitalization, etc.
8. desire for a quick, easy cure with a minimum of pain and frustration, and
9. a wealth of misinformation regarding health.[134]

Two additional phenomena that support continued use of folk health practices and practitioners are spontaneous remission and the placebo effect. The client improves in both cases and attributes improvement to the folk healer or remedy used. Yetiv[127] noted that approximately 80 percent of the effects of all medical practice may be due to placebo and that nontraditional healers are "able to offer the caring touch, the confidence in their healing powers" and are able to "concentrate more effectively on the placebo aspects of their contact with the patient."

Native Americans

Use of scientific and folk health care differs from culture to culture. Native Americans, for instance, differ from their Caucasian counterparts in terms of the conditions for which they seek professional care. Aches and pains and acute illnesses, which typically are self-limiting in nature, are considered by the Navajo to be part of life. For these conditions, no assistance is usually sought.[73]

Frequently, Native American clients will use both folk and professional health systems. In the choice of systems, a distinction is usually made by the Navajo

BOX 15–6

Similarities and Differences Between Folk and Scientific Health-Care Systems

SIMILARITIES

- Both systems employ similar diagnostic techniques including observation and listening.
- Both systems make use of verbal and nonverbal communication techniques.
- Both systems engage in the naming of illnesses and the creation of positive expectations.
- Both systems employ suggestion, interpretation, emotional support, and manipulation of the environment as therapeutic modalities.
- Both systems use medicinal substances and employ some form of laying on of hands in the care of the sick.
- Both systems are based on assymetric relationships between experts and laypersons.
- Both systems provide an explanation of disease, a rationale for treatment, and a rationale for social and moral norms.

DIFFERENCES

The Folk Health System	*The Scientific Health System*
• Takes into account the religious and social implications of disease	• Focuses primarily on the personal implications of disease
• Does not make a definite distinction between mental and physical illness	• Makes a definite distinction between mental and physical illness
• Oriented to the community	• Oriented to the individual
• Takes place in familiar surroundings	• Takes place in unfamiliar surroundings
• Emphasizes humanistic care	• Emphasizes impersonal care
• Emphasizes familiar, practical, and concrete facts	• Emphasizes abstract concepts
• Provides holistic care	• Provides fragmented care
• Emphasizes caring	• Emphasizes curing
• Stresses prevention	• Stresses diagnosis and treatment
• Emphasizes cultural support	• Does not emphasize cultural support
• Moderate cost for care	• High cost for care

and members of other tribes between symptoms amenable to modern therapy and the disharmony causing them. According to this view, only a folk practitioner can deal with the underlying cause of the illness, whereas the modern physician is capable of dealing only with the symptoms.[66] As expressed by one Otomi shaman, "The shaman removes the evil illness. The good illness that remains can be cured with medicine."[89]

Because expertise in treating illness is believed to come with age and experience, the youthful appearance of many physicians in Indian Health Service clinics run by the U.S. Public Health Service may be equated with lack of knowledge. To many Native Americans, the use of various diagnostic procedures is further proof that the physician does not know what he or she is doing.[120] These factors tend to limit Native Americans' use of these services until forced by the severity of illness to seek them out.

When Native Americans do make use of professional health-care services, compliance with recommendations may be less than desired. One possible explanation is the Native American client's need for group approval of actions taken. If a prescribed action appears not to make sense to a Native American's peers, approval is not given, and the client is likely to be noncompliant.[43] Professional interventions, then, need to fit the expectations of the client's social network. Such interventions will make sense and compliance will be more likely.

Asian Americans

Asian clients may use both Western and folk medical systems concurrently. However, they may be reluctant to inform either practitioner that they are seeing the other. In this way they avoid causing either physician to "lose face." This lack of knowledge on the part of either practitioner may result in drug overdose or adverse reactions due to interactions of drugs prescribed.[51] One area in which this is particularly pertinent is the treatment of hypertension. The physician may prescribe an antihypertensive drug while the traditional practitioner recommends a ginseng tonic. Ginseng itself is an antihypertensive, and the use of both medications might result in overmedication.[7]

Obtaining a health history from an Asian client who seeks professional care will require great tact and gentle probing. As in many cultures, the Asian is expected to be polite in interactions with others. Frequently, such courtesy involves responding to a question in the way one thinks the questioner wants one to respond.[135] This can result in the presentation of misinformation leading to inaccurate assessments and inappropriate interventions. When working with clients from Asian cultures, the health professional should be particularly careful to use the nondirective interview techniques described in Chapter 17, Care of the Individual Client.

Asian clients expect physicians to be able to make diagnoses based on history and physical findings rather than on complicated laboratory tests. The use of many involved or painful diagnostic procedures lessens the Asian client's respect for and confidence in the Western physician.[51] Another reason for female Asian clients to seek care from the traditional practitioner rather than the Western physician is their sense of modesty and discomfort with a health-care system consisting predominantly of male physicians.

While Asian clients use and have great respect for health professionals, there are certain practices common in Western health care that they are likely to resist. Among these are the drawing of blood, hospitalization, and surgical procedures. Blood is thought to be the source of the body's strength and is irreplaceable.[114,135]

Many Asians believe that hospitals are where people go to die.[7,51,53] Resistance to hospitalization is based on several factors. First, hospitals are considered unclean. Second, clients with little facility in English fear that no translator will be available. Hospital food is frequently unpalatable to Asian clients, and, finally, there is the belief that one's soul will become lost and be unable to return home.[51] Surgery is considered mutilating. The body is believed to be a gift from one's parents and ancestors and should, therefore, be maintained intact.[7]

A particularly problematic area among Asian clients is their nonuse of mental health services. Asian Americans use proportionately fewer mental health services, more frequently drop out of therapy, and, when they do seek assistance, present with more severe illness than their white, black, Latino, or Native American counterparts.[136] Failure to seek help with mental health problems stems from a variety of factors. The Asian client sees no separation of physical and mental illness and tends to somatize psychological stress. The failure of the Western mental health professional to treat somatic complaints as real rather than as an imaginary manifestation of mental stress may alienate the Asian client.[136]

Another complicating factor is the stigma attached to mental illness. Mental illness is frequently attributed to unlucky family inheritance, spirit possession, or misdeeds in past lives. Rather than risk stigmatization by seeking care, traditional Asian families will endeavor to conceal the condition, caring for the disturbed person at home. Professional services tend to be sought only after family resources are exhausted. When symptoms cease, treatment is usually discontinued and prolonged therapy is suspect.[136]

Black Americans

Many black clients tend to seek scientific health care for serious health problems while using folk health practices to deal with common complaints. Physicians are also not expected to be able to deal with some conditions, particularly those deriving from magic and evil spells.[28] The folk health system is also used for those diseases of magical origin not amenable to scientific medicine. Blacks do use the professional health system. However, research indicates noncompliance with treatment recommendations by as many as 75 percent of black women. Many possible reasons account for this noncompliance, some related to cultural expectations. One significant noncultural factor is a lack of funds to purchase medications prescribed. Other factors more closely related to the cultural situation include the impersonality of the professional system, long waits for service, immobilization due to feelings of powerlessness, and condescending attitudes exhibited by some health-care professionals. An additional factor in noncompliance is a lack of scientific information regarding illness and medications.[103]

American Latinos

Latino clients may experience a certain mistrust of the non-Latino physician. This mistrust is complicated by high fees, the physician's inability to cure illnesses of magical origin, and difficulties in communication. Hospitalization is viewed as the antithesis of good medical care, which should be able to treat any illness at home. Other barriers to Latino use of scientific health care include impersonality, unfamiliar procedures, lack of family participation in care, and the degree of control exerted by the professional. One further barrier is a fear of the relationships between health-care providers and government agencies. Many illegal aliens fear that health professionals are investigators for the Immigration and Naturalization Service.

The help of a physician may be sought by Latinos for illnesses of natural origin. However, a folk healer or witch is consulted for illnesses ascribed to unnatural causes. Efficiency on the part of the physician is not considered an admirable trait. Illness is perceived as a serious occurrence. Therefore, time should be taken to provide appropriate and effective treatment.

The use of folk health systems by Latinos varies considerably among groups. In several studies, participants indicated greater use of and trust in scientific medicine than in folk health care.[79,121,131] In one study, however, although only about 12 percent of subjects sought the services of a folk healer, 85 percent reported the use of folk remedies at home before seeking professional medical assistance. In this same study, use of folk health practices was not found to be associated with lower socioeconomic status or limited education.[121] In another similar study, 90 percent of subjects reported belief in both folk and scientific health practices.[131]

Appalachian Americans

The Appalachian client may experience a profound distrust of professional health care.[105] One modern-day healer expressed a fairly common sentiment among Appalachians in describing physicians as "trying to keep people from staying well. They want to cut and butcher. They want to give pills and shots. And they want to keep you from takin' something like bitters that's good for you. . . ."[105] In other words, there is a prevalent belief that physicians have a vested interest in keeping people ill. They are believed to be "conspiring with pharmaceutical manufacturers, hospital administrators, and government officials to keep people in poor health."[105]

There are other barriers to Appalachian use of professional health care besides this basic distrust. Some of these include difficulties in relating to strangers, the inflexibility of professional routines and schedules, and the impersonality of professional services.[81] Other barriers are cost and the fear of "being cut on." A further deterrent to the use of the health-care system is the overwhelming concern of the professional with health to the exclusion of other values held by the Appalachian client.[118] Scientific health care is generally sought only for childbirth, emergencies, or legitimization of disability claims.[24]

When the Appalachian client becomes ill, the normally independent and self-reliant person experiences a role reversal to dependence, expecting to be "taken care of." When professional care is sought, there is an expectation of immediate, on-the-spot assistance. The provision of medicine during the visit is considered appropriate. The giving of a prescription, however, may be seen as rejection.[87] When Appalachians do use medications, there is a potential for overdose in the belief that "if some is good, more is better."[87]

ASSESSING INDIVIDUAL CLIENTS

Up to now we have examined beliefs, attitudes, and behaviors typical of clients who adhere to traditional cultural patterns in each of the five cultural groups presented. It is important for community health nurses to recognize that the degree of a particular client's participation in folk health practices will vary. Social class and the concomitant degree of acculturation to the prevailing American culture are two of the factors that mediate the influence of folk health practices. Generally speaking, members of lower socioeconomic groups tend to adhere more closely to belief in and use of traditional health practices. Members of a cultural group who are part of the American middle class may continue to use the folk health system while expressing disbelief in its efficacy. Scientific medicine is also widely used by middle-class individuals. The upper class tends to use scientific medicine as a mark of prestige and may scoff at folk health practices.[80]

Acculturation is also associated with a number of factors in addition to social class. These include the amount of exposure to American culture, the closeness of kinship ties, the extent of family use of traditional practices, and the degree of familiarity with the English language.[80] Nurses working with clients from other cultures must ascertain for each client the extent to which he or she adheres to traditional health practices. The categories of information obtained in relation to the cultural group, which are presented in Box 15–7, can also be used to assess the influences of culture on the health of individual clients.

DIAGNOSTIC REASONING AND CLIENTS FROM OTHER CULTURES

Once client-specific data on cultural affiliation has been obtained, the nurse makes note of areas in which

BOX 15–7

Categories of Information Obtained in a Cultural Assessment

Human biology
- Genetic inheritance
  - Physical differences
  - Differences in normal physiologic values (for example, hematocrit, weight)
  - Common genetically determined illnesses
- Physiologic function
  - Attitudes to body parts and physiologic functions
  - Folk illnesses recognized by the group
  - Scientific diagnoses commonly found in the group

Environment
- Physical environment
  - Extent of physical isolation from other groups
  - Attitudes toward the physical environment
- Psychological environment
  - Attitudes to mental illness
  - Individual versus group goals
  - Authority and decision making
  - Attitudes to change
  - Relationships with the larger society
- Social environment
  - Interpersonal relationships
    - Family relationships
      - Family organizational structure
      - Family roles
      - Attitudes to children and child-rearing practices
    - Communication
      - Language
      - Importance of context to communication
      - Culturally prescribed reticence
      - Formality of address
      - Courtesy titles and epithets
      - Gestures
    - Beliefs and values
      - Value orientations
      - Value of material goods, success, competition
    - Religion and magic
      - Involvement of religious groups in health care
      - Influence of religion on health
      - Effect of religious sponsorship on use of health services
      - Incorporation of religious beliefs in health care
      - Beliefs in magical causes and treatment of illness
  - Economic status of group members

Life-style
- Food practices
  - Food preferences and consumption patterns
  - Food preparation
  - Symbolism and social value of food
- Life events
  - Conception and contraception
  - Birth
    - Beliefs and practices related to pregnancy
    - Beliefs and practices related to labor and delivery
    - Beliefs and practices related to the postpartum period
  - Death and dying
    - Attitudes toward death
    - Belief in an afterlife
    - Place of death
    - Preparation and disposal of the body
    - Grief and mourning
    - Knowledge of death and participation in mourning practices
    - Other consumption patterns

Health system
- Perceptions of health and illness and disease causation
- Folk health practitioners
  - Types of practitioners and services provided
  - Group attitudes to folk practitioners
  - Expectations of the client-practitioner relationship
- Folk health practices
  - Health-promotive and illness-preventive practices
  - Curative practices
- Relationships of folk and scientific health-care systems

Assessment of the individual client also includes identification of membership in a specific cultural group and the degree of adherence to group culture

the client conforms to the typical patterns and areas in which the client does not. This information can be useful in identifying underlying factors in a variety of client health problems identified as nursing diagnoses. For example, the nurse might make a diagnosis of "inadequate nutritional intake due to nonavailability of usual dietary components." Having made such a diagnosis, the nurse can then assist the client to incorporate foods as close as possible to the traditional diet to create a healthy diet.

Nursing diagnoses made at the population level can also be related to cultural factors. For example, the nurse might diagnose a "widespread lack of prenatal care due to failure to provide prenatal services acceptable to Asian clients." Or the nurse might find that clients receive prenatal care from traditional midwives within the cultural group. Efforts might then be directed toward incorporating these midwives into prenatal services provided in the scientific health-care system.

PLANNING AND IMPLEMENTING CARE FOR CLIENTS FROM OTHER CULTURES

As is the case with most clients in community health nursing, clients from other cultures will be largely responsible for implementing health-care activities suggested by the community health nurse. The nurse will enhance client compliance with these suggestions by encouraging both clients and their families to participate in planning health care.

Discuss the client's perceptions of problems, the usual plan of care, and any anticipated difficulties with the suggested plan.[7] It is important that the nurse and client engage in mutual goal setting, because nursing and family goals may not be perfectly congruent.[85] The plan of care can be adapted as much as possible to incorporate traditional health-care practices and to avoid introducing drastic changes in the client's life-style.

One aspect of a client's ability to act on advice is the question of who must give permission for such action. Sometimes a client cannot act on his or her own initiative because of cultural proscriptions. In such instances, nurses must identify the person responsible for health-care decisions and incorporate that person in planning for health care.

Community health nurses endeavor to integrate new health behaviors into the client's existing lifestyle as much as possible. This can be accomplished in several ways. The nurse can plan special diets around usual food preferences or tailor care to the client's normal routine. Other practices that may be revised in light of cultural practices are bathing and exercise. Incorporating family members whose role includes health care into the intervention plan is another way of providing culturally sensitive health care.

Another means of integrating new ideas into existing cultural patterns is the incorporation of folk health practices into the plan of care whenever they are not harmful to the client. Allowing the client to wear an amulet or drink herbal tea will not usually hurt and may actually benefit the client. The client's faith in the efficacy of folk remedies may go a long way to accomplish healing. When folk remedies are harmful, the nurse can explain the potential harm and assist clients to identify other actions that will meet the cultural need without harm.

Nurses may even incorporate folk healers into the plan of care, encouraging the *curandero,* medicine man, or elderly female practitioner to attend the client at home or in the health-care facility. Nurses may choose to participate in healing rituals if they and the client are comfortable with this role. When appropriate, the nurse may make referrals to a folk healer in place of or in conjunction with the usual plan of care. This may be warranted particularly when the client considers his or her condition to be the result of magical intervention. Table 15–7 presents several resources for nurses working to incorporate cultural variables into their care of clients.

Another practical consideration in nursing care for clients of other cultures is the need for advocacy. Nurses function as advocates when they interpret to other team members the sociodynamics influencing the client. They may provide information on cultural beliefs and practices to others caring for the client. They also fulfill an advocacy role in considering the cultural influences on target groups for specific health-care programs. Other avenues of cultural advocacy include fostering recognition of cultural differences among nurses and nursing students and recruiting members of other cultural groups into nursing.

EVALUATING CARE FOR CLIENTS FROM OTHER CULTURES

Evaluation of care provided to clients from other cultural groups should focus on both the outcomes of care and the delivery processes employed. In terms of outcomes, nurses should examine indicators of health status for individual clients and for subcultural groups. For example, has the nurse been able to improve the client's nutritional status without changing the client's cultural dietary pattern? Has a woman

TABLE 15–7. RESOURCES FOR NURSES WORKING WITH CLIENTS FROM OTHER CULTURES

Focus	Agency or Organization	Function
Native American	Administration for Native Americans 330 Independence Ave., SW Washington, DC 20201 (202) 245-7776	Policy formation, funds to promote social and economic development
	Indian Health Service 5600 Fisher's Lane Rockville, MD 20857 (301) 443-1083	Administers health program for American Indians
	U.S. Senate Select Committee on Indian Affairs SH-838 Hart Senate Office Bldg. Washington, DC 20510 (202) 224-2251	Policy formation
Asian	Asian-American Psychological Association c/o Dr. K. Sakamoto Dean of Academic Affairs 2325 Chester Blvd. Indiana University East Richmond, IN 47374 (317) 966-8261	Research, advocacy
Latino	Latino Family Life Education Project SIECUS New York University 32 Washington Square Place New York, NY 10003 (212) 673-3850	Training of professionals who work with Latinos
Healers and healing	American Acupuncture Association 42-62 Kissena Blvd. Flushing, NY 11355 (718) 886-4431	Legislation, public education
	American Association for Acupuncture & Oriental Medicine 1424 16th St., NW, Ste. 105 Washington, DC 20036 (202) 232-4495	Legislation, public education, regulation, research
	American Center for Chinese Medical Sciences c/o Jos. C. Hwang, Ph.D. 12921 Forest View Dr. Beltsville, MD 20705 (301) 572-4461	Information sharing between U.S. and China
	Association for Holistic Health P.O. Box 12407 La Jolla, CA 92037 (619) 535-0101	Sets standards, information on traditional and alternative forms of healing
	Center for Attitudinal Healing 19 Main St. Tiburon, CA 94920 (415) 435-5022	Public education on healing
	Friendly Contacts Association Box 1001 15 Myrtle Dr. Umatilla, FL 32784 (904) 357-9723	Research on healing and parapsychology
	G-Jo Institute 4950 S.W. 70th Ave. Davie, FL 33314 (305) 791-1562	Information on self-health technique based on traditional Oriental healing, acupuncture, and acupressure

(continued)

TABLE 15–7. (*Continued*)

Focus	Agency or Organization	Function
Healers and healing (*continued*)	International Foundation for Homeopathy 2366 Eastlake, E., #301 Seattle, WA 98102 (206) 324-8230	Public education
	Mandala Holistic Health P.O. Box 1233 Del Mar, CA 92014 (619) 481-7751	Education on holistic health practices
	National Association of Naturopathic Physicians 2613 N. Stevens Tacoma, WA 98407 (206) 752-2555	Research and education
	National Commission for the Certification of Acupuncturists 1424 16th Street, NW, Ste. 105 Washington, DC, 20036 (202) 232-1404	Administers certification examinations for acupuncturists
	National Council of Acupuncture Schools and Colleges P.O. Box 954 Columbia, MD 21044 (301) 997-4888	Sets standards for education of acupuncturists
	Natural Herbalist Assoc. c/o Bach Center 463 Rockaway Avenue Valley Stream, NY 11580 (516) 825-1677	Research and education
	Nurses in Transition P.O. Box 14472 San Francisco, CA 94114 (415) 282-7999	Fosters incorporation of holistic health practices in nursing
	Ohashi Institute 12 W. 27th St. New York, NY 10001 (212) 684-4190	Education on Japanese healing arts
	Psychic Science International Special Interest Group 7514 Belleplane Dr. Dayton, OH 45424 (513) 236-0361	Information on healing and other psychic phenomena
	Traditional Acupuncture Foundation American City Bldg. Suite 100 Columbia, MD 21044 (301) 997-4888	Public education on acupuncture and Oriental medicine, referral, legal information

from another cultural group had a successful pregnancy outcome? Have parents ceased giving potentially harmful tonics to their children?

The nurse should also evaluate the outcomes of health care for subcultural groups within the population. For example, the rising birth weights of babies born to Southeast Asian refugee women are an indication that better nutritional status and health care are a positive influence on the health of these women. Other areas that warrant attention are seen in the differences in cancer survival rates between blacks and whites, which indicate the inadequacy of care provided to blacks who have cancer. On the other hand, programs that contribute to declining rates of alcoholism among Native American youth are indicative of effective health care.

Attention should also be given to the way in which care is provided. Are health programs designed with cultural sensitivity as a central focus? Is the care that is provided to the individual client indicative of cultural sensitivity on the part of the particular community health nurse? Answers to these and similar questions are the focus of evaluation of the care provided to individuals from cultural groups other than that of the nurse.

CHAPTER HIGHLIGHTS

- Culture is the shared values, attitudes, and beliefs of a group of people that guide thought and action by members of the group. Race is a human classification system based on certain biological characteristics. Ethnicity is designation by self or others as a member of a distinct population group based on national characteristics.
- Culture is characterized by universality, uniqueness, stability, changeability, unconscious influence, and variability.
- Potential negative responses to people of other cultures include ethnocentrism, cultural blindness, cultural shock, cultural conflict, cultural imposition, and stereotyping.
- Ethnocentrism is grounded in the belief that one's own cultural beliefs and practices are superior to those of other cultural groups.
- Cultural blindness is a failure to acknowledge the existence of cultural differences.
- Cultural shock results in immobilization due to perceptions of overwhelming cultural differences.
- Cultural conflict occurs when one ridicules the beliefs and practices of another culture because of perceived threats to one's own beliefs and values.
- In cultural imposition one believes that everyone should conform to the tenets of one's own cultural group.
- Stereotyping occurs when one refuses to acknowledge differences among members of a cultural group.
- Cultural sensitivity is characterized by respect for others as individuals and for their culture, awareness of culturally prescribed beliefs and behaviors, modification of nursing care to fit cultural patterns whenever possible, and advocacy for clients from other cultural groups as needed.
- In assessing other cultures, community health nurses should view cultures in the context in which they developed, examine the underlying premises of cultural behavior, inquire into the meaning of behavior in the cultural context, and recognize the existence of intracultural variation.
- Considerations in cultural assessment related to human biology include potential genetic inheritance and factors related to physiologic function such as attitudes to body parts and functions, folk illnesses recognized by the cultural group, and common medical diagnoses experienced by the group.
- Aspects of the psychological environment to be considered in cultural assessment include cultural attitudes to mental illness, the preeminence of individual or group goals, modes of authority and decision making, attitudes to change, and the quality of relationships with the larger society.
- Social environmental factors addressed in cultural assessment include interpersonal relationships, acceptable demeanor, communication, beliefs and values, religion and magic, and the economic status of members of the cultural group.
- Life-style factors related to culture include dietary practices, beliefs and practices related to life events, and other consumption patterns.
- Aspects of cultural assessment related to the health system include cultural definitions of health and illness and perceptions of disease causation, folk health practitioners and practices, and the relationship of the folk health-care system to the professional health-care system.
- Plans for the care of clients from other cultures should be based on the client's culturally derived beliefs and values. As far as possible, interventions should incorporate aspects of the client's culture and minimize disruption of the client's usual life-style.

Review Questions

1. How does culture differ from race and ethnicity? (p. 282)
2. What are the six characteristics common to all cultures? Give an example of each characteristic. (pp. 282–283)
3. Describe at least four potential negative responses of nurses to people from other cultures and give an example of each type of response. (pp. 283–284)
4. Describe at least three characteristics of cultural sensitivity. (p. 285)
5. Describe four principles of cultural assessment. Give an example in which each principle has been violated. (pp. 288–289)
6. Describe three considerations in assessing the human biological component of a culture. Give an example of each. (pp. 290–295)
7. Identify at least five aspects of the environment to be considered in a cultural assessment. (pp. 295–307)
8. Describe at least three life events to be considered in a cultural assessment. Give an example of the effects of culture related to each life event. (pp. 309–314)
9. Describe three similarities and four differences between the folk and scientific health-care systems. Give an example of each. (pp. 326–330)
10. Describe four considerations in assessing the influence of folk health-care systems. (pp. 315–317)

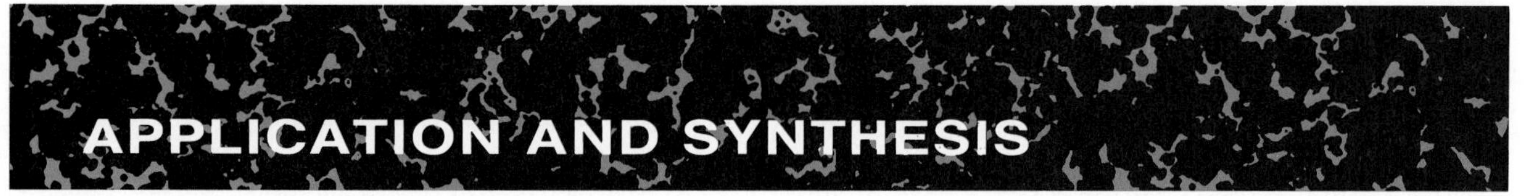

APPLICATION AND SYNTHESIS

In two weeks, the Ramirez family expect their fourth child. Mr. Ramirez works in an avocado grove for minimum wage. There is not enough money to pay the physician or the hospital, so Mrs. Ramirez is not receiving prenatal care. Although they seem pleased about the pregnancy, they have made no plans for the new baby and seem to have no interest in family planning after delivery.

Mr. Ramirez makes all the decisions for the family. The Ramirez family believe that good health and illness are gifts of God and there is very little that they can do to promote their health. All of their relatives are still in Mexico and they rarely communicate with any of them. They believe that the people around them are out to take their money if possible and have not made any friends in the rural neighborhood where they live.

Neither of the parents has ever attended school. The oldest child is in second grade, but is frequently absent when Mr. Ramirez needs his help in the groves. The public health nurse has talked to Mrs. Ramirez several times regarding the need for immunizations for the younger children, family planning, and prenatal care. Mrs. Ramirez has not attended any of the clinics even though she and her husband own an old truck and come to town regularly on Saturday to buy groceries.

1. Are the family roles depicted in this situation typical or atypical of the traditional Latino family?
2. What are the family's apparent values as evidenced by data in the case study?
3. How do the family's values conflict or coincide with those of the larger society?
4. What might the nurse do to provide culturally sensitive health care for this family?

REFERENCES

1. Bernal, H., & Froman, R. (1987). The confidence of community health nurses in caring for ethnically diverse populations. *Image, 19,* 201–204.
2. Melville, M. B. (1988). Hispanics: Race, class, or ethnicity? *The Journal of Ethnic Studies, 16*(1), 67–83.
3. Leininger, M. M. (1989). A new generation of nurses discovers transcultural nursing. *Nursing & Health Care, 8,* 38–45.
4. Zinn, M. B. (1982). Chicano men and masculinity. *The Journal of Ethnic Studies, 10*(2), 29–43.
5. Harris, M. (1975). *Cows, pigs, wars, and witches.* New York: Vintage Books.
6. Hollingsworth, A. O., Brown, L. P., & Brooten, D. A. (1980, November). The refugees and childbearing: What to expect. *R.N.,* 45–49.
7. Louie, K. B. (1985). Providing health care to Chinese clients. *Topics in Clinical Nursing, 7*(3), 18–25.
8. Leininger, M. M. (1977, March). Cultural diversities of health and nursing care. *Nursing Clinics of North America, 12,* 5–18.
9. Smith, E. J. (1977). Counseling black individuals: Some stereotypes. *Personnel and Guidance Journal, 55,* 390–396.
10. Brownlee, A. T. (1978b). *Community, culture, and care—A cross-cultural guide for health workers.* St. Louis: C.V. Mosby.
11. Kniep-Hardy, M., & Burkhardt, M. A. (1977). Nursing of the Navajo. *American Journal of Nursing, 77,* 95–96.
12. Fong, C. M. (1985). Ethnicity and nursing practice. *Topics in Clinical Nursing, 7*(3), 1–10.
13. United States Department of Commerce. (1990). *Statistical Abstract of the United States* (109th ed.). Washington, DC: Government Printing Office.
14. Rhodes, T. (1987). The urban American Indian. In T. E. Ross & T. G. Moore (Eds.), *A cultural geography of North American Indians* (pp. 259–273). Boulder, CO: Westview Press.
15. Ballas, D. J. (1987). Historical geography and American Indian development. In T. E. Ross & T. G. Moore (Eds.), *A cultural geography of North American Indians* (pp. 15–32). Boulder, CO: Westview Press.
16. United States Bureau of the Census. (1981). *1980 Census of population and housing. United States summary. Final population and housing counts.* Washington, DC: Government Printing Office.
17. Henderson, G., & Primeaux, M. (1981). The importance of folk medicine. In G. Henderson & M. Primeaux (Eds.), *Transcultural health care* (pp. 59–77), Menlo Park, CA: Addison-Wesley.
18. Santopietro, M. S., & Lynch, B. A. (1980, October). What's behind the inscrutable mask? *R.N.,* 55–62.
19. Sudden unexplained death syndrome in Southeast Asian refugees. (1987). *MMWR, 36* (ISS), 43SS–53SS.
20. Muecke, M. A. (1983a). Caring for Southeast Asian refugee patients in the U.S.A. *American Journal of Public Health, 73,* 431–438.
21. Medina, C. (1987). Latino culture and sex education. *SIECUS Report, XV*(3), 1–4.
22. Tuberculosis among Hispanics—United States, 1985. (1987). *MMWR, 36,* 568–569.
23. Magar, V. (1990). Health care needs of Central American refugees. *Nursing Outlook, 38,* 239–242.
24. Tripp-Reimer, T., & Friedl, M. C. (1977, March). Appalachians: A neglected minority. *Nursing Clinics of North America, 12,* 41–54.
25. Simmon, J. M. (1987). Health care of the elderly in Appalachia. *Journal of Gerontological Nursing, 13*(7), 32–35.
26. Brownlee, A. T. (1978a). The family and health care: Explorations in cross-cultural settings. *Social Work and Health Care, 4,* 179–198.
27. Tripp-Reimer, T. (1983). Nursing in the health professions. In D. B. Shimkin & P. Golde (Eds.), *Clinical anthropology: A new approach to American health problems?* Urbana-Champaign, IL: University Press of America.
28. Capers, C. F. (1985). Nursing and the Afro-American client. *Topics in Clinical Nursing, 7*(3), 11–17.
29. Andrews, M. M. (1989a). Culture and nutrition. In J. S. Boyle & M. M. Andrews (Eds.), *Transcultural perspectives in nursing* (pp. 333–355). Glenview, IL: Scott, Foresman.
30. Jackson, L. (1988). Acupuncture: An important treatment option. *Nurse Practitioner, 13*(9), 55–66.
31. Ross, M. (1981). Societal/cultural views regarding death and dying. *Topics in Clinical Nursing, 2*(10), 1–16.
32. Dicharry, E. K. (1986). Delivering home health care to the elderly in Zuni pueblo. *Journal of Gerontological Nursing, 12*(7), 25–29.
33. Randall-David, E. (1989). *Strategies for working with culturally diverse communities and clients.* Bethesda, MD: The Association for the Care of Children's Health.
34. Snow, L. (1981). Folk medical beliefs and the implications for the care of clients. In G. Henderson & M. Primeaux (Eds.), *Transcultural health care* (pp. 78–101). Menlo Park, CA: Addison-Wesley.
35. Andrews, M. M. (1989b). Transcultural perspectives in the nursing care of children and adolescents. In J. S. Boyle & M. M. Andrews (Eds.), *Transcultural concepts in nursing* (pp. 119–166). Glenview, IL: Scott, Foresman.
36. Gomez, G. E., & Gomez, E. A. (1985). Folk healing among Hispanic Americans. *Public Health Nursing, 2*(4), 245–249.
37. Hautman, M. A. (1979). Folk health and illness beliefs. *Nurse Practitioner, 4*(4), 23–34.
38. Rose, L. C. (1978). *Disease beliefs in Mexican American communities.* San Francisco: R. & E. Research Associates.
39. White, E. H. (1977). Giving health care to minority patients. *Nursing Clinics of North America, 12,* 27–40.
40. Gonzales, H. H. (1976). Health care needs of the Mexican-American. In *Ethnicity and health care* (pp. 17–34). New York: National League for Nursing.
41. Andrews, M. M., & Hanson, P. A. (1989). Religious beliefs: Implications for nursing practice. In J. S. Boyle & M. M. Andrews (Eds.), *Transcultural concepts in nursing* (pp. 357–382). Glenview, IL: Scott, Foresman.

for ethnic peoples of color. New York: Appleton-Century-Crofts.

120. Powers, W. K. (1987). *Beyond the visions: Essays on American Indian culture.* Norman: University of Oklahoma.
121. Marsh, W. W., & Hentges, K. (1988). Mexican folk remedies and conventional medical care. *American Family Physician, 37,* 257–262.
122. Goldwater, C. (1983). Traditional medicine in Latin America. In R. H. Bannerman, J. Burton, & C. Wen-Chieh (Eds.), *Traditional medicine and health care coverage* (pp. 37–49). Geneva: World Health Organization.
123. Finkler, K. (1983). Studying outcomes of Mexican spiritual therapy. In L. Romanucci-Ross, D. E. Moerman, & L. R. Tancredi (Eds.), *The anthropology of medicine: From culture to method* (pp. 81–102). New York: Praeger.
124. Mellinger, M. B. (1977). The spirit is strong in the root. *Appalachian Journal, 4,* 242–253.
125. Van Esterik, P. (1988). To strengthen and refresh: Herbal therapy in Southeast Asia. *Social Science and Medicine, 27,* 751–759.
126. Omura, Y. (1982). *Acupuncture medicine: Its history and clinical background.* Tokyo: Japan Publications.
127. Yetiv, J. Z. (1986). *Popular nutritional practices: A scientific approach.* Toledo, OH: Popular Medicine Press.
128. Hare, M. L. (1988). Shiatsu acupressure in nursing practice. *Holistic Nursing Practice, 2*(3), 68–74.
129. Weaver, M. T. (1985). Acupressure: An overview of theory and application. *Nurse Practitioner, 10*(8), 38–39, 42.
130. Lead poisoning-associated death from Asian Indian folk remedies—Florida. (1984). *MMWR, 33,* 638, 643–645.
131. Ailinger, R. L. (1985). Beliefs about treatment of hypertension among older Hispanic persons. *Topics in Clinical Nursing, 7*(3), 26–31.
132. Waterman, S. H., Juarez, G., Carr, S. J., & Kilman, L. (1990). *Salmonella arizona* infections in Latinos associated with rattlesnake folk medicine. *American Journal of Public Health, 80,* 286–289.
133. Leininger, M. M. (1981). Transcultural nursing: Its progress and its future. *Nursing & Health Care, II,* 365–371.
134. Cornacchia, H. J. (1976). *Consumer health.* St. Louis: C.V. Mosby.
135. Muecke, M. A. (1983b). In search of healers: Southeast Asian refugees in the American health care system. *Western Journal of Medicine, 139,* 835–840.
136. Flaskerud, J. H. (1987). A proposed protocol for culturally relevant nursing psychotherapy. *Clinical Nurse Specialist, 1,* 150–157.

RECOMMENDED READINGS

Geissler, E. M. (1991). Transcultural nursing and nursing diagnosis. *Nursing & Health Care, 12,* 190–203.

Describes current approaches to nursing diagnosis as bound by culture and discusses the lack of fit between nursing diagnoses and transcultural nursing.

Giger, J. N., & Davidhizar, R. (1990). Transcultural nursing assessment: A method for advancing nursing practice. *International Nursing Review, 37*(1), 199–202.

Presents a model for transcultural assessment based on communications, space, social organization, time, environmental control, and biological variation.

Giger, J., & Davidhizar, R. (1991). *Transcultural nursing: Assessment and intervention.* St. Louis: C.V. Mosby.

Discusses a theoretical framework and practical interventions for the care of clients from other cultural groups.

Randall-David, E. (1989). *Strategies for working with culturally diverse communities and clients.* Bethesda, MD: The Association for the Care of Children's Health.

Provides guidelines for assessing one's own cultural heritage and for working with culturally diverse communities and clients. Also addresses the use of interpreters.

Veatch, R. M. (1989). *Cross-cultural perspectives in medical ethics: Readings.* Boston: Jones and Bartlett.

Offers readings on the cultural implications of ethics.

Wing, D. M. (1989). Community participant-observation: Issues in assessing diverse cultures. *Journal of Community Health Nursing, 6*(3), 125–133.

Examines some of the issues presented by participant-observation techniques in cultural assessment of communities.

CHAPTER 16

Environmental Influences on Community Health

KEY TERMS

biological hazards
chemical and gaseous hazards
electromagnetic radiation
ionizing radiation
physical hazards
radiation
ultraviolet radiation

During much of history, human beings have been subject to the effects of the natural environment. Earthquakes, famines, floods, droughts, and other environmental calamities created upheavals in human society. Human progress has, to a certain extent, been measured in terms of capabilities for controlling the environment. In spite of, and sometimes because of, these capabilities, environmental factors still exert an impact on human health and welfare. Air, water, noise, radiation, waste, and noise present a variety of hazards to human health.

Community health nurses are concerned with the effects of environmental factors on the health of individuals, families, and communities. Interventions related to environmental concerns may occur at any of these levels. For example, a community health nurse may teach a family how to reduce the indoor air pollution in the home, or work for legislation to promote safe disposal of hazardous wastes. To engage in effective action at all levels, community health nurses must have an understanding of environmental influences on health.

LEARNING OBJECTIVES

After reading this chapter you should be able to:

- Summarize at least five national health objectives for the year 2000 related to environmental health.
- Identify three physical hazards to health arising from the environment.
- Describe three biological health hazards that may be present in the environment.
- Identify three chemical or gaseous hazards to human health arising from environmental conditions.
- Describe at least two health effects of environmental conditions on each of six human target organs or body systems.
- Identify two levels of nursing diagnoses related to environmental influences on health.
- Describe at least five primary preventive measures for health problems related to environmental conditions.
- Describe at least three secondary preventive measures for health problems related to environmental conditions.
- Describe at least three tertiary preventive measures for health problems related to environmental conditions.

ENVIRONMENTAL HEALTH HAZARDS

In recent years, greater attention has been given to the health risks posed by environmental conditions. Evidence of this attention can be found in the number of national health objectives for the year 2000 that focus on environmental health issues. Sixteen objectives related to environmental health were included in the objectives for the year 2000.[1] These objectives are summarized in Box 16–1.

Many environmental forces influence human health. Microorganisms such as bacteria, viruses, and fungi, for example, cause communicable diseases, and animals can even contribute to the spread of these diseases. Plants may contribute to accidental poisoning or to allergic reactions. Industry, vehicles, and buildings add to air and water pollution and excess noise. Climate and terrain contribute to natural disasters, which will be discussed in Chapter 29, Care of Clients in Disaster Settings. In addition, climate and terrain add to air and water pollution that have

BOX 16–1

National Health Objectives Related to Environmental Health

- Reduce asthma hospitalization to less than 160 per 100,000 population
- Reduce serious mental retardation among school-aged children to no more than 2 per 1000 children
- Reduce infectious waterborne disease and chemical poisoning outbreaks to no more than 11 per year
- Reduce the prevalence of blood levels exceeding 25 μg/dL in children aged 6 months through 5 years to zero
- Increase to 85% the proportion of people who live in counties that have not exceeded any air quality standard in the last 12 months
- Increase to 40% the proportion of homes tested for radon and found to pose minimal risk or modified to reduce risk
- Reduce toxic chemicals released into the air, water, and soil to less than 0.24 billion pounds of carcinogens and 2.6 billion pounds of other toxic chemicals defined by the Agency on Toxic Substances and Disease Registry
- Reduce the average number of pounds of municipal solid waste produced per person per day to no more than 3.6 pounds
- Increase to 85% the proportion of people who have access to drinking water that meets safe drinking water standards
- Decrease the number of lakes, rivers, and estuaries that do not support fishing and swimming to no more than 15%
- Perform testing for lead-based paint in at least 50% of homes built before 1950
- Increase to at least 35 the number of states in which 75% of local jurisdictions adopt construction techniques and standards that minimize indoor radon levels
- Increase to at least 30 the number of states requiring informing prospective buyers of the presence of lead-based paint and radon concentrations in all buildings offered for sale
- Clean up hazardous waste sites sufficiently to eliminate significant health risks identified
- Establish programs for dealing with recyclable materials and hazardous wastes in at least 75% of counties
- Establish and monitor plans to define and track sentinel environmental diseases in at least 35 states

(Source: U.S. Department of Health and Human Services[1])

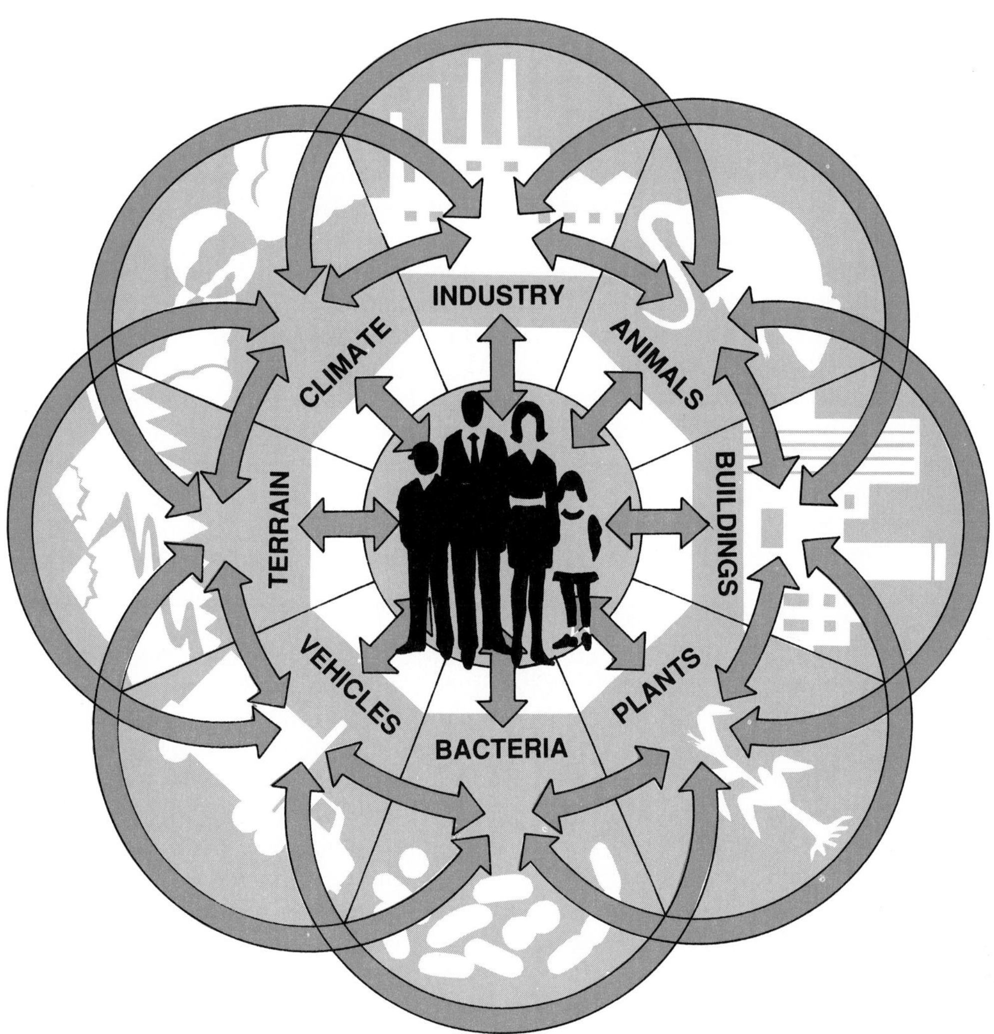

Figure 16–1. Selected environmental components that produce health hazards.

long-term effects on health. All of these facets of the environment give rise to environmental hazards that affect human health. Some of the environmental components that produce health hazards are presented in Figure 16–1. Health hazards arising from environmental conditions fall into three categories: physical hazards, biological hazards, and chemical and gaseous hazards.

PHYSICAL HAZARDS

Physical hazards to health arising from environmental conditions are those related to the physical objects and conditions that surround human beings. Physical hazards to be addressed here include radiation, lead and other heavy metals, and noise.

RADIATION

Radiation is energy in motion that occurs in the form of waves or particles.[2] Three forms of radiation can constitute health hazards. These are ionizing radiation, electromagnetic radiation, and ultraviolet radiation, a subtype of electromagnetic radiation.

Ionizing radiation is created when radioactive elements break up. Ionizing radiation occurs naturally in the soil and rock, and humans are exposed to this form of radiation daily. Exposure to natural ionizing radiation is greater in some parts of the country than in others depending upon the extent of radioactive elements found. Exposure to ionizing radiation may also occur as a result of some forms of technology. X-ray procedures, for example, are a form of ionizing radiation. Ionizing radiation also results from processes used to create nuclear power.

The health hazards of nuclear power were demonstrated by the effects of the bombing of Japanese cities that occurred at the end of World War II. These effects were demonstrated more recently in the morbidity and mortality that occurred as the result of the nuclear accident in Chernobyl, in the Soviet Union. In general, radiation from nuclear reactions is not a major source of radiation exposure for the public. In 1970, for example, fallout accounted for exposures of less than 10 millirems (mrems) per person per year (a rem is a measure of the biological damage produced in the human body by radiation), while nuclear power generation accounted for even less.[3] The recommended limit for exposure to ionizing radiation set by the National Academy of Sciences is 170 mrems per year, and most people are exposed to far less (100 mrems per year, on average).[2] There is evidence, however, to suggest that long-term occupational exposure to low levels of ionizing radiation may have cumulative health effects that culminate in increased incidence of cancer. In one study, the risk of death due to cancer increased by nearly 5 percent for every rem of radiation exposure incurred by employees of nuclear power plants. The findings of this study reinforce those of earlier studies.[4]

Some progress has been made in controlling occupational exposures to ionizing radiation. Figures from two surveys by the National Institute for Occupational Safety and Health (NIOSH) in 1972 and 1981 indicate that the proportion of facilities with potentially uncontrolled radiation exposure declined dramatically. This was particularly true for the primary metals industry, where about 15 percent of facilities had no controls for radiation exposure in 1972 compared to less than 1 percent without controls in 1982. Among health-care facilities, another major source of occupational exposure to ionizing radiation, more than 4 percent exercised no radiation controls in 1972 compared to less than 2 percent in 1981.[5]

For the general public, medical irradiation accounts for the greatest number of mrems of exposure to ionizing radiation (about 80 mrems per person per year). There is some question of the health effects of medical irradiation. In one study, for example, diagnostic X-rays were found to have no relationship to the incidence of leukemia and non-Hodgkin's lymphoma. There was a slight, though not significant, increase in the incidence of multiple myeloma in persons with multiple X-ray exposures.[6] There is also evidence that multiple X-ray procedures increase one's risk of breast cancer.[7] The findings of these and other similar studies underscore the need for keeping medical exposures to ionizing radiation to a minimum.[6]

Another concern related to radiation is the radiation exposure that may take place in the home. The source of ionizing radiation here is usually radon gas, a product of the breakdown of radium that is found in soil and in a variety of building materials, particularly pumice stone and granite that contain high levels of radium. Some evidence indicates that radon gas may enter indoor air from contaminated water in dishwashers, showers, and so forth.[8] Radon gas can be inhaled in free form or attached to dust particles. After being inhaled, the radioactive gas continues to decompose, releasing alpha particles that damage lung tissue, which may result in lung cancer. It is estimated that 20,000 lung cancer deaths among nonsmokers each year are due to radon exposure.[9] Ionizing radiation has also been implicated in chromosomal abnormalities and congenital defects, retarded growth and development in youngsters, and cancer of the thyroid.[7]

Electromagnetic radiation occurs in the form of waves created by disturbances in electric and magnetic fields that surround all matter. Forms of electromagnetic radiation include heat, light, and radio waves.[2] Electromagnetic radiation is produced by devices that generate electromagnetic fields such as video display terminals (VDTs) and microwave ovens.

The health effects of this type of radiation are not yet fully known, but there is some evidence that chronic exposure to microwave radiation may contribute to fatigue, headaches, blood dyscrasias, cataracts, memory loss, arrhythmias, decreased fertility, and genetic defects. VDTs have been suggested as sources of headache, eyestrain, visual disturbances, cataracts, and genetic defects.[2] In one study, however, no relationship was found between exposure to VDTs during pregnancy and risk of spontaneous abortion.[10] Some evidence suggests that the health effects of using VDTs are due not to the radiation produced, but to glare from the screen and other aspects of the work.[2]

Ultraviolet radiation consists of waves of light energy beyond the capability of the human eye to see. Ultraviolet radiation occurs naturally in sunlight and is created by fluorescent lights and sunlamps. Ultraviolet radiation has several positive uses including destroying pathogenic microbes and producing light that is less harsh and uses less energy than incandescent lighting. Ultraviolet light is also involved in producing vitamin D when human skin is exposed to sunlight. Unfortunately, ultraviolet light also results in sunburn, and exposure also contributes to the incidence of basal and squamous cell carcinomas and malignant melanomas. Over 500,000 cases of skin cancer are diagnosed each year and account for 2000 deaths annually in the United States. In 1989, for example, there were an estimated 27,000 cases of malignant melanoma with a fatality rate of over 22 percent.[11]

The potential for skin cancer due to exposure to ultraviolet radiation is increased by the destruction of the protective stratospheric layer of ozone surrounding the planet. Normally, the majority of ultraviolet rays from the sun are absorbed by dust and smoke particles in the atmosphere. Without the protective ozone layer it is estimated that up to 60 percent more skin cancers and 20,000 fatalities would occur annually in the United States. In addition, there would be an increase of 600,000 cases in the number of Americans with cataracts.[12]

LEAD AND OTHER HEAVY METALS

Other physical hazards to health arise from the presence of lead and other heavy metals in the environment. Lead may be present in soil, in water, and in the air, as well as in dust or paint chips in older dwellings painted with lead-based paint. Sources of lead in the air include vehicle emissions, stationary source fuel combustion (for example, burning coal to generate electrical power), industrial processes, and decomposition of solid wastes.[7] Lead in vehicle emissions was significantly reduced with the introduction of unleaded gasoline. From 1975 to 1982, for example, the amount of lead in gasoline decreased by 70 percent.[13] Similar declines have been noted in other sources of lead in the air until the amount of lead expelled into the air each year dropped from 147 million metric tons in 1975 to slightly more than 40 million metric tons in 1984.[7]

Elimination of lead-based paint from residential buildings began over 40 years ago.[14] These efforts contributed to a 37 percent decline in blood lead levels in the general population between 1976 and 1980.[15] Despite reduced lead levels in ambient air and reductions in blood lead levels, in 1984 approximately 5 percent of the American population lived in counties where lead levels in the ambient air were higher than allowable federal standards.[7] Older residences also remain a potential source of lead poisoning especially for young children. Approximately 42 million dwellings in the United States contain lead-based paint, and almost 2 million American children live in these dwellings.[14]

Young children are particularly at risk for lead poisoning because of their propensity to place objects that may be contaminated with lead-bearing dust in their mouths. Children may also ingest paint chips from peeling walls in deteriorating buildings. Painting over old surfaces with non-lead-based paint does not help, because as later coats of paint flake off, the older lead-contaminated layers peel as well.

Abatement procedures to remove lead-based paint in older homes traditionally consist of open-flame burning or sanding techniques with minimal cleanup of the resulting dust. This dust is heavily contaminated with lead and may present subsequent exposure risks. Recent research has indicated that neither traditional abatement methods nor modified methods incorporating better cleanup procedures are effective in reducing lead levels in house dust on a long-term basis,[14] so community health nurses working in older residential areas may still encounter clients with lead poisoning.

Exposure to lead and other heavy metals can also occur through drinking water. These metals enter water as it passes through soils containing lead, nickel, mercury, arsenic, cadmium, and other metals. This process is facilitated if water is acidified as a result of acid rain caused by chemical air pollution.[7] Metals are also leached into the water system from improper solid waste disposal.[16] Finally, lead and copper may be leached from lead and copper pipes in older homes. Again, acidification of water due to acid rain enhances leaching of metals from pipes.[7]

Lead interferes with red blood cell production and may cause damage to the brain, liver, and other vital organs. Typical symptoms of lead poisoning include headache, irritability, weakness, abdominal pain, vomiting, and constipation. In later stages, victims may exhibit convulsions, coma, and paralysis. Low-level exposure to lead in children can result in mental retardation. Treatment for lead exposure involves correcting dehydration and electrolyte imbalances and the use of chelating agents to facilitate urinary excretion of lead.[17]

Mercury poisoning manifests initially with listlessness and irritability. Recurrent rashes, photophobia, and a pinkish coloration of fingertips, toes, nose, hands, and feet are characteristic of the disease. Severe perspiration, pruritus, desquamation of hands and feet, and a burning sensation of hands and feet are also typical. Neurologic symptoms include neuritis, mental apathy, and loss of deep-tendon reflexes. Chelating agents and maintenance of nutrition and food and electrolyte balances are the key to therapy.[17]

Arsenic is used in both pesticides and herbicides and is found in water contaminated by runoff in agricultural areas. Arsenic is also found in the home in over-the-counter ant poisons and may be a source of accidental poisoning. Symptoms of acute arsenic poisoning include nausea, vomiting, diarrhea, severe burning of the mouth and throat, and acute abdominal pain. Chronic poisoning may manifest in weakness, prostration, muscle aches, desquamation and hyperpigmentation of the trunk and extremities, and linear pigmentation of fingernails.[18]

Cadmium poisoning can occur when acidic foods are prepared in cadmium-lined containers (for example, mixing lemonade in metal cans) or from contaminated drinking water. Symptoms of cadmium poisoning include nausea, vomiting, diarrhea, and prostration within 10 minutes of ingestion. Cadmium fumes can also be produced by some industrial processes and, when inhaled, cause a severe pneumonitis.[18]

NOISE

In addition to the physiologic effect of noise on hearing, evidence suggests that prolonged exposure to noise contributes to increased anxiety and emotional stress that may be manifested as nausea, headaches, and sexual impotence. Other effects include insomnia, skin problems, swollen ankles, increase in the incidence of minor accidents, heart trouble and hypertension, cardiac disrhythmias, and drug use. The psychological effects of noise can include irritability and depression. There is even some evidence to suggest that noise results in low birth weight in babies born to women exposed to consistently high noise levels.[19]

Hearing loss due to noise exposure is a serious problem in industry. Two studies by the National Institute for Occupational Safety and Health in 1972 and 1981 noted some attempts at noise control in various industries. However, the proportion of commercial enterprises without provisions for noise control ranged from 99 percent of auto repair services and garages to 21 percent of miscellaneous repair services. Other industries in which over half of the facilities did not control noise exposure include special trade contractors, general building contractors, apparel and other textile manufacturers, heavy construction contractors, printing and publishing, fabricated metal products, wood and lumber products, and air transportation.[5]

Exposure to noise outside the work environment is also a problem. Examples of noise sources that exceed the 80-decibel hearing-impairment threshold include buses, trucks, motorcycles, garbage trucks, trains, subways, recreational and off-road vehicles such as snowmobiles, motor boats, airplanes, and loud music.[3]

BIOLOGICAL HAZARDS

Biological hazards are those caused by living organisms in the environment. Biological hazards of concern to community health nurses include infectious agents, insects and animals, and plants.

INFECTIOUS AGENTS

Many infectious agents are transmitted by means of contact with an infected person. Others are transmitted by environmental means. Water is a primary means for environmental transmission of infectious agents. It is estimated that 80 percent of communicable diseases throughout the world is water-related. Approximately 2 billion people worldwide do not have access to safe water.[20] In the United States, sanitation and water treatment have limited the extent of waterborne infectious diseases, but transmission via contaminated water still occurs. In fact, there has been an increase in waterborne disease outbreaks in the United States since 1955. In 1980, 43 percent of community water systems were in violation of safe drinking water standards.[20]

In large part, contamination of drinking water supplies occurs via improper sewage treatment and improper solid waste disposal. Septic tanks may have leach lines that are too short to permit adequate filtration of water contaminated with human wastes before it enters the groundwater supply. Approximately 30 percent of the population use septic tanks to dispose of wastes, and 3.5 billion gallons of human waste are introduced into the soil and portions of it into groundwater each day.[21] Sewer systems prevent this sort of occurrence, but because of population expansion in many parts of the country, sewage treatment plants are inadequate to meet the demand for services. In some areas, untreated sewage contaminates water supplies. In San Diego, for example, untreated sewage from neighboring Tijuana, Mexico, contaminates both ground and surface water supplies, thus creating a biological health hazard.

Biological contamination of water supplies also occurs when solid wastes are improperly handled and rain water is contaminated as it flows through waste-disposal sites that breed bacteria, viruses, and other disease-producing microorganisms.[20] There is also potential for contamination of both drinking water and food supplies through the use of reclaimed water. Increased demands for water have led to an upsurge in waste-water recycling. This is particularly true in some parts of the country such as Southern California where waste-water reclamation programs are being developed or are already in operation in over 400 communities. Currently most of this water is used for crop irrigation, a use that not only provides needed water, but recharges groundwater basins and provides a nitrogen-rich fertilizer for crops. Because of its high nitrogen content, however, recycled waste water could contaminate drinking water supplies.[22] Use of waste water to irrigate food crops must be closely monitored to prevent contamination of fruits and vegetables with organic wastes.[23]

Chlorination assists in reducing the hazards of bacterial contamination of water, but water systems are occasionally recontaminated after chlorination due to surface water leaking into faulty pipes. Chlorination can produce its own hazards, though, because the chlorine can react with organic compounds that may be present in water to create carcinogenic compounds.[24] Currently, however, chlorination remains the most efficient and cost-effective mode of water treatment available.

Biological hazards also occur with improper disposal of medical wastes such as needles, syringes, and other objects contaminated with human blood or other secretions and excretions. While disposal of biological hazards from medical facilities is supposed to be strictly controlled, medical wastes have been found on beaches apparently washed ashore from ocean dumping. Contaminated medical wastes have also surfaced among ordinary solid wastes where they pose risks to waste-industry workers as well as contributing to the potential for biological contamination of water through solid waste disposal sites. In one study of waste-industry workers in Washington State, for example, 90 percent of workers reported medical wastes in the general waste stream. In another study, in New York City, multiple needle stick injuries were reported by sanitation workers.[25]

Finally, infectious agents can be transmitted through the air. This transmission is enhanced by technology when improperly cleaned air-conditioning units and heating systems provide breeding grounds for disease-causing microorganisms.[26] For example, contaminated heating and cooling systems have been implicated in the spread of Legionnaires' disease.[27]

INSECTS AND ANIMALS

As noted in Chapter 6, The Epidemiologic Process, insects and animals serve as reservoirs and vectors for a variety of communicable diseases that affect human beings. Insects such as flies, cockroaches, and mosquitoes, and animals such as rats transmit communicable diseases. Again, improper solid-waste disposal can provide a breeding ground for these and other insect and animal vectors.

The presence of large numbers of wild animals such as skunks, foxes, bats, coyotes, bobcats, and racoons increases the potential for transmission of rabies to humans. Large numbers of unimmunized domestic animals such as dogs and cats also present a biological health hazard for the human population.[27] In addition, animal feces provide breeding grounds for flies and other insects that transmit disease.

PLANTS

Plants can pose biological health hazards in two ways. First, many plants are poisonous and present the opportunity for accidental poisoning among small children. A variety of plants commonly found in homes and yards are potential poisons and account for almost 10,000 reports to poison centers annually.[17] Several of these common plants are included in Box 16–2. Plants also present a biological hazard for those individuals who have pollen allergies. Allergic responses to plant pollens may include mild to severe hay fever symptoms or asthma. Other plants such as poison ivy and poison oak produce severe dermatologic symptoms.

BOX 16–2

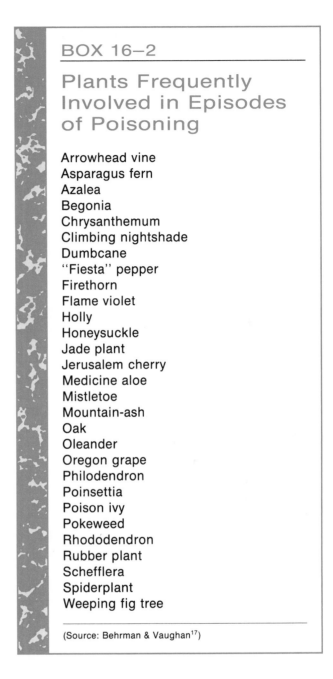

Plants Frequently Involved in Episodes of Poisoning

Arrowhead vine
Asparagus fern
Azalea
Begonia
Chrysanthemum
Climbing nightshade
Dumbcane
"Fiesta" pepper
Firethorn
Flame violet
Holly
Honeysuckle
Jade plant
Jerusalem cherry
Medicine aloe
Mistletoe
Mountain-ash
Oak
Oleander
Oregon grape
Philodendron
Poinsettia
Poison ivy
Pokeweed
Rhododendron
Rubber plant
Schefflera
Spiderplant
Weeping fig tree

(Source: Behrman & Vaughan[17])

CHEMICAL AND GASEOUS HAZARDS

The environment also provides opportunities for human contact with a variety of ***chemical and gaseous hazards***. These hazards are created by the effect of certain chemicals and gases on human tissue. These hazards can involve poisons and air and water pollution.

POISONS

Chemical poisons include insecticides, herbicides, fungicides, and rodenticides as well as a variety of household and industrial chemicals. The use of pesticides has been a primary factor in the increased agricultural production experienced in the United States, but their use has also contributed to the occurrence of a number of health-related effects.[28] Pesticide poisoning occurs through massive exposures such as when several thousand people died as a result of exposure to methyl isocyanate resulting from a leak at a chemical plant in Bhopal, India, in 1984. Poisoning also occurs with cumulative exposures among people who are exposed over a period of time. Pesticide use has been associated with increased incidence of lymphoma and leukemia among farmers, as well as mild reactions of dizziness and nausea.[28] Other health effects associated with pesticides include bladder cancer, neurotoxicity, and other cancers.[29]

Pesticides are used in large volume, and numerous exposures are reported to poison control centers every year. From 1960 to 1980 production of synthetic organic pesticides nearly doubled from 648 million pounds to 1,180 million pounds.[30] In 1987, more than 43,000 pesticide exposures were reported. Exposures can occur as a result of working with the chemicals or servicing and repairing equipment used to apply them.[29] Indirect exposure occurs through contamination of food and water that are then ingested by humans and by animal sources of human food. In particular, DDT is absorbed in body fat and is found in animals who consume treated vegetation. These animals, in turn, serve as a food source for humans, who are thus exposed to the stored DDT. While DDT use has been banned in the United States, it may still be present in foods imported from various other countries.

Chemical poisoning can also result from several household and industrial products and medications. Generally, such poisoning occurs in young children who ingest chemical compounds or medications improperly stored in the home. In 1984, more than 251,000 cases of poisoning were reported to 16 poison control centers nationwide. Over 87 percent of these cases were accidental, but approximately 5 percent involved attempted suicide. More than 64 percent of cases involved children under 5 years of age.[17] Accidental poisoning will be addressed in more detail in Chapter 20, Care of Children, and Chapter 31, Chronic Physical Health Problems.

AIR POLLUTION

Chemicals and gaseous materials add to air pollution, thus presenting additional hazards to human health. Both volatile chemicals and particulate matter contribute to the problem, and air pollution occurs in both indoor and outdoor, or "ambient," air. Pollution of the ambient air is measured in terms of the Pollutant Standards Index (PSI). PSI ratings between 100 and 200 are considered "unhealthful," ratings from 200 to 300 "very unhealthful," and levels over 300 "hazardous" to health.[3] Specific pollutants that are routinely monitored include carbon monoxide, ozone, sulfur oxides, volatile organic compounds, nitrogen oxides, lead, and particulates.

Some progress has been made in controlling pollutants in the ambient air. Between 1972 and 1978, the average number of days per year on which air pollution in 23 major American cities reached PSI levels considered "unhealthful" declined from 86 to 72.[3] From 1970 to 1986, carbon monoxide emissions in the United States decreased by 38 percent, sulfur oxide emissions by more than 25 percent, volatile organic compounds by 30 percent, and nitrogen oxide emissions by almost 30 percent.[30] Despite these declines, a recent World Health Organization report indicated that over 600 million people still live in areas where the average sulfur dioxide levels are above safety guidelines. The report of a 15-year monitoring project in 54 cities throughout the world indicated that sulfur dioxide pollution had declined by 5 percent per year in the developed areas of the United States and Europe, but had increased by 10 percent per year in Asian cities.[31] In 1984, over 32 percent of the U.S. population lived in counties where particulate levels in ambient air exceeded federal standards, while 61 percent lived in areas with excessive carbon monoxide levels and nearly 80 percent in areas with elevated levels of ozone.[7] Ozone levels in 1988 were the worst in a decade in the United States, and over 90 urban areas throughout the country violated Clean Air Act standards, some of them for the first time.[32]

Social factors such as widespread automobile use contribute to air pollution. Unfortunately, although vehicles produced today emit fewer hazardous and polluting substances, the number of autos on American roads has doubled from that of 20 years ago. Each vehicle also travels more miles than ever before and spends more time idling in traffic.[32] Automotive engineering appears to have made the greatest contribution to clean air possible without a complete revolution in the type of engine built.

Sources of ambient air pollution include technological processes used to manufacture consumer goods required to maintain the American standard of living. The level of emissions permissible by large industries is controlled under Clean Air Act standards, but contributions to air pollution are made by numerous small businesses such as dry cleaning and other processes and the use of nail polish remover, paints, aerosols, and other household products that are not controlled.

Pollutant emissions have a cumulative effect compounded by geographic features in some parts of the country. For example, in Los Angeles a persistent inversion layer, or increase of air temperature with increasing altitude, results in decreased dispersion of pollutants that would normally occur with air movements. The effect of the inversion layer is further compounded by the barrier to air movement presented by nearby mountains. In addition, sunlight interacts with particulate and gaseous matter to produce a photochemical smog.[13]

Ambient air pollution is normally dispersed by wind, but wind speed is slowed by the physical features of the earth's surface. The buildings of major urban areas reduce wind speed and thus hinder the dispersion of air pollutants.[13]

Health effects of air pollution include respiratory symptoms, eye irritation, fatigue, and headache. Occasionally, air pollution causes death. From 1880 to 1966, for example, there were 12 major air pollution episodes worldwide. Deaths per episode ranged from 20 to over 4700 fatalities that occurred during a 3-week period in London in 1952. Air-pollution-related mortality generally occurs in the elderly and those with chronic respiratory diseases. Air pollution can also result in increased nonfatal respiratory illness, particularly in children.[7] In one study, a 10 percent increase in upper and lower respiratory symptoms and a 30 percent increase in complaints of eye irritation occurred for each 0.1 parts per million (ppm) elevation in ozone levels.[33]

Air pollution causes acid rain, which contributes to chemical pollution of both groundwater and surface water supplies. As noted earlier, acid rain enhances leaching of a variety of compounds from soil and solid-waste disposal sites and from lead and copper pipes. Air pollution also produces a chemical reaction that depletes the stratospheric ozone layer and reduces the extent of atmospheric filtering, contributing to the adverse health effects of ultraviolet radiation.[13]

Indoor air pollution is also a cause for concern to community health nurses. Pollutants commonly found in household air include formaldehyde, carbon monoxide, carbon dioxide, nitrogen oxides, benzo(a)pyrene, asbestos, and other household chemicals.[26,34] Indoor air pollution tends to be most severe in newer buildings that have been designed, for reasons of energy conservation, to reduce air exchange with the outdoors.

Sources of indoor air pollution include contaminants such as formaldehyde, asbestos, organic dust, and fibrous glass particles released by structural components of buildings or by furnishings.[26] Other sources of pollution indoors include smoking, cooking, heating, cleaning with a variety of household products, and the use of personal hygiene products such as aerosol deodorants. The high cost of energy has also resulted in a shift to new forms of home heating that increase the number and types of pollutants present in dwellings. For example, the use of wood stoves or kerosene heaters, particularly in poorly ventilated areas, leads to the buildup of combustion products in the air.

Indoor air pollution is particularly serious in that most people spend over 90 percent of their time indoors. Those at particular risk for health effects of this type of pollution (children, the elderly, and the infirm) spend an even greater portion of their day inside. Health effects of indoor air pollution range from nose, throat, and eye irritation to respiratory impairment, heart disease, central nervous system damage, and a variety of cancers.[26,34]

WATER POLLUTION

Chemical pollution of both groundwater and surface water also results from sources other than acid rain. Some 17 chemical carcinogens have been identified in drinking water across the nation, and 33 hazardous chemicals have been identified in groundwater in states such as Pennsylvania, New York, New Jersey, Maine, Connecticut, Massachusetts, Hawaii, California, Arizona, and Delaware. Chemical contamination of groundwater is a particularly serious concern because groundwater comprises 96 percent of all freshwater in the United States[35] and is the source of drinking water for half of the American population.[21]

Manufacturing industries are major sources of chemical pollution of the water, but pollution also arises from mining operations, underground storage of chemicals, septic tanks, and the use of salt and de-icing chemicals on highways. Another source of contamination is the 7 million tons of sewage sludge containing both organic and inorganic chemicals produced in the United States each year.[21] Pesticides and fertilizers also find their way into the water supply to create chemical pollution. Health effects of chemical water pollution include bladder and colorectal cancers, central nervous system effects, skin irritation, alopecia, peripheral neuropathies, seizures, hepatitis and cirrhosis, infertility, congenital anomalies, developmental disabilities, anemia, renal failure, esophagitis, gastritis, stomach cancer, and heart disease.[36] In one study, contamination of drinking water with volatile organic chemicals was associated with increased incidence of leukemia in females, but not in males.[37]

HEALTH EFFECTS OF ENVIRONMENTAL HAZARDS

Physical, biological, chemical, and gaseous environmental hazards contribute to a variety of health problems and affect a number of target organs in the body. Target organs and systems include the central nervous system; respiratory, cardiovascular, gastrointestinal, genitourinary, reproductive, integumentary, hematopoietic, lymphatic, the metabolic/endocrine, and the musculoskeletal systems, as well as the eyes and ears.

Air pollution, for example, affects the respiratory system primarily, but may also produce cardiovascular, central nervous system, or hematopoietic effects. Air pollution also irritates the eyes and mucous membranes of the respiratory system. Water pollution can affect the gastrointestinal system, the skin, the liver, and the reproductive, hematopoietic, lymphatic, cardiovascular, and genitourinary systems. Pesticides can adversely affect the central nervous system and produce kidney damage, a variety of cancers, and chromosomal changes. Radiation can cause skin cancer, visual impairment, cataracts, and genetic mutations, as well as lung cancer and other cancers. Lead poisoning damages the central nervous system as well as the gastrointestinal system and can impair growth and development. Other metals and hazardous chemicals may cause cancers or central nervous system, gastrointestinal, and metabolic damage. Finally, high levels of noise not only compromise human hearing, but can contribute to gastrointestinal, dermatologic, central nervous system, cardiovascular, and psychological problems. Some of the effects of these environmental hazards are presented in Figure 16–2.

THE EPIDEMIOLOGIC PREVENTION PROCESS MODEL AND ENVIRONMENTAL INFLUENCES ON HEALTH

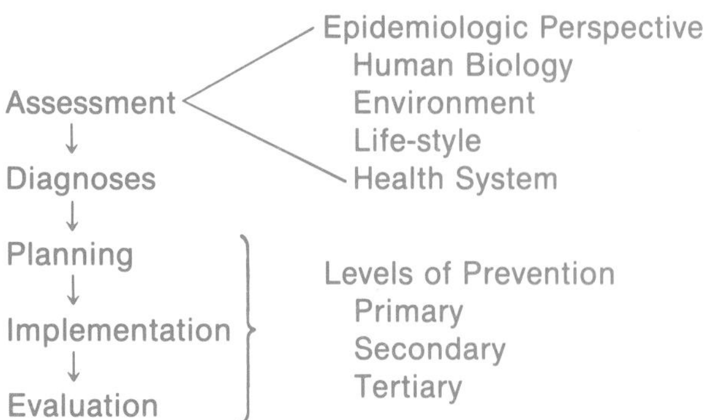

The epidemiologic prevention process model can be used by community health nurses to assess the existence of environmental health hazards and to plan, implement, and evaluate primary, secondary, and tertiary preventive measures to address these hazards. The model can be used with individuals, families, and population groups as the focus of care.

ASSESSING ENVIRONMENTAL INFLUENCES ON HEALTH

There are two aspects in assessing environmental conditions and their relationship to human health. The first involves identification of hazards present in the environment; the second involves assessment of the effects of those hazards on the health of individuals, families, and communities.

Part of the overall assessment of any client, individual, family, or community is a determination of environmental factors that may enhance or impair health. In doing a thorough assessment, the community health nurse would determine the existence of physical, biological, and chemical and gaseous hazards in the client's environment. The nurse would also determine increased susceptibility to the effects of environmental conditions on the part of the client. For example, the nurse might determine that air pollution is a serious problem in a particular community. The effects of air pollution will be more severe for older people, young children, and those with chronic respiratory conditions. For these clients, air pollution presents even more of a health hazard than it does for the general public.

In the assessment, the nurse would inquire about environmental factors discussed in this chapter. For instance, what is the potential for radiation exposure? Are certain families at greater risk because of high radon levels arising from the soil? Is noise a problem? If so, what are the sources of the noise? Is there potential for heavy metal poisoning either from lead-based paint in an older home or because of drinking water contamination? What infectious agents and communicable diseases are present in the community? Is there increased potential for exposure for some individuals and families within the community? Do insects and animals provide avenues for the transmission of these diseases?

Other questions would reflect the potential for poisoning through occupational or recreational exposure to pesticides and herbicides or through improper use or storage of chemicals and medications in the home. What is the quality of the air breathed? What particular pollutants, if any, are present in air or drinking water? Assessment of the environmental risks for individuals and families will necessarily entail knowledge of environmental conditions in the communities in which the clients live.

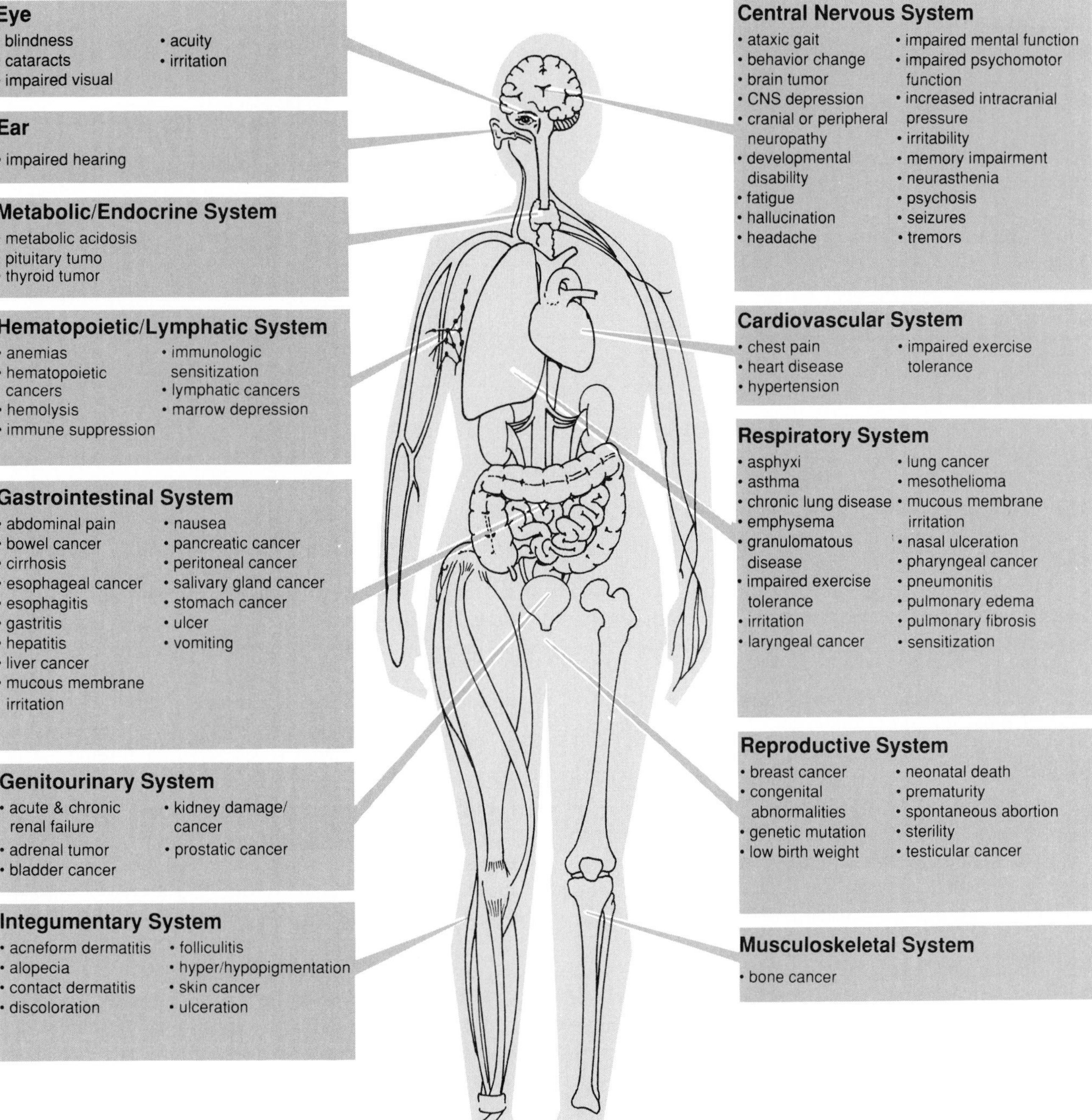
Eye
• blindness
• cataracts
• impaired visual
• acuity
• irritation
Ear
• impaired hearing
Metabolic/Endocrine System
• metabolic acidosis
• pituitary tumo
• thyroid tumor
Hematopoietic/Lymphatic System
• anemias
• hematopoietic cancers
• hemolysis
• immune suppression
• immunologic sensitization
• lymphatic cancers
• marrow depression
Gastrointestinal System
• abdominal pain
• bowel cancer
• cirrhosis
• esophageal cancer
• esophagitis
• gastritis
• hepatitis
• liver cancer
• mucous membrane irritation
• nausea
• pancreatic cancer
• peritoneal cancer
• salivary gland cancer
• stomach cancer
• ulcer
• vomiting
Genitourinary System
• acute & chronic renal failure
• adrenal tumor
• bladder cancer
• kidney damage/ cancer
• prostatic cancer
Integumentary System
• acneform dermatitis
• alopecia
• contact dermatitis
• discoloration
• folliculitis
• hyper/hypopigmentation
• skin cancer
• ulceration
Central Nervous System
• ataxic gait
• behavior change
• brain tumor
• CNS depression
• cranial or peripheral neuropathy
• developmental disability
• fatigue
• hallucination
• headache
• impaired mental function
• impaired psychomotor function
• increased intracranial pressure
• irritability
• memory impairment
• neurasthenia
• psychosis
• seizures
• tremors
Cardiovascular System
• chest pain
• heart disease
• hypertension
• impaired exercise tolerance
Respiratory System
• asphyxi
• asthma
• chronic lung disease
• emphysema
• granulomatous disease
• impaired exercise tolerance
• irritation
• laryngeal cancer
• lung cancer
• mesothelioma
• mucous membrane irritation
• nasal ulceration
• pharyngeal cancer
• pneumonitis
• pulmonary edema
• pulmonary fibrosis
• sensitization
Reproductive System
• breast cancer
• congenital abnormalities
• genetic mutation
• low birth weight
• neonatal death
• prematurity
• spontaneous abortion
• sterility
• testicular cancer
Musculoskeletal System
• bone cancer

Figure 16–2. Human health effects of environmental hazards.

Knowledge of the environmental risks present will guide the second aspect of the assessment—determination of the effects of these conditions on clients' health. In this phase of the assessment, the nurse would be alert to signs and symptoms of health problems related to environmental hazards. For instance, are people working in a particular building experiencing fatigue, eye irritation, increased respiratory illness, or other symptoms of indoor air pollution? Is a young child in a deteriorating older residential area exhibiting signs of lead poisoning? Have excessive noise levels resulted in hearing loss? Has the presence of carcinogenic chemicals in drinking water contributed to an increased incidence of cancer in community residents? In this aspect of client assessment, the nurse will engage in case finding to identify those individuals, families, or communities adversely affected by environmental hazards.

DIAGNOSTIC REASONING AND ENVIRONMENTAL INFLUENCES ON HEALTH

The two aspects of environmental assessment conducted by the community health nurse will give rise to two levels of nursing diagnoses. The first level reflects the presence of health hazards within the client's environment. For example, the nurse may make a diagnosis of "increased potential for lead poisoning due to lead-based paint in deteriorating older housing." Such a diagnosis would signal environmental risks for individuals who live in the area affected as well as for the community at large. In another instance, the nursing diagnosis may relate to risks experienced by a particular family, rather than the entire community. For example, the nurse might make a diagnosis of an "increased potential for poisoning due to the presence of young children and improper storage of household chemicals in the home."

The second level of nursing diagnosis reflects the presence of existing health problems related to environmental conditions. For example, the nurse might derive a diagnosis of "possible lead poisoning due to eating paint chips" in a young child. Or, the nurse might diagnose an "increased incidence of respiratory illnesses due to inadequate cleaning of air conditioning and heating units" in an energy-efficient office building.

As can be seen in the examples given, both levels of diagnoses may be made in relation to individuals, families, and groups or communities. For an individual or a family, diagnoses can reflect an increased risk of health problems due to specific environmental conditions or the identification of existing health problems related to those conditions. The same is true for diagnoses related to groups of people. The nurse may diagnose environmental conditions that pose risks for the entire community or existing health problems due to environmental factors.

PLANNING TO CONTROL ENVIRONMENTAL INFLUENCES ON HEALTH

Based on the findings of the nursing assessment and the nursing diagnoses derived from that assessment, the community health nurse will plan interventions to control environmental influences on health. These interventions can occur at the primary, secondary, or tertiary level of prevention.

PRIMARY PREVENTION

Primary preventive measures are directed toward modifying or eliminating environmental hazards or reducing the potential for exposure to them. Primary prevention can occur with individuals and their families or with groups of people. For instance, the community health nurse might discourage the use of industrial paints that may still contain lead for painting surfaces in a family's home. Or, the nurse may suggest that the family run the tap for a while before getting water for drinking or cooking and to use only cold water. The effects of acidified water in leaching lead and copper from pipes in older homes are enhanced by heat, so warm water or water that has been standing in sun-heated pipes for some time will contain higher levels of lead or copper than will cold water that has been allowed to run.[38] Another primary preventive measure directed toward the health of individuals and families would be education on the safe storage of medications and household chemicals to prevent accidental poisonings.

At the group level, community health nurses can engage in political efforts to minimize environmental hazards. For example, a nurse might campaign for a local ordinance that requires landlords to engage in lead-abatement procedures in older dwellings or a law that prevents improper disposal of hazardous wastes. Community health nurses can also educate the public regarding preventive measures. For instance, a nurse might be involved in developing a campaign to educate people on the appropriate disposal of hazardous household chemicals. Other primary preventive measures for individuals, families, and communities are presented in Table 16–1.

TABLE 16–1. PRIMARY PREVENTIVE MEASURES FOR SELECTED ENVIRONMENTAL HAZARDS FOR INDIVIDUALS, FAMILIES, AND COMMUNITIES

Environmental Hazard	Individual/Family	Community
Radiation	• Refer for assistance with testing and sealing a home against radon leaks • Encourage spending most of one's time in higher levels of the home	• Educate the public on the hazards of radon exposure and preventive measures • Engage in political activity to promote building standards that safeguard occupants in areas with high levels of natural radiation
	• Discourage overuse of diagnostic X-rays	• Educate the public about the hazards of overuse of diagnostic X-rays
	• Encourage adequate cleaning of door seals on microwave ovens and maintenance of safe distance while microwave is in operation	• Engage in political activity to promote and enforce safety standards for nuclear reactors
	• Discourage sunbathing • Encourage use of sun screen and protective clothing when outdoors	• Educate the public about the hazards of exposure to ultraviolet radiation
Lead and heavy metals	• Encourage families to remove lead-based paint from older homes • Encourage families to wash hands of small children as well as toys to remove lead contaminated dust • Encourage close supervision of small children	• Encourage communities to remove lead-based paint from older homes
	• Encourage families to use cold water to drink and cook with and to allow the tap to run for a few minutes	• Promote legislation to ban air pollution and acid rain to prevent pollution of water with heavy metals • Encourage policymakers to set and enforce standards for solid-waste sites to prevent metal contamination in water
Noise	• Encourage families to limit noise in the home • Encourage use of ear protection in high noise areas	• Promote noise-abatement ordinances
Infectious agents	• Promote routine immunization for all ages	• Educate the public on need for immunizations • Encourage policymakers to provide low-cost immunization services
	• Encourage good hygiene • Encourage washing fruits and vegetables before eating	
	• Encourage adequate refrigeration of food	• Encourage enforcement of regulations for food processing and food handlers
	• Encourage susceptible individuals to boil water for cooking and drinking in areas with unsafe water	• Promote adequate sanitation, waste disposal, and water treatment
Insects and animals	• Encourage immunization of family pets	• Encourage development and enforcement of immunization and leash laws
	• Refer for assistance in eliminating insects, rats, etc., from the home • Encourage use of insect repellent and protective clothing when outdoors	• Promote ordinances controlling insect breeding areas
Plants	• Eliminate poisonous house plants • Eliminate poisonous plants from the yard • Eliminate other hazardous plants (for example, poison ivy, plant allergens) from home environment • Encourage close supervision of small children	• Eliminate poisonous plants from recreational areas
Poisons	• Educate families on proper use and storage of household chemicals and medications • Encourage close supervision of children	• Educate public on hazards of household chemicals and medication • Promote legislation to limit use of hazardous chemicals in home and industry
Air pollution	• Encourage limiting physical activity on days with high air pollutant levels • Encourage car pooling	• Promote legislation to prevent air pollution
	• Discourage use of space heaters in poorly ventilated areas	• Promote legislation to develop safety standards for home heating devices

(*continued*)

TABLE 16–1. (*Continued*)

Environmental Hazard	Individual/Family	Community
Air pollution (*continued*)	• Encourage frequent cleaning of heater and air conditioning filters • Encourage opening doors and windows to permit air exchange • Encourage replacing asbestos insulation as needed	• Promote building standards that ensure adequate ventilation
Water pollution	• Encourage use of bottled water by high-risk persons in areas with heavily polluted water	• Promote legislation to prevent water pollution

SECONDARY PREVENTION

Secondary prevention with individuals and their families would be geared to identifying and resolving existing health problems caused by environmental conditions. For instance, community health nurses might be involved in screening for elevated lead levels or for hearing loss. They might also make referrals for testing of water supplies for clients who are concerned about potential contamination. When possible environmentally caused health conditions are identified, community health nurses might make referrals for medical diagnosis and treatment as needed. They might also make referrals for assistance with eliminating environmental hazards. For example, a nurse might be aware of lead-based paint in dwellings in some parts of town. He or she can screen young children in the area for elevated blood lead levels and make referrals for treatment for children with positive test results. The nurse might also make a referral for assistance in removing lead-based paint from the homes of affected children. Finally, the nurse would monitor children's responses to therapy and potential for continued exposure to lead.

Political activity might again be used as a secondary preventive measure at the aggregate level. For instance, a nurse might influence health-care policymakers to provide adequate access to diagnostic and treatment facilities for environmentally caused health problems. Or, a nurse might campaign for stricter standards for pollutant emissions in air and water. Potential secondary preventive measures for individuals, families, and communities are presented in Table 16–2.

TERTIARY PREVENTION

Community health nurses may need to work with individuals or families to prevent recurrence or complications of environmentally caused health problems. For example, a community health nurse might assist a family to find housing where exposure to lead is not a problem. Or, the nurse might provide parents with referrals for assistance in coping with the mental effects of long-standing lead poisoning in their children. Another tertiary preventive measure might involve suggestions for decreasing noise levels in the home to prevent further impairment of hearing.

Tertiary prevention might also be needed to deal with environmental problems at the aggregate or group level. An example of tertiary control measures at this level might include political activity to mandate standards that prevent the recurrence of a leak at a nuclear power plant or to pass a bond issue to renovate a water-treatment plant and prevent recontamination of drinking water with sewage. Other possible tertiary preventive interventions by community health nurses are presented in Table 16–3.

IMPLEMENTING ENVIRONMENTAL MEASURES

Implementing environmental control measures can involve both creating support for action to be taken and reducing resistance to action. The community health nurse may need to make individuals and families aware of the risks presented by environmental hazards. For example, the avid runner may not realize that vigorous exercise actually enhances the adverse effects of air pollution on lung tissue and may be unwilling to limit the amount of physical exertion on smoggy days. Or, a family may be not be aware of the need to wash children's toys frequently when there is potential for lead exposure.

In addition, the nurse may need to take steps to decrease resistance to action designed to modify environmental hazards. Resistance can arise from perceived barriers to action. The runner, for example, may be unwilling to reduce his or her exercise on days with elevated levels of air pollutants. Or, a landlord may be unwilling to replace lead or copper pipes with synthetics that will minimize the potential for heavy-metal poisoning. In the first instance, the nurse might suggest alternative exercises that the runner can perform indoors. In the second example, the nurse might

TABLE 16–2. SECONDARY PREVENTIVE MEASURES FOR SELECTED ENVIRONMENTAL HAZARDS FOR INDIVIDUALS, FAMILIES, AND COMMUNITIES

Environmental Hazard	Individual/Family	Community
Radiation	• Look for signs of radiation-caused health problems among clients and members of their families	• Monitor incidence of radiation-caused health problems
	• Refer for diagnosis and treatment as needed	• Promote accessibility of diagnostic and treatment facilities
	• Monitor effectiveness of treatment	• Monitor longevity to determine effects of treatment in groups of people
Lead and heavy metals	• Screen for elevated blood levels of heavy metals in persons at risk	• Promote accessibility of screening services
	• Observe for signs of heavy metal poisoning	• Monitor incidence of heavy metal poisoning • Educate the public on the signs and symptoms of heavy metal poisoning
	• Refer for diagnosis and treatment as needed	• Promote accessibility of diagnostic and treatment facilities
	• Monitor effects of treatment	• Monitor prevalence of complications due to heavy metal poisoning
Noise	• Screen for hearing loss in persons at risk	• Promote accessibility of screening services
	• Refer for diagnosis and treatment as needed	• Promote accessibility of diagnostic and treatment services
	• Monitor effects of treatment	
Infectious agents	• Screen for selected communicable diseases in high-risk persons	• Promote accessibility of screening services
	• Observe for signs of communicable diseases	• Monitor incidence of communicable diseases
Insects and animals	• Educate families about first aid for insect and animal bites	• Promote accessibility of treatment facilities for animal bites
	• Observe for signs and symptoms of diseases caused by insects or animals	• Monitor the incidence of diseases caused by insects or animals
	• Refer for medical assistance as needed	• Promote accessibility of diagnostic and treatment services for diseases caused by insects or animals
Plants	• Inform families of poison control center activities	• Educate the public about poison control center activities
	• Refer families for poison control center services as needed	• Promote community support of poison control centers
	• Refer for treatment of plant-caused allergies and other conditions	
Poisons	• Educate families about first aid for poisoning	• Educate the public about first aid for poisoning
	• Observe for signs and symptoms of poisoning	• Monitor the incidence of accidental poisoning
	• Refer families for poison control services as needed	• Promote access to poison control center services
Air pollution	• Observe for signs and symptoms of diseases caused by air pollution	• Promote legislation to reduce pollutant emissions
	• Refer for diagnosis and treatment as needed	• Promote access to diagnostic and treatment services
Water pollution	• Observe for signs and symptoms of water-related diseases	• Promote legislation to control water pollution
	• Refer for diagnosis and treatment of water-related diseases	• Promote availability of diagnostic and treatment services for water-related diseases

need to function as an advocate for the family, encouraging the landlord to take the needed action. Or, the nurse might assist the family to move to safer housing. If the family owns its own home, the nurse might refer members to agencies that will help with the cost of removing hazardous materials from the home. For example, some power companies will assist homeowners with the cost of installing nonasbestos insulation in homes.

Implementation of environmental controls at the aggregate level will also require developing support and measures to decrease or circumvent resistance to action. The community health nurse may engage in some of the political strategies described in Chapter

TABLE 16–3. TERTIARY PREVENTIVE MEASURES FOR SELECTED ENVIRONMENTAL HEALTH HAZARDS FOR INDIVIDUALS, FAMILIES, AND COMMUNITIES

Environmental Hazard	Individual/Family	Community
Radiation	• Remove or seal off radiation sources in homes to prevent further exposure • Assist clients to deal with effects of radiation-caused diseases	• Advocate steps to prevent recurrence of radiation exposures in the community • Promote community long-term treatment services for radiation-caused disease
Lead and heavy metals	• Refer families for help in removing lead-based paint and lead-bearing dust from homes • Encourage families to replace lead and copper pipes if possible • Encourage use of bottled water if needed to prevent subsequent exposure to waterborne metals • Provide assistance in dealing with long-term effects of heavy metal poisoning	• Advocate lead-abatement programs in older residential areas • Educate the public on the hazards of lead and copper pipes • Advocate legislation to promote reductions in water pollutants • Promote access to services needed to deal with effects of heavy metal poisoning
Noise	• Monitor for subsequent hearing loss • Assist client/family to adjust to hearing loss	• Advocate noise abatement legislation • Promote community programs for the hearing impaired
Infectious agents	• Encourage immunization • Encourage hygiene to prevent the spread of communicable diseases to other family members • Monitor for complications of communicable diseases • Maintain overall health status to prevent relapse	• Advocate access to immunization services • Educate the public to prevent the spread of communicable disease in the community • Promote access to long-term care for effects of communicable diseases
Insects and animals	• Assist clients to adjust to effects of diseases caused by insects and animals	• Promote access to long-term care as needed • Advocate eradication of insect and animal vectors to prevent the spread of disease
Plants	• Assist clients to live with long-term effects of plant poisoning or allergy	• Promote access to long-term care as needed
Poisons	• Assist clients to deal with effects of poisons • Encourage removing potential poisons from the home and proper storage of poisonous substances • Encourage better supervision of young children	• Promote access to long-term care for victims as needed • Advocate removal of potential poisons from the environment
Air pollution	• Assist clients to adjust to effects of pollution-caused diseases • Encourage activity limitation when air pollution is severe	• Promote access to long-term care services as needed • Advocate measures to prevent pollutant emissions
Water pollution	• Assist client to deal with long-term effects of diseases due to water pollution • Encourage use of bottled water by those at risk for recurrence of diseases due to water pollution	• Advocate measures to eliminate existing water pollution and prevent further pollution

12, the Political Process, to create public support for legislation related to environmental measures. Community health nurses may also be involved in educating the public regarding the risks posed by environmental hazards and in motivating people to take collective action to reduce those risks.

To influence individuals, families, policymakers, and the general public to implement primary, secondary, and tertiary control measures, community health nurses need to be knowledgeable about environmental issues. The agencies and organizations listed in Table 16–4 can serve as sources of information and assistance regarding environmental health for community health nurses and for the clients with whom they work.

EVALUATING ENVIRONMENTAL MEASURES

Community health nurses are also involved in evaluating the effectiveness of environmental control measures. Evaluation would focus on the effectiveness of primary, secondary, and tertiary preventive

TABLE 16–4. RESOURCES FOR PROMOTING ENVIRONMENTAL HEALTH

Agency or Organization	Function
Center for Atomic Radiation Studies P.O. Box 72 Acton, MA 01720 (617) 635-0045	Research, legal guidance after exposure, statistics, public information
Center for Disease Control Center for Environmental Health 1600 Clifton Rd. Atlanta, GA 30333 (404) 329-3291	Research, public information, policy formation
Citizens for Clean Air 32 Broadway New York, NY 10004	Legislative advocacy for clean air
Consumer Product Safety Commission 5401 Westbard Ave. Bethesda, MD 20207 (301) 492-6580	Research and public information on product safety
Environmental Action 1346 Connecticut Ave., N.W. Washington, DC 20036	Legislative advocacy on environmental issues
Environmental Protection Agency 401 M. St., S.W. Washington, DC 20460 (202) 382-2090	Policy formation; sets and enforces standards to protect the environment
Health Policy Advisory Center 17 Murray St. New York, NY 10007	Public information on occupational and environmental health
Ministry of Concern for Public Health 5495 Main St. Buffalo, NY 14221	Information on prevention of diseases due to environmental pollution, legislative advocacy
National Institute of Environmental Health Science P.O. Box 12233 Research Triangle Park, NC 27709 (919) 541-3345	Research on environmental hazards
Nuclear Regulatory Commission 117 H. St., N.W. Washington, DC 20555 (301) 492-7715	Regulates use of nuclear power; sets and enforces safety standards
Public Citizens, Inc. Health Research Group 2000 P. St., N.W., Suite 708 Washington, DC 20036 (202) 872-0320	Public information on toxic substances, food, drugs
Radiation Health Information Project c/o Environmental Policy Institute 218 D. St., S.E. Washington, DC 20003 (202) 544-2600	Advocacy and policy development to decrease exposure to ionizing radiation; monitors federal activities on radiation health
Sierra Club 530 Bush St. San Francisco, CA 94108	Legislative advocacy, public information on environmental protection
Toxic Project Clearinghouse Environmental Action Foundation 724 Dupont Circle Bldg. Washington, DC 20036	Information on toxic substances and exposure
U.S. Dept. of Agriculture Marketing & Inspection Service Food Safety & Inspection Service 14th & Independence Ave., S.W. Washington, DC 20250 (202) 447-7943	Inspection of meat and poultry

(*continued*)

TABLE 16–4. (*Continued*)

Agency or Organization	Function
U.S. House of Representatives Committee on Energy & Commerce Subcommittee on Health & the Environment 2415 Rayburn House Office Bldg. Washington, DC 20515	Policy formation related to energy and environmental health issues
Water Pollution Control Federation 2626 Pennsylvania Ave., N.W. Washington, DC 20037	Legislative advocacy

TABLE 16–5. SAMPLE QUESTIONS FOR EVALUATING PRIMARY, SECONDARY, AND TERTIARY PREVENTION OF ENVIRONMENTAL HAZARDS

Environmental Hazard	Primary Prevention	Secondary Prevention	Tertiary Prevention
Radiation	Have exposures to radiation been eliminated or reduced? Has the incidence of radiation-related illness been reduced?	Have those with radiation-caused diseases received adequate treatment? Have the effects of radiation exposure been minimized?	Have reexposures to radiation been reduced or prevented altogether?
Lead and heavy metals	Have environmental sources of exposure to heavy metals been eliminated? Has the incidence of heavy metal poisoning decreased?	Have blood levels for heavy metals decreased after treatment? Have long-term sequellae of heavy metal poisoning been prevented?	Has reexposure to heavy metals been prevented? Have lowered blood levels for heavy metals been maintained after treatment?
Noise	Have noise levels been reduced to prevent hearing loss? Has the incidence of hearing loss been reduced?	Have persons with hearing impairment received needed services? Has hearing been restored by means of hearing aids, etc.?	Has further deterioration of hearing been prevented?
Infectious agents	Has the incidence of communicable diseases declined? Has the proportion of persons immunized against immunizable communicable diseases increased?	Have individuals with communicable diseases been adequately treated?	Have recurrent cases of communicable diseases been prevented?
Insects and animals	Has the incidence of diseases spread by insects and animals decreased? Have insect and animal vectors been eliminated?	Have individuals with diseases spread by insects and animals been adequately treated?	Have recurrent episodes of diseases caused by insects and animals been prevented?
Plants	Have poisonous plants been removed from the environment? Has the number of cases of plant-related poisoning declined?	Has mortality due to plant poisoning been reduced?	Have recurrent plant poisonings been prevented?
Poisons	Has the incidence of poisoning decreased? Are hazardous substances disposed of appropriately?	Has poisoning mortality declined?	Have recurrent episodes of poisoning been prevented?
Air pollution	Has the level of pollutants in ambient or indoor air been reduced? Has the incidence of diseases due to air pollution declined?	Have individuals with diseases due to air pollution received adequate diagnostic and treatment services?	Has further contamination of ambient or indoor air been prevented?
Water pollution	Has the number of exposures to polluted water been reduced? Has the incidence of diseases due to water pollution declined?	Have individuals with diseases due to water pollution been adequately treated?	Have recurrent episodes of diseases due to water pollution been prevented? Has recontamination of water by pollutants been prevented?

measures related to individuals, families, and population groups. For example, the nurse might monitor blood lead levels of children in housing with lead-based paint to determine whether primary preventive measures have prevented initial elevation. For those children who already have elevated blood lead levels, evaluation would focus on the effects of chelating agents in reducing blood levels and the prevention of symptoms of lead poisoning, while evaluation of tertiary measures would be aimed at the effectiveness of abatement procedures in preventing blood lead levels from rising again after treatment. Similar approaches to evaluation of primary, secondary, and tertiary preventive interventions could be used for each of the environmental health problems addressed in this chapter. Evaluation at the aggregate level would focus on the extent to which national objectives for environmental health have been achieved. Possible foci for evaluating primary, secondary, and tertiary perventive measures for other environmental hazards are presented in Table 16–5.

CHAPTER HIGHLIGHTS

- Environmental conditions give rise to three types of health hazards: physical hazards, biological hazards, and chemical or gaseous hazards.
- Physical hazards to health arising from the environment include radiation, lead and other heavy metals, and noise.
- Ionizing, electromagnetic, and ultraviolet radiation affect human health. Ionizing radiation is created when radioactive substances break down into other substances that emit radiation in the process. Nuclear power, radon gas, and X-rays are potential sources of exposure to ionizing radiation. Health effects of ionizing radiation include a variety of cancers, genetic changes, and radiation sickness.
- Electromagnetic radiation consists of waves emitted from electric and magnetic fields surrounding matter. Electromagnetic radiation sources include VDTs and microwave ovens and similar devices. The health effects of electromagnetic radiation are only now being investigated but may include fatigue, headaches, blood dyscrasias, cataracts, memory loss, decreased fertility, and other conditions.
- Ultraviolet radiation is radiation from the portion of the light spectrum beyond the capability of the human eye to see. Health effects of ultraviolet radiation include sunburn, skin cancer, and cataracts.
- Lead and other heavy metals may be found in soil and in water. Lead may also be found in lead-based paint used in houses built before 1950. Lead and other heavy metals can result in poisoning and cause a variety of gastrointestinal, dermatological, and central nervous system disorders.
- Noise is a physical hazard that not only causes hearing impairment but also contributes to a variety of other physical and psychological health problems.
- Biological hazards include infectious agents that cause disease, insects and animals that spread disease, and plants that may result in poisoning or trigger allergic reactions.
- Chemical and gaseous hazards include poisons found in pesticides, herbicides, rodenticides, medications, and so on, as well as chemical and gaseous pollutants of air and water.
- Environmental health hazards affect almost every body system and organ. Some effects are merely irritating while others can be fatal.
- Community health nursing assessment of environmental influences on health focuses on determining the environmental risks affecting individuals, families, and communities and on identifying existing health problems related to environmental factors.
- Nursing diagnoses related to environmental health may reflect the presence of environmental risk factors or the existence of health problems caused by environmental conditions. Nursing diagnoses may be made related to individuals, families, and groups or communities.
- Planning to control environmental influences on health includes developing primary, secondary, and tertiary preventive measures to modify or eliminate environmental risk fac-

(continued)

tors or to deal with or prevent recurrence of existing health problems related to environmental conditions.

- Implementing environmental control measures can involve creating support for action related to environmental factors and decreasing resistance to action.
- Evaluating environmental measures focuses on the effectiveness of primary, secondary, and tertiary preventive measures in eliminating or modifying environmental risk factors and in preventing or ameliorating health problems related to environmental conditions.

Review Questions

1. Summarize at least five of the national health objectives for the year 2000 related to environmental health. (p. 344)
2. What are three physical hazards to health arising from the environment? Give an example of the effects of each on human health. (p. 345)
3. Describe three types of biological hazards to health that may be present in the environment. Discuss how each might adversely affect health. (p. 348)
4. What three types of hazards to human health are posed by chemical or gaseous materials? Give an example of the effect of each type of hazard. (p. 349)
5. Describe at least two health effects of environmental conditions on each of six human target organs or body systems. (p. 352)
6. What are the two levels at which nursing diagnoses may be made with respect to environmental influences on health? Give an example of a nursing diagnosis at each level. (p. 354)
7. Describe at least five primary preventive measures for health problems related to environmental conditions. (p. 354)
8. Describe at least three secondary preventive measures for health problems related to environmental conditions. (p. 356)
9. Describe at least three tertiary preventive measures for health problems related to environmental conditions. (p. 356)

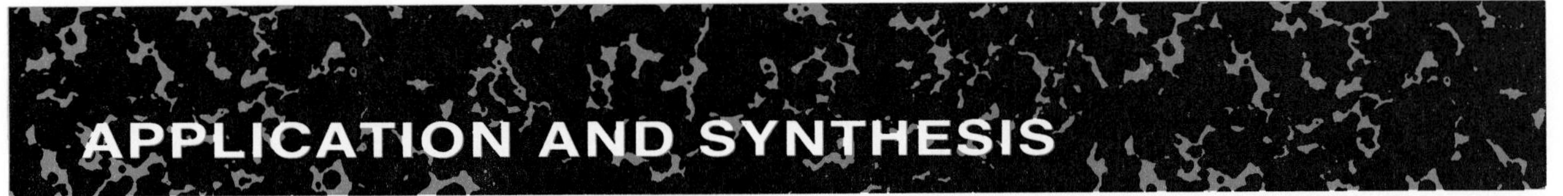

APPLICATION AND SYNTHESIS

Mary Jones, a community health nurse, is visiting a new client in a nursing home in an inner-city area in Los Angeles. As she is entering the nursing home, she notices that several of the residents are doing calisthenics in the yard. Some of the residents are sitting on the sidelines and appear quite short of breath. When Mary checks to be sure they are all right, they tell her that they usually have a hard time breathing when they exercise on smoggy days like today. The residents say that they usually try to continue their exercises because that is one of the few activities that gets them out of the building. They also enjoy the social aspects of the exercise sessions. Many of them state that they have always been active and want to maintain their strength and mobility as long as possible. They express fears of being bedridden and unable to care for themselves.

After Mary is sure that all of them will be all right, she goes on to see her client. When she enters the building, she notices that it is quite hot inside, even though all of the windows and doors are open. Although it is only 10 A.M., it promises to be one of L.A.'s scorching summer days. After seeing her client, Mary talks to the director about the heat in the building. The director tells her that the building is always hot and that the air conditioning has never worked properly. The last time the repairmen came to fix the air conditioning unit, they said it couldn't be repaired and would have to be replaced. The nursing home is run by a large national corporation, and the director says she has been told that they will have to wait until the next budget year (October) before there will be money available for a new air conditioner. Fortunately, the heating system is separate, so there will still be heat when the colder weather starts. The director says that staff members have been particularly careful about maintaining hydration in the residents during the hot weather, but many of the residents seem fatigued and listless with the heat.

1. What environmental hazards are present in this situation? What health effects, if any, are these hazards causing?
2. What human biological, life-style, social and psychological, environmental, and health system factors are interacting with hazards in the physical environment to contribute to problems?
3. What level(s) of prevention is(are) warranted in this situation? What might Mary do to intervene?

REFERENCES

1. U.S. Department of Health and Human Services. (1991). *Healthy people 2000: National health promotion and disease prevention objectives.* Washington, DC: Government Printing Office.
2. Pringle, L. (1983). *Radiation: Waves and particles/Benefits and risks.* Hillside, NJ: Enslow.
3. Council on Environmental Quality. (1981). *Environmental trends.* Washington, DC: Council on Environmental Quality.
4. Gibbons, W. (1991). Low level radiation: Higher long-term risk? *Science News, 139,* 181.
5. Trends of a decade—A perspective on occupational hazard surveillance, 1970–1983. (1985). *CDC Surveillance Summaries, 1985, MMWR, 34,* 15SS.
6. Boice, J. D., Morin, M. M., Glass, A. D., & Friedman, G. D. (1991). Diagnostic x-ray procedures and risk of leukemia, lymphoma, and multiple myeloma. *JAMA, 265,* 1290–1294.
7. Elsom, D. (1987). *Atmospheric air pollution: Causes, effects, and control policies.* New York: Basil Blackwell.
8. Radford, E. P. (1985). Potential health effects of indoor radon exposure. *Environmental Health Perspectives, 62,* 281–287.
9. Loken, S., & Loken, T. (1989). Radon: Detection and treatment. *Nurse Practitioner, 14*(11), 45–46, 48, 51.
10. Schnorr, T. M., Grawjewski, P. A., Hornung, P. A., Thun, M. D. (1991). Video display terminals and the risk of spontaneous abortion. *New England Journal of Medicine,* 324, 727–733.
11. U.S. Preventive Services Task Force. (1989). *Guide to clinical preventive services.* Baltimore: Williams & Wilkins.
12. Ralston, J. (1986). EPA estimates major long-term ozone risks. *Science News, 130,* 308.
13. Godish, T. (1985). *Air quality.* Chelsea, MI: Lewis.
14. Farfel, M. R., & Chisolm, J. J. Jr. (1990). Health and environmental outcomes of traditional and modified practices for abatement of residential lead-based paint. *American Journal of Public Health, 80,* 1240–1245.
15. U.S. Department of Health and Human Services. (1987). *Setting nationwide objectives in disease prevention and health promotion: The United States experience.* Washington, DC: Government Printing Office.
16. Edelstein, M. R. (1987). *Contaminated communities.* Boulder, CO: Westview Press.
17. Behrman, R. E., & Vaughan, V. C. (1987). *Nelson textbook of pediatrics* (13th ed.). Philadelphia: W.B. Saunders.
18. Poskanzer, D. C. (1980). Heavy metals. In K. J. Isselbacher, R. D. Adams, R. Braunwald, & R. G. Petersdorf (Eds.), *Harrison's principles of internal medicine* (9th ed) (pp. 965–967). New York: McGraw-Hill.
19. Clark, C. R. (1984). The effects of noise on health. In D. M. Jones & A. J. Chapman (Eds.), *Noise and Society.* New York: Wiley.
20. Page, G. W. III (1987). Water and health. In M. R. Greenberg (Ed.), *Public health and the environment* (pp. 105–138). New York: Guilford Press.
21. Loehr, R. C. (1989). Groundwater contamination—The problem and potential solutions. *National Forum, LXIX*(1), 26–28.
22. Fattal, B., Wax, Y., Davies, M., & Shuval, H. I. (1986). Health risks associated with wastewater irrigation: An epidemiological study. *American Journal of Public Health, 76,* 977–979.
23. Stover, M. (1989). What do a cow and a laundromat have in common? *Aqueduct, 55*(3), 28–29.
24. Shy, C. M. (1985). Chemical contamination of water supplies. *Environmental Health Perspectives, 62,* 399–406.
25. Turnberg, W. L., & Frost, F. (1990). Survey of occupational exposure of waste industry workers to infectious wastes in Washington state. *American Journal of Public Health, 80,* 1262–1264.
26. Briasco, M. E. (1990). Indoor air pollution: Are employees sick from their work? *AAOHN Journal, 38,* 375–380.
27. Benenson, A. S. (1990). *Control of communicable diseases in man* (15th ed.). Washington, DC: American Public Health Association.
28. Pope, K., & Olson, K. D. (1990). Pesticides and their control. *AAOHN Journal, 38,* 353–359.
29. McConnell, R., Anton, A. F. P., & Magnotti, R. (1990). Crop duster aviation mechanics: High risk for pesticide poisoning. *American Journal of Public Health, 80,* 1236–1239.
30. U.S. Department of Commerce. (1990). *Statistical abstract of the United States* (109th ed.). Washington, DC: Government Printing Office.
31. 600 Million live in cities with air pollution risk. (1987, July). *The Nation's Health,* p. 9.
32. McLoughlin, M. (1989). Our dirty air. *U.S. News & World Report, 106*(23), 48–54. (environment)
33. Raloff, J. (1991). Air pollution: A respiratory hue and cry. *Science News, 139,* 203.
34. U.S. Department of Energy. (1984). *Environment and power: Home weatherization & indoor air pollutants.* Washington, DC: U.S. Department of Energy.
35. Tangley, L. (1984). Groundwater contamination: Local problems become national issue. *BioScience, 34*(3), 142–148.
36. Buffler, P. A., Crane, M., & Key, M. M. (1985). Possibilities of detecting health effects by studies of populations exposed to chemicals from waste disposal sites. *Environmental Health Perspectives, 62,* 423–456.
37. Fagliano, J., Berry, M., Bove, F., & Burke, T. (1990). Drinking water contamination and the incidence of leukemia: An ecologic study. *American Journal of Public Health, 80,* 1209–1212.
38. Robbins, A. (1987, May–June). More than trees die from pollution caused by acid rain. *The Nation's Health,* p. 7.

RECOMMENDED READINGS

Gofman, J. W. (1981). *Radiation and human health.* San Francisco: Sierra Club.

Presents a comprehensive summary of research on the relationship of radiation to cancer and other diseases.

Moran, J. M., Morgan, M. D., & Wiersma, J. H. (1986). *Introduction to environmental science* (2nd ed.). New York: W.H. Freeman.

Provides an introduction to principles of environmental science. Addresses issues of air and water pollution, waste management, human population growth, and energy sources, and their effects on ecosystems.

Root, D. E., & Heard, S. R. (1987, May). Biological monitoring: Why do it? *Safety & Health*, 38–40.

Discusses screening procedures for routine monitoring of populations at risk for occupational exposure to hazardous substances.

U.S. Department of Health and Human Services. (1991). *Healthy people 2000: National health promotion and illness prevention objectives*. Washington, DC: Government Printing Office.

Presents national health objectives related to environmental health for achievement by the year 2000. Also describes the problems involved and provides baseline data for current environmental health problems.

Whelan, E. M. (1985). *Toxic terror*. Ottawa, MI: Jameson.

Contains research findings on many supposed environmental hazards including Love Canal, DDT, acid rain, hazards of nuclear power, and so on. Cautions against unfounded resistance and emotionalism in developing environmental policy.

UNIT FOUR

Care of Clients

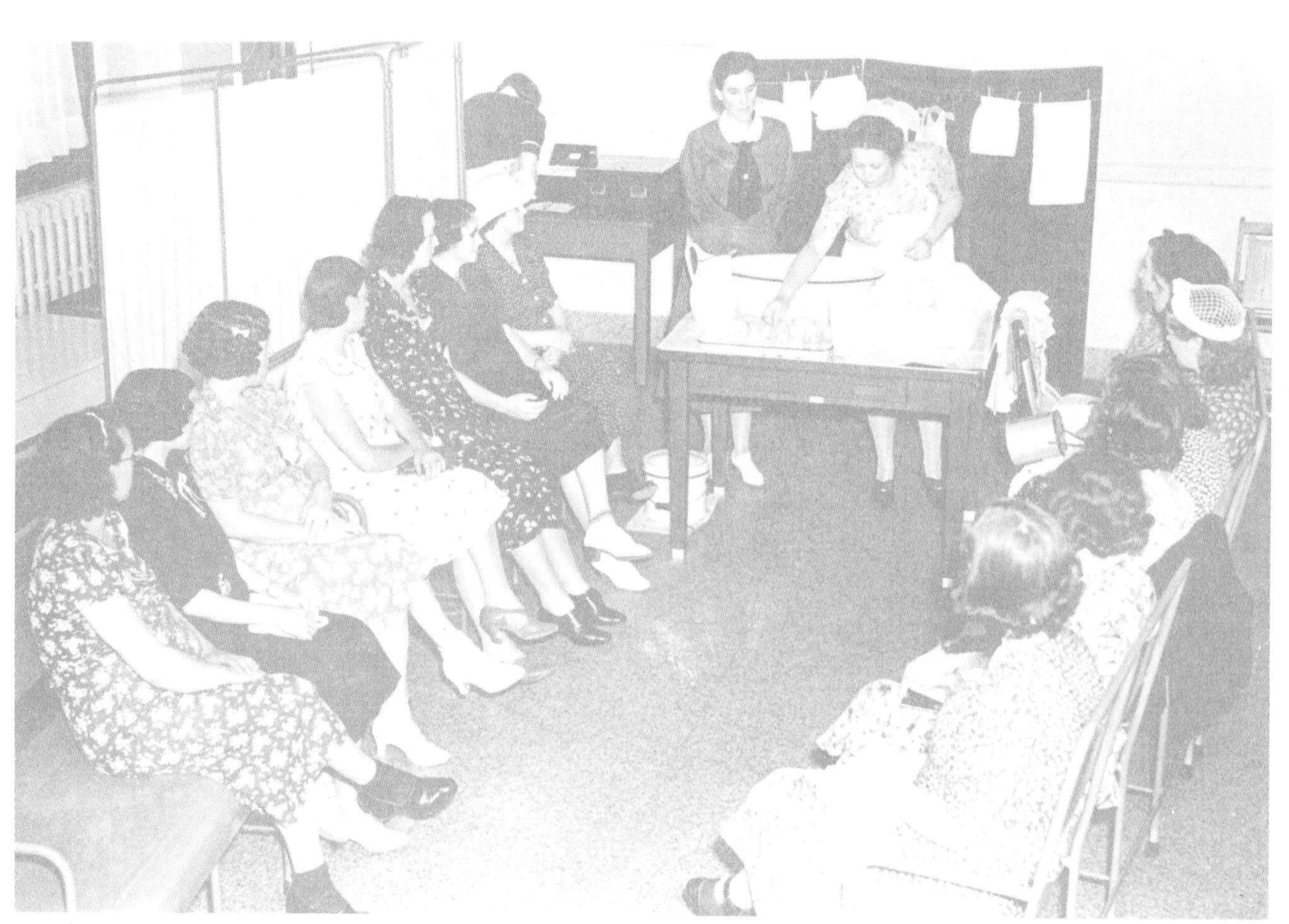

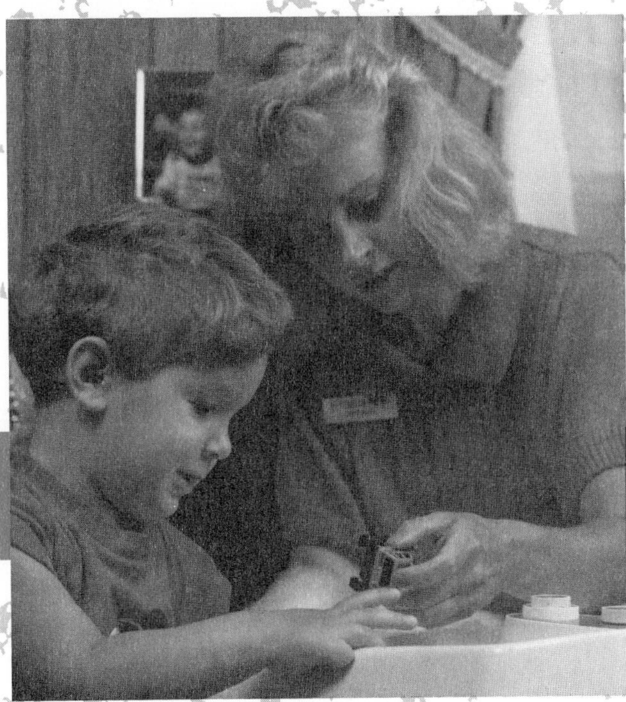

The essence of community health nursing is the care provided to clients to enhance their health. Community health nurses care for all types of clients: individuals, families, groups or communities, men, women, and children. They provide care to clients of all ages and from all racial, ethnic, and cultural groups, to both rich and poor.

In providing care to these diverse groups of clients, community health nurses employ the processes described in Unit Two and consider the influences on health discussed in Unit Three to design interventions to promote health, prevent illness, and resolve existing health problems. In this unit, the epidemiologic prevention process model will be applied to the care of diverse clients with diverse health needs.

Nursing care for an individual client will differ from that provided to families and groups. Chapter 17, Care of the Individual Client, Chapter 18, Care of the Family Client, and Chapter 19, Care of the Community or Target Group, address the unique health care needs of these three classifications of clients. In each chapter, specific areas for assessment are discussed, and considerations in planning, implementing, and evaluating nursing care for each type of client are addressed.

Age and sex contribute to differing needs for community health nursing services. These differences are addressed in Chapters 20 through 23. Care of children presents the community health nurse with the opportunity to influence clients' health status throughout their lives. Health promotion and prevention efforts with this age group can make a tremendous impact on the overall health of the population if children learn to engage in healthy behaviors. Youngsters today are subjected to a variety of health concerns such as drug and alcohol exposure, chronic illness, AIDS, psychological problems, and other conditions that community health nurses can help alleviate. These and other health concerns in young people are addressed in Chapter 20, Care of Children.

Both men and women experience unique health care needs. In part, these needs arise from sexual differences in susceptibility to specific health problems, but many arise out of social conditions that are amenable to change. The unique health-care needs of both men and women have frequently been ignored in developing health-care services, but they are of concern to community health nurses. These unique needs and their resolution are the focus of Chapter 21, Care of Women, and Chapter 22, Care of Men. The special needs of homosexual men and women are also considered in these two chapters.

The elderly population accounts for the greatest percentage of health-care expenditures in the United States. There is much that community health nurses can do to enhance the health status of this population group, to improve their quality of life, and to decrease health-care costs. Community health nursing activities designed to achieve these goals are presented in Chapter 23, Care of Older Clients.

As noted in Chapter 13, Economic Influences on Community Health, economic influences in society can significantly influence health status. One group for which this is particularly true is the homeless population. The number of homeless individuals and families in the United States is growing yearly, and society is only beginning to recognize the need to deal with this problem. Community health nurses should be in the forefront of efforts to meet the health-care needs of the homeless. These topics are the focus of Chapter 24, Care of Homeless Clients.

Each client classification addressed in this unit has unique health-care needs that can be addressed by community health nursing intervention. Through adaptation of the epidemiologic prevention process model, community health nurses identify these needs and plan, implement, and evaluate health-care interventions that will enhance both the health of the client and the overall health status of the population.

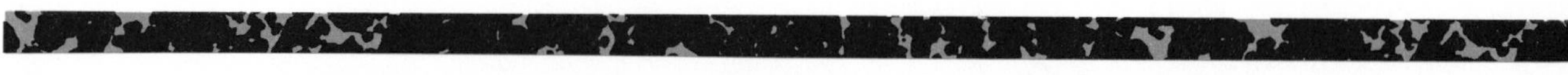

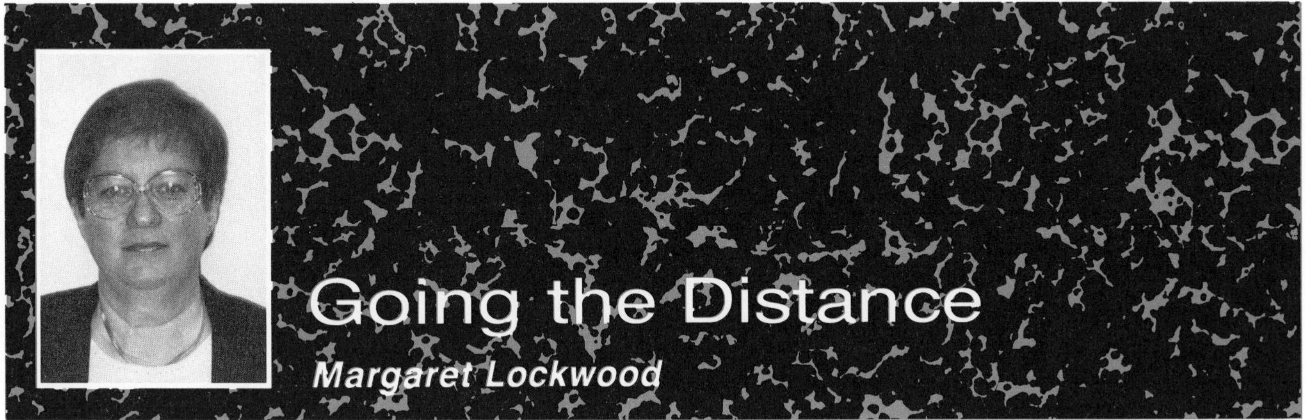

Going the Distance

Margaret Lockwood

Anne was the dearest 78-year-old lady I have ever had the privilege of caring for. She inspired and challenged me to practice nearly every role of special importance in client-oriented community health practice.

Anne was a survivor. At the age of 18 she had undergone a treatment for tuberculosis during which the physician answered a phone call and left Anne exposed to radiation for too long a time. Her left lung was destroyed, and her right lung was badly scarred. Consequently, Anne's health was seriously compromised the rest of her life. Bedfast for her last 25 years, she nevertheless managed to support herself by writing short articles for religious magazines.

I formed a very close relationship with Anne during the last 2 years of her life through daily home visits. She was living alone following the suicide of her youngest brother. This event proved so unsettling to Anne that she sometimes became delusional. The resulting stress and anxiety also caused chronic, severely irritating skin lesions.

My first challenge was to coordinate Anne's complex medication regimen for the skin lesions. This was quite a challenge, because Anne's arthritic hands couldn't easily grasp standard medicine containers, and her constant anxiety impaired her concentration and memory. I adopted the strategy of placing three small plastic tumblers on her fireplace mantle. In the first, I placed the pills she was to take when she awoke each morning; in the second, the pills she was to take with her main meal; and in the third, the pills she was to take at bedtime. The arrangement worked well. Still, I had to be watchful. When I once tried to set up a 2-day supply of medicine, Anne stayed awake all night worrying about what to do with the three "extra" tumblers!

Moreover, I arranged Anne's visits with a host of health-care providers and social-service agencies. There were visits to her general practitioner, dermatologist, podiatrist, ophthalmologist, optician, and dentist. There were visits from the community mental health social worker, the home health aide, and the Meals on Wheels volunteers. Not only did this sequence of visits and visitors require careful coordination, but each provider needed to be kept apprised of the others' actions. Through an ongoing process of consultation and collaboration, I was able to facilitate Anne's care and prevent duplicated efforts. In addition, I counseled Anne's relatives and friends about how to cope with her condition and about how to assist Anne to attain her highest level of independence.

My role as a community health nurse with Anne ceased after she developed a severe case of pneumonia and required the care of a long-term nursing facility. But I could not say goodbye. My love for her grew, and I became her closest friend over the course of her months of institutional care. Perhaps community health nurses cannot afford to become closely attached to their clients. But to me, community health nursing means going the distance with my clients to provide care in body, mind, and spirit. Certainly a spiritual bond developed between Anne and me which far surpassed any nurse/client relationship I have ever had.

CHAPTER 17

Care of the Individual Client

KEY TERMS

appraisal support
emotional support
genogram
informational support
instrumental support
interpretive paradigm
normative paradigm
review of systems

While the primary focus of community health nursing is the health of groups of people, community health nurses may seek to improve the overall health status of the population by providing health-care services to individual clients. The health status of individuals influences the health status of the families of which they are a part. In a similar way, the health status of individual members of society influences the overall health of the societal group.

Because community health nurses deal with a wide range of client conditions and factors that influence clients' health status directly or indirectly, their assessment of individual clients may be more comprehensive in some areas than that of nurses in other specialties. This is particularly true of the psychosocial and environmental aspects of assessment.

LEARNING OBJECTIVES

After reading this chapter you should be able to:

- Describe the use of a genogram to identify human biological factors influencing the health of an individual client.
- Identify at least three avenues for assessing the physiologic function of an individual client.
- Describe two aspects of an individual client's physical environment to be assessed.
- Identify at least three considerations in assessing the internal and external psychological environments of an individual client.
- Describe four components of social support to be addressed in assessing an individual client's social environment.
- Identify at least six life-style considerations to be addressed in assessing the health of an individual client.
- Describe four considerations related to the health system to be addressed in assessing an individual client's health status.
- Identify four considerations in planning nursing interventions to meet the health needs of individual clients.
- Describe outcome and process evaluation as applied to the care of an individual client.

ASSESSING THE INDIVIDUAL CLIENT

Assessing the individual client involves collecting data in each of the four aspects of Dever's epidemiologic perspective. These aspects include factors related to human biology, environment, life-style, and use of the health-care system. Appendix F, The Health Intervention Planning Guide–Individual Client, includes a tool that can direct data collection in each of these four areas.

Modes of data collection can include interviewing the client to obtain a health history and conducting some portions of a physical examination depending upon the client's situation. Additional data can be obtained by means of developmental testing or routine screening and laboratory tests. The type and amount of data collected will vary with the client's age and situation. The nutritional history obtained for a child, for example, may be much more detailed than that obtained for an adult client.

INTERVIEWING THE CLIENT

Because community health nurses are concerned with a broad range of factors that can influence a client's health, their approach to client interviews should be based on an interpretive paradigm rather than a normative paradigm. In the ***normative paradigm,*** the interview is constrained by specific rules governing the data to be obtained, and this may limit the interaction that takes place between nurse and client. The interview is oriented to tasks to be accomplished and may be guided by specific forms to be completed. The emphasis tends to be on physical issues, and the interview is usually highly structured.

Using an ***interpretive paradigm,*** on the other hand, the community health nurse takes a holistic approach to obtaining client-related data, and the interview is unconstrained by specific forms. The interview is largely unstructured, but addresses all aspects of the client's life and health status.[1] In this paradigm, the community health nurse most often elicits information through open-ended and nondirective questions that encourage the client to describe areas of concern. As potential areas for intervention are uncovered, the nurse might use direct questions to elicit additional information as needed. For example, the nurse might ask the client to describe his or her health status in general and then follow with questions about specific kinds of health problems. Or, the nurse might say, "Tell me more about your relationships with your family," and later ask specifically how often the client interacts with other family members. Judicious use of both directive and nondirective interviewing techniques will provide the community health nurse with an accurate picture of the client's health status and his or her perceptions of that status.

COMPONENTS OF THE ASSESSMENT

HUMAN BIOLOGY

Human biological factors addressed in assessing the individual client include the influence of genetic inheritance and maturation and aging on health, as well as the adequacy of physiologic function.

Genetic Inheritance

A client's genetic inheritance is determined in part by his or her race and sex and in part by familial characteristics inherited from previous generations. Information on the client's race and ethnic origin may suggest the potential for specific health problems. Clients descended from immigrants from Italy and several Mediterranean islands, central Africa, Asia, the South Pacific, and parts of India, for example, are at greater risk for thalassemia, a form of anemia, than those from other parts of the world.[2] Blacks of African descent, on the other hand, have a higher prevalence of sickle-cell disease.

The client's sex may also indicate a predisposition to certain health states. Hemophilia, for instance, occurs primarily in men,[3] whereas the circulatory difficulties of Raynaud's disease are more often found in women.[4]

In addition to racial or ethnic and sex characteristics that may predispose one to disease, the genetic inheritance unique to one's family can also influence the presence or absence of certain health problems. Obtaining the client's family history is one way to identify possible predispositions to disease inherited from prior generations. Information obtained in the family history should include the age and health status of family members as well as any history of illnesses that may have a genetic component. If family members are deceased, the cause and age at the time of death should be recorded, if known. The community health nurse should ask specifically about the presence of such conditions as cancer, heart disease, allergies, diabetes, kidney disease, hypertension, seizure disorders, emotional problems, and other chronic conditions in family members.[5] Notations about diseases identified in the family history should include the family member or members affected. Notation should also be made of the absence of specific diseases within the family configuration.[6] Family information can be described in a narrative format or diagrammed in a "genogram."

A ***genogram*** is an elaboration of one's family tree that provides information about genetic, medical, social, behavioral, and cultural aspects of one's family.[7] In a genogram, members of the client's family (as well as significant others in the client's life) are represented in a diagram similar to the one presented in Figure 17–1. Females are represented by circles and males by squares. The solid squares and circles represent members of the family who are deceased. In Figure 17–1, the client is a 36-year-old nonsmoking female with hay-fever-type allergies married to a 29-year-old nonsmoking male in good physical health. They have a 6-month-old son who also has hay-fever-type allergies, but no other health problems. The client's mother has hypertension and quit smoking 5 years ago. Her father has coronary artery disease and smokes. The client's paternal grandfather died at age 70 from a pulmonary embolus, and her paternal grandmother died of pneumonia at age 92. The client's maternal grandmother is alive at 92 years of age and has heart disease, while her maternal grandfather died at age 57 of a heart attack. The client has two brothers, ages 34 and 31, one of whom has allergies, but is otherwise in good health. The information in this genogram suggests that the client is at increased risk for cardiovascular diseases and for respiratory diseases due to passive smoking as a child. Based on this information, the community health nurse assessing this client would explore in depth any signs of cardiovascular or pulmonary disease. A genogram can also provide information related to the client's social network and interpersonal relationships. These additional uses of a genogram will be discussed later in this chapter.

Maturation and Aging

Another human biological consideration in assessing an individual is the client's age and level of maturation. The degree to which the client has accomplished the developmental tasks appropriate to his or her age is an important indicator of both physical and emotional health status. For children, the community health nurse would conduct an in-depth assessment of growth and development, examining the accomplishment of developmental milestones. Frequently, a developmental screening tool such as the Denver Developmental Screening Test is used for this portion of the assessment. Pediatric developmental assess-

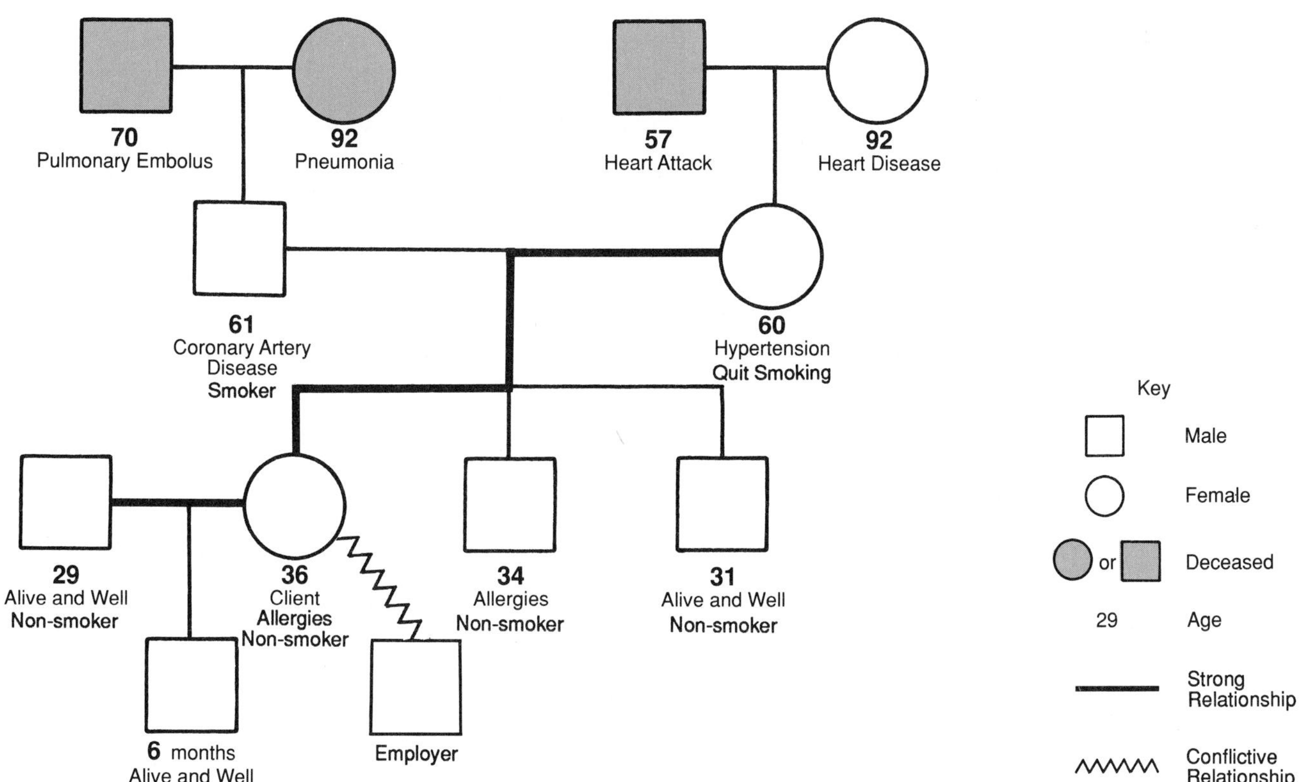

Figure 17–1. Sample genogram.

ment will be discussed in more detail in Chapter 20, Care of Children. For adult clients, the nurse would obtain information related to the accomplishment of developmental tasks appropriate to the client's age. Developmental characteristics of selected age groups are summarized in Table 17–1.

Assessment of maturation and aging should also focus on the occurrence of specific physiologic events appropriate to the age of the client. These events would include the eruption of the first tooth in a child, occurrence of "wet dreams" in preadolescent boys, or the onset of menstruation or menopause in

TABLE 17–1. DEVELOPMENTAL CHARACTERISTICS OF CLIENTS OF SELECTED AGES

Age	Developmental Characteristics
Birth to 1 month	*Neurophysical:* newborn reflexes intact, head lag present, follows objects to midline, responds to noise *Psychosocial:* regards human face, quiets when picked up
1 to 2 months	*Neurophysical:* follows objects 180°, holds head up in prone position, head erect and bobbing when supported in sitting position *Psychosocial:* vocalizes other than crying, smiles responsively
2 to 4 months	*Neurophysical:* newborn reflexes diminishing, sits well with support, rolls from side to side, grasps rattle *Psychosocial:* laughs aloud, initiates smiling, enjoys play activity
4 to 6 months	*Neurophysical:* reaches for and gets objects, puts objects in mouth, rolls over completely, supports own weight when standing, tooth eruption *Psychosocial:* turns to voice, begins stranger anxiety, strong attachment to mother
6 to 9 months	*Neurophysical:* sits alone, bounces, stands holding on, thumb-finger grasp *Psychosocial:* says "mama" or "dada," plays peek-a-boo and patty-cake, imitates speech sounds
9 to 12 months	*Neurophysical:* pulls to stand, creeps or crawls, walks holding on, sits from standing position, uses a cup with help *Psychosocial:* gives toy on request, speaks two to three words, gives affection, indicates wants
12 to 18 months	*Neurophysical:* scribbles, points to one or more body parts, uses a spoon, climbs and runs, plays ball, beginning bowel training *Psychosocial:* likes to be read to, 10-word vocabulary
18 to 24 months	*Neurophysical:* opens doors, turns on faucets, can throw or kick a ball, walks up and down stairs alone, day-time bowel and bladder control established *Psychosocial:* parallel play, 2- to 3-word sentences, imitates household tasks
2 to 3 years	*Neurophysical:* dresses with help, rides a tricycle, washes and dries hands *Psychosocial:* separates easily from mother, uses pronouns, perceives danger, understands sharing and taking turns
3 to 5 years	*Neurophysical:* dresses with decreasing supervision, hops on one foot, catches bounced ball, heel-to-toe walk *Psychosocial:* gives whole name, recognizes three colors, draws person with more than six parts, tells a story, operates from rules
5 to 10 years	*Neurophysical:* slowed physical growth, increasing motor coordination *Psychosocial:* beginning peer identification, forms friendships, learns more rules, begins sexual identification, increasing use of language to convey ideas, beginning understanding of cause and effect
11 to 14 years	*Neurophysical:* beginning pubertal changes, gawkiness *Psychosocial:* importance of peer group conformity, strong identification with sex-mates, learning one's role in heterosexual relationships, beginning to establish an identity, more abstract thought, negative attitude to family
15 to 18 years	*Neurophysical:* finishing pubertal changes and adolescent growth spurt, better able to handle the "new" body *Psychosocial:* Developing an independent identity, establishing relationships with members of the opposite sex, adopting an adult value set, movement away from family relationships
Early to late active adulthood	*Neurophysical:* beginning manifestation of aging process *Psychosocial:* developing and implementing career goals, establishing a family, becoming a productive citizen, assisting children to become independent, assisting older parents, cultivating friendships with age-mates, maintaining family relationships and learning new ones with spouses of children, grandchildren, establishing healthy routines, learning new motor skills, mastering complex financial dealings, formulating a philosophy of life
Late adulthood	*Neurophysical:* mobility limitations, sensory impairment, effects of chronic disease may manifest or become worse, decreased appetite *Psychosocial:* adjusting to retirement and to loss of family members and friends, keeping mentally alert, accepting help graciously, adjusting to reduced income, learning new family roles, preserving friendships, adjusting to declining strength and stamina, maintaining social interactions, adapting activities to diminished energy, preparing for death

women. Another area for consideration is whether the client looks his or her actual age. Clients who look older than their chronological age may be experiencing a variety of physical or emotional problems. For example, the 30-year-old mother who looks like she is 40 may be having difficulty coping with the needs of her young children. On the other hand, an older man who colors his hair and exercises may seem to be several years younger than he actually is. A 6-year-old who looks 10 may encounter unrealistic expectations on the part of parents or others who expect the youngster to act more grown up. Conversely, the 16-year-old who is mistaken for 12 or 13 because of a youthful appearance may engage in what he or she considers "adult" behaviors such as smoking or drinking to create an appearance of being older.

Physiologic effects of the aging process should also be considered in assessing the individual client. These effects will be addressed in greater detail in Chapter 23, Care of Older Clients.

Physiologic Function

Information obtained about the client's physiologic status should reflect existing illnesses or physical health problems, current evidence of disease, functional abilities, the client's past illness history, and findings derived from a physical examination and from selected tests. Information about physiologic status will also include an assessment of the client's immunization history.

The community health nurse will ask the client about the presence of existing illnesses or other physiologic conditions to identify the need for care related to those conditions. For example, the nurse might determine that the client is pregnant or that he or she has arthritis, hypertension, or diabetes. In addition to identifying the existence of these conditions, the nurse will also gather data on the effects of existing conditions on the client's life, the current status of these conditions, and what is being done about them. For example, how does the client feel about being pregnant? Is pregnancy causing any difficulties for the client? How far advanced is the pregnancy? Is the client receiving prenatal care? Or, how does arthritis affect the client's ability to function? What is the client doing for pain?

Information should also be obtained from the client about current signs and symptoms of conditions that may require nursing intervention. For example, if the client is experiencing symptoms of a possible pregnancy, the community health nurse can make a referral for a pregnancy test or for prenatal care. A review of systems (ROS) is an efficient way to elicit information about signs and symptoms of other conditions. The *review of systems* is a systematic approach to assessing the function of each organ system in the body. During the ROS, the community health nurse asks specific questions about symptoms related to each body system to identify areas in which nursing intervention may be required. In addition to identifying signs and symptoms of possible illness or other conditions, the community health nurse would explore the extent of the symptomatology; what, if anything, has been done about symptoms, and the effects of intervention. Areas addressed in the ROS are summarized in Table 17–2.

Functional abilities of clients are also assessed. Some of the areas to be addressed include clients' ability to dress and feed themselves, to carry out routine grooming activities, to communicate with others, to engage in housekeeping activities, and so on. Areas related to functional assessment are summarized in Table 17–3.

Information about the client's past health history may also help to determine areas in which nursing intervention is needed. For example, the woman who has a history of recurrent bladder infections may need education on wiping from front to back after urinating or defecating to prevent reinfection. Or, the adolescent with recurrent episodes of gonorrhea may need information about the use of condoms to prevent sexually transmitted diseases. A history of unusual injuries in a child might indicate potential child abuse or a need for safety education for parents and child. Specific information to be obtained about past health conditions includes the type of condition, when it occurred, the frequency of occurrence, what was done at the time, and the outcome of the condition.

The community health nurse may also obtain information about the client's physiologic status by means of physical examination or selected tests. Depending upon the setting and the client's circumstances, the nurse might do a complete physical examination or do only pertinent parts of an examination. On a routine newborn and postpartum home visit, for example, the community health nurse will probably do a complete routine physical on the newborn, but restrict examination of the mother to checking the breasts, fundus, episiotomy, and lochia. If, however, the mother complains of ear pain, the nurse would also examine the ears. In a tuberculosis clinic, on the other hand, the nurse's examination would focus on skin color, visual acuity, and other signs and symptoms of side effects and toxic effects of antituberculin drugs. In short, the extent of physical examination of the individual client by the community health nurse will vary with the client, client's needs, and the setting involved.

Community health nurses may also conduct a variety of screening tests that aid in determining the

TABLE 17–2. AREAS TO BE ADDRESSED IN A REVIEW OF SYSTEMS

Organ or System	Review Considerations
General	Weakness, fever, sweats, frequent illness, appetite
Integumentary	Lesions, growths, tumors, masses, excessive dryness or sweating, odors, pigmentation changes, pruritus, changes of temperature or texture, excessive bruising or scarring, decreased sensation, hair loss or brittleness, use of dyes or permanents, brittleness or peeling of nails, thickening
Head	Headache, past serious trauma, dizziness, syncope
Eyes	History of glaucoma, cataracts, infections, discharge, itching, lacrimation, pain, swelling around eyes, spots, flashes of light, visual impairment, loss of peripheral vision, double vision, sensitivity to glare, poor night vision, color blindness, photophobia, blurred vision, use of glasses, twitching
Ears	Pain, cerumen, infection, vertigo, ringing, care habits, hearing impairment, use of prosthetic devices, increased sensitivity to noise
Nose and sinuses	Discharge (character), epistaxis, allergies, pain over sinuses, postnasal drip, sneezing, crusting, painful nose breathing, mouth breathing, sense of smell
Mouth and throat	Sore throat or mouth, dry mouth, lesions, bleeding gums, burning sensation, toothache, loose or missing teeth, altered taste, difficulty chewing or swallowing, dentures or other devices, bad breath, bad taste in mouth, hoarseness, voice changes, pattern of dental hygiene
Neck	Node enlargement, swelling or masses, tenderness, limited range of motion, stiffness
Breast	Pain or tenderness, swelling, nipple discharge or changes, lumps, dimples, irritated skin, use of self-breast examination
Cardiovascular	Chest pain, dyspnea, palpitations, unusual respiratory patterns, orthopnea, confusion, high blood pressure, coldness of extremities, loss of sensation, exaggerated response to cold, exercise-induced peripheral pain, color changes, swelling, varicosities
Respiratory	Wheezing, bronchitis, pain with respiration, smoking, chronic or productive cough, hemoptysis, night sweats, shortness of breath with exertion, recent immobilization for nonrespiratory conditions
Hematolymphatic	Lymph node enlargement, easy bruising, petechiae, anemia, transfusion, excessive fatigue, radiation exposure
Gastrointestinal	Abdominal pain, excessive belching, anorexia, nausea, vomiting, food allergy, flatulence, bloating, diarrhea, jaundice, hemorrhoids, change in bowel habits, character of stool, constipation
Urinary	Character of urine, voiding pattern, retention, frequency, dribbling, incontinence, painful urination, polyuria, oliguria, pyuria, hematuria, flank, groin, low back, or suprapubic pain
Genital	Lesions, discharges, odors, pain, pruritus, STD, sexual activity, sexual satisfaction *Male:* prostate trouble, scrotal lumps, testicular self-exam, erection, pain with erection *Female:* menarche, menopause, menstrual problems, tenderness of vagina, pain with intercourse
Musculoskeletal	History of injury, muscle twitching or cramping, weakness, pain, inability to perform ADL, deformity, gait disturbances, walking aids, joint swelling or pain, stiffness, limited movement, crepitation, back pain, stiffness
Neurological	History of seizures, speech patterns, aphasia, stammering, cognitive changes in memory, orientation, phobias, hallucinations, unconsciousness, coordination, paralysis, tics, tremors or spasms, sensory deficit or tingling
Endocrine	Diagnosis of endocrine diseases, changes in skin pigmentation or color, hair distribution, intolerance to heat or cold, exophthalmos, goiter, hormone therapy, polydipsia, polyphagia, poluyuria, anorexia, weakness
Allergic/Immunological	Dermatitis, eczema, pruritus, urticaria, sneezing, vasomotor rhinitis, conjunctivitis, seasonal, patterns, treatment
Other	Any other physical signs or symptoms

(Source: Bowers & Thompson[5])

individual client's physiologic status. The types of tests obtained will vary with the age and circumstances of the client. For example, the nurse might check a child's hematocrit or hemoglobin at periodic intervals or determine blood lead levels in children who live in areas with potential for exposure to lead. Hearing tests might be done for an adult client who works in a high noise area, while vision screening would be appropriate for a client taking Ethambutol, an antituberculin drug that may cause visual impairment. Indications for routine use of specific screening tests are summarized in Table 17–4.

Finally, in assessing physiologic status, the community health nurse will ask clients about their immunization history. For a child, for example, the nurse would elicit information on the childhood im-

TABLE 17–3. AREAS FOR ASSESSMENT OF CLIENT FUNCTIONAL ABILITIES

Focus	Assessment Considerations
Self-care	Ability to dress self and maintain clothing Ability to bathe self, wash hair, brush teeth, shave Ability to care for nails and apply makeup Ability to use a toilet without assistance
Mobility	Ability to move around in the home Ability to sit or stand without help Ability to get around outside the home Ability to lift and carry objects
Communication	Ability to hear and speak Ability to dial a telephone Use of safety precautions in answering the door Access to emergency assistance
Eating	Access to grocery stores Ability to prepare food Ability to handle utensils and feed self Ability to chew and swallow food
Housekeeping	Ability to maintain a clean home Ability to dispose of garbage and trash Ability to do laundry Ability to maintain home repairs Ability to care for yard
Medications	Ability to take medications correctly Ability to open medication bottles Ability to see labels and directions Safe storage of medications
Community access	Availability of transportation Ability to drive safely Distance to church, stores, bank, doctor
Other responsibilities	Ability to care for others as needed (spouse, children, etc.) Ability to manage finances Ablity to care for pets

(Source: Bowers & Thompson[5])

munizations received. For adult clients, the nurse would focus on those immunizations relevant to the client's situation. For example, all adults should be asked about diphtheria and tetanus immunizations, while college students and women of childbearing age should be asked specifically about measles and rubella immunization since they are at particular risk for these diseases. Older adults should be asked whether they have received immunizations for pneumonia and influenza, and people in high-risk groups such as health-care providers and intravenous drug users should be questioned about hepatitis immunization. Additional information on immunizations for specific groups of clients is provided in later chapters of this book. Client assessment considerations related to human biology are summarized in Box 17–1.

ENVIRONMENT

Next, the community health nurse would assess for factors within the client's environment that may contribute to health or illness. These factors may exist within the client's physical, psychological, and social environments.

Physical Environment

Knowledge of the client's physical environment can assist in identifying client health problems or in determining factors contributing to them. Physical environmental factors to be considered relate to both the home and the larger environment. Areas for assessment in the home include the adequacy of the home for meeting the client's needs for shelter, for space, and for privacy as well as the presence of safety hazards within the home. Because of the growing numbers of homeless persons in the United States, the first question to be asked is whether the client has a place to live. If the answer is no, the nurse would then determine where the client seeks shelter and what effect homelessness has had on the client. Health-care needs of homeless clients are addressed in more detail in Chapter 24, Care of Homeless Clients.

TABLE 17–4. INDICATIONS FOR THE ROUTINE USE OF SELECTED SCREENING TESTS*

Screening Test	Indications for Use
ABO-Rh typing	Pregnant women (initial visit)
Blood lead level	Every few months in children at risk through age 6; adults at occupational risk
Blood pressure	Yearly, beginning at age 3; each visit for pregnant women
Breast examination	Every 1 to 3 years for women in high-risk groups aged 19 to 39; annually for all women aged 40 and older
Chlamydial testing	Periodically for all sexually active persons with multiple sexual partners (beginning in adolescence)
Dipstick urinalysis	Yearly for persons over age 65
Electrocardiogram	Every 1 to 3 years for those at risk from age 19 to 64; every year for those over age 65
Fasting plasma glucose	Every 1 to 3 years for those at risk from age 19 to 64; every year for those over age 65
Fecal occult blood/colonoscopy or sigmoidoscopy	Every 1 to 3 years for those at risk from age 19 to 64; yearly for those over age 65
Gonorrhea culture	Periodically for all sexually active persons with multiple sexual partners (beginning in adolescence), pregnant women (initial visit and 28 weeks)
Hearing	Initially at 18 months for high-risk infants; at age 3 for other children; all persons exposed to high noise levels (especially adolescents)
Height and weight	At birth, 2, 4, 6, 15, and 18 months, and when seen for immunizations to age 6; during periodic exams to age 18; every 1 to 3 years to age 65, then yearly; at each visit for pregnant women
Hemoglobin and hematocrit	Once during infancy; pregnant women (initial visit)
HIV testing and counseling	Every 1 to 3 years for those at risk from age 19 to 64; pregnant women in high-risk groups (initial visit and 28 weeks)
Mammogram	Every 1 to 2 years for women over age 35 with a family history of premenopausal breast cancer, and all women aged 50 to 75
Oral cavity exam	Every 1 to 3 years for those at risk from age 19 to 64; every year for those over age 65
Palpation for thyroid nodules	Every 1 to 3 years for persons at risk from age 13 to 64; every year for those over age 65
Pap smear	Every 1 to 3 years for sexually active females aged 18 or older
Rh(D) antibody	Pregnant women (28 weeks)
Rubella titre	Females of childbearing age lacking evidence of immunity; pregnant women (initial visit)
Skin exam	Every 1 to 3 years beginning at age 13 for persons at risk; every year for those over age 65
Testicular exam	Every 1 to 3 years for males aged 13 to 39 in high-risk groups
Total blood cholesterol	Every 1 to 3 years for those aged 19 to 64; yearly for those over age 65
Tuberculin skin test	Once for children between ages 2 and 6 and ages 7 to 12; yearly for household contacts who remain tuberculin negative or members of groups at risk and for persons at risk over age 65
Ultrasound exam	Pregnant women (36 weeks)
Urinalysis for bacteriuria	Once between age 2 and 6; every 1 to 3 years for persons with diabetes; pregnant women (each visit)
VDRL/RPR	Periodically for all sexually active persons with multiple sexual partners (beginning in adolescence); pregnant women (initial visit and 28 weeks)

* Indications for routine screening only; does not address use of tests with clients with a history of exposure or with signs and symptoms of disease.
(Source: U.S. Preventive Services Task Force. [1989]. Guide to Clinical Preventive Services. *Baltimore: Williams & Wilkins.)*

When the client does have a place of residence, the nurse would gather data on the size of the home and the number of people living there to determine the adequacy of the home for meeting the client's needs. Attention should also be given to features of the home that may impair or enhance the client's ability to function. If, for example, the client uses a wheelchair, is the home equipped with a ramp? Or, if the client is a small child, is there a fenced play area?

The home should also be assessed for safety hazards. Conditions that are considered hazardous will vary depending upon the age and health status of the client. For example, poisonous houseplants would be a safety hazard for a young child, but not for an adult, while inadequate lighting in a stairwell or loose throw rugs would present safety hazards for elderly clients. Specific areas for consideration in home safety for children and older adults are included in Appendix C, The Home Safety Assessment Guide.

The environment outside the home is also assayed to identify factors that enhance or impair the individual client's health status. Are there environ-

BOX 17–1

Considerations in Assessing Human Biological Factors Influencing the Health of Individual Clients

Genetic inheritance:
- Sex
- Race or ethnic origin
- Family history of diseases with genetic predisposition

Maturation and aging
- Accomplishment of developmental tasks
- Physical maturational events
- Effects of aging on health

Physiologic function
- Existing illnesses
- Current signs and symptoms of disease (review of systems)
- Functional abilities
- Past illness history
- Physical examination findings
- Results of screening tests
- Immunization history

mental pollutants that might present health hazards? How safe is the neighborhood? Is there a high incidence of crime in the area, and is the client at risk for victimization? If the client does not drive or have a car, is there transportation readily available? What services are available to the client in the immediate neighborhood? For example, are there grocery stores nearby, or must the client travel some distance to obtain food? Are there recreational opportunities appropriate to the client's age and economic status available in the neighborhood? The answers to these and similar questions will provide the nurse with direction for possible primary, secondary, and tertiary preventive interventions to enhance the client's health status. Areas to be addressed in assessing physical environmental influences on the client's health status are summarized in Box 17–2.

Psychological Environment

Information related to the client's psychological environment will reflect both the internal and external psychological environments. Elements to be considered in the internal psychological environment are the client's self-image and mood. Community health nurses would also explore with clients their approaches to dealing with stress and the effectiveness of those approaches. The self-image of clients will influence their perceptions of abilities to control events, including health-related events. Clients who have poor self-images may not see themselves as able to influence health outcomes and may be less motivated to take health-promoting actions for that reason.[8]

The nurse should also assess the mood of clients and ask about any significant changes that may indicate depression or the potential for suicide. Clients' abilities to cope with stress are also appraised. Does the client use appropriate coping mechanisms or are coping strategies maladaptive rather than adaptive? For example, the client who sleeps to avoid stress is engaging in a maladaptive behavior, while the client who reduces stress through physical activity or by

BOX 17–2

Considerations in Assessing Physical Environmental Influences on the Health of Individual Clients

Home environment
- Place of residence
- Adequacy of the home for shelter
- Adequate privacy
- Number of people in the home and adequacy of space
- Features that may promote or hinder function
- Presence of safety hazards

Larger Environment
- Safety of the neighborhood
- Availability of transportation
- Access to needed goods and services
- Access to recreational opportunities appropriate to the client's needs and financial status
- Presence of environmental pollutants that may influence health

actively seeking to eliminate sources of stress is coping adaptively. If emotional or psychiatric problems are suspected, the nurse might also conduct a mental status examination addressing the areas indicated in Box 17–3.

Assessment considerations related to the external psychological environment include recent significant losses or other major life events, sources of stress in the client's life, and the quality of the client's interpersonal interactions. Significant losses such as the death of a loved one or loss of a job may alter a client's ability to cope with the everyday stresses of life and may precipitate depression, substance abuse, family violence, or suicide. The nurse should identify the loss and the meaning of the loss to the client, as well as the client's progress through the grieving process and his or her ability to adjust to the loss. Other major life events, even positive ones such as obtaining a new job or getting married, create stress in the client's life that may stretch coping abilities beyond the client's capacity to adapt. The community health nurse would again explore with the client his or her perceptions of the event and its effects on the client's life, as well as what is being done to reduce the stressful effects of the event.

Other sources of stress should also be explored. Does the client juggle the multiple roles of employee, parent, participating citizen, and so on? Are there economic stresses present in the client's situation? Does the client's physical health status, or that of significant others, contribute to stress? Nurses should help clients identify which sources of stress can be eliminated or minimized and which will require adjustment on the part of the client.

The quality of the client's interpersonal relationships is another important aspect of assessing the external psychological environment. Any of several indirect, nonthreatening questions may elicit information in this area. For example, the nurse might ask, "Who do you talk to when you have a problem?" or "How would you describe your relationship with your family?" Again, a genogram might be used to elicit this information.[7] For example the genogram included in Figure 17–1 indicates that the client has a strong relationship with her husband and mother, but a troublesome relationship with her employer. The nurse would then explore with the client the factors that contribute to the troublesome relationship and what the client has done to try to improve the relationship. If the client seems to have multiple conflictive relationships, this may be an indication of ineffective interpersonal dynamics, and may warrant nursing intervention. Considerations in assessing both the client's internal and external psychological environments are presented in Box 17–4.

BOX 17–3

Considerations in a Mental Status Examination

General
- Overall behavior, posture, gait, gestures, facial expression, mannerisms, response to examiner
- Appearance, grooming, and hygiene; use of makeup

Speech patterns
- Loudness, flow, speed, quantity
- Level of coherence and logic

Emotional state
- Mood
- Affective reaction; congruence of affect and thought content

Preoccupations or special experiences
- Delusions
- Hallucinations or illusions
- Depersonalization
- Obsessions or compulsions
- Phobias
- Fantasies or daydreams

Sensorium or orientation
- Orientation to person
- Orientation to place
- Orientation to time
- Orientation to self

Memory
- Attention span
- Recall of remote past experiences
- Recall of recent past experiences
- Retention and recall of immediate impressions
- General grasp and recall

General intellectual level
- Level of general knowledge
- Ability to calculate
- Reasoning ability and judgment

Abstract thinking
- Ability to distinguish between similar abstract concepts (for example, idleness and laziness)
- Ability to interpret proverbs

Insight
- Ability to recognize the significance of the situation
- Client's explanation of symptoms and their cause

(Source: Wilson, H. S., & Kneisl, C. R. [1988]. *Psychiatric Nursing* (3d ed.). Menlo Park, CA: Addison-Wesley.

Box 17–4

Considerations in Assessing Psychological Environmental Factors Influencing the Health of Individual Clients

Internal factors
- Self-image
- Mood
- Ability to cope with stress
- Mental status examination as needed

External factors
- Significant losses experienced by the client
- Other major life events
- Sources of stress
- Quality of interpersonal interactions

Social Environment

Social environmental factors influencing the client's health should also be considered. Areas to be addressed include the client's economic status, social support network, and the effects of cultural, religious, and educational factors on the client's health.

Questions regarding the client's economic status would include the source of the client's income and how regular that income is. For example, some forms of occupation are seasonal in nature. If the client works in heavy construction and has little work during the winter, what does the client do for income during this time? Does he or she take on other jobs, rely on savings, or seek assistance from family members? Is the client's usual source of income some form of economic assistance program?

Other considerations reflect the adequacy of the client's income to meet personal needs. Is the client's income sufficient to provide for basic necessities? Is there money for "luxury" items? Finally, the nurse would explore the client's ability to handle finances and to budget income. Is the individual allocating income appropriately or does he or she need some help in establishing budgetary priorities? For example, an older client might be spending too much on items bought from door-to-door vendors because of an inability to resist sales pressure. Or, an adolescent mother may be buying expensive dresses for her baby daughter rather than taking the child for routine health care.

The adequacy of the client's social support network is another important consideration in assessing social environmental factors influencing health. Social support has been defined in terms of four components: emotional support, appraisal support, informational support, and instrumental support.[9] ***Emotional support*** involves providing evidence of esteem, affection, trust, and concern for the person, as well as serving as a listener who allows one to voice concerns and anxieties. ***Appraisal support*** is provided when the supportive person provides feedback or affirmation. For example, a friend may tell the client that he or she did the right thing in hospitalizing a teenage son or daughter for substance abuse. ***Informational support*** involves giving advice or suggestions, providing direction for action, or giving information. The friend who phones to let the client know about free hearing tests at the local mall, for example, is providing informational support. The last component of social support, ***instrumental support,*** usually involves providing material help such as money or items needed or giving labor or time in activities like mowing the lawn or providing transportation.

In assessing the client's social support network, the community health nurse would help the client identify the persons who provide each of the four types of social support, their availability, and the extent to which they meet the client's needs for support. There may be a variety of people who contribute to the client's social support including family, friends, neighbors, co-workers, and health-care professionals. During the assessment, the nurse may help the client identify gaps in social support as well as areas in which individuals in the client's support network could be better utilized.[10]

The client's culture should also be addressed as part of the assessment of the social environment. This will entail a cultural assessment as described in Chapter 15, Cultural Influences on Community Health. The community health nurse will identify the cultural group to which the client belongs and explore with the client the extent to which he or she adheres to the beliefs and practices typical of that cultural group. The nurse and the client would also identify the effects of those beliefs and practices on health.

The client's religion may also influence his or her health status. Religion may figure prominently in a client's ability to cope with stress. In addition, church groups to which the client belongs may enhance the client's social support network. The community health nurse would identify the client's religious affiliation, if any, and the extent to which the client adheres to religious beliefs and practices. The use of services provided by one's church or religious group should also be explored. For example, many churches provide transportation to members or have emergency assistance programs for food, housing, and so on, that may be of use to individual clients.

The client's educational level is the final component of the social environment to be assessed. The nurse would ask about the extent of the client's formal schooling, as well as gain an appreciation for the client's knowledge of health-related information. Generally speaking, more highly educated persons are more likely to know of and engage in health-promoting behaviors than less well-educated clients. However, even highly educated clients may have gaps in health-related knowledge. For example, a college degree does not often prepare one for parenthood or assist one to develop adequate parenting skills. The nurse will need to assess the individual client's knowledge regarding health and illness and use this information as a basis for planning health education as needed. Educational level and other aspects of social environmental assessment are summarized in Box 17–5.

LIFE-STYLE

Life-style factors play a major part in the development of many health problems. Areas to be addressed in assessing a client's life-style include occupation, consumption patterns, leisure activities, and other health-related behaviors.

Occupation

The client's occupation can often be a significant factor in many health problems. Considerations related to occupation include the type of work performed, features of the work that may present health hazards, and information about unemployment or frequent job changes. Knowledge of the type of work performed by the client may suggest the presence of certain job-related health problems. For example, the nurse dealing with a client who does word processing should be alert for problems of eye strain from video display terminals or musculoskeletal problems such as tendonitis related to keyboard use.

Other potential health hazards arising from one's occupation include the amount of stress generated by working conditions and interpersonal interactions at work, the use of repetitive movements that may contribute to muscle fatigue and injury, use of hazardous equipment, the potential for exposure to hazardous substances, noise, and vibration, and any other conditions, such as the potential for falls, that may contribute to illness or injury.

BOX 17–5

Considerations in Assessing Social Environmental Factors Influencing the Health of Individual Clients

Economic status
- Source of income and its regularity
- Adequacy of income to meet the client's needs
- Ability to handle financial transactions, budgeting

Social support network
- Sources of emotional, appraisal, informational, and instrumental support
- Use of available support
- Adequacy of the client's social support network
- Gaps in the availability of social support

Culture
- Cultural identification
- Degree of adherence to cultural norms
- Effects of cultural beliefs and practices on health

Religion
- Religious affiliation
- Adherence to religious beliefs and practices
- Membership in a religious group
- Availability and use of social support provided by religious groups

Education
- Formal educational level
- Health-related knowledge

If the client is unemployed, this information will assist in determining factors that may contribute to a lack of health care or otherwise impair the client's health. A history of frequent job changes could indicate emotional instability, alcoholism or other substance abuse, or difficulties with interpersonal relationships that may require nursing intervention.

Consumption Patterns

Areas for consideration related to consumption patterns include the client's diet and information on other habits such as the use of alcohol, tobacco, and drugs. Information on dietary patterns should reflect the client's food preferences, usual meal pattern (for example, does the client eat breakfast?), the amount of food consumed, and the usual mode of preparation. The nurse will also ask about who purchases and prepares food for the client and address any special dietary needs and the extent to which they are being met. For example, is a diabetic client's wife helping him to adhere to his diabetic diet, or does she maintain dietary patterns used before the client's diabetes was diagnosed? Or, is a nursing mother getting sufficient fluids and nutrients to support the nutritional needs of herself and her infant?

Information on other consumption patterns will reflect the substances consumed as well as the amount and frequency of consumption. Does the client drink alcohol? If so, how much and what kind of alcohol is consumed daily or weekly? It is important for the nurse to ask about other preparations that contain alcohol since clients may indicate that they do not drink, but consume large amounts of alcohol-containing preparations such as some cough syrups. Does the client smoke? If so, how long has the client been smoking, and how much does he or she smoke daily? Does the client use other forms of tobacco? How much coffee, tea, or caffeinated soft drinks does the client consume? What prescription or over-the-counter medications does the client use? Are these medications used appropriately? Does the client take any illicit drugs? Answers to these and similar questions may indicate health problems related to consumption patterns.

Leisure Activities

Knowing the types of leisure activities in which a client engages may give the community health nurse insight into the client's level of exercise and into stress-reduction mechanisms used by the client. Knowledge of leisure activities enjoyed by the client may also indicate the presence of risk factors for certain health problems. For example, does the weighlifter use proper body mechanics to avoid injury? Does the off-road vehicle enthusiast or avid bicyclist wear a helmet? What is the extent of the client's exercise? Are precautions taken to prevent exercise-related injuries? Does the client need to increase the amount of exercise obtained?

Other Behaviors

Information about other life-style behaviors can also help the community health nurse identify client health problems or the potential for developing problems. Nurses should obtain a sexual history that elicits information on the extent of a client's sexual activity and the number of sexual partners.[11] For clients with monogamous relationships who are relatively sure their partners are also monogamous, the nurse may merely ask about their preferences in sexual partners (males, females, or both), use of contraceptives if pregnancy is not desired, and if there are any problems related to sexuality. Questions about contraceptive use should reflect the client's perceived need for contraception, methods employed, if any, and the manner in which they are employed. For example, the nurse would determine that oral contraceptives were being used correctly or that a diaphragm is inserted properly.

For clients with multiple sexual partners, a more detailed sexual history is warranted including information on sexual practices such as anal intercourse, cunnilingus (oral stimulation of the vulva or clitoris), or fellatio (oral stimulation of the penis) that increase the risk of sexually transmitted diseases. Other practices such as sharing vibrators that may transmit diseases and use of condoms to prevent sexually transmitted diseases should be also explored.[11]

Other life-style behaviors should also be explored including the use of tattoos or acupuncture that might put clients at risk for blood-borne diseases such as hepatitis B and AIDS.[11] Finally, the nurse would ask the client about the use of safety devices such as seat belts or hearing protection in high noise areas. Considerations in assessing the individual client's life-style are summarized in Box 17–6.

HEALTH SYSTEM

The last component in the assessment of the individual client's health status reflects the client's use of the health system. The nurse will explore the client's attitudes toward health and definitions of health and illness, the client's usual source of health care, and the client's use of health-care services. How the client finances health care and perceived barriers to obtaining health-care services are other areas for consideration.

Client attitudes to health and definitions of health and illness will influence health-related behaviors as well as the types of health-care services sought by the client. When health is not valued by the client, he or she may be unlikely to engage in health-promotive or illness-preventive measures. For example, many people value going to work over preventive health care and may choose not to take the time off from work that would be needed for a routine dental checkup or to obtain a Pap smear. Others may feel that they just do not have the time, given their

BOX 17–6

Considerations in Assessing Life-style Factors Influencing the Health of Individual Clients

Occupation

- Current employment status
- Type of work done
- Presence of health hazards related to:
  - Stress
  - Interpersonal interactions at work
  - Potential for falls
  - Use of hazardous equipment
  - Exposure to hazardous substances
  - Exposure to noise or vibration
  - Repetitive activity
- Frequent job changes

Consumption patterns

- Information on dietary patterns including
  - Food preferences
  - Usual meal patterns
  - Amount of food consumed
  - Purchase and preparation of food
  - Special dietary needs
- Other consumption patterns
  - Extent of alcohol consumption
  - Smoking behavior
  - Extent of caffeine consumption
  - Use of prescription, OTC, and illicit drugs

Leisure activities

- Preferred leisure pursuits
- Extent of regular exercise
- Health hazards posed by leisure activities
- Precautions taken to prevent injury

Other behaviors

- Information on sexual activity
- Use of contraceptives
- Use of safety devices

other responsibilities, to get a "flu shot." Again, they value fulfilling their other responsibilities over maintaining their health. Similarly, if people define health as the ability to go to work and function adequately, they may avoid seeking care for minor problems until larger ones interfere with their ability to function.

The community health nurse should also inquire about the client's usual source of health care. Does the client see a health-care provider on a regular basis, or does he or she use an emergency room for necessary services? If the emergency room is used, why? Is the client unable to afford care from a regular provider? Does the client have Medicaid, but cannot find a provider who will accept Medicaid reimbursement? Or, does the client only seek care for health emergencies?

The nurse would also explore the extent to which clients engage in self-care activities and the appropriateness of self-care. Does the client adequately differentiate between conditions that can be treated at home and those that require professional assistance? The nurse might also discover that the client makes use of folk health providers described in Chapter 15, Cultural Influences on Community Health. Again, the nurse should explore the use of these services with the client and their effects on the client's health.

The nurse should ascertain the extent to which the client uses primary, secondary, and tertiary preventive services. Has the client obtained immunizations as needed? Does the client seek health-promotive and illness-preventive care, or does the client only seek care for existing health problems? Once acute health problems have been resolved, does the client seek help or engage in behaviors related to tertiary prevention? After being treated for gonorrhea, for example, does an adolescent client use condoms during sexual intercourse to prevent reinfection? Or, does the client hospitalized for diabetic acidosis become more compliant with his or her medical regimen?

Information is also obtained on the means used by the client to finance health-care services. Does the client have health insurance? If so, what insurance carrier is used, and what benefits are covered? Is the client covered under Medicare, Medicaid, or similar programs? Does the client have to pay for health-care services out of pocket, and, if so, is this a problem for the client?

Finally, the nurse would explore with the client any potential barriers to health-care services aside from the inability to pay for them. Does the client have problems with transportation? Is there a language barrier that interferes with the client's ability or willingness to seek services? Are health-care ser-

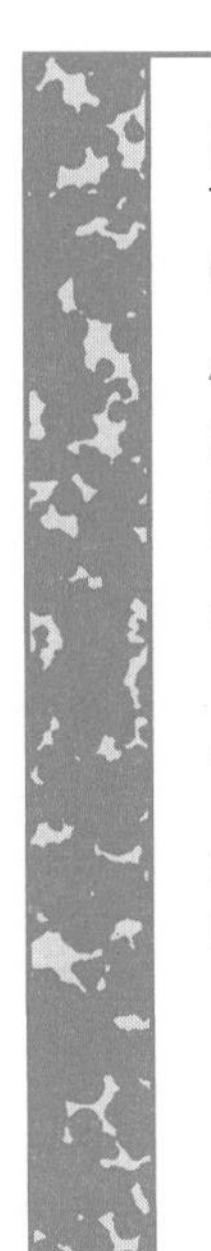

BOX 17–7

Considerations in Assessing Health System Factors Influencing the Health of Individual Clients

Attitudes to health and definitions of health and illness
Usual source of health care
Use of health services
- Use of primary preventive services
- Use of secondary preventive services
- Use of tertiary preventive services

Means of financing health care
Barriers to health care

vices that are needed by the client unavailable in the community? Health system considerations in assessing the individual client are summarized in Box 17–7.

DIAGNOSTIC REASONING AND THE INDIVIDUAL CLIENT

Based on the data obtained from the client assessment, the community health nurse derives nursing diagnoses. These diagnoses should reflect areas of strength that the nurse can reinforce or health problems that require nursing intervention. Nursing diagnoses can be organized in terms of the components of the assessment. For example, the nurse might diagnose strengths and health needs related to human biology, to the client's environment, to life-style, and to the health system. Box 17–8 presents sample nursing diagnoses in each of these areas.

PLANNING TO MEET CLIENT HEALTH NEEDS

Once the client assessment has been obtained and nursing diagnoses made, the community health nurse and client begin to plan to meet health needs. Considerations in this stage of the epidemiologic prevention process model include client participation in planning, prioritizing client needs, identifying intended outcomes, and designing nursing interventions to achieve those outcomes.

CLIENT PARTICIPATION IN PLANNING

Client participation in planning health-care interventions is always desirable, but nowhere more so than in community health nursing; this is because clients are more likely to retain autonomy and responsibility for their own health-care decisions and for implementing those decisions. Nurses could plan for solutions to client health problems without client input. When this is done, however, the client is less likely

BOX 17–8

Sample Nursing Diagnoses for an Individual Client

Human Biology
- Normal growth pattern for 1-year-old child due to adequate nutrition
- Recurrent ear infections due to bottle propping
- Diaper rash due to use of harsh detergent to wash diapers

Environment
- Strong maternal-child bond due to appropriate maternal parenting behavior and abilities to cope with stress
- Effective discipline due to mother's knowledge of child growth and development
- Potential safety hazard due to improper storage of household chemicals

Life-style
- Potential for respiratory difficulties due to parental smoking
- Overweight infant due to consumption of 40 ounces of milk per day

Health system
- Lack of regular source of health care due to inadequate financial resources

to follow through with the planned intervention. The client's input helps to assure that the plan of care meets his or her needs and fits the constraints of the situation. In addition, the client can provide information on solutions that may already have been attempted and on the outcome of those efforts. This information saves time that might otherwise be spent in devising solutions that have already been tried and have failed.

PRIORITIZING CLIENT NEEDS

As noted in Chapter 5, The Nursing Process, the first step in planning to meet client needs is prioritizing those needs. Here, too, the client's input should be sought. Client and nurse may have different perceptions of client needs and the priority that should be assigned to each. If the nurse proceeds to devise a plan of care for needs that the client does not perceive as a priority, the client is apt not to implement the plan of care. When client and nurse together agree on which needs will be addressed first, they can work more effectively to solve identified problems.

STATING INTENDED OUTCOMES

Planning to meet health-care needs involves delineating the expected outcomes of care. Outcomes are stated in terms of goals and objectives (see Chapter 5, The Nursing Process). Without specific goals and objectives, nursing care may not be appropriately directed, nor can the nurse accurately evaluate the effects of that care. Goals are broad statements of what is to be accomplished. Objectives are more specific, and they are stated in terms of the behaviors expected of the client or specific indicators of favorable changes in the client's health status as a result of nursing intervention. Objectives are developed for each of the client's identified needs. Client's needs for nursing care may reflect existing health problems, needs for health-promotive and illness-preventive actions, or reinforcement of client strengths. An objective related to one of the sample nursing diagnoses in Box 17–8 might be stated as: "The client's diaper rash will clear with a change to a milder detergent." An objective related to the nursing diagnosis of "safety hazard" might be: "Household chemicals will be stored in an area inaccessible to the child."

DESIGNING NURSING INTERVENTIONS

The development of specific outcome statements in client care objectives provides direction for the interventions needed to achieve those objectives. These interventions may occur at the primary, secondary, or tertiary level of prevention. The level of prevention at which activity occurs will depend on the client's health needs. If no health problems exist and the emphasis is on promoting health and preventing problems, primary prevention is in order. If the client has existing health problems that are in an acute phase, the focus of intervention will be on secondary prevention. When problems have been resolved, but there is a need to rehabilitate the client or prevent problem recurrence, implementation will take place at the tertiary level. The Health Intervention Planning Guide–Individual Client, included in Appendix F, may be used to direct the planning of nursing interventions at all three levels of prevention.

PRIMARY PREVENTION

Certain primary prevention measures should be considered with all types of clients. These are actions and behaviors that promote the client's general health and prevent illness. Areas for consideration with all clients are related to the four aspects of the epidemiologic perspective component of the epidemiologic prevention process model: human biology, environment, life-style, and health system.

Promotion of normal human development is one type of primary preventive activity related to human biology that is appropriate to all individuals. Opportunities for growth and development should be provided for all ages of clients, not just children. For the young client, however, such opportunities might include the provision of age-appropriate toys and acceptance and/or encouragement of age-appropriate behavior. For adolescents, opportunities to choose one's own course of behavior and to test one's values promote development. Adults and older persons also need opportunities to accomplish appropriate developmental tasks. For example, the older person may need an opportunity to discuss death and to prepare for that event.

Immunization is another primary preventive measure related to human biology. Again, this is an intervention appropriate to all age groups, not only children. Children should be provided with the basic immunization series. Previously unimmunized adults should also receive basic immunizations. Other adults with a history of prior immunization should receive boosters for certain immunizations (for example, diphtheria and tetanus) at periodic intervals.

Primary prevention can also be employed relative to aspects of the client's physical, social, and psychological environment. Physical environmental concerns would include provision of a safe environment. For the child, this means child-proofing a home and providing adequate supervision. For the adult client, primary prevention in this area might mean eliminating hazardous conditions from the work environment, while a safe home environment can be provided to the older client by emphasis on adequate lighting, installation of tub rails, or removal of throw rugs.

Assisting the client to develop an effective social network can be a primary preventive activity related to the social environment. Primary prevention related to the psychological environment might include activities that promote a strong self-image, adequate coping skills, and effective interpersonal relations. For example, community health nurses can encourage parents of young children to give praise and refrain from denigrating the child so as to promote a strong self-concept. Clients can also be taught effective coping skills to prevent health problems arising from stress.

Several general primary prevention measures are related to client life-style. The foremost of these is promoting adequate nutritional intake. Other measures related to life-style would include encouraging an appropriate balance between rest and exercise, promoting adequate hygiene, and encouraging moderate to no intake of caffeine and alcohol. One other area for primary prevention related to life-style is promoting consistent use of seat belts and other safety devices.

Primary prevention related to the health system would include fostering attitudes favorable to health and healthful behaviors. Another intervention in this area might be referral to a source of health care to meet needs for primary preventive services. General primary prevention activities related to human biology, environment, life-style, and the health system are depicted in Figure 17–2.

The kinds of primary preventive measures reviewed thus far could be applied to any individual client. Other aspects of primary prevention might be appropriate for some clients and not others. For example, primary prevention for people with hereditary

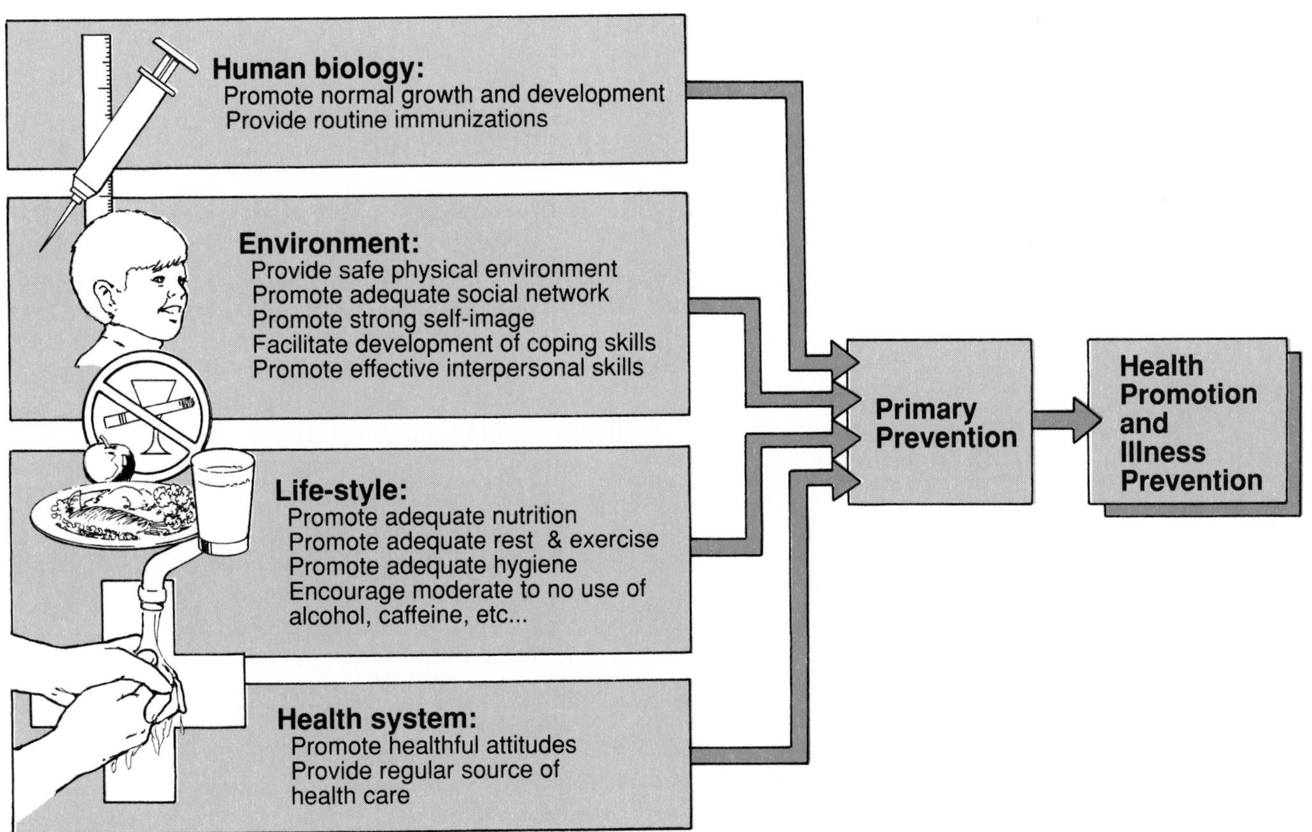

Figure 17–2. Primary prevention considerations for individual clients.

diseases might include genetic counseling. For a woman of childbearing age, primary prevention might include providing contraceptive services.

Control of risk factors for other health problems can also be a primary preventive measure. For example, blood pressure control in the hypertensive client is primary prevention for heart disease and stroke. Similarly, teaching a sexually active adolescent how to use a condom is a primary preventive measure for sexually transmitted diseases.

SECONDARY PREVENTION

The use of specific measures geared toward secondary prevention will depend upon the health problems experienced by the client. Again, problems might relate to human biology, environment, life-style, or use of the health system. For example, the client might have a problem related to physiologic function such as a bladder infection. Secondary prevention would be directed toward relieving the particular problem, in this case a urinary tract infection. Activities might include referral for treatment and encouraging the client to force fluids. If the community health nurse is functioning as a nurse practitioner, secondary prevention might also include prescription of antibiotics for the infection.

Secondary prevention activities might also be directed toward problems in other areas. For example, advocacy with a landlord would be a secondary preventive activity related to unsafe housing conditions. Similarly, referral for counseling would be an appropriate secondary preventive measure for the client with a drinking problem. Or, a referral for financial aid might resolve the problem of a lack of health care for an indigent client. In each instance, the measures employed by the nurse are directed toward resolving an existing health problem, but in each case activities are tailored to the client's needs and situation.

TERTIARY PREVENTION

Like secondary prevention, tertiary preventive activities are based on the nature of health problems experienced by the client. Tertiary prevention takes place once a health problem has been controlled or resolved and there is a need to return the client to normal function or to prevent a recurrence of the problem. For example, an adolescent may have been adequately treated for a sexually transmitted disease. Tertiary prevention in this instance would include education on the need for selective sexual activity and on the use of a condom to prevent reinfection. Similarly, for the woman who has three children and does not want any more, provision of contraceptive services would be a tertiary preventive measure.

IMPLEMENTING NURSING INTERVENTIONS

General implementation considerations include determining the approaches to be taken to carry out the plan of care and designating responsibility for various aspects of implementation. The nurse and client should decide together which aspects of the plan will be implemented by the client or by significant others in the client's life and which will be implemented by the nurse. The nurse may need to assist the client or significant others to develop the knowledge and skills needed to carry out the activities delineated in the plan of care.

Other approaches that may be used in implementing planned interventions are delegation and referral. Some aspects of the plan of care may be delegated to other individuals such as family members or ancillary health-care personnel. Again, the nurse has the responsibility for ensuring that these people have the knowledge, skill, and motivation needed to carry out the planned intervention. If referral is chosen as the means of implementing the plan, considerations of acceptablility, eligibility, and situational constraints must be addressed. These aspects of the referral process were discussed in some detail in Chapter 9, The Discharge Planning and Referral Process.

EVALUATING NURSING INTERVENTION

The last component of the epidemiologic prevention process model is the evaluation of care given and its effectiveness in meeting the client's needs. Both outcome evaluation and process evaluation should take place. Outcome evaluation involves determining whether interventions achieved the stated client-care objectives. If, for example, the stated objective was that the client would use an effective method of contraception, the nurse would need to determine whether the client is indeed using contraception and using it in an effective manner. If the objective was that the client would obtain a regular source of health care, the nurse would determine whether the client has found such a source and is using it.

In performing process evaluation, nurses examine the quality of their performance in providing care to clients. For example, was sufficient attention given to cultural considerations in planning interventions? Was the level of health education provided appropriately targeted to the client's level of understanding?

Based on the evaluation of the quality and outcomes of care, the nurse might make a variety of decisions about the client and his or her care. If all objectives have been met and the client's problems have been resolved, the nurse might decide to terminate the relationship with the client. The client could then be discharged from care with the understanding that further care can be provided should the need arise.

If objectives are being met, but the client continues to need support and assistance, the nurse might decide to continue the plan of care as originally designed. If, on the other hand, objectives are not being met, the problem may lie either in the plan of care or in its implementation. Process evaluation findings would help pinpoint the source of difficulty. If the implementation of the plan has not been accomplished as planned, the nurse might continue with the plan but improve its execution. However, if the problem lies with the plan itself, it may be advisable to start the planning process over again and devise a new approach to deal with the client's problems.

CHAPTER HIGHLIGHTS

- In assessing the health needs of individual clients, community health nurses frequently use an interpretive paradigm for interviewing clients. In this paradigm, the nurse takes a holistic approach to data collection, and the interview is unconstrained by specific forms.
- Human biological factors related to the individual client include genetic inheritance, maturation and aging, and the adequacy of physiologic function. Genetic influences on health arise from the client's race and sex as well as the genetic makeup inherited from prior generations of one's family. Inherited influences can be investigated using a genogram.
- The client's developmental level and the effects of the aging process on health should also be assessed.
- Information about the client's physiologic status can be gleaned from questions about existing illnesses and conditions, conducting a review of systems, asking about or observing functional abilities, inquiring about past health-related conditions, and conducting a physical examination and selected screening tests.
- Areas for consideration related to the client's physical environment include the size and condition of the home, the presence of any safety factors, and the influence of the larger environment on the client's health.
- Both the client's internal and external psychological environments should be assessed. Considerations related to the internal environment include the client's self-image and mood as well as his or her coping strategies and their effectiveness in dealing with stress. Considerations related to the external psychological environment include significant losses or major life events experienced by the client, sources of stress in the client's life, and the quality of interpersonal interactions.
- Social environmental factors to be assessed include the client's economic status, social support network, and the effects of cultural, religious, and educational factors on health. Social support is comprised of four components, each of which may be provided by different individuals. These four components are emotional support, appraisal support, informational support, and instrumental support.
- Life-style factors related to occupation that should be addressed in assessing the individual client include the type of work done, the presence or absence of health hazards posed by the work, and information about unemployment or frequent job changes.
- Information on consumption patterns of individual clients should focus on dietary patterns, including food preferences and amounts, meal patterns and preparation, and special nutritional needs, and also on the client's use of alcohol, medications, coffee, and tobacco.
- The community health nurse should explore leisure activities pursued by the client and potential health hazards posed. Other life-style behaviors to be addressed include sexual practices and use of contraceptives, as well as use of safety devices like seat belts and protection for one's hearing.
- Health system factors to be addressed in assessing the individual client include attitudes toward and definitions of health and illness; the client's usual source of health care; use of primary, secondary, and tertiary health-care services; the client's means of financing health care; and barriers to obtaining health-care services.
- Considerations in planning health care for individual clients include the need for client participation in planning, prioritizing client health-care needs, stating intended outcomes of care, and designing nursing interventions at primary, secondary, and tertiary levels of prevention to achieve those outcomes.
- Decisions must be made about who will implement the plan of care. Possible options include the client, significant others in the client's life, the community health nurse, or other health-care providers or agencies.
- Evaluation of the care given to an individual client will focus on both the outcome of care for the client and the performance of the caregiver.

Review Questions

1. Describe how a genogram can be used to identify human biological factors influencing the health of individual clients. Draw your own genogram. What genetic inheritance factors might influence your health? (p. 373)
2. Identify at least three avenues for determining physiologic functional status in an individual client. Give an example of each. (p. 375)
3. Describe at least two aspects of an individual client's physical environment to be assessed. Give examples of potential effects of these aspects of the environment on a client's health. (p. 377)
4. What are three considerations to be addressed in assessing the internal and external psychological environments of an individual client? Provide an example of each consideration and explain how factors in that area might influence health. (p. 379)
5. Describe the four components of social support and supply an example of each. (p. 381)
6. Identify at least six life-style considerations to be addressed in assessing the health status of an individual client. (p. 382)
7. Describe four considerations related to the health-care system to be addressed in assessing an individual client. (p. 383)
8. Identify four considerations in planning nursing intervention for an individual client. How might these considerations influence the outcome of nursing care? (p. 385)
9. What would be the foci of outcome and process evaluation of community health nursing care given to an individual client? (p. 388)

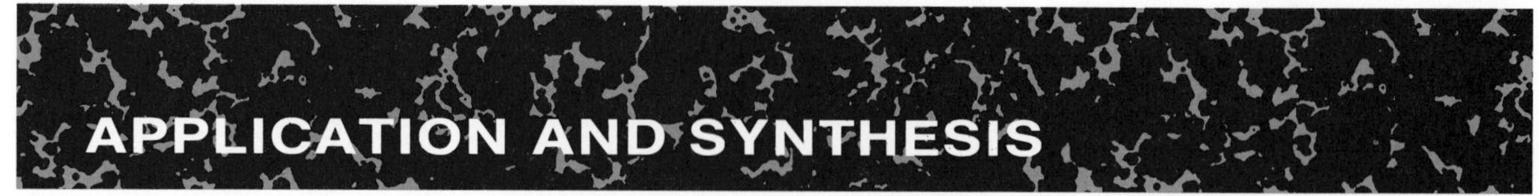

APPLICATION AND SYNTHESIS

Jeff is a 16-year-old client with diabetes mellitus. He has been referred to you for follow-up community health nursing services because of noncompliance with his diabetic diet and insulin injections. He was discharged from the hospital 3 days ago after being admitted in diabetic coma.

Jeff lives with his mother and two sisters in an apartment in a run-down area of town. Jeff's mother works, and Jeff is responsible for preparing his own breakfast and lunch and giving himself his insulin injection before going to school each morning.

Jeff's father died of a heart attack 3 years ago, and the family has some difficulty meeting their financial needs on the mother's income. Jeff tries to help with family finances by contributing part of the income from his after-school job at McDonald's. Because Jeff's father was in the military when he died, health-care services for the family are covered under their status as military dependents.

Jeff's school performance has been average, and he seems to get along well with school-mates. He is currently serving as vice-president of the sophomore class at the local high school. Before his father's death, Jeff was active in team sports at school, but now he feels like he needs to work instead of play sports. Jeff plans to attend college and major in business.

1. What factors in each of the four components of Dever's epidemiologic perspective are influencing Jeff's health? How adequate is your data base? What additional information would you want to collect? How might you obtain this information?
2. What are Jeff's health needs? Which of these needs would you address first? Why?
3. Develop a plan of care for Jeff's top two priority health needs. What are your goals and objectives for dealing with these needs? Write a SOAP note for each need. Be sure to include all four components of the plan of care in the "P" of your SOAP notes.
4. What criteria would you use to evaluate the status of Jeff's health-related needs? To evaluate your own performance in providing care?

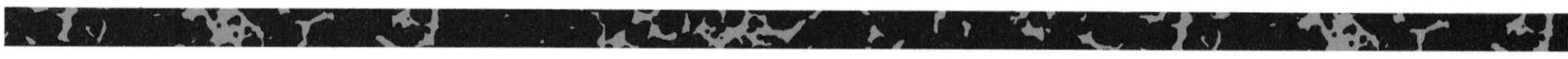

REFERENCES

1. Price, B. (1987). First impressions: Paradigms for patient assessment. *Journal of Advanced Nursing, 12*, 699–705.
2. Bunn, N. F. (1980). Disorders of hemoglobin structure, function, and synthesis. In K. J. Isselbacher, R. D. Adams, E. Braunwald, et al. (Eds.)., *Harrison's principles of internal medicine* (9th ed.) (pp. 1546–1554). New York: McGraw-Hill.
3. Nossel, H. L. (1980). Disorders of blood coagulation factors. In K. J. Isselbacher, R. D. Adams, E. Braunwald, et al. (Eds.), *Harrison's principles of internal medicine* (9th ed.) (pp. 1560–1562). New York: McGraw-Hill.
4. Strandness, D. E. (1980). Vascular diseases of the extremities. In K. J. Isselbacher, R. D. Adams, E. Braunwald, et al. (Eds.), *Harrison's principles of internal medicine* (9th ed.) (pp. 1181–1188). New York: McGraw-Hill.
5. Bowers, A. C., & Thompson, J. M. (1984). *Clinical manual of health assessment.* St. Louis: C. V. Mosby.
6. Grimes, J., & Burns, E. (1987). *Health assessment in practice* (2d ed.). Boston: Jones and Bartlett.
7. Herth, K. A. (1989). The root of it all: Genograms as a nursing assessment tool. *Journal of Gerontological Nursing, 15*(12), 32–37.
8. Pender, N. J. (1982). *Health promotion in nursing practice.* Norwalk, CT: Appleton-Century-Crofts.
9. House, J. (1981). *Work stress and social support.* Reading, MA: Addison-Wesley.
10. McGough, K. N. (1990). Assessing social support of people with AIDS. *Oncology Nursing Forum, 17*(1), 31–35.
11. Ungvarsky, P. (1988). Assessment: The key to nursing an AIDS patient. *RN, 51*(9), 28–33.

RECOMMENDED READINGS

Derdiarian, A. K. (1990). Effects of using systematic assessment instruments on patient and nurse satisfaction with nursing care. *Oncology Nursing Forum, 17*(1), 95–101.

Reports findings of a study of the effect of using a systematic approach to assessment on client and nurse satisfaction with care. Highlights the importance of systematic assessment.

Grimes, J., & Burns, E. (1987). *Health assessment in nursing practice* (2d ed.). Boston: Jones and Bartlett.

Provides direction for total health assessment of clients. Emphasizes the importance of cultural factors, values, attitudes, life-style, and health-related behaviors on physical and mental health.

Herth, K. A. (1989). The root of it all: Genograms as a nursing assessment tool. *Journal of Gerontological Nursing, 15*(12), 32–37.

Describes the use of a genogram to assess client health status. Provides a case-study example.

Price, B. (1987). First impressions: Paradigms for patient assessment. *Journal of Advanced Nursing, 12*, 699–705.

Presents normative and interpretive paradigms for interviewing clients to obtain health-related data. Reports research findings on the use of the two paradigms by nursing students in formulating client assessments.

CHAPTER 18

Care of the Family Client

Patricia Caudle
Susan Grover

KEY TERMS

binuclear family
cohabiting family
communication
communal family
coping strategies
crisis
defense mechanisms
extended family
external resources
family
family dynamics
family functions
family goals
family relationships
family structure
formal roles
homosexual family
informal roles
maturational crisis
nuclear conjugal family
role conflict
role overload
roles
single-parent family
situational crisis
step-family
social class
social system
subgroups
subsystem
suprasystem

The family, while changeable and as unique as its individual members, is the most enduring of social institutions. The family has been the basis for procreation, socialization, and continuation of cultures since the beginning of human history. As social norms have evolved over the centuries, many have predicted that the family would cease to exist as a social institution. This prediction, however, has not been realized. Despite periodic experimentation with communal living and other forms of social organization, the family unit of man, woman, and children is still the social unit most prevalent in society. Consequently, the family as a unit of service is an important consideration for community health nurses. Community health nurses contribute to the growth and health of the community and society through the assistance given to family groups. Knowledge of family health-care principles also prepares community health nurses to administer to individual family members, which will be examined in later chapters in this unit.

(*continued*)

LEARNING OBJECTIVES

After reading this chapter you should be able to:

- Describe at least five types of families and their characteristic features.
- Identify at least three characteristics of families.
- Describe at least six of the eight stages of family development and the developmental tasks to be addressed in each stage.
- Identify at least four considerations to be addressed in assessing family communication patterns.
- Describe the two central themes in assessing patterns of family dynamics.
- Differentiate between formal and informal family roles.
- Differentiate between maturational and situational crises.
- Describe the structure of a crisis event.
- Identify at least four principles of crisis intervention.

FAMILIES

The family is the basic social unit of American society. Defining family is difficult, however, because families can assume so many different forms. For the purposes of community health nursing, a ***family*** is a social system composed of two or more people living together who may be related by blood, marriage, or adoption, or who stay together by mutual agreement. Family members usually share living arrangements, obligations, goals, the continuity of generations, and a sense of belonging and affection.[1] This broad definition of family suggests that the principles of community health nursing applied to family clients must be flexible enough to meet the needs of many different family forms.

TYPES OF FAMILIES

NUCLEAR CONJUGAL FAMILIES

The ***nuclear conjugal family,*** or, more simply, the nuclear family, is composed of husband, wife, and children. Husband and wife are joined by marriage and their children are either biological offspring or adopted. The nuclear family is found in all ethnic and socioeconomic groups and is sanctioned by all religions. In the past, this type of family has been accepted as a social institution necessary to raise children properly. Today the high rate of divorce, increased sexual freedom, women's liberation, and the decreased social stigma attached to illegitimacy and alternative sexual life-styles have contributed to changes in the form of the family. The nuclear conjugal family is becoming less common in response to societal changes.[2] In fact, if the nuclear conjugal family is defined as a working husband, housewife, and one or more children, only about 10 percent of all households in the United States can be considered nuclear conjugal families.[3]

EXTENDED FAMILIES

The ***extended family*** is comprised of the family kin network such as grandparents, aunts, uncles, and cousins. Like the nuclear family, the extended family has been affected by societal change. In the past, members of extended families often lived in close proximity to the nuclear family. But owing to increased mobility and the enticement of better jobs in other areas, families are more likely to live away from their extended kin network. Thus, the extended family is now more likely to be a long-distance unit with whom the nuclear family corresponds and visits. This phenomenon has limited the social, economic, and emotional support formerly available to members of a nuclear family from older and more experienced relatives.

As time passes and circumstances change, the nuclear family may take extended family members into the home. This typically occurs as a consequence of early marriage of children where the newlyweds must live with parents or when adult children return home following a divorce, an economic setback, or some other life crisis. New living arrangements to incorporate extended family members into the nuclear family can also occur when aging parents can no longer live alone. The parent of a grown child may present adjustment problems for the nuclear family that has been separated from the parent for some time.

SINGLE-PARENT FAMILIES

The most common family unit to be encountered by community health nurses is the ***single-parent family.*** Single-parent families consist of an adult female or male and children. In 1988, over 10 million single-parent families were headed by women and nearly 3 million were headed by men. It is projected that, if current trends in marriage and divorce continue, by the year 2000 about 14 million single-parent families in the United States will be headed by women and about 4 million will be headed by men.[4]

STEP-FAMILIES

Step-families are increasingly evident in American society. A ***step-family*** is composed of two adults, at least one of whom has remarried following divorce or death of a spouse. Step-families can include children from either adult's previous marriage, as well as offspring from the new marriage. The extended kin network can include step-grandparents, step-aunts, uncles, and cousins, as well as an ex-spouse who is the biological parent of some of the children, but no longer a part of the household. Closely similar is the ***binuclear family,*** which exists when a child is a member of two nuclear households as a result of a joint-custody arrangement following the divorce of the child's parents.[2]

COHABITING FAMILIES

A ***cohabiting family*** consists of a man and a woman living together without being married.[5] Individuals who choose cohabitation range in age from teens to retired elderly persons. The reasons cited for preferring this arrangement include the desire for a "trial marriage," the increased safety of living with another, and financial necessity. Cohabitation is becoming more prevalent in the United States. In 1987, it was estimated that more than 2.3 million couples were cohabitating, and the number of cohabiting couples had quadrupled since 1960.[3]

HOMOSEXUAL FAMILIES

The ***homosexual family*** is a form of cohabitation that consists of a couple of the same sex who live together and share a sexual relationship. The homosexual family might include children and might resemble the traditional nuclear family in terms of the mutual support and sexual and economic interdependence of the couple involved. It may be difficult, however, for the homosexual family to stay together over time because of the lack of social sanction and support for their lifestyle.[6]

COMMUNAL FAMILIES

A ***communal family*** is made up of several adults and children living together, usually due to a common religious or ideological bond, or financial necessity.[5] Communal families typically resemble traditional extended families in qualities of affection and interdependence, rituals, migration, and influence or control.[7] Communal living can be more stressful than the typical nuclear family; this is because of crowding, because of more people and roles with which to deal, and a general lack of privacy for couples and children to resolve differences. Unlike the nuclear or cohabiting family, the communal family may not be able to continue over time because members tend to gravitate to the more traditional family forms.[3] The family types presented here are summarized in Table 18–1.

CHARACTERISTICS OF FAMILIES

Despite the outward variations in family form, all families share certain characteristics. Every family is a social system that has its own cultural values, specific functions, structure, and that moves through recognizable developmental stages.

FAMILY AS A SOCIAL SYSTEM

The family is a basic social system. A ***social system*** is a group of people who share common characteristics and who are mutually dependent upon one another. Because of this mutual dependence, community health nurses cannot work exclusively with

TABLE 18–1. TYPES OF FAMILIES AND THEIR CHARACTERISTIC FEATURES

Family Type	Characteristic Features
Nuclear conjugal family	Mother and father who are married with one or more biological or adopted children
Extended family	Kin network of the adult male and female of a nuclear family (for example, grandparents, aunts, uncles, cousins)
Single-parent family	One adult male or female with biological or adopted children
Step-family	Reconstituted or blended families created by a second marriage in which one or both spouses have children from a previous marriage and/or children of the new union
Binuclear family	A child (or children) who is part of two nuclear households as a result of divorce and joint custody
Cohabiting couple	A male and a female living together without marriage, with or without children
Homosexual family	A cohabiting couple of the same sex, with or without children
Communal family	Multiple adults and children in one household

individual family members because what affects one member will affect the entire family and vice versa.

The family is made up of members or ***subsystems,*** and it is part of a larger ***suprasystem,*** the neighborhood, community, nation, and the world. As a characteristic of family social systems, interdependence is mediated by a variety of factors. These factors include communication, roles, and the operation of subgroups within the family, all of which influence how the family solves everyday problems.

Communication, very simply, is the way that family members share meaning with each other.[8] Communication can be verbal or shown through gestures such as hugs or body language.

Roles are socially expected behavior patterns that are determined by a person's position or status within a family. Each person in a family occupies several roles by virtue of his or her position.[9] For example, the adult female in a family typically has the roles of wife, mother, cook, confidante, etc.

Alliances among family members create ***subgroups*** that may be very powerful. Subgroups can form horizontally (between members of the same generation) or vertically (between generations). For example, the parents are typically the powerful decision-making subgroup of the family. Or, a subgroup of mother and son may become aligned in such a way that father or older brother may be left out of close family interactions. Family communication, roles, and subgroups will be discussed in more detail later in this chapter.

FAMILY CULTURAL VALUES

A family's cultural values can greatly influence the way a family views health and the health-care system. A family's culturally mediated values and behaviors can either facilitate or impede a community health nurse's efforts to promote health and prevent disease. This subject was explored in detail in Chapter 15, Cultural Influences on Community Health.

STRUCTURE AND FUNCTION

Family structure is the organized pattern or hierarchy of members that determines how family members interact.[9] In other words, it is the way family members or subgroups are arranged to form a complete, interacting family unit. Components of a family's structure include the roles of each family member and how they complement each other and the family's value system, communication patterns, and power hierarchy. The power hierarchy typically places parents in charge of decision making for the family. A family's structure affects how a family functions.

Family functions are those activities that a family performs to meet the needs of its members. Members must be fed, clothed, housed, and given emotional support and guidance. Children must be socialized to societal and family cultural values and expectations. Members need economic security and mutual support as they adapt to changes in the environment and within the family.[10] All families, regardless of type, have in common these basic needs that require the family to function in ways that ensure family survival over time.

FAMILY DEVELOPMENT

Movement through developmental stages is characteristic of all families, regardless of their type. As the family expands and contracts, new role behaviors and communication skills are needed to cope with developmental crises and change. It has been postulated that each family passes through eight developmental stages beginning with family formation and continuing to the dissolution of the family.[11] During each stage, which is demarcated by acquisition of members and by the age of the oldest child, the family has certain developmental tasks or growth responsibilities that must be accomplished. Achievement of each developmental task is necessary for successful movement through subsequent stages.

Single-parent families experience developmental stages much like those of two-parent families. Single parents, however, may not establish or maintain a marriage. Their family adjustments are limited to dealing with added roles, socializing the children, encouraging education and separation of children from the family constellation, providing a healthful environment, and adjusting to the independence and eventual departure of the children to form families of their own.

Single parenthood that is precipitated by divorce or the death of a partner causes a pile-up of stressor events that can lead to crisis for many families.[12] The single parent must assume roles that were once fulfilled by the missing partner while continuing to perform his or her own roles.

Binuclear and step-families, created by remarriage of single parents, also experience predictable life-cycle stages. Their experience, however, is much more complex. There are many more adjustments to be made because there are more people involved in the transition. The central focus of family development is still the children, but at the same time the adults in the family are trying to adjust to each other. To sustain such families over a long period of time takes considerable compromise.[2]

TABLE 18–2. STAGES IN FAMILY DEVELOPMENT

Stage		Time Frame	Developmental Tasks
I	Beginning family	"Marriage" to birth of first child	1. Establish mutually satisfying marriage 2. Relate to kin network 3. Family planning
II	Early childbearing	Birth of first child plus 30 months	1. Establish stable family unit 2. Reconcile conflict in developmental tasks 3. Facilitate developmental tasks of members
III	Family with preschool children	Oldest child 2-½ to 5 years of age	1. Integrate 2d or 3d child 2. Socialize children 3. Begin separation from children
IV	Family with school-age children	Oldest child 6 to 13 years of age	1. Separate from children to a greater degree 2. Foster education and socialization 3. Maintain marriage
V	Family with teenage children	Oldest child 13 to 20 years of age	1. Maintain marriage 2. Develop new communication channels 3. Maintain standards
VI	Launching center family	From time first child leaves to time last child leaves	1. Promote independence 2. Integrate spouses of children into family 3. Restore marital relationship 4. Develop outside interests 5. Assist aging parents
VII	Family of middle years	From time last child leaves to retirement	1. Cultivate leisure activities 2. Provide healthful environment 3. Sustain satisfying relationships with parents and children
VIII	Family in retirement and old age	Retirement to death	1. Maintain satisfying living arrangements 2. Adjust to decreased income 3. Adjust to loss of spouse

(Source: Friedman.[10])

It is important to remember that, in addition to contributing to the accomplishment of the developmental tasks of the family unit, each family member is involved in accomplishing personal developmental tasks. These tasks can either parallel family tasks or be in conflict with them. The family must meet both individual and family developmental tasks to function as an effective unit. Thus, there may be conflict or stress when the accomplishment of a family task is in direct opposition to task achievement by the individual. The healthy family will develop effective mechanisms for dealing with this type of conflict when it arises. Table 18–2 lists the eight stages of family development and the developmental tasks to be accomplished at each stage.

THE EPIDEMIOLOGIC PREVENTION PROCESS MODEL AND CARE OF THE FAMILY

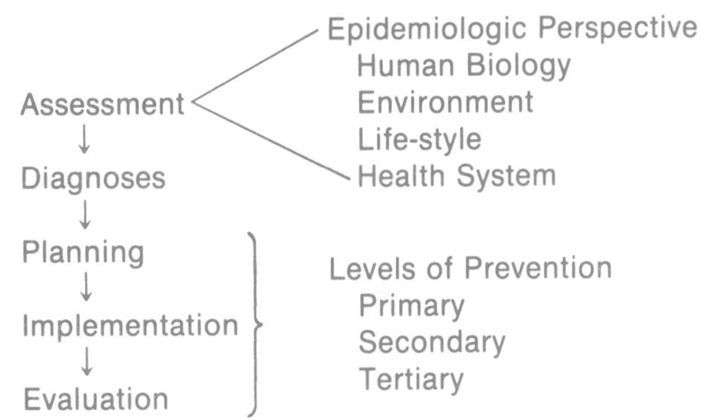

When working with families, the community health nurse's goal is to promote optimal health for each family member and for the family as a unit. The community health nurse can achieve this goal by using the epidemiologic prevention process model to facilitate care to family clients.

For the community health nurse to use the epidemiologic prevention process model with families, the nurse must first establish a relationship and ongoing interaction with the family. This entails open communication and trust that the nurse develops with the family over time by being reliable and honest. The relationship between the nurse and the family develops in the same way that individual relationships do. Initially, whether the nurse meets the family in the clinic setting or in the family's home, the nurse explains his or her role to the family. If the first meeting is in the family's home, the nurse will explain reasons for visiting and alleviate any discomfort the family may feel related to the presence of a stranger. Once an atmosphere of trust has been established, meaningful dialogue can occur.

Dialogue emphasizes the importance of two-way communication. In obtaining information about the family's health status, the nurse asks open-ended questions so that expanded discussion will occur. This allows the nurse to get a picture of areas that family members consider problematic. The nurse communicates both by speaking and listening and by being alert to nonverbal communications from family members.

The data gathered will be used to establish a contract with the family. A contract means that the family and the nurse have agreed to contribute to solving a problem that has been identified. For instance, the nurse might contract with the family to follow a low-calorie diet for one month after the family has clarified that one of their health problems is obesity.

The nurse should begin to focus on termination even in the assessment phase of the relationship with the family since the goal of nurse-family interaction is to enable the family to function independently. A plan established with the family that clearly denotes that the nurse's assistance will no longer be needed when the family has reached certain goals will facilitate family independence.

FAMILY ASSESSMENT

HUMAN BIOLOGY

When the community health nurse first encounters a family, assessment begins by gathering data to identify the physical needs of family members. Because individual physical assessment has been addressed previously (see Chapter 17, Care of the Individual Client), it will not be restated here. It is important to note, however, that the physical status of each family member should be weighed as part of the family assessment. The physical health status of each member affects how the family functions and how members relate to each other. For example, if a child has a chronic disease, the entire family must make adjustments to accommodate the youngster's special needs. The parents have to adjust their schedules to care for the child and ensure that the child is seen by appropriate health-care providers. Siblings can assume household chores and provide some measure of care for their ill brother or sister. Other family members can assist with care and offer emotional support for the parents and children.

Knowledge of the sex, age, and race of family members, as well as information related to genetic inheritance, can guide the nurse in identifying problems and planning family care. For example, knowing that there are several young children in the home, the nurse may emphasize safety precautions when interacting with the family. An elderly family is more likely to have members with chronic, debilitating illnesses and may need closer scrutiny for evidence of these problems. Or, a family's race may increase its members' risks for certain diseases such as sickle-cell disease among blacks and peoples of Eastern Mediterranean descent.

ENVIRONMENT

Physical Environment

The community health nurse's observational and interpretive skills are especially needed to assess the home environment. Within this setting, the family develops either functional or dysfunctional relationships. A chaotic, crowded, unsanitary, or unsafe home can contribute to physical and psychological health problems among family members.

To begin the assessment it is important to describe the home and its condition. Information such as the address, whether the family owns or rents the home, whether the home is big enough for the family, the presence of safety hazards, and family plans for fire or other disasters are all pertinent to the nurse's plan of care for the family. Box 18–1 lists several safety features that the nurse should take into consideration in assessing a family's physical environment. An example of a concise description of a home environment would be:

> Mrs. Turner, age 35, lives with her husband and 6 children in a run-down, single-family home. The home, consisting of 8 rooms (3 bedrooms) is well

BOX 18–1

Potential Physical Environmental Hazards for Families

- Absence of fire alarms in the home
- Peeling paint (especially lead-based paint in older homes)
- Broken furniture
- Loose throw rugs
- Broken stair railings (inside or outside the home)
- Broken stairs
- Broken porch floor boards
- Hazardous materials within children's reach
- Plumbing that does not allow for sanitary disposal of human wastes
- Toys in walkways
- Overcrowding
- Lack of a fire plan
- Lack of an earthquake, tornado, or other disaster plan
- Lack of a poison control plan (posted telephone numbers)
- Numerous house pets such as cats, chickens, or dogs
- Close proximity to a heavily traveled highway
- Lack of a fenced-in yard for small children

furnished and adequately heated. Health and safety hazards are presented by broken stairs and railings to the upstairs, peeling paint, and the lack of running water for the last 2 days. The owner has been notified of these conditions.

Information about the neighborhood should also be obtained. This includes physical characteristics such as the types of homes in the area, degree of industrialization, crime rate, and level of sanitation. Other important considerations include population density, common occupations of neighbors, availability of transportation, shopping facilities, health services, churches, schools, and recreational facilities. Each of these areas is assessed in relation to the specific needs of individual family members and of the family as a whole.

The community health nurse should note if there are any air, water, or noise pollution problems in the area that would increase the family's risks of disability and illness. It is important to determine what the sources of pollution are and the effects of pollution on the family.

After making this assessment, the community health nurse may want to question family members about perceptions of their environment. Does the family feel safe in this neighborhood? What are the hazards they perceive? Do they have an emergency plan if their safety should be jeopardized? Is the family aware of any existing pollutants in their neighborhood?

Psychological Environment

Communication Patterns. Communication patterns are an indicator of the psychological environment in which family members function. Both verbal and nonverbal modes of family communication should be considered, as should the listening ability of family members. How do members communicate values and ideas? When one family member talks, do others listen? Do they show anger or boredom while listening?

Mealtime is a good time to assess family interaction. It is here that the nurse can determine whether meals are a time of light conversation or heated argument, whether all family members eat together, and whether mealtimes contribute to family solidarity.

It is also important to assess the content of communications. Are they superficial or does the family engage in values clarification discussions? The type of statements made or questions asked tell the nurse a great deal about family interactions. For example, statements such as "You are wrong about that" and "Tell me more about your feelings" indicate different attitudes about interactions among family members. The latter, open-ended response facilitates communication, whereas the previous accusatory statement impedes it.

The feeling tone expressed in communication is another indicator of the psychological environment. Sarcastic and resentful statements could block further communication between family members. For example, a remark like "When are you ever going to use your head?" does not facilitate communication. Other types of one-way communication include repeated complaints, manipulation through covert requests, insulting remarks, lack of validation, and inability to focus on one issue.[10]

The nurse should ascertain what areas of communication are taboo (off limits) for family members. Typical areas include feelings, sexual issues, and religion. If certain topics are found to be taboo, the nurse may need to alter his or her approach to data gathering. For example, if one of the areas closed to discussion involves feelings, the nurse might try engaging in self-disclosure, thus acting as a role model. Another way to alter the approach is to gather data by examining areas related to the taboo issue. This may also help the nurse to identify the reason for resistance to communication about a specific area.

Communication patterns can influence the effectiveness of parenting, particularly in the area of discipline. Praise enhances the development of self-worth in the child, whereas negative or condescending communications restrict its development. More about communications and child discipline can be found in Chapter 20, Care of Children.

The nurse should be aware of several dysfunctional communication patterns that may be employed within families. For instance, messages may be passed from one family member to another in a chainlike fashion that does not allow for reciprocal discussion. Or, communication may isolate a family member, as when the mother and children exclude the father from their discussions. Another problematic pattern is the wheel in which a central person directs what communication will be passed between family members. By way of comparison, a successful pattern of communication is the "switchboard" in which there is reciprocal communication among all family members. Figure 18–1 illustrates these patterns of communication.

A final consideration is the degree of communication between the family and the suprasystem. Is the family open to new ideas and opinions from people outside the family? Are outsiders invited to participate in family discussions or are they expected to "mind their own business"?

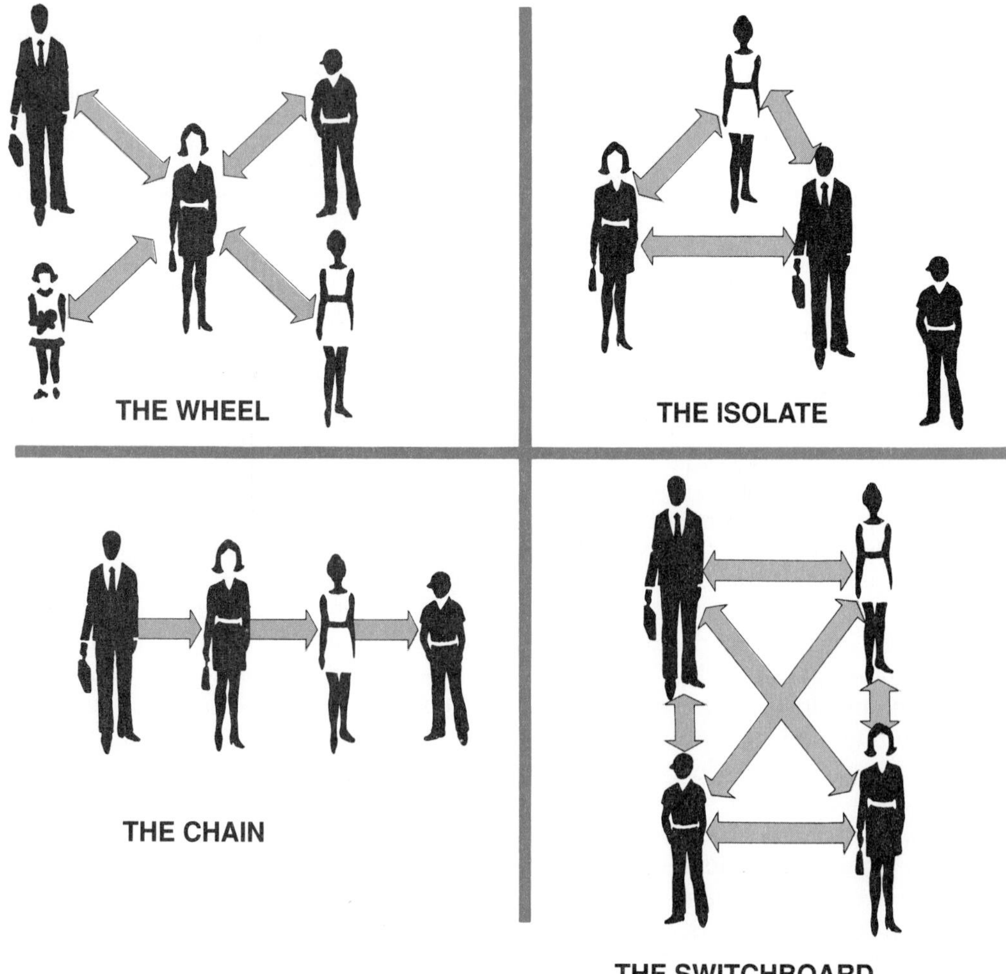

Figure 18–1. Family communication patterns.

Family Developmental Stages. As stated earlier, each family passes through developmental stages that have specific developmental tasks for the family to attain. The community health nurse should assess each family to determine the developmental stage the family is currently experiencing and whether or not developmental tasks of that and previous stages have been accomplished. For example, the Howard family is expecting the arrival of their second child. Their first child is 4 years old and has begun preschool this fall. The family developmental stage is that of the preschool family (Stage III of Table 18–2) and the tasks to be accomplished are: (1) to integrate the second child into the family; (2) to separate from the oldest child to a greater degree as he or she goes off to school; and (3) to socialize the children. The degree to which the Howards have achieved the tasks of the beginning family (Stage I of Table 18–2) and early childbearing (Stage II) will affect their ability to meet the tasks of Stage III. For instance, if the couple had been unable to establish a satisfying marriage, a task of Stage I, the second pregnancy may cause stress that will lead to the dissolution of the marriage.

Assessing the family's developmental stage will assist the community health nurse to provide anticipatory guidance that will help the family incorporate new members, adjust to the addition, and avert maturational crisis. Family maturational crisis will be addressed in some detail later in this chapter.

Family Relationships and Family Dynamics. Family relationships and family dynamics are areas of concern in the community health nurse's assessment of the family's psychological environment. ***Family relationships*** are those bonds between family members that create identifiable patterns such as subgroups or isolated members. ***Family dynamics*** describe the hierarchical patterns within the family. Power and leadership are the central focus for this area of assessment.

How does one assess relationships within the family? Initially, information regarding subgroups is compiled. For instance, the nurse may notice that there is a mother-daughter subgroup that has excluded the father from the decision-making process.

Communication within and between subgroups is then assessed in terms of both content (what is said) and process (who says it and how it is said). This is followed by identification of the relationship as supportive or close, demanding, maternal, and so on. Subgroups are described in terms of how they relate. For instance, one may describe the sibling group as one that shares feelings and actions, or they may be described as being alienated from each other.

Family dynamics are assessed by observing family leadership patterns. Who are the primary decision-makers? Who controls conversations? Is there a leader in the family? What leadership style does the leader employ? (See Chapter 11, The Change, Leadership, and Group Processes, for a discussion of leadership styles.) Do family members respect the leader? Do they respect each other? Respect requires that children view parents as individuals as well as parents. Likewise, parents need to learn to respect their children as individuals.

Family Emotional Strengths. A family's emotional strengths will become evident as the nurse observes interactions and communicates with family members over time. The nurse should look for evidence of family cohesion and the degree of sensitivity to others displayed by each family member. For example, the nurse might observe whether a mother anticipates the child's needs or whether there is a general feeling of warmth and caring. The nurse should also estimate the degree to which family members support and praise each other. The results of these observations will help the nurse to estimate how well the family is meeting the emotional and psychological needs of its members.

A positive self-image on the part of a family member is the result of daily family interactions that bolster the individual's feelings of self-worth. A child who is criticized too often may develop a poor self-image. The nurse can assess the self-esteem of each family member by observing nonverbal behavior as well as their communication patterns with others.

Coping Strategies. Identifying a family's coping strategies and defense mechanisms will enable the nurse to assist families to deal realistically with stress and crisis. ***Coping strategies*** are behaviors that help a family to adapt to stress or change and are characterized by positive problem-solving methods that lead to prevention or resolution of crisis situations.[10]

Defense mechanisms are tactics for avoiding recognition of problems. They may be used when the family cannot immediately determine how to solve a problem. Defense mechanisms are not considered problematic unless they interfere with coping. Examples of defense mechanisms include denial, rationalization, selective inattention, isolation, intellectualization, and projection.[10,13,14] Each of these defense mechanisms is defined in Box 18–2.

The use of coping strategies or defense mechanisms is seen most often when the family is faced with change. The community health nurse can assess how the family deals with change by observing behavior during life-change events or by obtaining information on how the family has dealt with a major move, job

BOX 18–2

Commonly Used Defense Mechanisms

Denial: ignoring threat-provoking aspects of a situation or changing the meaning of the situation to make it less threatening

Rationalization: giving a "good" or rational excuse, but not the real reason for responding to a situation with a particular behavior

Selective inattention: attending to only those aspects of the situation that do not cause distress or pain

Isolation: separating emotion from content in a situation so one can deal objectively with otherwise threatening or emotionally overwhelming conditions

Intellectualization: focusing on abstract, technical, or logical aspects of a threatening situation to insulate oneself from painful emotions generated

Projection: attributing one's own motivation to other people

(Source: Corsini, R. (Ed.) *Concise encyclopedia of psychology.* New York: Wiley, 1987.)

change, or loss of a family member in the past.[15] Working with a family in crisis will be discussed more fully later in this chapter.

Child-rearing and Discipline Practices. Another consideration in assessing the psychological environment of the family is that of child-rearing and discipline practices. Such practices have the potential either for causing psychological problems among family members or for strengthening a sense of right and wrong in each child.

The nurse should determine the type of discipline used, who administers it, and behavior that elicits disciplinary action. The nurse should also determine whether parents and other adults in the family support each other's decisions in matters of discipline. For instance, if the child is punished by the mother, does the child attempt to avoid punishment by manipulating the father? If so, are the adults able to discuss and support a joint decision? Ultimately, parents need to teach self-discipline, so it is important to assess whether they provide adequate role models for the child. For a more detailed discussion of discipline, see Chapter 20, Care of Children.

Roles. One of the most interesting aspects of the psychological environment is role enactment within families. Roles can take two forms—formal and informal. ***Formal roles*** are expected sets of behaviors associated with family positions such as husband, wife, mother, father, child, and so on. Examples of formal roles are those of breadwinner, homemaker, house repairman, chauffeur, child caretaker, financial manager, and cook. ***Informal roles*** are those expected behaviors not associated with a particular position. Informal roles influence the psychological environment within the family by determining whether, how, and by whom emotional needs are met.[10] Box 18–3 lists informal roles that may be present within any family group. The nurse identifies the presence or absence of these and similar informal roles and examines their effects on family function and cohesiveness.

Next, the nurse may want to assess for evidence of role conflict. ***Role conflict*** occurs when the demands of a single role are contradictory or when the demands attending several roles contradict each other. For example, a mother who works will experience role conflict when a business meeting she is expected to attend conflicts with her child's school play. Role conflict can also occur when one individual's definition of a role does not correspond with someone else's definition of the same role. For instance, a husband may expect that his wife should be responsible for all the cooking for the family, but the wife may work late and expect the husband to prepare an evening meal.

Role overload is another phenomenon that occurs in families when members assume multiple roles. ***Role overload*** occurs when an individual is confronted with too many role expectations at one time, even though these expectations do not contradict each other. For example, a mother with four children who returns to school and also has a part-time job may experience role overload in trying to meet the demands of housekeeping, cooking family meals, performing well on the job, and making straight A's.

Flexibility of family roles and mutual respect for individuality are also considered in the assessment of the psychological environment. Family roles often change when a family member is absent, ill, or incapacitated and cannot fulfill his or her usual roles. It is important to assess the ability of family members to take on these unfilled roles and make the necessary role adjustments. When the ill or absent member is ready to resume roles, a readjustment may again be

BOX 18–3

Informal Family Roles

- *Encourager:* praises others and is able to draw others out and make them feel that their ideas are important
- *Harmonizer:* mediates differences by use of humor and smoothing over
- *Blocker:* tends to be negative to all ideas
- *Follower:* passively goes along with the group
- *Martyr:* wants nothing for self but sacrifices for the sake of others
- *Scapegoat:* identified problem member, serves as a safety valve, relieving family tensions
- *Pioneer:* moves the family into unknown territory and new experiences
- *Go-between:* transmits and monitors communications among family members (often the mother)
- *Blamer:* fault-finder and dictator

(Source: Friedman.[10])

necessary. For instance, when Frank had his heart attack, Beth had to go to work and assume the breadwinner role. Now Frank is recovered and can return to work. Beth likes her job and does not want to quit. Assistance in adjusting to changes in roles can alleviate conflict and stress in this and in similar situations.

Role adjustments may also be required as the family progresses through its various developmental stages. For example, the parental role should be enacted differently with an adolescent child than with a preschooler. The nurse can assess the family's ability to adjust roles to the changing needs of its members and can also provide anticipatory guidance about adjustments that will be needed.

Family Goals. Family goals are an element of the psychological environment that may be difficult to assess because families often are not consciously aware of them. The nurse, however, can be aware of and observe for evidence of family goals; these include producing children and ensuring their survival, exchanging love and affective support, and providing economic survival or affluence.

Family goals are a function of family values and reflect a family's cultural background. Family goals also vary with a family's developmental stage, economic status, and the physical health of family members. Problems arise when there is disagreement on family goals. For example, the Gonzales family has worked hard to send their son to college (a family goal). Before his sophomore year, the son refused to return to school, preferring instead to work as a plumber's apprentice.

Social Environment

Social environment shares some of the influences of the psychological environment. For instance, relationships outside the family are the basis for a portion of personality development. Leadership ability of individual family members is developed in school and in cultural, social, and political organizations where family members have the opportunity to interact with others and to contribute to community endeavors. Family discussions of social, cultural, and political issues help to develop social awareness as children grow and encourage the children to become involved in community, county, state, and national politics or social movements. Areas for consideration in assessing the family's social environment include their religion, race and culture, social class and economic status, and external resources.

Religion. The influence of religious beliefs and practices on the health of the family can be assessed by asking specific questions about the importance of religion in family interactions and decision making and the role of religion for the family as a whole. For example, strong religious beliefs may prohibit the use of contraceptives, or health teaching may need to be modified in keeping with the family's religious convictions. Close affiliation with an organized church may also provide a source of emotional and/or material support for family members in time of need.

Culture. Family cultural information is an invaluable aid in building relationships and designing family interventions that will not conflict with cultural values. Does the family engage in cultural practices related to health? If so, are these practices helpful or harmful? What cultural factors will affect attempts to resolve family health problems? The nurse can compare the family's culture to that of the community in which they live and determine if there are differences present that may create problems for the family or the children of the family. Principles of cultural assessment discussed in Chapter 15, Cultural Influences on

Community Health, are applicable to assessment of the social environment of families.

Social Class and Economic Status. *Social class* delineations involve cultural groupings of people based on financial status, race, occupation, education, similar life-styles, language, or mutual consent.[1] In America, the lower social class is comprised of people with less money, less education, less access to resources such as health care, and, typically, people of color.

The family's social class is important to the extent that it affects life-style, interactions with the external environment, and the structural and functional characteristics of the family. Economic status is closely tied to social class and educational level. For instance, many single parents are members of lower socioeconomic groups, and most single-family households are poor. The single female parent in many of these families either works outside the home or accepts welfare for economic support of her family. Often the jobs available to such women are minimum wage, menial jobs that allow some flexibility so they can care for their children. The single female parent often has no other adult to share in family decision making and must call upon her children to carry out functions within the family that might have been her own if there were a male parent present.

The social class and economic status of a family can profoundly affect its health. Lack of financial resources can mean that the family does not have enough nutritious food, adequate shelter, or access to health care. The community health nurse can assess the family's social class and economic status and begin to make plans to assist the family through referral to community resources that will increase their access to food, better shelter, and health care.

External Resources. To assist families in dealing with social environmental stressors, the community health nurse will need to identify external resources available to the family. ***External resources*** include those materials or sources of assistance available to the family from the community. The nurse's assessment of the family's external resources may suggest ways of dealing with identified health problems. Questions that will elicit this information are those related to neighborhood sources of financial assistance, transportation, housing, health care, and education. The nurse should also investigate relational support systems such as kin networks, friends, and neighbors. Usually each community has service agencies that can assist families in need. For example, many poor families may be eligible for the *Women, Infants, and Children* (WIC) program, a federal supplemental food program that provides basic nutrition for pregnant women, young children, and breastfeeding women who are nutritionally deficient. Also, many churches offer food and clothing for the needy in their community.

LIFE-STYLE

The third component in the assessment phase of the epidemiologic prevention process model is the assessment of family life-style. Areas of focus here include family consumption patterns, rest and sleep patterns, exercise and leisure activities, and employment or occupational factors.

Family Consumption Patterns

A family's nutritional status can be assessed through physical assessment of each member and by observing the way in which the family selects, purchases, and prepares food. If any family members are nutritionally impaired, the nurse will need to determine the underlying causes. Is it lack of money to buy food? Does the person who prepares food lack information that would ensure good family nutrition? How is food prepared? Are there cultural patterns evident in food selection, preparation, and consumption? For instance, the excessive use of fried or high-fat foods sometimes seen among Latinos or families in the southern United States contributes to the increased incidence of atherosclerosis, heart disease, and stroke among members of these populations.

Other consumption patterns of interest to the nurse include the use of alcohol, drugs, medications, tobacco, and caffeine. Is the use of any of these substances causing a family member to be unable to carry out his or her role and functions within the family? Does the mother's smoking, for instance, aggravate the child's respiratory condition? Are prescription drugs being used as prescribed? Are there any side effects evident from the use of prescription drugs? Are over-the-counter (OTC) products used appropriately? The answers to these and similar questions will assist the nurse to identify problems arising from family consumption patterns.

Rest and Sleep

Family rest and sleep patterns may be a source of problems. For example, a new baby may sleep during the day and cry at night. This will adversely affect parents' rest and their subsequent performance the next day.

Another problem frequently encountered with respect to family sleep patterns is that of differing work schedules. If, for example, one parent works days and the other works nights, this situation may limit their opportunities to interact with each other and with their children. A parent's typical rest and sleep schedules may also require children to play at a neighbor's house during the day or find quiet pastimes at home. The nurse can assist the family in making decisions about how to deal with these and similar problems.

Exercise and Leisure

Regular exercise is necessary for good health. The earlier children are included in activities, the more likely they are to build lifetime habits of exercise. Exercise and leisure activities that include the entire family promote cohesion. Assessment in this area includes consideration of the type and frequency of exercise engaged in by family members. At times it is also helpful to plan leisure activities that are unique to certain members of the family. This allows for individuality among family members and promotes a balance between family togetherness and separateness that is needed for individual development. The nurse should explore whether there are exercise or leisure activities that include only the adults or only the children.

The nurse can also help the family to identify potential health risks involved in leisure activities. For instance, are safety helmets worn by all family members on bike trips? What are the safety rules when the family goes swimming? Is a backyard pool covered when not in use to prevent a child from going in alone or falling in accidentally?

High costs and low income may limit the activities that families can do together, but should not eliminate them. The nurse can help the family plan low-cost activities that will enhance family cohesion. For example, the family could take part in a picnic in the park followed by a game of ball or horseshoes.

Employment or Occupational Factors

Job-related factors that influence family health may present in three forms. First, the job might produce stress for the adult that results in illness. Second, the adult might be exposed to hazards that he or she brings home to other family members. Third, job-related problems and time constraints might interfere with family commitments.

Occupational or workplace stress can lead to a number of stress-related illnesses such as peptic ulcer and hypertension. Safety hazards within the work setting may cause injury and disability to the family breadwinner(s). The financial burden and stress that an occupation-related illness could cause has led to divorce and the dissolution of families, among other problems.

Sometimes substances to which a working parent is exposed not only threaten the parent, but may also inadvertently be brought home to other family members. For example, nurses and other health-care workers need to be aware that some infectious diseases may be transmitted to young children via clothing and shoes. Working with lead or other hazardous substances may also result in exposure of family members through contaminated clothing and other articles worn on the job.

Job-related family problems also might arise if a family member's work commitment conflicts with family commitments. For example, Dad may have to work late on the night the family was to attend a play, or a new job may interfere with family vacation plans. The nurse can assist family members to establish priorities and to plan quality time together. Chapter 5, The Nursing Process, describes the problem-solving process that will assist the nurse to help families set priorities and plan time together.

Household and Other Safety Practices

Safety practices such as seat belt use, use of infant safety seats, cribs with safe spacing between rails and proper mattress width, proper disposal of hazardous substances, safety education for children, and so on, are important considerations in family assessment. Are these life-style safety factors evident in the household? Who is the person most attentive to family safety issues? What family life-style behaviors contribute to health risks for members? Box 18–4 lists

BOX 18–4

Potential Family Safety Practices

- Consistent seat belt use
- Use of safety equipment such as eye and ear protection
- Use of infant safety seats
- Cribs with safe spacing between rails and proper mattress width
- Proper disposal of hazardous substances
- Safety education of children regarding:
  - Not talking to or going with strangers
  - How to cross the street safely
  - Use of seat belts and safety equipment such as helmets, goggles, and ear protection
- Safe use of appliances and craft equipment such as saws, glues, drills, etc.

several safety factors to be considered by the nurse assessing the family's life-style.

HEALTH SYSTEM

Family Response to Illness

Assessing the areas of human biology, environment, and life-style within the family should give the nurse a general idea of the health of the family and of the strategies family members use to remain healthy. But how do members deal with illness? Part of learning about this aspect of family life is determining who in the family decides when an ill family member should stay home from work or school and whether an ill member should receive health care. For example, in some families the mother decides who is ill and consults the father when she believes that the illness is severe enough to require the services of a health-care provider.

In some families, folk remedies or cultural health practices are used before consulting a health-care provider. The community health nurse will need to assess whether these practices are harmful to the sick family member and whether to encourage the family to seek professional assistance. Chapter 15, Cultural Influences on Community Health, provides more information on how the nurse can determine which cultural health practices may be harmful and how to help the family member choose other modes of care.

Use of Health-care Services

The accessibility, availability, and use of health-care services by family members need to be assessed by the nurse. Often there may be providers available for the mother and children because of federal and state programs. The father and other young adult males, however, are often excluded from these programs. The nurse may be asked to help the family find health care for excluded family members who become ill.

It is important to learn where family members go for health care and whether their choice provides any preventive health services or dental care. Many private medical doctors provide only sickness care, and the family will need information about where to go for preventive services such as immunizations, health teaching, and dental care.

Health care may be limited because of lack of funds to pay, language barriers, the distance of the health-care facility from the family and transportation limitations, and many other problems. The nurse will need to determine these deterrents to access and find resources within the community to help the family attain health care.

Occasionally, even when a family has health insurance, members are not able to take full advantage of this resource because they do not understand what services are covered (or not covered). The nurse can help them understand their insurance benefits or refer the family to resources in the community who can explain insurance benefits and how to use them.

An assessment tool is provided to assist in gathering family assessment data. This tool is included in Appendix G, The Health Intervention Planning Guide–Family Client.

DIAGNOSTIC REASONING AND THE FAMILY AS CLIENT

The data obtained during the assessment phase of the epidemiologic prevention process model enables the nurse to make informed decisions about how to intervene with families who need assistance. The best way to demonstrate how diagnostic reasoning progresses using the model is to present an example. Box 18–5 offers a case study that will serve as the basis for discussion of the use of the epidemiologic prevention process model with a family.

Mrs. Smith is pregnant and has hypertension. These are physical conditions that are affecting her ability to fulfill her roles as wife and mother. Mrs. Jones, the community health nurse, must assist Mr. and Mrs. Smith to choose health-care services that will provide affordable care. The question of affordability depends on whether the couple have health insurance. If they do not, Mrs. Jones can help them apply for assistance.

The psychological environment within the family is strained because of impaired communication between Mr. and Mrs. Smith and because of frequent quarrels between Mr. Smith and his son, Brian. Communication in the family may not have been effective before the pregnancy or may have deteriorated because of the unplanned pregnancy. A further evaluation of the communication pattern between father and son is needed to determine the best mode of intervention.

There is also a life-style risk factor evident in Mr. Smith's employment pattern. Holding down two jobs over an extended period of time will cause extreme fatigue and stress. Fatigue and tension can contribute to decreased safety precautions and increased risk of accidents. In addition, Mr. Smith is increasing his risk for stress-related illnesses such as hypertension and peptic ulcer. Box 18–6 lists sample nursing diagnoses for the Smith family based on the data contained in the case.

BOX 18–5

Family Nursing Case Study

Arlene Jones, R.N., a community health nurse, has been visiting the Smith family for a month. Mrs. Smith, age 30, is pregnant with her fourth child. The other children are ages 12, 10, and 6. This pregnancy was unplanned.

Mrs. Smith has been quite depressed and experiences frequent episodes of crying. She also has hypertension. Mrs. Smith has talked with the nurse about difficulties she is having with her husband and 12-year-old son, Brian. Mr. Smith is seldom home because he needs to hold two jobs to meet the family's financial needs. When he is home, his presence is characterized by frequent arguments with Brian. Brian is experiencing problems at school and is often truant. Mrs. Smith thinks her son's problems are due to his strained relationship with his father.

Mr. Smith has expressed concern about being able to provide for a fourth child. Perhaps for this reason, his relationship with his wife has deteriorated and there is little communication between them. Mrs. Smith is close to her neighbors and active in her church.

PLANNING AND IMPLEMENTING NURSING INTERVENTION

From the nursing diagnoses and the assessment data base, Mrs. Jones can compile a health status summary for the Smith family. Together, Mrs. Jones and the Smith family can give priority to identified health-care needs. Collaboration with the family is important. Without an agreement or contract with the family dealing with the needs most important to them, members may not enter into any of the planned interventions that involve their active participation.

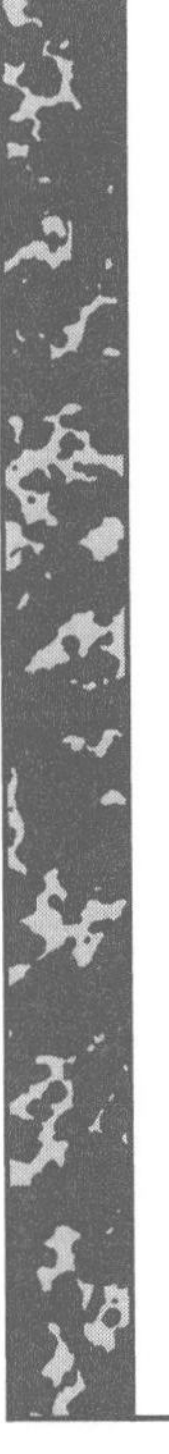

BOX 18–6

Sample Nursing Diagnoses for the Smith Family

1. Need for changes in family nutritional patterns due to mother's pregnancy and hypertension
2. Increased stress and anxiety due to poor communication patterns and frequent arguments
3. Inability to meet financial demands due to forthcoming birth of fourth child
4. Need for contraception to prevent subsequent pregnancies
5. Need for changes in family roles to accommodate addition of another family member

The health status summary for the Smith family might include the following needs and concerns:

1. Income inadequate to meet needs
2. Ineffective communication among family members
3. Anticipated role changes with the birth of a fourth child
4. Mrs. Smith's depression and hypertension
5. School truancy by the 12-year-old son
6. Mr. Smith's potential for stress-related accidents or diseases

Nursing interventions that may take place at primary, secondary, or tertiary levels of prevention must be designed for each health-care need. Goals and objectives for each need should be stated in measurable terms. The objectives should also state a date for attainment of expected outcomes. For example, Mrs. Jones has made a diagnosis related to the ineffective communication between husband and wife. The goal of intervention is to facilitate open communication and strengthen the marital bond. One objective that may promote goal achievement might be: "The Smiths will plan a weekend together without the children within the next month."

There may be several alternative solutions for each of the Smith family's identified problems. In an attempt to choose the most appropriate course of action, Mrs. Jones would mention these alternatives to the Smiths. Together, they would discuss the advantages and disadvantages of each alternative and select the most appropriate solution to each problem.

Not all of Mrs. Jones's goals need to be shared with the Smiths. It is appropriate for some goals to remain in the mind of the nurse.[16] For example, Mrs. Jones may feel that Mr. Smith is using an authoritarian approach with his son that is blocking communication between the two. She would not share the goal of changing Mr. Smith's approach because doing so might destroy the trust she has developed with the Smiths. Instead, she will work with the family to establish a communication pattern that is supportive of each member's needs, thereby changing the father's approach to his son without labeling the interaction "authoritarian."

PRIMARY PREVENTION

Planning primary preventive strategies for the Smith family requires that the nurse consider the data in the assessment. For example, based on the fact that the Smiths will soon be having their fourth child, the nurse can help them plan ahead for immunizations and other well-child services for the new baby.

The psychological environmental assessment revealed that the Smiths are in Stage IV (see Table 18–2) of family development, the family with school-aged children. Since they are also expecting a new baby, one of the tasks of Stage III will need to be repeated. The developmental tasks with which the Smiths may need assistance include the integration of a fourth child into the family, fostering education and socialization of the school-aged children, and maintaining the marriage. For the Smiths, the community health nurse will focus on anticipated role changes for each family member that will occur with the arrival of the new baby. For instance, she will plan to discuss with Mr. and Mrs. Smith such topics as who will get up with the baby at night, who will assist with household tasks, and the possibility of sibling rivalry.

Anticipatory guidance to develop new communication channels will be important to avert developmental crises as the son Brian enters adolescence. Allowing Brian to accept more responsibility and to have more freedom, while maintaining discipline, will set the pattern for the way his brothers and sisters will progress through adolescence.

Referrals for financial assistance in the form of WIC, Medicaid, and food stamps (depending on the family's eligibility) may decrease some of Mr. Smith's burden as sole breadwinner. Relieving the stress he is experiencing may prevent development of stress-related health problems.

SECONDARY PREVENTION

Secondary prevention is employed when Mrs. Jones plans meetings to give family members opportunities for mediated communication that will assist them to become more supportive of each other. With increased and enhanced communications, the family's power structure can be more equally divided and the changes in roles that will occur with the new baby can be planned.

With the resolution of the spousal communication problem and economic assistance, Mrs. Jones can look for a decrease in Mrs. Smith's depression. When this has occurred, Mrs. Jones will initiate dietary teaching related to Mrs. Smith's hypertension, an important secondary preventive measure.

Intervention to resolve the conflict within the father-son subsystem cannot begin until Mrs. Jones has gathered more data. However, because a behavioral problem and truancy have been identified, a referral can be made to the school counselor. The Smiths can meet with the counselor to determine how their son's problems can be resolved. After gathering more data about the block in communications between father and son, Mrs. Jones will facilitate communication between them by acting as a mediator to permit open communication. She can also help Mr. Smith become more accepting of the changes in his son and his son's developmental need to interact with his peers.

TERTIARY PREVENTION

Work with the Smiths to improve communications can also be considered a tertiary preventive measure. From this perspective, improved communications will prevent complications of family discord such as divorce. It will also prevent the recurrence of many of the family problems that have stemmed from poor communication between husband and wife. Another tertiary preventive measure might be a referral for contraceptive services to prevent another unplanned pregnancy.

EVALUATING NURSING CARE

Evaluation begins as the nurse examines the adequacy of the assessment data base and continues as he or she evaluates alternative approaches to meeting the family's health-care needs. The primary focus for post-intervention evaluation is the objectives of care. If these objectives were adequately developed, they are measurable and provide criteria for evaluating the outcome of the intervention. For example, Mrs. Jones set the following objectives for her intervention with Mr. Smith and Brian:

1. Mr. Smith will praise his son at least once a day.
2. Mr. Smith will agree to listen to his son for at least five minutes a day.

Mrs. Jones must then determine the means for collecting data to compare outcomes with the stated objectives. In this instance, Mrs. Jones could ask Mrs. Smith whether the desired communication pattern has been achieved. If the objectives are not met, an alternative solution can be attempted.

Evaluation is a continuous process throughout the nurse's relationship with the family. If evaluation is not planned at the same time as nursing intervention, it may be impossible to obtain the data needed to evaluate outcomes.

When Mrs. Jones finds that all goals and objectives have been achieved, she will terminate her relationship with the Smiths. Termination, like evaluation, should be planned and discussed early in the relationship. Termination is necessary because the goal of nursing intervention is to make the family independent.

Both the Smiths and Mrs. Jones may experience some degree of grief during the termination process. Resolution of that grief is necessary and, when achieved, will indicate growth. Mrs. Jones should leave the phone number and address of the health unit in case of a future need for services. If necessary, Mrs. Jones can refer the family to other agencies that may be of assistance.

THE EPIDEMIOLOGIC PREVENTION PROCESS MODEL AND CRISIS INTERVENTION

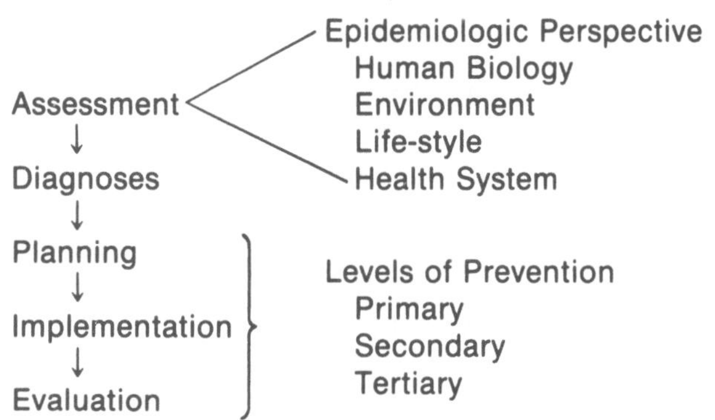

DEFINITION OF CRISIS

A family can view any situation as a crisis. What is a crisis for one family may not be a crisis for another. Moreover, some families function and thrive on daily crises and would deteriorate if crisis situations were eliminated from their lives. Assessment and intervention, then, must be based upon the family's perception of a crisis event.

A ***crisis*** occurs when a family faces a problem that is seemingly unsolvable. None of their methods of problem solving work. The problem becomes psychologically overwhelming, and anxiety and tension increase until the family becomes disorganized and unable to cope. A crisis state is unlikely to be sustained for more than 6 weeks because it is difficult to endure the high stress and tension associated with crisis without breakdown or change.[13] The result of a crisis can either be resolution, resulting in a healthier, more positive state of being, or a loss of well-being and a higher potential for recurrent crisis. Temporary relief can be gained from the use of defense mechanisms or environmental action or both.[14] Resolution and more permanent relief and growth require appropriate coping mechanisms.[10]

During periods of crisis, families are more susceptible to change and are usually more open to help when it is offered. This receptiveness affords the nurse the opportunity to produce change with very little intervention.

TYPES OF CRISES

There are two types of crises—maturational and situational. A ***maturational crisis*** is viewed as a "normal" transition point where old patterns of communication and old roles must be exchanged for new patterns and roles.[1] Every family experiences maturational crisis points, whether or not a crisis is actually experienced. Examples of transitional periods when maturational crises may occur are adolescence, marriage, parenthood, and one's first job. Such periods in life are usually predictable, so families can be prepared to use coping mechanisms that will assist them through each transition period.

All the transitional periods experienced by families have in common a change in roles or the addition of new roles, and crises occur when a family is unable or unwilling to accept new roles.[17] There may be a history of poor role modeling from parents that leaves children unprepared for new roles and unable to leave home successfully. There may be family members who are unable or unwilling to view one member in a new role. For example, it is sometimes difficult for parents to acknowledge that their teenage children need to make decisions for themselves.

A ***situational crisis*** can occur when the family

experiences an event that is sudden, unexpected, and unpredictable. Such events threaten either biological, psychological, or social integrity leading to disorganization, tension, and severe anxiety.[13] Examples include illness, accidents, death, and natural disasters.

Some crises may arise that contain elements of both situational and maturational crisis events. For example, a female may be going through the maturational transition of adolescence and encounter the situational crisis of an unwanted pregnancy. The multiplicity of crisis events further impairs the family's ability to cope.

FACTORS THAT INCREASE SUSCEPTIBILITY TO CRISIS

Why do some families go into crisis while others do not? Three factors seem to determine the occurrence of a crisis experience: the family's perception of the event, the family's coping mechanisms, and the presence or absence of situational support.[10]

The family's perception of the event may be distorted by previous experience with crises that were not growth producing. For example, there are crisis-prone families who have a chronic inability to perceive or solve existing problems. Their inability to cope with problems results in an exaggerated response to new changes, and crises occur for them that would be averted by other families.

The family's coping mechanisms represent internal family resources important to crisis resolution. Among these resources are cohesion or closeness among family members, open communications, use of humor, control of the meaning of the problem, and role flexibility.[10,14] The family's ability to cope lessens the impact of any crisis event. It is important to assess what degree of success has been achieved using these mechanisms in the past and whether the family is aware of the mechanisms used.

Situational support arises from external resources such as the extended family, community agencies, churches, neighbors, and friends of the family. The degree of security felt by family members in relationships with these support systems may be sufficient to avert crises.

STRUCTURE OF A CRISIS EVENT

In every crisis there are contributing factors that culminate in the crisis event. A hazardous incident of some sort triggers the sequence of events. Hazardous situations can arise from human biology as a result of aging, genetic factors, or illness; from the physical, psychological, or social environment; as a result of life-style patterns such as drug or alcohol use; or from health system problems such as lack of affordable medical care.

Such events are more broadly divided into three general categories of factors: a threat involving loss or danger of loss; the loss itself; or a challenge to master or perform well (for example, political aspirations, parenthood, and so on) that puts the family in a vulnerable position.[14] Regardless of its source, the hazardous situation is usually stressful and causes anxiety. The family experiences a reaction to the event characterized by depression or anger. Family members may use defense mechanisms, such as denial to ease their discomfort before beginning to use coping mechanisms that will help them deal constructively with the situation.

A precipitating event might occur that throws the family into acute anxiety and crisis. This event may be seemingly minor, but serves to tip the scales toward crisis. It overtakes coping mechanisms already stretched to the limits. For example, father's unemployment is a hazardous event that makes the family vulnerable to crisis. Because of the mother's job and other supports, members are not yet in crisis. Then the car breaks down! This last event is perceived by the family as overwhelming and pushes members beyond their ability to cope. A crisis has been born.

When coping mechanisms fail, the family resorts to different strategies. One person may laugh or cry a great deal; another might withdraw. Finally, the family is in full crisis, evidenced by inappropriate behavior and painful, stressful feelings. During this time they are unable to focus or concentrate and need clear, direct, precise direction. Figure 18–2 depicts the structure of a crisis event.

CRISIS INTERVENTION

ASSESSING THE CRISIS SITUATION

Interviewing during a crisis requires empathy, a calm demeanor, and a sensitivity to feeling tones that may not be readily apparent to others. Nondirective techniques are used. Inquiries and instructions need to be precise, concrete, and simple; a family in crisis is unable to focus and narrow the field to what must be done. Open-ended statements are used to encourage family members to speak spontaneously.

The primary concern during a crisis is the potential for physical danger that may be present within the family. Individual family members must be assessed for suicidal or homicidal tendencies. If there are indications that a family member is contemplating

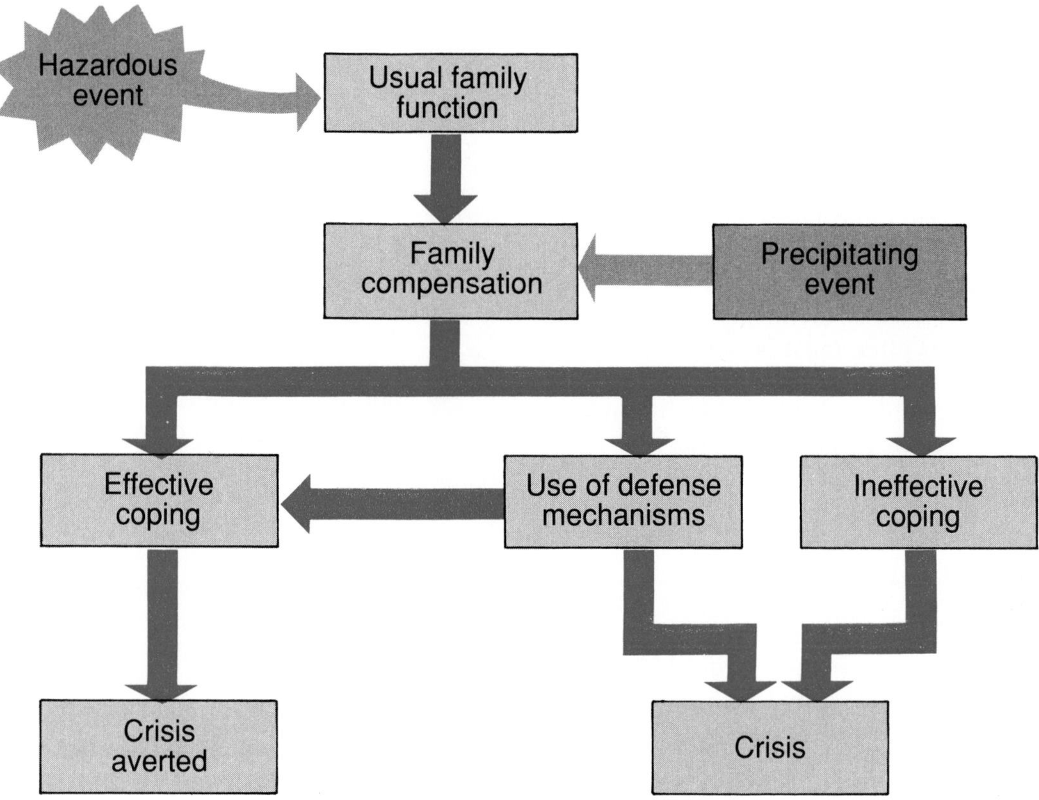

Figure 18–2. Structure of a crisis event.

violence to oneself or to others, immediate referral for psychiatric help is warranted.

Human Biology

Human biological factors such as aging, genetic factors, or illness can contribute to the crisis. For example, Mr. Simon is 74 years old and has to move into a nursing home because he can no longer buy his own groceries and cook for himself. He becomes very agitated and cannot make decisions.

The Psychological Environment

The initial step in assessing a crisis situation is to review the events leading to the crisis. This gives family members a chance to discuss their perceptions of the event and affords the nurse an opportunity to assess perceptions, defense mechanisms, and coping strategies. Detailed history is not necessary.[18] Just let them talk.

The nurse should determine if the family has ever experienced a similar event and how the family has reacted in the past. Past successful coping can be used to reassure members that they can cope with the current problem as well. Or, discussion of past events can be used to identify patterns that were not successful, and plans can be made to use alternative coping mechanisms.

The Social Environment

When family members have had an opportunity to discuss the situation and are emotionally open to exploring solutions, an assessment can be made of external resources arising from the social environment. Find out if there are extended family members nearby, agencies that have been helpful for the family in the past, clergy, church members, or friends that the family want near them now.

Sometimes social environmental factors such as unemployment, racial discrimination, or poverty can contribute to a crisis. For instance, Mr. Lloyd's son needs surgery so he can walk. Arrangements were made but had to be cancelled when Mr. Lloyd lost his job and his health insurance benefits. In this case, the community health nurse may want to determine whether there is an agency available that can help the family to obtain the care their son needs.

Life-style

Life-style factors such as alcohol or drug use can constitute the hazardous event, be a precipitating event, or can act as a defense mechanism for a family experiencing crisis. Alcohol and drug abuse can also impair a family's response to maturational and situational crises. The nurse must be alert to any evidence of alcohol or drug abuse and assist the family in seeking and obtaining counseling.

Health System

Assessment in this area includes determining whether the family has insurance coverage for counseling, emergency care, or hospitalization should these be required to deal with the crisis. Counseling and medical services for potentially suicidal family members, accident victims, or members with drug and alcohol problems often must be sought for families that do not have any insurance or money. Identifying local, county, and state resources for families in need is an important responsibility for the community health nurse.

DIAGNOSTIC REASONING AND CRISIS INTERVENTION

Often diagnostic reasoning and planning for crisis intervention occur at the same time. Working with a family in crisis requires expertise in quickly determining the family's needs, knowledge of resources available that can be used spontaneously or with very little delay, and the ability to teach problem solving. The case study in Box 18–7 will be used to illustrate how Mrs. James, a community health nurse, assisted the Robbins family during a crisis.

From this data, Mrs. James derives some nursing diagnoses. First, this is a situational crisis precipitated by son Bob's drinking and his argument with his father. There are also elements of a maturational crisis present because Mr. Robbins seems reluctant to accept Bob's new role as a young adult. Second, the family does not know how to deal with a teenage son who has a drinking problem. Third, son John is being left out of the discussions at a time when he is old enough to be a contributing member. Mrs. James also surmises that the family seems to have drawn together to help each other survive this crisis.

Intervention in a crisis situation is guided by several general principles. First, the nurse should listen actively and with concern to family members' perceptions of and feelings about the event. Second, the nurse should encourage open expression of feelings and help the family gain an understanding of the crisis event. The nurse should also help the client accept reality and explore new ways of coping with problems presented by the crisis situation. The nurse may also need to link family members with a social network that can assist them to deal with the crisis. The community health nurse will also engage in problem solving with the family and reinforce new coping strategies. Finally, the nurse will need to follow-up with the family after the crisis has been resolved to engage in primary prevention for future crisis events.[19]

BOX 18–7

Family Crisis Case Study

The Robbins family includes five members: Dad, 46; Mom, 43; Bob, 18; John, 16; and Debbie, 6 months. Bob will finish high school this year. He and his father seem to argue all the time about Bob's friends, Bob's drinking, and the way Bob drives. Last evening Bob and his father had a heated argument and Bob left the house in a rage. He drove away, squealing tires and swerving at the corner. When the community health nurse, Mrs. James, makes a visit the next morning, she finds the family in an agitated state. Bob did not come home last night. Dad has not gone to work and the family cannot seem to decide what to do to find Bob. They are worried that he may have had an accident.

During her assessment, Mrs. James discovers that part of the reason Mr. Robbins is so upset is related to his past experience with a similar crisis event. Mr. Robbin's brother died in an alcohol-related automobile accident 20 years ago, after an argument with his brother. It is obvious that Bob's leaving has had a tremendous impact on Mr. Robbins. Mrs. Robbins is trying to console her husband, but she too is very upset about Bob and the danger he may be in. John is sitting nearby pounding the arm of the chair because his parents will not listen to what he has to say about why Bob left. Debbie is sleeping.

Intervention with the Robbins family will focus on secondary prevention and is directed toward helping members to discuss and define the problem and to express their feelings concerning Bob. The nurse is an active listener and participates attentively, but the family must do the work. The emphasis is on bringing feelings out into the open. Mrs. James must be truthful, honest, and forthright. She does not give false reassurance about son Bob or his whereabouts following a heated argument with his father in which Bob stormed out of the house the previous evening and has not returned home.

It is important at this stage not to let the anxiety become contagious. If Mrs. James begins to experience anxiety, she should step out and perhaps make a phone call to maintain perspective.

Exploration of coping mechanisms already used enables the nurse to help the family examine ways to cope. Mrs. James's involvement will include helping the family to explore other options for dealing with the situation. The pros and cons of each of these alternatives should be discussed with the family.

Mrs. James would discourage Mr. Robbins from blaming himself or others for the problem. Suggestions are made about how to find Bob, and what to do once he is found. Mrs. James recommends the alcohol and drug rehabilitation center nearby. In addition, she refers the family for counseling with an experienced counselor.

Referral resources depend upon the location of the community health nurse and the family. A list of potential resources for families in crisis can be found in Tables 18–3 and 18–4.

PRIMARY PREVENTION TO AVERT CRISIS

Primary crisis prevention techniques are widely used by community health nurses because all families experience crises. Primary prevention includes providing anticipatory guidance related to common crises of family life and assisting families to develop effec-

TABLE 18–3. RESOURCES FOR NURSES WORKING WITH FAMILIES

Problem Area	Agency or Organization	Services
Emotional support	Emotions Anonymous P.O. Box 4245 St. Paul, MN 55104 (612) 647-9712	Self-help for families with emotional problems
	National Support Center for Families of the Aging P.O. Box 245 Swarthmore, PA 19081 (215) 544-5933	Support for families responsible for elderly persons
	Family Services Assoc. of America 7645 Family Circle San Diego, CA 92111 (619) 279-0400	Family/individual counseling
	National Mental Health Association 1021 Prince St. Arlington, VA 22314 (703) 684-7722	Advocates for the mentally ill
	Family Counseling Services of the Court System Local, County, Parish or State offices	Conciliation court
	Catholic Community Services Department of Family Services Local office	Marriage preparation, education for responsible parenthood, counseling
	Families Anonymous P.O. Box 528 Van Nuys, CA 91408 (818) 989-7841	Assistance with drug-abuse problems
	Families in Action National Drug Information Center 3845 Druid Hills Rd., Suite 300 Decatur, GA 31033 (404) 325-5799	Information on drug abuse
Nutrition	U.S. Department of Agriculture Food & Nutrition Service Supplemental Food Program Division Special Supplemental Food Program for Women, Infants, & Children 3101 Park Center Dr. Alexandria, VA 22302 (703) 756-3746	Administers WIC food supplement program for women, infants, and children

TABLE 18–4. RESOURCES FOR NURSES WORKING WITH FAMILIES IN CRISIS

Focus	Agency or Organization	Services
National	National Council on Child Abuse & Family Violence 1050 Connecticut Ave., N.W. Suite 300 Washington, DC 20036 (202) 429-6695	Information
	National Council of Community Mental Health Centers 6101 Montrose Rd., Suite 360 Rockville, MD 20285 (301) 984-6200	Information, resources referral
	American Cancer Society National Office 90 Park Avenue New York, NY 10016 (212) 736-3030	Information, public education
Local	County or Parish Mental Health Services	Crisis intervention, involuntary commitment
	Office of Counselor of Mental Health Superior Court	Counseling, crisis intervention
	Rape Crisis Centers	Counseling, advocacy
	Family Crisis Centers	Crisis intervention, counseling
	Police	Crisis intervention, referral, involuntary commitment
	Social Services	Crisis intervention, referral for financial assistance, counseling, other referrals

tive coping strategies to combat the stress of situational crises.

It is impossible, and sometimes undesirable, to prevent a crisis situation from occurring. However, the nurse can assist the family to prepare for and cope with the event. For example, the birth of a child or change of employment may be a very desirable event. Such an event will require changes in life-style and family adaptation that might precipitate a crisis. The nurse can assist the family to explore areas in which change will be required, avenues for accomplishing these changes, and strategies for dealing with the anxiety related to change. Through primary prevention implemented via anticipatory guidance, a potential crisis may be averted even though the stressful event takes place.

EVALUATING CRISIS INTERVENTION

The evaluation process in crisis intervention is continuous as the nurse assesses the family's progress through the crisis event. A more formal evaluation phase may also be used to review the entire process of intervention with the family. This will include a systematic review of the crisis, the coping mechanisms used (old and new), and the result achieved. The emphasis is on reinforcing learning and strengthening the family for future crises.

CHAPTER HIGHLIGHTS

- Families are an important unit of service in community health nurses' efforts to enhance the health of the population.
- Families can take many forms. Some of the types of families encountered by community health nurses include nuclear conjugal families, extended families, single-parent families, step-families, cohabiting families, homosexual families, and communal families.
- All families share certain characteristics. These include existence as social systems that exhibit communication, roles, and subgroupings; possession of unique cultural values, structure, and function; and passage through a series of developmental stages.
- The epidemiologic prevention process model can be used to identify family health needs and to plan, implement, and evaluate nursing care given to families.
- Human biological considerations in family assessment include the physical health and needs of family members as well as the age,

sex, race, and genetic inheritance of each member.

- Physical environmental considerations include the size and condition of the family's home and information about the neighborhood.
- Considerations related to the psychological environment include communication patterns, family developmental stage, family relationships and dynamics, emotional strengths, coping strategies, child-rearing practices, roles, and family goals.
- Considerations in the family's social environment include religion, culture, social class and economic status, and external resources available to the family.
- Health system considerations in family assessment include the family's response to illness and use of health-care services.
- Nursing intervention with families can take place at primary, secondary, and tertiary levels of prevention.
- Crisis occurs when a family is faced with a problem that is seemingly unsolvable. A crisis is an event defined as such by the family. What is considered a crisis by one family may not be a crisis for another family.
- Families may experience two types of crisis—maturational and situational. Maturational crises occur when families encounter normal transition periods in family development that require changes in roles or communication patterns.
- Situational crises occur with sudden, unexpected, unpredictable events that threaten the family's integrity and lead to disorganization, tension, and anxiety.
- Three factors that influence family equilibrium and the occurrence of a crisis are the family's perception of the event, the family's coping abilities, and the presence or absence of situational support.
- A crisis begins with a hazardous event that puts a family in a vulnerable position. Family members may use defense mechanisms or coping mechanisms to deal with the hazardous event. A precipitating event may overtake members' coping abilities and result in crisis and inappropriate behavior.
- General principles of crisis intervention include the following:
  a. The nurse needs to listen actively to family members' perceptions of and feelings about the crisis event
  b. Family members need to express feelings openly and gain understanding of the crisis event
  c. The family needs to accept the reality of the situation and explore new ways of coping
  d. The family may need to be linked to a supportive social network
  e. The family must engage in problem solving to develop new coping strategies
  f. New coping strategies will need to be reinforced
  g. Follow-up will be needed after the crisis itself has been resolved

Review Questions

1. List at least five different types of families. What are the characteristic features of each type? (p. 396)
2. Identify at least three characteristics of families. Give an example of each characteristic. (p. 397)
3. Identify at least six of the eight stages of family development. Describe at least two developmental tasks to be accomplished in each stage. (p. 399)
4. Describe four considerations to be addressed in assessing family communication patterns. Give an example of each consideration. (p. 401)
5. What are the two central themes in assessing patterns of family dynamics? Give an example of the influence of each. (p. 403)
6. How do formal family roles differ from informal roles? Give an example of each type of role. (p. 404)
7. Differentiate between maturational and situational crises. Give an example of each type. (p. 411)
8. Describe the structure of a crisis event. Identify points at which nursing intervention could occur. (p. 412)
9. Identify at least four principles of crisis intervention. (p. 414)

APPLICATION AND SYNTHESIS

You are a community health nurse, and you have received a request to visit the Miller family. On arriving at their home, you find that the family recently moved to your district from Georgia and that they have been married for only 18 months.

Sandy, age 26, is 3 months pregnant and does not have a source of prenatal care. She is an experienced elementary school teacher but needs a state credential to teach in this district.

Jim, age 30, is an engineer. This is his second marriage; Jane, age 13, is his daughter from his previous marriage. Jane resents Jim's marriage to Sandy. Jim does not understand why Jane and Sandy argue so much. Many of the couple's disagreements occur over discipline for Jane. Jane is particularly hard to handle after a weekend spent with her own mother. Jane refuses to obey Sandy or to help around the house.

During your visit, Jane arrived home from school. Sandy asked her to go to her room and change clothes. Instead, Jane flopped down on the floor to watch television. At this point, Sandy yelled, "Wait til your father comes home, young lady!" You and Sandy moved into the kitchen so you could talk away from the noise of the TV.

Sandy tells you that Jim is not happy about the pregnancy. He is worried about the effect of another child on an already stretched budget. Sandy is pleased about the baby, even though at present she is experiencing a lot of nausea and backaches. She has not mentioned this to Jim because she does not want him to think she complains a lot. When asked, Sandy tells you that she has not gotten prenatal care because of the cost. She also tells you that she and Jim have not discussed her need for care or made any plans for the new baby.

To add to Sandy's current problems, Jim has never assisted with housework. He feels that this is "woman's work." Sandy has been doing her best to keep up the house, but she resents Jim's attitude, especially since she has not been feeling well. She also resents Jim making the decision that she will not work until the baby starts first grade when she has not even been consulted.

1. What human biological, environmental, life-style, and health system factors are operating in this situation?
2. What nursing diagnoses might you derive from the data included in the case description?
3. What primary prevention measures would be appropriate with this family? Why?
4. What secondary intervention strategies would you employ to deal with existing health problems? What tertiary prevention might be warranted in this situation?
5. What client-care objectives would you set for dealing with this family? How will you go about evaluating the achievement of those objectives?

REFERENCES

1. Murray, R., & Zentner, J. (1989). *Nursing assessment and health promotion strategies through the life span* (4th ed.). Norwalk, CT: Appleton & Lange.
2. Bohannan, P. (1985). *All the happy families: Exploring the variety of family life.* New York: McGraw-Hill.
3. Levitan, S., Belous, R., & Gallo, F. (1988). *What's happening to the American family?* (Revised ed.). Baltimore: Johns Hopkins University Press.
4. U.S. Department of Commerce. (1989). *Statistical Abstract of the United States, 1989* (109th ed.). Washington, DC: U.S. Department of Commerce.
5. Macklin, E. (1980). Nontraditional family forms: A decade of research. *Journal of Marriage and Family, 42,* 905.
6. Scanzoni, J., & Szinovacz, M. (1980). *Family decision making* (Vol. 3). Beverly Hills, CA: SAGE Library of Social Research.
7. Scanzoni, L. (1976). *Men, women, and change: A sociology of marriage and family.* New York: McGraw-Hill.
8. Piercy, F., & Sprenkle, D. (1986). *Family therapy sourcebook.* New York: Guilford Press.
9. Nichols, M. (1984). *Family therapy concepts and methods.* New York: Gardner Press.
10. Friedman, M. (1986). *Family nursing: Theory and assessment* (2d ed.). Norwalk, CT: Appleton-Century-Crofts.
11. Duvall, E. (1977). *Marriage and family development* (5th ed.). New York: J. B. Lippincott.
12. Hill, R. (1986). Life cycle stages of types of single parent families: Of family development theory. *Family Relations, 35*(1), 19–29.
13. Aguilera, D. (1990). *Crisis intervention: Theory and methodology* (6th ed.). St. Louis: C. V. Mosby.
14. Leavitt, M. (1982). *Families at risk.* Boston: Little, Brown.
15. Schoolcraft, V. (1984). *Nursing in the community.* New York: Wiley.
16. Wright, L., & Leahy, M. (1984). *Nurses and families.* Philadelphia: F. A. Davis.
17. Hoffman, L. (1981). *Foundations of family therapy.* New York: Basic Books.
18. Sawicki, S. (1988). Effective crisis intervention. *Adolescence, 23*(89), 83–88.
19. Wilson, H. S., & Kneisl, C. R. (1988). *Psychiatric nursing* (3d ed.). Menlo Park, CA: Addison Wesley.

RECOMMENDED READINGS

Amundson, M. (1989). Family crisis care: A home based intervention program for child abuse . . . in Hawaii. *Issues in Mental Health Nursing, 10*(3/4), 285–296.

Describes an intensive home-based crisis interaction and family education program to prevent the out-of-home placement of abused children and to teach families new problem-solving strategies through intensive in-home intervention.

Duffy, M. (1987). Strategies for change: The one-parent family. *Family and Community Health, 10*(2), 11–21.

Examines family resources, health risks, and strategies for change for single-parent families.

Lerner, H., & Byrne, M. (1991). Helping nursing students communicate with high-risk families. *Nursing & Health Care, 12*(2), 98–101.

Provides several useful strategies for improving communications with high-risk families.

Norton, A., & Glick, P. (1986). One parent families: A social and economic profile. *Family Relations, 35*(1), 9–17.

Reports findings on the economic and social status of single-parent families.

Olds, D., Henderson, C., Chamberlin, R., & Tatelbaum, R. (1986). Preventing child abuse and neglect: A randomized trial of nurse home visitation. *Pediatrics, 78*(1), 65–78.

Presents the findings of a study of home visitation to unmarried, teenage, and low socioeconomic status clients and families with infants and its effects on the incidence of child abuse and neglect.

Olds, D., Henderson, C., Tatelbaum, R., & Chamberlin, R. (1988). Improving the life-course development of socially disadvantaged mothers: A randomized trial of nurse home visitation. *American Journal of Public Health, 78*(11), 1436–1445.

Sets forth research findings on home visits to pregnant women and the effects on return to school, employment, and subsequent pregnancies.

Risman, B. (1986). Can men "mother"? Life as a single father. *Family Relations, 35*(1), 95–102.

Examines findings of a study of experiences of single fathers regarding homemaking, parental roles, and their relationships with their children.

Stetz, K., Lewis F., & Primomo, J. (1986). Family coping strategies and chronic illness in the mother. *Family Relations, 35,* 515–522.

Contains the findings of a study of the types of coping strategies used by families in which the mother has a chronic illness.

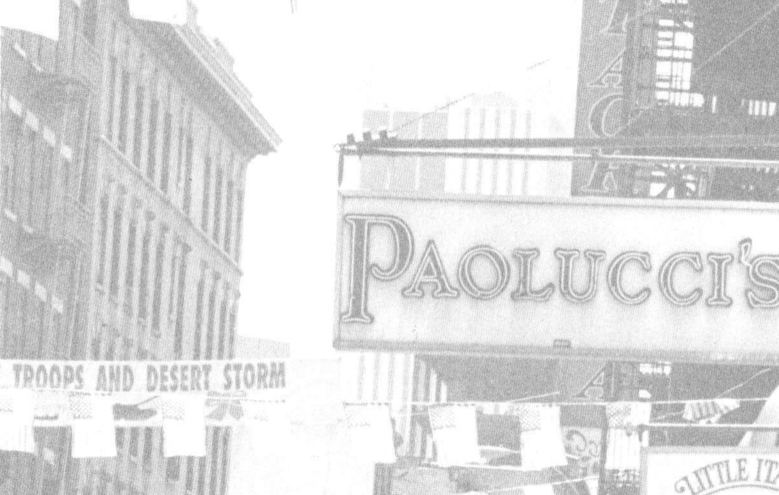

CHAPTER 19

Care of the Community or Target Group

KEY TERMS

age-specific death rate
Area Resource File (ARF)
cause-specific death rate
community assessment
crude death rate
forecasting
health index
key informant
participant observation
planning
screening
sensitivity
specificity
target group

When a community health nurse provides care to aggregates, the recipient of care—the client—may be an entire community or a subgroup within the community, called a target group. A ***target group*** can be either a particularly vulnerable subgroup within the population, such as the elderly, or a group with known health needs, such as people with AIDS. In either case, the nurse would apply the epidemiologic prevention process model to the care of the group rather than to specific individuals within the group. This chapter examines the application of the model to communities and target groups. The process used with both is the same, but information gathered will differ with the group addressed.

LEARNING OBJECTIVES

After reading this chapter you should be able to:

- Identify at least three purposes for assessing a community or a target group.
- Describe at least three factors that influence the scope of a community or target group assessment.
- Identify at least four considerations related to human biology to be addressed in a community or target group assessment.
- Describe at least six environmental factors to be considered in assessing a target group or a community.
- Describe at least four ways in which life-style factors can influence the health status of a community or target group.
- Identify three considerations in assessing the impact of the health-care system on the health of a community or target group.
- Describe two levels of nursing diagnoses related to the health status of a community or a target group.
- Describe at least three considerations in planning screening programs for communities and target groups.

(*continued*)

- Identify at least six tasks in planning health programs to meet the needs of communities or target groups.
- Describe the three levels of acceptance of a health-care program.
- Describe three types of considerations in evaluating a health-care program.

THE EPIDEMIOLOGIC PREVENTION PROCESS MODEL AND THE CARE OF COMMUNITIES AND TARGET GROUPS

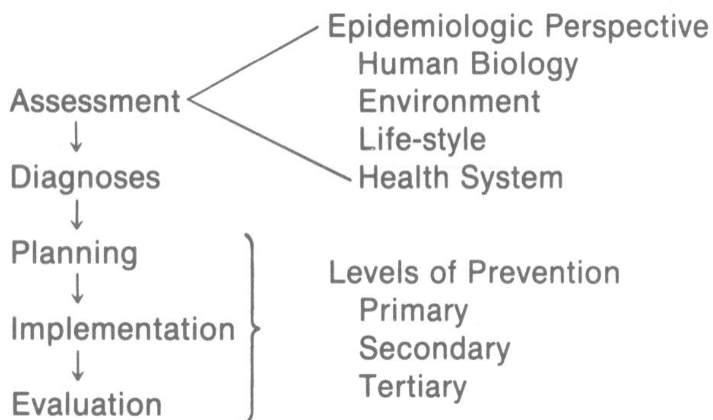

Community health nurses working with communities or target groups as clients use the epidemiologic prevention process model to identify client needs and to direct action to meet those needs. The process begins by assessing group needs and proceeds to a diagnosis of health problems. These steps are followed by the planning and implementation of health programs to meet the health needs of the group. The process concludes with an evaluation of the adequacy of those programs.

ASSESSING THE HEALTH OF COMMUNITIES AND TARGET GROUPS

Community assessment has been identified as one of the primary tasks of community health nurses.[1] ***Community assessment*** is the process by which data are compiled regarding a community's health status and from which nursing diagnoses are derived. Such assessment consists of the collection of two types of data: (1) data specific to the community or target group itself and (2) general information about particular problems of interest such as adolescent pregnancy, the incidence of AIDS, motor vehicle fatalities, and so on. General information is used to make comparisons between the community or target group and larger segments of society that aid in identifying strengths and weaknesses. General information collected might include state and national data on the extent of particular problems as well as information on factors contributing to those problems.

An accurate assessment is the basis of any community health endeavor and is essential to planning any program designed to meet health-related needs. Community or target group assessment provides a ***health index,*** a summary of a population's health status, which serves as a basis for planning to meet health-care needs. Without a clear picture of the health needs of the community or target group, health-care providers have no way of determining whether current programs are meeting health needs or how to go about planning programs that will.

PREPARING TO ASSESS THE HEALTH OF A COMMUNITY OR TARGET GROUP

Prior to beginning an assessment of the health status of a community or target group, the community health nurse should determine the purpose and scope of the assessment, the types of data to be collected, sources of data, and methods for data collection.

Determining the Purpose and Scope of the Assessment

The purpose for assessing a target group or community will determine the types of data to be collected, as well as the scope of the assessment. The first purpose of assessment is to determine the health status of a community or target group.[2] The nurse uses data derived from the assessment to develop community or target group diagnoses and then plans, implements, and evaluates programs designed to promote health and resolve existing health problems. For example, a community health nurse might assess the whole community or the target group of elderly persons within the community to determine what health-care needs exist, and then participate in designing programs to meet those needs. A second purpose for community assessment is to provide an understanding of the magnitude of a particular problem within the population and to identify factors contributing to its presence.[2] Assessment might be undertaken, for instance, to determine the extent of premature births in a community or in a target group such as migrant farm workers. Community or target group assessment can also be used to determine the health-related concerns of group members or to identify health-related resources available to the population and the extent to which those resources are used.[2] A final purpose of community or target group assessment might be to increase the awareness of policymakers of both health and nonhealth issues of concern to community members.[3] This awareness will allow policymakers to establish priorities among a variety of needs in allocating scarce resources.

The scope, or depth and complexity, of a community or target group assessment depends on a number of factors.[2] First, if the purpose of the assessment is to determine the group's health status, the assessment will need to be much more extensive than if the purpose is to obtain additional data about a known problem. Second, the size of the population will also affect the assessment. A small target group can be assessed in greater depth than can a community at large for the same expenditure of money and effort. Third, the time available for the assessment may limit its scope. If information is required within a specified period of time, the nurse may be limited in the depth of assessment possible. Fourth, a limiting factor may be the degree of expertise of those conducting the assessment. Fifth, the relationship between the cost and the perceived benefits of an in-depth assessment may also contribute to limitations on the scope of the assessment undertaken. Finally, the political environment within the community may affect the comprehensiveness of any assessment. If policymakers or group members do not place a high priority on health, they are unlikely to support an extensive assessment of health needs.

Selecting Data-collection Methods and Sources

When the scope of an assessment is limited by any of these factors, the community health nurse will need to decide what categories of data will be needed to accomplish the purpose of the assessment. In this chapter the focus will be on categories of data that would be collected in a comprehensive assessment of a community or a target group. In an assessment of lesser scope, the community health nurse must determine what categories of data are essential to accomplish the purpose of the assessment and what information may safely be left out.

A variety of methods will usually be used to collect the data needed for the assessment. Both quantitative and qualitative approaches should be used to assess the health status of communities or target groups.[4] *Quantitative* approaches involve the collection of numbers of events. *Qualitative* approaches focus on examination of perceptions of health, attitudes, and health concerns as voiced by members of the population. For example, in obtaining information on the use of health-care services by group members, quantitative methods would be used to gather data on the numbers of people who received care at various facilities; group members' perceptions of health-care services and their reasons for using or not using them would be more easily obtained using qualitative methods of data collection.

Quantitative data may be obtained by reviewing statistics compiled by health-care agencies and other sources at the local, state, and national level. For example, the nurse might obtain information on the racial composition of a community from published census figures, or the nurse might obtain figures on the incidence of child abuse from records kept by child protection agencies or from law-enforcement officials. The community health nurse might also obtain quantitative data by conducting surveys and compiling figures on the frequency of certain responses. For instance, the nurse might ask a sample of elderly persons how often they see a physician. The nurse might also obtain quantitative data through observations. As an example, the nurse might drive through the community noting each fire station on a map and then calculating the maximum distance of any point in the community from a fire station. This information would provide one indicator of the adequacy of protective services in the community.

Surveys and observations can also be used to obtain qualitative data about a community or target group. Community or group members can be asked about their attitudes to health and health-care services, for example, or about their perceptions of community health needs. It is important to remember that a diversity of community members should be approached for information because people's opinions and perceptions can vary greatly. This is particularly true of perceptions held by general residents of a community and the health-care providers within the community.[5]

Community health nurses might also conduct interviews with members of the community and with "key informants." ***Key informants*** are people who, because of their position in the community, possess information and insights about the community. Examples of key informants include public officials, school and health-care personnel, prominent business people, and local clergy. Again, it is important not to restrict interviews to these sources, but also to interview typical residents of the community because of the possible differences in perceptions of the community's health needs.

Participant observation is another means of gathering qualitative data. In ***participant observation,*** the community health nurse participates in the life of the community or target group making observations about health and health needs in the course of that participation. For example, the nurse might look for housing in the community and, in the search, observe housing conditions and determine rents typical of different areas of the community. Or, the nurse assessing the needs of the alcoholic population might attend meetings of an Alcoholics Anonymous (AA) group or spend time in a detoxification center.

Different methods of data collection are appropriate to different types of information. Appropriate methods for gathering specific data needed to assess the health of communities or target groups will be addressed later in this chapter.

Where does one find the information needed for a community or target group assessment? Prior to beginning an assessment, the community health nurse should identify several potential sources. Additional sources will usually be uncovered during the course of the assessment, but the nurse needs an identified starting point for data collection.

A wide variety of data sources provides the information required for community or target group assessment. Usually the local chamber of commerce can supply information regarding community size, history, industry, and facilities for transportation, communication, and recreation. Information about many population characteristics such as age, sex, race and language, income and educational levels, employment, and marital status can be obtained from the most recent census figures, as can some statistics related to housing. Similar information related to a particular target group may be less easy to find unless the group is one that is of interest to government officials or other agencies that gather statistics. For example, the nurse might be able to get information on people with certain types of cancer from a local cancer registry, or obtain information about older persons from the local office on aging.

Basic data from the most recent census can be found in most public and university libraries. More detailed census information is available from libraries designated as government document repositories. Libraries of large universities and large metropolitan areas are usually so designated. If there is no repository of government documents nearby, information can be obtained directly from the Bureau of Census located in Atlanta, Georgia. This office is also capable of providing recently collected data on microfiche prior to its publication in printed form.

Local school systems are good sources of information regarding the availability of educational facilities and immunization levels. Information regarding the presence of various religious groups in the community can be obtained from the yellow pages of the telephone directory, while further information on religious affiliation can be sought from local houses of worship.

The yellow pages are also an excellent source of information on the availability of health-care services and resources, transportation, and formal communication networks. In some communities, local agencies compile lists of referral resources for a variety of health-related services. A local Headstart program, for example, is required by federal standards to provide this type of information to parents of children enrolled.

Information on protective services can be obtained from the local government or police and fire departments. Statements of the adequacy of services can be validated in interviews with members of the community or target group or with insurance company representatives. The local health department can provide statistics related to births, deaths, and morbidity, as well as data on the availability and use of health resources and services. Information on water supply and waste disposal can also usually be obtained from health department sources.

Local government officials can provide information on the priority given to health-care programs in the budget. Many industries provide some forms of health-care services and would also have records of expenditures of this nature, as would insurance companies. Local voluntary and official health-care agencies can also be sources of information on health-care financing.

Area maps provide an idea of the size of the community and the presence or absence of recreational facilities. Maps can also provide information on thoroughfares that serve as links with the outside world.

Other possible sources of organized data include the local hospital association, local chapters of professional and business organizations, and voluntary agencies, such as the American Diabetes Association. Key persons in the community, both official and unofficial, can provide information as well. Specific sources of information will be addressed later in this chapter in relation to the categories of data that comprise a community or target group assessment.

There are some types of information, however, for which no records are available. Such information must be obtained by the nurse through personal observation and through contact with members of the community or target group. Community attitudes to health are one example of this type of data. Figures on the use of health-care services can provide a partial and indirect indication of attitudes, but nonuse may reflect the effects of cost or other barriers rather than a low priority given to health. The perceptive community health nurse derives information about attitudes based on the feeling tone of contacts with group members. For example, the nurse would note whether community members are receptive to suggestions regarding health practices and whether they would expend energy or resources to resolve an identified health problem.

COMPONENTS OF A COMMUNITY ASSESSMENT

Community health nurses can use Dever's epidemiologic perspective to guide the assessment of a total population or community. Human biological, environmental, life-style, and health-system factors influencing community health are examined.

Human Biology

Human biological factors influencing community health reflect specific physical attributes of community members. The first of these attributes relates to maturation and aging. Others reflect the genetic inheritance and physiologic function of community members.

Maturation and Aging. The composition of the population by age groups is an important indicator of probable health needs. Typically, there is an increased need for health services in areas with large numbers of the very young and the very old. Large numbers of women of childbearing age will increase needs for antepartal and family-planning services. Accident prevention is a major consideration in communities with large numbers of school-age and younger children. Information on the age composition of the population can be obtained from census figures for the census tracts that make up the community.

Another community factor related to maturation and aging is the annual birthrate, which provides information on the growth of the younger segments of the population. The annual birthrate is calculated on the basis of the number of live births during the year in relation to the total population of the community. As is true of several of the other rates discussed in Chapter 6, The Epidemiologic Process, the proportion of live births to the population is multiplied by 1000 to give the rate of births per 1000 persons. Birth statistics are usually compiled by local and state health agencies and can be obtained from these sources.

Age-specific death rates also provide valuable information regarding the health status of the community. An ***age-specific death rate*** is the number of deaths in a particular age group compared to the population within that group. Because of the relatively small number of deaths in some age groups, the multiplier used in calculating age-specific death rates is 100,000. Excess deaths (deaths over the number that would be expected for that age group in the general population) for any age group in the community would indicate the presence of health problems. Mortality statistics are available from state and local health agencies.

The average age at death also provides an indication of overall community health. If people in the community typically die at a relatively young age, this suggests the existence of health problems that are contributing to these early deaths. Native Americans, for example, have shorter expected life spans than the rest of the population because of the high incidence of such health problems as chronic disease and alcoholism, and also to high rates of homicide. A large proportion of the Native American population will die before age 45 compared to an average life expectancy of 75 years for the general public.[6] Information on age at death may be compiled by local health agencies, but may also be obtained by a review of death certificates or examination of obituaries published in local newspapers.

Genetic Inheritance. One feature of the genetic inheritance of the population is its distribution by sex. Many health problems such as obesity, hypertension, and various forms of cancer are more prevalent in one sex than in the other. Knowing the sex distribution in the community will sharpen the index of suspicion with regard to these problems. Knowledge of the composition of the population with respect to sex will assist the nurse to identify health needs and plan programs to meet them. For instance, knowledge that women constitute 79 percent of the population of a particular community might suggest the need for easily accessible detection programs for cancer of the cervix and breast.

The racial composition of the community is another important factor in assessment. Knowledge of the ethnicity and racial origin of the population will help to pinpoint health problems known to be prevalent in certain groups, such as sickle cell disease in blacks or diabetes in some Native American tribes. Data on both the sex and racial composition of the community population are available in census figures as well as from state and local agencies.

Physiologic Function. Information on physiologic function in the community is derived from morbidity and mortality data as well as other health status indicators such as immunization levels. Mortality rates of concern to the community health nurse include the crude death rate, cause-specific death rates, and death rates among specific segments of the population, such as the elderly, minority groups, and the homeless, to name a few.

The ***crude death rate*** reflects all deaths in the population regardless of age or cause of death and is calculated using the formula presented in Chapter 6, The Epidemiologic Process. The crude death rate presents a picture of the overall health status of the community, but it does not suggest the presence of specific health problems that may be contributing to deaths.

Cause-specific death rates, on the other hand, do provide information about specific health problems within the community. Cause-specific death rates are the number of deaths in the population attributable to specific conditions such as diabetes, heart disease, suicide, and so on. They are calculated in proportion to the total population using a multiplier of 100,000. When death rates due to specific causes are higher than those of populations with a comparable age composition, there may be a need for health-care programs dealing with these causes of death. Mortality statistics are compiled by state and local health departments. Information on mortality may also be available from other sources. For example, insurance companies or trauma centers might be able to provide information on motor vehicle fatalities, while homicide figures may be available from local law enforcement agencies.

The majority of health problems are nonfatal, and many existing health problems in the community are not brought to light by examining mortality statistics alone. For this reason, the nurse must consider morbidity as well as mortality rates. Morbidity rates reflect the extent of illness present in the community. The two morbidity statistics of greatest significance in community assessment are prevalence and incidence rates. Prevalence rates indicate the *total* number of cases of a particular condition at any given time. Incidence rates indicate the number of *new* cases of the condition identified over a period of time. For example, there may have been eight new cases of tuberculosis diagnosed in Clark County last month (incidence), but there are 39 people in the county who are currently under treatment for active tuberculosis (prevalence).

Local and state health departments compile statistics on the incidence and prevalence of certain reportable health conditions. These conditions include many communicable diseases, but may also include other conditions for which special surveillance programs are in place. For example, in some areas information is compiled on newly diagnosed cases of hypertension. For other conditions, the nurse may need to seek other sources of data. Cancer registries, for example, may be a source of information about the incidence and prevalence of certain forms of cancer, while local health-care facilities and providers may have figures related to the incidence of other conditions. For example, the local hospital may have data on the number of clients hospitalized for diabetes, myocardial infarction, and so on.

Immunization levels within the community also provide information on the physiologic function of community members. Information on immunization levels is usually extrapolated from immunization figures derived from school records. In areas where a large number of school-age children are not immunized, there are probably also large numbers of unimmunized younger children, and overall immunization levels in the general population are also likely to be low. School immunization records are not always an accurate indicator of high immunization levels, however. Because immunization is required for school entry in most places, school-age children may be immunized, while younger children remain unimmunized. For additional data on immunization levels, the nurse might want to examine the records of public immunization clinics as well as those of private physicians who provide immunization services.

Comparison figures on morbidity and mortality at state and national levels can be obtained from state health departments and from various federal publications, respectively. One publication that contains a great deal of information on morbidity and mortality statistics is the *Morbidity and Mortality Weekly Report* published by the Centers for Disease Control. National morbidity and mortality data can also be obtained from health and life insurance companies as well as specialty agencies concerned with specific health problems, such as the American Cancer Society or the American Heart Association.

Environment

Factors in the physical, psychological, and social environments also affect the health status of a community.

Physical Environment. Physical environmental factors affecting a community include its location, its type (for example, rural, urban, or suburban) and size, topographical features, and climate. Other physical factors to be assessed include the type and adequacy of housing in the community and considerations related to water supply, nuisance factors, and potential for disaster.

The location, climate, and physical geography or topography of the community will provide indications of some health problems likely to be identified in the course of the nurse's assessment. An area that is heavily wooded, for example, might increase the index of suspicion for problems such as Rocky Mountain spotted fever or Lyme disease. On the other hand, a dry, arid desert area would be more conducive to problems of heat exhaustion and sodium chloride loss.

Size and population density, as well as the type of community, are other factors that influence the type of health problems encountered. Certain health problems are more prevalent in urban areas than in rural ones and vice versa. Statistics indicate that suicide is more prevalent in urban communities, while one would expect a problem like rabies to occur more often in a rural area where wild animals are likely to be infected. Urban dwellers are less likely to encounter rabid animals because of regulations regarding vaccination of pets.

Housing is another important physical environmental factor. Inadequate, unsafe, or unsanitary housing conditions contribute to a variety of health problems including communicable diseases spread by poor sanitation, lead poisoning due to lead-based paint in older homes in poor repair, and unintentional injuries resulting from safety hazards. Overcrowding has been found to increase the incidence of a number of health concerns. Communicable diseases are spread more rapidly in crowded conditions, but the prevalence of stress-related conditions such as alcohol abuse, suicide, and other forms of violence increases with crowding as well.

The source of a community's water supply is another important physical environmental consideration. Are most residents supplied by local water systems or do they have independent wells? The nurse should investigate the potability, or drinkability, of the community's water. Is the community's water supply safe for drinking, or does it pose biological or chemical hazards to health? Moreover, the nurse should explore the presence or absence of fluoride in the water supply as an indicator of dental health.

Disposal of wastes is another area of consideration in assessing the physical environment of a community. The nurse should ascertain disposal methods for various types of materials. Of particular concern is the disposal of hazardous wastes. Do disposal methods ensure adequate safeguards for the health of the public, or is there potential for environmental pollution as a result of waste disposal? Concerns about hazardous waste disposal were addressed in Chapter 16, Environmental Influences on Community Health.

The nurse may also need to assess whether physical factors within the community contribute to accidental injuries. For example, there may be particularly dangerous intersections where motor vehicle accidents occur frequently, or there may be large numbers of swimming pools in the area that contribute to the incidence of drownings.

Nuisance factors such as insects, noxious plants, and other substances may provide physical health hazards or prove offensive to the senses, thereby decreasing the quality of life in the community. Nearby dairy farms, for example, might provide insect breeding grounds that contribute to the incidence of insect-borne diseases. Or there might be an airport that presents a noise hazard. Another consideration in terms of nuisances is the presence of various pollutants in the environment. The effects of pollution and the community health nurse's responsibility with regard to pollution were discussed in Chapter 16. In doing a community assessment, the nurse would obtain information related to the presence of environmental pollutants in the community being served.

The last factor to be addressed with respect to the physical environment is the potential for either natural or manmade disasters within the community. Is the community located on a major fault line and subject to earthquakes? Is there a chemical manufacturing plant close by that presents a potential hazard? Assessment of the potential for disaster and the community health nurse's role in planning for disaster response are addressed in more detail in Chapter 30, Care of Clients in Disaster Settings.

For the most part, information on the physical environmental characteristics of the community can be obtained through observation. For example, the nurse might drive through the community assessing its geographic features, nuisance factors, and the general adequacy of housing. Information about pollution, water supply, and waste disposal might be obtained from local government bureaus or the nearby public health agency. Data on population size and density are available from census figures or from local government agencies. This information, as well as information on the typical climate and geographic features, may also be available in local publications or from the chamber of commerce.

Psychological Environment. The psychological environment within the community influences the health of community members by increasing or mediating their exposure to stress and affects the ability of the community to function effectively. In addition, elements of the psychological environment may enhance or impede community action to resolve identified health problems. Some of the areas to be considered in assessing the psychological environment include the future prospects of the community, significant events in community history and the community's response to those events, communication networks existing within the community, and the adequacy of protective services. Other considerations in this area include evidence of psychological problems such as suicide and homicide rates and identifiable sources of stress within the community.

Information about community prospects contributes to the picture of the psychological climate within the community. If a community is a growing and productive one, for example, there is less likelihood of apathy regarding community problems than might be the case if the community is economically depressed and faltering. A community that is in decline or has multiple problems is also more likely to have multiple sources of stress that affect the health of its residents.

Likewise, knowledge of the community's history can provide insight into previous and current health problems and how the community has dealt with them. Historical information may also provide some clue as to how the community will deal with subsequent problems and where community strengths lie. For example, historical information on the cohesive response of community members to a past crisis suggests a strength that will enable the community to face future crises.

The psychological environment created by relationships between subgroups within the community should also be explored. Harmonious relations between groups indicate a psychological climate that is conducive to concerted community action to resolve identified problems. Tension and distrust between groups, on the other hand, may make resolution of community health problems more difficult. The community health nurse should be alert to unrest and conflict between groups within the community and the implications of such psychological tensions for the health of the community and its members.

The adequacy of protective services provided by law enforcement, fire, and other emergency personnel can profoundly influence the psychological climate of an area. Adequate protective services help to create a psychological environment that enhances feelings of personal safety and security. In areas where these services are inadequate to meet residents' needs, stress and insecurity are created and can negatively influence the health of the population. The nurse assessing the health of a community would obtain information about the availability and quality of police and fire services, as well as information on the availability and adequacy of legal services, services for victims of abuse, and consumer protection services.

Communication is an important contributing factor in the psychological climate of a community, so the nurse would also want to explore the communication network that exists there. Communication may take place via formal or informal channels. Formal channels include media such as radio, television, and newspapers, as well as the form that public announcements may take. Informal communications take place outside of these channels and may also influence the health of the community. For example, rumors about a particular religious or ethnic group may serve to exacerbate intergroup tension and strife. The degree of trust placed in official formal communications is another element of the psychological environment that may enhance or detract from community health.

Other indicators of the psychological environment in a community include annual incidence rates for homicide and suicide. Rates for specific subgroups within the community should also be examined, for there is usually considerable variation among different racial and ethnic groups. For example, both suicide and homicide rates are usually higher for minority group members than for the general population in most communities. Examination of these figures and their distribution in the population may help the nurse to identify factors contributing to poor psychological health in certain subgroups or in the population in general.

Finally, the nurse would want to identify common sources of stress within the environment. Widespread unemployment, lack of available housing, and crowded living conditions are examples of sources of stress in a community. These and other sources of stress serve to create a psychological environment that is not conducive to health.

Information on the psychological environment of the community will be obtained primarily through observations by the community health nurse and through interviews with area residents. Again, it is important to get a broad representation of community membership among the people interviewed.[5]

Social Environment. From the previous discussion it is clear that social and psychological environments are closely interrelated. Social environmental factors influence the psychological environment and have other effects on health as well. Considerations in assessing the social environment include information about community government and leadership, language, income and educational levels, marital status and family composition, and religion. Other areas to be addressed include transportation and the availability of goods and services needed by residents.

A community's government and power structure are important considerations in terms of planning and implementing programs designed to solve community health problems. Who holds the purse strings? How are decisions made? Who are the decision-makers in the community? The community health nurse should discover who are the formal and informal community leaders. In one isolated community, for example, no program was successful unless it first received approval from one elderly matriarch. It was she who controlled the community despite the presence of elected officials.

Information on the community's official leadership can be obtained from the mayor's office or from other local governmental agencies. Informal leaders may be more difficult to identify, but the nurse can ask key informants in the community (for example, school principals, clergy, and official leaders) who the informal leaders are. Other health-care providers and business leaders might also provide information on informal leadership within the community.

Language is another important social factor affecting the health of community members. The nurse should assess the degree to which language presents a barrier to health education or to the provision of other health-care services. Again, key informants in the community can provide the nurse with information about languages spoken. School teachers and principals, for example, will be knowledgeable about languages spoken by their students. The nurse may also derive this information from personal observation in the community. For example, the nurse may spend time observing in stores where large segments of the population shop or check for newspapers and radio and television broadcasts in languages other than English. Another aspect of language to be assessed is the use of colloquialisms by local residents.[7] Are there unique ways in which community members express themselves? Unfortunately, much of this information is gleaned by trial-and-error on the part of the nurse. However, the nurse can ask key informants about the use of colloquialisms and about their meaning.

Closely related to language are the cultural affiliations of community members. The nurse will need to assess the host of cultural factors within the community that affect its health status. (See Chapter 15, Cultural Influences on Community Health.) Information on cultural groups in the community can be obtained from key informants and through observation.

The average income of community residents also has bearing on a community's health status. Economic status influences the ability of residents to provide for basic necessities and to gain access to health-care services. In addition, the income of residents will influence the tax base of the community and the types of services that the community is able to provide its citizens. For example, when many residents are unemployed or have low incomes, they have less money to spend. Businesses take in less money and community revenues from sales and other taxes are decreased. Consequently, the community is less able to provide essential services for its citizens.

Income is closely related to educational level. Less well-educated people may have lower-paying jobs. They also tend to have less health-related knowledge, and, consequently, lower levels of health. Both income and educational levels are indicators of a community's standard of living and, indirectly, of its health status. The prevalence of several acute and chronic conditions in the population (for example, tuberculosis, pneumonia, and heart disease) tends to decline as income and educational levels rise. Information on income and educational levels can be obtained from census figures. This information may also be available from local government agencies or school districts.

In addition to determining the educational level of the population, the nurse will assess the community's educational resources. This information will enable the nurse to make diagnoses regarding the adequacy of community resources for meeting identified health needs. The telephone directory is a good starting place for obtaining information on educational facilities in the area. The nurse could then interview administrators of those facilities or review their brochures and other publications to determine the types of educational programs offered. Local school personnel can also provide information on educational opportunities in the community.

Religious affiliations within a community can either foster or impede health practices. The nurse should be aware of religious beliefs that may affect health or may influence the acceptability of health programs to community members. For example, some religious groups may be averse to the idea of providing on-site health-care services in high schools because of the fear that contraceptive services will be provided. (See Chapter 15, Cultural Influences on Community Health, for more information on the influence of religion on health.) Again, the telephone directory can provide a picture of the religious groups represented in the community, while the membership rosters of specific houses of worship can provide information on the number of people affiliated with each religious group.

Marital status and family composition are social environmental factors that might influence the health of communities. The nurse will determine the number of families in the community that consist of single parents with children or older persons living alone. Generally speaking, married individuals have lower death and illness rates than those who are unmarried, so information on marital status in the community can provide clues to overall health status. Information on marriage and family composition is available from census data for the community.

Accessibility of transportation is an important factor related to the use of health services and is, therefore, a necessary component of the nurse's assessment of the community. Transportation difficulties compound health problems in areas where there are large numbers of poor and elderly, the chronically ill or disabled, mothers with small children, and persons who are poorly motivated with respect to health. The nurse can obtain information on the number of families with cars from community census data. Information on other forms of transportation can be gleaned from the telephone directory and by contacting bus and taxi companies to determine routes, fares, and so on.

In addition, the community health nurse would obtain data on the types and adequacy of goods and services available to community members. Areas to be considered include the recreational programs available, the adequacy of local shopping facilities, prices for goods and services purchased locally, and the availability and accessibility of social service programs to meet the needs of community members. Much of this information can be obtained through participant observation. For example, the nurse might shop in local stores or look for recreational pursuits. Information is also available in the telephone directory on the number and types of stores and services available. Perusal of newspaper advertisements will also provide information on local prices. Finally, the nurse can contact personnel at local social service agencies to obtain information about the services offered.

Life-style

Life-style factors also influence the health status of a community and its members. Areas to be addressed in this portion of the assessment include community consumption patterns, occupations, leisure pursuits, and other health-related behaviors.

Consumption Patterns. Consumption patterns play a major part in the development of health or illness. In assessing consumption patterns in the community, the nurse would examine dietary patterns and the use of potentially harmful substances.

Information will be needed on the general nutritional level of community members and on specific dietary patterns. For example, the nurse might want to know the prevalence of overweight individuals in the population or the incidence of anemia in school-age children. Another area for consideration is any ethnic nutritional patterns that might influence health either positively or negatively. For example, movement away from traditional tribal foods to typical American dietary practices has contributed to obesity and a variety of chronic diseases among many Native Americans.[8] Information on dietary patterns may be obtained by interviews and surveys of community residents as well as by observation of foods purchased in grocery stores.

Use of harmful substances is another area for exploration. The nurse should determine the level of alcohol consumption within the community, both for the community at large and for specific target groups. The extent of both legal and illegal drug use may also merit investigation. The nurse would determine the types of substances abused and the typical sources of abused substances. Finally, the nurse would determine the number of residents who smoke and whether the number of smokers is increasing or decreasing. Indirect indicators of use of alcohol, drugs, and tobacco include the extent of sales of these items in the community. This information can be obtained from interviews with personnel in stores that sell these items or from information on related taxes collected. Information on substance abuse may be reflected in law enforcement agencies' records regarding arrests or accidents related to drugs and alcohol. Information can also be obtained on the number of admissions to drug and alcohol treatment facilities. Community self-help groups such as a local chapter of Alcoholics Anonymous may also provide information on the extent of substance abuse problems.

Occupation. In view of the large numbers of people within a community who are usually employed, it is important to assess types of occupations and health hazards involved. Persons in some occupational groups are at higher risk for certain health problems than those in other groups. For example, histoplasmosis is a frequent occurrence among people who work with birds (for example, poultry farmers), while black lung (pneumoconiosis) is prevalent among coal miners. Information about community businesses and industries is available from the local chamber of commerce. The numbers of people employed in specific occupations can be obtained from major employers in the area.

The nurse would also obtain information about other health hazards presented by jobs performed by community residents. Questions to be addressed include the potential for exposure to hazardous substances (for example, asbestos or chlorine gas), radiation, noise, or vibration, as well as the potential for injury due to falls or use of hazardous equipment. In addition to determining the potential for occupational injury or illness, the nurse would obtain figures on the extent to which such conditions occur. This type of information may be obtained from the illness and accident records of major employers or may be available from the state occupational health agency.

In addition to information about employment, the level of unemployment in the community provides an indication of possible health problems. Unemployment contributes to stress and to decreased income levels that affect access to health care as well as other necessary goods and services. Unemployment figures can be obtained from state or local employment offices.

Leisure Pursuits. Information about leisure activities prevalent in the community can also indicate the potential for certain kinds of health problems. For example, boating, waterskiing, and related recreational activities increase the risk of drowning and similar accidents. On the other hand, if watching television is the primary form of recreation, there may be increased potential for heart disease and other conditions associated with a sedentary life-style. The presence or absence of recreational opportunities in the community may also affect the psychological environment and the ability of community members to deal with stress effectively. Information on leisure-related exercise is usually obtained by means of interviews and surveys. To determine the extent of community interest in various forms of exercise, the nurse might also contact groups that offer exercise-related classes or sell related equipment. In addition, the nurse can observe for joggers or other exercise enthusiasts as he or she moves about the community. Information on recreational opportunities can be gotten from the telephone directory, from direct observation, and from events publicized in the newspaper or other means of communication employed in the community.

Other Behaviors. The community health nurse will also assess the prevalence of other health-related behaviors by community members. For example, the nurse would obtain information on the extent of seatbelt use in passenger vehicles or the use of safety devices in certain occupational settings. The nurse would also be interested in such behaviors as the extent of heterosexual and homosexual activity and use of condoms and other forms of protection against conception and sexually transmitted diseases. Two negative indicators of contraceptive use are the proportion of births that are illegitimate and the local abortion rate. In areas with a high prevalence of intravenous drug use, the nurse would also try to obtain information on the extent of needle sharing and other practices that contribute to the spread of diseases such as AIDS and hepatitis. Much of this information will only be available to the community health nurse through observation and through interviews of key informants in the community.

Health System

Health system factors can profoundly affect the health of a community. One of the primary influences arises from the availability or lack of health-care services. In assessing the community's well-being, community health nurses would obtain information on the type of health services available to residents. What types of primary, secondary, and tertiary preventive services are available? How adequate are these services to meet the needs of the people? The nurse would examine the availability and accessibility of specific types of services and how effectively they are used. For example, one might enquire as to the percentage of pregnant women who receive prenatal care and at what point in the pregnancy care usually begins. The nurse might also investigate the availability of services provided by emergency medical personnel and by emergency rooms or trauma centers. Other questions relate to the availability and accessibility of certain types of health-care providers. For example, there may be several physicians in town, but none of them provide prenatal services because of malpractice concerns.

Information on health-care services available in the community may be obtained from the telephone directory and from personal observation. Referral services provided by professional organizations or agencies such as local senior citizens groups can also supply information on health-care providers and facilities in the community. Health-care institutions are also a source of information on services provided, fees involved, and so on. Another source is the ***Area Resource File*** (ARF), a computerized, county-based data system containing information on available health professionals, facilities, and education as well as other information. The ARF is maintained by the Office of Data Analysis and Management of the Health Resources and Services Administration.[9]

The nurse would also determine to what extent available services are overused or underused. What factors contribute to overuse and to underuse? For example, emergency room services might be overused because many community members cannot afford a regular source of health care and seek care only in crisis situations. Conversely, the services of clinics and physicians might be underused because they are offered at inconvenient times or places or because people have no means of transportation to such services. Or, residents may simply not be aware of the need for or availability of certain services. Utilization figures can be obtained from health-care facilities and providers in the community.

Another area for consideration is the financing of community health care. Questions to be addressed include who pays for health-care services, the adequacy of funding sources to meet community health needs, the priority given to health-related concerns in planning community budgetary allocations, the extent of health insurance coverage among community members, and the availability of funds to pay for care for the indigent. (See Chapter 13, Economic Influences on Community Health.) Information on health insurance may be available from insurance agencies or major health-care facilities in the area. Health-care facility records may also contain data on the percentage of the population without health insurance. Information about recipients of Medicaid and Medicare benefits is available from the agencies that administer these programs.

Financing of health care can also provide an indirect indication of prevailing community attitudes toward health. For example, adequate health-care budgeting indicates that health is considered a public priority. Budgetary information can be solicited from public officials. Other considerations related to the health system include community definitions of health and illness and the use of culturally prescribed health practices and practitioners. (See Chapter 15, Cultural Influences on Community Health.)

A tool for assessing the health status of a community from the epidemiologic perspective of human biology, environment, life-style, and health system is included in Appendix H, the Health Intervention Planning Guide—Community Client.

COMPONENTS OF A TARGET GROUP ASSESSMENT

Similar factors are considered in assessing the health of a target group. Human biological, environmental, life-style, and health system elements influence the health of subgroups in the population as well as the total population.

Human Biology

In examining human biological factors, the nurse would obtain information on the age, race, and sex composition of the target group. Other necessary information in this category relates to the incidence and prevalence of specific health conditions among group members. For example, the incidence of alcohol abuse is particularly high among Native Americans, while tuberculosis is prevalent among Asian refugee groups.

Mortality data related to the group, such as the crude death rate, cause-specific death rates, and age-specific death rates, are also important. For example, the infant mortality rate for black males in 1988 was almost twice that for all infants.[10] Similarly, death rates due to motor vehicle accidents among Native Americans in New Mexico have been as much as four times higher than those of their Caucasian counterparts.[11]

Environment

Assessment of a target group would entail identification of special concerns in the physical, psychological, and social environment that influence the health of the group. For example, if preschool children are the target group, special attention would be given to home safety factors. Similar considerations would be appropriate to the assessment of the physical environment for a group of elderly clients.

In addition to concerns with the psychological environment discussed earlier, the nurse assessing a target group would examine the effects of attitudes toward group members on their health. For example, society's attitude toward drug abusers creates a psychological environment that makes resolution of the problem difficult. Because of the stigma attached to drug abuse and the potential for incarceration, drug abusers may not seek help for their problem. Nor are they likely to seek screening services for HIV infection despite their increased risk of infection via needle sharing and other practices. Social environmental concerns are similar to those considered in the assessment of a community.

Life-style

Specific life-style factors may also need to be considered in the assessment of a target group. For example, cultural factors might greatly influence the dietary patterns of some target groups such as Latinos. As noted earlier, were the target group drug abusers, the nurse would want to assess life-style practices such as needle sharing that put this group at higher risk for specific diseases such as AIDS and hepatitis. Similarly, sexual activity would be a more pressing concern were the target group adolescents rather than a group of preschoolers.

Health System

Specific health system factors can influence the health of some target groups more than others. For example, the unwillingness of many health-care providers to work in rural areas creates an influence on health not found in urban populations. Similarly, fear and anxiety on the part of some health-care providers may lead to their refusal to care for clients with AIDS, thereby further decreasing this population's access to necessary health-care services.

In assessing a target group, the nurse will often obtain data similar to that needed to assess the health of a community. Depending upon the particular target group, however, some of the data that would be obtained regarding a community may not be relevant. For example, information on employment and educational levels is not relevant to an infant target group. Likewise, there may be information specific to the target group that one would not necessarily obtain in assessing a community, as was the case with the information about needle sharing among a group of drug users. A general tool that can be used to assess the health status of a target group is provided in Appendix I, the Health Intervention Planning Guide—Target Group. The tool can be adapted to fit the needs of a particular target group to provide the information needed for the community health nurse to derive nursing diagnoses and to plan interventions to meet group health needs.

DIAGNOSTIC REASONING AND GROUP HEALTH STATUS

The collection of data on factors influencing the health status of a community or a target group is the first step in identifying group health needs. To be of any value, the data must be interpreted and analyzed to derive nursing diagnoses. In other words, assessment data are used to identify health-related needs that are amenable to nursing action. Community or group nursing diagnoses should reflect existing, emerging, and potential threats to the public's health[12] as well as community and group strengths or competencies.[13]

Community diagnoses have been described as possessing three characteristics.[14] First, diagnoses related to groups or communities are generated from assessment of the group as a total entity as well as assessment of group members. Second, community diagnoses imply intervention not through services to individuals in the group, but by creating change in the community. Finally, community diagnoses imply that the total group or community is the direct beneficiary of nursing care, while individuals are indirect beneficiaries.

The diagnostic reasoning process in formulating community diagnoses consists of three steps: identifying health risks present in the community, identifying characteristics of the community or group that are associated with risk, and specifying the health indicators that verify the existence of the risk or attendant problems.[15] The first step involves identifying environmental risks posed by conditions in the community that may contribute to health problems. These risks would be determined by an examination of the data collected regarding the physical, psychological, and social environments of the community.

The second step of the diagnostic reasoning process involves identifying characteristics of community or group members that make the members particularly vulnerable to the effects of the identified risk factors. Identification of community or target group member characteristics that make the members particularly vulnerable to risks would depend on the nurse's knowledge of characteristics associated with specific health problems. The nurse would compare data on community or target group assessment with findings in the literature that suggest associations between certain characteristics and vulnerability to specific kinds of health problems. For example, based on epidemiologic research, the nurse would know that being young, being black and male, and being unemployed are all characteristics associated with increased risk of suicide. If the community contains a large number of young black males who are unemployed, the nurse would recognize these as characteristics of a population at high risk for suicide.

In the third step of the diagnostic reasoning process, the community health nurse identifies existing health problems that validate the existence of risk in the population. The presence of health problems within the community or target group would be determined by comparisons of assessment data with various standards of health.

One type of standard that may be used in data analysis is the general health status of the state or the nation. For example, the community health nurse can compare data for the community or target group with data for the state or the nation as a whole. In doing so, the nurse might ask the following questions: How does this group stand in relation to the larger population on a variety of measures of health status? Is the local birthrate higher or lower than that of the state or the nation? How do death rates compare? For example, the southern region of Georgia is considered the "stroke belt" because the death rate for cerebrovascular accidents far exceeds that of the rest of the nation. Do morbidity rates for various illnesses exceed national and state rates? How do income and educational levels compare?

Another standard with which to compare present data is found in the history of the community or target group. How do current rates compare with those of a year ago? Five years ago?

Members' perceptions of areas of need are a third type of standard with which to compare the data gathered. What health problems are mentioned in interviews with group members? What problems are perceived by other health professionals and community or target group leaders? What are the expectations of the community or target group regarding these problems?

Completion of these three steps of the diagnostic reasoning process gives rise to a preliminary diagnosis of a vulnerable population group at risk for certain conditions.[16] Such a diagnosis would be stated in terms of the risk, the vulnerable population group, and the etiologic factors contributing to the risk.[15] As an example, a community health nurse might derive a nursing diagnosis of "increased risk of suicide among young black males due to unemployment and feelings of powerlessness."

A second stage of community diagnosis involves a comparison of the health-care needs posed by identified risks and the resources available to meet those needs. This may be referred to as a diagnosis of "need-service match" or mismatch.[16] Data for this level of nursing diagnosis would be found in the nurse's assessment of the health-care system. Using the previous example, if the community health nurse found community health-care resources inadequate to meet the needs posed by the increased risk of suicide in a vulnerable population, he or she would make a diagnosis of "need-service mismatch due to inadequate (or inaccessible) suicide prevention services."

The nurse might also make positive diagnoses related to the health status of a community or target group. For example, a preliminary diagnosis might indicate a vulnerable population group (for instance, children) at risk for certain health problems (such as communicable diseases). Examination of assessment data, however, might indicate that there are few problems with immunizable childhood diseases because of easy accessibility of immunization services and high immunization levels in the population. In this situation, the nurse's diagnosis might be a "need-service match due to accessibility and use of immunization services."

PLANNING TO MEET IDENTIFIED HEALTH NEEDS

Whenever a diagnosis of need-service mismatch is made, planning to meet the unmet need is warranted, and the community health nurse should become involved in planning health-care delivery programs to meet the identified needs of the population. Initiating health program planning frequently involves the use of the leadership skills described in Chapter 11, The Leadership, Change, and Group Processes. The process used in planning health programs is similar to that used to plan care for other types of clients but is somewhat more involved. Considerations in planning at the group level include priority setting, determining the level of prevention involved in meeting identified health needs, and developing health-care programs to meet those needs.

PRIORITY SETTING

Once nursing diagnoses have been derived, they must be assigned priority for intervention. The community health nurse, along with other health-care providers, must be able to set priorities that will allow for the best use of available resources. This is even more important when the client is a community or a target group than in the care of individuals or families, because care of communities and target groups usually necessitates a greater expenditure of resources than care of an individual. This frequently means that only the highest priority needs will be addressed because of limited resources available.

The criteria used to prioritize community or target group needs are essentially the same as those used in working with individuals and families: (1) the severity of the threat to the community's health, (2) the degree of the community's concern about the need, or (3) the extent to which meeting one need depends on meeting other needs.

It is likely that the priorities of the community or target group will involve needs that are easily perceived. Community health nurses may find that they must deal first with a need that they consider relatively minor, but which is of concern to the community, before tackling other more major problems. In other words, the nurse must establish credibility with the community before he or she can expect community support for subsequent efforts.

The American Public Health Association[17] identified five factors to consider in addition to those already addressed in determining priority of health needs. These five factors are:

1. the degree of special group concern
2. the extent of existing resources for dealing with the problem
3. the solvability of the problem
4. the need for special education measures relative to the problem, and
5. the extent of additional resources and policies needed

The community health nurse will probably need to consider all these factors in prioritizing needs identified in the community assessment.

DETERMINING THE LEVEL OF PREVENTION

Programs for meeting the health needs of communities or target groups may be needed at any of the three levels of prevention.

Primary Prevention Programs

Primary prevention programs are designed to promote the health of the population and prevent specific illnesses. An exercise program for senior citizens is an example of a health promotion program aimed at a target group. Community education programs on water safety or prevention of accidents in the home are primary preventive measures for a community. Other examples of primary prevention could involve educational programs of any kind designed to promote the public's overall health. For example, parenting classes for expectant couples could help prevent child abuse, while sex education in the school system could minimize problems of adolescent pregnancy and sexually transmitted diseases. Immunization programs are another example of primary prevention for a community or target group.

Secondary Prevention Programs

Secondary prevention involves identifying and resolving existing health problems in members of the community or target group. Specific secondary interventions may focus on screening programs or control programs for community health problems.

Screening Programs. One major area of program planning related to secondary prevention for communities and target groups is the development of screening programs. ***Screening*** is the preliminary examination or testing of a person to determine whether or not he or she might have a particular condition and whether further diagnostic testing is indicated. Screening procedures are not diagnostic. Instead, they serve to indicate the possibility that a particular disease or condition is present. Positive screening test results are always an indication of the need for further diagnostic procedures. Screening is frequently used with large population groups because it is considerably less expensive than conducting a battery of diagnostic tests when the majority of people can be expected to have negative results. Screening procedures are available and recommended for breast and cervical cancer, testicular cancer, colorectal cancer, skin cancer, hypertension, and diabetes. Screening may also be done for several sexually transmitted diseases such as syphilis and gonorrhea and for the human immunodeficiency virus (HIV) that causes AIDS. Screening for tuberculosis is also available. Another form of screening is the periodic health examination in which the person is examined for signs and symptoms of several common diseases.

There are several factors that need to be considered in decisions to implement large scale screening programs. These factors can be divided into three groups: (1) considerations regarding the condition that is being screened, (2) considerations regarding the test itself, and (3) considerations related to the target group for the program. Any condition for which screening is warranted should have several characteristics. First, the condition should affect a sufficient number of people to make screening cost-effective. Second, the condition should be a relatively serious condition. For example, although it would be cost-effective to screen for the common cold because of the number of people affected, the effects of colds are usually minor and thus do not justify screening. The third consideration is the availability of an acceptable treatment. It is not realistic, generally speaking, to screen for a disease for which there is no treatment. (A significant exception to this criterion is screening for HIV infection. In this case, knowledge of being HIV positive allows the infected individual to take precautions that can help limit the spread of the disease.) Fourth, there should be a significant preclinical period between the time of exposure and the development of clinical symptoms to allow for treatment before the person becomes symptomatic. Finally, early diagnosis and treatment need to make a difference. If the outcome is the same whether the condition is treated early or late in its course, there is no point in engaging in screening. If, on the other hand, earlier treatment increases the chances of being cured, as is the case in breast cancer, then screening is appropriate.

The second group of factors influencing decisions for mass screening relates to the screening test itself. These factors are the sensitivity and specificity of the screening test as well as the cost, ease of administration, and acceptability of the procedure. ***Sensitivity*** refers to the ability of the test to accurately identify those persons with the disease.[18] A sensitive screening test would be able to detect the presence of a condition even when very little of the indicator that the test reacts to is present. For example, if a screening test relies on the presence of a particular substance in the blood, a sensitive test would give a positive result even when a small amount of that substance is present. The ***specificity*** of a screening test reflects the extent to which it excludes those who do not have the disease.[18] A positive result on a highly specific test would indicate the potential presence of only one condition, rather than two or three possible conditions.

Other considerations with respect to the screening test itself are cost, ease of administration, and acceptability. Screening tests should be relatively inexpensive compared to specific diagnostic tests. They should also be easy to administer to large groups of people and not require expensive or sophisticated equipment to conduct the test. Finally, the test should be acceptable to those who are intended to participate in the screening. This means that the test should not be overly painful, embarrassing, or anxiety-provoking. The test should not have objectionable side effects. It would be unwarranted to screen people using a test whose potential side effects are worse than the symptoms of the disease in question.

Another consideration in deciding for or against mass screening projects is the population to be screened. The target group must be identifiable and accessible to screeners. If the target group for screening is not easily identifiable, screening programs may not reach those most in need. Adult women, for example, have been identified as being vulnerable to breast and cervical cancer, and this population can easily be screened for these conditions during the course of routine checkups for all adult women. If the appropriate target group is less easily identified or unlikely to come forward (for example, intravenous drug users or homosexuals), screening programs are less likely to be successful.

When conditions related to the illness, the screening test, and the target population are met, large-scale screening programs can prove worthwhile. When these conditions are not met, screening is unlikely to be effective in improving the health of communities. Disease, test, and target group considerations in planning large-scale screening programs are summarized in Box 19–1.

BOX 19–1

Disease, Test, and Target Group Considerations in Screening

Disease considerations

The disease affects a sufficient number of people to make screening cost-effective

The disease is relatively serious

There is an effective treatment available for the disease

There is a sufficient preclinical period to allow treatment before symptoms occur

Early diagnosis and treatment makes a difference in terms of outcome

Test considerations

The screening test is sensitive enough to detect most cases of the disease

The screening test is specific enough to exclude most other causes of positive results

The screening test costs little, is easy to administer, and has minimal side effects

Target group considerations

The target group is identifiable

The target group is accessible

Control Programs. Some of the same programs described as primary preventive measures may also be employed in secondary prevention designed to alleviate existing health problems. When a community or target group is already experiencing a high rate of sexually transmitted diseases, education on the transmission and prevention of STDs would be a secondary preventive measure. The intent of the program is to control an existing problem (a high rate of STD), rather than preventing a problem from occurring.

The kind of secondary prevention programs planned for a given community or target group will vary with the types of problems identified in the assessment. For example, if child abuse is prevalent in the community, parenting classes for abusive parents would be an appropriate secondary preventive measure. Similarly, if there is a high rate of hypertension among group members, clinics could be established to screen for, diagnose, and treat this problem. In another community, a program to enforce seat-belt legislation could be used as a secondary preventive measure for a high rate of motor vehicle accident fatalities.

Tertiary Prevention Programs

Tertiary prevention programs for communities or target groups are designed to prevent complications of identified problems or prevent the recurrence of a problem. For example, if a community is experiencing an epidemic of measles, mass immunization programs to control the epidemic would be used as a secondary preventive measure. When the epidemic is under control, a program designed to maintain immunity levels among community members would be a tertiary preventive measure designed to thwart future epidemics.

Tertiary prevention is also designed to prevent consequences of existing problems. For example, when an earthquake occurs and safe water supplies are limited, programs to conserve or to purify water will help to limit additional health effects of the earthquake that may arise from drinking contaminated water.

HEALTH PROGRAM PLANNING

Planning is a collaborative and systematic process used to attain a goal.[19] Planning is collaborative in the sense that persons who will be affected by the planned program need to be involved in its planning. It is systematic in that change is consciously and deliberately brought about.

Reasons for Planning

Until fairly recently, health-care programs were designed and implemented with little regard for principles of planning. Why the recent concern with planned efforts in terms of health care? For one thing, those in the health-care professions are coming to realize that there are limited resources available. Grassroots popular movements have done a great deal to curb government spending and have brought this realization home quite forcefully. Adequate planning helps to ensure that limited resources are used most effectively with the least waste possible.

A second concern is that consumers are demanding organized planning efforts into which they have some input. Gone are the days when taxpayers provided money on request. They now require adequate justification for the expenditure of tax dollars. Another consideration in the push for organized planning efforts is the psychological impact of planning. Systematic planning allows people to feel that they are in control. In an age when much of daily life seems dictated by circumstances beyond one's control, concerted efforts at program planning allow some degree of say over one's destiny. Finally, planning encourages health professionals and community members to take positive steps to ensure health rather than wait for events to dictate the future state of the community's health.

The Planning Process

The process of planning health-care programs for groups of people involves several discrete activities. These include selecting the planning group, developing planning competence, formulating a philosophy, establishing program goals, forecasting, developing alternative solutions, evaluating alternatives and selecting a solution, and developing program objectives. Other planning activities are identifying resources, delineating actions required to accomplish objectives, evaluating the plan, and planning for evaluation. These activities may or may not occur in the sequence in which they are presented here, but may occur simultaneously or in a slightly different order. What is important is that each one does occur at some point in the process.

Selecting the Planning Group. Those involved in planning should include key community or target group members expected to benefit from the program. Potential beneficiaries of the program need to feel a sense of "ownership" of the program to motivate its use.[7] For example, if the health need is one arising from adolescent sexuality (for example, high incidence rates for sexually transmitted diseases among teenagers), adolescents should be encouraged to provide input into planning a viable program to meet the need. They are the best judges of what will be acceptable to themselves and to their peers.

Other categories of persons to be included in the planning group depend, to a certain extent, on the type of problem to be solved. There are, however, some general guidelines that may prove helpful. It is wise, for instance, to involve diverse segments of the community whenever possible to provide a widespread base of support for the resulting program. Individuals who have the authority to deal with the problem should certainly be included in the planning group. Those in a position to promote acceptance of the program such as media representatives, key community leaders, and influential citizens should also be invited to participate.

Another group that should be involved are those who are going to implement whatever program is planned. For example, if the program will involve some type of educational campaign, local educators should be included in the planning process. Experts knowledgeable about the problem should also be included. These individuals can contribute to the group's understanding of the problem and provide knowledge of possible alternative solutions.

The last category of persons who should be involved in planning are individuals or groups who are likely to resist the program. This is one effective way of reducing opposition.[3] Once these people have contributed to a plan that is acceptable to them, they are usually committed to the program and will work toward its acceptance by others.

Developing Planning Competence. Once the planning group is assembled, the first step in program planning is developing necessary planning competencies. Few health professionals or consumers have any educational background or experience in program planning. For this reason, the community health nurse may find it necessary to educate members of the planning group in regard to planning processes and activities. It may also be necessary to prevent the group from engaging in activities for which an adequate foundation has yet to be provided. In doing so, the community health nurse will need to exercise well-developed skills in leadership and group dynamics addressed in Chapter 11, The Change, Leadership, and Group Processes.

Formulating a Philosophy. The next step, formulating a philosophy, is not often carried out as a conscious activity, but is an assumption on the part of group members. For example, there must be some type of commitment to adequate health care for prison inmates before a group would even consider planning a program to meet prisoners' needs. It is important, however, that the philosophies of various members of the planning group be compatible. Therefore, group members should be encouraged to verbalize their philosophies and to identify and deal with areas of conflict between philosophies.

Establishing Program Goals. Goals flow from the group's philosophy and describe the overall intent of the group with respect to the problem to be solved. Again, goals must be developed by the group as a whole to ensure consistency. Goals are usually stated in general terms as a desired ultimate outcome. In the prison example, a possible goal might be "to provide adequate health-care services for inmates." This goal, stated very generally, gives no indication of possible means of achieving the desired outcome. Objectives, on the other hand, are stated as specific expected outcomes that contribute in some way to realizing the goal. Objectives will be discussed more thoroughly later in this chapter.

Forecasting. The fifth step of planning is forecasting. ***Forecasting*** is a process whereby one predicts future events that may affect the solution to the problem at hand *and* also predicts what would take place if the problem were not solved. Forecasting should take place in the political, social, economic, technological, and health-related areas.

A high rate of illegitimate births to teenage mothers in a community can be used to illustrate the dimensions of forecasting. One consideration in this example is the impact of current and prospective political trends on the resources available to deal with this problem. For example, if school board members are averse to sex education in the schools, a sex education program may not be an effective approach to solving the problem. However, a change in the membership of the school board at the next election could make solution of the problem easier.

In terms of social forecasting, one can sometimes predict the effects of changes in social mores on the problem at hand. Past acceptance of sexual activity on the part of teens has contributed to the problem, while parental objections to contraceptive use by teens has compounded it. Concern related to AIDS may result in changes in adolescent sexual activity such as decreased sexual activity or the use of condoms. Both of these responses would decrease the number of illegitimate births, thus eliminating the need for community action.

If left unsolved, the problem will further complicate the social stresses currently prevalent in the community. How can teens assume the social roles required of parents when they are still hovering on the edge of childhood themselves? Adolescent parenthood has been shown to retard adolescents' achievement of social and economic independence.[6] Failure to solve the problem may also lead to more forced marriages, which contribute to stress in families.

Possible economic effects of the problem might also be forecast. Money to institute health-care programs designed to resolve the problem of adolescent pregnancy might be in short supply. At the same time, illegitimacy would increase the financial burden on individual families and on the community to provide for the needs of these citizens. For example, in 1985 public funds amounting to more than $16 billion were spent on the economic support of teenage mothers and their children.[6]

Technological advances can contribute to a solution to the problem to the extent that more effective means of contraception are being developed. On the other hand, teenagers who may have the potential for great technological contributions to society may be prevented from making them because of the need to support a young family.

The health-related effects of the program can also be forecast. If the problem remains unsolved, there will probably be increased demands for health-care services for illegitimate children as well as increased effects of stress on their health and that of their families. Conversely, adequate health care in the form of accessible contraceptive services could help to alleviate the problem.

Developing Alternative Solutions. The next step in the program planning process is developing alternative solutions to the identified health need. Here the planning group should be encouraged to exercise creativity in attempts to develop alternatives. A suggestion that appears absurd on first presentation may be found to be quite feasible on investigation. Inappropriate alternatives will eventually be eliminated during the next step of the planning process—evaluation of alternatives in terms of critical criteria for problem resolution.

Four obstacles have been identified that impede creative alternative solutions to health problems.[19] The first obstacle is making premature judgments before all possible options have been developed and discussed. The second obstacle is the search for a single answer when there are usually multiple potential solutions to problems. When group members seek a single answer, they are likely to accept the first one that seems feasible.

Assuming that alternatives are necessarily limited by situational constraints is the third obstacle. When people begin with the idea that something is "impossible because . . . ," they frequently leave undiscovered a number of alternatives that circumvent identified constraints. The final obstacle is thinking that the solution to the problem is solely the client's responsibility rather than that of the planning group. In this case, group members tend to withdraw from proposing alternatives and leave problem solution to a nebulous "they" who never materialize.

Evaluating Alternatives and Selecting a Solution. As noted in Chapter 5, The Nursing Process, one of the components in the planning stage of the nursing process is the development of critical criteria against which any solution to a particular problem must be weighed. Critical criteria for solutions are also required when the client is a community or target group rather than an individual or a family. Examples of critical criteria for solutions to community problems might be that such solutions fit within available budgetary resources, or that they are acceptable to ethnic or religious groups within the community.

Potential solutions to community problems should always be evaluated in terms of cost, feasibility, acceptability, availability of necessary resources, efficiency, equity, political advantage, and identifiability of the target group. Generally speaking, an alternative that costs less will be viewed more favorably, other factors being equal, than one that costs more. Or, one alternative may be selected over another because its implementation is more feasible. For instance, it is considerably easier to install a traffic light at an accident-prone intersection than to build a bridge to route one intersecting road over the other.

Potential solutions should also be evaluated in terms of their acceptability to policymakers, implementers, and the community. Policymakers are unlikely to approve an alternative that diminishes their power or authority, while implementers are certainly unlikely to accept a potential solution that requires them to work overtime or without pay if another alternative is available. Similarly, community members affected by the proposed program may find one alternative more acceptable than another for a variety of reasons.

Alternative solutions may also differ in terms of the resources needed to implement them. Generally speaking, an alternative that requires fewer resources or for which resources are already available is more likely to be endorsed than one that requires extensive or scarce resources. For example, a group seeking to improve the nutritional status of school children may select an alternative that makes use of existing facilities used to prepare meals for senior citizens rather than one that necessitates providing kitchen facilities in each school. Efficiency is a related criterion on which alternative solutions to a particular problem can be evaluated. An efficient alternative makes better use of available resources and is usually viewed more favorably in making planning decisions than an inefficient one.

Questions of equity also arise in evaluating alternative solutions to a problem. Alternatives that unfairly discriminate against one segment of the population are usually rejected. For example, one alternative to the problem of dealing with teen pregnancy might be to provide contraceptive services in the larger high schools. If, however, these schools tend to serve the upper-middle-class segment of the community while lower-class children attend smaller schools, this alternative would discriminate against a segment of the community also needing service.

Political consequences also need to be considered in evaluating the alternative solutions to specific problems. For example, an alternative plan that provides services to a highly vocal voting bloc might be viewed more favorably by politicians than one that serves a less politically involved minority group.

Finally, alternative solutions should be evaluated in terms of the identifiability of the target group. One potential solution for preventing the spread of AIDS might be to screen all prostitutes in the community for HIV infection. However, it is somewhat difficult to identify this group of people, since prostitution is an illegal activity in most places. It might be easier to screen everyone who requests services for sexually transmitted diseases because this group is sexually active and is also identifiable.

The community health nurse should assist the planning group to determine the relative weight to be given to each of these considerations in evaluating alternative solutions. Those considerations that are weighted most heavily become the critical criteria against which all potential solutions are evaluated.

The remaining considerations are those that are nice if they can be met, but not absolutely necessary. For example, if there is an unlimited source of funding for dealing with certain types of problems, cost might not be a critical criterion for selecting a solution to the problem in question. Or, it may be that criteria of cost, feasibility, and acceptability are considered critical and others are viewed as less important. Once the criteria have been established, the group can proceed to evaluate all of the potential solutions generated and select the one most appropriate to the situation.

Consideration of possible sources of opposition will also contribute to selection of the most appropriate alternative. If it is known that members of the community PTA would vigorously oppose a "sex fair" as a means of educating adolescents on sexual issues, another less threatening alternative would be more appropriate.

There are two basic types of opposition to proposed programs—rational and irrational. Rational opposition is based on sound reasoning and should be seriously considered, as it may prove beneficial to the planning effort. Rational opposition does pose problems to the extent that it lends support to irrational opposition and also tends to sway individuals who are undecided as to the merits of the planned program.

Irrational opposition can arise from several sources. It may result from a general attitude of conservatism in which only proven interventions are held to be acceptable. As a rule, conservatives usually discount innovative ideas as possible solutions and prefer to remain with more traditional approaches.

The second type of irrational opposition arises out of cultural patterns and social reactions to change in general. For example, agricultural change programs initiated by Peace Corps volunteers in India were considerably less successful than programs fostering small industries. The farmers were responding to centuries of culturally ingrained patterns of farming, while the small businessmen were engaged in pursuits that held no strong cultural connotations.

Opposition may also arise from perceptions that a particular course of action poses a threat to the power, prestige, or economic security of certain members in or outside of a group or community. For example, starting a clinic staffed by nurse practitioners to improve the accessibility of health care may be seen by local physicians as a threat to their economic security.

Another source of irrational opposition is usually unconscious in nature and results from feelings of overall vulnerability. This type of opposition is usually found in the same group of people, whatever the issue addressed. Because of their own personal insecurity, change of any type may be threatening to these individuals.

Additional sources of resistance to health-care programs include reluctance to spend money on health care, legal obstacles across jurisdictions, and unreasoning self-reliance. Reluctance to spend money can often be overcome by accurate documentation of the costs of the problem and the cost-effectiveness of problem resolution. For example, a county sheriff's department got council approval for a nursing clinic in the county jail by documenting the decrease in the cost of health care for prisoners when a nurse was available.

Jurisdictional obstacles can be combatted by including in the planning body persons with authority and prestige in the problem area. Pride or unreasoning self-reliance can also be an obstacle to utilization of health programs. For this reason, any alternative selected must be acceptable to the group for which it is designed. One method of accomplishing this is including members of the target group in the planning body.

Developing Program Objectives. Once alternative solutions have been evaluated in light of critical criteria and a solution selected, the process of planning a specific program based on that alternative begins. At this point, the planning group sets specific program objectives. Objectives are statements of specific outcomes expected to result from the program that contribute to the realization of the overall goal.

For objectives to be useful, they should meet several criteria. Perhaps the most essential of these is that the objective be measurable. A well-stated objective will include some means of measuring the outcome expected and evaluating the effectiveness of the effort. For example, if the overall goal is to improve children's nutritional status, one program objective might relate to hematocrit levels. It is not sufficient to state, however, that hematocrit levels will improve as no measure of the degree of improvement expected has been stated. A measurable objective could be that "75 percent of school-age children in the community (or target group) will have hematocrit levels within normal limits." A better objective would include a definition of normal hematocrit levels: "75 percent of school-age children in Clarksville will have hematocrit levels of 35 percent or greater." In this objective, a measure of the expected hematocrit level is specified as well as a measure of the number of children expected to achieve it. This objective is measurable.

A second criterion of good program objectives is the inclusion of a specific time frame within which the outcome is expected to occur. A time frame can easily be added to the previous objective to state that "a hematocrit reading of 35 percent or greater will be achieved in 75 percent of the school-age children in Clarksville within 6 months of initiating a food supplement program in the schools." As stated, this objective also meets several other criteria for program objectives. It is reasonable and practical to expect a significant increase in hematocrit levels after 6 months of an iron-rich diet. To expect it in 2 weeks would not be reasonable. It would also be unreasonable to expect that all of the children would achieve normal hematocrit levels as a result of the program. Seventy-five percent is reasonable.

The objective also meets the criterion of being within the competence of the planning group to accomplish. This would not be true, however, were the planners a group of electrical engineers. It is also legal, provided one has the permission of parents to provide nourishment to children in need of it and to obtain hematocrit levels. It fits the moral and value framework of the community and carries minimum unpleasant side effects. The latter would not be true, however, if the alternative chosen called for injectable iron preparations that are painful to administer. Finally, the objective, as stated, will probably be acceptable to those implementing the program, and it is hoped that it will fit within the budgetary limitations of the school system. Criteria for effective program objectives are summarized in Box 19–2.

BOX 19–2

Criteria for Effective Program Objectives

Measurability: The objective is measurable so as to determine whether it has been achieved.

Time specificity: The objective includes a statement of the time when it is expected to be accomplished.

Reasonability or practicality: The objective is practical and able to be met with a reasonable amount of effort.

Within group competencies: The objective is within the ability of the planning group to accomplish, given members' expertise and authority.

Legality: The objective does not violate any laws.

Congruence with community morals and values: The objective is consistent with the values and moral attitudes of implementers and members of the community or target group.

Carries minimal side effects: The objective has the fewest possible side effects, and these effects are acceptable to program beneficiaries.

Acceptability to implementers: The objective is acceptable to those who must work to accomplish it.

Fits budgetary limitations: The objective fits the community's budgetary limitations.

Identifying Resources. Once objectives have been established, the planning group can proceed to identify resources needed to implement the program. Resources include personnel, money, materials, and time. To continue with the previous example of improving the nutritional status of children, if the alternative selected was an iron-rich school meal program, there are a variety of resources required to institute such a program. Personnel needed include people to develop menus incorporating iron-rich foods palatable to school-age children and people to purchase, prepare, and serve the food as well as to wash dishes. Funds to purchase food and the equipment with which to prepare and serve it are also needed. Material resources needed would include the dishes, silverware, pots and pans, and cooking facilities. Other needs include the equipment and health-care personnel who will check hematocrit levels. Not only must the planning group decide what resources are required but they must also specify how these resources can be obtained. Will the PTA have a fund-raising drive? Will a grant proposal for federal assistance be submitted? The final consideration with respect to resources is that of time. The time needed to put the program into operation must be determined.

Delineating Actions to Accomplish Objectives. The next step in the planning process is delineating specific actions required to carry out the program. This is usually considered the "nitty-gritty" of planning, and many planning groups mistakenly jump immediately to this phase of activity. For planning to be effective, however, this step must be preceded by those discussed earlier.

In this phase of planning, the step-by-step details of the plan are developed. Using the example of the school meal program, some of the actions needed include presenting the problem and the proposed solution to the PTA, planning fund-raising projects, and purchasing equipment and supplies. In addition, the health department nutritionist would plan adequate menus. Advertisements for cooks and enlistment of parent volunteers to help prepare and serve food would be initiated, and so on, down to the last detail.

Evaluating the Plan. When the detailed plan has been constructed and specific activities delineated, the plan itself should be evaluated. Is the plan based on identified needs of the target group or is it unrelated to those needs? Is the plan flexible enough to adapt to changing circumstances in the foreseeable future? How efficient will the planned program be? Could program efficiency be improved by modification of the plan? Finally, how adequate is the plan? Have all constraints and contingencies been addressed? Answers to these and similar questions enable the planning group to evaluate the plan and to identify the need for any modifications before the plan is implemented.

Planning for Evaluation. The final component to be considered in program planning is planning for evaluation of program effectiveness. This may seem a bit premature because the program has not even started. However, it is essential. Unless planning for program evaluation is incorporated at this stage, the data needed for evaluating program outcomes will not be available when the time arrives for actual evaluation.

Planning for evaluation involves four considerations. The first of these is determining criteria upon which the program should be evaluated. The second consideration is the type of data to be collected and the means used to collect it. Determining the resources needed to carry out the evaluation is the third consideration in planning for evaluation. Finally, the planning group should determine who will evaluate the program. All of these considerations will be addressed in greater detail in the section dealing with program evaluation. At this juncture it is sufficient to reemphasize the point that planning for evaluation begins during program planning and not after the program has been implemented.

Effective health program planning involves all of the steps discussed up to now. When steps are ignored or bypassed, the program planned is likely to be less effective and its implementation may prove more difficult. The steps in the planning process are summarized in Box 19–3.

Nursing involvement in health-care planning is a relatively new phenomenon, and community health nurses may find themselves in need of assistance in this area. Selected sources of assistance with health-care programming are presented in Table 19–1.

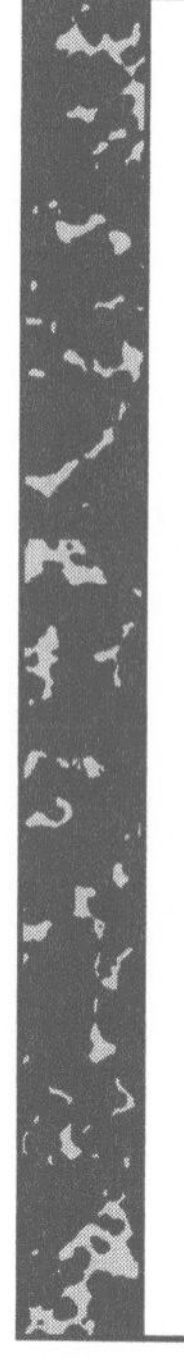

BOX 19–3

Steps in the Planning Process

- Selecting the planning group
- Developing planning competence
- Formulating a philosophy
- Establishing program goals
- Forecasting
- Developing alternative solutions
- Evaluating alternatives and selecting a solution
- Developing program objectives
- Identifying resources
- Delineating action to accomplish objectives
- Evaluating the plan
- Planning for evaluation

IMPLEMENTING THE PLAN

It is not enough for the planning group to devise a plan for a health-care program to meet identified health-care needs. The group must also ensure that the plan is implemented.[20] Implementing a health program involves several considerations. These include getting the plan accepted, performing the tasks involved in implementing the program, and use of strategies that foster implementation of the program as planned.

GETTING THE PLAN ACCEPTED

Acceptance of the planned program occurs at three levels. The first level is acceptance by community policymakers. If policymakers have been represented on the planning group, this level of acceptance should already have been achieved.

The second level of acceptance involves convincing those who are to implement the plan to implement it for everyday operation. Again, if program implementers have been adequately represented in the planning effort, this level is already partially achieved. It only remains for the implementers to actually convert the plan into an operational program.

Acceptance and participation in the planned program by members of the target group is the third level of acceptance. If, for example, the planned program involves providing contraceptive services to sexually active adolescents, the third level of acceptance will involve adolescents' participation in the program. Ac-

TABLE 19–1. RESOURCES FOR NURSES INVOLVED IN HEALTH PROGRAM PLANNING

Agency or Organization	Focus
American Health Planning Association 1110 Vermont Avenue, N.W., Suite 950 Washington, DC 20005 (202) 861-1200	Research, information on health planning
Forum for Health Care Planning 1101 Connecticut Avenue, N.W., Suite 700 Washington, DC 20036 (202) 857-1162	Advocacy, continuing education for planning
Health Policy Advisory Center 17 Murray St. New York, NY 10007 (212) 267-8890	Advocacy for health policy formation
Health Policy Council 1424 16th St., N.W., Suite 105 Washington, DC 20036 (202) 462-8805	Advocacy for health promotion

ceptance at this third level may require marketing the program to the intended target population.[21]

TASKS OF IMPLEMENTATION

Three basic tasks are involved in program implementation: activity delineation and sequencing, task allocation, and task performance. Necessary activities have been broadly outlined in plan development. Now they must be specified and subactivities identified. This involves identifying needed categories of action and the skills required for their performance. At this point, implementers would determine the appropriate sequencing of activities and might establish a time frame for their accomplishment.

Task allocation involves identifying the expertise of program implementers relative to the skills needed for effective implementation of the plan. Also at this point, responsibility is assigned for various activities delineated. Such assignments must be communicated to those involved, and they must be provided with whatever education or training is required for implementing the plan. Finally, the activities themselves are carried out and the planned program is put into operation.

STRATEGIES FOR IMPLEMENTATION

Program implementation can be enhanced if several specific implementation strategies are employed. The first of these strategies is to assign responsibility for coordination of the total effort to one person. Identifying preparatory steps to each activity and listing them in sequence also fosters implementation of the program as planned.

Another strategy that will enhance program implementation is periodic consultation with those implementing the program to address any difficulties that arise. Finally, the chances of implementing of the program as planned are enhanced when everyone involved is clearly informed of expectations and the time frame for meeting expectations.

Using the school meal program as an example, implementing the plan might involve designating the school nurse as the program coordinator, actually staging the PTA bazaar to raise funds after delineating all of the activities involved in doing so, hiring and training personnel, and developing menus. Other implementation activities would include purchasing food, supplies, and equipment, and preparing the meals.

PROGRAM EVALUATION

Evaluating the effects of health-care programs is an essential feature of the epidemiologic prevention process model as applied to the care of communities and target groups. Program evaluation is needed for many of the same reasons that a systematic process is used in program planning. Health-care providers recognize the limitation of available resources and must be accountable to the community members who use the program and particularly to the community members who pay for the program. They must be able to justify the program's existence and continuation. This can only be done by documenting the effectiveness of the program in solving the problem at hand.

Evaluation of a particular program may be undertaken for a variety of reasons. Some of these include justifying program continuation or expansion, improving the quality of service provided, determining future courses of action, or determining the impact of the program. Other reasons for evaluation might be a desire to call attention to the program, assess personnel performance, or to assuage political expectations. Evaluation is frequently conducted because it is required by a funding agency.

CONSIDERATIONS IN PROGRAM EVALUATION

Purpose Considerations

The purpose of the evaluation will influence all other aspects of the process. For instance, if the purpose of the evaluation is to justify continuing a program, the evaluation will focus on determining whether the program has a beneficial effect on the health of the population group for which it is designed. On the other hand, if the purpose is to decide whether programs are under- or overutilized, evaluation will focus on the number of persons served. In other words, the purpose of the evaluation will influence the types of data collected and how they are used.

Evaluator Considerations

The second area for consideration is who should conduct the evaluation. A number of choices are possible. The program can be evaluated by those who implement it or who benefit from it. Evaluation by people who are involved in the program has some disadvantages in that there is a certain amount of bias on the part of those with a vested interest in retaining the program. The advantage of an inside evaluator is familiarity with the program and knowledge of sources of data that will be needed.

Another possibility is to employ someone from outside the program to conduct the evaluation. This person is likely to be relatively objective in his or her approach to evaluation, but faces the disadvantage of not being well acquainted with the program and possibly being unable to identify appropriate sources of data. This alternative is also rather expensive.

The third option is the use of an academician to evaluate the program. Faculty members who have expertise in the program area are likely to be familiar with the general operation of the program but also remain relatively unbiased. Because college faculty are usually open to opportunities for research, it may also be possible to acquire their services for a lower fee.

Ethical Considerations

Ethical conflicts must be anticipated in program evaluation. Participation in the evaluation should be voluntary for staff and clients alike. This poses some problems in that staff members are sometimes unwilling to reveal information that reflects poorly on them or on the program that employs them. To circumvent this reluctance, the evaluator will need to have a variety of sources of data that provide an overall picture of the program and its effects.

Confidentiality is another issue. Persons who provide data need to be assured that their individual responses will not be identifiable. There is also the question of who will have access to the findings of the evaluation. Should findings be shared only with those involved in the program? With their supervisors? With funding agencies or regulatory bodies? The use to which findings can be put is also of concern. Can the evaluator publish the information? Will it be used to fire personnel?

Finally, the evaluator must consider the risks and benefits accruing from the evaluation. Is there potential for harm to the participants, either clients or staff? Do the anticipated benefits of the evaluation outweigh any possible risks?

Type of Evaluation

The last major consideration in evaluating a healthcare program is the type of evaluation to be conducted. There are two basic types of evaluation, each of which can be broken down into subtypes: outcome and process evaluation.

Outcome Evaluation. *Outcome evaluation* focuses on the extent to which program goals and objectives have been met, irrespective of how well-organized or how efficient the program was. Outcome evaluation documents the effects of the program and justifies decisions to continue, modify, or eliminate it. The two subtypes of outcome evaluation are evaluation of *effect* and assessment of *impact*.

A program's effect is the degree to which the specific program objectives were met. Using the previous example of the school lunch program, the effect of the program is evaluated when one determines whether 75 percent of the school-age children have a hematocrit level of 35 percent or greater within 6 months of the start of the program. If they do, the program can be considered effective. If not, the evaluator must determine to what degree the objective has been met and whether continuation of the program is warranted. For example, if the objective was achieved with 60 percent of the participating children, extending the program would probably be considered. If, on the other hand, only 20 percent of the children achieved normal hematocrit levels, alternative solutions to the problem may need to be considered.

The impact of a program is how well it serves to attain overall goals. If the goal was improving the nutritional status of school-age children, for example, the achievement of improved hematocrit levels does contribute to goal achievement. However, if the goal was to improve the children's learning ability through adequate nutrition, increasing hematocrit levels may or may not contribute to its achievement. In this case, one would need to know not only the hematocrit levels but also the amount of learning that has taken place in order to state that the program has had an impact on meeting the overall goal. One may find that hematocrit levels did indeed rise, but no improvement in learning ability has taken place. In this instance the program was effective in accomplishing its objective, but accomplishing the objective did not lead to achievement of the overall goal.

Process Evaluation. The second type of evaluation is *process evaluation.* Here one is concerned with the smoothness of operation of the program. Process evaluation examines program performance in terms of effort, efficiency, or organizational process.

The first aspect of process evaluation is *effort,* the amount of activity that has taken place or the effort expended in implementing the program. How many meals were served in the school meal program? How many person-hours were expended in carrying out the program? How many children participated? Obviously, this type of evaluation suggests little or nothing about the effectiveness of the program in meeting its objectives, but one may still wish to obtain this information for purposes of future planning. For example, if one knows how many children participated this year, one will have some idea of numbers to plan for next year.

Efficiency is a measure of the appropriateness of the use of resources. How efficiently was the program carried out? Was the food prepared well, but cold by the time it was served? Did the meals served fit the food preferences of school-age children? Were food and supplies purchased in quantities sufficient to save money and still prevent waste? Or, was uneaten food discarded at the end of each day? Cost-effectiveness is an important part of the efficiency aspect of program evaluation and is frequently used to justify continuance of a program.

Organizational process is the third aspect of performance evaluation. The concern in this type of evaluation is the structure and organization of the program. Organizational process may be a contributing factor in program efficiency. For example, the distance of cooking facilities from the serving area may be the main reason why food was cold when served. Or, it may be that the system for purchasing food and supplies results in a great deal of waste. For instance, if requisitions have to pass through a large bureaucratic system, program implementers may order greater quantities than are actually needed just to be sure they have sufficient supplies on hand at any given time.

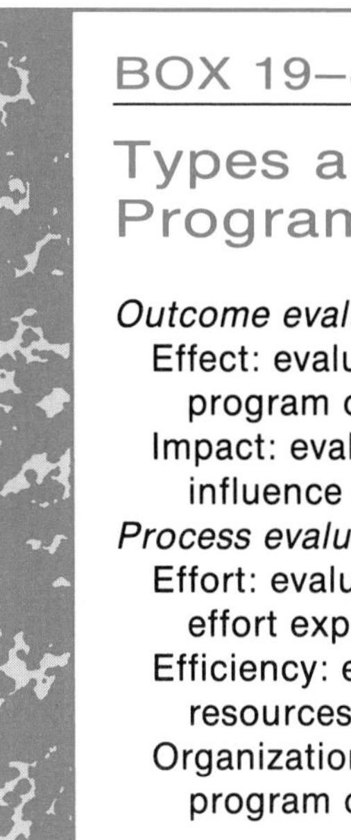

BOX 19–4

Types and Aspects of Program Evaluation

Outcome evaluation
- Effect: evaluation of achievement of program objectives
- Impact: evaluation of the program's influence on meeting overall goals

Process evaluation
- Effort: evaluation of the amount of effort expended in the program
- Efficiency: evaluation of the use of resources
- Organizational process: evaluation of program organization

The timing of the program is another consideration in organizational process evaluation. Was the school meal program instituted at a time when families in the area got pay raises sufficient to enable them to serve nutritious food at home, or were they all out on strike? In the first instance, the timing of the program is poor because it is no longer needed. Timing in the second instance is more appropriate.

Box 19–4 summarizes the types and aspects of program evaluation presented here. In designing a program evaluation, the community health nurse will need to decide which of the two types and five subtypes of evaluation are appropriate. A particular program can be evaluated with respect to any one aspect, a combination of several, or all five. The aspects selected will depend upon the purposes of the evaluation and the time and other resources available. Suggested guidelines for determining when to focus on product or process evaluation are presented in Table 19–2.

THE EVALUATION PROCESS

Like any other systematic process, evaluation takes place in a series of specific steps. Some of these steps, such as planning the evaluation, have already been completed as part of the total planning process. Other steps include collecting data, interpreting data, and using evaluative findings.

TABLE 19–2. GUIDELINES FOR DETERMINING TYPE OF EVALUATION

Use outcome evaluation when:	Use process evaluation when:
• Comparing outcomes of different programs • The program is sufficiently developed for outcome to be measured • The variables to be measured are well delineated • Justification for continuing the program is required	• A short-term project is involved • The program is in the early stages of operation • Quantitative or qualitative information is needed to guide decision making in implementing the program • Evaluation recommendations can be implemented and tested in an ongoing process • Unobtrusive measures are warranted • The program and its subjective value to participants are more important than the achievement of specific objectives

(*Source: Benner, P., & Meleis, A. (1975). Process or product evaluation?* Nursing Outlook, *23, 303–307.*)

Planning for Evaluation

Goals for the evaluation, evaluative criteria, the type of data needed, and appropriate methods of data collection were established as part of the planning process. Evaluative criteria and type of evaluation are based on the purpose of the evaluation. If the intent of the evaluation is to determine the extent to which objectives are met, evaluative criteria will be derived from the objectives. In the school meal program example, evaluative criteria related to program objectives would be hematocrit levels of children participating in the program. If the intent is to assess the efficiency of the program, evaluative criteria would include the amount of food wasted and the number of hours spent implementing the program.

Data needed to conduct the evaluation are determined and data-collection procedures established. Planning for evaluation also involves determining the necessary equipment and supplies. Items needed to evaluate accomplishment of the school meal program objectives would include parental consent forms for hematocrit testing, capillary tubes, lancets, a microcentrifuge, and so on. Other equipment and supplies would be needed to evaluate other aspects of the program.

Collecting Data

The evaluative criteria chosen influence the type of data collected and the manner in which it is collected. For the hematocrit criterion, data includes participating children's hematocrit levels, which need to be collected by testing blood samples at periodic intervals before and during the program. There needs to be a baseline level for each child from before the program to determine whether hematocrit levels have increased, so data collection related to evaluation must begin before the program itself starts. Data collection related to food wasted might include reviewing purchase orders and periodic observation of the amount of food discarded at the end of the day.

Interpreting Data

The next step in the evaluation process is interpreting the data collected. In this step, data are compared to the evaluative criteria. In evaluating the achievement of the objectives of the school meal program, the nurse would compare the children's hematocrit levels after starting the program with those obtained prior to the program. If there is an increase noted in most children, the program has been somewhat effective. The nurse would also determine how many of the children had now achieved a normal hematocrit level. If 75 percent or more of the children now have normal levels, the program has met its objective.

In examining data related to the efficiency of the use of supplies, the nurse would look at what percent of food purchased is actually consumed and what percent is wasted. If the criterion specified that less than

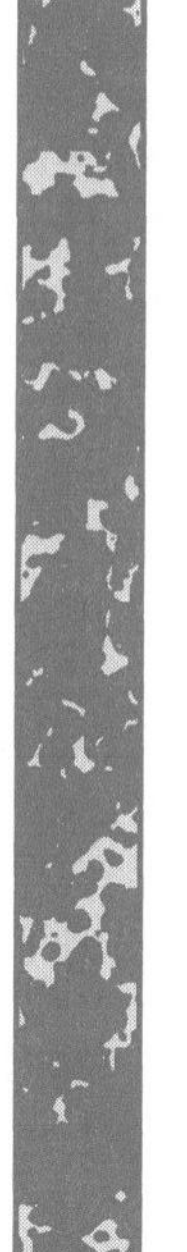

BOX 19–5

Steps in the Evaluation Process

Planning for Evaluation
- Setting evaluation goals
- Developing evaluative criteria
- Determining the data needed
- Establishing data-collection procedures
- Determining resources needed

Collecting data

Interpreting data

Using evaluative findings to make decisions to:
- Continue the program
- Modify the program
- Discontinue the program

5 percent of food and supplies purchased is wasted and the nurse finds that closer to 10 percent is actually wasted, the program is not operating as efficiently as planned.

Using Evaluative Findings

The findings of the evaluation are then used to make decisions about the program. There are basically three decisions that can be made based on evaluative findings: to continue, to modify, or to discontinue the program. If the nurse finds that the program's objectives are being achieved, he or she may decide to continue the program. If the nurse finds that only a few children are participating in the program, the nurse may decide either to stop the program or take steps to increase participation. For example, perhaps the menu needs to be changed to include nutritious foods that are more acceptable to the target group. Looking at program efficiency, if the nurse finds that 10 percent of the food purchased is being wasted, various waste-control practices may need to be instituted. The use of evaluative findings and the other steps in program evaluation are summarized in Box 19–5.

CHAPTER HIGHLIGHTS

- The epidemiologic prevention process model may be used to direct community health nursing care for communities or target groups.
- A target group may be a particularly vulnerable subgroup within the population or a group with known health needs.
- Community assessment is the process whereby data are compiled regarding a community's health status and from which nursing diagnoses are derived.
- Tasks involved in preparing for a community or target group assessment include determining the purpose and scope of the assessment and selecting data-collection methods and sources.
- Factors related to maturation and aging considered in assessing a community include the age composition of the population, the annual birthrate, age-specific death rates, and the average age at death.
- Human inheritance factors in assessing a community include the racial and sexual composition of the population. Factors related to physiologic function of community members include the crude and cause-specific death rates, morbidity rates, and immunization rates.
- Physical environmental factors to be assessed include the community's location, size and type, topographical features, and climate. Other factors to be addressed include the type and adequacy of housing, water supply considerations, nuisance factors, and potential for disaster.
- Factors in the psychological environment that may affect a community's health status include future prospects of the community, significant events in the community's history, communications, the adequacy of protective services, suicide and homicide rates, and identifiable sources of stress.
- Social environmental factors such as community government and leadership, language, income and educational levels, marital status and family composition, religion, transportation, and the availability of goods and services also influence a community's health status.
- Life-style factors to be addressed include community consumption patterns related to food and potentially harmful substances; typical occupations of community members and attendant health hazards; leisure pursuits; and other behaviors such as seat-belt use.
- Health system factors include the health-care services available and the extent to which they are used, how health care is financed, and community definitions of health and illness.
- Information gathered for a target group assessment is similar to that for a community assessment, but may vary in terms of the relevance of certain information to a particular target group.
- Community nursing diagnoses occur at two levels: identification of vulnerable populations at risk for certain health conditions and the degree of fit between the population's health needs and services available.

(continued)

- Planning to meet identified community or target group health needs involves setting priorities among needs, determining the level of prevention needed, and developing health programs to meet identified needs.
- Steps in the program planning process include selecting the planning group, developing the group's planning competence, formulating a philosophy, establishing program goals, forecasting, and developing and evaluating alternative solutions. Other tasks in program planning include developing program objectives, identifying resources, delineating actions to accomplish program objectives, evaluating the plan, and planning for evaluation.
- Implementing the plan involves getting it accepted at three levels: acceptance by policymakers, acceptance by implementers, and acceptance by members of the target group.
- Three basic tasks in implementing a health-care program are delineating and sequencing activities and allocating and performing planned activities.
- Considerations in program evaluation include the purpose of the evaluation, who should conduct the evaluation, ethical concerns in evaluation, and the type of evaluation to be conducted.
- Outcome evaluation focuses on the program's effect, the degree to which objectives were met; and the program's impact, the contribution of the program to goal accomplishment.
- Process evaluation focuses on the amount of effort expended in implementing the program, the efficiency of the program, and its organizational processes.
- The program evaluation process includes planning for the evaluation, collecting and interpreting data, and using evaluative findings to make decisions to continue, modify, or discontinue a program.

Review Questions

1. Describe at least three purposes for assessing a community or a target group. (p. 422)
2. Identify at least three factors that influence the scope of a community or target group assessment. Give an example of the influence of each factor. (p. 423)
3. List at least four considerations related to human biology to be addressed in a community or target group assessment. Explain how each could affect the health of a community. (p. 425)
4. Describe at least six environmental factors to be considered in assessing a target group or a community. Give an example of the influence of each factor on the health of a community. (p. 426)
5. Describe at least four ways in which lifestyle factors can influence the health status of a community or a target group. (p. 430)
6. What are three considerations in assessing the impact of the health-care system on the health of a community or target group? (p. 431)
7. Describe two levels of nursing diagnoses related to the health status of a community or a target group. Give an example of a diagnosis at each level. (p. 434)
8. Describe at least three considerations in planning screening programs for communities or target groups. (p. 435)
9. Identify at least six tasks in planning a health program to meet the needs of communities or target groups. (p. 437)
10. What are the three levels of acceptance of a health-care program? (p. 442)
11. Describe three types of considerations in evaluating a health-care program. (p. 444)

APPLICATION AND SYNTHESIS

You are the community health nurse assigned to Clark City, a small town in New Mexico with a population of 3000. You have just arrived in town and have been given the task of assessing the health needs of the community and developing a plan to meet those needs.

During your assessment, you obtained the following information: Clark City is a small town run by a city council and a mayor. Most of these officials are administrators of the local copper mines or owners of large chicken farms in the area. The town is in a largely rural area, and lies 50 miles from Tucumcari. The surrounding countryside is hot and arid.

The ethnic composition of the town is 80 percent Caucasian of European ancestry and 20 percent Latino, primarily of Mexican descent. Fifty percent of the town's population is under 8 years of age. There are very few elderly persons in the community, because Clark City is a relatively new town that grew up around copper mines discovered in the last 20 years. The birthrate is 30 per 1000 population. Approximately 10 percent of all births are premature, and the neonatal death rate is 50 per 1000 live births. Only about 10 percent of the women receive prenatal care during their pregnancies.

The major industries in the area are copper mines and chicken farms, which employ approximately 85 percent of the adult men and 50 percent of the women. The majority of the Latino population works on the chicken farms. The remaining 15 percent of the adult males and another 20 percent of the adult females are employed in offices and shops in the town. The unemployment level is 0.5 percent, far lower than that of the state and the nation.

The average annual family income is $8000, and 75 percent of the population is below the poverty level. Nearly one-third of those below the poverty level receive some form of aid such as Medicaid, AFDC, and so on.

The predominant religion among the Caucasian population is Methodist, and among the Latino group it is Roman Catholic. There are two Methodist churches in town, one Catholic church, and a small Southern Baptist congregation.

Many of the Latino group subscribe to folk health practices. They frequently seek health care from a local *yerbero* (herbalist). They may also drive to a nearby town to solicit the services of a *curandera* (faith healer). Close to one-third of the Latino population speaks only Spanish.

The average educational level for the community is tenth grade. For the Spanish-speaking group, however, it is only third grade. Educational facilities in the town include a grade school and a high school. The high school also offers adult education classes at night. There is a Head Start program that enrolls 50 children, but no other child-care facilities are available.

There is a high incidence of tuberculosis in the community, and anemia and pinworms are common problems among the school-age children. Several of the men have been disabled as a result of accidents in the mines.

The only transportation to Tucumcari is by car or by train, which comes through town morning and evening. About half of the families in town own cars.

There is one general-practice physician and one dentist in the town. The nearest hospital is in Tucumcari, and the funeral home hearse is used as an ambulance for emergency transportation to the hospital. The driver and one attendant have had basic first aid training. The county health department provides family planning, prenatal, well-child, and immunization services one day a week in the basement of the larger of the two Methodist churches. In addition to yourself, the staff consists of a physician, one licensed practical nurse, a masters-prepared family nurse practitioner, and a nutritionist. The well-child and immunization services are heavily utilized, and immunization levels in the community are high among both preschoolers and school-age youngsters.

1. What are the human biological, environmental, life-style, and health system factors influencing the health of this community?
2. What community nursing diagnoses might you derive from this data?

3. What are the health problems evident in the case study? Which are the three most important problems for this community? Why have you given these problems top priority over others?
4. Select one of the three top priority problems and design a health program to resolve it. Be sure to address:
   a. the level of prevention involved
   b. who should be involved in the planning group and why
   c. additional information you would need, if any, and where you would obtain that information
   c. goals and objectives for the program
   d. resources needed to implement the program.
5. How would you gain acceptance of your program?
6. How would you go about implementing the program?
7. How would you conduct outcome and process evaluation of the program?

REFERENCES

1. American Nurses' Association. (1984). *A guide for community-based nursing services.* Kansas City, MO: American Nurses' Association.
2. Higgs, Z. R., & Gustafson, D. D. (1985). *Community as client: Assessment and diagnosis.* Philadelphia: F. A. Davis.
3. Josten, L. E. (1989). Wanted: Leaders for public health. *Nursing Outlook, 37,* 230–232.
4. Ruffing-Rahal, M. A. (1985). Qualitative methods in community analysis. *Public Health Nursing, 2,* 130–137.
5. Ruffing-Rahal, M. A. (1987). Resident/provider contrasts in community health priorities. *Public Health Nursing, 4,* 242–246.
6. United States Department of Health and Human Services. (1991). *Healthy people 2000: National health promotion and disease prevention objectives.* Washington, DC: Government Printing Office.
7. Cook, H. L., Goeppinger, J., & Brunk, S. E., et al. (1988). A re-examination of community participation in health: Lessons from three community health projects. *Family and Community Health, 11*(2), 1–13.
8. Toma, R. B., & Curry, M. L. (1980). North Dakota Indian traditional foods. *Journal of the American Dietetic Association, 76,* 589–590.
9. Stambler, H. V. (1988). The Area Resource File—A brief look. *Public Health Reports, 103,* 184–188.
10. United States Department of Commerce. (1991). *Statistical abstract of the United States* (110th ed.). Washington, DC: Government Printing Office.
11. Bernstein, E., & Wallerstein, N. (1988). ASAP: An alcohol and substance abuse program developed for adolescents in New Mexico. *Border Health, IV*(4), 17–24.
12. McCreight, L. (1989). The future of public health. *Nursing Outlook, 37,* 219–225.
13. Goeppinger, J., & Baglioni, A. J. (1985). Community competence: A positive approach to needs assessment. *American Journal of Community Psychology, 13,* 507–523.
14. Hamilton, P. (1983). Community nursing diagnosis. *Advances in Nursing Science, 5*(3), 21–36.
15. Muecke, M. A. (1984). Community health diagnosis in nursing. *Public Health Nursing, 1,* 23–35.
16. Porter, E. J. (1987). Administrative diagnosis—Implications for the public's health. *Public Health Nursing, 4,* 247–256.
17. American Public Health Association. (1961). *Guide to a community health study.* New York: American Public Health Association.
18. Valanis, B. (1986). *Epidemiology in Nursing and Health Care.* Norwalk, CT: Appleton-Century-Crofts.
19. Archer, S. E., Kelly, C. D., & Bisch, S. A. (1984). *Implementing change in communities: A collaborative approach.* St. Louis: C. V. Mosby.
20. Sofaer, S. (1988). Community health planning in the United States: A postmortem. *Family and Community Health, 10*(4), 1–12.
21. Courtney, R. (1987). Community practice: Nursing influence on policy making. *Nursing Outlook, 35,* 170–173.

RECOMMENDED READINGS

Finnegan, L., & Ervin, N. E. (1989). An epidemiological approach to community assessment. *Public Health Nursing, 6,* 147–151.

Applies the epidemiologic triad to assessment of a community's health needs. Provides a case study illustrating the application of the model to community assessment.

Goeppinger, J., & Baglioni, A. J. (1985). Community competence: A positive approach to needs assessment. *American Journal of Community Psychology, 13,* 507–523.

Describes a study using Cottrell's model of community competence to assess community health status. Examines four factors in community competence in healthy communities: democratic participation style, crime, resource adequacy and use, and decision-making interactions.

McLemore, M. M. (1991). Nurses as health planners. In B. W. Spradley (Ed.), *Readings in community health nursing* (4th ed.) (pp. 201–208). Philadelphia: J. B. Lippincott.

Sets forth the health planning process and suggests strategies to promote nursing involvement in health program planning.

Muecke, M. A. (1984). Community health diagnosis in nursing. *Public Health Nursing, 1,* 23–35.

Addresses the historical development of the concept of community diagnosis. Reviews the diagnostic process as used with communities and provides a case study illustrating application of the concept.

Nettle, C., Laboon, P., & Jones, S. N., et al. (1989). Community nursing diagnosis. *Journal of Community Health Nursing, 6*(3), 135–145.

Describes the use of Gordon's typology of health patterns to assess the health status of a community. Provides a tool to guide data collection in terms of the model.

Porter, E. J. (1987). Administrative diagnosis—Implications for the public's health. *Public Health Nursing, 4,* 247–256.

Reports findings of a study on the diagnostic reasoning process used by community health nursing administrators in making decisions on program changes.

Valdiserri, R. O. (1988). The immediate challenge of health planning for AIDS: An organizational model. *Family and Community Health, 10*(4), 33–48.

Applies principles of program planning to the problem of dealing with AIDS in communities.

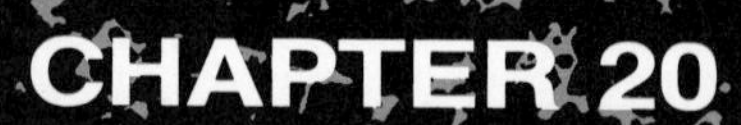

CHAPTER 20

Care of Children

KEY TERMS

anticipatory guidance
attention deficit hyperactivity disorder (ADHD)
development
developmental milestones
downward comparison
fetal alcohol syndrome (FAS)
growth
low birth weight
reactivity pattern
very low birth weight

One of the most effective ways to improve the health status of a community is to maintain and enhance the health of its children. Children who receive effective health-care services, particularly health-promotive and illness-preventive services, are less likely to develop a variety of acute and chronic health problems. Even when working with children with physical, mental, and emotional health problems, community health nurses endeavor to promote the child's ability to reach his or her fullest potential. The importance of community health efforts to improve the health of the nation's children is seen in the fact that 49 of the national health objectives for the year 2000 directly address the health needs of children and another 37 objectives address those needs indirectly.[1] Some of these objectives are summarized in Box 20–1.

Goals for primary prevention for children include promoting normal growth and development, developing positive parent-child relationships, preventing health problems, and developing strengths and resources. When children are ill or have existing health problems, the community health nurse also works toward goals related to secondary and tertiary prevention. Goals of secondary prevention reflect efforts to accurately diagnose health and treat health problems. Tertiary prevention goals in the care of children include restoring function and preventing problem recurrence, preventing complications, adapting to any long-term effects of illness, and minimizing the effects of health problems on the child and his or her family. Community health nursing goals in the care of children are summarized in Box 20–2.

Community health nurses encounter children in a variety of settings. The focus of this chapter is community health nursing activities with children seen in the home or in the clinic or office setting. Pediatric care in acute-care settings is addressed in detail in many pediatric nursing textbooks, while care of the child in the school setting is addressed in Chapter 26, Care of Clients in the School Setting.

LEARNING OBJECTIVES

After reading this chapter you should be able to:

- Identify at least five problems of particular concern to community health nurses working with children.
- Differentiate between growth and development and describe how one would assess each.
- Identify at least three safety considerations in assessing infants, toddlers and preschool children, and school-age children.
- Describe at least five areas to be addressed in assessing the psychological environment of the child.
- Identify at least three life-style considerations in assessing the health status of a child.
- Describe at least five primary preventive measures appropriate to all children.
- Identify at least three approaches that may be taken in providing secondary preventive care for children with existing health problems.
- Describe three tertiary preventive considerations in the care of children with existing health problems.

HEALTH PROBLEMS OF CONCERN IN THE CARE OF CHILDREN

In addition to concerns for health promotion and illness prevention, there are several specific health problems that are of concern to community health nurses caring for children. Some of these problems include infant mortality and low birth weight, congenital anomalies, human immunodeficiency virus (HIV) infection, chronic illness, fetal drug and alcohol exposure, and child abuse.

INFANT MORTALITY

The United States ranks eighteenth in the world in terms of infant mortality rates, far higher than many

BOX 20–1

Summary of Selected National Health Objectives for the Year 2000 Related to the Health of Children

- Reduce the infant mortality rate to no more than 7 per 1000 live births.
- Reduce growth retardation among low-income children aged 5 and under to less than 10%.
- Reduce to less than 10% the prevalence of mental disorders among children and adolescents.
- Reverse to less than 25.2 per 1000 children the rising incidence of abuse of children younger than 18 years of age.
- Reduce the rate of deaths due to motor vehicle accidents to no more than 5.5 per 1000 children aged 14 or younger.
- Reduce the prevalence of blood lead levels exceeding 15 μg/dL and 25 μg/dL among children aged 6 months through 5 years to less than 500,000 and zero, respectively.
- Reduce the prevalence of serious mental retardation in school-age children to less than 2 per 1000 children.
- Increase to at least 30% the proportion of those over age 6 who engage regularly in light to moderate activity for at least 30 minutes daily.
- Reduce the initiation of smoking behavior to no more than 15% of people under age 20.
- Reduce iron deficiency to less than 3% among children aged 1 through 4.
- Achieve access to high-quality and developmentally appropriate preschool programs for all disadvantaged children and children with disabilities.
- Increase use of occupant protection systems in motor vehicles to at least 95% of children aged 4 and under.
- Increase to at least 90% the proportion of children under age 2 who have completed a basic immunization series.
- Increase to at least 80% the proportion of children aged 2 through 12 who have received all of the screening and immunization services and at least one counseling service recommended by the U.S. Preventive Services Task Force.
- Increase to at least 85% the proportion of people aged 10 through 18 who have discussed human sexuality with their parents or received information through another parentally approved source
- Enact in 50 states laws requiring new handguns be designed to minimize the likelihood of discharge by children.
- Increase to at least 80% the proportion of babies under 18 months of age who receive recommended primary care services.
- Increase to 50 the number of states that have service systems for children with or at risk for chronic and disabling conditions.

(Source: U.S. Department of Health and Human Services. (1980). *Promoting health/preventing disease: Objectives for the nation.* Washington, DC: Government Printing Office.

BOX 20–2

Goals of Community Health Nursing Care for Children

Goals for Primary Prevention:
- Promote normal growth and development
- Develop positive parent-child relationships
- Prevent the occurrence of health problems
- Develop strengths and resources

Goals for Secondary Prevention:
- Promote accurate diagnosis of existing health problems
- Facilitate treatment for existing health problems
- Eliminate existing health problems

Goals for Tertiary Prevention:
- Restore function and prevent problem recurrence
- Prevent complications of existing conditions
- Promote adjustment to chronic conditions

other developed countries.[2] In 1987, the infant mortality rate in the United States was 10 deaths for every 1000 live births. Infant mortality is even higher for some segments of the population. Nearly 18 of every 1000 black babies and 12 of every 1000 Native American babies die before they are a year old. While current infant mortality rates are the lowest in history in this country, the rate of decline has slowed considerably in the last decade. Primary causes of death in the neonatal period (the first 30 days of life) are congenital anomalies, respiratory distress syndrome and other consequences of prematurity, and the effects of maternal complications during pregnancy. Post-neonatal infant mortality is most often due to sudden infant death syndrome (SIDS), congenital anomalies, injuries, and infections.[1]

LOW BIRTH WEIGHT

Low birth weight among those infants who survive also presents problems. ***Low birth weight*** is a weight less than 2500 grams at birth, while ***very low birth weight*** is a birth weight of less than 1500 grams. In 1987, almost 7 percent of all babies had low birth weights and over 1 percent were of very low birth weight. Again, figures are worse for certain segments of the population. For example, nearly 13 percent of black babies have low birth weight, while almost 3 percent are of very low birth weight.[1]

Low birth weight is associated with younger and older maternal age, poor maternal weight gain, multiparity, lack of prenatal care, and substance abuse. As much as 30 percent of low birth weight may be due to smoking.[1] Despite increasing public knowledge of the effects of smoking during pregnancy, nearly one-fourth of women continue to smoke while pregnant.[3]

Effects of low birth weight include lower IQ, cerebral palsy, seizure disorders, and blindness. Approximately one-fourth of very low birth weight babies will exhibit moderate to severe disabilities, while 2 to 4 percent of low birth weight babies will be affected.[1] In addition, very low birth weight children have been found to have problems in school and with hyperactivity.[4]

CONGENITAL ANOMALIES

While many children with congenital anomalies die in utero or during infancy, modern medical technology has increased the number of children with anomalies who survive. In recent years, there has been an increasing prevalence of several congenital abnormalities in newborns. These abnormalities include anomalies of the central nervous system (hydrocephalus, encephalocele), eye (congenital cataract), cardiovascular system (ventricular and atrial septal defects, tetralogy of Fallot, pulmonary and aortic valvular stenosis, patent ductus arteriosus), cleft lip and palate, and anomalies of the gastrointestinal system (intestinal atresia, tracheoesophageal anomalies), genitourinary system (renal agenesis and hypoplasia), and musculoskeletal system (club foot), as well as chromosomal abnormalities (Down's syndrome, trisomy 13, trisomy 18). During the period from 1979 to 1987, the prevalence of some of these anomalies increased by as much as 10 to 29 percent.[5]

HIV INFECTION AND AIDS

Other areas of concern are HIV infection and the growing number of AIDS cases in children. As of September 1990, over 2600 cases of AIDS had been diagnosed in youngsters under 13 years of age. Of these children, 83 percent were born to mothers with or at risk for HIV infection, 9 percent had been transfused or received other infected donor tissues, and 5 percent had hemophilia or other coagulation disorders. Risk factors for 3 percent of the children with AIDS were undetermined.[6]

A high proportion of infants born to HIV-infected mothers are themselves infected. In one study, 30 percent of infants born to mothers with known HIV infection were found to be infected. Forty percent of these infected infants died within 18 months of birth.[7] An estimated 1500 to 2000 HIV-infected infants were born in 1989.[8] With the increasing incidence of HIV infection among women of child-bearing age, there will be continued increase in the number of children with HIV infection and with symptomatic AIDS.

CHRONIC ILLNESS

Children also suffer from a variety of chronic illnesses including asthma, various forms of cancer, diabetes, hypertension, juvenile arthritis, and seizure disorders, to name a few. As many as 10 percent of youngsters may exhibit signs and symptoms of asthma at some point during childhood. Asthma has both physical and psychosocial effects on the child and contributes to a significant number of school days lost for children affected.[9]

The most commonly encountered cancers in children include acute lymphocytic leukemia, brain and central nervous system tumors, neuroblastomas, soft-tissue sarcomas, Wilms' tumors, non-Hodgkin and Hodgkin lymphomas, and acute granulocytic leukemia. From 1977 to 1980, approximately 130 malignant tumors were diagnosed per 1 million children under age 15. While the prognosis varies with the type of cancer involved, roughly one-third of these children die of their disease. Risk factors for malignant neoplasms include environmental exposures to carcinogens, viral exposures (for example, the Epstein-Barr virus that causes infectious mononucleosis), genetic characteristics, and other existing conditions such as some congenital anomalies, immunodeficiency states, and chromosomal anomalies.[10]

Insulin-dependent (Type I) diabetes mellitus occurs in approximately two out of every 1000 school children.[11] The incidence of insulin-dependent diabetes is higher in Caucasian children of European descent and lower in black and Asian children. Type I diabetes also appears to be less common among Native Americans and Polynesians, groups that have high incidence rates for Type II diabetes, formerly known as adult-onset diabetes.[12]

Hypertension in children most often occurs as a result of an underlying organic problem such as renal disease or coarctation of the aorta.[13] Essential hypertension (hypertension due to no discernible organic cause) does occur in children, however. Approximately 3 percent of children in the United States have hypertension and can be effectively treated. Routine blood pressure measurements starting at 3 years of age are recommended to identify youngsters with hypertension.[14]

Juvenile arthritis is a collection of syndromes that have in common chronic arthritis beginning in childhood. Although precise incidence and prevalence are unknown, it is estimated that approximately one in every 2000 American children may be affected. This amounts to about 35,000 youngsters in the United States.[15] Arthritis in children can affect single or multiple joints, and virtually any joint may be involved. Anywhere from 10 percent to over 50 percent of children with various forms of juvenile arthritis will have severe joint involvement during their lifetime.

Approximately 5 percent of children will experience at least one seizure sometime during their childhood.[16] Most seizures experienced by children are a manifestation of underlying acute systemic or central nervous system diseases such as meningitis and encephalitis, metabolic disturbances such as hypoglycemia and hypocalcemia, or intoxications. Some children, however, experience recurrent seizures that constitute a seizure disorder or epilepsy.[17] Prevalence rates for grand mal seizures range from 2 to 3 per 1000 children.[18] Approximately 75 percent of these children obtain good seizure control with antiepileptic drug therapy,[19] but the disease is still a frightening one for both parents and children.

The presence of these and other chronic illnesses in children creates special needs for community health nursing care. These illnesses may also necessitate creative approaches to general health promotion and illness prevention in these youngsters.

ATTENTION DEFICIT HYPERACTIVITY DISORDER

Attention deficit hyperactivity disorder (ADHD) affects as many as 10 percent of school-age boys[20] and somewhat fewer girls. ***Attention deficit hyperactivity disorder*** is a condition characterized by poor attention span, impulsive behavior, and hyperactivity.[21] Hyperactive children frequently have difficulties with school performance, peer interactions, and unacceptable behavior. There is also some evidence that hyperactivity in childhood is a risk factor for later development of antisocial disorders and criminal behavior.[22] Attention deficit with associated hyperactivity is frustrating for the children affected and for everyone who interacts with them. Approximately 1 to 2 percent of school-age children receive psychostimulants as treatment for ADHD, yet only about two-thirds of these children show improvement of problematic behaviors. Compliance training and behavior modification have been shown to be effective with some children.[23]

FETAL ALCOHOL AND DRUG EXPOSURE

Fetal alcohol syndrome (FAS) is a condition resulting from maternal alcohol consumption during pregnancy and is characterized by growth retardation, facial malformations, and central nervous system dysfunctions that may include mental retardation. In 1987, 2 babies in every 10,000 live births exhibited evidence of fetal alcohol syndrome. Incidence of FAS is even higher in some segments of the population. From 1981 to 1986, FAS incidence rates for Native American infants were 33 times higher than for whites, while those for black infants were 7 times higher than for their white counterparts.[1] Long-term effects of FAS include inability to hold down a job, impulsivity, social withdrawal, poor judgment, and mental retardation.[24]

Even those infants exposed to moderate amounts of alcohol during pregnancy may have long-term effects. Approximately 2 percent of infants exposed to less than an ounce of alcohol a day have anomalies due to the teratogenic (deformity producing) effects of alcohol.[25] In 1988, about 20 percent of pregnant women continued to drink throughout their pregnancies.[26]

Fetal drug exposure also has adverse effects on children. Use of cocaine during pregnancy, for example, increases the incidence of stillbirth, low birth weight, and congenital malformations.[27] Fetal drug exposure has also been shown to result in neurological abnormalities and developmental delays[28] and increased risk of sudden infant death syndrome (SIDS). In one study, the incidence of SIDS in babies born to drug-abusing mothers was nearly eight times that of infants born to nonabusing mothers.[29]

CHILD ABUSE

Child abuse is another area of serious concern to community health nurses. In 1987, nearly 16 of every 1000 children under age 18 was the victim of neglect, while the incidence of physical abuse among this group was almost 6 per 1000 children. Incidence rates for sexual abuse and emotional abuse were somewhat lower (2.5 and 3 per 1000 children, respectively). Increasing incidence of all forms of child abuse has been noted since 1980, and in 1986 1.6 million children experienced some form of abuse or neglect.[1] Child abuse is addressed in detail in the section on family violence included in Chapter 34, Violence.

Evidence of all of the problems discussed above highlights the need for community health nursing services to children. Such services can help to prevent the occurrence of these and other problems affecting children and to minimize their effects on both the child and the child's family.

THE EPIDEMIOLOGIC PREVENTION PROCESS MODEL AND CARE OF CHILDREN

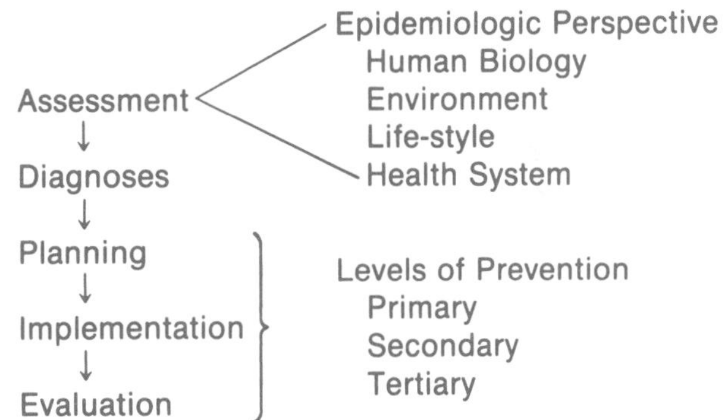

The epidemiologic prevention process model provides a framework for community health nursing efforts to accomplish the goals of primary, secondary, and tertiary prevention in the care of children.

ASSESSING THE HEALTH NEEDS OF CHILDREN IN THE COMMUNITY

As always, the use of the model begins with assessing the client's health status to identify the need for nursing intervention. Assessment of children should be thorough, but it is not necessary to obtain all of the assessment data in the first encounter with the child. Data collected during a first encounter will depend upon the child and the situation. If the child is basically well, more data may be collected than if the child is ill at the time of the initial encounter. With an ill child, one would obtain data related to current problems and defer gathering additional data until a later time. Over time, however, the nurse will elicit information on factors in each of the four areas of Dever's epidemiologic perspective.

HUMAN BIOLOGY

Human biological factors that may influence a child's health include maturation and aging, genetic inheritance, and physiologic function.

Maturation and Aging

Assessing Growth. *Growth* is an increase in body size or change in the structure, function, and complexity of body cells until a point of maturity. Growth parameters considered in the nurse's assessment of the child include weight, height, and head and chest circumferences. With respect to height and weight, the nurse assesses the child in relation to normal values for the child's age and in comparison to the child's own previous growth pattern. Height and weight should be plotted on a graph at periodic intervals to establish the child's growth pattern. Plotting also facilitates comparisons to age norms. Height and weight are also examined in relation to each other and to other growth parameters. Plotting a child's height in relation to his or her weight is demonstrated in Figure 20–1. Marked deviations from normal values for the child's age, changes in previous growth patterns, or marked incongruence among growth parameters are indications of a need for further evaluation.

Head circumference is another indicator of growth that is usually measured and plotted on a graph until 1 to 2 years of age. Head circumference is measured at the largest diameter of the head with the tape measure circling the forehead and the occipital bulge as indicated in Figure 20–2. Head circumference is always evaluated in conjunction with chest circumference measured at the nipple line as indicated in Figure 20–2. The ratio between head and chest circumference changes dramatically in the first year of life. At birth, head circumference is approximately three-fourths of an inch greater than chest circumference.[30] By 1 year of age, the two measurements are approximately equal. Beyond 1 year of age, chest circumference should exceed head circumference, and the difference in the two measurements will increase with increasing age until adult proportions are reached.[31]

A marked departure from the expected ratio between head and chest circumference may indicate neurological, cardiovascular, or respiratory problems. For example, an overly large head might indicate hydrocephaly, while a small head may be related to microcephaly or poor bone growth of the skull. A large chest might be due to respiratory difficulties or cardiac enlargement. A small chest, on the other hand, could reflect malnutrition or other causes of poor bone growth.

The nurse assesses the child in terms of these

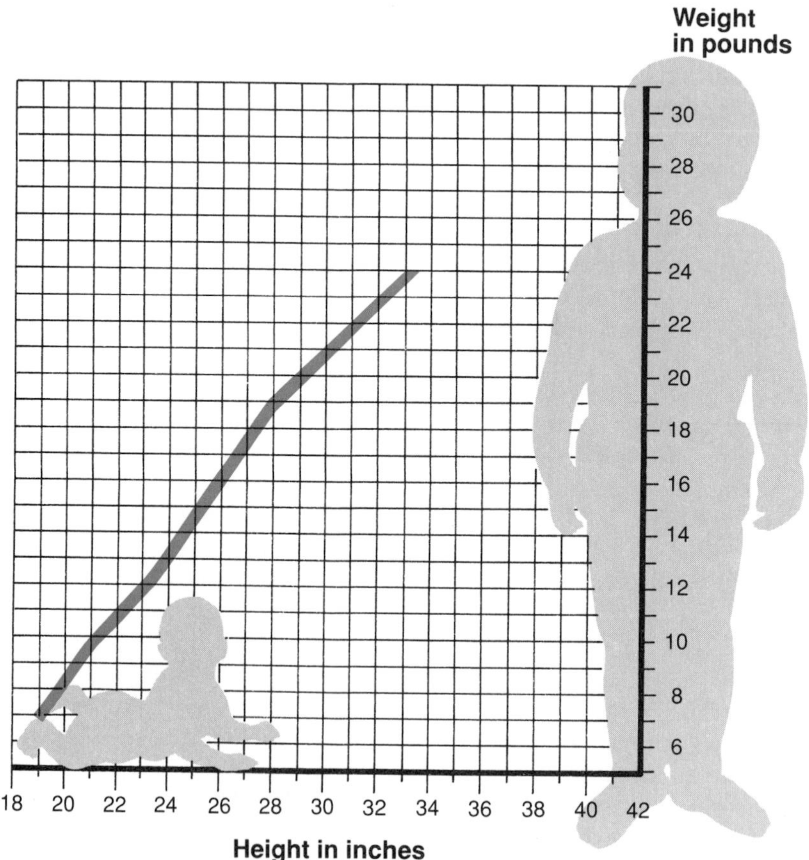

Figure 20–1. Plotting height in relation to weight.

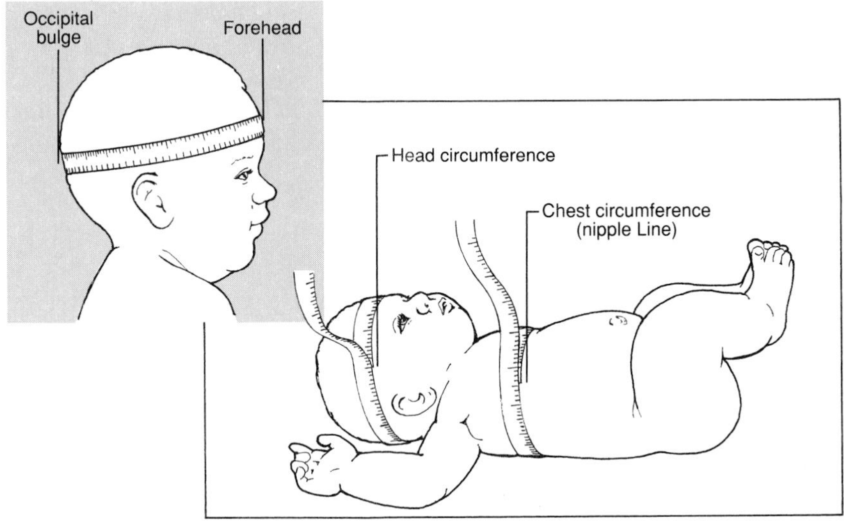

Figure 20–2. Measuring head circumference and chest circumference.

growth parameters, noting deviations from age norms or changes in the child's own growth pattern. Such deviations or changes are examined to determine whether they indicate the presence of health problems. For example, deviation from age norms may be related to metabolic or hormonal disorders, poor feeding, overfeeding, neglect, or familial characteristics, to name a few underlying factors. Unexpected changes in the child's previous growth patterns may result from either physical or emotional causes. General guidelines for assessing growth patterns in children are presented in Table 20–1.

Assessing Development. *Development* is a process of patterned, orderly, and lifelong change in structure, thought, or behavior that occurs as a result of physical or emotional maturation. The community health nurse assesses the child's development in terms of ***developmental milestones,*** which are critical behaviors expected at specific ages. Developmental assessment may be approached in a number of ways. The most widely used tool for assessing the development of children from birth to age 6 is the Denver Developmental Screening Test (DDST). This test provides a gross measure of the child's fine motor and

TABLE 20–1. GENERAL PARAMETERS FOR ASSESSING GROWTH IN CHILDREN OF SELECTED AGES

Age Group	Assessment Parameters
Neonate (birth to 30 days)	• Median weight of a full-term infant: 7 to 7¼ pounds • Loss of several ounces in first few days • Return to birth weight by 10 days of age • Median length at birth: 19¾ to 20 inches
Infant (1 to 12 months)	• Doubles birth weight by 4 to 5 months of age • Triples birth weight by 1 year of age • Gains 10 inches in length by 1 year of age • Head circumference increases by about 4¾ inches (12 cm) by 1 year of age
Toddler and preschool child (2 to 5 years)	• Quadruples birth weight in the second year of life • Gains 5 inches in height in the second year of life • Gains 3 to 5 pounds per year from age 2 to age 5 • Grows 1½ to 2½ inches per year from age 2 to age 5 • Head circumference increases by 1 inch in the second year
School-age child (6 to 12 years)	• Gains 3 to 5 pounds per year through age 10 • Grows 1½ to 2½ inches per year through age 10 • Boy: Gains 15 to 20 pounds per year through age 12 Grows 4½ to 5 inches per year through age 12 • Girl: Gains 20 to 25 pounds per year through age 12 Grows 5 to 6 inches per year through age 12

(Source: Lathrop.[30])

gross motor development, personal-social development, and language development. Although the test is easy to administer and can indicate problem areas related to the child's development, it is *not* a diagnostic tool and does not give an indication of the possible causes of developmental delays. The DDST is also useful as an aid in providing parents with anticipatory guidance regarding their child's behavior. (Test kits, score sheets, and directions for performing a DDST can be purchased from DDM, Inc., P.O. Box 6919, Denver, CO 80203-0911.)

An abnormal DDST should be repeated in 2 to 3 weeks. If results on the retest are similar, a more in-depth developmental assessment is warranted. In addition to retesting, the nurse would also explore factors that may be contributing to delayed development. For example, if the child is not given the opportunity to engage in certain activities, a developmental delay may occur. Mothers who will not let their children feed themselves because of the "mess" may be contributing to a delay in personal social development on the part of the individual child. Similarly, if the child always gets what he or she wants by pointing, language development may be delayed. Other potential reasons for developmental delay include neurological deficits, mental retardation, or neglect.

The DDST is a useful tool for assessing the development of children from birth through age 6. The development of older children should also be assessed. There are a few assessment tools available for use with older children, but these are less widely used and less well known than the DDST. For children over age 6, a general assessment in terms of accomplishment of specific milestones for their age is probably sufficient. Major developmental milestones for various age groups were presented in Chapter 17, Care of the Individual Client.

Genetic Inheritance

Two intrinsic genetic factors that influence the health of the child are the child's sex and racial background. Male and female children and children of different racial groups tend to experience different types of health problems. For example, the nurse would want to direct more attention to a review of systems related to the urinary tract in school-age girls than in boys because urinary tract infections occur more frequently in girls than in boys in this age group.[32] Similarly, screening tests for sickle cell anemia would be routinely conducted on a black newborn, but not a newborn of European Caucasian descent.[33]

Other information about genetic inheritance is obtained from the family history discussed in Chapter 17, Care of the Individual Client. A family history of insulin-dependent diabetes, for instance, alerts the nurse to the need for careful assessment in this area. Finally, the nurse should be alert to physical or developmental findings that suggest the presence of genetic disorders such as Down's syndrome and Turner's syndrome.

Physiologic Function

Information on various aspects of the child's physiologic functioning can be obtained from the history of present and past health problems, the review of systems, the physical examination, the results of routine screening tests, and a review of the child's immunization status. The review of systems is very similar to that presented in Chapter 17 but is tailored to the age of the child. For example, the nurse would not need to ask questions related to sexual activity when the client is an infant. Similarly, questions about urinary tract function for an infant would center around the number of wet diapers and any strong odor to the child's urine.

Physical examination of a child is also somewhat different from that of an adult. Differences are found primarily in the way the exam is conducted and in the findings. Most examiners adopt a head-to-toe approach when systematically examining an adult. This is not particularly appropriate with young children. With children, the nurse will want to start the exam with noninvasive techniques and leave invasive procedures, such as the examination of ears and throat, until last. Similarly, different techniques may need to be adopted to examine the ears of a child or the abdomen of a ticklish child. The exam will also take place at a slower rate because of the need for extensive explanation and reassurance for the child.

There are also differences in what is considered normal and abnormal in the findings of a pediatric physical. For example, normal values for vital signs vary considerably in young children compared to those for adults. Also, some findings that would be considered definitely abnormal in an adult are perfectly normal in children of certain ages. One such finding is a positive Babinski's reflex in an infant. This is an expected response, and a negative Babinski's reflex at this age would be an abnormal finding. It is beyond the scope of this book to describe all of the differences in physical findings between children and adults. Community health nurses working with youngsters should, however, become familiar with these differences so as to perform accurate assessments of children's health status.

Assessing physiologic function will also involve obtaining information about current and past condi-

TABLE 20–2. COMMON PHYSICAL HEALTH PROBLEMS IN CHILDREN AND ORGAN SYSTEMS AFFECTED

Organ System	Commonly Encountered Problems
General	Anemia, communicable diseases, fever, failure to thrive, physical abuse
Cardiovascular system	Murmurs
Gastrointestinal system	Abdominal pain/appendicitis, colic, constipation, diarrhea, food allergy, spitting up, vomiting
Integumentary system	Abrasions, bruises, burns, diaper rash, eczema, impetigo, lice and scabies, monilial infection, other rashes, swollen lymph nodes
Musculoskeletal system	Congenital hip displasia (CHD), fractures, scoliosis, sprains and other muscle injuries
Neurological system	Headache, hearing loss, visual problems, speech problems, delay
Respiratory system	Allergic rhinitis, asthma, bronchitis, bronchiolitis, croup, otitis media, pharyngitis, pneumonia, upper respiratory infection
Urinary system	Bed wetting, urinary tract infection

tions experienced by the child. Of particular concern are the types of conditions discussed at the beginning of this chapter. The nurse should ask about the presence of these conditions or any other diagnosed health problem. In addition, the nurse would also be alert to the signs and symptoms of a variety of problems that commonly occur in children. Some of these common problems are included in Table 20–2.

Information about the child's physiologic function may also be obtained by means of several routine screening tests performed at periodic intervals. Indications for the use of several routine screening measures are included in Box 20–3. In many states, screening for phenylketonuria (PKU) and thyroid dysfunction occurs at birth. Early intervention in these two conditions can prevent lasting consequences such as mental retardation, so early diagnosis is important and warrants routine screening of all newborns. Other screening tests are performed at intervals throughout childhood. Hematocrit or hemoglobin levels are usually tested at 6 months and 1 year of age and yearly thereafter. Another blood test routinely performed on children in high-risk groups is for sickle cell disease. Sickle cell screening is recommended for black children at birth. Routine screening for tuberculosis is conducted in areas with a high incidence of this disease. The Mantoux intradermal test is recommended and is usually given before 1 year of age and periodically thereafter depending on the incidence of TB in the community. Formal testing of vision and hearing can begin at 3 to 4 years of age, when children are old enough to understand and to cooperate in testing. Prior to that time, gross assessment of hearing and vision is performed as part of the physical examination. Blood pressure measurement is also recommended yearly, starting at age 3, because of the number of children

BOX 20–3

Typical Schedule for Routine Screening of Children

Age	*Screening tests*
Birth	PKU, T4
6 months	Hematocrit or hemoglobin, lead
9 months	Tuberculin skin test (PPD)
1 year	Hematocrit or hemoglobin, sickle cell (for blacks), lead
2 years	Hematocrit or hemoglobin
3–4 years	Hematocrit or hemoglobin, lead, blood pressure, hearing, vision, dental
5–6 years	Hematocrit or hemoglobin, lead, blood pressure, hearing, vision, dental, urinalysis (for girls)
7–8 years	Hematocrit or hemoglobin, lead, blood pressure, hearing, vision, dental
9–10 years	Hematocrit or hemoglobin, lead, blood pressure, hearing, vision, scoliosis, dental
11–12 years	Hematocrit or hemoglobin, lead, blood pressure, hearing, vision, scoliosis, dental

(Source: U.S. Preventive Services Task Force.[33])

TABLE 20–3. RECOMMENDED SCHEDULE FOR CHILDHOOD IMMUNIZATIONS

Immunization	Recommended Schedule
Diphtheria, pertussis, and tetanus (DPT)	2, 4, 6, and 15 months, with a booster at school entry
Hemophilus influenzae Type B (HIB)	2, 4, 6, and 15 months
Measles, mumps, and rubella (MMR)	15 months (12 months or sooner in case of an epidemic) with a booster at school entry
Oral polio	2, 4, and 15 months, with a booster at school entry
Tetanus, diphtheria (Td)	Every 10 years after initial DPT series

(Source: California State Department of Health Services, Immunization Unit. [1990]. Summary of Pediatric Immunization Recommendations. *Sacramento: California State Department of Health Services.)*

who are found to be hypertensive. The final routine screening procedure for children is a urinalysis for little girls at age 4 or 5.[33]

The nurse should also assess the child's immunization status. Has the child received immunizations appropriate to his or her age? Guidelines for childhood immunizations are summarized in Table 20–3. For the very young infant, the nurse would also want to explore the mother's immune status since immunity in the newborn is derived from transplacental transfer of maternal antibodies. If the mother has had chicken pox, for example, the child will probably have some protection against this disease. This is also true for diseases against which the mother has been immunized.

ENVIRONMENT

Environmental factors can have a profound impact on the health status of children. This is particularly true because children have less ability to control their environment than do adults. The community health nurse will examine factors in the physical, psychological, and social environments that may affect the health of the child.

Physical Environment

Safety hazards are a major factor in the physical environment that influences the health of children of all ages. Safety concerns are related to the child's physical surroundings and the child's ability to gain access to dangerous substances. The nurse should assess both the presence of hazardous conditions in the child's environment and the child's knowledge of safety-related behaviors.

The community health nurse also would assess the knowledge of and adherence to safety practices among parents and other caretakers. Areas for consideration relative to caretaker practices include the amount of supervision provided for the child and parental use of safety devices. Child safety practices in both the home and the child-care environment should be considered if they are different.

Considerations in assessing child safety factors will vary with the age of the child. Specific questions related to safety assessment for infants, toddlers and preschool children, and school-age children are presented in Table 20–4.

For the infant, the nurse would assess parental safety practices, sleeping arrangements, and toys. The nurse should determine whether parents are aware of the potential for falls and the danger in leaving an infant unattended on an elevated surface. The use of safety belts in high chairs, swings, strollers, and infant seats should also be explored. The safety of sleeping arrangements should be addressed as well. Areas to be considered are the spacing between crib slats, use of plastic film to cover mattresses, and the use of nontoxic paint on crib surfaces. The nurse should also make sure that there are no cords dangling from drapes near the crib in which the child could become entangled and thus strangle. Toys should be soft with no sharp edges and should not have small parts that can be detached and swallowed. Care should also be taken that toys with small parts belonging to older siblings are kept out of the infant's reach.

Safety concerns for the toddler or preschool child include supervision of play activities, use of safety equipment, safety education, the extent to which the home or child-care center has been "child-proofed," toy safety, and playground safety.

Considerations in child-proofing include covering electrical outlets, eliminating dangling electrical cords, and appropriate storage of sharp objects or hazardous substances. Sharp objects should be locked away as should any poisonous substances. Placing these items up high is not a sufficient precaution, as children rapidly learn to climb and can devise ingenious methods of obtaining objects placed out of reach. Locks or child-proof latches should be used on drawers or cabinets where hazardous substances are kept, and children should be closely supervised at all times.

Access to medications and other potentially poi-

TABLE 20–4. QUESTIONS FOR ASSESSING ENVIRONMENTAL SAFETY FOR CHILDREN OF SELECTED AGES

Age Group	Assessment Questions
Infant (birth to 1 year)	• Is the child left unattended on elevated surfaces? • Is an approved car seat restraint used consistently? • Do parents routinely fasten safety straps in high chairs, strollers, swings, and infant seats? • Do parents use flame-retardant sleepwear? • Does the infant have his or her own crib? • Is plastic film that might suffocate the child left on or in the crib? • Are there dangling drapery or other cords near the crib in which the child could strangle? • Are slats on the crib sufficiently close together that the child cannot get his or her head stuck? • Has nontoxic paint been used on crib surfaces? • Are bumper pads used to prevent injury? • Are soft pillows removed from the bed? • Do mobiles or toys have sharp surfaces or small parts that can be swallowed? • Are toys free of strings that could choke the child? • Are siblings' toys with small parts kept out of the infant's reach? • Do parents refrain from giving a bottle in bed or propping a bottle?
Toddler (age 2 to 3 years)	• Are car seats used consistently? • Is the child adequately supervised during waking hours? • Do parents check the infant periodically during naps? • Has the environment been child-proofed so that: –electrical outlets are covered? –sharp objects and poisonous substances are locked away, not just placed out of reach? –medications and other hazardous substances are kept in appropriate containers? –safety latches or locks are on cabinets used to store hazardous items? –child-resistant containers are used correctly? –dangling electrical cords have been eliminated? –stairs are gated? –bathroom doors are kept closed to prevent the child from falling in the toilet? • Have parents inspected play equipment for hazards? • Is the surface below playground equipment padded in some way? • Are toys appropriate to the child's age and ability? • Do parents leave the child unattended in the tub? • If the family has a pool, is it adequately fenced?
Preschool child (3 to 6 years)	• Has the home been child-proofed as above? • Are pot handles turned away from the edge of the stove? • Are car seats or seat belts used consistently? • Is play equipment safe? • Are toys used appropriately, with adult supervision as needed? • Is the child adequately supervised at all times? • Has the child been given safety education regarding: –talking to or going with strangers? –crossing the street? –fire safety? –water safety?
School-age child (6 to 12 years)	• Is play equipment safe? • Are sports and play activities well supervised? • Are sports activities age-appropriate? • Are seat belts used consistently? • Has the child been given safety education regarding: –sports? –bicycling? –water safety? –opening the door to strangers or letting others know one is home alone? –correct use of medications? • Does the child know how to swim? • Is a helmet used consistently for bike riding? • Are firearms kept in the home? If so, are they locked up? Is ammunition kept locked in a separate place from guns?

sonous items should be prevented. While deaths from poisoning have decreased significantly over the last few decades, an estimated 1.4 million poisonings occurred among children under 5 years of age in 1983 alone. Approximately 90 percent of such poisonings occur in the home.[34] Potential poisons include medications, cleaning agents, paints, and paint-removal substances. The Poison Prevention Packaging Act of 1970 requires child-resistant containers for 15 categories of products. Ever since the implementation of this legislation, poisonings from products in these categories have declined. Poisonings related to unregulated products have increased, however. Possible causes for the still overwhelming numbers of unintentional child poisonings include failure to use child-resistant packages correctly, improper storage of potential poisons, ignorance of first aid measures for poisoning, and failure of some pharmacies to use child-resistant packaging.[34]

Toys are another safety concern for children in this age group. In 1983 over 594,000 toy-related injuries occurred to youngsters under the age of 15.[35] Many of these injuries resulted from physical impact with, or ingestion of, the toy. The primary factors involved in toy-related injuries are selection of toys inappropriate to the child's age and improper use of the toy. In conjunction with the U.S. Consumer Product Safety Commission, the Toy Manufacturers of America has developed guidelines for the selection and use of toys that the community health nurse can pass on to parents to enable them to make their child's environment a little safer. These guidelines are included in Box 20–4.

Playground safety is another area of concern. From 1983 to 1987 over 300,000 emergency room visits for children under 4 were due to injuries from playground equipment. Thirty-eight percent of these injuries occurred at home and 29 percent in recreational areas. The nurse should assess the safety of any playground equipment in the home or day-care environment. Some considerations include the ground surface on which equipment is placed and the state of repair of equipment. Energy-absorbing mats, wood chips, or sand under equipment reduce the likelihood of injuries due to falls. Concrete, asphalt, or packed earth, however, are very dangerous. The nurse should also determine whether equipment is properly anchored and free of obstructions. Equipment should also be in good repair and children should be supervised in its use.[36]

Safety assessment for school-age children should include considerations of playground safety described above and the correct and appropriate use of toys. Other considerations include supervision of sports activities and seeing that such activities are appropriate to the age and development of the child. Elementary school children, for example, should not engage in contact sports such as football. Youngsters of this age should be taught safety rules for sports and bicycling. Seat-belt use and the ability to swim are other important areas for assessment.

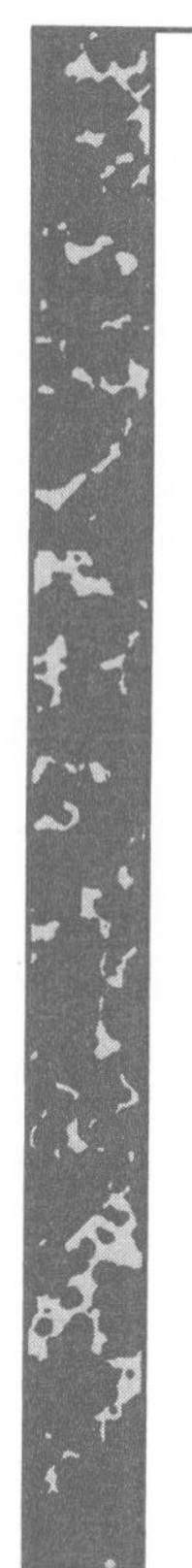

BOX 20–4

Guidelines for Toy Selection and Use

- Select toys appropriate to the child's age, ability, and interest.
- Establish ground rules for playing with the toy.
- Select toys with clear instructions for parents and child on use of the toy.
- Select toys that are sturdily constructed.
- Avoid toys with small parts for young children.
- Avoid toys that propel or shoot objects.
- Supervise use of toys with electrical heating elements (use recommended for children over 8 years of age only).
- Consider the environment in which toys are used.

(Source: Toy Safety.[35])

A major concern with this age group is exposure to firearms. The nurse should explore whether firearms are present in the home, or in the homes of friends, and how access to firearms is controlled. Guns should be kept away from all children, while youngsters in early adolescence should be taught how to handle them correctly.

Psychological Environment

There are nearly 3 million seriously emotionally disturbed children in the United States, and approximately two-thirds of these children do not receive treatment.[37] Community health nurses should routinely assess children for evidence of emotional problems and should explore factors in the psychological environment that may contribute to those problems. The child's psychological environment is a product of forces within and outside the child. Areas for consideration related to the psychological environment include the child's reactivity patterns, parental expectations and discipline, parental coping abilities, parent-child interaction, and the child's self-image. The nurse should also give consideration to the potential for child abuse within the family or child-care environment.

Reactivity Patterns. Children react differently to their environment based on their individual temperament. These differences in response are the child's reactivity patterns.[38] ***Reactivity patterns*** are a set of typical responses to environmental stimuli displayed by a particular child. These patterns are part of the child's internal psychological environment. Reactivity patterns may persist throughout life and may influence the way others react to the child, thereby affecting the child's self-image and ability to interact meaningfully with others.

There are nine areas in which children's reactivity patterns may differ. These are the child's activity level, rhythmicity, approach to new situations, adaptability, intensity of reaction, distractibility, attention span, threshold of response, and mood. The characteristic features of differences in these reactivity patterns and their implications for the child's interactions with others are presented in Table 20–5.

The nurse can determine the child's reactivity patterns or typical patterns of response to his or her environment by means of the client interview and by observation. In the interview, either the child or caretaker—in the case of a young child—can be asked how the child responds in each of the areas addressed. The nurse will be able to determine reactivity patterns by also observing the child. For example, perseverance can be seen in the child who repeatedly returns to an activity when told "no" or when a hand has been slapped. Similarly, response to new situations can be gauged on the basis of the child's response to the nurse as a stranger or to the environment of the clinic or office.

Knowledge of a child's reactivity patterns can suggest some potential problems that the child may encounter in his or her interactions with the outside world. Such knowledge will also aid the nurse in designing interventions to assist families to adapt to

TABLE 20–5. CHARACTERISTIC FEATURES AND IMPLICATIONS OF DIFFERENCES IN REACTIVITY PATTERNS AMONG CHILDREN

Reactivity Pattern	Characteristic Features	Implications
Activity level		
Active	• Curious and motivated to learn new things • Always into something • Doesn't always consider consequences of action • Gets dirty frequently	• Responds rapidly to new ideas or directions • Needs close supervision • Need to channel energy productively • Delay dressing for important occasions until the last minute
Placid	• Slow to react • Frequently late • Needs more time to complete activities	• Need to encourage interaction with environment • May need to be awakened early to get to school on time • Need to allow extra time for activities • Need to allow time for child to respond
Rhythmicity		
Regular	• Tends to eat, sleep, defecate, etc., at the same time each day • Responds poorly to schedule changes • Schedule may not coincide with that of family members	• Predictable behavior allows planning • Need to maintain a regular schedule • Easier to toilet-train • Need to adjust family schedules to accommodate child • Need to accept fussiness related to schedule changes
Irregular	• Eating, sleeping, and other habits unpredictable • Responds well to schedule changes	• Unable to plan daily schedule • More difficult to train • Need to maintain flexibility in family schedules • May need relief of caretaker to carry out other duties

(*continued*)

TABLE 20–5. (*Continued*)

Reactivity Pattern	Characteristic Features	Implications
Approach to new situations		
Adventurous	• Accepts new ideas and people easily • Willing to try new things • Frequently unaware of danger	• Need to caution on talking to strangers • Need for close supervision • Need to discuss consequences of action • Need to provide safe "adventures"
Shy	• Slow and cautious in new situations • May have difficulty meeting new people • May have difficulty adjusting to new situations	• Less likely to engage in dangerous activities • Needs advance warning of changes • Needs extra time to adjust to change • Need to reinforce similarities to previously encountered situations • Need to implement changes slowly
Adaptability		
Adaptable	• Adjusts easily to changes in situation	
Rigid	• Adjusts poorly to changes in situation	• Need to assist child to adjust to changes • Need to accept and deal with child's feelings of anger and frustration • Need to introduce changes slowly if possible
Intensity of reaction		
Intense reaction	• Reacts strenuously to stimuli • Cries with little stimulus • Emotionally wearing for caretakers • Difficult to know when there is cause for concern	• Need to accept and legitimize child's expression of feelings • Need to arrange respite for primary caretaker • Need to help child express emotion in appropriate ways • Need not to ignore in case of serious injury
Moderate	• Slow to anger • Easy to soothe and comfort	• Need to be aware of subtle signs of distress • Need to encourage child to express feelings
Distractibility		
Easily distracted	• Easily distracted from current activity	• Use distraction to halt unacceptable behavior • Need to promote task accomplishment by removing distractions or refocusing attention • Needs frequent reminders • Provide extra time for task completion • Acknowledge small accomplishments
Persevering	• Perseveres in current activity despite distractions	• May need to remove child from temptation • May need help in recognizing futility of efforts • May need help in dealing with failure
Attention span		
Long	• Can work at the same activity for extended periods • May bore others with continued attention to a "dead" topic	• May need to be made to stop one activity to move on to others • May need to set time limits on activities • Need to help child understand others may not have same level of interest
Short	• Easily bored with an activity	• Needs to be kept busy to avoid mischief • Need to refocus attention on task accomplishment
Threshold of response		
High	• Requires extensive stimulus to react	• Need to be aware of subtle signs of distress • Need to watch for extreme reaction when threshold is reached
Low	• Requires minimal stimulus to react • Emotionally wearing for caretakers	• May need to help child channel reaction in productive ways • Need to arrange respite for primary caretaker
Mood		
Happy	• Basically happy with life	• May need to be sure child is not taken advantage of
Unhappy	• Unhappy with most of life • Frequently critical of others or situation • Emotionally wearing for caretakers	• Need to accept feelings of discontent • Need to help child be less critical of others or express criticism in socially acceptable ways • Need to arrange respite for primary caretaker

their youngsters' reactivity patterns or to aid children in adapting patterns to better fit the world around them.

Parental Expectations. Many of the difficulties in relationships between parents and children, and between the father and mother regarding their children, stem from unrealistic beliefs about things that children should and should not do. Community health nurses can help prevent such difficulties by assisting parents to develop realistic expectations of children's behavior. For example, it is unrealistic to expect a 3-year-old not to wet the bed occasionally. The community health nurse can explain to parents that the depth of a child's sleep at this age is such that urges to empty one's bladder are not sufficient to wake the child and so accidents occur. Similarly, the negativism of a 2-year-old is normal behavior, not evidence of deliberate disobedience. The nurse should explore with parents their expectations of children's behavior to determine whether these expectations are realistic in light of the child's age and developmental level, as well as his or her physical status.

Discipline. Discipline is frequently an area of concern for parents and children alike. Many parents need assistance in knowing when and how to discipline children appropriately. The nurse should assess parental approaches to discipline and the appropriateness of disciplinary measures used. The nurse should also determine the extent to which parents adhere to the principles that should guide discipline. These principles and related assessment questions are presented in Box 20–5.

Discipline can take any of several forms, and the community health nurse should ascertain the approach taken to discipline and the effectiveness of that approach. Verbal discipline is very effective with some children. When verbal discipline is used, the nurse should make sure that parents are focusing on the child's behavior and not the child. The idea should be conveyed that it is the *behavior* that is unacceptable, not the child. Physical punishment, such as spanking, may be used, but the nurse should ascertain that it is used with caution. Children should not be hit with anything other than the hand and then only where no damage can occur (for example, on the buttocks). The nurse should also be sure that parents refrain from using too much force even in spanking.

Removal of privileges is another effective means of discipline. When parents use this approach to discipline, the nurse should determine that the "punishment fits the crime" whenever possible and that the child is helped to see the connection between his or her behavior and the restriction imposed. For example, if a young child has purposefully broken another child's toy, he or she can be made to give up a similar toy for a period of time. Another effective method of discipline is "time-out." Time-out effectively stops the behavior and affords the child an opportunity to contemplate its consequences. Whatever the form of discipline used, the nurse should ensure that it is employed in a way that leads to the accomplishment of its purposes.

Parental Coping Skills. The ability of a child's parents to cope with the stresses and frustrations of parenthood and everyday life is another factor that influences the child's psychological environment. Parents who are unable to cope with their own frustrations are likely to take some of their frustration out on the child. Even when this is not so, children are sensitive to the atmosphere around them and may feel insecure and uncertain in a situation in which parents are under obvious stress.

Three basic approaches can be taken to cope with the stresses of parenthood. The first of these is to change the situation that is creating stress. If a child's behavior is creating stress, the parent can attempt to alter the child's behavior. Or the parent can temporarily remove oneself from the situation by hiring a babysitter and going shopping.

The second approach is to change one's attitude toward the situation. Parents may stop to consider that they will only have their children at home for a few more years or that their own children could be twice as bad (like the Smiths' child) and so decide that the situation is not as bad as it first seemed. Finally, parents can change their response to the situation. This may occur when the parents channel their frustrations into a floor-scrubbing spree or other activity, or decide that it isn't worth worrying about.

Community health nurses should assess whether parents use any of these three methods of coping and the effectiveness of their use. In addition, community health nurses can identify ineffective parental coping mechanisms that may contribute to a psychological environment that is not conducive to the child's physical or emotional health. Parents can be asked what stressors they perceive in their lives and how they deal with stress.

Parent-child Interaction. The quality of interaction between parent and child is another important factor in the child's psychological environment. In assessing this area, the nurse would observe the pattern of interaction that occurs between parent and child in the nurse's presence. Do parents relate well to the child, or do they scream and yell over minor misbehavior? Do parents convey a sense of concern for the child and his or her welfare, or do they ignore the child

BOX 20–5

Principles of Effective Discipline and Related Assessment Questions

Principle 1: Determine what is important.

- Have parents determined what behaviors are never acceptable?
- Is there good rationale for this determination?
- Do parents say "no" automatically?

Principle 2: Be consistent.

- Are parents consistent in what is considered unacceptable behavior?
- Do parents allow children to wear them down until they let unacceptable behavior pass?
- Do parents agree on what behavior is unacceptable, or can children manipulate parents?
- Have parents determined situations in which certain behaviors, otherwise allowed, are not acceptable?
- Have parents explained to children the reason for the difference in what is allowable at some times and not at others?

Principle 3: Never act in anger.

- Do parents control their anger before disciplining children?
- Do parents use a "cooling off" period when needed?
- Have parents explained the reason for the cooling off period so children will learn appropriate ways of dealing with anger?

Principle 4: Allow time for compliance.

- Do parents allow time for children to comply with directions, or do they expect instant obedience?
- Do parents respect children's need to complete a task in which they are engaged before complying with parental instructions?

Principle 5: Set limits ahead of time.

- Do parents establish rules of behavior prior to disciplining certain behaviors on the part of the child?
- Do parents use knowledge of child growth and development to anticipate children's behavior?
- When children engage in unacceptable behavior that is not addressed in previously established rules, do parents give a warning before instituting punishment?

Principle 6: Be sure the child understands the rules.

- Are parents clear on what behavior is expected of the child and what behavior is unacceptable?

Principle 7: Prevent rather than punish unacceptable behavior.

- Do parents take steps to prevent unacceptable behavior before it occurs, rather than punishing it afterwards?
- Do parents remove sources of temptation for young children?
- Do parents provide adequate supervision for children?

Principle 8: Be sure that discipline is warranted.

- Do parents ascertain the facts of a situation before punishing children?
- Are parental expectations warranted given the developmental level of the child?
- Have rules been clearly established and made clear to the child?
- Do parents attempt to determine the reason for the child's behavior and explain what is wrong when the child's intentions were good?

Principle 9: Be sure that discipline is meaningful.

- Do parents make sure that the child understands the reason for punishment?
- Do parents explain how the child can correct his or her behavior?
- What form of discipline do parents use?
- Is the form of discipline used effective in modifying the child's behavior?

unless the behavior impinges on the parents' level of comfort? Answers to these and similar questions will provide the nurse with a picture of typical interactions between parent and child.

In the child with a chronic illness or disability, the quality of parent-child interactions may be profoundly influenced by the parents' response to the child's condition. These children tend to have higher incidence rates for emotional problems than do healthy children.[39] The community health nurse can assess the parental response to the child's condition and identify any problem areas that may adversely affect the child's emotional status.

Parental responses to chronic illness or disability in their children usually occur in four stages: disbelief, anger, demystification, and conditional acceptance.[39] The community health nurse should assess the stage of parental response and the effects of that response on interactions with the child.

In the stage of disbelief, the parent exhibits denial of the condition. If prolonged, this denial could result in unrealistic expectations of the child and frustration for the child who is unable to meet those expectations.

In the second stage, anger, the parent begins to understand the implications of the child's condition for the parent and for other family members. The parent is faced with additional duties and responses that he or she may not be willing to assume. Feelings of anger related to the disruption of life caused by the child's condition may be turned against the child and may be exhibited in emotional or physical abuse. Other feelings that may be experienced in this stage are guilt, anxiety, and depression.[39] These feelings may also interfere with healthy parent-child interactions. Guilt, for example, can lead to attempts to "make up to the child for his or her condition" that interfere with appropriate discipline for the child or encourage the child to manipulate parental behavior by playing on that guilt. Anxiety may contribute to an attitude of overprotectiveness on the part of the parent, and the child may not be allowed opportunities for development appropriate to his or her age and health status. Depression can result in parental immobilization and consequent neglect of the child.

In the demystification stage, parents actively seek information about the child's condition. In addition, they begin to cope with the problem through a mechanism called "downward comparison."[39] ***Downward comparison*** is a coping strategy in which one compares one's own situation to that of others whose circumstances are worse. In this stage, parents also begin to develop a sense of control over the situation, which they can communicate to the child, thus decreasing the child's level of fear and anxiety and improving the child's self-image.

The final stage is conditional acceptance, when parents incorporate the child's condition into their view of reality. Parents and child accommodate to the condition and normalize family life as much as possible. Parents also exhibit control of the problem by developing contingency plans to deal with potential problems. In addition, family members may come to see positive effects of the child's condition such as drawing the family closer together. Parents who have accepted the child's condition foster the child's ability to develop as normally as possible.

Each of the stages of parental response presented here are normal. When parents fail to proceed to later stages, however, their response may have adverse effects on interactions with the child and on the child's psychological environment. The community health nurse should identify any problems resulting from parental response to chronic illness or disability in the child.

Self-image. Another area to be addressed in relation to the child's psychological environment is the child's self-image. The nurse can determine the child's self-perceptions by asking the child to "Tell me about yourself." A similar approach would be to ask the child to describe things that he or she does well. A child who has difficulty answering this question may not have a very strong self-image. For younger children who cannot easily articulate their feelings about themselves, nurses might watch for self-punishing behavior (for example, slapping oneself or saying "I'm dumb").

Child Abuse. Inability to cope with life's stresses is one of the primary contributors to child abuse, a growing area of concern for community health nurses. The community health nurse should be alert to evidence of actual or potential child abuse. While child abuse has both physical and psychological effects on children, it is factors in the psychological environment that place families at risk for the occurrence of abuse. Guidelines for child abuse assessment include considerations of parent characteristics and role expectations, child characteristics and behavior, and environmental stressors.[40] Parental characteristics that increase the potential for child abuse include a history of abuse or parental abandonment when they themselves were children, feelings of hostility to or alienation from their own parents, and physical or emotional health problems experienced by the child's parents. Unrealistic parental expectations of the child, verbalizations of hostility or disappointment in the child, parental expectations that the child will always understand the parents' feelings, and a belief that the child does not love the parents enough are also parental indicators of potential for abuse.

Characteristics of the child may also signal potential for abuse. Such characteristics include prematurity, early separation from parents, developmental disability, obvious differences from siblings, difficulty concentrating, and inappropriate ways of expressing needs. The nurse should also be aware of environmental stressors such as financial pressures, social isolation, alcoholism or drug abuse, spousal abuse, and poor school performance that may indicate a potential for abuse.

Community health nurses should also be alert to signs of actual abuse or neglect. Some of these include evidence of obvious injury; torn, stained, or bloody underwear; an enlarged anal opening; signs of malnutrition and poor hygiene; and failure to thrive. Nurses should also be suspicious of stories that are inconsistent with injuries presented or with the child's stage of development and of inappropriate behavior on the part of adults in the situation (for example, belligerence, being overly concerned, or refusal to allow diagnostic tests). Children may also display unusual behavior such as being excessively withdrawn or extremely passive. Abused children may also cling to parents with unusual force or be remarkably detached from them.[41]

The nurse should be alert to families at risk for child abuse and work to help them develop positive parenting skills as described in this chapter. The development of such skills may help to prevent abuse or to eliminate it in families where it already exists. The problem of child abuse and potential nursing interventions will be addressed in more detail in Chapter 34, Violence.

Social Environment

Factors in the child's social environment that contribute to health or illness should also be assessed. In younger children, the nurse might observe interactions with others in the environment, including the nurse. Parents can also be asked about the child's interaction with siblings and with peers. The nurse should determine whether such interactions are normal for the child's age. For example, parallel play (play alongside of, rather than with, other children) is to be expected of toddlers, while sharing and interactive play would not be expected to occur until preschool years. Competitive games and activities with rules are normal interactive behaviors for school-age children.

Older youngsters can also be asked about their friends and what kinds of things they do together. In addition, parents may offer their perspective on how the child interacts with age-mates at school and in other settings.

Another area for assessment related to the child's social environment is an exploration of family culture and its effects on children's health. Other social factors within the family environment may also influence the health of the child. For example, a father's unemployment may mean a lack of available health care for children, or, in some cases lack of money for adequate nutrition, housing, and other necessities. Prejudice in the social environment may also affect children. For example, they may be subjected to ridicule by other children at school because of their dress, physical appearance, family culture, or religion.

LIFE-STYLE

Life-style factors can be important contributors to health or illness in children. Areas of primary concern include nutrition, rest and exercise, child-care, and school performance.

Nutrition

Childhood growth and appropriate development are facilitated by adequate nutrition. Pediatric nutrition is an area of concern for the community health nurse. In a 1984 study by the Centers for Disease Control (CDC), 1.8 percent to 8.7 percent of children of various ages and ethnic groups were found to be below the 5th percentile for weight-versus-height comparisons. From 3.9 percent to 13.7 percent were found to be above the 95th percentile. In another study, 24 percent of 11- to 14-year-olds were found to be overweight compared to only 15 percent of the same population in 1973. Similar results have been found with 6- to 11-year-olds.[42]

In the 1984 study, 1 percent to 35 percent of children of various ages and ethnic groups were found to be anemic. Hematocrit levels tended to be lower for children under 1 year of age and for Native American children than for other groups. As indicated by the figures presented here, many American children are poorly nourished.

Much of the malnutrition found among children in this country is due to inadequate knowledge of nutrition on the part of parents. The community health nurse should assess parental knowledge of child nutritional needs as well as nutritional practices related to children. Nutritional status should be assessed in relation to the child's age and nutritional needs. Specific questions related to assessment for children of different ages are included in Table 20–6.

Rest and Exercise

Another area for consideration with respect to life-style factors and their influence on child health is the ratio of rest to exercise. With infants, the nurse would assess sleeping patterns and the length of periods of sleep and periods of wakefulness. One problem that

TABLE 20–6. QUESTIONS FOR ASSESSING THE NUTRITIONAL STATUS OF CHILDREN OF SELECTED AGES

Age Group	Assessment Questions
Infant (birth to 1 year)	• Is the child breast- or bottle-fed? • If breast-fed, –How often does the child nurse? –How long does the child nurse? –Does mother alternate breasts? –Is mother's nutritional intake adequate? –Does the child seem satisfied? • If bottle-fed, –How often does the baby eat? –How much formula is consumed in 24 hours? –What type of formula is used? Is it iron-fortified? –Do parents prepare formula correctly? –Do parents use appropriate feeding techniques? (for example, not propping the bottle) –Does the infant tolerate the formula well? • Is the infant gaining weight? • At what point did parents introduce solids? (recommendations are for cereal at 6 months, followed by vegetables, fruits, and meat) • How much solid food does the baby eat? • Do parents use individual foods rather than less nutritious combination foods (like vegetable and beef combinations)? • Is one new food introduced at a time? Over several days? • Has the child started eating table food? (usually occurs at about 9 months of age) • Is the child weaned from the bottle by 1 year?
Toddler and preschool child (2 to 5 years)	What foods is the child eating? • How much food is the child eating? • Is the child's diet well-balanced? • Are finger foods and variety encouraged? • Are nutritious snacks provided? • Is the child given small portions initially and allowed to ask for more to enhance independence? • Is the child's growth pattern normal for his or her age?
School-age child (6 to 12 years)	• Is the child's diet well-balanced? • Is junk food avoided? • Are snacks nutritious? • How much does the child eat? • Is the child overweight or underweight? • Is the child's height within normal limits for his or her age?

may become evident at this point is the child whose schedule does not coincide with that of the rest of the family, so the nurse should be sure to ask when sleep periods occur. The nurse would also want to note whether the child appears to be sleeping more or less than would be expected at that age.

Activity level should also be assessed. Is the child normally active or listless and apathetic? Lethargy may be a sign of a variety of physical health problems including acute illness, hypothyroidism, and anemia. Hyperactivity should also be noted. Hyperactivity in young infants is a frequent after-effect of drug exposure during pregnancy.

Child-care Outside the Home

Child-care outside the home is a factor in the health of a child that coincides with a family's dual wage-earner life-style or with a single parent life-style when the parent works. The nurse assessing factors influencing the child's health should determine who cares for the child and where. Other questions that the nurse might want to ask about child-care arrangements are presented in Box 20–6.

School Performance

The last area for consideration with respect to life-style relates to school-age children. The nurse will want to obtain information on the child's response to the school environment and on performance in school. Children can be asked how they like school. Information on performance can be obtained from both children and parents. Areas of academic and interpersonal strength and weakness should be identified, and the nurse should also try to gain some insight into family attitudes toward education because these will influence the child's performance. Do parents assist the child with learning tasks? What are parental expectations with regard to school perfor-

BOX 20–6

Questions for Assessing the Adequacy of Child-Care Arrangements

- Who cares for the child?
- Where does child-care take place?
- Are child caretakers qualified to care for children?
- Have parents requested references from private child caretakers other than family members?
- Is there more than one adult in the child-care setting?
- Have parents inspected the child-care premises for potential safety hazards?
- Do parents "drop in" to witness the quality of care provided to children in the child-care setting and the extent of supervision of children's activities?
- Do parents investigate unusual stories reported by children?
- Have parents made contingency plans for care of the child when he or she is ill or when the child caretaker is unavailable?
- Are child-care facilities licensed if appropriate?

mance? Are they too high or too low? What efforts, if any, are being made to assist the child with problems related to school performance? The child's ability to interact with peers and any school behavior problems should also be determined.

HEALTH SYSTEM

Health system factors to be assessed with respect to the health of the child are similar to those for any individual client discussed in Chapter 17, Care of the Individual Client. Areas for consideration include attitudes of the child and the family to health and health care, the usual source of health care, and use of health-care services. Particular consideration should be given to the use of primary preventive services related to immunization and dental care.

The nurse should also explore parental knowledge of the care of minor illness in the home. Do parents know not to give aspirin to children? Does the caretaker know how to take a child's temperature? Are parents aware of when to take a child for medical care? Another related question is the type of illness care practices employed by the family. Are any of these practices potentially harmful? Appendix J, Child Health Assessment Guide, contains a tool that may be used by the community health nurse to assess the health needs of children.

DIAGNOSTIC REASONING AND THE CARE OF CHILDREN

Based on the data gathered in the assessment of the child, the community health nurse derives diagnoses or statements of the child's health status and health-care needs. Both positive and problem-focused nursing diagnoses should be made based on the child's situation. Diagnoses may reflect the need for primary, secondary, or tertiary preventive measures. For example, a positive nursing diagnosis related to primary prevention might be: "Immunizations up-to-date due to high parental motivation and access to health-care services." On the other hand, a problem-focused nursing diagnosis related to immunizations might be: "Lack of appropriate immunizations for age due to lack of transportation to immunization clinic." Another problem-focused nursing diagnosis related to primary prevention might be: "Potential for child abuse due to unrealistic parental expectations of child, parental stress, and poor parental coping abilities."

Nursing diagnoses related to secondary prevention are necessarily problem-focused because secondary prevention is warranted when actual health problems exist. Examples of nursing diagnoses at this level might include: "Need for medical evaluation and treatment due to possible otitis media" or "Need for referral to child protective services due to probable child abuse." Nursing diagnoses at this level might reflect physical, psychological, or social problems affecting the child's overall health status.

At the level of tertiary prevention, nursing diagnoses would focus on the need to prevent complications of existing problems or to prevent the recurrence of problems. For example, the nurse might derive a nursing diagnosis of a "need for education on proper infant feeding techniques due to practice of propping bottle" to prevent recurrent middle ear infections. Or the nurse might diagnose a "need for emotional support due to imminent death of child" for a child with AIDS. The intent in this latter diagnosis is to direct nursing care to preventing family complications of a terminal illness.

PLANNING NURSING CARE FOR CHILDREN

As in the care of any individual client, planning nursing care for children involves prioritizing needs, developing criteria for approaches to meeting those needs, evaluating alternatives, and selecting a course of action. Developing objectives for care and planning specific interventions related to needs for primary, secondary, and tertiary prevention are also required.

Client participation in planning is desirable. Most often this participation will include the child's parents or other caretakers. However, it is important for the nurse to remember that participation by the child in planning for his or her own care is also important. Even young children can be involved in some of the decisions about their care, particularly when problems can be addressed by relatively simple interventions. For example, if the school-age child is anemic, he or she may be given a choice of iron-rich foods to be included in the diet. Similarly, if the problem is one related to behavior, the child may have some ideas of strategies that will help to alter that behavior.

Whatever interventions are selected should be appropriate to the problems identified as well as to the age and developmental level of the child. For example, toys designed to enhance motor development should be challenging but not beyond the child's capability to use. If such strategies are not capable of implementation by the child, frustration will result. As another example, it may be appropriate to make a preadolescent responsible for soaking a sprained ankle periodically, but this would not be appropriate for a first-grader.

Nursing intervention for the health problems of children will include primary, secondary, and tertiary preventive measures. In dealing with the well child, emphasis will be placed on primary prevention—health promotion and prevention of illness. Initial intervention for the acutely ill child will be geared to secondary prevention for the illness, with later attention to primary and tertiary prevention. For the child with a chronic illness, the initial focus of care may be either secondary or tertiary prevention depending upon the child's status. Primary prevention with this child would not be neglected, however.

One general measure that cuts across all three levels of prevention is the provision of access to health-care services for health-promotive, illness-preventive, restorative, and rehabilitative care. The community health nurse may be instrumental in referring children and their parents to appropriate sources of health care. The nurse may also need to refer families for financial assistance with health-care needs.

PRIMARY PREVENTION

Primary preventive activities are designed to promote the health of the child and to prevent illness. Major considerations in primary prevention include promoting growth and development, nutrition, safety, immunization, dental care, and support for parenting.

Promoting Growth and Development

To develop properly, the child needs an environment conducive to growth and development. Community health nurses can assist parents in creating such an environment. One of the ways in which this assistance may be provided is in the form of anticipatory guidance. ***Anticipatory guidance*** is the act of providing information to parents regarding behavioral expectations of children at a specific age before the child reaches that age.

Such information allows parents to engage in activities that will promote development and to cope with some of the more negative aspects of that development. For example, the community health nurse might warn parents who have a child about to turn 2 of the negative behavior typical of this age group. Parents need to know that this negativism is an attempt on the child's part to become autonomous and is a normal behavior. They should be assisted to deal with this behavior in such a way that autonomy is fostered while the child's safety is ensured and discipline is maintained. The community health nurse can also reinforce the consistent use of the principles of discipline presented earlier.

Most parents are concerned about their child's development and ability to accomplish developmental milestones. Parents can be told when to expect the child to perform various activities, but should also be informed that children develop at different rates. Toilet training is a common parental concern. Many parents attempt toilet training before the child is physically ready. The nurse can inform parents that toilet training is not appropriate until the child is walking. It is not until this time that sufficient sphincter muscle development has occurred to permit the child to control defecation. Parents can be encouraged to look for signs that a child is ready to begin toilet training, such as squatting behaviors, hiding behind furniture, or pulling at their clothing when they feel the urge to defecate. Children may also demonstrate readiness by displaying curiosity about parents' eliminative behavior.

When the child has begun to demonstrate some of the signs of readiness for toilet training, parents should determine patterns of defecation and urination and should time trips to the bathroom to coincide with these patterns. If the child normally defecates after a meal, then meals should finish with a trip to the toilet. Children should not be left unattended in the bathroom and should not be encouraged to play during this time. Two to 3 minutes on a "potty seat" is sufficient. If the child is successful in defecating or urinating on the potty seat, he or she should be praised. Accidents, however, should be ignored. Parents should also be aware that early in the training process, children have very limited sphincter control. When a child indicates a need to go to the bathroom, they mean "now!" Parents who tell the child to "wait" are inviting trouble, and accidents that occur in these situations are not the child's fault, but the parents'.

Teething is another developmental concern for parents. Children are frequently irritable when cutting their first teeth. Parents can be encouraged to provide safe teething objects for the child. Teething objects that can be placed in the freezer are comforting. Parents can even place an ice cube inside a washcloth to make a cold, hard surface for children to teeth on. The nurse should discourage the use of commercial teething preparations as these may cause irritation to the gums.

Promoting growth and development in children with chronic illnesses or disabilities should also be a concern for the community health nurse. Parents may need to be encouraged to allow their youngster to engage in behaviors that will facilitate the child's development. For example, the parents of a blind child may need to be reminded that the child can use other senses to compensate for his or her lack of vision and should be encouraged to engage in activities appropriate to his or her age, rather than over protecting the child. Parents may also need to learn about specialized activities they can do to facilitate the child's development. Information on these types of activities can be obtained from a variety of agencies and organizations that address the needs of children with specific conditions or special needs. Some of these agencies and organizations are included in Table 20–7.

Providing Adequate Nutrition

Childhood growth and appropriate development are facilitated by adequate nutrition. Here again, the primary function of the community health nurse will be educating the parents to provide adequate nutrition for their children. The nurse may also provide referrals to food supplementation programs such as the Women, Infants, and Children (WIC) program.

Much of the malnutrition found among children in this country is due to inadequate knowledge of nutrition on the part of parents. The community health nurse can help to alleviate such problems by educating parents on the nutritional needs of children at various ages. Parents should be told that children under 6 months of age should be maintained on breast milk or formula alone, because early introduction of solid foods contributes to food allergies and overweight in later life.

When foods are introduced, parents need to be aware that they should introduce new foods slowly to allow for identification of food allergies. They should give a new food for several days without introducing any other new substance to allow time for the development of allergic symptoms. Juices can be introduced between 4 and 5 months of age with the exception of orange juice, which may cause some allergies. Parents should be cautioned against using adult apple juice as it has not been pasteurized and may contain bacteria that can cause severe diarrhea in infants. Solid foods should be introduced at about 6 months of age beginning with easily digestible cereals such as rice cereal.

Once the baby has been able to tolerate several different types of cereal, parents can begin to introduce an array of vegetables, beginning with yellow vegetables and progressing to green. Vegetables should be introduced before fruits to avoid the development of a preference for the sweeter fruits and later resistance to eating vegetables. After the child is eating a variety of cereals and vegetables, fruits can be introduced followed by meats. Again, parents should start with the more easily digested meats such as lamb.

Parents can either prepare pureed foods themselves or purchase commercially available baby foods. If using commercially processed foods, parents should be taught to evaluate food products for their nutritive value. They should be made aware that they should buy plain items rather than combinations of foods. For example, vegetable and meat should be purchased separately and mixed if desired, rather than buying the vegetable and meat combination. This is both more economical and more nutritious for the baby. Plain fruits should be purchased over the baby desserts as these merely add unneeded calories and expense.

Parents also need an understanding of the eating habits of children. The nurse should encourage parents to provide nutritious meals and snacks for youngsters of all ages and to avoid offering junk food. Parents should also avoid food fads such as the use of raw milk and other "natural" foods that may actually be harmful to children (examples of potentially harmful foods are raw eggs and unpasteurized honey).

Many children begin eating finger foods at 8 to 9 months of age. Parents should see that children are carefully supervised to prevent choking on small

TABLE 20–7. RESOURCES FOR FAMILIES OF CHILDREN WITH SPECIAL NEEDS

Problem Area	Agency or Organization	Services
Arthritis	American Juvenile Arthritis Organization 1314 Spring St. Atlanta, GA 30309 (404) 872-7110	Advocacy for children with arthritis
Asthma	National Asthma Center 875 Avenue of the Americas New York, NY 10001	Information on asthma
	National Foundation for Asthma, Inc. P.O. Box 50304 Tucson, AZ 85703 (602) 624-7481	Outpatient treatment
Birth defects	Association of Birth Defects in Children 3526 Emerywood Lane Orlando, FL 32806 (305) 859-2821	Information, public education on hazards of prenatal drug use; research, statistics
	March of Dimes Birth Defects Foundation 1275 Mamaroneck Ave. White Plains, NY 10605 (914) 428-7100	Research, public information
Blindness	Braille Institute 741 Vermont Avenue Los Angeles, CA 90029 (213) 663-1111	Training in Braille
	Carroll Center for the Blind 770 Centre St. Newton, MA 02158 (617) 969-6200	Rehabilitation and training for the blind
	Leader Dogs for the Blind 1039 Rochester Rd. Rochester, MI 48063 (313) 651-9011	Trains dogs for the blind
	National Association for Visually Handicapped 305 E. 24th St. New York, NY 10010 (212) 889-3141	Counseling, books, information
Cancer	Candlelighters Foundation 2025 Eye St., NW Washington, DC 20006 (202) 659-5136	Self-help group for parents of children and adolescents with cancer
	United Ostomy Association 1111 Wilshire Blvd. Los Angeles, CA 90017 (213) 255-4681	Mutual aid, support, information
Cystic fibrosis	Cystic Fibrosis Foundation 6000 Executive Blvd., Suite 309 Rockville, MD 20852 (301) 881-9130	Research, family assistance
Diabetes	Association of Insulin-dependent Diabetics c/o Juvenile Diabetes Foundation International 60 Madison Ave. New York, NY 10010 (212) 889-7575	Self-help group, education, workshops
	Juvenile Diabetes Association 23 E. 26th St. New York, NY 10010 (212) 889-7575	Research, public information
Down's syndrome	National Association for Down's Syndrome P.O. Box 63 Oak Park, IL 60303 (312) 543-6060	Parental support

(*continued*)

TABLE 20–7. (*Continued*)

Problem Area	Agency or Organization	Services
Epilepsy	National Epilepsy League 6 N. Michigan Avenue Chicago, IL 60602	Research, public information
Growth disorders	Human Growth Foundation 4930 W. 77th St., Suite 150 Minneapolis, MN 55435 (612) 831-2780	Research, education on growth disorders
Handicapped	Association of Maternal Child Health and Crippled Children's Services 275 E. Main St. Frankfort, KY 40621	Research, education, advocacy for handicapped children
	Easter Seal Society for Crippled Children and Adults 2023 W. Ogden Avenue Chicago, IL 60612	Public information, research, assistance
	Shriner's Hospital for Crippled Children P.O. Box 25356 Tampa, FL 33622 (813) 885-2575	Assistance in the care of handicapping conditions
Hemophilia	National Hemophilia Foundation Room 903 25 W. 39th Street New York, NY 10018	Research, public information
Liver disease	Children's Liver Foundation 28 Highland Ave. Maplewood, NJ 07040 (201) 761-1111	Research, parental support, education, public information
Mental retardation	Association of Retarded Citizens P.O. Box 6109 Arlington, TX 76005 (817) 640-0204	Political advocacy, public education
	Mental Retardation Association 211 E. 300 South St., Suite 212 Salt Lake City, UT 84111 (801) 328-1575	Advocacy, prevention, research, public education
	National Association of Retarded Citizens 2501 Ave. J Arlington, TX 76011 (817) 261-4961	Political advocacy
	Pilot Parents 3610 Dodge St., Suite 101 Omaha, NE 68131 (402) 346-5220	Support for parents of mentally handicapped children, education
Multiple sclerosis	National Multiple Sclerosis Society 205 E. 42nd Street New York, NY 10017	Research, public information
Muscular dystrophy	Muscular Dystrophy Association 810 7th Avenue New York, NY 10019 (212) 586-0808	Medical services, research
Phenylketonuria	PKU Parents c/o Dale Hillard Eight Myrtle Lane San Anselmo, CA 94960 (415) 457-4632	Support of parents of children with PKU, education
Respiratory diseases	Children's Lung Association of America 150 Pond Way Roswell, GA 30076 (404) 993-5859	Research, education, promote legislation
Sickle cell disease	National Association for Sickle Cell Disease, Inc. 945 S. Western Ave. Los Angeles, CA 90006	Research, public information, aid

pieces of food. Table foods may also be started at about this age, and children may begin drinking from a cup at mealtime (retaining the bottle at nap or bedtime). Parents can try any table food to see how a child responds. They should, however, be sure that their children are getting a well-balanced diet and that they are carefully supervised to prevent choking. If small vegetables such as peas or lima beans are provided, parents might want to mash them since children have been known to put such small objects into any bodily orifice, including the ears, the nose, and the vagina.

Many parents become concerned over the apparent loss of appetite that occurs with toddlers. Community health nurses need to reassure parents that this is a normal phenomenon resulting from the slower rate of growth that occurs at this age. Again, the primary concern should be the quality of what is eaten rather than the amount. Parents may want to arrange several small meals and nutritious snacks throughout the day rather than the usual three meals. Toddlers and preschoolers also react well to foods that can be eaten "on the go" because they are much more interested in playing than eating. Small portions and colorful meals will also tempt a flagging appetite.

School-age children should receive well-balanced diets that provide them with sufficient energy to engage in all of their activities in and out of school. At this age, children tend to be very strongly influenced by what their peers are doing and eating, and parents may need to insist on nutritious foods without making the child feel too different from his or her peers.

Besides providing parents with information on nutritional needs and eating habits of children at various ages, the community health nurse may be called upon to provide assistance in budgeting for adequate nutrition. In this area the nurse can assist parents in the development of lower-cost menus that provide adequate nutrition. Nurses may also be involved in referring parents to sources of financial assistance with nutrition. They may refer mothers with young children to the WIC program or suggest applying for other food supplement programs that may be available in the community.

Special attention may be needed in meeting the nutritional needs of children with chronic conditions or disabilities. For example, the parents of a young child with diabetes may need to adapt family dietary patterns to accommodate the child's diabetic diet. Or the parents of a child with a cleft lip and palate may need assistance in learning feeding techniques to prevent aspiration of food. Based on an assessment of parents' (and children's) knowledge of special dietary needs, the nurse may educate parents or help them develop the skills needed to meet the nutritional needs of their children. Information on resources to help parents deal with routine and specialized dietary needs can be obtained from the agencies listed in Table 20–8.

Promoting Safety

Adequate supervision is the major primary preventive measure for promoting the safety of children of all ages. The community health nurse can educate parents regarding safety hazards and measures to keep children safe. Infants and young children should never be left unsupervised, even for short periods, unless they are sleeping soundly in a crib or are otherwise confined, as in a playpen. Even then, frequent checks by parents are indicated.

Children, even when securely restrained, can somehow manage to climb out of high chairs or strollers. Even small children can tip over swings and infant seats. For these reasons, as well, children should not be left unattended. Parents should also be taught not to leave infants alone on elevated surfaces from which they might fall. Care should also be taken that young children are not left unsupervised, even for a few minutes, in the bath.

Another primary preventive measure is instructing parents on the need for consistent use of safety devices such as seat belts and restraints in cars, strollers, high chairs, infant seats, and swings. Parents can also be encouraged to insist on the use of safety helmets for any child over 6 months of age in any form of wheeled conveyance. Helmets are particularly important for older children riding bicycles or skateboards.

The community health nurse should also instruct parents about age-appropriate toys and the need to examine toys frequently for sharp edges, damage, or other conditions that might present safety hazards. Parents can also be encouraged to establish rules for the appropriate use of toys and for toys that are not to be used without adult supervision.

Parents may also need assistance in providing safety education for their children. The community health nurse can inform parents of safety issues to be addressed with children of specific ages and assist parents with ways of presenting this information to their children. Areas that should be addressed include watching for cars, crossing streets, talking to strangers, answering the phone or the door, playing with fire, and poisonous substances. Children should also be taught safety rules for sports and bike riding, water safety, and safety with firearms.

Child-proofing the home is another area of primary prevention for the young child. This involves placing hazardous objects where children cannot get access to them and eliminating other safety hazards

TABLE 20–8. RESOURCES FOR CHILDHOOD NUTRITION

Agency or Organization	Services
La Leche League 9616 Minneapolis Ave. Franklin Park, IL 60131 (312) 455-7730	Assistance with breast feeding; public information
Society for the Protection of the Unborn through Nutrition 17 N. Wabash, Suite 603 Chicago, IL 60602 (312) 332-2334	Education, public information on prenatal nutrition
U.S. Department of Agriculture Food and Consumer Services Food and Nutrition Services 3101 Park Center Drive Alexandria, VA 22302 (703) 756-3276	Administers food programs for the needy
U.S. Department of Agriculture Food and Consumer Services Home Nutrition Information Service 6505 Belcrest Rd. Hyattsville, MD 29782 (310) 436-7725	Public information on food use, management, and problems in human nutrition
U.S. Department of Agriculture Food and Nutrition Service Child-care Food Program Park Office Building, Room 512 3101 Park Center Drive Alexandria, VA 22302 (703) 756-3590	Funds for food programs in child-care centers

from the environment. Safety instruction for parents should be geared toward the age and developmental level of the child. Before the child begins creeping, parents need to think of plugging electrical outlets and keeping small objects out of the reach of young children. Stairways should be inaccessible, as should sharp objects and medications of all kinds. Because children learn at a surprisingly early age to climb to reach an objective, sharp objects and poisons should be in areas with sturdy locks or latches that the child cannot open, rather than placed out of reach.

Parents should also be discouraged from putting toxic substances in unlabeled or usually innocuous containers. The child who sees liquid in a soda bottle may drink it, even if it tastes as bad as bleach or gasoline. Special attention should be given to supervising the activities of young children when visiting friends or relatives whose homes may not be childproofed.

Dealing with firearms is an important safety consideration for school-age children. Parents should be encouraged to eliminate firearms or to make them inaccessible to children, never to leave a gun loaded, and to store ammunition apart from weapons. As noted earlier, preadolescent youngsters should be taught the principles of gun safety, and all children should be discouraged from pointing even toy guns at other people. Resources that may be used by the nurse or the family for promoting various aspects of child safety are presented in Table 20–9.

Immunization

Immunization is a particular concern of the community health nurse working with children and their families. In addition to providing protection for the individual who is immunized, maintenance of high immunization levels in the community leads to smaller numbers of susceptible persons and less risk of exposure for those who are not immunized. Unless otherwise contraindicated, a child's immunizations should be begun at 6 to 10 weeks of age. All children should have a primary series of DPT (diphtheria, pertussis, and tetanus) vaccine consisting of two doses with intervals of 1 to 2 months between doses followed by a third dose 6 to 12 months after the second. Oral polio immunization should be initiated at the same time; it consists of two initial doses 6 to 8 weeks apart and a third dose at about 15 months of age. Booster doses of oral polio vaccine and DPT should be provided just prior to entry into kindergarten or first grade. Subsequent boosters of tetanus and diphtheria vaccine are recommended at 10-year intervals.

More frequent boosters are not necessary and may contribute to increased frequency and severity of adverse reactions.[43]

Immunization for measles, mumps, and rubella (MMR) should take place at about 15 months of age, and a booster may be given prior to school entry or at junior-high entry. In areas with a high incidence of measles, immunization can be given as early as a few months of age, but should be repeated sometime after 1 year of age. Immunization for diseases caused by *Hemophilus influenzae* type B (Hib) can be given as early as 2 months of age, and parents of all young children should be encouraged to obtain this immunization.[33] There is no reason why a child cannot receive several vaccines at one time if this is needed to update the child's immunization status. According to the CDC, polio, MMR, and DPT vaccines may be given simultaneously.[43] Hib vaccine can also be given in conjunction with other vaccines.

The community health nurse will be able to inform parents regarding the schedule for immunizations and refer them to an appropriate provider. In addition, the nurse should inform parents of the expected side effects of immunizations and interventions to minimize them. Parents should also be informed about the signs and symptoms of unusual reactions.

Immunization is of particular concern for children with immunodeficiency problems. For example, live virus vaccines such as oral polio are usually contraindicated for children with AIDS. Inactivated polio vaccine (IPV) should be given both to the child with AIDS and to his or her siblings. Measles immunization may be considered in children with AIDS since measles in individuals who have AIDS can be extremely serious, and the benefits of immunization outweigh its risks. Immunization for pneumococcal pneumonia and annual influenza immunization should be provided for children with chronic illnesses or disabilities, including those with AIDS.[44] Hepatitis B vaccine may be given to children who have been exposed to hepatitis B.

Dental Care

Dental health is another area of concern in primary prevention with children. Dental hygiene should begin as soon as the first tooth erupts. At this time parents can be encouraged to rub teeth briskly with a dry washcloth. Later, parents can begin to brush the child's teeth with a soft toothbrush. Older chil-

TABLE 20–9. RESOURCES FOR PROMOTING CHILD SAFETY

Agency or Organization	Services
American Association of Poison Control Centers c/o Dr. Ted Long Arizona Poison and Drug Information Center Health Science Center, Room 3204K 1501 Campbell Hall Tucson, AZ 85725 (602) 626-7899	Information, development of standards, education, statistics
American National Red Cross 17th & D Streets Washington, DC 20006 (202) 737-8300	Classes in water safety, child-care, first aid, home alone, child/infant CPR, and preparation for parenthood
Boy Scouts of America 1325 Walnut Hill Lane Irving, TX 75015-2079 (214) 580-2000	Personal Health Decisions educational program
National Safety Council 444 N. Michigan Ave. Chicago, IL 60611 (312) 527-4800	Assistance with accident prevention information
United Cerebral Palsy Association 710 Plaza, Suite 804 New York, NY 10001 (800) USA 1 UCP	Passenger and home safety education
U.S. Consumer Product Safety Commission 5401 Westbard Ave. Washington, DC 20207 (301) 492-6800	Federal regulation of consumer products

dren can be taught to brush and floss their own teeth with adult supervision. Use of a fluoridated toothpaste should be encouraged in areas with unfluoridated water, while parents can give vitamins with fluoride to infants in such areas.

Community health nurses can instruct parents to wean infants from the bottle before a year of age to prevent bottle-mouth syndrome. The use of sugarless snacks and rinsing the mouth after eating—when brushing is not possible—can also be encouraged. Finally, community health nurses should encourage parents to obtain regular dental checkups for children and to get prompt attention for dental problems. Financial assistance may be needed for such services for low-income families. In such cases, the community health nurse should make a referral for Medicaid in those areas where dental care is covered.

Support for Parenting

Another major consideration in primary preventive activities for child health is that of support for parenting. As noted earlier, unrealistic parental expectations of children, excessive parental stress, and poor parental coping skills may contribute to child abuse. These conditions also create a psychological environment that is not conducive to health for either parents or children. Such conditions can be modified by community health nursing support in the parenting role. Parents can be assisted to develop realistic expectations of child behavior through anticipatory guidance and help with skills related to communications and discipline. The community health nurse can also help parents to identify children's reactivity patterns and develop approaches to dealing with children that minimize some of the negative aspects of specific patterns. Some of these approaches were discussed earlier in this chapter.

In addition, community health nurses can engage in activities that will minimize parental stress. This may involve referral for financial assistance, arrangement of respite care, assistance with finding work or adequate housing, or whatever is required to meet family needs. At the same time, the nurse can assist the parent to identify coping strategies that work for them. Parents may also need assistance in problem-solving skills to decrease their own stress levels.

Support for parenting is particularly needed by parents of children with chronic or terminal illnesses or disabilities. Parents may need assistance or referral in dealing with feelings of guilt and anxiety engendered by the child's condition. In addition, the community health nurse may provide assistance in developing new child-care skills necessitated by the child's condition. Referral to groups of parents with children who have similar problems may provide parents with avenues of emotional, social, and material support.

Another area in which the community health nurse may be able to support parents of children with serious health problems is respite care. Parents need to be able to maintain their own lives and care for other children, in addition to meeting the needs of the ill child. The nurse may need to encourage parents to take some time for themselves. Frequently, this entails assisting parents to obtain respite care so they can be sure the child's needs are adequately being met while they are away.

Parents and other family members also need to be encouraged to maintain a family life that is as normal as possible. The ill or disabled child should be incorporated into family activities whenever possible, and family members should be encouraged not to let the child's condition become the focus of family life.[39] Family members should be assisted to discuss problems posed by the child's condition and to engage in active problem solving to resolve those concerns. Other avenues for providing support to parents of chronically ill or disabled children include giving information about the child's condition and its treatment, providing emotional support, focusing on positive aspects of the situation, encouraging use of existing support networks, and helping families to expand sources of support.[39]

Families of terminally ill children will need additional support in coming to terms with the eventuality of death. The nurse can determine the family's stage in the grief process and design interventions that will help them successfully pass through these stages. The stages of grief are similar to those described earlier in parental response to a chronic illness. Referrals for counseling or for hospice services may also be helpful in working with families of terminally ill children.

Other Primary Preventive Activities

Additional primary preventive measures may be warranted for children with specific illnesses. For example, parents of children with AIDS and other immunosuppressed conditions should be taught how to minimize exposure to opportunistic infections. Special intervention may also be warranted to create a healthy self-image in children with chronic conditions or disabilities. For example, the physically handicapped child can be helped to develop skills such as artistic ability that will contribute to a positive self-image. Primary preventive interventions employed by community health nurses in caring for children are summarized in Box 20–7.

BOX 20–7

Primary Preventive Interventions in the Care of Children

Promoting growth and development
- Provide anticipatory guidance to parents
- Assist with accomplishment of developmental tasks
- Provide assistance with developmental concerns

Promoting adequate nutrition
- Educate parents regarding children's nutritional needs
- Provide assistance in meeting nutritional needs

Promoting safety
- Encourage parents to provide adequate supervision of children
- Educate parents regarding safety concerns appropriate to the child's age
- Eliminate hazardous conditions from the environment
- Assist parents to provide safety education appropriate to the child's age and health status

Immunization
- Educate parents regarding the need for immunization and immunization schedules
- Refer parents to immunization services
- Educate parents about side effects of immunizations
- Modify immunization practices or provide additional immunizations for children with special needs

Dental care
- Encourage adequate dental hygiene
- Encourage regular dental checkups

Support for parenting
- Assist parents to develop realistic expectations of children
- Take action to minimize parental stress
- Assist parents to develop effective coping strategies and learn child-care skills
- Assist parents to deal with the special needs of children with chronic illnesses or disabilities
- Assist parents to deal with feelings of guilt, anger, and frustration engendered by a chronic or terminal condition in a child
- Arrange respite care as needed for parents of children with chronic conditions or disabilities

SECONDARY PREVENTION

Secondary prevention is geared toward resolution of health problems currently experienced by the child. Activities are directed toward screening for conditions, care of minor illness, referral for diagnostic and treatment services, and dealing with illness and treatment regimens.

Additional Screening Procedures

While many screening tests are routinely conducted as part of the assessment of a child's health status, assessment data may indicate a need for additional screening tests. As part of secondary prevention aimed at detecting existing health problems, the nurse can either conduct or make referrals for these additional tests. For example, lead screening may be indicated for children who live in areas with high lead levels in ambient air or who reside in areas where lead-based paint was used. Blood lead levels would also be obtained for children who exhibit signs of lead poisoning (see Chapter 16, Environmental Influences on Community Health).

Other screening tests may be warranted by assessment data. Children who are at risk for HIV infection should be referred for screening. Children at risk include those born to mothers who are intravenous drug users or partners of intravenous drug users or of bisexual males and children who have been transfused. Children who exhibit signs of immunodeficiency or opportunistic infections associated with AIDS (see Chapter 31, Communicable Disease) should also be referred for screening. Similarly, screening for hepatitis B antibodies may be conducted for children who have been exposed to the disease.

Care of Minor Illness

Many of the health problems experienced by children can be treated by parents at home. However, many parents are quite inexperienced in dealing with minor childhood ailments. They may require help in determining when illness can be dealt with at home and when the assistance of health-care professionals is required. The community health nurse can educate parents on the signs of illness in children, appropriate measures to be taken at home, and when to seek medical intervention. Common areas of concern that the nurse will want to address are teething, fever, diarrhea and constipation, vomiting, and rashes. Parents should be acquainted with what is normal and what is abnormal as well as what home remedies are appropriate and what might be harmful.

Besides providing such information, the community health nurse will frequently be called upon to assess a child's health status and recommend appropriate interventions or make a referral for medical assistance. Potential interventions for minor problems in children and indications for referral for medical assistance are addressed in Appendix K, Nursing Interventions for Common Health Problems in Children.

Referral

Community health nurses frequently encounter health problems in children that require further diagnostic evaluation and treatment. Unless the nurse is also a nurse practitioner, he or she will most probably refer the family to another source of diagnostic and treatment services. Referrals made should be appropriate to the condition suspected and to the circumstances of the situation. Considerations in making referrals and the referral process were addressed in Chapter 9, The Discharge Planning and Referral Processes.

In addition to making referrals for diagnosis and treatment services, the nurse may also educate parents and children about probable diagnostic and treatment procedures. For example, if the nurse suspects that a child may have hepatitis, he or she will explain the need for diagnostic blood tests to the parent (and to the child, if the child is old enough to understand) and will describe the typical treatment for hepatitis.

Referrals may be made for assistance with physical, psychological, or social health problems. In the case of child abuse, for example, the nurse might make a referral for evaluation and treatment of the physical effects of abuse on the child. At the same time, the nurse may refer both the perpetrator and the victim of abuse (or other family members) for psychological counseling. Finally, the nurse may refer for assistance those families whose social factors create stress and contribute to the potential for abusive behavior. Sources of assistance for nurses and families dealing with child abuse are presented in Table 20–10. General counseling resources are included in Table 20–11.

TABLE 20–10. RESOURCES FOR NURSES AND FAMILIES DEALING WITH CHILD ABUSE

Agency or Organization	Services
Child Abuse Listening Mediation, Inc. P.O. Box 718 Santa Barbara, CA 93102 (805) 682-1366	Abuse hotline, child-care, parental support, public information
Childhelp, USA, Inc. 6463 Independence Ave. Woodland Hills, CA 91370 (818) 347-7280	Public education, residential and after-care programs
Local Child Protective Services or law enforcement agencies	Investigate suspected abuse, foster placement
National Committee for Prevention of Child Abuse 332 S. Michigan Ave., Suite 950 Chicago, IL 60604 (312) 663-5320	Political advocacy, public education
Parents Anonymous 6733 S. Sepulveda, Suite 270 Los Angeles, CA 90045 (213) 410-9732	Self-help group for abusive parents and potential abusers
Village of Childhelp P.O. Box 247 14700 Manzanila Park Rd. Beaumont, CA 92223 (714) 845-3155	Residential program for abused children and their families

TABLE 20–11. COUNSELING AND HEALTH EDUCATION RESOURCES FOR FAMILIES

Area	Agency or Organization	Services
Counseling	American Academy of Child and Adolescent Psychiatry 3615 Wisconsin Ave., N.W. Washington, DC 20016 (202) 966-7300	Research
	American Association for Marriage and Family Therapy 924 W. Ninth St. Upland, CA 91786 (800) 854-9876	Referral for family counseling
	American Association of Psychiatric Services for Children 1725 K St., NW, Suite 1112 Washington, DC 20006 (202) 659-9115	Referral for child counseling
	Association for Children and Adults with Learning Disabilities 4156 Library Rd. Pittsburgh, PA 15234 (412) 341-1515	Public information
	National Consortium for Child Mental Health Services 1424 16th St., NW, Suite 201A Washington, DC 20036 (202) 462-3755	Public information
	National Society for Autistic Children 1234 Massachusetts Ave., NW Suite 1017 Washington, DC 20005-4955	Research, advocacy, public information
	National Sudden Infant Death Syndrome Foundation, Inc. 8240 Professional Place, Suite 205 Landover, MD 20785 (301) 459-3388	Research, public information, parental support
	Parents of Suicides c/o Bergen/Pasaic TCF P.O. Box 373 Englewood, NJ 10731 (201) 894-0042	Support for parents and siblings of young suicide victims
Health Education	Council for Sex Education and Information Box 72 Capitola, CA 95010	Information on sexuality
	International Council of Sex Education and Parenthood 5010 Wisconsin Ave., NW Washington, DC 20016 (202) 885-8534	Curricula and materials for sex education
	National Center for Education Materials and Medica for the Handicapped Ohio State University Faculty for Exceptional Children Columbus, OH 43210 (614) 422-7596	Bibliographies of education aids for the handicapped
	National Parents Resource Institute for Drug Education 100 Edgewood Ave., Suite 1002 Atlanta, GA 30303 (404) 658-2548	Information on drug abuse in youth; help in developing support groups
	Sex Information and Education Council of the U.S. 80 5th Ave., Suite 801 New York, NY 10011 (212) 929-2300	Public information and advocacy for sex education

Dealing with Illness and Treatment Regimens

When an illness requiring medical intervention has been diagnosed, the community health nurse may engage in several secondary preventive interventions related to the diagnosis and its treatment. These interventions include educating parents and children about the condition and its treatment. For example, parents of a child with a newly diagnosed case of diabetes may need information on diet, exercise, and the effects of infection on insulin needs, as well as instruction on how to give insulin. Or parents of a child with otitis media may need directions on the use of the antibiotic prescribed. Parents and children should also be given information on the side effects of medications or treatments. For example, parents should be warned about the potential side effects of radiation therapy for cancer and educated on ways to minimize these consequences as much as possible.

Secondary prevention may also entail informing parents and children about what to expect regarding a chronic disease and its treatment. For example, they should be informed that diabetes or essential hypertension can usually be controlled with therapy, but will not be cured, and that the child will probably need to take medication for the rest of his or her life. On the other hand, parents should be informed that symptoms of an ear infection should abate within a day or so of starting antibiotic therapy, but that medication should be completed.

The community health nurse may also be responsible for monitoring the effect of treatment and the child's health status between visits to a physician. In addition, the nurse will observe the child for evidence of medication side effects or other adverse effects of therapy. For example, the nurse may observe a child with ADHD to determine whether medication results in diminished hyperactivity or whether the child exhibits any medication side effects.

Monitoring compliance with a treatment regimen is another secondary preventive measure in the care of children with acute and chronic conditions. The community health nurse will need periodically to assess the child's or family's compliance with medication or other treatments. If noncompliance occurs, the nurse will need to determine factors contributing to noncompliance and plan interventions that will enhance compliance. For instance, if parents have not been giving their child prescribed antiepileptics because they cannot afford them, the nurse may make a referral for financial assistance or help the family budget their income more effectively. If, on the other hand, parents stopped giving antibiotics prescribed for the child's otitis media because the child got better, the nurse will educate them on the need to finish the prescribed medication.

Secondary prevention for children with conditions like arthritis, cancer, or other illnesses that cause pain will include interventions for pain control. Parents and children may need to be encouraged to use pain medications before pain becomes uncontrollable, or they may need suggestions for dealing with side effects related to pain medication.

TERTIARY PREVENTION

As is the case with secondary prevention, tertiary prevention will be geared toward the particular health problems experienced by the child. Generally, there are three aspects to tertiary prevention with children: preventing a recurrence of problems, preventing further consequences, and, in the case of chronic illness or disability, promoting adjustment.

Preventing Problem Recurrence

Community health nurses may educate parents and children to prevent the recurrence of many health problems experienced by children. For example, the parent may need information on the relationship of bottle propping to otitis media to prevent subsequent infections. Similarly, education about the need to change diapers frequently, to wash the skin with each diaper change, and to refrain from using harsh soaps to wash diapers may help to prevent further episodes of diaper rash.

Preventing Consequences

Tertiary prevention related to preventing further consequences of health problems is most often employed with children with chronic conditions. For example, the child with diabetes will need attention to diet, exercise, medication, and so on to control the diabetes and prevent physical consequences of the disease itself. At the same time, attention must be given to promoting the child's adjustment to the condition and normalizing his or her life as much as possible. Nursing interventions would be geared toward convincing the child to stick to one's diet and promoting the child's social interactions with peers.

The nurse might also need to intervene to prevent or minimize the consequences of the child's condition for the rest of the family. For example, the nurse might need to point out to parents that in their concern for the child with a chronic heart condition, they are neglecting the needs of siblings. Or tertiary prevention for an infant with AIDS may entail educating parents on the disposal of bodily fluids and excreta to prevent infection of other family members. Tertiary prevention may also extend to helping the child and his or her family deal with death if the child's condition is terminal.

Tertiary prevention may entail a wide variety of

activities on the part of the nurse, from education on how to deal with a specific condition to referral for assistance with major medical expenses. Nurses may also need to act as advocates for children with chronic conditions. The example that most readily comes to mind is the need for advocacy for children with AIDS who are still well enough to attend school.

Emotional support by the nurse is a very important part of tertiary prevention for children with chronic conditions. Parents' and children's feelings about the condition need to be acknowledged and dealt with. The nurse can also reinforce positive activities on the part of parent or child. Again, this support may need to extend to support as families go through the grieving process. Grieving will probably occur with most chronic illnesses, even those that are not terminal, and the nurse should be prepared to reassure families that their feelings of grief are normal and to support them through this process.

Promoting Adjustment

The community health nurse may also engage in activities that are designed to return the child and family to a relatively normal state of existence. For children with chronic illnesses or disabilities, this means restoring function as much as possible, preventing further loss of function, and assisting the child and his or her family to progress through the stages of family response to chronic illness discussed earlier in this chapter. The community health nurse might accomplish this by encouraging the family to discuss problems posed by the child's condition and to view the condition in the most positive light possible. The nurse should also encourage the family to normalize family life as much as possible. For example, if the Little League activities of a sibling have been curtailed because of an exacerbation of the child's illness, parents should make an attempt to reinstitute those activities as soon as the youngster's condition is stable. Or the family can be encouraged to call on members of their support network to take the sibling to baseball practice and games.

IMPLEMENTING NURSING CARE FOR CHILDREN

Planned nursing interventions may be implemented by the nurse, by family members, or by the child. The nurse should be certain that the child or family members are motivated and capable of carrying out planned care activities. This might necessitate interventions by the nurse to improve motivation or to help the child or family members develop the skills needed to implement the plan. The processes involved in motivating and educating people to take action were addressed in Chapter 11, The Change, Leadership, and Group Processes, and in Chapter 7, The Health Education Process.

During the implementation phase of nursing intervention, the nurse should check frequently with the child and the family to determine that the plan is indeed being implemented. If it is not, the nurse would assess reasons for noncompliance and plan interventions to facilitate implementation. The nurse should also determine whether the family is experiencing any problems with implementation. Perhaps the nurse has arranged for physical therapy for a handicapped child, but visits by the therapist are interfering with the mother's work schedule. In this case, the nurse might explore the options for providing therapy in the school or in a day-care setting instead of the home.

EVALUATING NURSING CARE FOR CHILDREN

The effectiveness of nursing interventions for the child is assessed in the same manner that care of any individual client is evaluated. Some of the questions that might be addressed are: Has intervention fostered the child's growth and development? Is the child's nutrition adequate for normal needs? Is the child up-to-date on his or her immunizations? Are there physical or psychological hazards present in the child's environment? Is the child receiving health care as needed? Have acute health-care problems been resolved?

The community health nurse would also examine the extent to which care has contributed to the adjustment of the child and family to existing chronic disease or disability. Are parents comfortable and adequately prepared to parent a child with special needs? Do they perform this role adequately? Have complications of the child's condition been prevented?

The community health nurse would identify criteria that would provide the answers to these and similar questions. Data would then be collected relative to the criteria to determine whether nursing intervention has resulted in an improved health status for the child and whether specific client care objectives have been met. If, for example, the child is anemic, the criteria used to evaluate nursing interventions related to this problem might include hemoglobin or hematocrit levels and the number and type of iron-rich foods in the child's diet. Evaluative data would be used to modify the plan of care or to determine the appropriateness of terminating services.

CHAPTER HIGHLIGHTS

- Care of children presents community health nurses with significant opportunities to influence the future health of the general population.
- Problems of particular concern in the care of children include infant mortality, low birth weight and congenital anomalies, HIV infection and AIDS, chronic illness, attention deficit hyperactivity disorder, and child abuse.
- Human biological concerns in assessing children include assessment of growth parameters and developmental milestones, exploring genetic inheritance, and assessing physiologic function in terms of present and past illnesses, signs and symptoms of illness, immunization status, and the results of other screening tests.
- Assessment considerations related to the physical environment focus on the presence or absence of safety hazards in the home or child-care environment.
- Areas to be addressed in assessing the psychological environment include the child's reactivity patterns and parental responses to them, parental expectations of the child, discipline, parental coping skills, parent-child interactions, and the child's self-image. The nurse should also assess the situation for evidence of actual or potential child abuse.
- Life-style considerations in the assessment of children include nutrition, rest and exercise, child-care outside the home, and school performance.
- Primary preventive measures appropriate to all children include promoting growth and development, providing adequate nutrition, promoting safety, immunization, dental care, and support for parenting. Other primary preventive measures may be necessitated by the child's health status.
- Secondary preventive measures for children with existing health problems may include additional screening tests, care of minor illnesses, referral, and assisting the child and his or her family to deal with illness and treatment regimens.
- Concerns in tertiary prevention for children with health problems include preventing the recurrence of problems, preventing consequences of existing problems, and promoting adjustment to long-term problems.
- Evaluation of community health nursing care focuses on the achievement of the objectives of primary, secondary, and tertiary preventive measures.

Review Questions

1. Describe at least five problems of concern to community health nurses working with children. (p. 454)
2. Differentiate between growth and development. How would you go about assessing each? (p. 458)
3. What are three safety considerations in assessing the physical environment of the infant? Toddlers and preschool children? School-age children? (p. 462)
4. List at least five areas to be addressed in relation to the child's psychological environment. Describe how factors in each of these areas might affect the child's health. (p. 464)
5. Identify at least three life-style considerations in assessing the health status of a child. Give an example of the influence of each on a child's health. (p. 470)
6. What are five primary preventive measures appropriate to all children? What modifications might be needed in these measures when caring for a child with a chronic or terminal illness or a disability? (p. 473)
7. Describe at least three approaches in providing secondary preventive services to a child with existing health problems. Give an example of the use of each. (p. 481)
8. What are the three considerations in tertiary preventive measures for children with existing health problems? Give an example of each consideration. (p. 484)

APPLICATION AND SYNTHESIS

You have received a referral to visit Mrs. Davis, a 24-year-old mother with a newborn baby. There is also another child in the family, Mandy, who is 3. Mother's pregnancy and delivery were uneventful, and mother and baby were discharged after 2 days in the hospital. When you make your home visit, Mrs. Davis tells you that the baby is spitting up an ounce or so of formula after each feeding but had gained almost a pound at her 2-week visit to the pediatrician yesterday. Otherwise the baby is doing well.

When you first arrive in the home, Mandy is sitting with her back to you watching cartoons on television. The TV is rather loud and she doesn't seem to be aware that a visitor has arrived. While you are talking to Mrs. Davis, Mandy turns around and sees you. She picks up her rag doll and comes to lean against her mother's knee with her thumb in her mouth. She seems to be rather pale compared to her mother's coloring.

Mandy pulls at her mother's sleeve to get her attention. When Mrs. Davis continues to tell you about the baby spitting up, Mandy hits the infant with her doll. Mrs. Davis scolds her and then tells you that Mandy used to be a very good girl, but ever since they brought the new baby home, she has been throwing tantrums and sucking her thumb.

1. What human biological, environmental, life-style, and health system factors are influencing the health of these two children?
2. What screening tests and immunizations should these two children have had?
3. Based on the data presented above, what are your nursing diagnoses?
4. How could you involve members of the family in planning to resolve the problems identified?
5. What primary, secondary, and/or tertiary preventive measures might you employ with this family?
6. How would you go about evaluating the effectiveness of your nursing interventions?

REFERENCES

1. United States Department of Health and Human Services. (1991). *Healthy people 2000: National health promotion and disease prevention objectives*. Washington, DC: Government Printing Office.
2. Johnson, P. A. (1990). A national health insurance program: A nursing perspective. *Nursing & Health Care, 11*, 416–418, 427–429.
3. Novello, A. C. (1990). Surgeon General's report on the health benefits of smoking cessation. *Public Health Reports, 105*, 545–549.
4. McCormick, M. C., Gortmacher, S. L., & Sobol, A. M. (1990). Very low birth weight children: Behavior problems and school difficulty in a national sample. *Journal of Pediatrics, 117*, 687–693.
5. Edmunds, L. D., & James, L. M. (1990). Temporal trends in the prevalence of congenital malformations at birth. *CDC Surveillance Summaries, MMWR, 39*(SS-4), 19–23.
6. United States Department of Health and Human Services. (1990, October). *HIV/AIDS Surveillance*. Washington, DC: U.S. Department of Health and Human Services.
7. Hutto, C., Parks, W. P., & Lai, S., et al. (1991). A hospital-based prospective study of perinatal infection with human immunodeficiency virus type I. *Journal of Pediatrics, 118*, 347–353.
8. Karon, J. M., & Dondero, T. J. (1990). HIV prevalence estimates and AIDS case projections for the United

States: Report based upon a workshop. *MMWR, 39*(RR-16), 1–31.
9. Ellis, E. F. (1987). Respiratory allergy. In R. E. Behrman & V. C. Vaughan (Eds.), *Nelson textbook of pediatrics* (13th ed.) (pp. 494–501). Philadelphia: W. B. Saunders.
10. Leventhal, B. G. (1987). Neoplasms and neoplasm-like structures. In R. E. Berhman & V. C. Vaughan (Eds.), *Nelson textbook of pediatrics* (13th ed.) (pp. 1079–1110). Philadelphia: W. B. Saunders.
11. Sperling, M. A. (1987). Diabetes mellitus. In R. E. Behrman & V. C. Vaughan (Eds.), *Nelson textbook of pediatrics* (13th ed.) (pp. 1248–1262). Philadelphia: W. B. Saunders.
12. Greenberg, R. E. (1987). Diabetes mellitus. In R. A. Hoekelman, S. Blatman, & S. B. Friedman, et al. (Eds.), *Primary pediatric care.* (pp. 1214–1220). St. Louis: C. V. Mosby.
13. Ruley, E. J. (1987). Acute hypertension. In R. A. Hoekelman, S. Blatman, & S. B. Friedman, et al. (Eds.), *Primary pediatric care* (pp. 1538–1542). St. Louis: C. V. Mosby.
14. United States Department of Health and Human Services. (1988). *Report of the Joint National Committee on the Detection, Evaluation, and Treatment of High Blood Pressure.* Washington, DC: Government Printing Office.
15. Gewanter, H. L. (1987). Juvenile arthritis. In R. A. Hoekelman, S. Blatman, & S. B. Friedman, et al. (Eds.), *Primary pediatric care* (pp. 1326–1332). St. Louis: C. V. Mosby.
16. Huttenlocher, P. R. (1987). The nervous system. In R. E. Behrman & V. C. Vaughan (Eds.), *Nelson textbook of pediatrics* (13th ed.) (pp. 1274–1330). Philadelphia: W. B. Saunders.
17. Bresnan, M. J., & Kinkol, R. J. (1987). Seizure disorders. In R. A. Hoekelman, S. Blatman, & S. B. Friedman, et al. (Eds.), *Primary pediatric care* (pp. 1467–1477). St. Louis: C. V. Mosby.
18. Hirtz, D. G. (1989). Generalized tonic-clonic and febrile seizures. *Pediatric Clinics of North America, 36,* 365–382.
19. Pellock, J. M. (1989). Efficacy and adverse effects of antiepileptic drugs. *Pediatric Clinics of North America, 36,* 435–448.
20. Schachar, R., & Wachsmuth, R. (1990). Hyperactivity and parental psychopathology. *Journal of Child Psychology and Psychiatry, 31,* 381–392.
21. Wender, E. H. (1987). Attention deficit disorders. In R. A. Hoekelman, S. Blatman, & S. B. Friedman, et al. (Eds.), *Primary pediatric care* (pp. 671–679). St. Louis: C. V. Mosby
22. Mannuzza, S., Klein, R. G., Konig, P. H., & Giampino, T. L. (1989). Hyperactive boys almost grown up. *Archives of General Psychiatry, 46,* 1073–1079.
23. Johnson, C. M., Yehl, J. F., & Stack, J. M. (1989). Compliance training in a child with attention deficit-hyperactivity disorder—A case study. *Family Practice Research Journal, 9*(1), 73–80.
24. Bower, B. (1991). Alcohol's fetal harm lasts a lifetime. *Science News, 139,* 244.
25. Henderson, R. W. (1989). *Fetal alcohol syndrome.* Pediatrics Update 1989, San Diego, CA.
26. Serdula, M., Williamson, D. F., & Kendrick, J. S., et al. (1991). Trends in alcohol consumption by pregnant women. *JAMA, 265,* 876–879.
27. Bingol, N., Fuchs, M., & Diaz, V., et al., (1987). Teratogenicity of cocaine in humans. *Journal of Pediatrics, 110,* 93–96.
28. Piazza, S. F., Lanza, B., & Dweck, H. S. (1989, Spring). Neurological abnormalities and developmental delays in infants of substance abusing mothers. *Pediatric Research,* 260A.
29. Ward, S. L. D., Bautista, D., & Chan, L., et al. (1990). Sudden infant death syndrome in infants of substance abusing mothers. *Journal of Pediatrics, 117,* 876–881.
30. Lathrop, J. (1989). *Milestones: Growth and development guide.* Milwaukee: Maxishare.
31. Gundy, J. H. (1987). The pediatric physical examination. In R. A. Hoekelman, S. Blatman, & S. B. Friedman, et al. (Eds.), *Primary pediatric care* (pp. 63–109). St. Louis: C. V. Mosby.
32. Gonzales, R., & Michael, A. (1987). Urological disorders in infants and children. In R. E. Behrman & V. C. Vaughan (Eds.), *Nelson textbook of pediatrics* (13th ed.) (pp. 1147–1169). Philadelphia: W. B. Saunders.
33. United States Preventive Services Task Force. (1989). *Guide to clinical preventive services.* Baltimore: Williams & Wilkins.
34. Update: Childhood poisonings—United States. (1985). *MMWR, 34,* 117–119.
35. Toy safety—United States, 1983. (1984). *MMWR, 33,* 697.
36. Playground-related injuries in preschool-aged children—United States, 1983–1987. (1988). *MMWR, 37,* 629–632.
37. Rooney, E. (1990). Corporate attitudes and responses to rising health care costs. *AAOHN Journal, 38,* 304–311.
38. Pilletteri, A. (1987). *Child health nursing: Care of the growing family* (3rd ed.). Boston: Little, Brown.
39. Austin, J. K. (1990). Assessment of coping mechanisms used by parents and children with chronic illness. *MCN, 15,* 98–102.
40. Broome, M. E., & Daniels, D. (1987). Child abuse: A multidimensional phenomenon. *Holistic Nursing Practice, 1*(2), 13–24.
41. Leatherland, J. (1986). Do you know child abuse when you see it? *RN, 49*(3), 28–30.
42. Shear, C. L., Freedman, D. S., & Burke, G. L., et al. (1988). Secular trends of obesity in early life: The Bogalusa heart study. *American Journal of Public Health, 78,* 75–77.
43. ACIP: Diphtheria, Tetanus, and Pertussis: Guidelines for vaccine prophylaxis and other preventive measures. (1985). *MMWR, 34,* 405.
44. ACIP: General recommendations on immunization. (1989). *MMWR, 38,* 205–227.

RECOMMENDED READINGS

Alexander, M. M., & Brown, M. S. (1979). *Pediatric history taking and physical diagnosis for nurses* (2nd ed.). New York: McGraw-Hill.

Describes techniques for taking a pediatric history and conducting a physical examination on a child.

Behrman, R. E., & Vaughan, V. C. (1987). *Nelson textbook of pediatrics* (13th ed.). Philadelphia: W. B. Saunders.

Presents diagnostic signs and symptoms and medical treatment of major pediatric disorders.

Ferholt, J. D. L. (1980). *Clinical assessment of children: A comprehensive approach to primary pediatric care.* Philadelphia: J. B. Lippincott.

Sets forth a complete assessment of the health status of a child including obtaining a history, conducting a physical examination and screening procedures, assessing development, and interpreting findings.

Foster, R. L. R., Hunsberger, M. M., & Anderson, J. J. T. (1989). *Family-centered nursing care of children.* Philadelphia: W. B. Saunders.

Provides a foundation for pediatric nursing care.

Hoekelman, R. A., Blatman, S., & Friedman, S. B., et al., (Eds.). (1987). *Primary pediatric care.* St. Louis: C. V. Mosby.

Discusses primary care for pediatric practice. Addresses both health promotion and treatment of illness.

Pilletteri, A. (1987). *Child health nursing: Care of the growing family* (3rd ed.). Boston: Little, Brown.

Offers a basic understanding of the nursing of children within the context of the family.

Rose, M. H., & Thomas, R. B. (Eds.). (1989). *Children with chronic conditions: Nursing in a family and community context.* Orlando, FL: Grune & Stratton.

Contains a general overview of nursing care for children with chronic conditions and describes specifics of care for children with selected conditions. Addresses community attitudes and adaptation to children with chronic conditions, as well as family responses.

Whaley, L. F., & Wong, D. L. (1988). *Nursing care of infants and children* (3rd ed.). St. Louis: C. V. Mosby.

Provides a basic foundation for the nursing care of children.

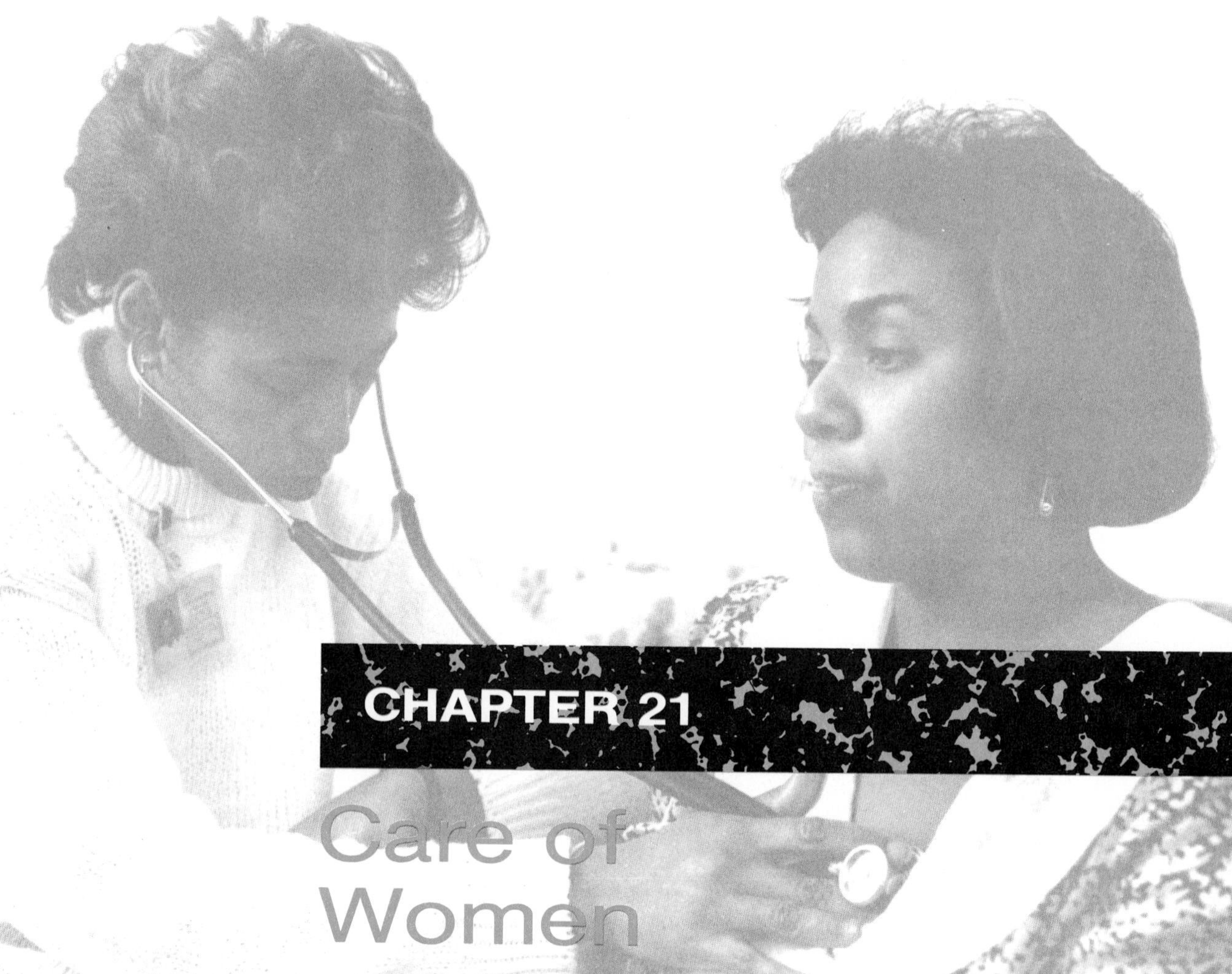

CHAPTER 21

Care of Women

Patricia Caudle
Susan Chen

KEY TERMS

homophobia
infertility
menarche
menopause
osteoporosis
patriarchy

Women have unique health-care needs, not only because of their anatomy and reproductive functions, but also because of their vulnerability within society. Traditionally, women have been wives and mothers; submissive to males and, yet, an essential member of the family. Community health nurses working with women have opportunities not only to improve the health status of women but also women's abilities to care for themselves and their families.

The importance of improving the health of women in the United States is reflected in the national health objectives for the year 2000. Seven of these objectives address issues specifically targeting the health needs of nonpregnant women.[1] These objectives are summarized in Box 21–1.

In this chapter the epidemiologic prevention process model will be applied to the care of adolescent, young adult, and middle adult women. The health needs of older women are the focus of Chapter 23, Care of Older Clients.

LEARNING OBJECTIVES

After reading this chapter you should be able to:

- Describe at least two factors to be considered in assessing the influence of each component of Dever's eidemiologic perspective on the health of women.
- Identify at least four health problems common to women.
- Describe at least three specific considerations that are unique in assessing the health needs of the lesbian client.
- Identify at least five general concerns in primary prevention for women.
- Describe three areas for consideration in secondary preventive activities in the care of women.
- Describe two dimensions of secondary prevention of physical abuse of women.
- Describe at least two actions that the community health nurse can take to provide more sensitive and effective care to the lesbian client.

BOX 21–1

Summary of National Health Objectives Related to Women's Health

- Increase to at least 80 percent the proportion of women 40 years and over who have ever had a clinical breast examination and a mammogram.
- Increase to at least 95 percent the proportion women 18 years and over with uterine cervix who have ever had a Pap test, and to at least 85 percent those who have received a Pap test in the preceding 1 to 3 years.
- Increase to at least 90 percent the proportion of perimenopausal women counseled about the benefits and risks of estrogen replacement therapy to prevent osteoporosis.
- Reduce physical abuse of women by male partners to no more than 27 per 1000 couples.
- Reduce rape and attempted rape of women aged 12 and older to no more than 108 per 100,000 women.
- Reduce to less than 10 percent the proportion of battered women and their children turned away from emergency housing due to lack of space.
- Reduce iron-deficiency to less than 3 percent among women of childbearing age.

(Source: U.S. Department of Health and Human Services[1])

FACTORS AFFECTING HEALTH CARE FOR WOMEN

American women remain comparatively disadvantaged in society at large and in the health-care delivery system. Women have higher rates of diagnosed illness than do men.[2] Women use the health-care system more frequently than do men owing to factors related to human reproduction. Women need to seek health-care services during pregnancies and to obtain the means to prevent pregnancies. Women are also more likely to require medical intervention as a result of rape, physical assault, or battering by spouses. Not only are they more often recipients of health care for themselves, but women are frequently given the responsibility for obtaining health care for children. Finally, because women, as an aggregate, live longer than men (life expectancy of 78 years compared to 71 years for men),[3] they are more likely to live the latter portion of their lives in a nursing home.[4]

Women not only use health-care services more often than men but they are often more hard-pressed to pay for these services. More women live in poverty than do men. Salaries for females are still about 60 percent to 70 percent of those earned by males in comparable jobs. Women are also less likely to be covered by medical insurance as a job benefit because they are more likely to hold part-time jobs. More women than men are heads of single-parent households and are the sole support of their children. For all of these reasons, women are more likely to be dependent on such programs as Medicaid and Medicare.[4]

These conditions are the result of social traditions and age-old prejudices that have been legitimated through religion, law, and culture. Not surprisingly, the health-care system reflects and perpetuates many sexist attitudes and beliefs within the culture at large.[5,6] At the turn of the century, men and some women believed that a woman's primary functions were procreation and taking care of the home and family. As a result of a prevailing culture of sexism, physicians tended to perceive women as creatures totally controlled by their womb, ovaries, and hormones. Everything from headache to arthritis in women was attributed to sexual disorders.[5] This tradition lingers today to the extent that discussions of women's health issues are limited to reproductive and gynecologic concerns.

During the formative years of America's health-care system, physicians converted female reproductive functions into medical conditions and encouraged women to depend on a male-dominated profession for care. According to one observer, "Pregnancy and menopause became diseases, menstruation a chronic disorder, and childbirth a surgical event."[7] Because of prevailing paternalistic attitudes, it also became normal for physicians to withhold information about medical conditions and to treat women as if they were intellectually, emotionally, and physically inferior to men.[6,8] Regrettably, many women are still subjected to such treatment, especially women who are poor, uneducated, or members of minority groups.

COMMUNITY HEALTH NURSING AND WOMEN'S HEALTH

The legacies of past sexism still linger, but change is possible. Community health nurses are in a unique position to assist women to deal with the problems they are experiencing. As women (and most nurses are women), community health nurses experience many of the same problems as their female clients, and both are learning ways to change or cope with the existing system. As citizens and professionals, community health nurses work for change through efforts to raise awareness of women's issues through political processes (see Chapter 12, The Political Process). And, too, the nurse's knowledge of the health-care system, social welfare systems, and other community resources can be shared with clients.

Community health nurses contribute to women's health as advocates, counselors, providers of direct physical care, case finders, teachers, and researchers. They are concerned with the well-being of women within the context of lived experience. Each woman is viewed as a whole person with physical, psychological, and social needs, none of which can be ignored in favor of a preoccupation with a single problem.

Community health nurses advocate and encourage the same attributes that today's women are demanding: independence, control over one's body, egalitarian relationships, cooperation rather than competition, personal experience as an important source of information, demystification of health care that leads to empowerment of women, and holism.[9] These demands have evolved out of the women's movement and reflect the social expectations of women who want to control their own lives and to be independent within a male-dominated society and health-care delivery system.

THE EPIDEMIOLOGIC PREVENTION PROCESS MODEL AND THE CARE OF WOMEN

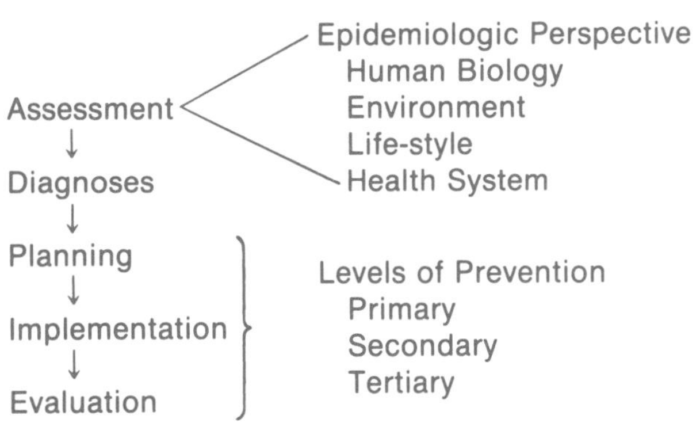

ASSESSING THE HEALTH NEEDS OF WOMEN

Use of the epidemiologic prevention process model with the female client begins with an assessment of health status. Factors influencing health status are examined according to the four epidemiologic components of the model: human biology, environment, life-style, and health system. Aggregates of women, like other groups within communities, can be assessed as described in Chapter 19, Care of the Community or Target Group.

HUMAN BIOLOGY

Human biological factors are of concern to the community health nurse assessing the female client. The nurse would obtain information related to the genetic inheritance, maturation and aging, and physiologic function.

Genetic Inheritance

Women are prone to a number of genetically related or genetically linked conditions. For example, cancers of the breast have been shown to occur more frequently among women whose mothers, sisters, aunts, or grandmothers have had similar cancers. Similarly, diseases of the thyroid gland seem to occur more frequently among women than among men.[10]

Maturation and Aging

Maturational events affect women throughout their life. Two that are of particular interest are menarche in the adolescent and menopause in the middle-age to older adult woman.

Menarche. *Menarche,* the first appearance of menstrual flow in the adolescent female, usually occurs between 12 and 13 years of age, but is considered within normal limits unless it occurs before or during the eighth year or after age 18. Menarche that occurs too early (age 8 or younger) is associated with precocious puberty, an anomaly of the endocrine system. Delayed menarche (after age 18) is also a signal that the endocrine system is not functioning properly. Both early and late onset of menses is cause for referral for medical evaluation.

The onset of menarche seems to depend on an individual's fat-to-muscle ratio (leaner individuals have later menarche), the individual's weight-height ratio (taller, thinner girls have later menarche), and her genetic predisposition (girls usually imitate their mothers for age of onset of menses if other factors are consistent with onset).[11]

Prior to and after menarche, girls experience predictable body changes. These body changes have

TABLE 21–1. STAGES OF SEXUAL MATURATION IN GIRLS

Stage	Pubic Hair Characteristics	Breast Characteristics
1	None present	Preadolescent
2	Sparse, straight, lightly pigmented, present on the medial border of the labia	Increase in areola diameter, breast and papilla elevated as a small mound
3	Darker pigmentation, increased amount, hair beginning to curl	Enlargement of breast and areola, no contour separation between breast and areola
4	Hair is dark and curly, abundant, but less in amount than as an adult	Areola and papilla form a secondary mound separated from the contour of the breast
5	Adult female inverted triangle; hair distribution spread to medial aspects of thighs	Nipple projects, areola forms part of general breast contour

(Adapted from Litt, I. R., & Vaughan, V. C. [1987]. Growth and development during adolescence. In R. E. Behrman & V. C. Vaughan (Eds.), Nelson textbook of pediatrics *[13th ed.] [pp. 20–22]. Philadelphia: W.B. Saunders.)*

been described by Tanner and associates as occurring in five stages. For instance, girls who are in Tanner Stage III usually display an increased amount of dark, curling pubic hair and breasts that are enlarged and have no contour separation between the breast and the areola. It is during Tanner Stage III that menarche occurs. With menarche, further changes will occur in the appearance of the young female. Her weight, disposition of body fat, breasts, and hair growth patterns will change to those of an adult over a period of 4 to 5 years. The stages of sexual maturation in girls are summarized in Table 21–1.

These body changes have the potential to create physical or psychological problems for the adolescent. Community health nurses will encounter many young women before, during, and after menarche. Assessment of each 8- to 12-year-old female should include the client's stage of sexual maturity, knowledge of menstruation, and preparation for the event. If menarche has occurred, other considerations related to menstruation may include menstrual regularity, extent and duration of flow, and the experience of dysmenorrhea, or painful menstruation. The nurse would also inquire about signs and symptoms of premenstrual distress (premenstrual syndrome) such as depression, irritability, nervousness, tension, inability to concentrate, breast tenderness, bloating, edema, fatigue, headache, and food cravings.[12] Symptoms of premenstrual distress may be severe and require medical referral or may be less severe and respond to dietary changes and exercise.

Menopause. In assessing older women, the nurse should determine whether menopause has occurred. ***Menopause*** is the cessation of menstruation that occurs with advancing age. Most women experience menopause and its physical and emotional effects between 41 and 59 years of age. The onset of menopausal symptoms and menopause are somewhat determined by heredity. The client's mother's history of menopause will often reveal the pattern the client can be expected to experience.[13]

Physical effects of menopause can include hot flashes or flushes accompanied by perspiration and chills; menstrual irregularity consisting of greater flow and longer times between periods; and vaginal dryness and atrophy. Other effects may be redisposition of body fat, headache, dizziness, insomnia, depression, anxiety, and nervousness and irritability.[14] Each individual responds to these changes differently. Some women are very uncomfortable and others are not. The nurse must assess each individual female according to symptoms she describes.

Another concern during the perimenopausal years is osteoporosis. ***Osteoporosis*** is a common metabolic bone disease characterized by a loss of bone minerals that weakens bones so that fractures occur more easily.[15] Although bone mineral loss begins to occur in the fourth decade of life, the loss is gradual until menopause. At menopause, bone loss is accelerated because of declining estrogen levels.

Physiologic Function

The client's physiologic function is assessed in terms of considerations presented in Chapter 17, Care of the Individual Client. Special considerations in assessing the female client include pregnancy, infertility, and the presence or absence of specific illnesses such as reproductive cancers and sexually transmitted diseases.

Pregnancy. Pregnancy is one of the most prevalent problems related to human physiology in the adolescent girl. In 1986, births to unmarried teenagers of all races accounted for about half of births to unmarried women.[16] However, this percentage represents only a portion of teen pregnancies because it does not include those pregnancies that are terminated either

TABLE 21–2. FUNDAL HEIGHT AT SELECTED WEEKS OF GESTATION

Weeks of Gestation	Fundal Height
12	At the level of the symphysis pubis
16	Halfway between symphysis pubis and umbilicus
20	At the level of the umbilicus
20–26	Height of fundus in centimeters correlates with weeks of gestation
36–40	1 cm below the xiphoid process until lightening occurs, then decreases; varies with the weight of the baby and maternal parity

(Adapted from Olds, S., London, M., & Ladewig, P. [1988]. Maternal-newborn nursing: A family-centered approach *[3rd ed.]. Menlo Park, CA: Addison-Wesley.)*

through spontaneous or therapeutic abortions. It has been estimated that 40 percent of teen pregnancies end in therapeutic abortion.[17] It is also important to note that about 20 percent of teen pregnancies occur among those who already have one child.[18]

Pregnancy is more often associated with complications, prematurity, and fetal and maternal mortality among adolescents than among older women. The pregnant teen requires close monitoring of both physiologic and psychologic status during and after pregnancy.

Pregnancy also occurs in young adult and middle adult women, of course, and should be an area for exploration in assessing the female client. Information regarding potential current and past pregnancies is solicited and any related problems should be identified. If the client is pregnant, the nurse will want to assess fetal growth as well as maternal health. Fetal growth patterns are assessed by measuring fundal height during each visit. The fundal height should increase steadily until just before delivery. Consult Table 21–2 for the expected fundal height at selected weeks of gestation.

Evidence of complications such as pregnancy-induced hypertension and gestational diabetes should also be sought. For example, signs of pregnancy-induced hypertension include increased blood pressure (140/90 or greater or a rise of 30 mm Hg in systolic or 15 mm Hg in diastolic levels over the baseline blood pressure), proteinuria (1+ or greater protein in a clean catch specimen), and edema (sudden, excessive weight gain or swelling of the hands and face).[19] Gestational diabetes can be suspected if there is a family history of diabetes, history of miscarriage, history of babies weighing 9 pounds or more, the pregnant woman is overweight, or there is positive glycosuria, polyuria, polydipsia, polyphagia, or recurrent monilial infection.[19] Table 21–3 lists some of the most common complications of pregnancy and their signs and symptoms.

Infertility. There is an increasing incidence of infertility among American women. ***Infertility,*** the inability to conceive and have a child, occurs in approximately one out of six couples in the United States, and the rate of infertility has tripled in the last 20 years.[20] Causes of infertility among women include the occurrence of sexually transmitted diseases that damage fallopian tubes, environmental toxins affecting ova, and a tendency to postpone pregnancy until the late 30s or early 40s. Women aged 38 and older tend to ovulate less frequently than younger women, thereby becoming less fertile than they would have been in their 20s.

Infertility can have serious consequences for the individual and the couple who are unable to conceive. Some of these consequences are enumerated in Box 21–2. The community health nurse can assess the client's desire to have children and any attempts made to conceive. Data collected should include the ages of the female and her partner; her menstrual

TABLE 21–3. SIGNS AND SYMPTOMS OF COMPLICATIONS OF PREGNANCY

Complication	Signs and Symptoms
Gestational diabetes	Polyuria, polydipsia, polyphagia, obesity, large baby, glycosuria (may be asymptomatic)
Iron-deficiency anemia	Fatigue, pallor, hemoglobin below 11 mg/dL, history of poor dietary iron intake
Pregnancy-induced hypertension	B/P 140/90, 30 mm Hg rise in systolic pressure or 15 mm Hg rise in diastolic pressure; edema (especially of face and hands); proteinuria (convulsions in severe form)
Hyperemesis gravidarum	Severe vomiting, retching, dehydration, starvation, infant small for gestational age
Rh sensitization	Rh-negative mother, Rh-positive father
Abruptio placenta	Vaginal bleeding
Premature labor	Strong uterine contractions prior to the 35th week of gestation

(Adapted from Olds, S., London, M., & Ladewig, P. [1988]. Maternal-newborn nursing: A family-centered approach *[3rd ed.]. Menlo Park, CA: Addison-Wesley.)*

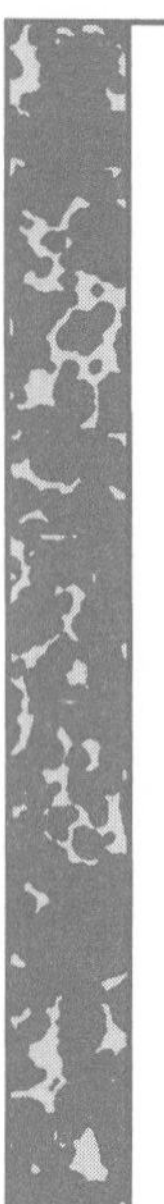

BOX 21–2

Consequences of Infertility

- Feelings of guilt, especially among women, who are usually the focus of the search for a cause
- Expense of diagnostic and other procedures
- Obsession with the inability to conceive
- Disapproval and pressure from family to adopt or try other methods to conceive
- In some cultures, perceptions of the female as less than a woman

history (especially information about irregular periods); a medical history that includes information on mumps in the partner, pelvic inflammatory disease in the woman, reproductive or abdominal surgery or serious illness in either partner, dysmenorrhea or dyspareunia; forms of contraception used in the past (especially use of an intrauterine device, or IUD), diethylstilbestrol (DES) exposure of either partner in utero, and whether or not either partner has ever achieved a pregnancy.[12] These data will form the basis for nursing intervention to be discussed later in this chapter.

Illness. Assessment of physiologic function also includes the collection of data related to the presence or absence of physical illness. The community health nurse would obtain a complete health history and physical examination, looking for signs and symptoms of illness. Areas for particular concern with the female client are evidence of reproductive cancers and possible sexually transmitted diseases.

Reproductive cancers (cancers of the breast, uterus, cervix, or ovaries) occur frequently among women. In 1986, the death rate for cancer of the breast ranged from 18 per 100,000 women aged 25 to 44 to 180 per 100,000 women aged 85 years and older. Genital cancer occurred at the rate of 7 per 100,000 women aged 35 to 44 and 108 per 100,000 women aged 85 years and older.[16] When detected early, these types of cancers can be cured, and their detection is an important component in assessing the health of a female client.

Assessment of each woman should include present and past medical history, family history of breast, uterine, or ovarian cancer, and the woman's use of early detection procedures such as self-breast examination, biannual or annual mammograms (depending on the age of the client), annual Pap smears (for early detection of cervical cancer), and annual pelvic examinations (for early detection of uterine or ovarian abnormalities). Cancer and cancer detection are discussed more fully in Chapter 31, Chronic Physical Health Problems.

Problems of sexually transmitted diseases will be addressed in detail in Chapter 30, Communicable Disease. Here, however, we will consider some of the implications of acquired immunodeficiency syndrome (AIDS) as it relates specifically to women.

AIDS is a viral disease that destroys the body's immune system, causing the person with AIDS (PWA) to succumb to opportunistic infections. AIDS is caused by the human immunodeficiency virus Type I and Type II (HIV-1 and HIV-2). For a person to become infected, the virus must enter the bloodstream. The pathways of transmission that have been identified include sexual contact with an infected person, use of infected needles, use of infected blood or blood products, or transplacentally (where the virus enters the fetus from the mother's infected blood by crossing the placental barrier).[21,22] The person infected by HIV may not manifest symptoms of AIDS for 2 to 10 years or more, but can pass the disease on to others.[23]

Although once thought to be a disease primarily affecting male homosexuals, AIDS has proven to be nondiscriminatory with respect to gender. The number of women infected through heterosexual contact has shown a consistent increase since 1985, while the percentage of cases among men has decreased.[24] It is estimated that by the year 2000, the worldwide number of women with AIDS will begin to equal that of men.[25] In New York City, AIDS is the number-one killer of women (especially black and Latino women) aged 25 to 49.[26,27]

These statistics do not convey the anguish this disease has caused women. AIDS is a physical threat with a tremendous social impact. Single women must enter relationships cautiously and be assertive enough to explore the sexual history of a potential partner. Women are reluctant to do this for fear it may interfere with the relationship.[26] If a woman can convince a male partner to use them, condoms are generally protective, but not foolproof. The only absolute way to avoid HIV infection is to have a mutually monogamous relationship with an uninfected person or to practice sexual abstinence.[21]

Women with AIDS typically lack the support systems that male homosexuals have been able to build. Often women with AIDS are ostracized and isolated.

Minority women may even avoid treatment for AIDS-related conditions for fear that if it is known that they have AIDS, their children will be taken from them.

Women who are HIV infected carry a burden that men do not share. An infected pregnant woman can transmit HIV to her unborn child. Perinatal AIDS cases rose 38 percent between 1988 and 1989. This percentage increase was greater even than the percentage increases recorded among homosexual men and intravenous drug users.[24] Infants born with AIDS are usually very ill and have a very short life. For instance, in California the median survival time from diagnosis to death for infants and children was just over 6 months. Of the children in the study, 75 percent died within 16 months of diagnosis.[28] For a woman who has dreamed of motherhood and who values children highly, this can be a nightmare. Many of these pregnancies occur during the dormant period of HIV infection, before symptoms of AIDS appear in the mother. Imagine the devastation felt by a mother on learning that her baby is infected with a fatal disease and that she is the cause. Women in these circumstances need assistance to cope.

Because women usually assume care-giver roles within families, they suffer when family members contract and die of AIDS. When a family member is terminally ill, the commitment to care for that individual can be emotionally draining, not only because of the pain and eventual death of the individual, but also because of the ever-present fear of contracting the disease. Women who assume a care-giving role need a strong support system to assist them in working through the fears associated with this role. To provide such assistance, the community health nurse needs to be tactful when eliciting information related to the potential for AIDS in the female client or in family members. Table 21–4 presents some assessment inquiries that can be made by the community health nurse.

TABLE 21–4. ASSESSING AIDS RISK

Question	Response Indicating Risk
• Did you receive a blood transfusion prior to 1984?	Yes
• Are you monogamous?	No
• Is your partner monogamous?	No
• Do you and your partner use a latex condom and nonoxynol-9?	No
• Do you engage in anal intercourse?	Yes
• Do you engage in oral-genital or oral-anal intercourse?	Yes
• Have you or your partner ever used IV drugs?	Yes
• Do you use crack?	Yes
• Have you or your partner ever tested positive for HIV?	Yes
• Do you share syringes with others for injecting vitamins or other medications?	Yes

ENVIRONMENT

Physical, psychological, and social environmental factors also influence the health of women. They are exposed to physical environmental hazards both at home and in the work setting. In the home there are household chemicals used to clean, inhalants such as powders and sprays, and potential for falls related to stools, stairs, and throw rugs. The effects of the workplace on women's health will be covered later in this chapter during the discussion of the occupational component of women's life-style. Here we will focus on the effects of psychological and social environmental factors on the health of women. Areas of particular concern relate to perceptions of and attitudes toward sexuality, life goals, violence and abuse, and abilities to cope with life. Because psychological and social factors tend to be inseparably related in these areas they will be addressed together.

Sexuality

Psychological and social environmental factors interact with physiologic factors and those related to maturation and aging to create a number of health problems for women. Teenagers are often confused and unsure about themselves and their place in life. Psychological factors surrounding menarche, sexuality, identity development, pregnancy, and so on will influence the teen's health status.

Many young girls will be embarrassed to discuss menstruation even while they have a number of misconceptions and fears about it. It is crucial that the teen be adequately prepared for the event or she may develop negative feelings toward menstruation that will continue throughout her reproductive years. In assessing the adolescent girl, the nurse would obtain information related to attitudes and anxieties about menstruation as well as knowledge of menstrual physiology and hygiene. Social factors such as family and cultural attitudes and knowledge and parental educational level will also affect family readiness to assist the young girl to deal with the physical, emotional, and practical issues posed by menarche.

Menopause, at the other end of the reproductive spectrum, also has social environmental implications. In American society, menopausal women have been considered relatively useless and are not held in high esteem.[29] Women have been barred from productive work on the basis of their menopausal symptoms. Society's lack of regard for the older woman adds to her emotional symptoms, thereby limiting her abilities to cope with physical and psychological changes occurring at this time.

Identity formation is a major task of adolescence. Women derive their sense of identity from relationships.[30] Essential to effective relationships and identity formation is the formation of a sexual identity and orientation and choosing types and frequency of sexual expression. Stereotypical male views of female sexuality and sexual identify can hinder the formation of a healthy sexual identity in the female.

Each female, including the adolescent female, has a right and responsibility to choose her sexual life-style, whether she chooses heterosexuality, lesbianism, bisexuality, or celibacy. Because of societal and family beliefs and attitudes, however, women may encounter strong psychological pressure to conform to stereotypical female notions of female sexuality. In doing an assessment, the nurse should explore the client's sexual preferences in a nonjudgmental fashion and should support the client in the sexual life-style chosen. Additional assessment considerations in working with lesbian clients are presented later in this chapter.

Sexual activity by women, especially teenagers, may have a variety of psychological precursors. For instance, the adolescent may think, if she is still a virgin at age 15, that there is something wrong with her. Or, if she perceives her mother as asexual or "Madonna-like," she may rebel and seek sexual outlets totally unlike those of her mother. The nurse will want to assess the client's knowledge and attitudes about her sexual identity and about sexual activity. Sexuality for women is more than a biological drive. Sexual activity may be an attempt to define personal and sexual identity as well as a means of communicating with others. For women, sexuality is a total experience of emotions, relationships, and life experiences.[31]

There is much evidence that both psychological and social factors contribute to the problem of adolescent pregnancy. Psychological theories of the cause of teenage pregnancy include beliefs that (1) the pregnancy meets a psychological need and is intentional, (2) pregnancy is an expression of ambivalent feelings about parents, (3) pregnancy is a form of rebellion or a response to loneliness, (4) pregnancy may be an attempt to bolster personal feelings of self-worth, or (5) pregnancy is a bid for attention. The problem with these theories is that they are based on studies of white teenagers, many of whom were under psychiatric care. Other theories of teen pregnancy include ideas that (1) teens enter into a sexual relationship in search of love and become pregnant accidentally, (2) teens become pregnant to have a baby to love and love them, and (3) teens seek pregnancy to punish their parents.[32]

A number of social factors may also contribute to intended or unintended pregnancy. This is particularly true in the case of adolescent pregnancy. Sexual experimentation by adolescents is expected, but may come as a shock to parents who have not recognized their son or daughter as a sexual being. Unfortunately, American teenagers are becoming sexually active earlier than was previously the case. In 1970 less than 29 percent of girls aged 15 to 19 participating in the National Survey of Family Growth reported having premarital sexual activity compared to more than 50 percent in 1988.[33] Such early sexual activity exposes the teen to increased risks for unwanted pregnancy and sexually transmitted diseases.

There are several social theories related to adolescent sexual activity and resultant pregnancy. Learned sexual behavior through interaction and identification with peers, family, and cultural groups is one such theory.[32] Peer pressure or a need for status and popularity may be the motivation for sexual activity that results in pregnancy.

Some authorities believe that teen pregnancy is a reaction to the dominant American culture in which teens are dependent and have no meaningful role in society.[32] Furthermore, given the cultural stereotype of woman's role and function as that of procreation, the teen who seeks pregnancy may be attempting to fulfill her cultural destiny.

Teens must also negotiate the differences between what society says and does with respect to sexuality. At one level, teens see parents resisting school-based sex education because it is perceived as promoting promiscuity. At another level, teens are exposed to images and messages in the entertainment media in which sexual innuendo and sexual acts are frequently portrayed without even hinting that such activity could lead to pregnancy or STDs. To condemn simultaneously the female who becomes pregnant out of wedlock yet tacitly condone such media exposure presents teens with conflicting messages about proper sexual conduct.

Finally, a lack of information and knowledge about sexuality, reproduction, and the use of contraception are regarded as causative factors in unwanted pregnancy, particularly among teenagers.[32] Ultimately, the causes of unintended pregnancy are as complex and as varied as the many women who become pregnant. Research that can capture the essence of the meaning of the pregnancy for the pregnant woman as she experiences it may reveal more causative reasons that have not been identified as yet. Community health nurses need to assess the social factors that promote unprotected intercourse by individual clients and by groups in society with an eye toward controlling the problem of unwanted pregnancy. Chapter 10, The Research Process, describes how such projects can be conducted.

Psychological and social environmental considerations also influence women's decisions to use contraceptives. Several of these factors are listed in Box 21–3. Psychological factors include personal tastes and preferences, perceptions of sexuality and sexual activity, and the attitudes of significant others, particularly the partner, toward contraception. Social factors influencing contraceptive decisions focus on career and economic considerations in the choice of when to have children, and one's cultural and religious attitudes toward sexuality and sexual activity. Other factors include one's value system and knowledge of sexuality and contraception, which are, in turn, influenced by one's educational level. Knowledge of these factors will enable the community health nurse to counsel each woman for a contraceptive method appropriate to her unique situation. An excellent resource for contraceptive information is *Contraceptive Technology, 1990–1991* (see the Recommended Readings at the end of this chapter).

BOX 21–3

Psychological and Social Factors in Decisions to Use Contraceptives

Psychological factors:
- Choice of when to have children
- Perceptions of sex and sexual activity
- Personal tastes and preferences
- Perceived risks and benefits of specific contraceptive methods

Social factors:
- Attitudes of significant others
- Culture
- Value system
- Educational level
- Religious beliefs
- Economic status
- Knowledge of sexuality and contraceptive methods

(Source: Hatcher, R., Stewart, F., Trussell, J., et al.[12]; Schober[46])

Life Goals

Self-actualization and the accomplishment of one's life goals are important considerations in assessing the effects of psychological and social environmental factors on women's health. In assessing the female client, the community health nurse should question the client about her life goals, her plans for achieving them, and factors that may interfere with their attainment. Life goals may include, but are not limited to, finishing one's education, getting married and having three children who grow up to be professionals, being the best high school math teacher, or enjoying a comfortable retirement.

Movement toward retirement as a life goal for middle-aged adult women may present a host of psychological factors that can affect health. Loss of productive work life may result in diminution of self-esteem and onset of depression. As women move toward retirement age, they may find themselves shunted to less challenging jobs, which may also contribute to lower feelings of self-worth. Community health nurses can help at this time by assisting women to plan for retirement and for activities to replace work as a foundation for self-esteem. To provide such assistance, the nurse will need to assess the woman's attitudes to work and retirement and the contribution that productive work makes to her self-esteem.

Social factors related to approaching retirement may affect the health status of the middle-aged adult woman. The woman who is nearing retirement needs to be aware of and plan for the financial shortfalls that are likely to occur with retirement. Leaving the work force means living in poverty for many older people, and women comprise 72 percent of all older poor.[4] Retirement assets are usually tied to lifetime income. Women who worked for low pay and poor benefits will neither have pensions nor full Social Security benefits. About 80 percent of retiring women are in this situation. Social Security retirement benefits are the only income for 60 percent of unmarried women over 65. Of people who receive minimum Social Security benefits, 85 percent to 90 percent are women.[4] A divorced woman may draw Social Security from her ex-husband's account if they were married at least 10 years.[34] The nurse will assess the woman's potential for retirement income and use such data to assist the woman to adjust her personal savings and investments to assure a more secure financial future.

Violence and Abuse

Abuse of women is the product of many psychological and social environmental factors, and it fosters a psychological environment detrimental to women's health. Psychological dependence on males and poor self-esteem on the part of both the victim and the abuser are some of the psychological causes at work. Feelings of shame and worthlessness may hamper the woman's ability to seek help while in an abusive situation.

The community health nurse also assesses clients for evidence of violence. Violence against women is a pervasive, under-recognized, and culturally condoned phenomenon in American society. Women, especially single women between the ages of 16 and 24, are more likely to be victims of violence than are women of other ages. Minority and poor women are more often victims of violence than white middle- and upper-class women. The most common acts of violence against women are rape, assault, robbery, incest, and sexual and physical abuse.[4] Current statistics show that 3 million to 4 million women are beaten each year by husbands, ex-husbands, boy friends, or lovers.[35,36] Assault and domestic violence are often directed against women just because they are women.[37]

Domestic violence such as wife abuse is rarely a one-time event. By the time injuries are identifiable as inflicted by a batterer, a woman may have been abused for several years.[38] If the woman does not ask for help or injuries are not discovered, battering usually increases in severity and frequency. Violence against women in its most deadly form is reflected in homicide statistics. In 1985, 30 percent of female homicide victims were killed by a husband or boy friend.[35,38]

Many causative factors have been postulated for domestic violence and abuse of women. Some are deeply rooted in cultural beliefs that have existed for centuries. Several underlying factors are reviewed here to demonstrate that wife abuse is not a new or simple problem.

Some of the oldest teachings on how wives should be treated are found among the writings of the world's religions, specifically Judaism, Christianity, and Islam. Many of these tenets support ***patriachy,*** a hierarchical arrangement of society and family in which the leader is always male. These religious beliefs support the inferiority of women, depicting them as the "private property of men."[39]

Until 1899, in the United States, men had the legal right to beat their wives in order to maintain their authority. Even with legislation to prevent wife abuse, domestic squabbles today are often viewed by police and courts as private matters, and intervention does not always occur.[35]

The socialization of female children also contributes to patterns of violence. Many females are raised to be dependent on males for approval, to be inferior and inadequate. They have been taught that they have little control over what happens in their lives. Males often are taught to be aggressive, domineering, and independent.[11] Where these conditions exist, the dichotomy between male and female socialization extends to form a sexist family structure where men dominate and women submit. Such an arrangement encourages husband-to-wife violence.[40]

Other factors contributing to violence against women include a sociocultural tolerance of family violence and violence against women that is sustained by the media; childhood experiences of abusive situations that serve as role models for future generations; and economic insecurity resulting in female dependence on men.[11] Social factors such as lack of equal access to employment, housing, and resources can trap women in an abusive situation that they might otherwise flee.

Economic insecurity has also been implicated as the basis for the increase of battering of pregnant women. The addition of another child may be perceived by the male as a further strain on a limited budget. Feelings of frustration and inadequacy cause the violence to escalate.[41]

The plight of abused women in the United States has improved somewhat in the last few years. The women's movement stimulated a national "battered women's movement" by the 1970s. Wife abuse and violence against women was identified as a social and political issue, not merely a private domestic concern.[35] Among the accomplishments of the battered women's movement was the passage of the Family Violence Prevention and Services Act of 1984 that earmarked federal funds for programs to protect women. Today there are over 1200 formal shelters, hotlines, and safe-home networks for victims of abuse throughout the country.

The movement continues to work for changes in the criminal justice system so abusers are punished and battered women gain the right to be protected. Where there are still law enforcement agencies that see domestic violence as a private matter and practice a policy of nonintervention, such attitudes are being increasingly challenged by studies that demonstrate that arrest is the best deterrent to repeated violence.[35]

Probably the most influential occurrence creating change in law enforcement attitudes toward wife abuse was a Connecticut class action suit that was brought against a police department for its failure to protect victims of domestic violence. This case resulted in a multimillion dollar payment to the victims.[35]

Suits, injunctions, and the use of lawyers to help protect victims against abuse cost money. Unfortunately, the legal system still does not offer much in the way of protection for low-income and minority women. In addition, many lawyers, judges, and

TABLE 21–5. MYTHS AND TRUTHS ABOUT ABUSED WOMAN

Myth	Truth
Battering occurs in a small percentage of the population.	An estimated 3 million to 4 million women are beaten annually. Battering often goes unreported.
Violence among family members is a private matter and it is a man's right to keep his woman in line.	Violence is not allowable in society. No one has the right to beat or rape a woman.
The abuse is not that bad or the woman would leave. It is easy to leave an abusive situation.	Home is not unbearable all the time. Home offers comfort, memories, and shelter for the children. Economic insecurity. Many women are economically dependent on the abuser and have nowhere to go. The woman's culture or religion may prohibit separation or divorce. The legal system may also make it hard to leave an abusive situation. Women may fear the loss of their children or further abuse if they leave. Women endure abuse to keep the family together for the sake of the children.
Women tend to become helpless in abusive situations.	Abused women come to believe that they are worthless and that they have no one to turn to but the abuser. Health-care workers perceive women as powerless and themselves as "rescuers."
Abused women are masochistic and enjoy being abused.	Abused women may feel that they deserve abuse, but they do not enjoy being abused.
Alcohol causes wife abuse.	Sober men do more damage than those who are drunk. Alcoholism is used as an excuse for abuse.
Battering is limited to minorities and the poor.	Abuse of women occurs in all socioeconomic and racial groups.
Women provoke men to beat or rape them.	Abusers and rapists lose control because of their own inadequacies, not because of the woman's behavior.
Batterers and abused women cannot change.	Batterers and abused women can be resocialized and can learn more effective ways to interact and relate to others.

(Source: Griffith-Kenney[43]; King & Ryan[38]; Diehm & Rose[35])

health professionals believe myths that have surrounded violence against women. Table 21–5 presents some of the myths and truths associated with abuse of women.

Community health nurses assessing female clients should be alert to evidence of physical or sexual abuse. Bruises, burns, fractures, or other injuries that are poorly explained or recurrent may suggest abuse. Since battered women are frequently afraid or ashamed to admit to being beaten, the nurse may need to suggest tactfully the possibility of battering as a cause for such injuries. Exploration of such areas will require an atmosphere of trust that is free of value judgments on the part of the nurse.

In assessing a potentially abused woman, the nurse will need to ask the client about depression, the possibility of suicide, and her risk of being killed by her partner.[38] Another important consideration is the woman's willingness to leave the situation. Many women in such situations continue to hope that their partner will change or are fearful that the partner will hunt them down and further injure them if they try to leave. Another common fear is that the partner will attempt to win custody of children if the woman leaves.

Abilities to Cope

The final area for consideration related to psychological and social environments and their effect on women's health is the client's ability to cope with life. This is influenced by a number of factors. Learned coping skills are an important facet of the client's psychological makeup that the nurse will want to assess. How does the client normally handle adversity? What factors in the environment strengthen her ability to cope?

Here the nurse would explore the strength of the client's social support network. Does the client have family or friends on whom she can call for material or emotional assistance? Is the client plugged into the social services network to receive support as needed? Is the client even aware of the existence of such a network and its operation?

Another area for consideration is economic factors that may affect the client's ability to cope. What is the client's financial status? What is the source of her income? Is it sufficient to meet her needs? Income is frequently based on educational level, so information about the client's education will assist the nurse to identify potential problem areas in coping skills.

LIFE-STYLE

Life-style factors also affect the health of women clients. Areas of particular concern include consumption patterns, occupation, sexual life-style, and attendant concerns with fertility control.

Consumption Patterns

The nurse assesses consumption patterns of the female client in the same terms as assessing any client. Specific areas for consideration include diet, smoking, and substance abuse. Dietary concerns may be particularly problematic among women, many of whom are obese or overweight or who engage in fad diets to obtain or maintain a fashionably slim figure. Fad dieting is especially prevalent among adolescent females who also have high incidence rates for eating disorders such as bulimia and anorexia nervosa.

Smoking is another consumption pattern that is problematic for women. While the number of male smokers has declined rather dramatically in the last few years, the number of women who smoke has increased, leading to corresponding increases in lung cancer and heart disease among women. The nurse assessing the female client would obtain data about smoking including the number of years the client has smoked as well as the number of cigarettes or other forms of tobacco smoked per day. Motivation to quit smoking should also be explored as part of the assessment.

Substance abuse among women is the third area of concern related to consumption patterns. While women still tend to abuse alcohol and drugs less often than men, the incidence of such problems among females is increasing. Problems of drug and alcohol abuse are addressed in Chapter 33, Substance Abuse.

Occupation

Occupation is another life-style factor that has profound effects on the health of many women. Most women in the paid labor force continue to work in traditional "women's jobs" such as nursing, teaching, the garment industry, and secretarial/clerical and service jobs. While considered "women's work," these jobs are not without health risks. Physical risks arise from chemicals, radiation, infectious disease, noise, vibration, and repetitive movements.

As more women enter the world of "men's work" such as heavy industry, construction, mining, and factory work, they face a different set of physical hazards. Health risks arise from heavy lifting, use of dangerous machinery, and tools that were designed for larger men rather than smaller women.[6] Minority women are at higher risk than white women for job-related injury because they often take jobs that others will not. Their economic need prevents them from saying no or quitting.

High-tech employment, once touted as safe, also entails health risks. The scrupulously clean area needed to produce a computer chip or to work with computers contains threats to human reproduction posed by radio-frequency or microwave radiation, video display terminal radiation, arsine, and chlorine gases.[42] Some of the physical hazards encountered by women in the work setting are presented in Table 21–6. Working women today face essentially the same physical hazards as working men. They have the same risks for reproductive failure, respiratory ailments, skin disorders, and cancer.[6] The health risks of the work setting will be discussed in more detail in Chapter 27, Care of Clients in the Work Setting.

The psychological environment of the workplace can be as detrimental to women's health as its physical hazards. For instance, studies have shown that it is not the female administrator who suffers the most from stress and depression, but women in the more traditional positions of secretary and clerk. It is postulated that stress is intensified by the lack of freedom to control one's work that secretaries and clerks experience. The "dead end" quality of these jobs with little possibility of advancement may decrease incen-

TABLE 21–6. PHYSICAL HAZARDS BY TYPE OF OCCUPATION

Type of Occupation	Hazards
Clothing, laundry, and textile work	Chemicals, dyes, solvents, synthetic and cotton dust and fiber, bleaches, heat, contamination from dirty clothing
Hospital workers, nurses, laboratory assistants, X-ray technicians	Infection, lifting and falls, radiation, chemical hazards
Service work, waitress, airline stewardess	Noise, lifting, falls
Teachers and child-care workers	Respiratory infections, viruses, influenza, noise
Clerical and secretarial work	Chemicals from copy and correction fluid, noise, poor lighting and chair design, sedentary work, repetitive-use syndrome

(Source: Albino & Tedesco[6]; Davis, Marbury, Punnett, et al.[44])

tive. In addition, the low salaries available for secretaries and clerks add stresses related to financial insecurity.[30]

Social factors in the work environment also affect women's health. The world of work for women differs from that of men in several ways. First, more jobs are open to men than to women. In addition, those jobs that are open to women often provide unequal pay and levels of benefits compared to men in similar jobs. Finally, until a 1991 Supreme Court ruling, women were more often barred from work based on reproductive capacities than were men. Childbearing has also been blamed for women's late entry into the work force and women's lack of training and education.[6]

Once having gained entry into the workplace, women frequently continue to have primary responsibility for maintaining the household and caring for children. This role proliferation adds tremendous stress to a woman's life and often leads to feelings of frustration, inadequacy, anxiety, and depression.[43] In addition, family responsibilities tend to lower a woman's market value as an employee.[4]

There are no uniform policies for paid maternity leave for women[4] despite federal mandates for a minimum of 4 months (unpaid) leave for childbirth. Consequently, when a woman must have time off from work because of pregnancy, she must often take it without pay.

Child care is another social environmental factor that creates problems for the working woman. Employer or community assistance with child care is practically nonexistent. Invariably, women must find quality child care on their own. If children are sick, it is usually the mother who stays home, often without pay, to care for them.[4,6]

Disproportionate pay between traditional women's jobs and such "men's work" as road construction is a strong incentive for women to seek such jobs.[42] Women who enter male-dominated jobs often feel pressure to prove they are equal to men in ability. They may not speak out against safety hazards because they do not want to appear weak or "unable to take it."[44] Sexual harassment is another problem that may be encountered by women in the work setting. Although there are laws prohibiting such abuse, women may not complain because they need work so badly.

It is important to note that minority women must contend with a higher degree of discrimination and lack of job opportunity than white women. They are particularly subject to dead-end jobs and hazardous jobs with low pay and few benefits.[4,44] Minority women are less likely to finish high school, more likely to become head of a single-parent household, and more likely to have job-related illnesses than their white counterparts.

It would seem that the increased number of stressors in the lives of working women would cause increased incidence of diseases such as peptic ulcer or coronary artery disease. Studies in this area, however, suggest that there is no difference in stress-related disease rates for women who work in the home and those who work outside the home.[4,6,43] Illness is more closely associated with multiple roles and family stressors than with the workplace. In addition, it seems that being a housewife is just as stressful as working outside the home.

Sexual Life-style and Fertility Control

Assessment of the female client's sexual life-style may provide information related to potential health problems. For example, clients who are not sexually active and those who engage in homosexual activity have no need for contraceptive assistance, while the heterosexually active client who is not ready to have children may need such services. Information about the client's sexual activity may also suggest what form of contraception is most appropriate for those clients who do not wish to become pregnant. For example, the client with multiple sexual partners may prefer to use a barrier method of contraception rather than birth control pills to provide protection against sexually transmitted diseases as well as pregnancy.

Every woman from menarche to menopause has a right and responsibility to choose a method of fertility control that is effective, safe, and compatible with her life-style. The right to information on contraception and access to birth control agents are mandated by Title X of the Public Health Services Act and Titles V, XIV, and XX of the Social Security Act.[18] The decision to use contraceptives reflects personal feelings about sexuality, one's self-concept, sense of autonomy and control, one's value system, the relationship with the significant other, and the personal, social and political power of women.[32,45,46]

The ideal contraceptive method would be absolutely safe, 100 percent effective, easy to use, immediately reversible, free, and readily accessible to all. It would be acceptable to all religious and social groups and its use would be independent of coitus.[45–47] No single method available today meets all these criteria. In addition, there is no single method today that will meet the needs of an individual woman throughout her fertile years. The nurse should assess the need for contraception and biological and other factors that influence the need for contraceptive services. Information about various forms of contraception available to clients is presented in Table 21–7.

TABLE 21–7. TYPES OF CONTRACEPTION AND RELATED CONTRACEPTIVE METHODS

Type of Contraception	Related Contraceptive Methods
Abstinence	Abstinence from sexual intercourse
Barriers	Condom, diaphragm, cervical sponge, cervical cap
Fertility awareness	Basal body temperature, cervical mucus changes, position of cervix
Hormonal	Oral contraceptives, Norplant Progestosert (IUD) injections, postcoital contraception
Intrauterine device	Copper T, Progestosert, Paragard
Sterilization	Tubal ligation (female), vasectomy (male)

HEALTH SYSTEM

Lack of attention to women's health needs, lack of illness-prevention and health-promotion resources, health insurance discrimination, and lack of support for the informal care-giver in the home are health-care system issues that adversely affect women.

As noted earlier, the medical system tends to focus on female reproductive problems, frequently to the exclusion of other health problems faced by women. Failure to recognize and deal with physical abuse is just one example of failure of the health-care system to meet the needs of women. By and large, the health-care system has only recently come to recognize the special health needs of the female client.

Services provided by the health-care system tend to focus on secondary and tertiary prevention of injury and disease. Few efforts are made to provide preventive health care, particularly for women. On a more personal level, those preventive health services that are available are not always offered at a time when busy working women can take advantage of them. Compounding this problem is the lack of provision for child care while women seek preventive health-care services.

Another handicap for women is the cost of health care. Women are less likely than men to have health insurance, and they are more likely to work in part-time jobs or jobs that do not offer this benefit. Many insurance companies will not insure single women because of the likelihood of pregnancy and the more frequent occurrence of diagnosed disease among women than among men. Single women are also less likely to be able to pay the monthly insurance premiums. This situation is particularly hard on divorced and separated women with children who are already faced with financial deficits.[4,48] For information on economic assistance from Medicaid refer to Chapter 13, Economic Influences on Community Health.

Another problem for working women attributable to the health-care system is the lack of support for the informal care-giver. Women may be forced to quit their jobs to care for a sick child or elderly family member but cannot expect the financial support that might be available for institution-based care of the loved one.[4]

The health-care system has provided some services to deal with health problems posed by menopause. These have consisted primarily of hormone supplementation. Lately, however, there has been some controversy over the role of hormone replacement in endometrial cancer. At present, many health-care providers, weighing the risks of osteoporosis and fractures that are prevented by hormone replacement against the risks of endometrial cancer, feel that the benefits of replacement therapy outweigh the risks.[49] Considerations in assessing health system influences on the health of women are summarized in Table 21–8. A guide for assessing factors unique to the health status of women is included in Appendix K, Health Assessment Guide—Adult Female.

SPECIAL FOCUS: ASSESSING THE LESBIAN CLIENT

Lesbians are a segment of the female population with whom the community health nurse will knowingly or unknowingly come in contact. According to a study by Kinsey in 1953, an estimated 10 percent of the general population is homosexual. This means that there may be upwards of 10 million gay women in the United States. Lesbians have specific health-care needs that nurses can be sensitive to and assist with. For this section, the terms "lesbians," "gay women," and "homosexual women" will be used to indicate women whose preferred sexual partner is another woman. The term "straight" will be used to refer to women who prefer heterosexual intimacy.

The American Psychiatric Association recognizes that homosexuality is neither a choice nor a psychiatric disorder; it is a normal variant and an inherent part of a person's identity.[50] Sexual orientation is not chosen; it is discovered.[51] Being a lesbian means that a woman's primary affectional and sexual preferences are for other women. Lesbians exist in all cultures, races, religions, and classes. They cannot be identified by appearance, assumed role, or mannerisms.[52] Lesbians are at high risk for misunderstanding and discrimination because they share the homosexual label with men, yet they have much in common with heterosexual women.

In examining lesbianism from Dever's epidemiologic perspective, the goal is for the nurse to become better able to meet the lesbian client's needs by gain-

TABLE 21–8. ASSESSING HEALTH SYSTEM INFLUENCES ON WOMEN'S HEALTH

Health Concern	Related Assessment Questions
Need for secondary prevention—screening	• Have you ever had a Pap smear? When? What were the results? • Have you ever had a mammogram? When? What were the results? • When was your last eye examination? What were the results? • Have you had an ECG? When? What were the results? • Have you had a TB skin test? When? What were the results? • Have you had a breast examination? When? What were the results? • Have you had any recent blood tests? What were they for? What were the results?
Need for respite	• Is there anyone who can relieve you so you can have a break from caring for your children (elderly parents)?
Access to health care	• Do you have health insurance? • If yes, do you know what services are covered? • Where do you usually go for health care? • How do you usually pay for health care? • Are health-care services provided at a time that is convenient for you? • Do you have transportation to receive health-care services? • Are child-care services available while you seek health care? • Are there any barriers that prevent you from getting the health care you need? If so, what are they?

ing greater understanding and insight into the similarities and differences between lesbians and the heterosexual population. Using this knowledge, the nurse will then be able to formulate a more sensitive and effective plan of care for the client.

HUMAN BIOLOGY

There are no differences in the maturational or aging processes between homosexual and heterosexual women. While it is sometimes assumed that the needs of lesbians are similar to those of gay men, their needs are actually quite different.[51] There have been no medical problems identified that are specifically attributable to being a lesbian,[53] but there are some differences in morbidity between gay and heterosexual women that need to be addressed.

From a gynecologic viewpoint, the woman who engages in sexual activity exclusively with other women is at significantly lower risk for sexually transmitted diseases, including gonorrhea, syphilis, herpes, or AIDS, than her heterosexual counterpart.[51,53–55] Pelvic inflammatory disease is highly unlikely. A lesbian will rarely need treatment for genital trauma, and she may have a lower incidence of sexual dysfunction than her heterosexual counterpart.[55] While the mode of transmission for monilial or nonspecific vaginitis infections is not necessarily sexual, the lesbian is less likely to develop such an infection.[53] Because 50 percent to 70 percent of all lesbians remain childless, they are at above-average risk for developing mammary and endometrial cancer.[55]

There is little research available on women's diseases, and even less specific information on the risks of transmission of diseases between lesbian partners. One study of sexually transmitted disease in lesbians determined that gay women who had been sexually active exclusively with other women did not contract gonorrhea, herpes, or chlamydia. It is conceivable that a herpes virus-shedding lesion on the lips or genitals of a lesbian could cause the herpes infection to occur in her lesbian lover. There has also been one report that hepatitis B had been transmitted from a nurse to her lesbian lover. The incidence of all of these diseases rises sharply if the lesbian has had recent heterosexual contact.

Should the lesbian client develop symptoms of disease, it is important for the nurse to obtain a medical history pertinent to those symptoms. If the symptoms indicate a possible sexually transmitted disease, then information about any recent heterosexual contacts should be elicited. Treatment is diagnosis-dependent and identical to that for heterosexual women; when an infection occurs, the woman should be counseled to stop activities that are uncomfortable until the infection is treated.

Routine Pap smears are as important for the lesbian client as for heterosexual women. Studies have shown that lesbians have cervical dysplasia and carcinoma in situ. The incidence of these cervical disorders rises sharply if the lesbian has had several heterosexual lovers, just as for her heterosexual counterpart. The screening interval for Pap smears should be determined on an individual basis depending on risk factors. Most lesbians need a Pap smear at least annually.[53,55]

ENVIRONMENT

The environmental issues of concern are the social and psychological environments that the lesbian deals with on a daily basis. A woman cannot be a lesbian without problems.[56] The discrepancy between socially prescribed behaviors and homosexual needs automatically sets up a conflict between the lesbian and her environment. Society tends to react to lesbianism almost exclusively as a sexual behavior and not as a sociocultural identity.[57] Thus, lesbians are identified in unidimensional terms. ***Homophobia,*** an irrational fear, hatred, or intolerance of homosexuals, encompasses a belief system that justifies discrimination against gays. The routine conflict with the environment, coupled with homophobia, and religious, legal, familial, and economic constraints, all combine to make life more difficult for the homosexual woman.

Social Environment

From a religious perspective, most Christian denominations advocate sexual activity only in the context of procreation. Most—especially fundamentalist denominations—consider homosexuality biologically unnatural, sinful, and condemned by the Bible. Homosexual feelings, no matter how weak, are undesirable. Many religious organizations are active socially and politically against homosexuals and gay rights groups. Consequently, the community health nurse should explore with the lesbian client any guilt feelings or feelings of abandonment she may be experiencing as a result of attitudes and values of the religious denomination to which she may belong.

Homosexuals are denied legal sanction for their pairings and are often discriminated against in housing, employment, or social services.[57] They are denied the right to serve in the military or to be named as beneficiaries of some insurance policies. Oftentimes homosexuals are denied the right to make or to have input into medical decisions for their incapacitated partner because they are not "blood relatives." In the event of the death of a partner who has left no will, lesbians have no rights to inheritance. The community health nurse can assess for any legal problems the couple may be having and determine whether some legal counseling may be needed.

Many women realize and act upon their same-sex preferences after they are married and have children. Their fitness as mothers is often questioned in the courts if their sexual preference becomes known. Because of the threat of custody battles and the inherent difficulties of adoption, many lesbian couples are opting to have their own children, either by artificial insemination or through the participation of a gay or straight male partner. This decision must involve careful planning and negotiation on the part of the lesbian (and possibly her partner) to ensure acceptance by the biological family, the health-care provider, and both gay and nongay society.[58] A guideline for the community health nurse to use in assessing the lesbian couple's adaptation to parenting can be found in Table 21–9.

TABLE 21–9. ASSESSING THE ADAPTATION OF LESBIAN COUPLES TO PARENTHOOD

Adaptive Task	Assessment Questions
Acceptance of pregnancy	• What is the response of the partner to the pregnancy? • What is the response of the couple's families, social network, and support system to the pregnancy? • What is the legal relationship of the biological father to the baby? • Does the partner plan a long-term legal or social relationship as a co-parent (for example, through adoption)?
Binding-in	• How was the pregnancy achieved? • Did the partner have a role in the pregnancy? • Are the characteristics of the biological father known, if donor insemination was used? • Has the couple expressed a sex preference for the baby? If yes, do they agree? • How will the couple's support system view the sex of the baby? • What are the couple's views of the baby? Are they congruent?
Safe passage	• If donor's sperm was used to achieve pregnancy, what health screening criteria were used to select donor sperm (for example, was the donor screened for HIV infection)? • Does the couple plan to use natural childbirth methods during delivery? Will the partner serve as the pregnant woman's coach? • Will the couple feel comfortable acknowledging their relationship to prospective birth attendants?
Self-giving	• What do the couple perceive as the costs and benefits (emotional, legal, economic, and social) of having this baby? • How do the couple replenish each other's emotional reserves?
Maternal role development	• How will the tasks of the maternal role be allocated? • Who are the couple's role models for the maternal role? Are these role models adequate? • Will the couple have assistance in developing the facets of the maternal role? From whom? • Will the child call one of the partners "mother"? Which one?
Co-parent role development	• How is the pregnancy affecting the couple's relationship? • What will the child call the co-parent?

(Adapted from Wismont, J., & Reame, N.[58])

Other social issues facing the lesbian client are the lack of social outlets or places other than bars to meet other gay women, particularly outside of large metropolitan areas. This can be a contributing factor in substance abuse and poor self-esteem.[59] Economically, like women generally, lesbians usually earn lower wages than their male counterparts. Those with children from a prior marriage have particularly little disposable income or time to engage in social activities. Also, because homosexuality is such a taboo subject, women in general are socialized to have a negative view of homosexuality and there are few visible role models to refute that view. Many lesbians, consequently, begin with a very negative self-image that they must strive to change.

Psychological Environment

Psychological factors affecting lesbians are closely entwined with social factors. A woman who realizes that she has a same-sex orientation has three basic choices. She can live openly as a lesbian, thereby setting herself up for potential rejection by her family, loss of her job or professional reputation, and societal labeling and abuse. The second choice is to deny her identity and put her energy into fulfilling the accepted female role. Third, she can live a lesbian life but maintain a heterosexual appearance.

The lesbian who does not live openly as a lesbian must deal, on a daily basis, with the fear that someone will discover who she really is. This involves the complex task of vigilance about how she looks and acts, where she is, who she is with, and what she says. This task has no parallel and is not duplicated in the experience of the nonlesbian woman.[60] This means that the lesbian must constantly monitor her responses and change pronouns to misrepresent the identity of her partners. She must hide from co-workers, family, or friends important life events such as new relationships or the breakup of old ones.[56,61]

An important emotional event the lesbian goes through is the "coming out" experience. A lifelong process, coming out can be roughly defined as a woman's realization and admission to herself and to others of her same-sex orientation. While the process of coming out usually occurs in the tumultuous years of the late teens and early 20s, it can happen at any phase in the lesbian's life. Coming out usually (but not always) includes stages of denial, decreased self-esteem, learning, growth, and, eventually for some, self-acceptance.[62] Once the initial coming out is accomplished, the question of how open to be with others becomes a constant underlying source of pressure or tension.[63]

How does a woman discover her sexual orientation? She can begin having vague feelings that she is somehow different from others as early as age 4 or 5.[59] The feelings turn into suspicions during the teen years. At this point, 80 percent of women with lesbian feelings will begin to date, have heterosexual experiences, and try to pass as "straight." Fifteen percent to 35 percent will marry and will have children. Two-thirds of those marriages eventually end in divorce as the woman begins acknowledging her sexual orientation.[56] After a woman "comes out," homosexual behavior becomes predominant, and the lesbian typically begins to search for a supportive community.[64]

The coming-out process deals also with the contradictory feelings of excitement and relief at having found an inner answer to guilt, sadness, and anger about what the lesbian is losing or giving up.[56] She must come to terms with any guilt she experiences for being different and for not fulfilling her role in the heterosexual life-style to which she has been socialized. She may also mourn the loss of her relationship with a husband or male lover, the fact that she will not fulfill parental expectations of a wedding and grandchildren, and that she will never be totally socially acceptable. Additionally, it has been found that many women go through the coming-out process without the influence or support of the lesbian subculture, thereby adding isolation to the difficulty of the task.[56] The community health nurse should assess for feelings of guilt or depression among lesbians who have recently declared their preference.

From a mental health perspective, while mental health is of concern among lesbians, they are no more likely to be diagnosed with psychiatric disorders than heterosexual women.[52] Their level of social and psychological functioning is indistinguishable from that of their heterosexual counterparts. The community health nurse must be aware, however, of the medical and psychological implications of the emotional stresses that arise from the moral and social stigma of being lesbian. As a result of these stresses, lesbians are more likely to abuse substances such as alcohol and nonprescription drugs than heterosexual women.[55] As many as one in four lesbians has attempted suicide at least once for reasons of fear or social discrimination, lack of self-acceptance, or conflicts with partners.[56]

LIFE-STYLE

Consumption Patterns

Lesbianism does not cause alcohol or substance abuse, but there does seem to be a relationship between the two. Although empirical research that adequately assesses factors accounting for the increased incidence of alcoholism among lesbians is almost nonexistent,[57] data from the late 1960s found that lesbian women are five to seven times more likely to use alcohol excessively, to be alcoholics, or to become dependent upon nonprescription drugs than are heterosexual women.[65]

There have been several theories advanced to explain this phenomenon. Some researchers speculate that because lesbians live under conditions of increased stress and limited social alternatives, they are more vulnerable to the use of alcohol as a coping mechanism.[57] The use of alcohol (or other drugs) could be construed as an attempt to alleviate emotional pain and bolster self-esteem.

The nurse can assist the lesbian client by being alert to cues that would indicate patterns of substance abuse, by not assuming that the alcoholism is related to sexual preference, by respecting the woman's reluctance to enter a traditional treatment program, by being familiar with gay resources in the community, and by involving the significant other in the treatment plan.[55,57]

Occupation

For the majority of lesbians, disclosure of sexual preference in the work setting could lead to being passed over for promotion, subtle or overt harassment, or termination, particularly if they work with children or young women. As was mentioned under psychological factors, the ever-present fear of discovery adds immeasurable anxiety and tension to the inherent stress of work.

In spite of this, the economic and occupational achievements of lesbians are similar to those of their heterosexual counterparts. While they exhibit more job instability, lesbians earn the same level of income and work productively, and many tend to be high achievers. They often display a greater degree of assertiveness and aggressiveness in their jobs.[64] One study found that a higher concentration of lesbians had some college education, and that 50 percent to 60 percent were in semiprofessional or managerial positions, a statistic that is higher for lesbians than for women in general.[51]

HEALTH SYSTEM

The basic difference in the way the lesbian interacts with the health-care system centers around the issues of acceptance and confidentiality. When the lesbian client senses discomfort or disapproval on the part of the health-care provider, she is more likely to hide her sexual orientation for fear of receiving judgmental, nonsupportive, or suboptimal care. Such repercussions might include treatment that is nonresponsive or callous; the woman may find that her partner is either not allowed to visit (because she is not blood kin) or harassed or that the partner is not allowed input into treatment decisions.

Potential repercussions of loss of confidentiality also arises when sexual orientation is revealed to health-care providers. As noted earlier, disclosure could negatively affect the client's status at her place of employment, with her family, or with the remainder of the health-care team if she was not previously "out" to those persons. A phenomenon that is seen among lesbians as a result of their lack of trust in the conventional medical system is that substantial numbers are more holistic in their approach to health, choosing alternative forms of health care.[53]

Most lesbians believe that their care providers are not well-versed on lesbian health-care issues, and many are put off by questions about marital status, birth control, and sexual activity. Such issues put the woman in the constant position of having to decide whether to withhold information about her sexuality or to be honest.[55] Yet there is no routine or comfortable way for the client to reveal her lesbianism.[60] Consequently, the lesbian may be subjected to unwarranted lectures on birth control, prescriptions for contraceptives, and treatment for sexually transmitted diseases, or may be denied the support of her partner when she needs her the most.

There are several suggestions that could be of value to community health nurses assessing lesbian clients. First, nurses need to examine their own attitudes toward sexuality and homosexuality. Although it is not necessary to sanction homosexual behavior, it is not ethical to discriminate against or deny the gay client supportive professional care that will assist in strengthening her self-esteem and realizing optimal wellness. As one observer has noted, "passing moral judgments is not a nursing function: such judgments can only impede the ability to give quality care."[66] If the nurse is unable to provide such care, the client should be referred to another provider.

Further suggestions are not to record a client's sexual preference on the record without her approval,[53] to provide an atmosphere of openness and tolerance, and—of the utmost importance—involve the partner or designated other in the plan of care.

Another peculiar problem arises when the practitioner automatically assumes the client is heterosexual. Assessment questions can be less alienating if differently phrased. Non-sex-typed pronouns such as "lover" and "partner" can be used. Questions such as "Are you sexually active?" and "Do you use contraceptives?" are more appropriate than "When was the last time you had intercourse?" or "What kind of birth control are you using?" A question such as

"Who would you like contacted in an emergency?" can also go a long way toward helping the lesbian client feel more comfortable.

A lesbian client is more likely to be satisfied with her care if she is able to safely disclose her sexual orientation to health-care providers.[67] Additionally, studies show that while most lesbians are more comfortable with female health-care providers,[60] it is more important to have a caring, knowledgeable, non-judgmental provider, regardless of sex or sexual preference.[55]

DIAGNOSTIC REASONING AND CARE OF WOMEN

Based on information obtained during client assessment, the nurse develops nursing diagnoses that direct further interventions. These diagnoses reflect both positive health states and potential or existing health problems and the factors contributing to them. Nursing diagnoses might relate to health problems experienced by an individual woman such as "role overload due to employment, single parenthood, and lack of a social support network." Or diagnoses may be made at the aggregate level regarding the health needs of groups of women. An example of a nursing diagnosis at this level might be a "need for adequate and inexpensive child care due to the number of single-parent working women and a lack of affordable child-care." Box 21–4 presents some nursing diagnostic statements for women, both individual and aggregate.

BOX 21–4

Sample Nursing Diagnoses for Individual Female Clients and Female Aggregates

Individual client:

- Strong social support system owing to close relationship with parents and siblings.
- Lack of knowledge of menarche in adolescent attributable to mother's discomfort with discussing sexuality.
- Hot flashes and menstrual irregularity due to menopause.
- Guilt over inability to conceive.
- Potential for HIV infection stemming from IV drug use.
- Potential for repetitive-use syndrome due to assembly-line job.

Aggregates:

- Potential for assault due to lack of safe transportation from factory to home for female workers.
- Inadequate access to health-care owing to lack of health services after working hours.
- Potential for occupational injury in construction industry attributable to lack of safety equipment scaled to women's smaller stature.
- Potential for unwanted pregnancy stemming from lack of contraceptive counseling for women of childbearing age.

PLANNING AND IMPLEMENTING HEALTH CARE FOR WOMEN

In planning to meet the identified health needs of female clients, the community health nurse incorporates the general principles of planning discussed in Chapter 5, The Nursing Process. It is important to keep in mind the unique needs of the female client. Participation by the client in planning for health care is particularly important in view of the passive and dependent role expected of the female client by health-care providers of the past. Women need to be encouraged to be active participants in health-care decision making. Both community health nurses and their female clients may need additional resources in dealing with the woman's identified health-care needs. Several sources of assistance with specific kinds of problems are presented in Table 21–10.

Planning and implementing plans of care for groups of women also needs to be based on considerations of women's unique circumstances. Services should be offered at times when women, especially working women, can take advantage of them. Provision for transportation and child-care services during appointments might also need to be considered. Financing of such programs can also be problematic, given the lower earning capacity of many women, and political activity to ensure program funding may need to be part of the planning process. Planning to

TABLE 21–10. RESOURCES FOR NURSES AND THEIR FEMALE CLIENTS

Focus	Agency or Organization	Services
AIDS	Mothers of AIDS Patients (MAP) 3403 E. Street San Diego, CA 92101 (619) 234-3432	Support group formation, information
Childbirth	American Society for Psychoprophylaxis in Obstetrics 1840 Wilshire Blvd., Suite 204 Arlington, VA 22201	Information
	Childbirth Education Foundation P.O. Box 5 Richboro, PA 18954 (215) 357-2792	Public information
	Childbirth Without Pain Education Association 20134 Snowden Detroit, MI 48235 (313) 341-3816	Public information
Fertility and fertility control	American Academy of Natural Family Planning 615 S. New Ballas Rd. St. Louis, MO 63141 (314) 569-6495	Public information
	American Fertility Society 2131 Magnolia Ave., Suite 201 Birmingham, AL 35256 (205) 251-9764	Referral for fertility services, information, research
	Association for Voluntary Surgical Contraception 122 E. 42nd St. New York, NY 10168 (212) 573-8350	Information, research
	Barren Foundation 4100 N. Marine Dr. Chicago, IL 60613 (312) 281-2826	Research, information, support group for infertile couples
	International Planned Parenthood Foundation 18–20 Lower Regent St. London SW1Y 4PW England	Research, education about family planning, sex education
Sexuality	Council for Sex Information and Education Box 72 Capitola, CA 95010	Information on sexuality
	Daughters of Bilitis 1209 Sutter St. San Francisco, CA 94109	Social advocacy for lesbians, public information
	Dignity-National 755 Boylston Boston, MA 02116	Counseling and support for Roman Catholic homosexuals
	Dykes and Tykes New York Chapter Box 621 Old Chelsea Station New York, NY 10011	Social and legal help for homosexuals and their children
	Gaia's Guide 115 New Montgomery St. San Francisco, CA 94105	Provides a nationwide listing of local resources for lesbians
	Gay Activist Alliances New York Chapter 399 Lafayette St. New York, NY 10011	Classes, public information, legal help

TABLE 21–10. (*Continued*)

Focus	Agency or Organization	Services
Sexuality (*continued*)	Integrity/San Francisco P.O. Box 6444 San Francisco, CA 94150 (408) 268-3378	Counseling and support for Episcopalian homosexuals
	Metropolitan Community Church Box 1757 New York, NY 10011 (212) 691-7428	Social support, counseling, advocacy for Christian homosexuals
	National Gay Task Force 80 Fifth Avenue New York, NY 10011 (212) 741-1010	Civil rights advocacy for homosexuals
	Sex Information and Education Council of United States 80 Fifth Avenue, Suite 801 New York, NY 10011 (212) 929-2300	Public information, education on sexuality
Violence and abuse	Batterers Anonymous 1269 North E. Street San Bernardino, CA 92405 (714) 355-1100	Self-help group for male abusers
	Emerge 18 Hurley Street, Suite 23 Cambridge, MA 02141 (617) 547-9870	Counseling for men to prevent abuse of women
	Feminist Alliance Against Rape P.O. Box 21033 Washington, DC 20009 (202) 686-9463	Education about rape, self-defense
	National Coalition Against Domestic Violence P.O. Box 34103 Washington, DC 20043-4103 (202) 638-6388 (800) 333-SAFE (7233)	Hotline, safe haven information
	Rape Crisis Center P.O. Box 21005 Washington, DC 20009	Information on crisis intervention for victims of rape

meet the health needs of women clients may involve developing primary, secondary, or tertiary preventive interventions.

PRIMARY PREVENTION

Primary preventive measures for the female client generally include health education, health appraisal, modifying risk factors, providing a healthy environment, and developing adequate coping skills. Specific needs of female clients include preparation for menarche, sexuality education, fertility control, and prenatal care. Other primary preventive measures for women include preparation for menopause, facilitating access to care, primary prevention in the work setting, preventing STDs, and developing coping skills and assertiveness.

Preparation for Menarche

Traditionally, the health-care system has not been concerned with menarche unless there is pathology involved. Many potential problems can be avoided, however, with preventive care. For instance, negative feelings toward menstruation, premenstrual tension, emotional lability, the tendency to overeat just before menses, and water weight gain are all controllable with diet, rest, and exercise.

Preventing problems surrounding menarche and menstruation is an important consideration for community health nurses working with preteens and teenagers. The community health nurse can provide direct care, counseling, and teaching in a school-based clinic, in the home, or through community health agencies that offer guidance and information at this time.

Nurses can teach parents to explain menstruation to their daughters or may provide the explanation themselves if parents are unwilling or uncomfortable in doing so. Nurses can also assist girls in the practical aspects of menstruation; for example, how to use tampons or sanitary napkins, the potential dangers inherent in tampon use, and effective hygiene. They can also provide opportunities for girls to discuss fears and anxieties related to this physiologic change. Instruction on dealing with premenstrual tension or menstrual cramps may also be needed.

Sexuality Education

The community health nurse can provide anticipatory guidance, teaching, and counseling concerning sexuality for adolescent and preadolescent girls. Such issues as giving up one's virginity, romantic love and sex, pregnancy, and contraception can be discussed in a nonthreatening atmosphere that may serve to increase self-confidence and dispel myths related to sexuality. In addition, the nurse may prepare the teen for her first pelvic examination, explaining the procedure in terms that will decrease fear and embarrassment. These actions require that nurses be comfortable with their own sexuality and that they be adequately informed about sexual issues.

Community health nurses may also need to educate older women about sexuality and assist them in the formation of healthy sexual identities. This frequently involves correcting past misinformation. Women may also need assistance with sexuality issues during pregnancy. Changes in libido can be discussed and practical suggestions for more comfortable sex as the pregnancy progresses may be helpful. Nurses can also function as advocates for older clients who are attempting to meet their sexual needs, while reassuring them that sexual activity by older persons is a normal phenomenon.

Advocacy and reassurance may also be required by the lesbian client. Community health nurses may need to take an active role in societal changes that protect the rights of lesbian women and assure their freedom of choice in their sexual life-style. Advocacy for these clients is particularly needed in the realm of health-care services. Lesbian clients may need support and reassurance in the process of "coming out." This is particularly true of the adolescent homosexual who is doubly confused and anxious in the process of developing a sexual identity.

Fertility Control

Primary prevention related to fertility control usually involves contraceptive education and referral for contraceptive services. In the case of a nurse practitioner, the community health nurse may also provide the physical examination and dispense various contraceptive methods.

The nurse and client together will select the type of contraceptive best suited to meet the client's needs based on her sexual life-style. It is important to remember that some clients neither want nor need contraceptives. The client may wish to become pregnant. Even if this does not seem to be a wise decision to the nurse in light of client circumstances, it *is* the client's decision. Lesbian clients also have no need of contraceptives. However, they are frequently badgered by health-care professionals regarding contraception to the point that they are forced to reveal their sexual preferrence at the risk of disapproval and discrimination on the part of the health-care provider.

Prenatal Care

Community health nurses are frequently actively involved in the provision of prenatal care to pregnant women. Initial activity frequently involves case finding and referral to a source of care. Nurses may also be involved in monitoring the status of the client during and after the pregnancy and, in the case of the nurse midwife, may actually deliver the baby.

Counseling at the point of recognition of the pregnancy should include the options available to the woman including termination of the pregnancy, adoption, or keeping the child. Women may choose different options depending upon their age, marital status, and life-goals. The community health nurse should be prepared to support the client's decision regardless of the option chosen and the nurse's personal value system.

Direct care in the form of prenatal teaching and physical care during the pregnancy are other avenues of primary prevention. The goal of care is a healthy infant and mother. Therefore, instruction in the areas of life-style such as nutrition, rest and exercise, avoidance of teratogens, and so on, is important. Careful assessment for signs of impending complications is also essential.

Home visits to the pregnant women can be used to assess environmental conditions and their suitability for mother and infant. What provisions have been made for the child? Will the birth of the child present an economic strain on the mother and family? How involved is the father of the child? Answers to these questions will assist the nurse to identify potential health problems posed by the pregnancy.

The nurse can assist the pregnant client to deal with common discomforts of pregnancy such as nausea, vomiting, heartburn, constipation, hemorrhoids, urinary frequency, backache, vaginal discharge, and so on. Referral to such programs as WIC can enhance the eligible client's nutritional status. The nurse can also teach and counsel the client regarding clothing, sexual activity, childbirth preparation, baby supplies, signs of labor, danger signs and fertility control after delivery. In addition, the nurse can encourage the client to voice feelings and concerns about the pregnancy and to explore role changes that will occur with the birth of the child.

Primary prevention of child abuse and problems with the new infant can be started during the last trimester of pregnancy through anticipatory guidance and education in parenting skills. This form of primary prevention can prevent potentially serious problems for the infant. Parenting skills were discussed more fully in Chapter 20, Care of Children.

Preparation for Menopause

Primary prevention is also warranted for the middle-aged adult woman in anticipation of menopause. The community health nurse can be of assistance in helping women to accept and cope with menopause and the physical changes that occur with age. Anticipatory guidance, counseling, and referral may be needed depending on the individual's response to the event. These interventions should be geared to allowing the client to make informed decisions regarding medical regimens, nutrition, and exercise.

Preparation for menopause and the changes it causes should begin early in the woman's life. Dietary and exercise habits affect bone structure and the immune system. Community health nurses can help mothers and daughters to adopt a diet high in calcium, protein, complex carbohydrates, and vitamins, and one that is low in fat. The nurse can also encourage exercise patterns that include aerobic exercises that place moderate stress on bones so minerals are retained and osteoporosis is delayed indefinitely. These measures will greatly enhance health and slow the aging process.

Diet and exercise programs for the prevention of osteoporosis are especially important for the teenage girl. Teens have the poorest nutritional habits of any group studied. In addition, they tend to drink and smoke, both of which contribute adversely to bone structures leading to osteoporosis. They are also among the most difficult to convince that preventive measures will help them in later years.

Primary prevention among women who are nearing menopause will include anticipatory guidance on what to expect as changes occur and information about their options in estrogen replacement therapy. Counseling and teaching should be temporized to be of benefit to all women whether or not they have symptoms that require estrogen replacement. Diet and exercise, avoidance of caffeine and alcohol, and encouragement to quit smoking are also helpful.

Facilitating Access to Care

A primary preventive intervention requiring political activity is facilitating adequate access to health-care services for women. Action is needed to ensure the availability of such services and the financial resources that allow women to take advantage of them. Again, advocacy may be required on the part of the nurse to ensure that ancillary services such as transportation and child care are also available to women who need them.

Primary Prevention in the Work Setting

The psychosocial environment of the work setting can be changed by means of several strategies.[68] These strategies include educating and socializing women to expect wage equity and to believe that their work is as important as a man's; promoting legislation to prevent job discrimination; educating women about their rights (a useful guide is *A Working Woman's Guide to Her Job Rights*),[69] and encouraging women to challenge sexual harassment. Additional strategies include political support for women running for office, influencing the legislative process, and promoting collective bargaining, mentoring, and networking among women. A final strategy is active participation in organizations working for changes to benefit women.

The community health nurse working in the occupational setting can provide primary preventive care for women by identifying and understanding stressors affecting women in the work setting, counseling regarding work options, encouraging women to report safety hazards (or the nurse can report them personally), encouraging organization of women in the work setting, fostering personal preventive measures such as the use of protective devices, and keeping a log of jobs and exposure to hazardous materials and health changes.[43,44] Another major contribution can be made by community health nurses who have clients experiencing role proliferation. These nurses can assist clients to plan for efficient use of time, to use outside help when possible, and to let go of minor household duties that can wait. Single parents particularly need help in this area.

Preventing STDs

For women the chief route of exposure to sexually transmitted diseases (including AIDS) is sexual intercourse with a heterosexual or bisexual carrier of infection. Consequently, safer sex practices, monogamous relationships with an uninfected partner, or abstinence are the primary means of preventing infection.

Knowing that use of a condom reduces the risk of AIDS and other STDs does not mean that a woman will insist that her partner use these devices.[70] Some women do not want to relinquish control by relying on a man's behavior to protect them from disease or pregnancy.[27] The community health nurse can suggest that the woman use a diaphragm and nonoxynol-9 spermicidal jelly, which will offer a measure of protection from gonorrhea and chlamydia if used correctly.

The community health nurse should teach and counsel regarding STDs in a realistic and nonjudgmental way. Specific information about unsafe sexual practices such as rectal sex and the increased risk of AIDS must at times be explicit. Nurses should let clients know that they are comfortable with the information and that they are properly informed.

Adolescent females may be particularly difficult to reach with education on STDs. Strategies for educating adolescents include recognizing the teen as a sexual being; teaching skills such as condom or diaphragm use needed to reduce risk; instructing in a manner that gives the teen a sense of personal control; using concrete, simple terminology; employing visual aids as much as possible; involving the teen in the learning process through games and other strategies.[71] Other strategies include making use of role-play and decision-making exercises that help teens rehearse safe-sex scenarios. Peer counseling is also effective because teens are more likely to rely on peers for information and role models than they are to seek adult advice.

Developing Coping Skills and Assertiveness

Primary prevention for female clients also involves assistance in the development of coping skills and assertiveness. Community health nurses can help families to raise their children so little girls are no longer taught to be dependent and passive, but assertive and in control. Boys must be taught that abusiveness, violence, and over-controlling behavior are not acceptable ways of acting.[35] Societal norms, at present, make these changes in socialization of children very difficult. Even if the family does succeed in raising children this way, schools (from elementary through college) still reward girls who are passive and boys who are aggressive.[35] Community health nurses can begin some more permanent changes in these attitudes by increasing the awareness of parents and teachers about this issue and encouraging them to change the way they view girls and boys.

Older women can also be assisted by the nurse to develop skills in assertiveness. Interventions can be designed to improve women's self-esteem and to teach them how to cope with life stress in effective ways. These strategies along with political activity are effective primary preventive measures for abuse and violence against women. Prevention of family violence and abuse will be addressed in more detail in Chapter 34, Violence. Primary preventive care measures for women are summarized in Box 21–5.

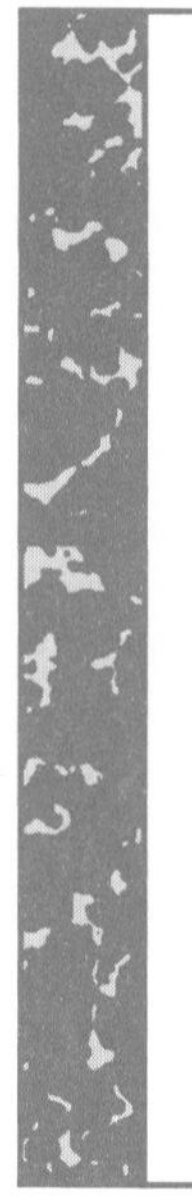

BOX 21–5

Considerations in Primary Preventive Care for Women

- Preparation for menarche
- Sexuality education
- Fertility control
- Prenatal care
- Preparation for menopause
- Facilitation of access to health care
- Primary prevention in the work setting
- Development of coping skills and assertiveness

SECONDARY PREVENTION

Secondary prevention focuses on screening and diagnosis and treatment for existing health problems.

Screening

Screening procedures specifically recommended for women include those used to detect breast and cervical cancer and sexually transmitted diseases. Women should, of course, also be screened for other health problems such as hypertension, diabetes, and skin cancers. Screening procedures routinely recommended for women are included in Box 21–6.

Community health nurses can be particularly effective in educating women on the need and procedure for regular breast self-exam (BSE). The nurse can demonstrate the techniques involved in BSE and recommend that women examine their breasts monthly about 1 week after their menstrual period or, in the case of menopausal women, on the same day of each month. Nurses can also recommend periodic mammography and Pap smears for detection of breast and cervical cancers, respectively. Community health nurses may also refer clients to agencies that provide

BOX 21–6

Routine Screening Procedures Recommended for Women

Pap smear
TB skin test
Chest X-ray
Mammogram
Vision test
Hearing test
Serum cholesterol test
Serum glucose test
Blood pressure screening
Urine test for bacteria, glucose, and protein
Testing for chlamydia, gonorrhea, syphilis, and genital herpes

such services as well as educating them on the need for screening.

Women at risk for sexually transmitted diseases should be screened periodically for such diseases as gonorrhea, syphilis, and HIV infection. Women in high-risk groups include those with multiple sexual partners, intravenous drug users, and those who have sexual contact with IV drug users or bisexual men. Pregnant women in these high-risk groups should be particularly encouraged to undergo screening for STD. This subject will be discussed in more detail in Chapter 30, Communicable Disease.

Diagnosing and Treating Existing Problems

Community health nurses would refer women clients for medical or social assistance with any identified health problems. Problems unique to female clients for which secondary prevention may be required include infertility, fertility control, menopause, and physical abuse.

Infertility. Treatment for infertility generally requires referral to a fertility specialist. The role of the community health nurse with respect to infertility will center around case finding, referral, and support during a fertility workup. The nurse can also assist the client and her significant other in considering alternative options such as adoption, artificial insemination, or in vitro fertilization. The nurse may also refer couples to self-help groups for assistance in dealing with the problems of infertility.

Fertility Control. Helping women who are having difficulty using a contraceptive method is another aspect of nursing care at the level of secondary prevention. Some women discover that they cannot use the method they have chosen and just stop using it. This can lead to unwanted pregnancy. The nurse can counsel, teach, and refer as needed to help each woman or couple find the best way to control fertility or to plan for children. Occasionally, secondary prevention in this area may entail presenting the client with options for dealing with the problem of an unintended pregnancy.

Menopause. Once menopause has occurred, referral to a physician or nurse practitioner for estrogen replacement therapy can take place if the client expresses discomfort related to hot flashes or has risk factors predisposing her to osteoporosis. These risk factors include being white, having a small skeleton and lean body, leading a sedentary life-style, and poor diet, decreased calcium intake, fair complexion, thin skin, and sparse hair.[72]

If the client decides to be evaluated for estrogen replacement therapy, the nurse should describe what to expect during the initial visit. Generally, this will include a complete history and physical, and several laboratory tests including a fasting blood glucose, complete blood count, blood lipids, liver function tests, and a Pap smear. Some physicians will also do an endometrial biopsy to determine the potential for endometrial cancer. This is a painful procedure for the client and should be discussed by the nurse to alleviate fear and to assist the client to cope with the procedure.[72]

Menopause may cause vaginal dryness and discomfort during sexual intercourse. The nurse can counsel women concerning longer foreplay and the use of vaginal lubricants to relieve the problem.

Some women also experience a decreased sexual desire. The community health nurse can help the client explore some of the contributing factors in this experience such as depression, a feeling of being at the end of the reproductive years, and the acceptance of a new phase of life. Self-help groups for women who are having similar problems are extremely helpful during this stage of life. If there is no such group in the local community, the nurse can start one by inviting clients to meet and begin discussions.[73]

Physical Abuse. Secondary prevention related to physical abuse of women has two dimensions. The first of these is dealing with the physical and psychological effects of physical abuse, and the second is dealing with the source of the problem itself. Recognizing the problem is a prerequisite to either dimension of treatment. Women clients should be asked in a caring and sensitive manner about any violence in their lives. Careful recording of the history and of information regarding old and new injuries is important in the diagnosis of abuse. Such a record may reveal a pattern the woman is unwilling or unable to admit to the nurse. If there is evidence of abuse, it is unethical for the nurse not to confirm this diagnosis with the client.[38] Allowing the woman to describe what is happening to her through open-ended questions is therapeutic and can serve as the first step in stemming the cycle of abuse.

It is important that the nurse convey to the client that she does not deserve to be abused and that the nurse is sorry that this has happened to her.[38] These are critical statements that are needed to reveal to the client that someone cares and that she is not worthless, helpless, or deserving of abuse.

It is not easy for a community health nurse to intervene in an abusive relationship. Inherent in such situations are reasons to fear that intervention will not be successful, that the woman may become depressed and suicidal or resent the nurse for interfering in a private family matter, or that the male abuser may punish the woman or the nurse. Such fears have kept health professionals from pursuing evidence and attempting to help women in abusive situations.[38]

When the nurse is able to work through and conquer personal fear and is able to identify a client in an abusive relationship, the nurse should encourage the client to discuss the circumstances of her abuse. It is important that the client realize the danger inherent in her situation.[74]

Once the diagnosis of abuse is made, the primary goal is to assist the woman to reestablish a feeling of control and to empower her to change the situation. Supportive counseling and reassurance are essential. The nurse should let the woman work out her problems at her own pace. Each woman has the capacity to change when she is ready. The nurse must realize that the victim will feel ambivalence in the love-hate relationship she has with her partner. The nurse should support realistic ideas for change and assist the client in changing unrealistic ideas. The nurse should help the client to clarify her beliefs about the situation. The nurse should also help to identify myths about abuse that the client may have internalized. For example, if the victim believes that she deserves the beatings, the nurse can assure the client that her partner is totally responsible for his own actions.

The nurse can help the client explore alternative plans for solutions to her problem. What are her personal supports? Is there anyone to whom she can go for help? The client may want to go home. If the client can do this without risk of suicide or homicide, the nurse should help her plan strategies for managing at home and provide her with resources for assistance or escape should the need arise. If necessary, however, the community health nurse can also help the woman to plan for a quick getaway. The client will need to accumulate extra money, collect necessary documents like birth certificates and immunizations records for children, pack a change of clothing, and carry a few emergency supplies.[11] If the client has children, she should take them with her if she leaves or risk losing them to the abuser if he should claim that the client abandoned them.[11]

It is important to remember, however, that the nurse should avoid becoming another controller in the life of the client. The physically abused woman needs every opportunity to develop independence. Nurses tend to want to rescue victims in order to stop the violence. They cannot make decisions for the woman. While nurses can provide information on shelters and other resources, they must allow the woman to make the call.

Nurses should be familiar with the resources that they recommend. Are they reliable? Will they assist the woman to become independent while providing a safe haven for her and her children?

Community health nurses can also provide assistance in referrals for medical care for injuries and for counseling to deal with contributing factors and psychological effects of abuse. Such services may be needed for children as well as the woman. The woman should also be cautioned that her children may resist being removed from their home and/or father. If this should be the case, the community health nurse can help her cope with grief and hostility on the part of the children. The client may also need help in dealing with her own grief over the loss of a significant relationship.

TERTIARY PREVENTION

As with all clients, tertiary prevention in the care of women focuses on rehabilitation and preventing the recurrence of health problems. Areas in which tertiary prevention are particularly warranted for the female client include pregnancy, abuse, and STD. Tertiary prevention may also be needed to deal with some of the effects of menopause.

Tertiary prevention with respect to pregnancy involves the use of an effective contraceptive to prevent subsequent pregnancies. Again, the nurse may be involved in education, counseling, and referral for contraceptive services.

In the case of abuse, tertiary prevention will necessitate the rebuilding of the woman's life and that of her family. This may involve developing new financial resources as well as ways of coping with problems. The woman will need to become self-sufficient. Again, referrals to a variety of agencies to help with employment skills and to provide counseling may be of assistance.

Women can also be helped to prevent recurrence of sexually transmitted diseases or to cope with the life changes necessitated by a diagnosis of AIDS. Tertiary prevention related to STDs will be discussed more fully in Chapter 30, Communicable Disease.

EVALUATING HEALTH CARE FOR WOMEN

Health care provided to women should be evaluated using the evaluative process described in Chapter 5, The Nursing Process. Once more, it is important to evaluate both the quality of the care given and its outcomes. Because of the dependent role of many women, it is particularly important that they play an active role in evaluating the health care they are given.

CHAPTER HIGHLIGHTS

- Women have been somewhat disadvantaged in the past with respect to access to health care to meet their unique needs.
- Human biological considerations in assessing the health status of women include the maturational events of menarche and menopause and changes in physiologic status such as pregnancy, infertility, and illness.
- Factors to be addressed in assessing the influence of psychological and social environments include factors related to female sexuality, the woman's life goals, and violence and abuse of women.
- Life-style factors of concern in assessing the health needs of women include consumption patterns related to diet, smoking, and substance abuse; occupation and related factors; and the woman's sexual life-style.
- Health system factors that particularly influence women's access to health-care services include the relative lack of primary preventive services for women, the cost of care, and lack of support for informal care-givers.
- Lesbian clients have special health-care needs related to each of the four areas of Dever's epidemiologic perspective. These needs must be addressed by the community health nurse assessing the health status of the lesbian client.
- Nursing diagnoses related to the health status of women may be made with respect to individual women or to groups of women.
- Planning to meet the health-care needs of women may include efforts at the primary, secondary, and tertiary levels of prevention.
- Primary preventive concerns in the care of women include preparation for menarche, sexuality education, fertility control, prenatal care, preparation for menopause, facilitating access to health care, primary prevention in the work setting, preventing STDs, and developing coping skills and assertiveness.
- Special areas for consideration in secondary preventive activities for women include screening and diagnosis and treatment of existing conditions, particularly problems of infertility, fertility control, menopause and physical abuse.
- Evaluation of nursing care for women focuses on the outcome of care as well as the quality of the care given.

Review Questions

1. Describe at least two human biological factors, two environmental factors, two life-style factors, and two health system factors that influence the health status of women. (p. 493)
2. Identify at least four health problems common to women. (p. 494)
3. Describe at least three specific considerations that are unique in assessing the health needs of the lesbian client. (p. 504)
4. Identify at least five general concerns in primary prevention for women. (p. 511)
5. Describe three areas for consideration in secondary preventive activities in the care of women. (p. 514)
6. What are the two dimensions of secondary prevention of physical abuse of women? (p. 515)
7. Describe at least two actions that the community health nurse can take to provide more sensitive and effective care to the lesbian client. (p. 512)

APPLICATION AND SYNTHESIS

Susan is a 25-year-old wife and mother of two girls. She is pregnant for the third time. You have scheduled a home visit with her following a referral from the community clinic where she is receiving prenatal care. According to the referring agency, Susan does not always keep her appointments, and the baby is small for gestational age. The prenatal clinic requests that you teach nutrition and encourage her to keep her appointments.

When you arrive at the home, Susan is reluctant to allow you inside. She turns her face away and will not look at you as she answers your questions.

Because you know that every woman has the potential for being a victim of physical abuse, you ask Susan if someone has hurt her. In a nonthreatening, caring, and sensitive manner you say, "I see many women in my practice who are in a relationship with a person who hits or abuses them. Did someone hurt you?" Susan begins to cry and says, "My husband hit me last night." She allows you to come in, and you observe that she has a black eye and a swollen jaw. Her two small children are thin and poorly clothed. The house, though neat, is sparsely furnished.

In speaking with Susan, you find out that her husband works in a local factory and has been denied a promotion and a raise in the last week. He seems to blame Susan for becoming pregnant again and causing more financial worries. Susan tells you that she has been missing appointments at the prenatal clinic because of her black eye and the lack of transportation when her husband is at work.

1. What are the human biological, environmental, life-style, and health system factors operating in this situation?
2. What are your nursing diagnoses in this situation?
3. How would you address the two dimensions of secondary prevention of physical abuse of women in this case?
4. What other secondary preventive measures seem to be warranted in this situation?
5. What primary and tertiary preventive interventions might be appropriate in working with Susan?
6. How will you evaluate whether intervention has been successful?

REFERENCES

1. U.S. Department of Health and Human Services. (1991). *Healthy people 2000: National objectives for health promotion and disease prevention.* Washington, DC: U.S. Government Printing Office.
2. Gentry, J. (1987, July/August). Social factors affecting women's health. *Public Health Reports Supplement,* 8–9.
3. National Center for Health Statistics. (1990). *Health, United States, 1989.* Hyattsville, MD: United States Public Health Service.
4. Leslie, L., & Swider, S. (1986). Changing factors and changing needs in women's health care. *Nursing Clinics of North America, 21,* 111–123.
5. Abrums, M. (1986). Health care for women. *Journal of Obstetrics, Gynecologic, and Neonatal Nursing, 15*(3), 250–255.
6. Albino, J., & Tedesco, L. (1984). In A. Rickel, M. Gerrard, & I. Iscoe (Eds.), *Social and psychological problems of women: Prevention and crisis* (pp. 157–172). New York: Grune & Stratton.
7. Ehrenreich, B., & English, D. (1973). *Complaints and disorders: The sexual politics of sickness* (p. 6). New York: The Feminist Press.
8. Church, O., & Poirier, S. (1986). From patient to consumer: From apprentice to professional practitioner. *Nursing Clinics of North America, 21*(1), 99–109.
9. Webster, D., & Lipetz, M. (1986). Changing definitions: Changing times. *Nursing Clinics of North America, 21,* 87–97.
10. Rakel, R. (Ed.). (1987). *Conn's current therapy.* Philadelphia: W.B. Saunders.
11. Griffith-Kenney, J. (Ed.). (1986). *Contemporary women's health: A nursing advocacy approach.* Menlo Park, CA: Addison-Wesley.
12. Hatcher, R., Stewart, F., Trussell, J., et al. (1990). *Contraceptive technology, 1990–1991* (15th ed.). New York: Irvington Publishers.
13. Neeson, J., & Stockdale, C. (1981). *The practitioner's handbook of ambulatory OB/GYN.* New York: Wiley.
14. Jones, J., Cox, A., Levy, E., & Thompson, C. (1984). *Steps to better health for women: Common problems and what to do about them.* Reston, VA: Reston.
15. Coralli, C., Raisz, L., & Wood, C. (1986). Osteoporosis: Significance, risk factors, and treatment. *The Nurse Practitioner, 11*(9), 16–35.
16. U.S. Department of Commerce. (1990). *Statistical Abstract of the United States 1990* (110th ed.). Washington, DC: Bureau of the Census.
17. Kantrowitz, B. (1990, Special Issue on Teens). Homeroom. *Newsweek,* 50–54.
18. Travis, C. (1988). *Women and health psychology: Biomedical issues.* Hillsdale, NJ: Lawrence Erlbaum.
19. Varney, H. (1980). *Nurse-midwifery.* Boston: Blackwell Scientific.
20. Leiblum, S. (1988), Infertility. In E. Blechman & K. Brownell (Eds.), *Handbook of behavioral medicine for women* (pp. 116–125). New York: Pergamon Press.
21. Perdew, S. (1990). *Facts about AIDS: A guide for health care providers.* Philadelphia: J.B. Lippincott.
22. Ulene, A. (1987). *Safe sex in a dangerous world.* New York: Vintage Books.
23. Peterman, T., & Petersen, L. (1990). Stalking the HIV epidemic: Which tracks to follow and how far? *American Journal of Public Health, 80,* 401–402.
24. Update: Acquired Immunodeficiency Syndrome—United States, 1989. (1990). *MMWR, 39,* 81–86.
25. Women and AIDS: The crisis mounts. (1991). *The APA Monitor, 22*(2), 30.
26. Lester, B. (1989). *Women and AIDS.* New York: Continuum Books.
27. Mays, V., & Cochran, S. (1988). Issues in the perception of AIDS risk and risk reduction activities by Black and Hispanic women. *American Psychologist, 43,* 949–957.
28. Pediatric AIDS in California. (1990, September). *California AIDS Update, 3*(8), 93–97.
29. Weiss, K. (Ed.). (1984). *Women's health care: A guide to alternatives.* Reston, VA: Reston.
30. Wood, C. (1989). The reality of women's health. *Nursing Times, 85*(48), 54–55.
31. Kitzinger, S. (1983). *Women's experience of sex.* New York: Putnam's.
32. Fogel, C., & Woods, N. (1981). *Health care of women: A nursing perspective.* St. Louis: C.V. Mosby.
33. Premarital sexual experience among adolescent women, United States, 1970–1988. (1991). *MMWR, 39,* 929–932.
34. Morrissey, S. (1986). Aging. In J. Griffith-Kenney (Ed.), *Contemporary women's health: A nursing advocacy approach* (pp. 377–394). Menlo Park, CA: Addison-Wesley.
35. Diehm, C., & Ross, M. (1988). Battered women. In S. Rix (Ed.), *The American woman 1988–1989* (pp. 292–302). New York: W.W. Norton.
36. National Clearinghouse on Domestic Violence. (1981). *Wife abuse in the medical setting: An introduction for health personnel.* Rockville, MD: National Clearinghouse on Domestic Violence; Monograph, Series 7.
37. Kimbrough, C. (1990, May 31). Rights groups battling violence against women. *Arkansas Gazette,* p. 10B.
38. King, M., & Ryan, J. (1989). Abused women: Dispelling myths and encouraging intervention. *Nurse Practitioner, 14*(5), 47–58.
39. Eisler, R. (1987). *The chalice and the blade.* San Francisco: Harper & Row.
40. Anderson, C. (1982). Violence against women. In L. Sonstegard, K. Kowalski, & B. Jennings (Eds.), *Women's health: Volume 1, Ambulatory care* (pp. 221–245). New York: Grune & Stratton.
41. Bullock, K., McFarland, J., Bateman, L., & Miller, V. (1989). The prevalence and characteristics of battered women in a primary care setting. *Nurse Practitioner, 14*(6), 47–56.
42. Rose M. (1988). Reproductive hazards for high-tech workers. In S. Rix (Ed.), *The American woman 1988–1989* (pp. 277–285). New York: W.W. Norton.
43. Murphy, D. (1986). Occupational health hazards. In J. Griffith-Kenney (Ed.), *Contemporary women's health: A nursing advocacy approach* (pp. 419–431). Menlo Park, CA: Addison-Wesley.
44. Davis, L., Marbury, M., Punnett, L., et al. (1984). En-

vironmental and occupational health. In Boston Women's Book Collective, *The new our bodies, ourselves* (pp. 77–98). New York: Simon & Schuster.

45. Bell, S. (1984). Birth control. In Boston Women's Health Book Collective, *The new our bodies, ourselves* (pp. 220–262). New York: Simon & Schuster.
46. Schober, M. (1986). Contraception. In J. Griffith-Kenney (Ed.), *Contemporary women's health: A nursing advocacy approach* (pp. 450–465). Menlo Park, CA: Addison-Wesley.
47. Seaman, B. (1984). Contraception, 1984. In K. Weiss (Ed.). *Women's health care: A guide to alternatives* (pp. 9–33). Reston, VA: Reston.
48. Davis, K. (1988). Women and health care. In S. Rix (Ed.), *The American woman 1988–1989* (pp. 162–204). New York: W.W. Norton.
49. Jennings, B. (1982). Physiology and life stages of the menstrual cycle. In L. Sonstegard, K. Kowalski, & B. Jennings (Eds.), *Women's health: Volume 1, Ambulatory care* (pp. 101–138). New York: Grune & Stratton.
50. Owen, W. (1980). The clinical approach to the homosexual patient. *Annals of Internal Medicine, 93,* 90–92.
51. Williamson, M. (1986). *Contemporary women's health: A nursing advocacy approach* (pp. 279–296). Menlo Park, CA: Addison-Wesley.
52. Bell, A., & Weinberg, M. (1978). *Homosexualities: A study of diversity among men and women.* New York: Simon & Schuster.
53. Johnson, S., Guenther, S., Laube, D., & Kettel, W. (1981). Factors influencing lesbian gynecologic care: A preliminary study. *American Journal of Obstetrics and Gynecology, 140*(1), 20–28.
54. Bernhard, L., & Dan, A. (1986). Redefining sexuality from women's own experience. *Nursing Clinics of North America, 21,* 125–135.
55. Johnson, S., & Palermo, J. (1984). Gynecologic care for the lesbian. *Clinical Obstetrics and Gynecology, 27,* 724–731.
56. Schafer, S. (1976). Sexual and social problems of lesbians. *Journal of Sex Research, 12,* 50–69.
57. Anderson, S., & Henderson, D. (1985). Working with lesbian alcoholics. *Social Work, 30,* 518–525.
58. Wismont, J., & Reame, N. (1989). The lesbian childbearing experience: Assessing developmental tasks. *Image: The Journal of Nursing Scholarship, 21,* 137–141.
59. Lewis, L. A. (1984). The coming-out process for lesbians: Integrating a stable identity. *Social Work, 2,* 464–469.
60. Stevens, P., & Hall, J. (1988). Stigma, health beliefs, and experiences with health care in lesbian women. *Image: Journal of Nursing Scholarship, 20,* 69–73.
61. Groves, P. (1985). Coming out: Issues for the therapist working with women in the process of lesbian identity formation. *Women and Therapy, 4*(2), 17–22.
62. Deevey, S. (1989). When mom or dad come out: Helping adolescents cope with homophobia. *Journal of Psychosocial Nursing, 27*(10), 33–36.
63. Berg-Cross, L. (1982). Existential issues in the treatment of lesbian clients. *Women and Therapy, 1*(4), 67–83.
64. Saghir, M., & Robins, E. (1980). Clinical aspects of female homosexuality. In J. Marmor (Ed.), *Homosexual behavior: A modern reappraisal* (pp. 280–295). New York: Basic Books.
65. Saghir, M., Robins, E., Walbran, B., & Gentry, K. (1970). Homosexuality: IV. Psychiatric disorders and disability in the female homosexual. *American Journal of Psychiatry, 127*(2), 65–72.
66. Lawrence, J. (1975). Homosexuals, hospitalization, and the nurse. *Nursing Forum, 14,* 305–317.
67. Dardick, L., & Grady K. (1980). Openness between gay persons and health professionals. *Annals of Internal Medicine, 93,* 115–119.
68. Opie, N. (1986). Employment discrimination. In J. Griffith-Kenney (Ed.), *Contemporary women's health: A nursing advocacy approach* (pp. 396–417). Menlo Park, CA: Addison-Wesley.
69. U.S. Department of Labor. Women's Bureau. (1983). *A working woman's guide to her job rights.* Leaflet 55. Washington, DC: U.S. Government Printing Office.
70. Brandt, A. (1988). AIDS in historical perspective: Four lessons from the history of sexually transmitted diseases. *American Journal of Public Health, 78,* 367–371.
71. Janke, J. (1989). Dealing with AIDS and the adolescent population. *Nurse Practitioner, 14*(11), 35–41.
72. Ladewig, P. (1985). Protocol for estrogen replacement therapy in menopausal women. *Nurse Practitioner, 10*(10), 44–47.
73. Graham, E. (1986). Menstruation and menopause. In J. Griffith-Kenney, *Contemporary women's health: A nursing advocacy approach.* Menlo Park, CA: Addison-Wesley.
74. Campbell, J. (1986). Nursing assessment for risk of homicide with battered women. *Advances in Nursing Science, 8*(4), 36–51.

RECOMMENDED READINGS

AIDS in women—United States. (1991). *MMWR, 39,* 845–846.

Discusses the increasing incidence of AIDS among women and its implications for women's health in the future.

Bohn, D. (1990). Domestic violence and pregnancy: Implications for practice. *Journal of Nurse Midwifery, 35,* 86–98.

Presents the problem of physical abuse of pregnant women. Addresses effective nursing interventions in abusive situations.

Collins, J. (1990). Health care of women in the workplace. *Health Care for Women International, 11*(1), 21–32.

Examines women's health at work, specifically why women have particular health needs. Highlights historical and social influences on women's health.

Hatcher, R., Stewart, F., Trussell, J., et al. (1990). *Contraceptive technology, 1990–1991* (15th ed.). New York: Irvington Publishers.

Provides the latest information on reproductive health, contraceptive methods, pregnancy and family planning, and global trends in family planning.

Keleher, K. (1991). Occupational health: How work environments can affect reproductive capacity and outcome. *The Nurse Practitioner, 16*(1), 23–37.

Compiles research data on how the work environment can affect reproductive capacity and outcome. Also includes taking occupational and reproductive histories and guidelines for counseling women regarding occupational hazards.

Kirschstein, R. (1991). Public health policy forum: Research on women's health. *American Journal of Public Health, 81,* 291–293.

Discusses the mission, policy statement, and relevance of the new Office of Research on Women's Health of the National Institutes of Health.

Kjervik, D. (1990). Ethical and legal dilemmas of battered women. *Journal of Professional Nursing, 6*(5), 253.

Inquires into the ethical and legal dilemmas faced by battered women.

Sanford, N. (1989). Providing sensitive health care to gay and lesbian youth. *The Nurse Practitioner, 14*(5), 30–47.

Describes useful approaches in assisting homosexual youth. Emphasis is on education and support.

Sherwen, L. N., Scoloveno, M. A., Weingarten, C. T. (1991). *Nursing care of the childbearing family.* Norwalk, CT: Appleton & Lange.

Offers a family-centered approach to maternal-newborn care. Emphasis is on each family member's psychological adaptation to pregnancy. Also highlights the importance of designing care based on a family's cultural background.

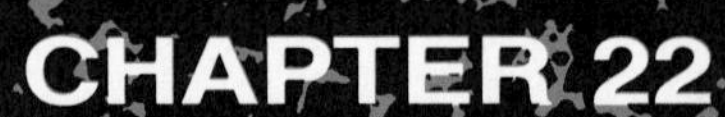

CHAPTER 22

Care of Men

Edward A. Herzog

KEY TERMS

antisocial personality disorder
barrier
countertransference
denial
empathy
hydrocele
juvenile conduct disorder
posttraumatic stress disorder
reframing
socially prescribed norms

The male client possesses physical and physiological characteristics that distinguish him from his female counterpart. As important, however, are the psychosocial differences between the male and the female client that may affect how the male client responds to nursing care. A male, for instance, may react differently from a female to caring overtures by the nurse. Although it is commonly thought that men are "less emotional" than women, a male may respond with a surprising depth of emotion to perceived threats to his well-being. Research suggests, for instance, that men may respond to cardiovascular disease more "emotionally" than women, exhibiting greater degrees of depression and other emotional responses to potential loss.[1]

Moreover, there are clear differences between men and women in the epidemiology of certain health problems and health-related behaviors. These epidemiological and behavioral differences are reflected in gender differences in life expectancy, which is 78.3 years for women but only 71.3 years for men.[2] The gap in life expectancy between men and women is an ironic reflection of the fact that our health-care system—created by and still largely controlled by men—apparently does not serve men's health-care needs well. A closer look at national health-care policy objectives would seem to confirm this view. Currently, there are no specific national health objectives targeted exclusively toward men. The current objectives for the year 2000 do not even address the prevention of or screening for testicular or prostatic cancers.

This chapter investigates some of the physiological, psychosocial, and health system differences that the community health nurse might encounter when providing care for adult male clients.

LEARNING OBJECTIVES

After reading this chapter you should be able to:

- Describe three factors that may influence male clients' responses to care by community health nurses.
- Identify at least four factors that may contribute to aggression against the community health nurse by a male client.
- Describe at least five considerations in assessing the effects of human biological factors on the health of men.
- Identify at least three environmental influences on men's health.
- Describe four areas for consideration in assessing life-style factors influencing men's health.
- Identify at least two effects of the health-care system on the health of male clients.
- Describe at least three factors that contribute to adverse health effects for male homosexual clients.
- Identify at least four areas for primary prevention with male clients.
- Describe at least four secondary prevention considerations for male clients.
- Identify at least three areas of emphasis in tertiary prevention for male clients.

NURSES WORKING WITH MALE CLIENTS

Working with male clients may present the community health nurse with some problems not as regularly encountered when working with female clients in community settings. For example, the male client may make romantic overtures toward the female nurse, may resist health teaching efforts or health examinations, or may be reluctant to accept the nurse's guidance. The male client may be unusually prone to noncompliance, may use humor in a manner the nurse finds inappropriate, or may make derogatory comments that are focused on the nurse's gender (whether female *or* male). In order to work with male clients, the nurse needs to understand how the male client's attitudes—and the nurse's response to these attitudes—can positively or negatively influence nursing care.

SOCIALLY PRESCRIBED NORMS

Socially prescribed norms are expectations society holds concerning human behavior. Socially prescribed norms concerning men include various beliefs about male strength, achievement, and power. Men tend to be socialized to behave according to these expectations and, as a result, may engage in "compensatory, aggressive, risk-taking behaviors that may predispose them to illness, injury, and even death."[3]

When working with male clients, it may be very beneficial for community health nurses to respond to these socially prescribed norms in two ways: (1) by avoiding reinforcing stereotypical and counterproductive images of masculinity and (2) by giving men permission to behave according to alternative role images (for example, to be caring toward oneself). This latter strategy can be accomplished by giving the male clear permission to have and to talk about health concerns.[4] For example, the nurse could state, "I know that some men think that men should not talk about what bothers them, but men have the same right to talk about their health concerns as anyone else."

Moreover, the nurse can guide and support the male in understanding the effect that acting out socially prescribed norms about male roles can have on health. For example, the nurse could state, "I wonder if being a man has made you act tough even when it hurts to do so. Your talking about it now shows that you are not afraid to challenge how you've been taught to act, and I think this is very helpful."

The nurse could also directly confront life-style choices that adversely affect the male client's health and that are the result of efforts to act out socially prescribed roles. For instance, the nurse could note that taking the risk of drinking and driving may be a way of appearing strong in order to fulfill one's role image but that doing so presents a great and unnecessary danger.

Because society has tended to define male and female as opposite sets of characteristics (men tough, women soft), it may be quite helpful for community health nurses to begin a process of redefining both women's and men's roles in our society. Community nurses can do this through their educational efforts and by supporting and encouraging the efforts made by male clients to see themselves in ways less stereotypical and more conducive to happiness and good health.

COUNTERTRANSFERENCE

Countertransference is the tendency to respond to clients based on one's own emotions. The management of countertransference can be especially important in caring for male clients, whose behavior and values may be sufficiently different from the nurse's own that they incite especially strong emotional reactions. When this behavioral tendency is allowed to influence a nurse's judgment, it may have either a positive or negative effect on client care.

If a female nurse, for example, perceives an elderly male client as "cute and gentle," she may find herself going out of her way to meet his health-related requests. She may visit him more often and for greater periods than his health-care needs require. In this instance, the nurse's affectionate feelings have colored her judgment of the client's circumstances and led her to behave differently toward him than toward other clients (though perhaps no harm is done).

In another case, a female nurse may find herself working with a recovering male alcohol abuser who insists on calling her his "honey," despite her requests that he not do so. In this instance, the nurse will likely feel embarrassment and resentment and may react by reducing both the frequency and duration of her visits. Although this client's health-related requests are no more unreasonable than the elderly man's, the nurse might require that the recovering alcoholic "be more self-sufficient" and respond by minimizing his legitimate needs. Here, the nurse's emotional reactions (and quite likely her values pertaining to alcohol abuse) have caused her to distort her view of the client. In this instance the result is likely to be more detrimental to the client. Of course, nurses are not always female, but male nurses are likely to behave similarly under comparable circumstances.

The risk of countertransference, then, is that it can insidiously erode the quality of nursing care provided to clients. To reduce this effect, it is essential that the community health nurse (1) recognize and label his or her own feelings about a client, (2) consider the possibility that these feelings are altering the nurse's view of the client, and (3) evaluate the client's care with the aim of identifying the effect that the nurse's emotions may be having. One method for doing this is to compare one's feelings and nursing care for clients who are of objectively similar circumstances. If there are variations in how the nurse sees or cares for these clients, it is likely that countertransference is unduly affecting client care.

Another method to thwart countertransference is to use one's colleagues as sounding boards and points of comparison. A nurse can become more self-aware, more objective, and more effective in his or her care by discussing personal views with other nurses, actively seeking their feedback about performance, and by observing other nurses' behavior as a basis for comparison.

EMPATHY

Empathy is the capacity to see things from another's perspective, and to sense how that person feels. This capacity develops when one stops to consider how a situation might seem to the client and to consider how the client's differing values and beliefs affect his or her views and responses. Consider the case of the male cardiac client who insists on shovelling snow despite the attendant risk to his health. The nurse who fails to empathize will likely assume that the client has a knowledge deficit and proceed to "educate" him about the risks of strenuous physical activity. When the client continues to shovel snow, the nurse is likely to become frustrated and angry and presume that the client doesn't care about his health.

An empathetic nurse encountering the same cardiac client shovelling snow asks, "Why might he be doing this?" Further inquiry reveals that the client understands that shovelling is dangerous "for some heart patients" but that he feels he won't be hurt by it and will in fact become stronger as a result. The nurse senses that the client is using denial as a means to deal with his fear of dying and also pauses to consider the male client's view of the world. In the client's view, "men are men," and shovelling the snow is a manly activity. *Not* shovelling the snow would, in effect, be like saying "I am not a man anymore," a prospect that the client cannot face. The empathetic nurse takes these insights about the client's behavior and sets about helping him deal more effectively with his fears and his need to perceive himself as still very much a man. She talks with him about what it was like to have had a heart attack, and she helps him "open up" about fear by pointing out that most heart attack victims—even the most masculine—are very frightened. She also conveys her empathy by noting that it is hard for many men to talk about fear, although all men experience it.

The empathetic nurse also understands that this male client's compromised cardiac status has left him feeling powerless, so the nurse helps him regain a sense of power. The nurse does this by ***reframing*** his view of the situation—that is, explaining it in different terms. For example, instead of the heart attack being a crippler and snow shovelling being a way to prove it isn't, the nurse suggests that the heart attack is an enemy, and the way to beat an enemy (and beating an enemy is certainly a masculine thing to do) is by countering its every move. The heart attack destroys some heart muscle, but the client can counter by resting and engaging in limited exercise to strengthen the remaining muscle. The nurse uses an analogy: When the enemy destroys half your bridge, do you then drive across that bridge to show your enemy he can't hurt you or do you do whatever it takes to repair the bridge so your enemy loses his advantage? As a result, the client sees the situation a little differently. By following nursing recommendations, he is a man fighting heart disease rather than snowfall, and his image of himself as masculine is preserved.

MALE CLIENTS AND PERSONAL SAFETY

In most client-care settings, the community health nurse often works apart from colleagues and in locations that are not "home turf." Understandably, a community health nurse may experience a degree of concern from time to time regarding personal safety. This is especially true when working with male clients. It is relatively rare for female clients to behave toward a community health nurse in a physically threatening or sexually inappropriate manner, and the same is true of most male clients. Under some circumstances, however, some males may represent potential safety risks to community health nurses—whether the nurse is male or female.

Males are more likely to behave in aggressive or socially inappropriate ways if they

1. belong to subgroups that lack norms against aggressive behavior (drug abusers, gang members);
2. come from backgrounds that supported antisocial behavior (abusive parents);

BOX 22–1

Nurse Safety When Working With Male Clients

1. Travel in pairs where feasible, especially when serving the higher-risk male clients or when working in high-risk environments.
2. Arrange to visit and conduct care of males when trusted client relatives or others are present in the immediate vicinity.
3. Behave in a calm, controlled, capable manner when interacting with male clients so as to convey that you feel secure (not vulnerable) yet not a threat to the client himself.
4. Present yourself in such a manner that the male client perceives you as an ally worth protecting rather than as an authority figure, source of inappropriate gratification, or contributor to the client's problems.
5. Dress in a manner that clearly identifies you as a health-care worker. Because community nurses are often held in high regard by the communities they serve, being recognized as a community "friend" can reduce aggression toward the nurse and increase the likelihood that others will offer assistance if needed.
6. State clear expectations about acceptable and unacceptable behavior when male clients "test limits" with provocative behavior. Back up those expectations by withdrawing from the nurse/client relationship when necessary.
7. Terminate the visit immediately when a male client's behavior starts becoming threatening or when risk elements are noted.
8. Avoid allowing your own denial mechanisms to cause you to underestimate the risks in working with a male client.
9. Position yourself so that you can access safety resources readily (exits, equipment bags that can serve as shields, for example).
10. Obtain training in basic self-defense techniques. (Local police departments or the local YMCA/YWCA are often good sources of either training referrals or training itself.)

3. abuse substances (especially alcohol) that impair impulse control and alter judgment;
4. feel powerless to meet their needs or to effect positive changes in their lives (for example, are unable to obtain work or sexual outlets);
5. are unable to express their feelings or needs verbally (for example, the angry client acting out his anger because he cannot or has not expressed it verbally); and
6. have neurological or psychiatric disorders that impair their reasoning ability, perceptions, or impulse control (such as schizophrenia or dementias).

Although the actual risk of injury or harm to the typical community nurse working with male clients is quite small (usually smaller than the risk of injury while driving to work), it clearly benefits the nurse to provide for his or her own safety in an active and thoughtful manner. Behaviors and practices that the community health nurse can adopt that enhance personal safety are described in Box 22–1.

THE EPIDEMIOLOGIC PREVENTION PROCESS MODEL AND CARE OF MEN

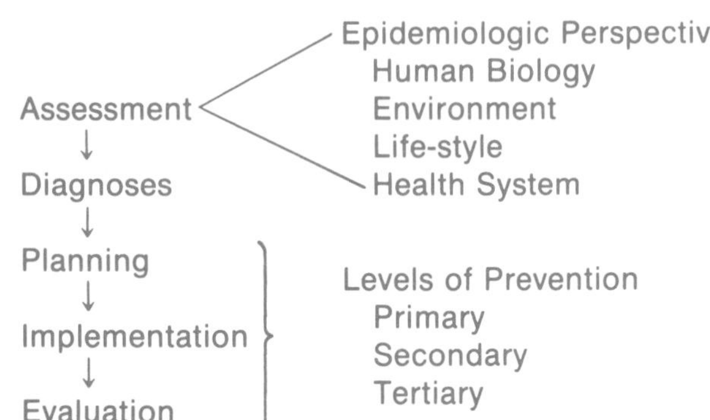

Men differ from women in their patterns of physical health disorders and health-related needs. These differences are attributable to (1) the physiologic differences between men and women (testicular cancer in men, for example); (2) the differences in health-related habits and health-seeking behavior between men and women (for example, men have fewer contacts with health-care providers than do women); and (3) psychosocial and life-style differences between the sexes (for example, men consume more alcohol and are more likely to resolve conflicts by resorting to violence). The epidemiologic prevention process model provides a useful framework for the community health nurse to account for these differences when assessing and working with men as individuals or as aggregates.

ASSESSING THE MALE CLIENT

HUMAN BIOLOGICAL FACTORS

Genetic Contributions

Genetic factors play a significant role in the physical health of male clients and are an important area for nursing assessment relative to cardiovascular disease, hypertension, and cerebrovascular disease. Genetic factors also may play a role in testicular and prostatic cancer (and cancer generally), as well as tendencies toward alcoholism and violence. Genetic factors may also influence a man's psychological health. They are, for example, suspected as a contributing factor in various mood disorders (which, in turn, often precipitate suicide among males).

The community health nurse assesses potential genetic contributions to a client's health status by obtaining a family history of the occurrence of physical and psychological disorders. It may be necessary to interview both the client and older family members and relations to secure an accurate picture of genetically mediated health problems.

Physiologic Function

Cardiovascular and Cerebrovascular Disorders. Morbidity and mortality rates for cardiovascular disorders, particularly for ischemic heart disease, are significantly higher among men than among women. In 1987, age-adjusted death rates for all forms of heart disease for white males were double those for white females, with ischemic heart diseases producing a mortality rate for white males more than double that for white females. Nonwhites, both male and female, had still higher mortality rates in these areas than whites, but also demonstrated a similar sex-differentiated pattern.[2] The death rate for coronary heart disease among black men ages 35 to 44 is about six times that of black women.

Given these figures, it is essential that the community health nurse assess the cardiovascular status of male clients. Assessment would include checking blood pressure, pulse, and respirations, as well as auscultating for abnormal heart sounds (such as murmurs) and sounds suggesting pulmonary congestion.

Death rates for cerebrovascular disorders among both black and white males are about 10 percent higher than for females of either race.[2] Consequently, it is important for the community health nurse to assess for two readily identifiable risk factors: hypertension (through blood pressure measurement) and carotid artery occlusion (through auscultation for cardiac bruits). Nurses should also assess for signs or be alert to reports of alterations in cognitive functioning such as confusion, impaired memory, or disorientation. Similarly, the nurse should be alert for other neuromotor changes such as weakness, facial asymmetry, ataxia, or changes in speech.

White males have a higher incidence of hypertension than do white females (44.8 percent vs. 34.2 percent). Among blacks, however, the rates of hypertension for both sexes are about equal (roughly 50 percent for both men and women).[2] The community health nurse needs to monitor the blood pressure of male clients on a regular basis to detect consistently elevated pressures (above 140 systolic or 95 diastolic for males over 40, and above 130 systolic or 90 diastolic for males under 40).

Cancers. The incidence and mortality rates for all cancers combined are significantly greater among men than among women.[2] The leading causes of cancer death among men include (in decreasing order of deaths produced) lung cancer, colorectal cancer, pancreatic cancer, leukemia, cancers of the brain and central nervous system (CNS), stomach cancer, and prostate cancer. Cancers that present the greatest threat to an individual male client's life include (in decreasing order of lethality) testicular cancer, Hodgkin's disease, leukemia, cancers of the brain and CNS, and skin cancer.[5]

Cancer incidence rates per 100,000 population that are greater for men than for women include colorectal cancer (approximately 50 percent greater), pancreatic cancer (25 percent greater), and lung and bronchial cancer (approximately 150 percent greater). Morbidity rates for respiratory cancers among white males are double those of white females, and for black males the rates are more than triple those for black females.[2]

Most of the theories offered to explain gender differences in cancer rates focus on life-style factors. Explanations include the higher rates of tobacco and alcohol consumption among men, higher exposure to dietary carcinogens (for example, from eating larger amounts of well-cooked meat), greater exposure to occupational carcinogens, physiological and psychosomatic differences in males' immune responses, and different patterns of health promotion and maintenance among males.

In addition to assessing for cancer risk factors related to life-style, the community health nurse should carefully note any symptoms that might suggest impairment or change in a particular organ. Changes of particular importance in the male client would include respiratory difficulty (persistent coughs, blood-tinged sputum, shortness of breath, coughing on exertion), changes in bowel or bladder habits (persistent diarrhea, bloody or dark tarry stools, ribbon-shaped stools), diminished activity tolerance, and unexplained changes in either weight or appetite.

Reproductive System Disorders. A variety of disorders involving the male reproductive system may also be encountered by the community health nurse. The prostate gland, for example, is subject to infection (prostatitis), carcinoma, and also to nonmalignant hyperplasia (benign prostatic hyperplasia). The testes and surrounding structures also are prone to carcinomas and inflammatory diseases.

The symptoms of prostatitis, an inflammation of the prostate, typically include urinary flow restriction in association with fever, burning on urination, and perineal pain. The condition may also be accompanied by pyuria or hematuria. Prostatitis often accompanies cystitis. The condition may result as a consequence of sexually transmitted diseases and may develop into a chronic, recurring form. Because of this risk, it is especially important for the community health nurse to assess for the symptoms of this condition.

Benign prostatic hyperplasia (BPH) commonly occurs in men over age 50, usually presenting with signs and symptoms of urinary flow restriction (urinary frequency, hesitancy, terminal dribbling, bladder fullness or distension, or urinary incontinence). Nurses should assess male clients over the age of 50 for these symptoms and facilitate follow-up evaluation.

Prostate cancer occurs in several forms and has recently surpassed lung cancer as the leading cancer in males.[6] It is most common in men over age 50. Prostate cancer is slow to develop, is often asymptomatic until late in its course, and is prone to metastasis. The 5-year survival rate for this condition is approximately 62 percent.[2] As a result, it is important that the community health nurse working with males over age 50 assess for signs of bladder obstruction, hematuria, and pyuria and encourage males to obtain annual rectal examinations.

Testicular cancer is the most common malignancy in white males between the ages of 15 and 24.[6] While the primary symptom of this disorder is a mass within one of the testes, research has shown that only 30 percent of young men are familiar with testicular self-examination (TSE) techniques, and less than 10 percent actually perform TSE.[7,8] Research has also indicated that very few physicians teach TSE.[9] Although the prognosis for most forms of testicular cancer is quite good when detected early (an 80 percent survival rate after 5 years for some common forms),[10] the lack of TSE results in late detection of many such tumors. (The discussion of secondary prevention measures will review TSE techniques).

Epididymitis, or inflammation of the epididymis, is the most common form of intrascrotal inflammation. It usually presents as painful swelling within the scrotum and is frequently accompanied by urethritis. Complications include infertility, abscesses, and testicular atrophy. The condition may be idiopathic or result from sexually transmitted pathogens (most frequently, *Chlamydia trachomatis* and *Neisseria gonorrhoeae*).[11] Assessment by the community health nurse should include a review of the client's sexual habits for factors that would increase the risk of acquiring this infection (frequent sexual partners, failure to use condoms) in addition to assessing for the presence of signs or symptoms.

A ***hydrocele*** is an abnormal collection of fluid within the tunica vaginalis of a testicle or along the spermatic cord. Males with this disorder typically note a swelling and may report that they have found a scrotal mass. The pain and discomfort associated with this condition can be considerable.[10] Community health nurses assess for this disorder by asking whether the male client has noted any changes in his scrotum or has experienced scrotal pain.

Other Disorders. **Inguinal hernia.** Occurring almost exclusively among men, this disorder is relatively common. Usual symptoms include lower abdominal or groin pain upon straining (when lifting and sometimes during bowel movements). While typically manageable on a symptomatic level, inguinal hernias require surgical repair in about 8 percent of cases.[2] In some cases herniation of the intestine through the inguinal canal(s) may lead to bowel obstruction and necrosis, a life-threatening situation. For this reason, the community health nurse working with a male client who is diagnosed with an inguinal hernia should carefully assess for the presence of persistent pain in the inguinal area, particularly if accompanied by persistent intestinal symptoms such as abdominal rigidity, pain, and cramping.

Tourette's syndrome. Tourette's syndrome is a fairly rare neurological disease of unknown etiology. The condition typically begins in childhood and may continue throughout life. Tourette's affects males three times more frequently than females. The disease is characterized by highly distressing and often socially debilitating symptoms that include involuntary movements and facial tics, as well as involuntary vocalizations consisting of grunts, barks, and—occasionally—obscenities.[12] Assessment involves the detection of characteristic vocal or motor tics, which are generally readily detected as they cannot be suppressed or concealed by the client.

Maturation and Aging

Because maturation and aging play a significant role in many health risks and problems experienced by male clients, the community health nurse needs to assess these factors when providing care. Certain physical disorders are associated with advanced age in men: cardiovascular disease, cerebrovascular disease, prostate cancer and hypertrophy, and hypertension. Other physical health concerns are more frequently associated with younger male clients: trauma, violence, and testicular cancer.

Physical sexual maturation in the male typically begins between ages 10 and 13 years and is completed between ages 14 and 18 years. At age 10 years the adolescent male is devoid of pubic and underarm hair and has genitals in proportion to their childhood size. As development progresses, there is first an enlargement and reddening or darkening in the color of the scrotum, accompanied by sparse growth of light-colored, straight pubic hair at the base of the penis. Subsequently, there begins an enlargement of the penis and further growth in the size of the scrotum and testes, accompanied by the growth of darker, curly coarse pubic hair that begins to spread out from the base of the penis. Next the penis and testes enlarge in girth, with further spread of the pubic hair (though still less than in adults).[13]

In the final period of development the genitals reach adult proportion, and there is continued spread of pubic hair. During this genital development more generalized changes take place: Underarm hair develops, followed in many males by hair on the upper legs and later on the lower legs. Most males begin to develop chest hair growth in late adolescence, but this is highly variable. Facial hair can become evident at any time during adolescence but is most typical after age 15. As the adolescent male approaches adulthood he experiences an increase in muscle mass, resulting in a broadening of the shoulders relative to the waist; this, too, is highly individualized. It should be noted that the adolescent male is typically very concerned with his sexual and physical development, often comparing himself to other males and many times experiencing anxiety about the possibility that his development is delayed or inadequate. In some cases this anxiety can be sufficient to cause social impairment or serious emotional distress, and the community health nurse should make a special effort to be supportive and accepting. The community health nurse can also benefit the adolescent male client by offering information and reassurance about the normal patterns and variations in growth and development. In the majority of adolescent males a degree of transient gynecomastia (enlargement of the breasts) occurs. This is variable in degree, but can be a source of significant concern to the adolescent; again, reassurance, explanation, and acceptance are of benefit.[14]

During this period the adolescent becomes increasingly concerned with the values of his peers and is increasingly focused on achieving acceptance from his peer group. He is prone to value peers over parents at this stage, and his attitudes are more reflective of peers than family. He often experiences uncertainty about his identity, and may engage in a variety of behaviors that, although perhaps disconcerting to his family or other adults, are necessary experiments in determining what type of person and life he will incorporate into his self-concept. Hormonal changes result in increased growth and libido, confronting him with the possibility of new (and perhaps anxiety-provoking) roles; these changes are also mirrored in the behavior of his peers, upon which he tends to model his own behaviors and choices.

The adolescent male may feel embarrassed about the physical and emotional changes he experiences. For example, he may have spontaneous and ill-timed erections, or nocturnal emissions. His physical development and social circumstances, coupled with peer pressure and a desire to conform, may lead to varying degrees of sexual activity, presenting the risks of unwanted pregnancy and sexually transmitted diseases. It is not unusual for some of the adolescent male's sexual exploration to involve sexual contact with other males; approximately 50 percent of all males have had such contact at some point, and there is no correlation between such sexual activity and later sexual orientation (though the adolescent may again experience significant anxiety, guilt, or shame about this experimental behavior).

Over time, the adolescent male's preoccupation with sexual performance and activity as the major parameters of a relationship are increasingly replaced by romantic attributes and genuine caring; initially these romantic views are often stereotypic and exaggerated, but this also changes as he progresses through early adulthood. Again, the nurse's role involves assessing the young male's development relative to existing norms and providing education about growth, development, sexuality, and related risks and safety precautions—and providing reassurance and guidance relative to the changes he is experiencing.

Psychological maturity—or the lack thereof—is a significant contributing factor to trauma, substance abuse, and suicide. Additionally, certain health-related life experiences can also be viewed from a maturational perspective, particularly divorce (married males tend to live longer than divorced or never-married males) and retirement (which can result in a higher risk of isolation or depression), both of which are associated with poorer health and higher risk of suicide. Divorce is discussed more fully as a sociological factor later in this chapter.

The nurse assesses the male client's maturational level by observing his behavior, or through interviews that elicit information about the client's concerns, interests, habits, and judgment. The nurse may also gather assessment data about a client's maturity level from indirect sources such as reports from significant others and other health-care professionals.

ENVIRONMENTAL FACTORS: PSYCHOLOGICAL AND SOCIAL

Psychological and Social Factors as Barriers

It is difficult to draw a clear line between psychological and social factors as they influence the male client's health. Both categories of factors are tightly interwoven and help shape one another, sometimes quite subtly. In many instances, psychological or social factors can act as a ***barrier,*** or obstacle, to health-promoting behaviors.

For example, men experience social pressures to conform to images of a masculine role that sometimes conflict with health. Socialized to view the male role as strong or invulnerable, a man may have difficulty admitting health-related frailties to a community health nurse. Similarly, men who believe that taking physical risks is fundamental to their masculinity may experience more frequent health impairment from trauma. As seen from these examples, as societal messages about male roles become internalized by men, they become psychological factors influencing male health behaviors.

Socially prescribed norms especially influence how men cope with stress ("don't cry" or "keep it inside") and thus affect male health by limiting the manner in which men experiencing stress can cope with it. For this reason, assessment by the community health nurse would focus on determining how a male client views himself and the masculine role, and would include assessing the client's ability to cope with stress and his access to support systems.

Men may also have a stronger psychological need than women to see themselves as healthy and even invulnerable. Because men tend to value strength and endurance more than women, they are more likely to conceal or suppress pain and other perceived indicators of frailty. An example of this state of mind can be seen in the male post-myocardial infarction client who resumes shovelling snow against the recommendations of health-care professionals and his family, and who continues it despite the return of the now-familiar angina. As a result of this need for strength in his self-image, the male client minimizes the importance of the problem. Consequently, when shovelling snow causes further angina, he may seek health care less readily and use it less effectively than would a female client in a similar situation.

Conversely, it should be noted that male values of strength and endurance do not always adversely affect a male client's health. Some men who value strength actually may be more motivated to exercise and maintain a higher level of general fitness and to seek preventive health care to preserve their sense of themselves as strong and invulnerable.

The male client may also be prone to other psychological or social barriers to health care. One such barrier relates to male-female modesty and intimacy. Many men find it exceedingly difficult to submit to physical assessment by, or even relate information about certain physical functions to, female nurses or other female health-care professionals. This is particularly true of the older male client, who has grown accustomed to examination by male physicians and may hold more traditional views of male-female role behaviors. If a man believes men to be inherently stronger physically, he may experience greater difficulty admitting to a female that his stamina has decreased or that his pain has exceeded his tolerance. When faced with making disclosures of this sort to a female community health nurse, or with the prospect of having intimate aspects of his person examined by a female nurse, he may opt to conceal his need for this form of health care or to avoid the contact altogether.

Another psychological barrier to men's health is the male client's inconsistent response to feelings attending a health problem. For example, a man who values strength may exercise regularly, but he may avoid having a swelling in his groin examined because he cannot cope effectively with the fear that the swelling may represent a threat to his sexuality.

A closely related barrier is the difficulty many

men experience in disclosing their feelings, particularly if those feelings run counter to traditional notions of masculinity (for example, that a man should be in control of his feelings or remain unaffected by them). Feelings that men typically find to be difficult to express include fear, anxiety, and sadness. The male client may have significant difficulty disclosing these feelings to female and male nurses alike, or in asking for assistance from others in coping with feelings. Consequently, a male client may suffer needlessly as a result.

Anger

Anger is a common response to loss or frustration. It is particularly significant for the male client if unexpressed or blocked, because anger can become directed toward the self and predispose the client toward suicide. Also, when inappropriately expressed, anger can be the genesis of physical violence. Both of these outcomes relate directly to major health issues of the male client. Some men perceive anger as an unacceptable emotion and suppress, deny, or externalize it. Others view anger as an emotion that is caused by others, and as a result they believe they are justified in converting their anger to violence.

Assessment by the community health nurse should include determining how the client views and manages his anger (specifically whether he expresses it verbally or acts it out physically), obtaining a history of trauma that might represent anger (for example, hand fractures from punching walls or a history of unexplained vehicle accidents), and evaluating the client's ability to control his impulses to act out his anger.

When working with male clients whom the nurse suspects to be easily prone to anger, the nurse should be alert for signs of developing anger such as reddening of the face, rising volume and pressure of speech, angry facial expressions, and increasing physical activity (pacing, slamming doors). It may be helpful for the nurse to state his or her observations ("You seem angry") to prompt verbal expression of the client's anger, as this both increases the nurse's understanding of the client and (in most instances) reduces the likelihood that the client will express his anger physically.

Violence and Trauma

Violence and trauma are often the effects of psychological and sociological factors. A male's socially reinforced aggressiveness and cultural role models that promote risk-taking are frequently cited explanations for the significantly greater trauma-related morbidity and mortality rates among males. ***Juvenile conduct disorder,*** involving a pattern of chronic antisocial behavior during childhood, is approximately four times more common in males than in females. ***Antisocial personality disorder,*** characterized by a chronic pattern of irresponsible and antisocial behavior that frequently involves criminal acts, is known to be three times more common among men than among women. Both of these disorders predispose males to higher risks of trauma through physically violent behavior, involvement in dangerous activities such as drug dealing, retribution from intended victims or coconspirators, and exposure to prison-based violence when incarcerated.[12]

The death rate from homicide is two-and-a-half times greater for white males than for white females, and four times greater for black males than for black females. Death rates from motor vehicle accidents are at least double for males than for females, and the distinction is even greater (approximately 3 to 1 males vs. females) among those aged 15 to 34 years.[2]

Suicide

Although some sources report that females attempt suicide more frequently than do males, males are much more likely to be successful in their suicide attempts. Among white males, the death rate for suicide for all ages is four times that of females. These figures are more dramatic when the two age groups at highest risk are compared. Males 15 to 24 years of age are almost five times as likely to die of suicide than females in the same age group, and males over 75 are eight to nine times as likely to die from suicide as their female counterparts.[2]

It is important for community nurses to appreciate the often-concealed prevalence of suicide in a community. Suicide claims more lives annually than many of the diseases that health-care professionals combat so effectively. The death rate for suicide in white males of all ages (20.1 per 100,000 population), for example, is greater than that of diabetes, liver disease, colorectal cancer, pneumonia, or AIDS.[2] Because suicide is such a high source of mortality for males, it is important that the community health nurse directly address the issue with those male clients most at risk (Box 22–2).

Clients who appear to be at risk for suicide should be directly but emphatically questioned about this possibility. For example, a nurse could state, "It would not be unusual for a person who's been through what you have to be thinking about suicide. Is that something you have considered?" Suicide assessment would further include distinguishing thoughts about suicide from actual intent and plans to initiate it, determining the client's access to lethal means of suicide (guns, heights, drugs), and the presence or absence of support persons who can ensure

BOX 22–2

Male Clients Presenting a Risk of Suicide

- Clients 15 to 24 years of age or over age 65
- Clients with chronic physical or mental disorders (particularly those that are progressively debilitating or that lead to deterioration in function)
- Clients who are depressed, or who feel hopeless or helpless
- Clients with a recent history of significant loss (death of a family member, end of a marriage)
- Clients who are intoxicated
- Clients with a history of recent or remote suicides among peers or family members
- Clients with impaired impulse control

the client's safety. It is important that the community health nurse not allow his or her own denial of the reality of suicide to limit assessment of this important threat to a male client's well-being.

Military Veterans

Military service, whether during war or during times of peace, can powerfully influence a man's identity and view of the world around him. Many military veterans continue to base their network of friends and their social activities in veterans organizations and among peers who are also veterans. As a result of this ongoing military identity, veterans sometimes demonstrate military-based behaviors in civilian settings, such as using military slang that is unfamiliar to civilians.

Another behavior sometimes seen among veterans is claiming entitlement to services. This behavior may provoke a negative reaction in community health nurses, who may view attitudes of entitlement as inappropriate, self-centered, or needlessly demanding. It is important to realize that the armed forces do reward military duty by providing various benefits (entitlements) after discharge. Consequently, a veteran's attitude of entitlement may simply reflect his military values and expectations.

Community health nurses working with veterans exhibiting this attitude may find it helpful simply to remind the veteran of the differences between the military and civilian worlds so that expectations become more realistic and misunderstandings are avoided. Nurses working with veterans, whether on an individual level or on an aggregate basis, also may benefit from familiarizing themselves with the Veterans Administration health-care system to assist in their referrals and other efforts to meet the clients' health-care needs.

Veterans who have experienced combat may suffer from an insidious and debilitating disorder that requires exceptional understanding and patience on the part of the nurse. ***Posttraumatic stress disorder*** (PTSD) is caused by exposure to traumatic events with which an individual is profoundly unable to cope. This disorder is characterized by disturbances in sleep (insomnia, nightmares), poor interpersonal relationships, modulation of emotions, vivid recollections of the traumatic episode, and by periods of profound depression. Other reactions may include rage, homicidal impulses, and suicidal tendencies. Although this disorder can occur equally readily in men or women under the same circumstances (for example, as a result of childhood sexual abuse), the much greater involvement in military combat by men and the resulting disproportionate exposure to the severe trauma of war (particularly the Vietnam War) has led to a significant number of American men with PTSD. As a measure of the magnitude of this problem, some have estimated that more Vietnam veterans have died from suicide since the war (over 100,000) than died from combat injuries during the conflict, and that over a half million Vietnam veterans may suffer from this disorder.[15]

Community nurses often encounter undiagnosed cases of PTSD, and they can be of tremendous value by case-finding and by helping PTSD sufferers to seek or accept treatment. Community health nurses should assess clients who have experienced major psychological or physical trauma for the signs and symptoms of PTSD. These can occur at any time after the trauma, ranging from days to years later. Nurses should also assess for health issues frequently accompanying PTSD, including substance abuse, violence, and risk of suicide.

Divorced Men

Divorce is one of the most significant stressors a person can experience, and it frequently has a significant effect on physical and psychological health. Divorced men in particular have been shown to experience increased morbidity and mortality as compared to married men. Males may respond to divorce or its aftermath with intense anger, a profound sense of loss, or significant depression. Suicidal behavior occasionally occurs as the male reacts to the divorce as an assault against his self-image and self-worth, or homicidal behavior if he directs his anger about his own behavior toward his ex-spouse instead.

Assessment appropriate to the issue of divorce would include evaluating the client's style of coping with stress; for example, drinking alcohol as contrasted to talking with support persons. The nurse would also assess the client's access to support personnel of adequate quality as well as the client's psychological responses such as depression, suicidal behavior, and anger. Given the impact of divorce on physical health, it would also be important to assess for stress-related physiological health problems such as exacerbation of hypertension, infectious illnesses, and cardiovascular disturbances.

Sexually Abused Males

Although society tends to think of males as abusers rather than victims, the incidence of sexual abuse of male children is surprisingly high, with studies reporting ranges of 3 percent to 30 percent.[16] Male children and adolescents typically experience significant shame and have great difficulty reporting sexual abuse and dealing with its psychological and social effects. Sexually abused males typically experience the same negative societal and professional responses that female sexual abuse victims might encounter (such as "blaming the victim" or disbelief). Additionally, many male victims of abuse either experience—or at least fear—accusations that they are homosexual. As a result, maintaining confidentiality is essential to the nursing care of the male victim of sexual abuse.

Assessment should focus on symptoms of abuse: persistent acting-out behavior, aggression, and withdrawal from family members or peers. Many males, like females, do not disclose or deal with their abuse until years later as adults.[16] Community health nurses can facilitate the disclosure of abuse by the male victim through education, supportive behavior, empathy, and actively conveying acceptance (abuse victims typically fear rejection and/or punishment).

LIFE-STYLE FACTORS

Occupation

Although the increase in the number of women in the American work force has been significant, most hazardous occupations (such as mining or agriculture) are still performed by men. In 1987 over 1750 individuals, most of them male, died from health disorders clearly linked with specific occupational hazards: coal-worker's pneumoconiosis, asbestosis, silicosis, and malignant neoplasms such as mesothelioma.[2] Males are also exposed to workplace toxins such as lead, resulting in impaired fertility and sexual functioning, anorexia and gastrointestinal distress, and (rarely in adults) encephalopathy.[10,17] Other occupational hazards that men typically face more frequently than women include exposure to chemical agents, physical agents (temperature extremes, sunlight), mechanical agents (vibration, repetitive-use syndromes), and psychosocial agents (stress and burnout, role models of poor health habits such as smoking).[18]

Assessment of occupational health pertaining to the male client would include determining the physical, chemical, and psychosocial hazards existing in the client's work environment. Whenever possible, the community nurse would collaborate with the occupational health nurse in determining which risks would be most likely in a given work setting, and in using that data to determine which health disorders or needs would be appropriate for further evaluation. For example, a nurse working with a male client who had been a coal miner for two decades would consult with occupational health nurses or other professionals to determine that "black lung" (pneumoconiosis) is a significant occupational hazard for miners. The community nurse would use this information to assess the client's respiratory function and activity tolerance. Additional assessment recommendations are presented in Chapter 27, Care of Clients in the Work Setting.

Consumption Patterns

Five times as many males as females are described as heavy users of alcohol (those consuming more than an ounce of pure alcohol each day). The incidence of alcohol use by males aged 12 to 25 is 5 percent to 40 percent greater than for females. Alcohol abuse is widely known for its negative affect on physical and emotional health. For example, at least 40 percent of all traffic fatalities involve alcohol. With respect to drug abuse, males over age 18 use marijuana and cocaine twice as frequently as do females. Drug abuse is strongly correlated with criminal behavior, physical trauma, and homicide, all of which are significant social and health risks disproportionately evident among males.

Assessment by the community health nurse for alcohol abuse includes observation for signs of intoxication (slurred speech, ataxia, unexplained behavioral changes), the presence of an alcohol odor on the client's breath, or evidence of empty alcohol containers. It is also important to assess the client's family history and social circumstances for evidence that alcohol use is prevalent or supported by others. The nurse should also assess the client for the possible presence of depression, as this disorder may either predispose to, or result from, alcoholism.[19]

When assessing for physiologic changes suggesting substance abuse, the nurse should look for unexplained sedation or hyperactivity, dilated or constricted pupils, or elevated vital signs. The community health nurse also should be observant for signs that a client who abuses substances may be experiencing withdrawal: elevated vital signs, hallucinations (particularly tactile and visual forms), irritability, unexplained pain, diaphoresis, psychomotor restlessness or hyperactivity, delirium, and seizures. It is also helpful to assess the client's knowledge of the risks attendant to substance abuse, as well as his motivation to alter his behavior. Detailed assessment information concerning drug and alcohol use appears in Chapter 33, Substance Abuse.

Cigarette smoking is considered the single most preventable cause of death in American society.[2] Thirty-one percent of males over age 18 are smokers compared with 26.7 percent of females (although males who do smoke report smoking less frequently than do females).[2] Males clearly dominate in the use of chewed forms of tobacco and experience an increased risk of oral cancers as a result. Assessment would focus on determining the form and frequency of the client's tobacco use, his knowledge of the health-related risks of smoking, and the client's motivation to quit smoking.

Leisure

Men and women increasingly share similar leisure patterns in American culture. Nevertheless, men still tend to be more active in competitive contact sports and, more often than women, to choose leisure activities involving some degree of physical risk (skydiving, white-water rafting, rock climbing). Moreover, males also tend to choose leisure activities associated with alcohol consumption. For these reasons, men experience relatively greater incidence of recreation-related trauma. Community health nurses should assess male clients' leisure pursuits relative to their risk of producing injury. The nurse should also assess the client's understanding of the risks involved in his leisure behaviors, and his knowledge and use of safety techniques or equipment to reduce health risks (for example, eye shields and helmets during contact sports and bicycling).

Sexuality

Once separated by a double standard that encouraged sexual activity by men while discouraging it for women, male and female sexual behavior has grown to have more similarities than differences in many respects. Consequently, the psychosocial aspects of the sexually related health needs of men and women are very similar. For male clients, the differences often involve their physiology. For example, while cystitis is less common in men, males do develop prostatitis and urethritis. Community health nurses should assess male clients' sexual behaviors as they relate to health in a manner similar to that used for female clients, determining the client's knowledge and use of safer sexual practices, the presence or absence of symptoms of sexually transmitted diseases, and the presence of behaviors that may increase the risk of sexually related disorders.

HEALTH SYSTEM FACTORS

Men tend to define health very differently from the way women define it, often viewing health as the ability to complete certain functions rather than as the presence or absence of specific symptoms. For example, a man who is obese, hypertensive, and diabetic may nonetheless feel in good health because he is able to perform what he considers to be necessary role functions at work and home. Moreover, males tend to have fewer contacts with the health-care system than do women, perhaps because of psychological and sociological factors such as a reluctance to see themselves as needing assistance. This is all the more surprising in that the majority of physicians are male, so male clients typically would have little difficulty obtaining services from someone of the same gender.

The American health-care system tends to focus on health from an illness perspective, with relatively little attention afforded to prevention. This state of affairs parallels the health-seeking behaviors of many male clients, who tend to focus on their health only when symptoms are significant enough to interfere with role function. Consequently, the relative lack of concern in prevention seen among many males is reinforced by the prevailing attitudes and operation of the health-care system.

As is true of the population at large, men who are unemployed or employed in low-paying or part-time jobs typically lack health insurance and, therefore, experience a barrier to health-care services. Men who are employed, however, may also find it difficult to access health-care services because their work hours conflict with those of health-care providers.

Community nurses should assess male clients for self-images (for example, invulnerability) that reduce the motivation to utilize health-care services. Nurses should also assess male clients for other factors that serve as barriers or motivators relative to accessing the health-care system, such as work hours, value placed on health, ability to function in important roles despite health problems, and financial resources such as insurance.

SPECIAL FOCUS: ASSESSING THE GAY MALE CLIENT

Approximately 4 percent to 10 percent of males are believed to be homosexual in their sexual orientation, a rate thought by some to be twice that of females. Male homosexuals (gay men) are at increased risk of experiencing certain health problems compared to heterosexuals, may have different health-care needs, and may benefit from different approaches to nursing care. Appendix L, Health Assessment Guide—Adult Client, can be modified to direct assessment of the homosexual client.

Although earlier perspectives on homosexuality held that it was the result of the Devil's influence, hostility toward the opposite sex, incomplete psychological development, inadequate parenting, or some noxious environmental influences (for example, being sexually assaulted), current theories focus instead on prenatal hormonal imbalances or choices an individual makes based on his or her own personality. Although the origins of homosexuality are not yet known, it is certain that there exists a range of sexual orientations among individuals, with many being neither exclusively heterosexual nor exclusively homosexual. Research also suggests that most homosexually oriented persons do not differ in any psychological, physical, or social respect from their heterosexual peers. These views often conflict with those held by some people, and these conflicts may significantly affect the health behavior and status of gay men. The following discussion examines male homosexuality by following Dever's epidemiologic model.

HUMAN BIOLOGICAL FACTORS

Although research findings are inconclusive, some studies suggest that there may be genetic or physiologic origins for homosexual orientations. These include an imbalance in the amounts of male and female hormones during the prenatal period, or an abnormality in the estrogen feedback response of gay men.[20] Homosexual activities are associated with significantly higher risks of selected physical health disorders. A major concern relative to the health of gay men is that of sexually transmitted diseases (STDs), in particularly HIV and AIDS. Gay clients experience a significantly greater risk of STDs because of the nature of their sexual practices and physiology. For example, anal-receptive intercourse readily traumatizes the highly vascularized intestinal mucosa, leading to increased susceptibility to entrance of infectious organisms. For this reason the community health nurse needs to assess carefully the safety of the sexual practices of gay clients, the client's experience of symptoms suggesting STDs, and the client's history of exposure to high-risk sexual partners.

ENVIRONMENTAL FACTORS

The social environment of gay men, once believed in some cases to be the cause of homosexuality, is now known for its likelihood of negatively affecting this client subgroup. Beliefs that gay men are psychiatrically ill, deviants, sinners, or criminals have been, and continue to be, anything but rare in American culture. The American Psychiatric Association considered homosexuality to be a psychiatric disorder up until 1974, and many states maintain laws against homosexual activities to this day. Gay men live in a social environment that often considers their behavior as highly unacceptable and that discriminates against them in both overt and covert ways. Gay males experience significant amounts of social stigmatization. They may fear loss of career potential or jobs, shunning by heterosexual peers, or loss of civil rights. Rarely are homosexual relationships legally recognized; this results in discrimination in awarding health-care benefits, distributing communally acquired property, and enacting of inheritance and child custody rights. Consequently, gay men may prefer to conceal their sexual preferences to avoid experiencing discrimination in work or social settings. As a result, it is essential that community health nurses make a special effort to establish a high degree of trust to enhance their effectiveness in assessing the health-related behaviors and concerns of this population. Nurses should emphasize the confidential nature of the nurse-client relationship and convey empathy regarding the stigma faced by gay men.

Psychologically, gay men may find themselves unable to access the usual support systems heterosexual men use to cope with health and social concerns. This may result in increased stress in some circumstances, though the research suggests that most gay men adjust well to their circumstances and are no less uncomfortable in their circumstances than are their heterosexual male counterparts. However, one psychological factor is known to be a great concern for gay men—fear and anxiety related to encounters with homophobia and other potentially dangerous responses to their sexual orientation. Homophobia is an irrational fear of homosexuality that may manifest itself through discriminatory behavior, demeaning or derogatory comments and humor, or actual physical assaults. Some homophobics feel they have a right to assault homosexuals owing to their belief that homosexuals are criminals or deviants.

An additional source of fear for gay men is physical assault and robbery. This may be because aggressors believe gay men will be less able to resist or less willing to report crimes because of their desire to maintain the secrecy of their life-style. Finally, gay men may feel compelled to conceal their sexual orientation from the heterosexual world to such an extent that they experience significant isolation; they cannot reveal their romantic joys or losses, nor share their longing for children, nor display the routine forms of affection accepted between members of the opposite sex. This latter problem is more acute for gay men than for lesbians because people are more likely to perceive hugs, hand-holding, or dancing between men as homosexual (and therefore unacceptable) behavior than between females.

As a result of these psychological factors, community health nurses should assess the gay male client's coping skills and access to support systems, his self-esteem (it is difficult to maintain self-esteem in the face of widespread societal rejection), and his preferences relative to privacy and confidentiality.

LIFE-STYLE FACTORS

Many myths exist regarding the life-styles of gay men. Beliefs commonly held by society at large are that gay men are very different from heterosexual men in nonsexual matters as well as sexual ones; that they have very different longings and romantic needs; and that they are highly promiscuous. In reality, the majority of gay men maintain life-styles not significantly different from those of their heterosexual male counterparts. Even "cruising," the active seeking of new and varied sexual partners, is shunned by at least 40 percent of gay men.[21] Furthermore, cruising is almost always limited to gay social settings only, with no effort being made to "seduce" heterosexuals into homosexual life-styles (another myth). However, for those gay men who do engage in frequent changes of sexual partners, there is clearly a greater risk of STDs.

Many gay men desire to become parents and to succeed in this role; the children raised by gay men are as well-adjusted (and rarely more prone to homosexuality themselves) as those raised by a heterosexual couples. Gay men work in all occupations, and contrary to popular conjecture they do not disproportionately enter careers usually associated with females. In terms of social habits, some research suggests that gay men may have more close friendships and interpersonal support than do heterosexual men.[21] In addition, while a small number of gay men may behave in an overtly or even exaggeratedly feminine manner, the great majority do not appear physically or behaviorally different from heterosexual men. Finally, no clearly established difference has been shown in the consumption patterns of gay men, especially with respect to substance abuse.

In terms of nursing assessment and client lifestyle, the major area for assessment involves sexual behaviors. It is beneficial to stress the rationale for seeking this information, emphasizing that the community nurse's concern is based solely in the client's health risks and needs. Factors to evaluate include patterns of sexual activity, sexual exposure, and knowledge of sex-related risks and safety procedures. Bisexual men with female spouses may be even more concerned with privacy and confidentiality issues in order to maintain their concurrent heterosexual relationships; this may require significant amounts of reassurance and empathy from the nurse.

The occupational risks and concerns experienced by gay men relate primarily to avoiding discrimination and rejection in the workplace. No clearly established occupational health risks pertain to homosexual life-styles. It should be noted, however, that in occupational settings where masculine roles are stereotypical and exaggerated (for example, steel mills), there may be an increased incidence of acting out of homophobic thinking, resulting in an increased risk to a gay man's safety due either to assault or failure to provide assistance. Nursing assessment should focus on such potential safety risks and should consider the possibility that gay men who are unable to accept their sexual orientation may themselves enact exaggerated masculine roles—and experience the related safety risks these behaviors may entail.

HEALTH SYSTEM FACTORS

Gay men may encounter homophobia among health-care workers, and the perception of homophobia represents a significant barrier to health care. Even when the health-care provider, whether an individual or an institution, is devoid of homophobia, various circumstances may threaten the gay client and act as a health barrier. For example, assessment questions about birth control practices, if answered truthfully, might have the effect of requiring that a client disclose his homosexuality. For the client who fears loss of health-care benefits (due to assumed higher risk of AIDS for all gay men), this is very much a situation to be avoided. To best serve gay clients it will be necessary to ensure that American health-care institutions and personnel do not in any way discriminate or limit services to this population. Unless American society is able to overcome its biases and its homophobic responses (now heightened by the AIDS epidemic), the health-care system may remain as much a threat to gay men as it is a benefit. Community health nurses can improve these circumstances by challenging their own prejudices and subconscious fears, by seeking to enlighten themselves about homosexuality and sexuality in general, by actively conveying acceptance of all persons, and by working to make all assessments and interventions sexually neutral (neither presuming nor eliciting a particular sexual orientation) wherever feasible.

DIAGNOSTIC REASONING AND CARE OF THE MALE CLIENT

Community health nurses use data from their client assessments to identify health needs and determine appropriate nursing diagnoses. Nursing diagnoses for individual male clients may relate to educational deficits (for example "increased health risk due to lack of knowledge of TSE technique"), to barriers to health-care utilization (for example, "failure to cope with stress related to belief that men should not need help in coping"), to consequences of specific health problems (for example, "pain due to overuse of strained ligaments," or "diminished self-esteem due to lost erectile functioning related to prostatectomy"). Nursing diagnoses may also relate to males as aggregates. For example, many young adult males living in poverty might merit the community health nurse's diagnosis of "increased health risk related to socioeconomic pressures to participate in drug use and sales."

PLANNING AND IMPLEMENTATION

PRIMARY PREVENTION

Although it is difficult to generalize about male clients' attitudes to health-promotion activities, there are some commonly encountered patterns of health behavior among men. One such behavior is a tendency to view exercise as sufficient to compensate for unhealthy behaviors such as a high intake of fats in the diet. Men also tend to attribute greater significance to health changes they can sense than to those they cannot (for example, they can sense pain, but not elevated blood pressure). Because men tend to rate their health as very good or excellent more often than women,[2] they may feel they do not need to be actively involved in health-promotion activities. They may also err in their health appraisal efforts, stemming from a tendency to believe that their past athletic or current work activities may provide for their present health needs ("When I was a teenager I would run all day." "I work hard all day in the fresh air. What could be healthier than that?")

One technique that can be used to promote positive behavioral change is reframing, which was discussed earlier in the chapter and which focuses on helping the client to see the same situation in a different light.[22] A second technique for promoting change involves emphasizing alternate ways of coping with anxiety or fearfulness. Education, of course, is a crucial aspect of any primary prevention strategy. Education is perhaps most effective when teaching is initiated with school-age male youngsters, as this is the stage when lifelong health values and habits are forming. Health promotion by the client's family members is known to be a significant motivator and predictor of client compliance and outcomes, and involvement of family members in educational efforts and treatment planning is usually of significant benefit.

Primary prevention for health concerns specific to male clients focuses on increasing the client's use of health-promoting behaviors in the areas of cardiovascular and cerebrovascular disorders, hypertension, cancer, occupational disorders, substance abuse, violence and trauma, suicide, and posttraumatic stress disorder.

Cardiovascular disorders involve education as a major primary prevention measure. The community health nurse provides education in home, school, or occupational settings, and emphasizes knowledge of risk factors and preventive strategies. The nurse also emphasizes methods to produce behavioral changes, recognizing that knowledge alone does not determine behavior. For example, most male clients *know* the importance of limiting fat-derived calories, but they fall short in being able to change their behavior because they lack understanding of their own behavioral dynamics (such as eating more when anxious).

Cerebrovascular disorders also involve education as a major preventative strategy. The community nurse educates clients about the relationship between other health problems, such as hypertension and diabetes, and cerebrovascular disease. The nurse educates and motivates the client to maintain a weight and blood pressure appropriate to his age in order to control hypertension and minimize the risk of developing some forms of diabetes.

Hypertension can be minimized for many male clients by promoting a weight appropriate for the client's body build, and by promotion of regular exercise. A diet that excludes excessive sodium may have preventative value as well. For some clients, knowledge and use of stress-management techniques such as stress compensators (relaxing walks, vacations) or relaxation techniques (progressive muscle relaxation, guided imagery) may assist in minimizing hypertensive changes. It is helpful to focus on the fact that the hypertensive client is typically asymptomatic, as this feature encourages ***denial*** (a way of responding to fear) and avoidance (which are already prominent among many male clients). Again, it is helpful to link efforts to control hypertension with the client's own values about health, such as invulnerability or physical activity. For example, the nurse could take advantage of the client's interest in sports by noting famous athletes with hypertension.

Primary prevention interventions for cancer include education regarding recognizing and limiting exposure to carcinogens in the workplace (such as chemicals and sunlight), around the home, or in the diet. The possibility of a link between stress and immune system functioning supports the promotion of effective stress-management techniques. Life-style choices such as smoking and consuming large amounts of meat are believed to have a significant effect on an individual's risk of cancer. Ascribing healthy behaviors to masculine role images can increase cancer-preventative behaviors in male clients by tying such behaviors to male values such as strength and power. For example, a nurse could state, "Men do what makes them strong, not what makes them weak, and smoking weakens the body." It may also be helpful to reframe male clients' poor health habits as being the result of manipulation by advertisers (for example, "I wonder whether eating all that meat might be because all your life the commercials have made eating meat seem like the right thing to do").

Primary prevention interventions for substance abuse focus on education at all age levels regarding the risks of substance abuse and on alternate means of coping with stress. Also important are efforts to assist males to redefine their social roles in healthier ways so that, for instance, teenage males do not feel as compelled to drink or to behave as their peers might wish. In addition, a community health nurse's activities that help reshape societal norms held by males, such as the anti-drinking publicity campaign undertaken by Mothers Against Drunk Driving, are also appropriate primary prevention measures.

Trauma and violence are complicated issues with many potential levels of nursing interventions. Primary-level interventions include educating male children on methods of coping with their feelings and countering social demands to take unnecessary risks or to participate in unhealthy behaviors. Teaching males nondestructive ways to express their feelings and initiating political activity on behalf of safety-related legislation (motorcycle helmet laws, enforcement of driving under-the-influence statutes) are also appropriate as primary prevention interventions.

Important nursing interventions related to sexually abused male clients include educating key persons about the realities of male sexual abuse (school teachers, case managers, school nurses), and detecting families at risk. It is also important to facilitate referrals to treatment agencies specializing in sexual abuse of children or adults. Finally, while pairing male nurses with male clients for the purposes of providing care for issues involving male sexuality can be a very helpful strategy, this may not be the case with the child or adolescent male abuse victim, who may instead feel more secure working with a female nurse.

Community health nursing interventions appropriate for the angry client include role-playing a situation that prompts anger so as to identify effective responses to that situation. It is also important to identify and support alternative responses to situations that provoke anger and to find more constructive ways of expressing anger.[23]

Primary prevention measures for suicide include helping a male client to avoid or cope with such feelings of despair, hopelessness, or anger. Interventions that help a male avoid or cope with such feelings include role-modeling, teaching disclosure of one's feelings, and prompting expression of a client's concerns through the use of empathy and acceptance. Also helpful are interventions designed to promote self-esteem and a positive self-image. Such interventions should begin with young males, prior even to school age. The community nurse can promote the use of mental health resources that provide services to individuals or groups. Nurses can also educate families, children, workers, and other groups about the risk of suicide, factors that contribute to its occurrence, and appropriate ways to detect and respond to persons within their midst who are at increased risk of becoming suicidal. Males should be educated about their high degree of risk, especially those males who are younger than 24 and over age 65.

Posttraumatic stress disorder (PTSD) involves primary prevention of a more immediate sort—aiding the male victim to express his feelings about the traumatic experience in a supportive and accepting environment. By aiding the client to work through his feelings about the trauma rather than being overwhelmed by them, the community health nurse can prevent or minimize the severity of this disorder. However, in that PTSD is a complex psychological disorder, the community health nurse usually works in an adjunctive capacity with more expert or specialized providers within the mental-health-care system. Vietnam veterans with PTSD may benefit greatly from referral to peer-run "Vet Centers" and other support groups. A list of these is available from the Veterans Administration or local veterans organizations. Nurses should also understand that Vietnam vets with PTSD, and veterans in general, are distrustful of government-related providers. For this reason a veteran may respond more favorably when the nurse relates to him as an individual rather than as an agent of a health-care organization. A willingness to accept the veteran and a high level of trustworthiness are characteristics highly valued by Vietnam vets.

Primary prevention interventions relating to adolescent factors include aiding the adolescent to reevaluate images he holds regarding the male role; assisting the client to express his feelings through role-modeling; teaching communication and social skills; conveying empathy and acceptance; and raising issues experienced by most male adolescents. Nurses can also intervene at the primary level by promoting effective parent-child relationships via education about growth and development and communication skills, provided to both the client and his family.

Primary prevention measures for newly divorced men include referrals to peer support groups, encouragement of socialization and activities, and referral to mental health professionals when indicated (some mental health agencies sponsor special programs for newly divorced persons). It is also helpful for the community health nurse to provide support, assist the client to express his feelings, and guide him in coping with periods of crisis that may ensue.[24]

For the gay or bisexual male client, providing education to increase the safety of sexual practices is an extremely important primary prevention measure. Community health nurses can perform a very valuable function by promoting safer sexual practices such as condom use and encouraging clients to reduce the number of sexual partners. These efforts are enhanced by conveying openness, showing acceptance of the client, and displaying an intent to address issues in a confidential and professional manner. Community health nurses sometimes find themselves ill prepared to meet the needs of homosexual clients due to a poor understanding of homosexuality. Some sources of information for nurses and services for homosexual clients are listed in Table 22-1.

Community health nurses may sometimes find themselves in a position wherein a health-promoting intervention (such as reporting an adolescent substance abuser) may also have repercussions within the client's family or result in the client becoming enmeshed in the criminal justice system. The nurse should remember that it is not his or her actions that produce these consequences; rather, it is the actions of the individual that have led to such an outcome. Instead of experiencing guilt, the nurse should reframe nursing actions so that they can clearly be perceived as health promoting.

SECONDARY PREVENTION

Secondary prevention involves the earliest possible detection of health needs, using the assessment techniques described earlier in this chapter. It also encompasses the actual treatment of the health needs or disorders themselves. Secondary prevention roles for community health nurses working with male clients are appropriate for all disorders discussed in this chapter via special efforts to assess male clients in high-risk categories such as agricultural workers (trauma, skin cancer), teenagers (trauma, suicide, substance abuse), gay or bisexual males (AIDS), and those over age 50 (prostate cancer, cardiovascular disorders).

Community health nurses may also participate in health-screening activities by providing or encouraging the client's use of health measures such as blood pressure screening and cardiovascular risk-assessment programs in public, educational, or occupational settings. Nurses can also facilitate the offering and use of screening examinations by other health-care professionals within the community, such as rectal examinations and blood testing for prostate cancer and chest X-rays for lung cancer. Early detection of both prostate and testicular cancer are very important areas for secondary prevention by community health nurses.

One intervention that facilitates detection of testicular cancer is teaching testicular self-examination technique (TSE), which was touched upon earlier in this chapter. Because testicular cancer occurs primarily in young men, the community health nurse can often educate and motivate clients efficiently (and minimize individual embarrassment in the process) by working with groups of males in school or work settings.

The TSE technique involves a gentle but thorough palpation of each testis, repeated monthly and akin to the procedure for breast self-examination. The male client should rotate each testis gently, moving his fingers so that all portions of the organ are palpated. He should feel uniform smoothness, without indentations, lumps, or dissymmetry within an individual testis. Abnormal findings, along with any other changes noted since the last TSE, should be promptly reported to his physician. It is helpful for the nurse to inform the client that it is normal for one

TABLE 22–1. RESOURCES FOR ASSISTING HOMOSEXUAL CLIENTS

Agency or Organization	Services
Council for Sex Information and Education Box 72 Capitola, CA 95010	Information on sexuality
Dignity-National 755 Boylston Boston, MA 02116	Counseling and support for Roman Catholic homosexuals
Dykes and Tykes New York Chapter Box 621 Old Chelsea Station New York, NY 10011	Social and legal help for homosexuals and their children
Gay Activist Alliances New York Chapter 399 Lafayette St. New York, NY 10011	Classes, public information, legal help
Integrity/San Francisco P.O. Box 6444 San Francisco, CA 94150 (408) 268-3378	Counseling and support for Episcopalian homosexuals
Metropolitan Community Church Box 1757 New York, NY 10011 (212) 691-7428	Social support, counseling, advocacy for Christian homosexuals
National Gay Task Force 80 Fifth Avenue New York, NY 10011 (212) 741-1010	Civil rights advocacy for homosexuals
Sex Information and Education Council of United States 80 Fifth Avenue, Suite 801 New York, NY 10011 (212) 929-2300	Public information, education on sexuality

testis to be larger than the other, and that the client may encounter other intrascrotal structures apart from the testes themselves, so that the client, for example, will not presume the epididymis is an abnormal finding. The ideal source of instruction for this technique would be direct guidance by a physician or nurse practitioner during a physical examination. Referrals to these providers are an appropriate form of secondary intervention.

Younger male clients may experience even more embarrassment about sexually related issues than their older counterparts, and significant attention to averting this embarrassment and anxiety is indicated. Humor may be a very helpful tool in that it is a common coping mechanism used by younger males in this age group for dealing with anxiety. Three-dimensional models, slides, and other teaching devices can be quite beneficial by giving the anxious male client something to focus on other than the (usually) opposite-sex nurse. Assignment of male nurses to this population may also reduce clients' hesitancy or embarrassment, as can creating an environment where male clients can feel free to face and voice their fears about their own mortality.

The community health nurse is not usually directly involved in the detection and screening of prostate cancer. Detection is usually achieved by digital (rectal) examination or by ultrasound examination. In addition, blood screening for a prostate-specific antigen promises to be more effective than rectal screening alone at early identification of prostate cancer.[25] Early detection of prostate cancer can also be aided by psychosocial-oriented nursing interventions. For example, education about the risk of this disorder among older males helps counter the denial experienced by many men (due to a need to perceive oneself as invulnerable, perhaps), and informing the client of the importance of annual digital (rectal) examinations increases health-promoting behavior. Many times such teaching can be effectively enacted with male clients in work or social settings (for example, a senior citizen's organization). It is important to stress the very positive prognosis that accompanies early detection so as to help motivate the client by compensating for the uncomfortable—but necessary—rectal examination.

Community health nurses do participate in the treatment of other illnesses experienced by male clients. In the case of ischemic and certain other cardiac disorders, for example, stress has been shown to impact negatively on treatment outcomes, in some cases leading to a threefold increase in mortality (for post-myocardial-infarction clients, for example). Treatment programs that identify high-stress clients during hospitalization, that track and reduce their stress levels after discharge, and that provide prompt assistance from nurses in the community when episodes of increased stress occur can result in significant reduction of the stress-related mortality experienced by post-myocardial-infarction clients.[26]

Prostatitis is another disorder with implications for secondary prevention by the community health nurse. Prostatitis is usually responsive to a regimen of antibiotics, and education about the nature of the disorder (particularly when sexually transmitted) and its treatment is the major area of nursing intervention. In that it is a personally intimate and uniquely male phenomenon, however, there is likely to be embarrassment and avoidance on the part of the male client. The nurse can manage this response pattern by being straightforward and matter-of-fact when discussing the issue, and by noting that, while perhaps embarrassing, the disorder is not unlike having cystitis or other common infections. In effect, the nurse is using reframing. Interventions for prostatitis also apply to the rarer epidymititis.

Benign prostatic hyperplasia, or BPH, also involves the nurse at the secondary level of prevention. Here the nurse can educate the male client about his risk of this disorder, and by being straightforward and professional in demeanor, the nurse can reduce the client's embarrassment about assessment questions and examinations used to screen older male clients for this disorder. An important part of the detection process involves noting that rectal examinations are an essential examination for early detection of BPH as well as prostatic cancer. The nurse should instruct the client that, while this examination may not be pleasant to experience, it in effect serves double duty—and is therefore doubly valuable. In terms of treatment, community health nurses may find themselves assisting the client with postoperative catheter care at home, and interventions to reduce embarrassment apply here as well.

Nurses can assist male clients with mild inguinal hernias to succeed in conservative treatment strategies and avert the need for surgery. One intervention involves education and encouragement to motivate the client's compliance with wearing supportive trusses, limiting exertion, and using proper body mechanics (to reduce straining and increased intra-abdominal pressure). Inguinal hernias involve both an intimate area of the body and an image of weakness rather than power. As a result many men may delay treatment for this disorder because of embarrassment or fear of surgery. Nurses can assist the client by helping him to overcome his embarrassment and reframing his interpretation of this disorder as a weakness. By being open and up-front about this condition the nurse can demonstrate that it does not require embarrassment, and in fact for many males is part of being a man. These interventions also promote compliance with conservative treatment approaches.

TERTIARY PREVENTION

Tertiary prevention for male clients is directed at those disorders that influence the client in some ongoing manner or that have a likelihood of recurrence. The goals of tertiary prevention are to assist the client in coping with the continuing manifestations of his illness, and to reduce the likelihood of future episodes of an illness. To this end, it is useful to group tertiary prevention measures into care directed toward those disorders that affect a male's sexual functioning or sexual identity or as they present a threat to notions about male strength. Tertiary prevention measures also would be directed at supporting a client's compliance with a long-term course of treatment.

One area for tertiary prevention measures by the community health nurse involves those disorders that affect the male client's sexual functioning or sexual identity such as testicular and prostate cancers or any male reproductive system disorder. Male clients with testicular or prostate cancer may face significant emotional distress owing to the effect that surgical treatment may have on their sexuality. Prostate cancer is treated by surgical removal of the gland in most instances. Although the prognosis is often excellent when discovered early,[10] the surgery itself may result in impotency (though recent nerve-sparing surgical techniques have reduced this problem).[6] Similarly, the treatment for testicular cancer is surgical removal of the affected testes followed by hormonal therapy.[10] These treatments, along with their side effects (loss of fertility, emasculation), can have a profound impact on the client's self-image and psychosocial functioning.

An important area of tertiary prevention in this regard involves encouraging the male client to join support groups. Interaction with other men who have experienced the same problems can be very effective in facilitating the client's adjustment to a treatment that has so tangibly affected his sense of masculinity. On a one-to-one basis, the nurse can be accepting, supportive, and facilitative of the male client's expression of his feeling of loss.

Some disorders may affect the male client's sense of strength; this is particularly true of cardiovascular disorders. The heart is a symbol of masculine strength for some men. Consequently, cardiovascular disorders not only can leave residual symptoms and physiological impairment but can also threaten a male's self-image. Males with cardiovascular disease often benefit from interventions that support their self-image as masculine, and by discussing their feelings about their illness. As noted elsewhere, stress-management training also can have a significant positive effect on the outcome of a male client who has cardiovascular disease. These interventions are essential to promote the client's adjustment and compliance with treatment.

Of course, community health nurses should also support and reinforce the male client's positive responses to cardiac rehabilitation efforts initiated in other treatment settings. Foremost among these would be weight control, limiting intake of saturated fats, maintaining regular exercise, compliance with follow-up examinations and medications, and control of other disorders that exacerbate cardiovascular disorders (hypertension, diabetes).

In the case of some chronic disorders—especially those producing no overt symptoms—male clients tend to be lax about complying with long-term treatment recommendations. This is especially true for male clients with hypertension. Interventions that help the male client understand the importance of controlling this disorder and that build on his perceptions of masculinity are very helpful. Maintaining a regimen of antihypertensive medications may be especially difficult for male clients owing to side effects that interfere with what the client judges to be necessary masculine roles. Examples of such side effects could include impotence, dizziness, and decreased tolerance for physical activity. Nurses can assist the male client by teaching ways to compensate for these side effects, thereby helping him to maintain a sense of control over his own circumstances. In cases where the side effects are not manageable and are affecting the client's masculinity (impotence), collaborating with the client's physician or assisting the client to discuss the problem with the physician can lead to acceptance of the treatment for hypertension.

Male clients with Tourette's syndrome often experience significant decreases in their self-esteem because of the social embarrassment they encounter as a result of their singular vocal mannerisms and behavioral tics. Interventions that promote self-esteem can be very beneficial; in particular the use of empathy, an accepting attitude, and referral to support groups for those with this disorder are very helpful for this purpose. Also, assisting the client to cope with medication side effects may promote increased compliance and improved symptom control.

Preventing recidivism in instances of substance abuse is a major tertiary intervention in working with male clients. Interventions that decrease the likelihood of recidivism include encouragement of the client's use of therapeutic support groups (Alcoholics Anonymous), and education regarding factors that predispose the client to continued substance abuse (poor coping skills, co-dependent relationships, maintaining social contacts with abusers). It is also important for the community health nurse to consider the client's family and significant others when caring for the substance-abusing male. Families and significant others can be either enablers of substance abuse or corrective forces leading to its elimination. Education of family and support persons as to those behaviors that produce improvement and those that permit further substance abuse is essential, and referrals to family treatment and support services are also of value. Finally, substance abuse can also negatively affect self-esteem, and the interventions described for Tourette's syndrome may also benefit the substance abuser.

EVALUATION

As when working with other individual clients or aggregates, community health nursing plans and interventions are evaluated by determining the degree to which client goals have been met. It is also important to determine whether the interventions were efficient. Could the same results have been accomplished with less expense of time or other resources?

The community health nurse also needs to consider the client's reaction to nursing interventions. Is the client satisfied with the nurse's efforts and with the manner in which interventions were planned and implemented as well as with their results? The goal of evaluation is to ensure that client needs are met and to improve the nurse's abilities; inviting the critique of one's clients and colleagues is an excellent source of feedback.

CHAPTER HIGHLIGHTS

- Males differ in both their physiology and their psychology. They tend to see health in terms of role functioning and symptomatology, and they exhibit differing patterns of health-promotion behavior and health-care utilization.
- Men are typically more prone to exhibit denial, aggression, and avoidance. They often have a need to fulfill societally prescribed masculine roles such as strength, power, risk-taking, and invulnerability. These attitudes may become barriers that interfere with male health.
- Men may have difficulty expressing feelings, particularly if the feelings seem contrary to masculine roles. They also may experience significant reluctance to address issues involving physical or interpersonal intimacy, and as a result they may experience poorer health.
- Men have a higher incidence and mortality of cardiovascular and cerebrovascular disorders, hypertension, cancer (in particular lung and colorectal). Men also have a higher incidence of Tourette's syndrome and inguinal hernias.
- Physical disorders that occur only in men include prostatitis (infection of the prostate gland), benign prostatic hyperplasia (growth of the prostate leading to impaired urinary flow), prostatic and testicular cancer, and hydrocele (fluid buildup within the scrotum).
- Education concerning the impact of life-style on health is a major intervention with male clients because of the much higher mortality rates for trauma, suicide, homicide, and alcohol-related health problems. Guiding males to adjust their views of masculine roles is an important way to alter the risk-taking behavior and sense of invulnerability that diminish male health.
- Nursing interventions that allow men to disclose and discuss their feelings are health-promoting because they enable males to cope more effectively with stress and health matters.
- Nursing interventions to reduce embarrassment and reluctance to deal with issues involving physical and interpersonal intimacy include being empathic, matter-of-fact, and straightforward in one's approach; actively conveying acceptance and support; and using humor where appropriate.
- Men often respond well to peer pressure and support. Primary prevention in group settings (school, occupational, or social) can be very effective in influencing male health behaviors. On a secondary intervention level, males often respond well to the support and guidance available in peer support groups.
- Case finding is an important role of community health nurses, especially in the areas of substance abuse, sexual abuse, and homicidal and suicidal tendencies on the part of the client.
- Countertransference (being unduly influenced by one's emotional response to a client) can be aroused by male behavior, and it can interfere with the nurse's objectivity and effectiveness. Active self-awareness and management of one's feelings are essential countermeasures.
- Male clients may present a greater safety risk to the nurse owing to societal role stereotypes, aggressiveness, and poor modulation of anger. Safety interventions for the nurse include using people and objects/structures to serve as inhibitors of male aggression, being clear about limits on client behavior, terminating contacts immediately when the risk of danger is suspected, and conducting oneself in a safety-conscious manner.
- Men are sometimes the victims of sexual abuse as children. Teaching those in contact with children to identify such abuse and facilitating the male's disclosure of such abuse so that specialized treatment may be arranged are important nursing interventions.

Review Questions

1. Describe three factors that may influence male clients' responses to care by community health nurses. Give at least one example of ways that the community health nurse might influence each factor to enhance the effectiveness of nursing care. (p. 524)
2. Identify at least four factors that may contribute to aggression against the community health nurse by a male client. (p. 525)
3. Describe at least five considerations in assessing the effects of human biological factors on the health of men. (p. 527)
4. Identify at least three environmental influences on men's health. (p. 530)
5. Describe four areas for consideration in assessing life-style factors influencing men's health. (p. 533)
6. Identify at least two effects of the health-care system on the health of male clients. (p. 534)
7. Describe at least three factors that contribute to adverse health effects for male homosexual clients. (p. 535)
8. Identify at least four areas for primary prevention with male clients. How might the community health nurse be involved in each? (p. 537)
9. Describe at least four secondary prevention considerations for male clients. Give an example of at least one community health nursing intervention related to each consideration. (p. 539)
10. Identify at least three areas of emphasis in tertiary prevention for male clients. How might the community health nurse be involved in each? (p. 541)

APPLICATION AND SYNTHESIS

You are a community health nurse working with a hypertensive, diabetic, middle-aged single mother for the past year. Her 17-year-old son has had hand surgery and has been added to your caseload for wound and cast care. On your next meeting with the mother you discover that she is very upset about her son's behavior. He broke his hand when he punched a wall in a fit of anger, and the necessary care has hurt the family's very limited finances. The mother reports that she believes her son is drinking, and she is especially angry and upset about this because her ex-husband had deserted the family largely because of his own alcohol abuse. While the mother answers a phone call you attempt to speak to the son. He seems wary but does concede he punches walls when angry. His view at present is that "It's no big deal—the cast will handle it." When asked about alcohol, he replies, "It's what we do . . . a little doesn't hurt anyone." When you begin to address the risks involved in this behavior, he cuts you off by angrily retorting, "It's none of your damn business! Get lost and leave me alone!"

1. What environmental and sociological factors are influencing the son's behavior?
2. What actual and potential health issues are raised by the life-style of the son and his past and present family situation?
3. What countertransference issues are likely relative to this situation, and how should they be addressed?
4. What primary interventions are indicated for the health risks present in the son?
5. What secondary interventions are indicated for the health issues present in the son?
6. How should the nurse respond to the client's denial and anger?
7. How should the nurse's interventions be evaluated?

REFERENCES

1. Rankin, S. (1990). Differences in recovery from cardiac surgery: A profile of male and female patients. *Heart and Lung: Journal of Critical Care, 19*(5), 481–485.
2. National Center for Health Statistics. (1990). *Health, United States, 1989.* Hyattsville, MD: Public Health Service.
3. Forrester, D. (1986). Myths of masculinity: Impact upon men's health. *Nursing Clinics of North America, 21*(1), 15–23.
4. DeHoff, J., & Forrest, K. (1984). Men's health. In J. Swanson & K. Forrest (Eds.), *Men's reproductive health.* New York: Springer.
5. Friman, P., Finney, J., & Leibowitz, J. (1989). Years of potential life lost: Evaluating premature cancer death in men. *Journal of Community Health, 14*(2), 101–105.
6. Martin, J. (1990). Male cancer awareness: Impact of an employee education program. *Oncology Nursing Forum, 17*(1), 59–64.
7. Blesch, K. (1986). Health beliefs about testicular cancer and self-examination among professional men. *Oncology Nursing Forum, 13*(1), 29–33.
8. Rudolf, V., & Quinn, K. (1988). The practice of TSE among college men: Effectiveness of an educational program. *Oncology Nursing Forum, 15*(1), 45–48.
9. Goldenring, J. (1986). Equal time for men: Teaching testicular self-examination. *Journal of Adolescent Health Medicine, 7*(4), 273–274.
10. Berkow, R. (Ed.). (1987). *The Merck manual of diagnosis and therapy.* Rahway, NJ: Merck & Co.
11. Kaler, S. (1990). Epididymitis in the young adult male. *Nurse Practitioner, 15*(5), 10–16.
12. American Psychiatric Association. (1987). *Diagnostic and*

statistical manual of mental disorders (3rd ed. rev.). Washington, DC: Author.

13. Rew, L. (1989). Promoting healthy sexuality. In R. Foster, M. Hunsberger, & J. Anderson (Eds.), *Family-centered nursing care of children* (pp. 692–698). Philadelphia: W. B. Saunders.
14. Coody, D. (1989). Nursing strategies: Altered endocrine function. In R. Foster, M. Hunsberger, & J. Anderson (Eds.), *Family-centered nursing care of children*. Philadelphia: W. B. Saunders.
15. Mullis, M. (1984). Vietnam: The human fallout. *Journal of Psychosocial Nursing, 22*(2), 27–31.
16. Rew, L., & Esparza, D. (1990). Barriers to disclosure among sexually abused male children. *Journal of Child Psychiatric Nursing, 4*(1), 120–127.
17. Cunningham, M. (1986). Chronic occupational lead exposure. *AAOHN Journal, 34*(6), 277–279.
18. Ossler, C. (1986). Men's work environment and health risks. *Nursing Clinics of North America, 21*(1), 25–36.
19. Loosen, P., Drew, B., & Prange, A. (1990). Long-term predictors of outcome in abstinent alcoholic men. *American Journal of Psychiatry, 147*, 1662–1666.
20. Kaplan, H., & Saddock, B. (1988). *Clinical psychiatry* (pp. 222–223). Baltimore: Williams & Wilkins.
21. Davies, J., & Janosik, E. (1991). *Mental health and psychiatric nursing: A caring approach* (pp. 382–384). Boston: Jones and Bartlett.
22. Johnson, G., & Werstlein, P. (1990). Reframing: A strategy to improve care of manipulative patients. *Issues in Mental Health Nursing, 11*, 237–241.
23. Chitty, K., & Maynard, C. (1979). Dealing with anger: Guidelines for nursing intervention. *Journal of Psychosocial Nursing and Mental Health Services, 17*(6), 36–41.
24. Beal, G. (1989). Helping men cope with divorce. *Journal of Psychosocial Nursing and Mental Health Services, 27*(8), 30–32.
25. Catalona, W., Smith, D., & Ratliff, T., et al. (1991). Measurement of prostate-specific antigen in serum as a screening test for prostate cancer. *New England Journal of Medicine, 324*(17), 1156–1161.
26. Frasure-Smith, N. (1991). In-hospital symptoms of psychological stress as predictors of long-term outcome after acute myocardial infarction. *American Journal of Cardiology, 67*(3), 121–127.

RECOMMENDED READINGS

Abraham, I., & Krowchuk, H. (1986). Unemployment and health: Health promotion for the jobless male. *Nursing Clinics of North America, 21*(1), 37–47.

A thoughtful review of the impact of joblessness on the psychosocial and physical health of the individual, the family, and the community. Provides an overview of issues and addresses specific nursing interventions for preserving health during unemployment. This issue of Nursing Clinics *focuses on male health issues and is an excellent resource.*

Allen, D., & Whatley, M. (1986). Nursing and men's health: Some critical considerations. *Nursing Clinics of North America, 21*(1), 3–13.

Compares the women's and men's health movements and healthcare delivery for each gender. Addresses the political elements and their impact on individual health. Offers a broad-based, objective, and comprehensive view of both men's and women's health.

Ewedemi, F., & Linn, M. (1987). Health and hassles in older and younger men. *Journal of Clinical Psychology, 43*(4), 347–353.

Details research that evaluates the connection between daily stressors (hassles), compensating events (uplifts), and health status.

Foreman, M. (1986). Cardiovascular disease: A men's health hazard. *Nursing Clinics of North America, 21*(1), 65–73.

Provides an excellent overview of cardiovascular health dynamics and issues concerning male clients, including well-known contributing disorders (for example, hypertension) as well as lesser-known theories about the impact of noncardiac male physiology on the cardiovascular system. Includes recommendations.

George, J., & Quattrone, M. (1988). Opposite sex RN's in the emergency department. *Emergency Nurse Legal Bulletin, 14*(4), 2–4.

Discusses the issue of male RN–female client relative to (charges of) inappropriate sexual behavior by the RN. Reviews legal and liability issues regarding caring for clients of the opposite sex.

Greer, S., Dickerson, V., & Schneiderman, L. (1986). Responses of male and female physicians to medical complaints in male and female patients. *Journal of Family Practice, 23*(1), 49–53.

Reports research addressing the impact of both staff and patient gender on quality of care.

Millon-Underwood, S., & Sanders, E. (1990). Factors contributing to health promotion behaviors among African-American men. *Oncology Nursing Forum, 15*(5), 707–712.

Sets forth findings suggesting that positive attitudes about cancer prevention and early detection, coupled with knowledge of early warning signs, are associated with higher motivation and participation in health promotion. Includes thoughtful recommendations/comments.

Pinch, W., Heck, M., & Vinal, D. (1986). Health needs and concerns of male adolescents. *Adolescence, 21*(84), 961–969.

Surveys health-related habits and perceived needs of male college freshmen and notes prevalence of both positive health habits (exercise), problem areas (stress and substance abuse), and needs for information about sexual health. Helpful but perhaps limited overview for those working with college-age males.

Swanson, J., Swenson, J., Oakley, D., & Marcy, S. (1990). Community health nurses and family planning services for men. *Journal of Community Health Nursing, 7*(2), 87–96.

Reports survey of community health nurses on knowledge and services they provide males regarding family planning, noting that fewer provided such services to males; also that there were notable knowledge gaps regarding male contraception and most community health nurses felt unprepared to serve male family-planning needs. Implies males are perhaps underserved relative to females.

Thomas, S. (1990). Theoretical and empirical perspectives on anger. *Issues in Mental Health Nursing, 11,* 203–216.

Thorough review of theories on anger with a focus on clinical application. Clearly and interestingly presented. Excellent review of clinical implications; well-chosen summaries of important research. Concise and informative, with thoughtful recommendations for practice.

Wallen, J., Roddy, P., & Meyers, S. (1986). Male-female differences in mental health visits under cost-sharing. *Health Services Research, 21*(2), 341–350.

Research report suggesting that co-pay requirements may reduce needed health-care utilization, especially among males. Also notes that hospitalizations for males increased after co-pay began, but not so for females. Raises concerns about the impact of economic factors on health outcomes especially for male clients.

Wiesmeier, E., Forsythe, A., & Sundstrom, M., (1986). Sexual concerns and counseling needs of normal men attending a university student health service. *College Health, 35*(7), 29–35.

Research survey reports regarding male sexually based worries and desire for assistance with these concerns. Highlights the higher-than-suspected amount of sexual concerns among young men, with limited recommendations regarding clinical management.

CHAPTER 23

Care of Older Clients

KEY TERMS

activity theory
continuity theory
disengagement theory
free-radical theory
error theory
human needs theory
immunological theory
interpersonal theory
intrinsic mutagenesis theory
neuroendocrine theory
psychoanalytic theory
social network
somatic mutation theory
theory of psychosocial development

The number of elderly people (those age 65 or older) in the United States doubled between 1950 and 1980 to reach 25.5 million. During this same period, the number of persons over 85 years of age quadrupled to 2.2 million people. By the year 2030, it is estimated that the elderly will comprise approximately 21 percent of the nation's population compared to only 12 percent today.[1]

In part, the growth in the elderly as a percentage of the population is due to a lower birth rate and fewer young persons than in previous years. However, another major contributing factor is increased longevity. Improvements in medical treatment and the use of advanced medical technologies to sustain life have resulted in a life expectancy of 71 years for men and 77 years for women.[2] Although life expectancy has increased, the quality of life for the elderly is often questionable. In working with older adults, individually or as an aggregate, community health nurses must be concerned with quality-of-life concerns as well as longevity.

This emphasis on quality of life can be seen in the focus of the national health objectives for the year 2000 addressing the health needs of the elderly. A major thread throughout these objectives is a reduction in activity limitations that impair the quality of life for older persons.[3] Selected objectives dealing with the health needs of this population are summarized in Box 23–1.

LEARNING OBJECTIVES

After reading this chapter you should be able to:

- Identify four myths related to aging.
- Describe at least five theories of aging.
- Describe at least two changes in each body system that occur as a normal result of the aging process.
- Identify three major themes in assessing physical environmental factors influencing the health of older clients.
- Describe at least four considerations in assessing the influence of life-style factors on the health of older clients.
- Identify at least six areas for primary prevention in the care of older clients.
- Describe secondary preventive nursing interventions for at least four common health problems among older clients.
- Identify at least three factors related to older clients that may influence the community health nurse's approach to health education.
- Describe four considerations unique to older clients that influence the evaluation of nursing care.

BOX 23–1

Summary of Selected National Health Objectives Related to Older Persons

1. Reduce to no more than 90 per 1000 people the proportion of individuals aged 65 and older who have difficulty in performing two or more personal-care activities.
2. Reduce deaths among people aged 70 and older due to motor vehicle accidents to no more than 20 per 100,000 population.
3. Reduce deaths among people aged 65 through 84 due to falls and related injuries to no more than 14.4 per 100,000 population.
4. Reduce hip fractures among people aged 65 and older so hospitalizations for fractures are no more than 607 per 100,000 population.
5. Reduce to no more than 20% the proportion of people aged 65 and older who have lost all of their natural teeth.
6. Increase length of healthy life to at least 65 years.
7. Reduce significant visual impairment among people aged 65 and older to no more than 70 per 1000 population.
8. Reduce epidemic-related pneumonia and influenza deaths among people aged 65 and older to no more than 7.3 per 1000 population.
9. Increase to at least 30% the proportion of people aged 65 and older who engage regularly in light to moderate physical activity.
10. Increase to at least 80% the proportion of people aged 65 and older who receive home food services if needed.
11. Increase to at least 60% the proportion of people 65 and older using the oral health-care system each year.
12. Increase to at least 95% the proportion of women aged 70 and over with uterine cervix who have ever received a Pap test.
13. Increase to at least 50% the proportion of people aged 50 and older who have received fecal occult blood testing in the preceding 1 to 2 years.
14. Increase to at least 90% the proportion of perimenopausal women who have been counseled about the benefits and risks of estrogen replacement therapy.

MYTHS OF AGING

Aging is a normal human phenomenon. Although much research has been conducted recently on the aging process, aging itself remains a mystery surrounded by myths.[4] Among the myths surrounding aging are beliefs that aging is a time of tranquility and that aging is synonymous with senility. For many older adults, however, aging is a time of increased problems and decreased resources for dealing with those problems. Moreover, senility is not an inevitable consequence of aging. Many older persons retain their mental faculties well beyond the ninth decade of life.

Another myth is that old age is a time of reduced productivity. This is misleading. Many older adults remain productive throughout life. Societal factors, however, may limit opportunities for older adults to demonstrate their productivity. For example, many older adults are forced to retire at a specific age despite continued abilities to perform their jobs capably. Continued productivity among older persons is seen among those who do continue to work as well as among those who channel their energies into other areas after retirement. Retirees may continue to contribute to society through volunteer activities, artistic endeavors, or other pursuits.

Older persons are also thought by many to be resistant to change—again, a myth. Resistance to change tends to be a lifelong characteristic, not one developed with advancing age. Persons who have been relatively resistant to change throughout life will probably continue to resist change in their older years, while those who have welcomed change will probably continue to do so.

A final myth is that aging is purely a matter of chronology, a uniform process that progresses at the same rate and with the same results for all. The truth, however, is that aging affects each individual differently, and the outcomes of aging may be very different from one individual to another.

THEORIES OF AGING

Aging and circumventing aging are topics that fascinated humankind long before Ponce de León's search for the fountain of youth. Science cannot fully explain why aging occurs, but several theories have been advanced to explain the process. These theories tend to fall into stochastic, genetic, psychological, or sociological categories.

STOCHASTIC THEORIES

Stochastic theories of aging are based on assumptions that the cumulative effects of environmental assaults eventually become incompatible with life.[5] One of these theories, the ***somatic mutation theory,*** holds that prolonged exposure to background radiation of several types results in cell mutations that will eventually lead to death.

The ***error theory,*** a second stochastic theory, is based on the belief that environmental changes interfere with cell function and reproduction, thus causing errors in reproduced cells. These errors multiply in a geometric progression until cells are no longer viable.

GENETIC THEORIES

Genetic theories of aging are based on the assumption that aging is a part of the developmental process with differences in that process genetically programmed from conception.[5] ***Neuroendocrine theory*** holds that aging is the result of functional decrements in neurons and their hormones. In one version of this theory, for example, changes in the hypothalamic-pituitary system, over time, lead to changes in other body systems, possibly due to diminished responsiveness of neuroendocrine tissue to various signals.

Intrinsic mutagenesis theory is another genetic theory in which it is believed that each person has a genetic constitution that regulates the replication of genetic materials. Over time, regulatory activity diminishes, creating mutations in cells that result in the effects of aging.

A third genetic theory of aging is the ***immunological theory,*** which holds that aging is an autoimmune process. As cells change with age, the body's immunological mechanisms perceive them as foreign bodies and destroy them. Finally, the ***free-radical theory*** of aging is based on the belief that most physiological changes of aging are due to damage caused by the action of free radicals, which are highly chemically reactive by-products of metabolism. Generally speaking, these free radicals are rapidly destroyed by protective enzyme systems. Over time, however, it is believed that those radicals not destroyed accumulate to cause cell damage. Despite the stochastic and genetic theories of aging and related research, the physiologic processes involved in aging and the variability of this process among individuals remain unexplained.

PSYCHOLOGICAL THEORIES

A number of theories have also been advanced to explain the psychological aspects of aging.[6] Jungian ***psychoanalytic theory*** regards aging as a time of developing self-awareness through reflective activity. Harry Stack Sullivan's ***interpersonal theory,*** another psychological theory of aging, is developmental in nature. Maturity, in this theory, involves the development of satisfactory interpersonal relationships. The loss of these relationships over time is believed to result in a loss of interpersonal security and the consequent psychological aspects of aging.[7]

In Abraham Maslow's ***human needs theory,*** physical aging and environmental changes contribute to difficulty in meeting basic human needs. These difficulties contribute, in turn, to the psychological effects sometimes seen with age. The greater the difficulty in meeting basic needs, the greater the impact of aging.[8] Maslow's hierarchy of human needs is presented in Box 23–2. Finally, in Erik Erickson's ***theory of psychosocial development,*** the degree of success experienced in accomplishing the developmental tasks in stages 1 through 7 influences the accomplishment of the tasks of the older adult in stage 8.[9] The developmental tasks of each of Erickson's eight stages are presented in Box 23–3.

SOCIOLOGICAL THEORIES

Sociological theories have also been advanced to explain the effects of aging. The first of these is ***disen-***

BOX 23–2

Maslow's Hierarchy of Human Needs

Survival needs: oxygen, food, water, sleep, sexual activity
Safety and security needs: protection from physical hazards, emotional security
Love and belonging needs: affection from others, ability to feel and express affection for others, group identification, companionship
Esteem and recognition needs: sense of self-worth, recognition of accomplishments by others
Self-actualization needs: achievement of person potential
Aesthetic needs: order, harmony, and achievement of spiritual goals

(Source: Maslow[8])

BOX 23–3

Erickson's Stages of Psychosocial Development

Stage 1: Trust vs. mistrust
Focuses on developing a sense of trust in oneself and others
Stage 2: Autonomy vs. shame and doubt
Focuses on the ability to express oneself and cooperate with others
Stage 3: Initiative vs. guilt
Focuses on purposeful behavior and the ability to evaluate one's own behavior
Stage 4: Industry vs. inferiority
Focuses on developing belief in one's own abilities
Stage 5: Identity vs. role confusion
Focuses on developing a clear sense of self and plans to actualize one's abilities
Stage 6: Intimacy vs. isolation
Focuses on developing one's capacity for reciprocal love relationships
Stage 7: Generativity vs. stagnation
Focuses on creativity and productivity and developing the capacity to care for others
Stage 8: Ego identity vs. despair
Focuses on acceptance of one's life as worthwhile and unique

(Source: Erickson[9])

gagement theory. In this perspective, the older person recognizes death as inevitable and so begins a process of withdrawal from society that permits the individual to enjoy old age and to prepare for death without causing social disruption when death occurs.[6]

Activity theory, on the other hand, posits continued engagement with society and the assumption of new roles and responsibilities by the older person. In ***continuity theory,*** one's behavior becomes more predictable with age.[6] For instance, the conservative person becomes more conservative and the adventurous person becomes more adventurous. Also, a change occurs in roles and relationships as the older adult becomes more concerned with introspection and self-reflection.

Some of the sociological theories are unsatisfactory in certain respects.[10] For example, disengagement theory fails to account for individual variations in the desire to disengage and the influence of the degree of one's involvement with society throughout life. The theory also fails to address the effects of a societal structure that mitigates against the involvement of older adults. Activity theory, on the other hand, does not account for the influence of other factors, such as economic and health status, that limit one's ability to engage in many of the expected activities of retirement (travel and hobbies, for example).

Developmental theories such as those of Erickson and Sullivan also discount the effects of health and economic status on one's ability to accomplish developmental tasks in later life. Similar concerns can be voiced with respect to other theories of aging discussed here. Although nurses need a theory base for gerontologic nursing practice, it may be advisable to adopt more than one theory in working with older persons.[10] Nurses must assess the individual needs of each client and select a theoretical perspective that

TABLE 23–1. SELECTED THEORIES OF AGING

Perspective	Theory	Description of Theory
Stochastic	Somatic mutation theory	Cumulative exposures to background radiation cause cell mutations incompatible with life
	Error theory	Aging is the cumulative effects of errors in cell reproduction
Genetic	Neuroendocrine theory	Aging is due to the effects of diminished response of neuroendocrine tissue to stimuli
	Intrinsic mutagenesis theory	Genetic regulatory activity diminishes over time, resulting in cell mutations that eventually lead to cell death
	Immunological theory	Aging is an autoimmune process
	Free-radical theory	Aging is due to the accumulation of free radicals, by-products of cell metabolism that interfere with cell function
Psychological	Psychoanalytic theory	Aging leads to a focus on introspection and self-reflection
	Interpersonal theory	The psychological effects of aging are due to the loss of satisfactory interpersonal relationships and consequent loss of interpersonal security
	Human needs theory	Difficulty in meeting basic human needs results in the psychological effects of aging
	Theory of psychosocial development	The degree of success achieved in developmental tasks in earlier stages affects one's response to aging
Sociological	Disengagement theory	Recognizing death as inevitable, the older person begins to separate from society in order to provide for the continuity of the social order
	Activity theory	Interaction with society continues with assumption of new roles and responsibilities
	Continuity theory	Previous personality traits become more pronounced with age and behavior becomes more predictable

best fits those needs. Theories of aging are summarized in Table 23–1.

THE EPIDEMIOLOGIC PREVENTION PROCESS MODEL AND CARE OF OLDER CLIENTS

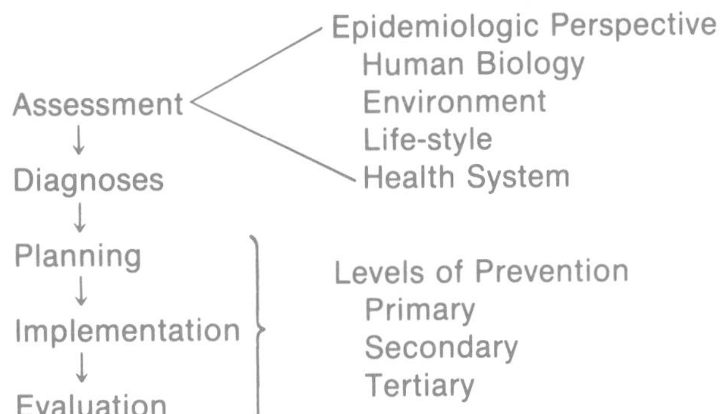

Epidemiologic Prevention Process Model can be used to design nursing interventions to meet the health-care needs of older clients. Using the model, the community health nurse conducts an in-depth assessment of the older client's health status; derives nursing diagnoses from the data obtained; plans and implements primary, secondary, and tertiary preventive care; and evaluates the effects of nursing intervention.

ASSESSING THE HEALTH STATUS OF OLDER CLIENTS

Effective nursing care for older clients requires an accurate assessment of the client's health status. Human biological, environmental, life-style, and health system factors may influence that health status. Consequently, the community health nurse would explore factors in each of the four areas of Dever's epidemiologic perspective.

HUMAN BIOLOGY

Maturation and Aging

Aging affects the function of all body systems. Many of the changes brought about by the aging process are contributing factors in health problems frequently experienced by older persons.

Integumentary Changes. Normal changes in the integumentary system include decreased skin turgor and perspiration and increased pigmentation. The hair thins, and nails grow more slowly. The thinning of scalp hair predisposes older individuals to sunburn. Sclerosis and loss of subcutaneous fat result in loss of skin elasticity and wrinkling. Concerns over body image due to increased skin pigmentation, loss of hair, and wrinkling may make some older adults susceptible to the claims of quackery in these areas. Nurses may want to explore what types of creams, lotions, or other treatments clients are using on hair and skin, as some of these products can cause damage and most are ineffective and expensive. Loss of skin elasticity also contributes to drooping lower eyelids and increased potential for conjunctivitis. Consequently, the nurse should be sure to assess the client's conjunctivae for signs of irritation.

Dry skin and increased skin fragility are other changes that may cause itching and contribute to skin injuries. Dry, itching skin may also contribute to loss of sleep at night. Decreased perspiration in older persons may predispose them to the effects of hyperthermia[11] and heat stroke.

Cardiovascular Changes. Reduced cardiac reserves due to less efficient pump action of the heart results in a decreased ability to meet oxygen needs, leading to diminished physical abilities. Increased fatigue and diminished contractility of vessels resulting in orthostatic hypertension may predispose clients to falls. Systolic blood pressure rises, and the pulse pressure widens in the older adult,[12] creating an increased risk for myocardial infarction. Peripheral vascular changes also include varicose veins and venous stasis.

Respiratory Changes. Structural changes in the respiratory system reduce the efficiency of the respiratory process. As alveolar sacs enlarge and lose their elasticity, they may rupture and fuse with adjacent sacs, resulting in greater residual volume. Arteriole changes lead to reduced gas exchange, and skeletal changes produced by osteoporosis and kyphosis can restrict chest movement, thus lowering vital capacity. All of these changes result in less efficient gas exchange and greater difficulty in meeting oxygen needs. Furthermore, slower mucous transport, reduced cough strength, and dysphagia increase the client's susceptibility to respiratory infection and choking due to aspiration of food.[13]

Gastrointestinal Changes. Gastrointestinal system changes also affect the older adult's ability to maintain usual body function. As teeth wear down, the client may be less able to chew food properly. Decreased volume and acidity of saliva result in less moisture added to food and intolerance to some foods.[12] Decreased salivation also results in dry mouth. Loss of taste buds may contribute to poor appetite and malnutrition.

As muscles in the mouth, cheeks, and tongue atrophy, older persons begin to require more time to eat and to speak. Thinning of the esophageal wall and a reduction in protective mucin, along with reduced peristalsis, may contribute to a sense of fullness or heartburn after eating. Reductions in hydrochloric acid content and enzyme production within the stomach may lead to decreased vitamin B_{12} levels and pernicious anemia. Calcium deposits within the lumen of arterial vessels may reduce the blood supply to the intestines and contribute to intestinal problems. Decreased muscle strength in the intestines can lead to formation of polyps and diverticuli. Many of these changes along with restricted activity, less sleep, and less dietary fiber contribute to constipation.

Urinary Changes. In the urinary system, a reduction in the number of nephrons in the kidney results in a decreased ability to concentrate urine and a need to urinate more frequently. Renal arteriole constriction due to arteriosclerosis leads to decreased filtration. In younger persons, the kidneys automatically lower filtration rates at night. In older persons, however, decreased filtration rates have already reduced kidney efficiency so that this physiologic change no longer occurs. For this reason, many older persons normally experience one to two episodes of nocturia per night. More frequent episodes of nocturia are cause for concern because urinary tract infection is a common occurrence among older clients, especially older women due to the decreased acidity of the urethra and bladder base.[12]

Reproductive Changes. The reproductive system in both male and female clients is also subject to the effects of aging. In the female, ovarian atrophy leads to an increased potential for development of cysts. Aging also brings about further reductions in progesterone and estrogen levels begun in the fourth and fifth decades of life, respectively. Other reproductive changes in the female include reduction in uterine size and thickness of uterine walls, loss of subcutaneous fat in external genitalia,[6] loss of pubic and axillary hair, and drooping of breast tissue.

In the male, there is a decrease in the number of sperm produced and changes in the size and shape of sperm, resulting in decreased potential for fertilization. Decreased testosterone levels also occur.[14] Erectile impotence is not a normal consequence of aging. However, erections may take longer to achieve and the refractory period between erections is prolonged in older males.[12]

For both men and women, a reduction in the frequency of intercourse seems to result in lowered response levels. Clients who maintain sexual activity on a regular basis do not appear to experience any loss of libido. The extent of activity, however, is highly dependent on one's psychology and on conditions in the social environment. The sexual changes that occur with aging may have a detrimental effect on a client's self-image.

Musculoskeletal Changes. In the musculoskeletal system, reductions in muscle tone and size usually lead to avoidance of heavy activity. Decreased range of motion in joints affects posture, gait, balance, and skeletal flexibility, thus increasing the potential for falls and injury. The kyphosis that occurs with aging leads to diminished stature and poor use of respiratory muscles, which predisposes clients to respiratory infection. Breakdown of chondrocytes in joint cartilage leads to osteoarthritis with consequent pain, reduced mobility, and a diminished ability to accomplish activities of daily living.

Neurological Changes. Neurological changes also occur with age. The slower pace of electrical impulses in the brain reduces sensory ability and slows reaction times, thus increasing the potential for injury. Increased reaction time affects mental as well as physical responses. Intelligence is not diminished, but increased reaction time leads to decreased performance in mental skills.

Changes in sensory function are particularly noticeable in older clients. Problems with vision may result from changes in focal accommodation, cataracts, and decreased color sensitivity. Older persons also take longer to adapt to changes in light, which makes nighttime activities such as driving and moving about the home in darkness particularly dangerous. Reduction in lacrimation results in dry eyes and, combined with lid inversion or the drooping of eyelids mentioned earlier, contributes to irritation and conjunctivitis.

Hearing becomes less acute, particularly for higher-pitched sounds. Cerumen becomes more tenacious and tends to block the ear canal, further reducing the ability to hear. Hearing loss can result in social isolation and withdrawal from interpersonal interaction. Reductions in the senses of taste and smell may add to loss of appetite and lead to inadequate nutrition. Because eating is also a social function, loss of appetite may further impair social interaction. Finally, reduced sense of touch can increase an older person's potential for injury. Common physical changes due to aging and their implications for health are summarized in Table 23–2.

Physiologic Function

In addition to assessing clients for commonly occurring age-related changes and their effects, community health nurses should assess older clients for the presence of acute and chronic illnesses. Although most older persons are in basically good health, 86 percent of those over 65 have one or more chronic conditions.[15]

Assessment for the presence of acute and chronic conditions is best done using a systems approach. The nurse should examine the client for signs and symptoms of the conditions included in Box 23–4. Nurses should keep in mind that, when assessing clients for signs of these conditions, symptomatology may differ markedly in younger and older persons. For example, older persons with pneumonia may not exhibit pain or fever, but only confusion and restlessness. Similarly, emphysema may present with weakness, weight loss, and loss of appetite. Tuberculosis may not exhibit the classic symptoms of fever and night sweats, but only anorexia, weakness, and hemoptysis.[16]

Cardiovascular problems are also frequently encountered in the elderly. Myocardial infarction in the older person can occur without symptoms or with only jaw pain or a vague indigestion. Congestive heart failure is also seen relatively frequently, manifesting with confusion, insomnia, wandering at night, peripheral and presacral edema, cough, distended neck veins, and rapid increase in weight. Other cardiovascular problems to be considered include hypertension, angina, and anemias. Hypertension may be evidenced by a dull headache, difficulties with memory, and epistaxis. Angina may only be signaled by a vague discomfort after meals.

Anemia may be related to iron-deficient diet, chronic blood loss, or inability to absorb vitamin B_{12} (pernicious anemia). The nurse should assess the client for weakness and fatigue and, in the case of pernicious anemia, for sore tongue and numbness and tingling of the extremities. A thorough diet history should also be obtained and evidence of any bleeding (for example, bleeding gums or occult blood in the stool) should be sought.

Urinary incontinence may, on occasion, be due to fecal impaction, so a history of constipation should trigger suspicion of this problem. In men, urinary incontinence may be due to prostatic hypertrophy, whereas in women stress incontinence may be related to sequelae of childbirth or perineal muscle weakness.[12] Bladder infection is the most common cause of fever in older adults, and signs and symptoms of bladder infection should always be looked for in older clients presenting with fever.[16] Reproductive problems in older females may include vaginitis with dis-

TABLE 23–2. COMMON PHYSICAL CHANGES OF AGING AND THEIR IMPLICATIONS FOR HEALTH

System Affected	Changes Noted	Implications for Health
Integumentary system	Decreased skin turgor, increased sclerosis and loss of subcutaneous fat lead to wrinkles	Lowered self-image
	Increased pigmentation	Lowered self-image
	Thinning of hair	Lowered self-image, risk of sunburn to scalp
	Dry skin	Itching, risk of injury, insomnia
	Decreased perspiration	Hyperthermia, heat stroke
Cardiovascular system	Less efficient pump action and lower cardiac reserves	Decreased physical ability
	Thickening of vessel walls, replacement of muscle fiber with collagen, connective tissue, and calcium	Elevated blood pressure, varicosities, venous stasis
Respiratory system	Decreased elasticity of alveolar sacs, skeletal changes in chest	Decreased gas exchange, decreased physical ability
	Slower mucous transport, decreased cough strength, dysphagia	Increased susceptibility to infection and increased risk of aspiration
Gastrointestinal system	Wearing down of teeth	Difficulty chewing
	Decreased saliva	Dry mouth, difficulty digesting starches
	Loss of taste buds	Decreased appetite
	Muscle atrophy of cheeks, tongue, etc.	Difficulty chewing, slower to eat
	Thinned esophageal wall	Feeling of fullness/heartburn after meals
	Decreased peristalsis	Constipation
	Decreased hydrochloric acid and enzyme production in stomach	Pernicious anemia
Urinary system	Decreased number of nephrons and decreased ability to concentrate urine	Nocturia
Reproductive system	*Female:* ovarian atrophy	Ovarian cysts
	Decreased estrogen and progesterone	Menopause, osteopososis
	Changes in external genitalia	Lowered self-image
	Male: decreased testosterone	Fatigue, weight loss, decreased libido, lowered self-image
Musculoskeletal system	Decreased muscle size and tone	Decreased physical ability
	Decreased range of motion with changes in gait, posture, balance, and flexibility	Increased risk of falls
	Kyphosis	Lowered self-image, increased risk of respiratory infection
	Breakdown of chondrocytes in joint cartilage	Osteoarthritis, joint pain
	Osteoporosis	Increased risk of fractures
Neurological system	Diminished hearing, vision, touch, and increased reaction time	Increased risk of injury, social isolation
	Decreased ability to problem-solve	Difficulty adjusting to new situations

charge or vaginal soreness and itching. Vaginal prolapse may also occur as evidenced by protrusion, low back pain, and pelvic pulling.

Hiatal hernia is seen in 67 percent of persons over age 60[16] and usually involves chest pain and a feeling of fullness immediately after meals. Many older clients also experience diverticulosis accompanied by pain, constipation, and nausea and vomiting.

Osteoporosis is a common musculoskeletal problem among older women. This condition causes increased porosity and fragility of bones, contributing to 1.3 million fractures annually. Eighty-four percent of the 200,000 hip fractures in the United States each year occur in persons over 65 years of age. Wrist fractures and compression fractures of the spine are also common occurrences.[17] The potential for osteoporosis increases with chronically low calcium intake, lack of exercise, smoking, alcohol abuse, and in those who are underweight.

Problems commonly encountered in the neurological system include cerebrovascular accidents, Parkinson's disease, and acute or chronic organic brain disease. Ten percent of persons over 65 years of age have Alzheimer's disease.[17] This condition frequently

BOX 23–4

Common Physical Health Problems among Older Clients

Cardiovascular system
- Angina
- Atherosclerosis
- Congestive heart failure
- Hypertension
- Myocardial infarction

Gastrointestinal system
- Constipation
- Diverticulosis
- Fecal impaction
- Gall bladder disease
- Hemorrhoids
- Hiatal hernia

Hematopoietic system
- Anemia

Integumentary system
- Basal cell carcinoma
- Decubitus ulcers
- Herpes zoster infection
- Squamous cell carcinoma

Musculoskeletal system
- Arthritis
- Hip and other fractures
- Osteoporosis

Neurological system
- Alzheimer's disease
- Cerebrovascular accident
- Organic brain syndrome
- Parkinson's disease

Reproductive system

Female:
- Breast cancer
- Cervical cancer
- Vaginitis

Male:
- Benign prostatic hypertrophy
- Impotence
- Prostatic cancer

Respiratory system
- Emphysema
- Influenza
- Pneumonia
- Tuberculosis

Urinary system
- Bladder cancer
- Incontinence
- Urinary tract infection

presents with memory loss and disorientation, leading to confusion and sometimes to wandering. Some clients with Alzheimer's become severely depressed or begin to hallucinate. As the disease progresses, clients become more and more in need of complete care.

ENVIRONMENT

The second major component of a thorough assessment of the older adult is an evaluation of environmental factors influencing health. Physical, psychological, and social environmental factors may all affect the health of the elderly.

Physical Environment

Physical environmental concerns with older clients include the adequacy of housing, the existence of safety hazards in the home or community, and the availability of necessary goods and services. The community health nurse will assess the adequacy of living conditions to meet clients' needs. For example, do living arrangements provide adequate space? Is there provision for privacy for the older person? Are living quarters adequately heated and ventilated? The nurse would also note whether there are adequate facilities for food storage and preparation.

A major concern in the assessment of the older client's physical environment is the presence of safety hazards. The community health nurse would note the presence of stairs, rugs, or other objects that might lead to falls and injuries. The nurse would also assess the adequacy of lighting and the presence or absence of tub rails and other safety features. Because of poor circulation, many older clients frequently feel cold and may use space heaters or kerosene stoves that present safety hazards. (See Appendix C, Home Safety Assessment—Older Adult.)

The neighborhood is another area of concern. Are fire and police services adequate to meet the needs of older clients? Is the neighborhood safe? Is there transportation available if needed? Finally, does the older person have access to shopping facilities and health-care providers within a reasonable distance?

Psychological Environment

Examination of factors in the psychological environment includes assessing the client's psychological health status and related problems. A psychological assessment involves considering the client's cognitive and affective status. Both cognitive and affective status are addressed by the mental status examination described in Chapter 17, Care of the Individual Client. In assessing the client's cognitive status, the nurse would evaluate long- and short-term memory and orientation, powers of concentration and judgment, and ability to engage in mathematical calculations. Considerations in the assessment of affective status include the presence of depression, dementia, and saddened mood states.[18] Commonly noted psychological problems among older adults include confusion, depression, and grief. Information to be obtained in assessing clients for depression include anniversary dates; recent changes in relationships; changes in physical health status; alterations in mood or behavior; depressive symptoms such as depressed affect and apathy; history of depression; and recent losses or crises.[19]

It is important to keep in mind that sensory deficits may interfere with the assessment of psychological status and that such deficits must be compensated for in order to obtain an accurate assessment. To compensate for sensory deficits, the nurse should face the client, eliminate background noise, provide good lighting, speak clearly and slowly, and keep questions short.

The nurse should also try to reduce the client's anxiety, as this may also interfere with obtaining an accurate picture of the client's abilities. The nurse can help to reduce anxiety by establishing rapport, explaining the purpose of the psychological evaluation, providing privacy, and limiting distractions. Other factors that may affect a psychological assessment include the client's use of medications, communication impairments, ethnic and cultural differences, and language barriers. Nurses may want to validate their findings regarding an older client's psychological status with family members to be sure that findings are consistent with typical behavior and not the product of the present situation.

The client's psychological status may be affected by abuse by family members. This is an area in which the nurse's careful observation, assessment, and documentation are essential. Nurses should assess clients for signs of both physical and psychological abuse or neglect. Signs of physical abuse would include injuries with questionable explanations, poor hygiene, and poor nutritional status. Psychological abuse is more difficult to determine, but the nurse should observe family interactions with the client. Some signs of abuse or neglect might include social isolation, lack of needed assistance with activities of daily living, evidence of tampering with the client's finances, and failure to assist the older person to maintain his or her independence. Failure of family members to visit institutionalized clients may also indicate neglect, a milder form of elder abuse. While most states do not yet have laws requiring mandatory reporting of the abuse of older persons, community health nurses may be called upon to present testimony in abuse cases. For this reason, the nurse should carefully document all findings when assessing the client, including reports by the client and significant others explaining bruises, burns, or other possible indicators of abuse.

Social Environment

The third component of environmental assessment for the older client is the assessment of social functioning. To accomplish this the nurse would assess the client's social network and assess the extent of available social support. The client's ***social network*** is "the web of social relationships that surrounds a person including number and frequency of contacts, the presence of a confidant, the durability of the network, geographical proximity, and reciprocity (mutual helping)."[18] Social support includes emotional, instrumental, or financial assistance that the client receives from the social network.[18]

In assessing the client's social network, the community health nurse will identify those persons with whom the client has frequent contact and whom the client feels able to call on for assistance. The nurse would also explore with the client the types and adequacy of support available from members of the social network.

Institutionalization is another important consideration in the social assessment of the client. For many clients there is a need to determine whether institutional care is appropriate. Families caring for older members may need assistance in making such a determination. There is also a need to decide what type of institution is appropriate based on the extent of self-care in which the client can engage. Is placement in a nursing home appropriate? Or would the client do as well or better in a retirement community? Whatever the choice, the institutionalized client will need assistance in adjusting to altered living circumstances. Nurses should assess the extent of the client's adjustment to the institution and attempt to assist in that adjustment.

LIFE-STYLE

The third aspect of the epidemiologic perspective in the assessment of the older client is that of life-style. Considerations to be addressed in this portion of the assessment include diet, exercise, leisure pursuits, and retirement; adjustment to reduced income; personal habits including medication use, sexuality, and the client's level of independence and ability to perform activities of daily living. With respect to diet, the nurse should assess eating patterns and the adequacy of nutritional intake. The nurse should also evaluate compliance with specific dietary recommendations. Many clients need to restrict sodium intake or increase calcium. The older client with diabetes may or may not comply with a diabetic diet. Particular attention should also be given to the amount of fluid and fiber in the diet.

Nurses should also explore with clients how foods are prepared and by whom. Many older clients have inadequate diets because they are not physically able to prepare some foods. Other problems impeding nutrition include lack of adequate cooking facilities, difficulties in chewing or swallowing, or poor dietary habits throughout life. In addition to assessing dietary intake, therefore, the nurse needs to identify factors contributing to poor nutritional status.

Exercise is another life-style factor addressed in a comprehensive assessment. Half of the older persons in one study did not engage in regular exercise.[20] Many older clients mistakenly believe that their need for exercise diminishes with age. Again, the nurse should assess not only the extent of exercise but also factors that impede adequate exercise such as pain, fatigue, and weakness.

Leisure pursuits and adjustment to retirement are other factors to be considered in life-style assessment. Many older persons who have worked all their lives find adjustment to retirement difficult. This is particularly true if they have not cultivated other interests during their working life. The nurse should assess the types of leisure activities in which clients engage as well as their satisfaction with these activities.

Another adjustment that is required in retirement is living on a reduced income. Nurses working with older clients should assess the adequacy of the client's income. Nurses can also assess clients' abilities to budget their money and to prioritize expenditures appropriately.

One of the consequences of most chronic illnesses is the need for prolonged use of medication. Consequently, community health nurses assessing older clients with chronic illnesses need to assess medication use carefully. Older persons consume 25 percent of all drugs used in the United States. Eighty-five percent of the noninstitutionalized elderly use an average of two to three prescription drugs daily in addition to a variety of over-the-counter medications.[21] The number and the variety of drugs increase the potential for drug toxicity and drug interactions. Each year over 200,000 older adults are hospitalized for drug reactions, with 163,000 experiencing serious impairment.[22]

Nurses need to assess older clients to determine what medications they take, when and how these medications are taken, and the client's knowledge of side effects and signs of toxicity. Nurses should also explore with clients their use of nonprescription drugs and acquaint them with those that are contraindicated by their health status or because of other medications they are taking. Clients should also be assessed for signs of side effects or toxicity.

Nurses should determine the extent to which clients engage in other personal habits such as smoking, drinking, and caffeine consumption as well as the extent of motivation to change such habits. Nonsmoking and moderate alcohol intake were two of seven factors found to be highly predictive of healthy aging in one study.[23] Despite the evidence that nonsmoking promotes health, 43 percent of older persons in another study either were or had been smokers.[20] Caffeine consumption is another personal habit to be addressed in life-style assessment.

Alcohol abuse is one more concern that may be identified in the elderly population. The findings of the Surgeon General's Workshop on Health Promotion and Aging[1] indicated that the prevalence of alcoholism among older adults is approximately the same as that in the general population (roughly 8 percent). Because of metabolic changes, detoxification of alcohol, as well as other substances, is slowed, making the older person increasingly susceptible to the toxic effects of alcohol. Older individuals may also take a number of medications that interact with alcohol, thus increasing the dangers of abuse. Alcohol contributes to deleterious effects on a number of body systems that may already be impaired by age and chronic disease. For example, a definite dose-response relationship exists between the amount of alcohol ingested and blood pressure. For the client who is already hypertensive, alcohol abuse compounds the problem and impedes hypertension control.[1]

The meeting of sexual needs is another important, but often overlooked, component of the assessment of social function. As noted earlier, older clients continue to have sexual needs. These may be fulfilled by a spouse if the couple is afforded the privacy necessary for sexual activity. For example, if older parents live with their children, their opportunities for sexual intimacy may be somewhat limited. The same may be true of older people in institutional settings. For clients who have no living spouse or whose spouse is unable to meet these needs, alternative methods of meeting sexual needs include masturbation and fantasizing.

Because most older people grew up in an era when sexuality was not a topic for discussion, they may find it difficult to talk about such needs with the nurse. Before addressing such intimate issues, the nurse should first develop a rapport with the client. The nurse should also assure clients that sexual problems are not uncommon. For the older male client, the nurse should be aware that many of the medications taken for chronic illnesses, especially antihypertensives, may cause impotence.

Nurses should assess clients for problems with sexuality and identify any underlying factors. Nurses should also explore clients' satisfaction with their sexlife. Another consideration in assessing this area is the potential for exposure to sexually transmitted diseases. Although STDs are primarily found in adolescents and young adults, older persons who are sexually active may be exposed as well. Nurses should also assess the environment of the older person to see whether it is conducive to sexual intimacy if this is desired. Finally, nurses should be aware of the potential for sexual abuse of older clients, particularly in institutional settings.

Client independence and the ability to perform basic activities of daily living are the last areas for consideration in life-style assessment. Areas to be addressed include both personal and instrumental activities of daily life.[18] Personal activities include feeding, bathing, dressing, transfers (getting in or out of a chair or bed), continence, and ambulation. The General Accounting Office of the federal government estimates that 6.5 million older persons currently need help with such personal activities and that by the year 2020 this number will more than double to 14.3 million.[24] Instrumental activities include housekeeping, shopping, taking medications, using transportation, using the telephone, cooking, and managing money. The nurse should evaluate the client's abilities in each of these areas. Problems should be identified and factors contributing to them should be explored.

HEALTH SYSTEM

Health system factors also influence the health of older clients. In assessing these factors, the community health nurse would ascertain whether the client has a regular source of health care. Are health services sought to promote health as well as cure illness? Does the older client have adequate financial resources to afford health care? To what extent are health services used effectively? In addition to determining the source and adequacy of the client's health-care funds, the community health nurse will explore the distance to health facilities used and the means of transportation used to get there. Health system factors and other factors affecting the health of older clients can be assessed using the Health Assessment Guide for the Older Client included in Appendix M.

DIAGNOSTIC REASONING AND HEALTH-CARE NEEDS OF OLDER CLIENTS

Based on the data derived from the in-depth assessment of the older client's health status, the community health nurse derives nursing diagnoses or statements of health-care needs that require nursing action. Nursing diagnoses may be derived relative to each of the areas of assessment described above. For example, the client may have problems related to the normal aging process such as constipation or dry skin. There may also be nursing diagnoses related to existing chronic or communicable diseases.

In addition, the client may encounter factors in the physical, psychological, or social environment that give rise to nursing diagnoses. For example, a nursing diagnosis related to the physical environment might be "safety hazard due to loose handrail on stairs." Problems of "feelings of worthlessness since retirement" or "social isolation due to death of family and friends" are samples of nursing diagnoses related to the psychological and social environments.

Life-style factors may also give rise to nursing diagnoses. For instance, the diagnosis "shortness of breath due to emphysema and smoking" indicates the contribution of smoking, a life-style behavior, to a physiologic problem. The nurse may also derive nursing diagnoses reflecting health system factors such as "lack of health promotion services due to inadequate finances."

PLANNING NURSING CARE FOR OLDER CLIENTS

Community health nurses must be particularly mindful to involve clients and their families in the planning of care. Because older clients are particularly vulnerable to loss of independence, their involvement in planning their own health care is an important way to foster their sense of independence. Client involvement in planning is also likely to enhance compliance with the plan. Planning to meet the health-care needs of older clients may take place at the primary, secondary, and tertiary levels of prevention.

PRIMARY PREVENTION

As with other groups of clients, the most cost-effective means of providing health care to older clients involves primary prevention—preventing health problems before they occur. Areas of concern in planning health promotion for older clients include nutrition, hygiene, safety, immunization, rest and exercise, maintaining independence, and preparing for death.

Nutrition

Adequate nutrition is important for the older person to maintain health and prevent disease and further effects of existing chronic conditions. In a recent study, having a normal weight was found to be one of seven factors that were predictive of healthy aging.[23] Nurses can assist older clients in choosing a diet that will help them attain and maintain a normal body weight.

Adequate nutrition for health promotion frequently entails a reduction in caloric intake. Caloric needs decrease roughly 7.5 percent for each decade after 25 years of age.[4] Recommended daily caloric intake for women aged 50 to 75 years is approximately 1800 calories, whereas for women over 75 the recommendation is for 1600 calories. For men, approximately 2400 calories per day are recommended from age 50 to 75 years, dropping to 2050 calories daily after age 75.[25] Of course, specific caloric needs will vary from person to person, and the nurse should assess the needs of each individual client.

Despite reduced caloric needs, older adults continue to require a balance of all other nutrients. Nutritional deficits are most frequently noted for calcium, iron, vitamins A and C, and the B vitamins riboflavin and thiamine, as well as for dietary fiber. Community health nurses can promote the health of older clients by encouraging diets high in these nutrients as well as other essential nutrients.

Older persons are frequent targets for food faddists promoting supplements. Nurses can assist clients to obtain adequate nutrition by educating them regarding a well-balanced diet and can discourage expenditure of limited finances on dietary fads. Nurses can also educate clients as to the harmful nature of some food fads.

Hygiene

Promoting adequate hygiene is another aspect of health maintenance in the older adult. Skin care can be maintained by periodic bathing with mild soaps and the use of lotions to prevent drying and cracking of the skin. Clients should be discouraged from using water that is too hot and from using alcohol or powders that may further dry or irritate skin. Nails can be protected by a weekly manicure including a massage with oil and shaping with an emory board. Dry and split nails can also be prevented by advising the clients against keeping their hands in water or by wearing protective gloves while performing household cleaning chores.

Adequate hygiene and hydration can protect the older client's remaining teeth and prevent dry mouth. Special toothpastes (such as Sensodyne®) may be needed by clients who have sensitive gums. Toothbrushes should be firm enough to clean teeth, but not so hard as to injure gums. Clients should be encouraged to use a softer toothbrush on their own remaining teeth than they use on dentures.

Community health nurses can also educate older clients on the care of their hair and protection from sunburn. Hair should be brushed and combed daily with a weekly shampoo and monthly conditioning. Care should be taken in the use of dyes or permanent solutions that may irritate fragile skin. Wearing a hat while outdoors will prevent sunburn due to thinning hair.

Wearing apparel may be another area for client education to promote health. Properly fitted clothing and shoes can prevent skin irritation and breakdown. Close-toed shoes and low heels are recommended for everyday wear. Shoes should always be worn with stockings and socks should be changed daily.

Safety

Three aspects of safety should be addressed when planning primary preventive measures for older clients: elimination of environmental hazards, home and neighborhood security, and prevention of elder abuse and neglect. Plans can be made to ensure the interior and exterior repair of the client's home. Modifications can be planned to accommodate special needs. For example, graduated ramps can replace steps to facilitate access by wheelchair or walker.

The community health nurse can also plan to educate older clients on home safety, and plans can be made to eliminate safety hazards in the home. All areas of the home, especially stairs, should be well lighted and furniture should be placed so as to prevent falls. Because many elders experience nocturia, they may need to be encouraged to keep a nightlight burning to avoid disorientation or falls in the dark. Or, the client can keep a flashlight close to the bed for nighttime use as needed.

Clients should be encouraged to keep electrical cords as short as possible and to tack them along baseboards to prevent tripping over them. If throw rugs must be used, they should be of the nonskid variety. Bathrooms can be equipped with tub rails or seats and hand-held shower fixtures to make bathing safer and less arduous for the older person.

The use of space heaters and other portable heating devices should be discouraged because of the danger of burns and residential fires. Nurses should also encourage clients or their landlords to install smoke detection devices, as the elderly are particularly likely to be trapped by a fire and need sufficient warning to get out. To prevent burns, community health nurses can encourage clients to use electric blankets rather than hot water bottles in cold weather.

Older clients should also be warned about the potential for hypothermia. Persons over 60 years of age account for about half of deaths due to hypothermia each year. Clients with hypothyroidism and those using sedative-hypnotic drugs are particularly at risk for hypothermia and should be cautioned accordingly. Nurses should make sure that these and other elderly clients have an adequate caloric intake and that the homes of older persons are adequately heated.[26]

Promoting home and neighborhood security are also of concern. Older clients should be cautioned to be careful about admitting strangers into the home and to refrain from walking alone in high-crime areas. Doors and windows should have secure locks, and cars should be locked even when kept in the garage.

In many neighborhoods, police and fire personnel can be notified of homes where older persons live. If this is the case, the nurse can encourage clients to provide such notification. Clients can also arrange for "disaster signals" to neighbors. For example, if neighbors don't see the kitchen window shade raised by a certain time in the morning, they may decide to investigate.

Motor vehicles are a cause for concern in the safety of older adults. Although many older persons would like to retain their independence and continue to drive, they may not be able to do so safely because of a variety of sensory impairments. When this type of situation occurs, the nurse can encourage older clients to find other ways of remaining mobile and maintaining their independence. Perhaps they can be encouraged to drive in the daytime, but not at night. Or the nurse might acquaint the older client with local bus routes and schedules. Many local organizations will frequently provide transportation at little or no cost to older people. Or the older adult can be encouraged to ride along with a younger friend.

Motor vehicles are also problematic when older people are pedestrians. In many areas the bulk of pedestrian fatalities occur among elderly individuals. In areas where there are large numbers of elderly, nurses can campaign for traffic signals at heavily used crossings, strict enforcement of speed limits, and public awareness of the presence of older adults.

The last area of concern in promoting the safety of older clients is preventing abuse and neglect. Elder abuse and neglect frequently occur when those caring for elderly clients are unable to cope with the resulting stress. Providing support for these caretakers, teaching positive coping skills, and providing periodic respite care may help to prevent abuse. Assisting older clients to maintain their independence may also help prevent the development of a potentially abusive situation.

Immunization

Immunization of older adults is a special safety issue. Many adults in the United States, particularly older adults, have never been immunized for tetanus and are also unprotected against diphtheria. In the last few years, two-thirds of cases of tetanus have occurred in persons over 50 years of age.[27] Current Immunization Practices Advisory Committee (ACIP) recommendations for adult immunization indicate a need for completion of the primary series of diphtheria and tetanus toxoids and boosters every 10 years.[27] Annual immunization for influenza is recommended for all healthy adults over 65 years of age.[28] Immunization against pneumococcal pneumonia is also recommended for older persons.

During the period from 1972 to 1981, over 80 percent of deaths due to influenza occurred among people aged 65 or older, yet in the 1987 Behavioral Risk Factor Surveillance, only 32 percent of those over 65 reported having been immunized.[28] These figures indicate a need for community health nurses to plan education for older clients regarding the need for immunization. Older clients may also need to be referred to sources of inexpensive immunization. For example, many local health departments offer influenza and pneumococcal immunizations free or for a small charge.

Rest and Exercise

Many people believe that the need for exercise decreases with age. However, older people need exercise as much as their younger counterparts. In one study, lack of regular exercise was found to be one of the factors that significantly increased the probability of hospitalization in people over age 65. In this same study, half of the participants did not engage in regular physical activity.[20] Community health nurses should encourage older clients to engage in moderate exercise on a regular basis. Encouraging clients to elevate the legs and refrain from crossing the legs will help to prevent venous stasis and skin breakdown.

Older clients also need adequate rest. Older people tend to sleep fewer hours at night than when they were younger. They continue to need rest, however, so daily activity patterns may need to be planned to accommodate an afternoon nap. Clients should also be encouraged to arrange activities to allow for rest periods throughout the day.

Maintaining Independence

Because of physical and economic limitations, it is sometimes difficult for older persons to maintain their independence. Decreased income and physical inability to care for oneself sometimes force older clients to give up their own residence and live with family members. Whatever the living arrangements of the older client, community health nurses should assist them to maintain the highest degree of independence possible. Some older clients may be able to continue to live alone if referred to supportive services such as homemaker aides, transportation services, and Meals-on-Wheels. When older persons are living with family members, the nurse can encourage family members to foster independence in the client. This may mean encouraging them to assign specific roles within the household to the older family member.

Life Resolution and Preparation for Death

One of the developmental tasks to be accomplished by the older adult is preparation for death. This entails developing a personal set of goals and the ability to view one's life as having been meaningful and productive. Reminiscence is one way of accomplishing life resolution and achieving positive feelings about one's own life. The community health nurse must recognize and foster the older client's need to reminisce and should encourage other family members to do so as well. This is sometimes difficult given the nurse's busy schedule and the number of clients who need to be seen. However, nurses should be able to find some time during interactions with older clients to listen to these reminiscences and to help clients reflect upon their lives.

Preparation for death usually also entails a number of practical activities involved in getting one's affairs in order. Older clients may need to make decisions about funeral arrangements or the disposition of their belongings. Both nurses and family members should be encouraged to listen to clients in their reflections on such matters, rather than putting them off with assurances that they "won't die for a long time yet." Nurses may also need to refer clients for legal assistance with wills, burial plans, and other financial arrangements. Many communities have low-cost legal aid services available to elderly clients. Primary preventive interventions for older clients are summarized in Table 23–3.

SECONDARY PREVENTION

Secondary preventive measures are undertaken when health problems have occurred and primary prevention is no longer possible. As noted earlier, older clients experience a variety of health problems related to the effects of aging. They are also subject to problems stemming from chronic and communicable diseases. Secondary prevention for communicable diseases and chronic conditions are addressed in detail in Chapter 30, Communicable Disease, and Chapter 31, Chronic Physical Health Problems.

Skin Breakdown

Because of the fragility of older skin, skin breakdown is a common difficulty. The initial plan of care should be to prevent skin breakdown using the primary preventive strategies discussed earlier. Extremities should be inspected regularly for evidence of skin breakdown, and any breakdown noted should be cleansed properly and examined for signs of infection. Adequate dietary intake will contribute to maintaining skin integrity and to healing when breakdown does occur. Care should also be taken to relieve pressure on bony prominences by frequent changes of position. When skin breakdown has already occurred, the nurse should make sure that the area is kept clean and dry. If healing does not occur, the client should be referred to a physician for evaluation.

Constipation

Constipation is another common problem in older clients. Again, the primary consideration is prevention through adequate fluid and fiber in the diet as well as adequate exercise. But when constipation does occur, the nurse can suggest the use of mild natural laxatives such as prune juice. Clients should be cautioned against the overuse of laxatives. Bulk products such as Metamucil® or stool softeners should also be used with caution.

If necessary, the nurse or a family member can administer an enema. Nurses working with older clients who are constipated should determine agency policy regarding whether an enema requires a physician's order. If an order is required, the nurse can call the physician to request the authorization. Care should be taken that the enema solution is not too hot and that the client is close to the toilet, as poor sphincter control occurring with age may result in the inability to hold the enema. Again, overuse of enemas

TABLE 23–3. PRIMARY PREVENTION STRATEGIES FOR OLDER CLIENTS

Area of Concern	Primary Prevention Strategies
Nutrition	• Educate clients regarding nutritional needs • Promote caloric intake adequate to meet energy needs • Encourage well-balanced diet high in nutrient content (especially calcium, iron, and vitamins A and C, riboflavin and thiamine, and fiber) • Discourage participation in food fads • Maintain hydration
Hygiene	• Periodic bathing with mild soaps • Use of lotion to prevent drying of skin • Keep hands out of water or wear gloves • Maintain oral hygiene with good toothbrush • Maintain hydration to prevent dry mouth • Brush and comb hair daily • Weekly shampoo with mild soap, monthly conditioning
Safety	• Wear hat to protect scalp from sunburn • Wear properly fitted clothes and shoes • Use electric blanket rather than hot water bottles • Provide adequate lighting, especially on stairs • Use a nightlight at night and keep a flashlight handy • Place furniture to prevent falls • Keep electrical cords short and tack along baseboards • Eliminate throw rugs if possible or use nonskid type • Install tub rails and other safety fixtures • Discourage use of space heaters, kerosene stoves, etc. • Install smoke alarms • Notify police and fire personnel of older person in home • Promote adequate and safe heating and ventilation of home • Provide door and window locks and keep car locked • Don't admit strangers to home • Ride with others or use a bus rather than drive if senses are impaired • Use care in crossing streets • Promote family coping abilities and relieve stress to prevent abuse of older persons
Immunization	• Encourage adequate immunization for diphtheria and tetanus • Provide annual influenza immunization • Provide pneumonia vaccine
Rest and exercise	• Encourage moderate exercise on a regular basis • Arrange activities to accommodate rest periods as needed
Maintaining independence	• Provide support services that allow clients to live independently if possible • Encourage family members to foster independence • Encourage client participation in health-care planning • Advocate for client independence as needed
Life resolution and preparation for death	• Encourage reminiscence • Assist client to discuss death with family members • Assist client to put affairs in order

is contraindicated. Fecal impaction that is unrelieved by enema should be referred to the physician.

Urinary Incontinence

Urinary incontinence is a particularly distressing problem for some older adults. Incontinence occurs in approximately 30 percent of women over age 60 and may result in social withdrawal because of fear of embarrassing accidents in public. For clients with incontinence, not only are there the problems of hygiene and odor, but self-image is threatened by the inability to control one's bodily functions. Clients with stress incontinence should be referred for a urological consultation. Nursing interventions that may help urinary incontinence include encouraging clients to void frequently and teaching them Kegel pelvic floor exercises. Bladder training may also help to resolve the problem. Biofeedback techniques have been found to relieve both urinary and fecal incontinence in older adults.

In some instances, incontinence becomes a chronic problem. For clients in this situation, the nurse needs to assure that skin, clothing, and linens remain clean and dry. Sanitary pads, disposable underpants, or panty liners may prevent clothing and linens from becoming wet and may increase the client's confidence in going out in public. Frequent changes in such sanitary aids should be encouraged to prevent skin breakdown.

For bedfast clients, ready availability of a bedpan or urinal, or assistance to a bedside commode at frequent intervals, may reduce the frequency of linen changes. A bedside commode may also be of use to clients who are able to get up but have mobility limitations. The community health nurse may help arrange for the purchase or rental of these devices from durable medical equipment companies.

Sensory Loss

Planning to provide adequate lighting is particularly important in compensating for loss of visual acuity. If clients wear glasses, nurses should make sure that the degree of correction is appropriate and that glasses are kept clean. Nurses and clients should also take care that when glasses are removed they are placed in a safe, but accessible, location.

The use of large-print books, a magnifying glass, or books on tape can assist older clients to continue reading as a leisure activity. Taking medications may also be hampered by loss of visual acuity. When clients have difficulties reading medication labels, the nurse can color-code the labels. Colors used should be easily distinguishable, as there may be a loss of color discrimination with age, particularly with the colors blue, green, and violet.[29]

The community health nurse can also suggest several measures that will help to compensate for diminished hearing. Speaking clearly (not loudly) and at a lower pitch will improve the older client's ability to hear. Properly functioning hearing aids will also help some clients. Clients who are concerned about the unsightliness of old-fashioned hearing aids can be assured that there are many less noticeable devices available today. Speech should be slower, as many older persons have problems hearing rapid speech and have difficulty discriminating several specific sounds, among them *s, z, t, f, g,* and *th.*[29] These auditory problems can be overcome by the use of multisensory input (for example, using visual as well as auditory techniques in teaching older clients).

Eliminating background noise may also enhance the older person's ability to hear. Nurses working with older clients should always obtain feedback to be sure that clients have accurately heard and interpreted verbal messages. For clients living alone or others who must be able to use a telephone, the nurse can suggest voice-enhancement devices that enable older people to hear better.

Because of older clients' diminished sense of touch, nurses should discourage clients from using hot water for bathing and from wearing open-toed shoes. Clients should be encouraged to check extremities periodically for injuries and to use extreme caution in working with sharp or other potentially harmful objects.

Decreased senses of smell and taste pose problems for older adults in that they may lead to diminished appetite. Older individuals can be encouraged to add additional spices and herbs to flavor foods. However, care should be taken that such condiments are not contraindicated (for example, additional salt for the client with hypertension or chili pepper for the client with an ulcer). Loss of the sense of smell is also problematic in that older clients may not be as easily able to tell when foodstuffs are spoiled or may not be able to smell smoke or a gas leak. Nurses may want to encourage clients using gas for cooking or heating periodically to check that pilot lights remain lit. They should also encourage the purchase of small amounts of perishable foods and rapid use before they spoil. Smoke detectors are also necessary devices in the homes of older clients.

Mobility Limitation

Related problems for older clients involve limitation of mobility and consequent impairment in the ability to carry out activities of daily living. Nurses can explore options for assisting older clients to perform activities of daily living (ADL). Referral to a home-care agency that has homemaker services may help with tasks such as housekeeping and grocery shopping. Home-care agencies may also provide assistance with personal-care services such as bathing or hair washing. There are also a number of mechanical devices that make it easier for older clients to care for themselves (for example, special devices for clients with arthritis that make it easier to open jars or reach objects on shelves).

For clients who need outside assistance but do not have insurance coverage or cannot afford special services, volunteer services may be available through local churches or other social groups. Students workers are sometimes a good source of assistance with instrumental activities. Both high school and college students may be willing to provide services for small fees or for a room. The community health nurse can also explore service projects undertaken by sororities or fraternities at local colleges or universities that may provide assistance for older clients.

The nurse may refer clients who cannot cook for themselves to a Meals-on-Wheels program. For clients who are mobile, a referral for a lunch program at the local senior citizen center may be more appropriate. Such centers may also provide assistance with transportation to and from the center, for shopping, and for physician appointments.

Pain

The management of chronic pain is another common problem among older adults. For clients with arthritis, pain may be controlled with the use of anti-inflammatory and analgesic agents such as aspirin. When a mild analgesic is not effective, stronger medication may be prescribed by the physician. Nurses should evaluate the appropriateness of any pain medication being taken by clients and should educate clients on the correct use of medications. They may also need to caution clients regarding overuse of some medications and discourage the use of medications that are contraindicated by the client's condition. For example, clients taking anticoagulants should not take aspirin for pain, because aspirin further increases clotting time and may lead to serious bleeding.

Clients with arthritis pain may do better if they do not attempt strenuous activity immediately after awakening when joints tend to be stiff and sore. Clients can be helped to plan activities for when their pain is at a minimum. Warm baths or soaks may also help to relieve pain. For other forms of pain, medication may again be used and the nurse should monitor its effectiveness in relieving pain. Nurses should also educate clients as to the adverse effects of specific pain medications and make sure that clients are familiar with the symptoms of adverse effects.

Confusion

Confusion is a problem encountered in some older clients. Confusion may be either a transient or a persistent condition. Transient confusion frequently occurs in new situations or in the dark. It may also occur when clients are moved away from familiar surroundings as might occur following a move to a residential community or a nursing home. In this case, confusion may be referred to as "relocation trauma."[30] Relocation trauma may even occur when the client is moved from one hallway or one bed to another.

Continuing confusion is sometimes called *dementia,* a global impairment of intellectual functioning that may include such symptoms as failing attention, failing memory, and declining mathematical ability.[30] Confusion is a frequent side effect of many medications, and nurses should monitor a client's state of orientation with respect to medication use. Other nursing interventions include improving sensory input, preventing malnutrition and dehydration, and preventing falls.

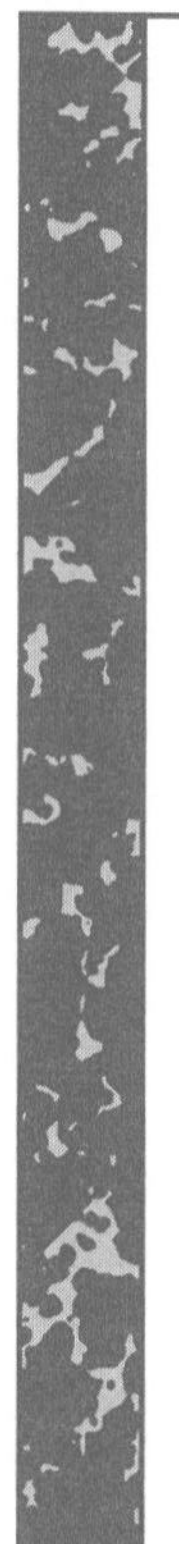

BOX 23–5

Principles of Reality Orientation

- Provide a calm environment without excessive stimulation
- Establish and maintain a regular routine
- Phrase questions and answers clearly and concisely
- Speak directly to the client
- Provide clear instructions or directions
- Provide frequent reminders of date, time, and place
- Refocus the client on reality and prevent rambling speech
- Be firm, but gentle
- Be sincere
- Be consistent

(Source: Forbes & Fitzsimons[7])

In working with confused older clients, the nurse should plan for consistent intervention to reorient clients to their environment. Reality orientation interventions are based on several general principles that can be found in Box 23–5.

Confusion is a symptom frequently encountered in clients with Alzheimer's disease. While Alzheimer's is no longer considered a natural part of aging, its cause is, as yet, not well understood. It is, however, a debilitating disease that places a heavy burden on the client and his or her family. Nurses working with families of clients with Alzheimer's will need to provide a great deal of support. Families may need to consider nursing home placement and may need help in making arrangements. They may also need assistance in dealing with the guilt engendered by their inability to care for a family member, especially a spouse, at home.

For families who choose to care for the client with Alzheimer's at home, the nurse can help arrange home care or respite care. Nurses can also encourage families of clients who wander to use an identification kit similar to that used for identifying lost children.

Such kits can be purchased at low cost through the *One in a Million* program of the American Red Cross.

Depression

Depression is another area in which the nurse working with older clients may need to take action. Mild transient depression is a relatively normal phenomenon for most people. Depression may occur with the loss of familiar people and places or on anniversaries of those losses. It is normal, for example, for the older person to become somewhat depressed on the anniversary of a spouse's death or on the deceased person's birthday. In these instances, nurses can help clients to recognize their depression as a normal feeling. Encouraging them to discuss the loved one and to relive happy memories while acknowledging their feelings of sadness may help to alleviate the depression.

Severe depression, on the other hand, requires referral for counseling or other forms of therapy. Severe depression may be marked by continued inattention to personal hygiene, failure to take part in normal activities such as dressing or combing one's hair, and by poor appetite. Depression may also be signaled by withdrawal from interaction with others. Again, the nurse should encourage the client to ventilate feelings regarding the cause of the depression, but should also refer the client for additional help as needed.

Social Isolation

Social isolation is a relatively common problem among older adults, especially the "old elderly." Isolation may stem from a variety of circumstances mentioned earlier, including sensory deficits, communication difficulties, and loss of mobility.

Loss of family and friends is a significant contributor to social isolation in the elderly. As spouses and other family members or friends die, the social support system for the older person is reduced. In this instance, nurses can help older clients to establish new social support systems by helping them get involved with other groups. Referral to an active senior citizens center may be appropriate. Many religious groups also have a variety of social activities for older persons. Special-interest groups that incorporate people of all ages may provide an avenue for social interaction. For example, there may be a local bridge club or garden club that may be of interest to a particular client. The nurse can also encourage remaining family and friends to include the older person in their activities.

Loss of family and friends also leads to the problem of grief. Grief may also be engendered by anticipation of the client's own death, particularly when the client has a terminal illness. The nurse can assist clients to deal with grief by exploring with them their feelings about death. Acceptance of possible anger may be necessary as well. Clients can be assisted to deal with their own feelings of anger and depression regarding death.

If the client is willing, referral to a pastor or other source of spiritual counsel may be appropriate. Family and friends should be encouraged to talk with the client about his or her impending death and the client should be allowed to make arrangements for disposition of personal property or plans for burial. As much as possible, dying clients should be allowed to continue in accustomed roles and should have control over decisions affecting their own life or death. If the client has a living will, the nurse should see that a copy of the will is placed in the client's record and that the will is adhered to by both family members and health-care professionals.

Abuse and Neglect

Abuse or neglect of older persons is another problem for which nursing intervention may be required. Nurses should be alert to situations that have potential for abuse. Dependent elders who place a serious burden on caretakers or who were abusive parents themselves are at risk for abuse and neglect. Other situations in which potential for abuse is increased include reduced social status, other sources of stress for care-givers (for example, unemployment or illness in other family members), and family dysfunction.[25]

Resolving an abusive situation may require assisting caretakers to develop adequate mechanisms for coping with the frustrations of caring for an older adult. Persons in abusive situations can also be referred for counseling. Respite care can also help to reduce the burden of care of an older family member, and the nurse may need to help families arrange for such care. Removal of the older person and nursing home placement may also reduce the potential for abuse. Finally, in situations where abuse cannot be controlled, the nurse may arrange for placement of the older person in a temporary shelter while arrangements are made for other care.

Alcohol Abuse

Abuse of alcohol may warrant referral for a variety of services. Initially, the nurse may need to refer the client to a detoxification facility. Because of their diminished capacity to detoxify alcohol and other substances, older clients are at high risk for complications during detoxification and should be in a facility where adequate supervision is possible. Once detoxification has been accomplished, the client should be referred for ongoing counseling for his or her drinking problem. Referral to such groups as Alcoholics Anonymous may also be appropriate. Families with older alcoholics may also need assistance in dealing with the problem, and referral to Al-Anon may help.

Older clients and their families should also be educated regarding the effects of alcohol and its potential for interaction with medication. Overuse of preparations containing alcohol should be discouraged as well.

Inadequate Financial Resources

Another common problem of older adults is inadequate financial resources. Many older people have reduced incomes that may not be sufficient to meet their needs. Nurses can refer clients to sources of financial assistance as appropriate. Clients who are receiving minimal Social Security benefits may be eligible for Supplemental Security Income (SSI) that also entitles them to Medicaid benefits. Referrals may also be made for food stamps and other general assistance programs. Some utility companies provide reduced rates for older adults, something that the client can inquire about. Moreover, in some places the Area Office on Aging may provide free food from government surpluses. The nurse should become familiar with other local sources of financial assistance for older persons and make referrals to these agencies as appropriate.

The community health nurse may also be of assistance to older persons living on reduced incomes by helping them to prioritize expenditures and budget their income accordingly. The nurse may also provide information about lower-cost foods that provide adequate nutrition. Clients should be encouraged to buy staple goods in quantities that will reduce prices. Perishable foods, however, should only be purchased in quantities that can be used before spoiling. The nurse may also encourage several older clients to buy items in bulk and split the costs to reduce expenditures for each individual.

Chronic Illness

As noted earlier, older persons experience a variety of chronic illnesses. Among these are arthritis, heart disease, hypertension, diabetes, and chronic lung conditions. Secondary prevention for these conditions would include screening for specific diseases, diagnosis, and treatment. Community health nursing involvement in secondary prevention for these illnesses includes referral for medical services as needed, as well as supportive therapy during treatment. Community health nurses frequently educate clients regarding their conditions and the treatment recommended. Older persons may need instruction regarding their medications and possible side effects. In addition, the nurse will monitor clients for treatment effects and for side effects and toxic effects of medications. They may also educate clients in other forms of symptom relief—for example, warm soaks for arthritic joints. Clients may also need emotional support in dealing with their disease and its effects.

Communicable Diseases

Older clients are at higher risk than younger people for communicable diseases such as influenza and pneumonia. Primary prevention of these diseases through immunization is desirable, but when this fails, the community health nurse may be involved in referring clients for medical care for these conditions as needed. Nurses will also instruct clients in self-care during illness and monitor the effects of communicable conditions on health status. The nurse working with older clients with these diseases should be particularly alert to signs of complications as these are more common in older individuals than in their younger counterparts. Controlling fever and maintaining hydration are two particularly important aspects of secondary prevention for communicable diseases in the elderly.

Advocacy for Older Clients

Many times nursing interventions for older clients will involve advocacy. Advocacy may take place at the individual or aggregate level. At the individual level, the nurse may encourage family members to respect the client's need for privacy or allow the client to make his or her own health-care decisions. Advocacy may also be needed in interactions with other health-care providers. Advocacy may also involve encouraging families to allow the client as much independence as possible. Intervention on behalf of the abused client is also a form of advocacy.

At the aggregate level, nurses can see that the needs of the older population are made known to public policymakers. They can become politically active to see that the needs of this group are being met by governmental agencies. They may also need to work with nongovernmental agencies to ensure that the needs of older clients are met. For example, community health nurses might work with a coalition of religious groups to provide shelter for abused elders, or they might help a group of older adults establish some type of cooperative buying effort to decrease expenditures. There may also be a need to point out the needs of older persons to transportation authorities. Table 23–4 summarizes secondary preventive activities that may benefit older clients.

TABLE 23–4. SECONDARY PREVENTION FOR COMMON PROBLEMS IN OLDER CLIENTS

Client Problem	Secondary Preventive Measures
Skin breakdown	• Inspect extremities regularly for lesions • Keep lesions clean and dry • Eliminate pressure by frequent changes of position • Refer for treatment as needed
Constipation	• Encourage fluid and fiber intake • Discourage ignoring urge to defecate • Encourage regular exercise • Encourage regular bowel habits • Use mild laxatives as needed, but discourage overuse • Administer enemas as needed, discourage overuse • Administer bulk products or stool softeners as indicated
Urinary incontinence	• Refer for urological consult • Encourage frequent voiding • Teach Kegel exercises • Assist with bladder training • Encourage use of sanitary pads, panty liners, etc., with frequent changes of such aids • Keep skin clean and dry, change clothing and linen as needed • Offer bedpan or urinal frequently or assist to bedside commode at frequent intervals
Sensory loss	• Provide adequate lighting • Keep eyeglasses clean and hearing aids functional • Eliminate safety hazards • Use large-print books or materials • Use multisensory approaches to communication and teaching • Avoid using colors that make discrimination difficult • Speak clearly and slowly, at a lower pitch • Eliminate background noise • Assist clients to obtain voice enhancers for phone, etc. • Use additional herbs and spices, but use with discretion • Purchase small amounts of perishable foods • Check pilot lights on gas appliances frequently • Encourage the use of smoke detectors
Mobility limitation	• Provide assistance with ambulation, transfer, etc. • Assist clients to obtain equipment such as walkers, wheelchairs, etc. • Install ramps, tub rails, etc., as needed • Promote access to public facilities for older persons • Assist clients to find sources of transportation • Make referrals for assistance with personal-care or instrumental activities
Pain	• Plan activities for times when pain is controlled • Encourage warm soaks • Encourage adequate rest and exercise to prevent mobility limitations
Confusion	• Apply principles of reality orientation
Depression	• Accept feelings and reflect on their normality; encourage client to ventilate feelings • Refer for counseling as needed
Social isolation	• Compensate for sensory loss; enhance communication abilities • Improve mobility; provide access to transportation • Assist client to obtain adequate financial resources • Refer client to new support systems • Assist client to deal with grief over loss of loved ones
Abuse or neglect	• Assist caretakers to develop positive coping strategies • Assist families to obtain respite care or day care for older members • Refer families for counseling as needed • Arrange placement in temporary shelter • Assist families in making other arrangements for safe care of older clients
Alcohol abuse	• Identify problem drinking by older clients • Refer for therapy; Alcoholics Anonymous or Al-Anon as appropriate • Observe for toxic effects of alcohol ingestion • Maintain hydration and nutrition
Inadequate financial resources	• Refer for financial assistance • Assist with budgeting and priority allocation • Educate for less expensive means of meeting needs • Function as an advocate as needed

TABLE 23–5. TERTIARY PREVENTION STRATEGIES FOR OLDER CLIENTS

Client Problem	Tertiary Prevention Strategies
Inadequate nutrition	• Educate clients regarding nutritional needs • Promote caloric intake adequate to meet energy needs • Encourage well-balanced diet high in nutrient content (especially those with prior deficits) • Discourage participation in food fads • Maintain hydration
Skin breakdown	• Periodic bathing with mild soaps • Use of lotion to prevent drying of skin • Keep hands out of water or wear gloves • Elevate legs and refrain from crossing legs • Wear loose-fitting clothing and properly fitted shoes • Inspect extremities regularly for lesions • Relieve pressure on bony prominences by frequent change of position
Constipation	• Encourage fluid and fiber intake • Discourage ignoring urge to defecate • Encourage regular exercise • Encourage regular bowel habits • Use mild laxatives as needed, but discourage overuse • Administer enemas as needed, discourage overuse • Administer bulk products or stool softeners as indicated
Sensory loss	• Provide adequate lighting • Keep eyeglasses clean and hearing aids functional • Eliminate safety hazards • Use large-print books or materials • Use multisensory approaches to communication and teaching • Avoid using colors that make discrimination difficult • Speak clearly and slowly, at a lower pitch • Eliminate background noise • Assist clients to obtain voice enhancers for phone, etc. • Use additional herbs and spices, but use with discretion • Purchase small amounts of perishable foods • Check pilot lights on gas appliances frequently • Encourage the use of smoke detectors
Confusion	• Apply principles of reality orientation
Abuse or neglect	• Provide support for victim and caretakers • Assist families to obtain respite care or day care for older members • Refer families for counseling as needed • Monitor family situation closely • Assist families in making other arrangements for safe-care of older clients as needed • Promote self-image of victim and abuser • Foster independence of victim and abuser
Alcohol abuse	• Provide support for abstinence • Refer to support group • Provide support to family in dealing with problem • Provide assistance in dealing with stress • Promote positive self-image
Accidental injury	• Eliminate safety hazards from environment • Encourage use of safety aids • Provide supervision for confused older person
Social isolation	• Assist client to build social support network • Refer to church or other groups for social activities • Provide means of transportation

TERTIARY PREVENTION

Tertiary preventive activities for older clients focus on preventing complications of existing conditions and preventing their recurrence. Tertiary prevention for the individual client will depend upon the problems experienced by the client. For example, tertiary prevention for an abused older client may include long-term counseling for family members, while that related to financial inadequacies may involve assistance with budgeting.

TABLE 23–6. SOURCES OF ASSISTANCE FOR OLDER CLIENTS AND THEIR FAMILIES

Problem Area	Agency or Organization	Services
Aging	American Society on Aging 833 Market St., Suite 516 San Francisco, CA 94103 (415) 543-2617	Advocacy, legislation, policy formation, information on resources
	Gerontological Society 1835 K Street, NW, Suite 305 Washington, DC 20006 (202) 466-6750	Research on aging and care of the elderly
	National Geriatrics Society 212 W. Wisconsin Ave. Milwaukee, WI 53203 (414) 272-4130	Research and public education on care of older persons
	National Institute on Aging 9000 Rockville Pike Bethesda, MD 20892 (301) 496-1752	Research on aging
	Western Gerontological Society 833 Market St., 5th Floor San Francisco, CA 94103 (415) 543-2617	Research, information
Airway disease	American Lung Association 1740 Broadway New York, NY 10019 (212) 245-8000	Research, information, antismoking programs
	Emphysema Anonymous, Inc. P.O. Box 66 Ft. Myers, FL 33902 (813) 334-4226	Self-help group
Alcohol abuse	Al-Anon Family Group Headquarters P.O. Box 182 Madison Square Station New York, NY 10159 (212) 481-6565	Help for families with alcoholic members
	Alcoholics Anonymous 468 Park Avenue South New York, NY 10016 (212) 686-1100	Self-help group for alcoholics
Alzheimer's Disease	Alzheimer's Disease & Related Disorders Association 70 E. Lake Chicago, IL 60601 (312) 853-3060	Research, advocacy, public education, family support
Arthritis	Arthritis Foundation 3400 Peachtree Rd. Atlanta, GA 30326 (404) 266-0795	Public information
	Arthritis Rehabilitation Center 1234 19th St., NW Washington, DC 20036 (202) 223-5320	Diagnostic and treatment services
	Arthritis Society 920 Young St., Suite 420 Toronto, Canada M4W 3J7 (416) 967-1414	Professional training, research, information
Diet and nutrition	Local Meals-on-Wheels	Hot lunch delivered to home

(*continued*)

TABLE 23–6. (*Continued*)

Problem Area	Agency or Organization	Services
Diet and nutrition (*continued*)	Local senior citizens centers	Low-cost meals
	Area Office on Aging	Distribution of surplus foodstuffs
Cancer	American Cancer Society 777 Third Ave. New York, NY (212) 371-2900	Research, information, rehabilitation
	Cancer Care, Inc. One Park Ave. New York, NY 10016 (212) 679-5700	Social work assistance, counseling, home management, financial assistance, bereavement counseling
	United Ostomy Association 1111 Wilshire Blvd. Los Angeles, CA 90017 (213) 255-4681	Mutual aid and support, information
Death and dying	Concern for Dying 250 W. 57th St., Room 831 New York, NY 10107	Individual care, help for families with dying members
	Hospice Education Institute P.O. Box 713 5 Essex Square, Suite 3B Essex, CT 06426 (203) 767-1620	Public and professional education on hospice, death, and dying
	International Institute for the Study of Death P.O. Box 8565 Pembroke Pines, FL 33084 (305) 435-2730	Support dialogue on death
	Living/Dying Project P.O. Box 357 Fairfax, CA 94930	Counseling for terminally ill
	Make Today Count, Inc. P.O. Box 303 Burlington, IA 52601 (319) 753-6521	Self-help group for those with serious illnesses
Dental problems	International Academy of Geriatric Dentistry 2 No. Riverside Plaza Chicago, IL 60606 (312) 432-2341	Research in geriatric dentistry
Diabetes	American Diabetes Assoc. 1 W. 48th St. New York, NY 10010	Research, information
Health Promotion	National Center for Health Promotion and Aging ℅ National Council on Aging 600 Maryland Ave., SW Washington, DC 20024 (202) 479-1200	Information and materials on health promotion programs for older adults
Hearing loss	Alexander Graham Bell Association for the Deaf 3417 Volta Place, NW Washington, DC 20007 (202) 337-5220	Assistance to hearing-impaired adults and children, public education, policy formation, advocacy
	American Speech-Language-Hearing Association 10801 Rockville Pike Rockville, MD 20852 (301) 897-5700	Research, public information on prevention of communication problems

TABLE 23–6. (*Continued*)

Problem Area	Agency or Organization	Services
Hearing loss (*continued*)	Deafness Research Foundation 55 E. 34th St. New York, NY 10016 (212) 684-6556	Public education on deafness, research; sponsors National Temporal Bone Bank
	Hearing Industries Assoc. 1800 M St., NW Washington, DC 20036 (202) 833-1411	Research and public education about hearing aids
	National Association of the Deaf 814 Thayer Ave. Silver Spring, MD 20910 (301) 587-1788	Advocacy, public education, legislation
Heart disease	American Heart Association 7320 Greenville Ave. Dallas, TX 75231 (214) 750-5300	Research, information
	Council on Arteriosclerosis of American Heart Assoc. 7320 Greenville Avenue Dallas, TX 75231 (214) 750-5300	Coordinates research on arteriosclerosis; provides information
	Mended Hearts, Inc. 7320 Greenville Ave. Dallas, TX 75231 (214) 750-5442	Assistance to persons having heart surgery
Home care/nursing homes	American Association of Homes for the Aging 1050 17th St., NW, Suite 770 Washington, DC 20036 (202) 296-5960	Advocacy, technical assistance to nursing homes and institutions
	Americans for Better Care 913 Tennessee No. 2 Lawrence, KS 66044 (913) 842-3088	Legislation and advocacy for nursing home residents
	CHAP Program of the National League for Nursing 100 Columbus Circle New York, NY 10014	Accredits home health-care agencies
	International Council of Homehelp Services Postbus 13020 NL 3507 LA Utrecht, Netherlands	Trains family members in care of handicapped; public education, research
	National Council for Home Caring 67 Irving Place New York, NY 10003 (212) 674-4990	Research, public information
Menopause	International Menopause Society 8 Avenue Don Bosco B1150 Brussels, Belgium	Research, information
Safety	American National Red Cross One-in-a-Million Program 17th & D Streets Washington, DC 20006	Client identification kit for use with confused or disoriented clients who may become lost
Social welfare	American Association of Retired Persons 3200 E. Carson St. Lakewood, CA 90712	Advocacy, cooperative buying programs for insurance and medications

(*continued*)

TABLE 23–6. (*Continued*)

Problem Area	Agency or Organization	Services
Social welfare (*continued*)	Gray Panthers 3635 Chestnut St. Philadelphia, PA 19104 (215) 382-3300	Advocacy for needs of older persons
	Health Care Financing Administration Administration on Aging 330 Independence Ave, SW Washington, DC 20201 (202) 245-0724	Identify elder needs, coordinate federal assistance to elderly
	Medicare Hospital Insurance Medicare Supplemental Medical Insurance Meadows East Bldg. 6325 Security Blvd. Baltimore, MD 21207 (310) 594-9000	Reimburses for services under Medicare
	National Indian Council on Aging P.O. Box 2088 Albuquerque, NM 87103 (505) 766-2276	Advocacy for older American Indians and Alaskan Natives
	National Support Center for Families of the Aging P.O. Box 245 Swarthmore, PA 19081 (215) 544-5933	Support for families caring for elders; public education
	Social Security Administration 6401 Security Bldg. Baltimore, MD 21235 (301) 594-3120	Administers Social Security and Medicare programs
	U.S. House of Representatives Select Committee on Aging Subcommittee on Health and Long-Term Care H2-377 House Office Bldg. Annex II Washington, DC 20515 (202) 226-3381	Policy formation, legislation
	U.S. Senate Committee on Labor and Human Resources Subcommittee on Aging SH-404 Hart Senate Office Bldg. Washington, DC 20510 (202) 224-3239	Policy formation, legislation
Visual impairment	Christian Record Braille Foundation, Inc. P.O. Box 6097 Lincoln, NE 68506 (402) 488-0981	Free books and magazines (Braille and large-type) records and cassettes
	Eye Bank for Sight Restoration, Inc. 210 E. 64th St. New York, NY 10021	Provides donor tissue for corneal transplants
	John Milton Society for the Blind 475 Riverside Dr., Room 832 New York, NY 10115 (212) 870-3335	Christian literature (Braille and large-type), records
	Local Lions Club	Provides eyeglasses
	National Association for Visually Handicapped 305 E. 24th St. New York, NY 10010 (212) 889-3141	Counseling, information, books

In many instances, tertiary preventive measures are similar to those used for primary prevention. For example, primary and tertiary prevention for constipation both involve increasing fluid and fiber intake and exercise. Similarly, primary preventive measures to prevent skin breakdown can also be used to prevent a recurrence of the problem. Examples of tertiary prevention measures used with older adults are presented in Table 23–5.

In planning health care to meet the needs of older clients, the nurse will frequently make referrals or obtain assistance for clients from outside agencies. Some sources of assistance for older clients and their families are presented in Table 23–6. In making referrals for older clients, the nurse should consider carefully the client's ability to follow through on the referral. The nurse should also explain carefully to the client what services may be provided by the referral agency and how to go about obtaining those services. In some instances, it may be necessary for the nurse to make arrangements for the client if the client is not able to do so. For instance, some social service agencies will make arrangements to visit a client's home if the client is unable to get to them.

IMPLEMENTING NURSING CARE FOR OLDER CLIENTS

Nurse and client together implement the plan of care. Some activities of implementation may also be carried out by members of the client's family or by significant others. The extent of responsibility of each will depend on the client's level of function and the ability of the client or others to carry out the actions required.

Frequently, implementing the plan of care involves educating the client (or significant others). Health education for older clients is based on the general principles of teaching and learning discussed in Chapter 7, The Health Education Process. There are also some unique considerations in implementing an educational plan for the older adult.

Sensory losses need to be taken into consideration when teaching the older client. Strategies to circumvent hearing loss include using a lower-pitched voice; facing the client while speaking; employing nonverbal teaching techniques; using clear, concise terminology; and having client use a hearing aid when possible. The effects of hearing loss can also be minimized by limiting background noise, reemphasizing important points, and supplementing verbal with written materials.[31]

The use of glasses, a magnifying glass, and large print may help to minimize visual deficits. Learning can also be enhanced by visual materials using black lettering on white or yellow paper and providing adequate lighting and eliminating glare in the learning environment.

In implementing health education plans for the older client, the nurse may need to repeat material more frequently.[29] Because of decreases in short-term memory, it may take longer for an older client to learn new material. Once material is learned, however, older clients will retain it as well as younger ones. With age, memory for information that is heard is better than that for information seen, so multisensorial presentation of information is desirable.[31] Multiple repetitions, reinforcement of verbal content with written materials, and the use of memory aids (for example, a calendar for taking medications) may also assist learning in the older client.

Because response times are longer for older people than for their younger counterparts, lessons should proceed at a slower pace and the nurse should allow increased time for responses on the part of the client. Self-paced instruction is helpful. Motivation to learn can be heightened by increasing client participation in the lesson and by setting easily attainable, progressive goals that enhance success and satisfaction. Irrelevant material can confuse clients and should be eliminated from the presentation.

Endurance may be somewhat limited in the older client, so teaching sessions should be kept short (10 to 15 minutes per session). Lessons should be scheduled at times of the day when the client is rested and comfortable. Health education for the older client should not be time-limited, as the client may need more or less time to learn specific material. Again, learning should be broken down into small, progressive steps so that periodic success will motivate the client to further effort. The teaching–learning process should also allow for rest periods as needed.

EVALUATING NURSING CARE FOR OLDER CLIENTS

The last aspect of the use of the epidemiologic prevention process model with older clients is evaluation. Evaluation should include an assessment of the current status of all identified health problems and the effectiveness of nursing interventions in resolving them. Evaluation should also consider the overall health status of the client and the quality of his or her life.

Some specific constraints need to be considered in evaluating the effectiveness of nursing intervention with the elderly.[18] One of these is that the etiology of some problems may lie in other problems caused by aging itself and that these problems may not be capable of complete resolution. In this case, the nurse should evaluate the extent to which the effects of the problem on the client's life have been ameliorated. For example, it will not be possible to eliminate arthritis pain. The nurse and client can, however, evaluate the extent to which nursing interventions have limited the effects of pain on the client's ability to perform ADL.

The second consideration is that the prognosis for one problem may be affected by the presence of other problems. For instance, the existence of a terminal condition may make pain control increasingly difficult. In some cases, orientation and alertness might need to be sacrificed so as to control pain with the use of more powerful analgesics.

Evaluation must also take into account the possibility that one problem may diminish while another gets worse. Again, the example of pain control in terminal illness may lead to increasing confusion and disorientation that will entail other nursing interventions. Finally, the nurse and client must consider that deterioration in one area might lead to the development of additional problems that will need to be addressed. For example, decreased mobility will lead to greater potential for constipation and skin breakdown. Therefore, while the status of individual problems needs to be assessed, there is a need to allow for a give-and-take or a realistic assessment of the ups and downs that may be involved in the care of the older person.

CHAPTER HIGHLIGHTS

- The number of elderly people in the United States is increasing dramatically. This population is in need of community health nursing services to improve the quality, as well as length, of life.
- Aging is a normal human phenomenon surrounded by myth. Some of the myths associated with aging include beliefs that aging is a time of tranquility; that aging is synonymous with senility; that older persons are less productive than younger persons; that older persons are resistant to change; and that aging is a uniform process with similar outcomes for all people.
- Theories of aging may be categorized as stochastic theories, genetic theories, psychological theories, and sociological theories. Stochastic theories include somatic mutation theory and error theory. Genetic theories of aging include neuroendocrine theory, the intrinsic mutagenesis theory, the immunological theory, and the free-radical theory.
- Psychological theories of aging include Jungian psychoanalytic theory, Sullivan's interpersonal theory, Maslow's human needs theory, and Erickson's theory of psychosocial development.
- Sociological theories of aging include disengagement theory, activity theory, and continuity theory.
- Aging results in changes in each body system. These changes may contribute to a variety of health problems experienced by the elderly. In assessing human biological factors influencing the health of older clients, the community health nurse would assess both the effects of aging and the presence of physical health problems unrelated to the aging process.
- Physical environmental considerations in assessing the older client include the adequacy of housing, the presence of safety hazards in the home or community, and the availability of necessary goods and services.
- Assessment of the client's psychological environment entails consideration of the client's mental status and sources of stress for the client. One area of stress to which the nurse should be particularly alert is abuse or neglect of the older person.
- Areas of concern in relation to the older client's social environment include the adequacy of the client's social network and considerations related to institutionalization.
- Life-style concerns in assessing the health of older clients include nutrition, exercise, leisure pursuits and retirement, adjustment to reduced income, personal habits and medication use, sexuality, and level of independence and ability to perform activities of daily living.
- Health system assessment with respect to the older client would address the client's usual source of health care and the adequacy of care for meeting the client's health needs. Barriers to the use of health-care services would also be explored.
- Areas for consideration in planning primary preventive interventions for older clients include nutrition, hygiene, safety, immunization, rest and exercise, maintaining independence, and life resolution and preparation for death.
- Secondary preventive interventions may be required for a variety of health problems experienced by older clients. Some common conditions for which nursing intervention may be required include skin breakdown, constipation, urinary incontinence, sensory loss, mobility limitations, pain, confusion, and depression. Other common problems for which nursing intervention may be required are social isolation, abuse and neglect, alcohol abuse, inadequate financial resources, chronic illness, and communicable diseases. Advocacy is another secondary preventive measure that may be needed by older clients.
- Tertiary prevention with older clients is geared toward preventing recurrence of health problems or preventing complications of existing conditions.
- Implementing health-care plans for older clients frequently entails educating the client or significant others. Special considerations in implementing health education for older persons include the effects of sensory losses, the need to repeat material more often, the need to slow the pace of the lesson, and the need to limit educational sessions to prevent fatigue.

Review Questions

1. What are four common myths related to aging? What is the reality related to each myth? (p. 550)
2. Describe at least five theories of aging. Be sure to identify the category theory to which each theory belongs. (p. 551)
3. Describe at least two changes in each body system that occur as a normal result of the aging process. What are the implications of these changes for the health of older clients? (p. 555)
4. What are the three major factors in assessing the physical environment of an older client? (p. 557)
5. Describe at least four considerations in assessing the influence of life-style factors on the health of older clients. Give an example of the influence on health of factors in each area. (p. 559)
6. Describe at least six areas for primary prevention in the care of older clients. (p. 561)
7. Describe at least one secondary preventive measure for each of four common health problems encountered among older clients. (p. 563)
8. Identify at least three factors related to older clients that may influence the community health nurse's approach to health education. What nursing interventions might modify the influence of these factors? (p. 575)
9. Describe four considerations in evaluating the effects of nursing care that are unique to older clients. (p. 575)

APPLICATION AND SYNTHESIS

Jessica MacDonald is a 68-year-old black woman who has been referred for community health nursing services following her discharge from the hospital. She was hospitalized after being found unconscious in her room by her 50-year-old daughter. A diagnosis of diabetes mellitus was made, and Mrs. MacDonald was placed on 15 units of NPH insulin daily. She and her daughter were instructed on injection technique and a diabetic diet at the hospital.

Mrs. MacDonald lives with her daughter and son-in-law and their three teenage boys (ages 18, 15, and 13). They live in a lower-class neighborhood and the son-in-law works at the local textile plant. His income is barely enough for the family to live on. Mrs. MacDonald doesn't know how she will pay her hospital bill. She is on Medicare and has a small Social Security income, but she does not have any supplemental health insurance.

Mrs. MacDonald's vision is failing, probably as a result of undiagnosed diabetes of long-standing. She hears well, but is 80 pounds overweight, so is unsteady on her feet. The family lives in a second-floor apartment and there is no handrail on the stairs outside the apartment. Mrs. MacDonald tries to help out around the house because her daughter works. She says she doesn't want to be a burden to her daughter and her son-in-law. Mrs. MacDonald's husband died of a heart attack 8 months ago, and she came to live with her daughter then. Mrs. MacDonald's daughter says that her mother's presence has caused some friction among the boys because the two younger ones now have to share a room.

1. What are the human biological, environmental, life-style, and health system factors influencing Mrs. MacDonald's health?
2. What nursing diagnoses can be derived from the information presented in the case study? Be sure to include the etiology of Mrs. MacDonald's problems where appropriate. How would you prioritize these diagnoses? Why?
3. How would you go about incorporating client participation in planning interventions for Mrs. MacDonald's health problems?
4. List at least three client-care objectives that you would like to accomplish with Mrs. MacDonald.
5. Describe some of the primary, secondary, and tertiary prevention strategies that would be appropriate in resolving Mrs. MacDonald's health problems. Why would they be appropriate?
6. How would you evaluate your nursing intervention? What criteria would you use to evaluate care?

REFERENCES

1. Surgeon General's workshop on health promotion and aging. (1989). *MMWR, 38,* 385–388.
2. National Center for Health Statistics. (1990). *Health, United States, 1989.* Hyattsville, MD: United States Public Health Service.
3. United States Department of Health and Human Services. (1991). *Healthy people 2000: National health promotion and disease prevention objectives.* Washington, DC: Government Printing Office.
4. Diekelmann, N. (1977). *Primary health care of the well adult.* New York: McGraw-Hill.
5. Christofalo, V. J. (1988). An overview of theories of bi-

ological aging. In J. E. Birren & V. L. Bengston (Eds.), *Emerging theories of aging* (pp. 118–127). New York: Springer.

6. Ebersole, P., & Hess, P. (1990). *Toward healthy aging: Human needs and nursing response* (3rd ed.). St. Louis: C. V. Mosby.
7. Forbes, E. J., & Fitzsimons, V. M. (1981). *The older adult: A process for wellness.* St. Louis: C. V. Mosby.
8. Maslow, A. (1968). *Toward a psychology of being* (2nd ed.). New York: Van Nostrand Reinhold.
9. Erickson, E. (1963). *Childhood and society* (2nd ed.). New York: W. W. Norton.
10. Archbold, P. G. (1981). Ethical issues in the selection of a theoretical framework for gerontologic nursing research. *Journal of Gerontological Nursing, 7,* 408–411.
11. Hogstel, M. (1989). The integumentary system. In V. Burgraff & M. Stanley (Eds.), *Nursing the elderly: A care plan approach* (pp. 48–75). Philadelphia: J. B. Lippincott.
12. Kain, C. D., Reilly, N., & Schultz, E. D. (1990). The older adult: A comparative assessment. *Nursing Clinics of North America, 25,* 833–848.
13. Reed, E., & Stanley, M. (1989). The respiratory system. In V. Burgraff & M. Stanley (Eds.), *Nursing the elderly: A care plan approach* (pp. 129–149). Philadelphia: J. B. Lippincott.
14. Eliopoulos, C. (1990). *Health assessment of the older adult* (2nd ed.). Redwood City, CA: Addison-Wesley.
15. Paremski, A., Schams, K. H., & Yurkovich, P. (1988). A conceptual model for CNS practice. *Journal of Gerontological Nursing, 14*(2), 14–17.
16. Carroll, M., & Brue, L. J. (1988). *A nurse's guide to caring for elders.* New York: Springer.
17. Diseases of the older woman. (1988). *Women's Health, 88*(1), 22–25.
18. Lekan-Rutledge, D. (1988). Functional assessment. In E. S. McConnell & M. A. Matteson (Eds.), *Gerontologic nursing: Concepts and practice* (pp. 57–91). Philadelphia: W. B. Saunders.
19. Keane, S. M., & Sells, S. (1990). Recognizing depression in the elderly. *Journal of Gerontological Nursing, 16*(1), 21–25.
20. Lubben, J. E., Weiler, P. G., & Chi, I. (1989). Health practices of the elderly poor. *American Journal of Public Health, 79,* 731–734.
21. Steffl, B. (1989). Discharge planning and the elderly. In V. Burgraff & M. Stanley (Eds.), *Nursing the elderly: A care plan approach* (pp. 17–35). Philadelphia: J. B. Lippincott.
22. Many adverse drug reactions found in elderly patients. (1989, April). *The Nation's Health,* p. 6.
23. Guralnik, J. M., & Kaplan, G. A. (1989). Predictors of healthy aging: Prospective evidence from the Alameda County study. *American Journal of Public Health, 79,* 703–708.
24. Elderly needing help to double. (April, 1989). *The Nation's Health,* p. 5.
25. McConnell, E. S., & Matteson, M. A. (1988). Psychosocial problems associated with aging. In E. S. McConnell & M. A. Matteson (Eds.), *Gerontologic nursing: Concepts and practice* (pp. 481–527). Philadelphia: W. B. Saunders.
26. Hypothermia prevention. (1988). *MMWR, 37,* 780–782.
27. Adult immunization: Knowledge, attitudes, and practices—DeKalb and Fulton Counties, Georgia, 1988. (1988). *MMWR, 37,* 657–661.
28. Influenza vaccination levels in selected states—Behavioral Risk Factor Surveillance System, 1987. (1989). *MMWR, 38,* 124, 129–133.
29. Kim, K. K. (1989). Patient education. In V. Burgraff & M. Stanley (Eds.), *Nursing the elderly: A care plan approach* (pp. 36–47). Philadelphia: J. B. Lippincott.
30. Burnside, I. M. (1981). Psychosocial issues in nursing care of the aged. *Journal of Gerontological Nursing, 7,* 689–694.
31. Fox, B. (1988). Geriatric patient education: Issues and answers. *The Journal of Continuing Education in Nursing, 19,* 169–173.

RECOMMENDED READINGS

Bremer, A. (1989). A description of community health nursing practice with the community-based elderly. *Journal of Community Health Nursing, 6,* 173–184.

Reports findings of a study of community health nursing activities with elderly clients in community settings.

Butler, R. R. (1990). The tragedy of old age in America. In P. R. Lee & C. L. Estes (Eds.), *The nation's health* (3rd ed.) (pp. 363–373). Boston: Jones and Bartlett.

Describes problems encountered by the elderly in the United States and myths and stereotypes regarding the aged. Addresses the question of responsibility for the care of the elderly.

Collinsworth, R., & Boyle, K. (1989). Nutritional assessment of the elderly. *Journal of Gerontological Nursing, 15*(12), 17–21.

Details findings of a study on the types of indicators used by nurses to identify nutritional needs of older clients.

Eliopoulos, C. (1990). *Health assessment of the older adult* (2nd ed.). Redwood City, CA: Addison-Wesley.

Sets forth in-depth assessment of older clients. Provides several assessment tools for use with older clients.

Estes, C. L., & Wood, J. B. (1990). The non-profit sector and community-based care for the elderly in the U.S. In P. R. Lee & C. L. Estes (Eds.), *The nation's health* (3rd ed) (pp. 374–381). Boston: Jones and Bartlett.

Addresses issues of social justice and equity in allocation of resources for care of the elderly. Discusses effects of cost-containment efforts on care for low-income elderly.

Hewner, S. J. (1986). Bringing home the health care: Nurses make a difference. *Journal of Gerontological Nursing, 12*(2), 29–35.

Focuses on providing care for elderly clients in their homes.

Kain, C. D., Reilly, N., & Schultz, E. D. (1990). The older adult: A comparative assessment. *Nursing Clinics of North America, 25,* 833–848.

Examines the assessment of physical health status in older clients. Focuses in-depth attention on the special needs of both older men and women.

Philips, H. T., & Gaylord, S. A. (1985). *Aging and public health.* New York: Springer.

Explores the biological, environmental, and psychosocial aspects of aging within the framework of public health priorities.

Ruthven, W. B. (1984). Nursing diagnosis in the community: Case management for the homebound elderly. In M. J. Kim, G. K. McFarland, & A. M. Lane (Eds.), *Classification of nursing diagnoses: Proceedings of the fifth national conference.* St. Louis: C. V. Mosby.

Describes the use of the diagnostic reasoning process with older clients in community settings. Ties nursing diagnosis to documentation in the problem-oriented record.

Scitovsky, A. A., & Capron, A. M. (1990). Medical at the end of life: The interaction of economics and ethics. In P. R. Lee & C. L. Estes (Eds.), *The nation's health* (3rd ed.) (pp. 382–388). Boston: Jones and Bartlett.

Discusses ethical implications of high-cost, low-return health care for elderly persons, particularly the gravely ill, but not terminal, client.

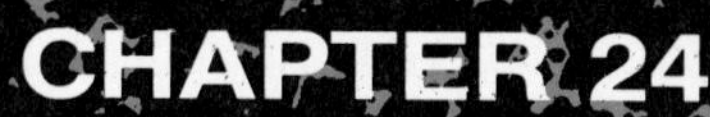

CHAPTER 24

Care of Homeless Clients

KEY TERMS

deinstitutionalization
gentrification
means-tested income transfers
non-institutionalization
structural unemployment

A paradox exists in many American cities today. In many areas, developers were overly optimistic about the market for new homes and overbuilt to the point that these new homes stand vacant without buyers or renters. In these same cities, however, a growing number of people live on the street because they have no other place to go.

Who are these people who make up the growing homeless population? Contrary to popular belief, most of those who are homeless are not the stereotypical "skid row bum," a perpetually drunk male vagrant inhabiting a rundown district of a large city. Today, homeless individuals include families, single women with children, and the elderly as well as single adult males. Most of them are poor, but some are not. Many have low educational levels, but some are well-educated. Many are mentally ill, but, again, many are not. Blacks, Hispanics, and Native Americans are all overrepresented among the homeless and constitute approximately 50 percent of the homeless population in the United States.[1] Children of minority group members comprise as much as 75 percent of the young homeless population in some areas.[2] Box 24–1 highlights the circumstances of homelessness for two women and their families.

Community health nurses may encounter homeless clients in a variety of ways. The nurse may be approached by homeless individuals asking for work, shelter, or food while making home visits to other clients. Or the nurse may provide health-care services in shelters for the homeless. Community health nurses may receive requests for service for the homeless from local merchants in whose doorways homeless people sleep encounter homeless clients in clinics or when following up on contacts to communicable diseases. Additionally, community health nurses may participate in task forces mounted by local governments or religious groups to address the problem of homelessness. Wherever they encounter homeless clients, community health nurses must be prepared to assist the homeless individual to deal with a variety of health and social needs.

LEARNING OBJECTIVES

After reading this chapter you should be able to:

- Identify at least three physiologic problems common among homeless individuals.
- Describe at least three social environmental factors that contribute to homelessness.
- Identify two life-style factors that influence the health of homeless clients.
- Describe two ways in which health system factors contribute to homelessness.
- Describe at least three approaches to primary prevention of homelessness.
- Identify at least three areas in which secondary preventive interventions may be required in the care of homeless individuals.
- Identify at least two strategies for tertiary prevention of homelessness at the aggregate level.
- Describe two considerations in implementing care for homeless individuals.
- Identify the focus of evaluation for care of homeless clients.

BOX 24–1

Two Homeless Women

Angela

Angela is a good-looking woman in her late 30s. She and her 6-year-old daughter are staying temporarily at a shelter for homeless women with children. She has a college education and had her own business in New York. She has been divorced for a year, but her ex-husband still beat her regularly, so she decided to take her daughter and move to California. She sold her business and left without letting her ex-husband know what she was doing.

When Angela arrived in California she used the money from her business to buy inventory and rent a place to begin again. She used the little money left over to pay the rent on a small apartment. After living in the apartment for a week, she discovered that the building housed an illegal drug lab run by the building's owner and that most of the other tenants were substance abusers. She decided that this was not an appropriate environment for her child, so she left. She was afraid to ask the landlord for her money back for fear that he would think she was going to the police. She had no other funds, so she and her daughter were homeless.

Angela was very close to her parents, but her father had recently had heart surgery and her parents could barely afford their mortgage payments. Angela did not think she could ask them for help. Fortunately, Angela knew that there were usually shelters available for homeless women with children, so she contacted the health department and was referred to the shelter.

Nancy

Nancy is also staying in the shelter. Nancy is in her early 30s and is tall, gaunt, and emaciated. She describes living for a year in a Volkswagen with her boyfriend and her 7-year-old son.

Nancy and her boyfriend were drug abusers and occasionally gave drugs to her son when he began to "snivel about being hungry." Nancy and her boyfriend worked odd jobs, but used the bulk of their income to support their drug habit.

Nancy's son was enrolled in public school but was frequently absent, and his school performance was poor. When school personnel began to investigate his absences, his circumstances were discovered, and he was placed in a foster home. Nancy voluntarily entered a drug detoxification center, but had no place to go when she was discharged. The social worker at the center made arrangements for Nancy to stay at the women's shelter. Nancy is currently trying to regain custody of her son.

THE MAGNITUDE OF HOMELESSNESS

There are no exact figures on the number of homeless persons in the United States, but estimates range from 250,000 to 3 million.[1,3] Approximately 33,000 homeless people can be found in the Los Angeles area alone,[4] while close to 15,000 haunt the streets of New York City. Homeless individuals can be found in almost any major city, in affluent suburbs, and in rural areas, and the number of homeless nationwide is growing each year.

Who are the homeless? According to the National Governors' Association, a homeless individual is "an undomiciled person who is unable to secure permanent and stable housing without special assistance."[5] The homeless are by no means a homogeneous group. Recent literature speaks to the difference in the composition of the homeless population of today compared to that of several years ago. In the past, homeless individuals were typically adult males. Today, however, the homeless population can be subdivided into four distinct groups: the chronically mentally ill, street people, chronic substance abusers, and the situationally homeless.[5,6]

The chronically mentally ill may become homeless because of their inability to cope with normal activities of life such as maintaining a residence. Or they may be abandoned by family members who can no longer cope with the effects of mental illness on the family. Chronic substance abusers frequently become homeless because they are too intent on their addiction to attend to the activities needed to maintain a residence (for example, paying the rent). Street people are those who are chronically homeless and who have lived on the street for some time (for example, runaways and "bag ladies"). Finally, the situationally homeless are people who have encountered an event that overextends their resources and results in sudden homelessness. Examples of such events include unemployment, eviction, or a recent move to a new area where housing is unavailable or unaffordable.

In the past, most homeless individuals were males over the age of 45. Today, however, two-thirds of the homeless are under 40, with an average age of 35 to 40[1] and 20 to 25 percent of them are women.[1,3,4,7] In one study in Washington State, 54 percent of homeless individuals were children under age 6. Generally, about 10 percent of the homeless are over age 60. It is thought that the underrepresentation of the elderly in counts of the homeless is not because few elders become homeless, but because of high mortality among homeless elderly persons.[5]

Many more families are becoming a part of the homeless population, which in the past was comprised primarily of single individuals. It is estimated that families with children constitute as much as 35 percent of the homeless population nationwide.[8] In the 1990 census, attempts were made to determine the number of homeless. Results of these efforts are not yet available, but difficulties encountered in data collection suggest that the figures derived will still largely underrepresent the actual extent of the homeless population in the United States.

THE EPIDEMIOLOGIC PREVENTION PROCESS MODEL AND CARE OF HOMELESS CLIENTS

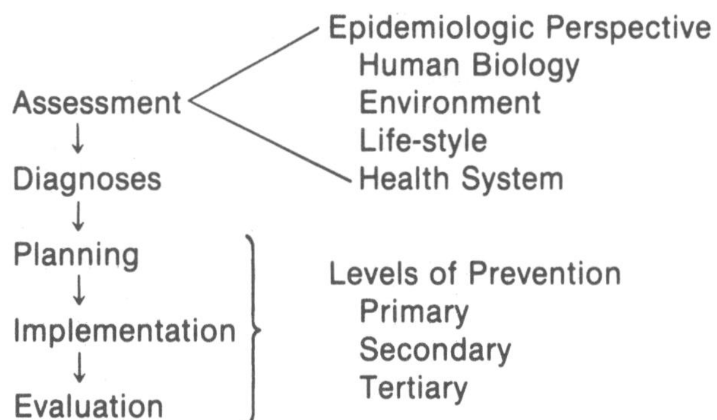

Efforts of community health nurses to resolve problems of the homeless can be guided by use of the epidemiologic prevention process model. Nurses can use the model to identify factors contributing to homelessness and the effects of homelessness on health, and to plan, implement, and evaluate interventions to resolve some of these problems.

ASSESSING HEALTH NEEDS OF HOMELESS CLIENTS

The first step in the use of the model is assessing the health status of homeless clients and the factors that influence their health. The community health nurse examines factors in the client's situation that contribute to homelessness as well as the health effects of their homeless state.

HUMAN BIOLOGY

There are no human biological factors that contribute to a state of homelessness. Homelessness, however, has differential effects on health based on maturation and aging. Homelessness also adversely affects physiologic function in a variety of ways.

Maturation and Aging

Age is a biological factor that exacerbates the health effects of homelessness for both the young and the elderly. In one study, 49 percent of homeless children had acute or chronic health problems. In addition, homeless children were four times more likely than youngsters in the general population to have their health rated as fair or poor, rather than good. While few of the children were below the 5th percentile of weight for height, 35 percent were over the 95th percentile, indicating a reliance on high-calorie foods with relatively low nutritional value.[2] In other studies, 5 percent of homeless children exhibited serious growth failure, while 25 percent were anemic.[8]

At particular risk of health problems stemming from homelessness are the elderly. All of the usual problems of the elderly discussed in Chapter 23, Care of the Older Client, are intensified by homelessness. The homeless elderly are particularly susceptible to the effects of communicable diseases, exposure, burns, and trauma due to alcoholic, physical, or mental impairment or assault.[5]

Physiologic Function

Homeless persons are particularly vulnerable to a variety of health problems that are compounded by their lack of income and residence. A study of the homeless in Los Angeles found that they were three times more likely to report fair or poor health status, 50 percent more likely to report physical disability, and twice as likely to have been hospitalized compared to the general population.[4] Similar results have been noted in other studies.[2,6]

The health problems encountered among the homeless population are many and varied. Accidental and violence-related trauma is a common occurrence, as are skin diseases and ulcerations.[1] Upper respiratory infections and influenza are easily spread among poorly nourished persons congregating in crowded shelters and food lines. Infestations of lice are prolonged by the inability to shower or wash clothes. Extensive walking and standing in line for prolonged periods, coupled with an inability to recline, leads to venous stasis and edema that contribute to foot and leg ulcerations and cellulitis.[3] Such problems are further complicated by poorly fitted or rundown shoes.

Other problems seen among homeless individuals include hypothermia; burns from sleeping on hot grates in an effort to keep warm; hypertension; neurological diseases; injuries and poisoning (including food poisoning); circulatory diseases; gastrointestinal disease; and chronic respiratory problems. Prevalence rates for tuberculosis are up to 300 times higher than those of the general population with a rate of 1700 cases per 100,000 homeless individuals.[1]

Chronic health problems are compounded by the homeless person's difficulty in following a prescribed treatment regimen. For instance, exposure to cold will exacerbate the effects of chronic respiratory diseases, while an unstable diet places the diabetic at higher risk. In addition, because insulin syringes are highly valued by IV drug users, the homeless person with diabetes faces the risk of being attacked for the syringes in his or her possession. The homeless person with diabetes also might be tempted to sell the syringes.[3]

Physiologic problems experienced by homeless children include respiratory and ear infections, dental problems, poor vision, musculoskeletal problems, abdominal pain and ulcers, seizures, sickle cell disease, trauma, and renal disease. In addition, these children are less likely to be adequately immunized. For instance, 27 percent of children in one study were not up to date on their immunizations, and 21 percent of those under age 5 had not been immunized against measles.[2]

Problems frequently encountered among the homeless elderly include hypothermia, malnutrition, parasitic infestations, peripheral vascular disease, and tuberculosis. Other common conditions are cardiac disease, diabetes, hypertension, and pulmonary disease.[5]

The community health nurse working with a homeless individual would be particularly alert for these commonly encountered health problems. In addition, the nurse would assess the client for the presence of any other chronic or communicable diseases.

ENVIRONMENT

Physical, psychological, and social environmental factors contribute to homelessness. Environmental factors also influence the effects of homelessness on health.

Physical Environment

An actual lack of housing units in a community may be one factor that contributes to homelessness. In communities where housing is scarce, whatever housing units are available may be unaffordable for the poor and the elderly.

Physical environmental factors also contribute to the effects of homelessness on health. Exposure to cold, even in the mildest climates, can lead to hypothermia. This is particularly true when people are lying on concrete or are clothed in wet garments.[3] Overcrowding and poor sanitary conditions in shelters contribute to the spread of communicable diseases among a population that is already debilitated by exposure and poor nutritional status.

Psychological Environment

Psychological factors can lead to homelessness when people are unable to cope with the demands of daily life and have limited support systems. Estimates of the extent of psychiatric illness in the homeless population vary. In several studies, the portion of the homeless population with recognizable mental illness varied from 27 percent to 90 percent.[3,6,8,9,10] Mentally ill persons tend to swell the homeless populations of large urban areas. This may be due in part to a migration of individuals with psychiatric illness from rural to urban areas. Large metropolitan centers have been shown to be more tolerant of bizarre behavior than rural areas. In rural areas, mentally ill persons tend to be cared for by family members and are less likely to become homeless. Homeless mentally ill persons in rural areas, on the other hand, are frequently incarcerated for unusual behavior or encouraged to move on.[11]

Homeless women seem to exhibit greater evidence of mental disorders than homeless men. In one study, two-thirds of homeless women exhibited personality disorders and had difficulties parenting their children. Many of these women themselves grew up in dysfunctional homes.

Homelessness, in turn, influences an individual's emotional health. Suicide and depression are psychological health problems common among homeless adults.[1] Children, too, are at risk for mental health problems influenced by homelessness. For instance, over half of the homeless children in one study were clinically depressed, while 60 percent displayed marked anxiety. In addition, 47 percent of these children exhibited developmental delays.[1] Similar findings have been noted in other studies, with homeless children displaying greater degrees of anxiety, depression, developmental delay, learning problems, repeated grade failure, and poor school performance than other children.[8]

Social Environment

Social environmental factors play a major role in the development of homelessness and in its effects on the health of homeless individuals and families. Changes in family structure and support, widespread unemployment, poverty, and urban redevelopment are some of the societal conditions that contribute to homelessness. As noted by one observer, "Poverty may beget homelessness, but it seems to do so more often when social and economic conditions limit housing resources or when they promote population mobility."[7]

In some cases, homelessness may occur as a result of a breakdown in family ties. Mobility within the population has led to the breakup of extended family systems. This, in turn, results in a restricted social support network for families facing psychological and/or economic crises. High unemployment rates in some areas have led large numbers of individuals and families to move to other parts of the country in search of work. Others have fled countries plagued by poverty and violence.[5] In one study, 13 percent of the homeless population gave a recent move to the area as a reason for their homelessness.[2] Many of these people arrive in a new locale to find the job market closed and a lack of available low-cost housing. Without an established social support network, they have no recourse but to live in cars, on the street, or in "welfare hotels."

Increases in poverty and consequent homelessness in the United States are, in part, the result of declining family income. Between 1973 and 1985, the poorest 20 percent of the population experienced more than a 32 percent decline in family income. These declines are the result of several social environmental factors. Some of these factors include changes in government assistance programs and increased taxes.[12]

Changes in government programs to assist the poor have contributed to increased poverty and homelessness in two ways. First, the level of assistance provided has not kept pace with the rate of inflation. Consequently, individuals and families receiving aid fall deeper into poverty.[12] In Alaska, for example, which has a high level of benefits, the total income of families receiving assistance only brings them to 89 percent of the poverty level income. In Alabama, with some of the poorest benefits, people on public assistance subsist on incomes that are 46 percent of the poverty level.[13] Thus a family of four living on public assistance in Alabama might have a total annual family income of just over $5000. Such an income may preclude obtaining adequate housing.

Second, budgetary cutbacks have actually reduced benefits in some instances and increased eligibility requirements so that fewer of the working poor are eligible for aid. At the same time, taxes paid by the poor have increased. Families at the poverty level in 1985, for example, saw roughly 10 percent of their total income going to pay for taxes. Recent tax reforms have somewhat decreased the tax burden on the poor but not sufficiently to offset declines in income.[12]

A further problem with the current system of

public assistance is a need for persons to rid themselves of most of their resources in order to be eligible for help. In some instances, this also means breaking up family units and suffering the degradation often involved in the application and verification processes. When family members do obtain work in an attempt to add additional income, assistance benefits are frequently reduced by a similar amount, placing these families in a no-gain situation from which escape is impossible.[13]

Unemployment is another major social factor contributing to homelessness. While many people remain employed, there has been a shift in the job market from relatively well-paid manufacturing jobs to lower-paid employment in service industries (for example, janitorial work).[14] This phenomenon is referred to as ***structural unemployment*** because it arises from changes in the nation's economic and occupational structure such as the shift from heavy to light industry and from manufacturing to service occupations. The emergence of high-technology occupations requires new sets of skills that many displaced workers do not have. Such changes in the structure of the job market have resulted in a situation in which approximately 8 million people are seeking jobs despite the creation of 20 million new jobs since 1970.[13]

The percentage of homeless people who are jobless varies from group to group. In some studies, as many as 93 percent of the homeless population is unemployed,[2] while in others many of the homeless were working or had worked recently.[4] Whether employed or not, almost all homeless individuals and families in these studies had low incomes.

Finding employment is difficult for most homeless individuals. Those with mental illness find it hard to maintain a job, if they can get one, because of their instability. Homeless single women with children, who account for almost half of homeless families,[2] have problems of child care while they work.

Even those homeless persons with employable skills in areas where jobs are available may have difficulty negotiating the employment process. Lack of transportation may make it difficult to go to an interview or to get to work when a job is found. In addition, job application and interviews take time, which may prevent the individual from securing food or shelter for the night when these are only obtained after long waits in line in competition with many other homeless persons. Moreover, the homeless person may also find that he or she is penalized for working by reduction or even loss of assistance benefits.

Homelessness is not necessarily correlated with the social factor of low educational levels. In various populations of homeless persons, those with at least a high school education comprise one-fifth to two-thirds of the group.[1,3,4]

Loss of affordable housing for low-income individuals and families is a major contributing factor in homelessness. Eviction is a common precipitating cause[5] and may result from inability to pay one's rent or mortgage. Furthermore, the redevelopment of urban areas with a consequent loss of many low-cost housing units also fosters homelessness.[7] This process, called ***gentrification,*** occurs when more affluent members of society move into and rehabilitate areas inhabited by the poor.[10] Since 1970 over 1 million single-room occupancy units, one-half of the available supply, have been lost, eliminating many low-cost housing alternatives.

The cost of housing in relation to income is another factor contributing to homelessness among the poor. The amount of family income spent on housing has steadily increased over the last few years. In 1970, some 2 million families spent more than 70 percent of their income on housing. By 1983, this figure had risen to 3.7 million.[7] High housing costs leave little money available for other needs and often lead to an inability to afford housing of any kind.

Other social factors that contribute to homelessness in certain populations are divorce or separation and flight from abuse.[2] Many women and their children are forced from their homes by abusive partners/fathers, while another sizable group of homeless individuals are teenage runaways fleeing abusive home situations.[3]

The effects of homelessness on health status are compounded by social factors such as lack of transportation and residential requirements for public assistance programs.[4,6] Lack of transportation limits the ability of the homeless to secure housing, employment, and health care, among other things. In addition, in most areas, a permanent address is required for persons to be eligible for financial assistance as well as other forms of aid. Persons living on the street or in rundown automobiles are most in need of assistance but have no hope of meeting residency requirements. Recently, homeless persons applying for assistance in some jurisdictions have been allowed to use the address of a shelter as a mailing address even though they may no longer be living there.

Crime is another effect of homelessness. Homeless men are twice as likely to report arrest as a comparable group of non-homeless. They are also more likely to report multiple arrests.[6] Often the arrests of the homeless are for theft of items sold to purchase food or shelter. The homeless are also at risk for robbery and assault. This is particularly true of homeless women and the elderly, who are less able to protect themselves and their belongings than homeless adult men.

Provision of shelter for the homeless may create problems in and of itself. The number of shelter beds available is often unequal to the needs of the population, especially in areas with large numbers of homeless. Competition for beds often results in intimidation of women and older persons in an attempt to force them to give way to stronger and more dominant males.[5] Unless shelters are segregated by age or sex, or special shelters provided for homeless women, families, and the elderly, these groups may be prevented from making use of available shelter resources.

LIFE-STYLE

Substance abuse is a life-style factor that may contribute to homelessness when the abuser is unable, because of his or her addiction, to meet, or even care about, needs for shelter. Substance abuse may also lead to expenditure of money for alcohol or drugs that could be used for shelter. Substance abusers comprise about 30 percent of the overall homeless population, but the percentage of substance abusers has been found to be as high as 58 percent of the homeless in some studies. Most of these persons abuse alcohol, but there is a significant portion who abuse other drugs as well.[1] Cocaine use, in particular, has contributed to the increase in homelessness in many American cities.

Prostitution is a life-style that may arise as a result of homelessness in an effort to earn enough money for food and shelter. Prostitution is particularly prevalent among adolescent runaways who find no other way to earn enough money to support themselves.[3]

Prostitution and intravenous drug abuse among some members of the homeless population place this group at risk for communicable diseases such as AIDS and hepatitis B. AIDS in and of itself may be a contributing factor in homelessness when persons with AIDS lose their jobs and their ability to provide shelter for themselves or their families. In many instances, avenues of assistance such as shelters and nursing homes that might otherwise assist terminally ill people may be closed to people with AIDS because of fear of the disease.

Homelessness also influences life-style factors related to nutrition and rest, further compounding the health problems of this population. Inadequate nutrition among the homeless is a life-style factor leading to ill health. Even those homeless persons housed in shelters rarely have access to kitchen facilities. Some shelters do provide meals, but they are rarely adequate to meet the nutritional needs of those served. This is particularly true in the case of homeless children who frequently exhibit anemia or serious growth failure.[8] The inability to rest frequently places homeless individuals at greater risk for a variety of health problems and worsens existing health conditions.[3] For example, the inability to lie down to rest may lead to venous stasis and contribute to leg and foot ulcers. These adverse effects on circulation are made worse if the homeless individual smokes. Smoking also intensifies the effects of respiratory infections contracted from others in crowded shelters.

HEALTH SYSTEM

Deinstitutionalization of the mentally ill is a major health system factor in the growing number of homeless people. ***Deinstitutionalization*** is the process of discharging large numbers of mentally ill persons from mental institutions in an attempt to enable them to live in the least restrictive environment possible. This move was prompted by recognition of the appalling conditions prevalent in many institutions for the mentally ill. While the intent of deinstitutionalization was laudable, the results were not. Unfortunately, there was no concurrent move to provide the community services needed for the mentally ill to live in non-institutional settings. Many deinstitutionalized persons were virtually left to fend for themselves. Without the social or personal resources to provide adequate care for themselves, many of the deinstitutionalized became part of the homeless population.

A related social phenomenon is ***non-institutionalization*** of the mentally ill. This refers to a lack of hospitalization of persons with mental problems who are in need of care.[5] Often, particularly in urban areas, people with mental illness are not hospitalized until they have deteriorated to the point where they are a danger to themselves or others. Such tolerance of deviant behavior prevents mentally ill individuals from obtaining help when they need it and when they could most easily benefit from it.[11]

Health system factors may also contribute to homelessness when overwhelming medical bills cause an individual or family to be unable to continue to afford paying rent or making mortgage payments. In fact, in one study, medical bills were one of several reasons given for homelessness in the group studied.[2] The effect of medical expenses on one's ability to provide shelter is particularly noticeable in the case of clients with catastrophic illness. These are clients who are already at risk for a variety of health problems and in whom homelessness further complicates their needs.

More often than causing homelessness, however, health system factors make it more difficult for homeless individuals to obtain health care and to prevent or resolve health problems. Financial costs are one barrier to health care for the homeless. In some studies, homeless individuals are up to nine times less likely to have any form of health insurance compared to the general population.[4] More than half of the homeless report no regular source of health care.[2,4]

Cost is not the only barrier to health-care access. Other problems include lack of transportation, long waits for service (which may mean missing a meal at the soup kitchen or being unable to obtain shelter for the night), insensitivity of health-care providers to the needs and circumstances of the homeless, and fragmentation of services.[3] Homeless individuals and families frequently have neither the expertise nor the energy to complete the processes involved in registration or application for services. Lack of preventive care is a particular problem among this population.

Few pregnant homeless women receive prenatal care. These women and their offspring are at higher risk for complications of pregnancy than is the general population.[1] In addition, babies born to mothers in welfare hotels for the homeless have twice the risk of low birth weight and twice the rate of infant mortality compared to non-homeless counterparts.[8]

Preventive care is also lacking for young children. Homeless youngsters use emergency room services as a regular source of health care two to three times more frequently than the general pediatric population, suggesting a focus on crisis care rather than prevention. These children are also less likely to receive immunization, particularly measles immunization.[2]

Mental health services for the homeless population are also lacking. Some observers have noted a mismatch between traditional community mental health services and the needs of the homeless population. Comprehensive services are seldom offered at one location, and mental health services seldom address the social factors contributing to homelessness.[10]

DIAGNOSTIC REASONING AND THE HEALTH NEEDS OF HOMELESS CLIENTS

Based on the assessment of the health status of homeless clients and factors contributing to that status, nursing diagnoses may be derived at any of several levels. At the individual client level, the community health nurse may make diagnoses related to the existence of homelessness. As discussed before, the diagnostic statement will include underlying factors if identifiable. Examples of nursing diagnoses at this level might be "homelessness due to inability to pay for shelter" or "homelessness due to mental illness and inability to care for self."

Other kinds of diagnoses made at the individual or family level might relate to specific health problems resulting from or intensified by homelessness. As an example, the nurse might make a diagnosis of "statis ulcers due to excessive walking and standing and inability to lie down at night." Another possible diagnosis might be "malnutrition due to inability to afford food and lack of access to cooking facilities."

Nursing diagnoses may also be made at the group or community level. For example, the community health nurse may diagnose a significant problem of homelessness in the community. Such diagnoses might be stated as an "increase in the homeless population due to recent closure of major community employer" or an "increase in the number of homeless families due to unemployment and reductions in public assistance programs." Diagnoses may also be made at the aggregate level relative to specific problems engendered by homelessness. For example, the nurse might note "increased prevalence of tuberculosis due to malnutrition and crowding in shelters for the homeless" or "increased incidence of anemia among homeless children due to poor nutrition."

PLANNING TO MEET THE HEALTH NEEDS OF HOMELESS CLIENTS

Planning done to meet the needs of homeless clients should focus on long-term as well as short-term solutions to problems. Planning should also reflect the factors contributing to the needs of the homeless in a particular locale. For example, if most of the homelessness in one community is due to unemployment, long-term interventions would most likely be directed toward improving employment opportunities in the area or increasing the employability of those involved. If, on the other hand, a significant portion of homelessness in the area is due to mental illness and inability to care for self, attention would be given to providing supportive services for the mentally ill.

Planning should address the underlying factors contributing to homelessness as well as its health consequences. For example, providing shelter on a nightly basis may decrease the risk of exposure to cold for homeless persons but does nothing to relieve homelessness. In planning to meet the health needs of homeless clients, community health nurses may work independently or in conjunction with other health-care and social service providers. When planning to address factors contributing to homelessness, however, the community health nurse will frequently be part of a group of government officials and concerned citizens who have assumed responsibility for dealing with the overall problem of homelessness.

Efforts to alleviate homelessness and its consequences may take place at the primary, secondary, or tertiary level of prevention. Community health nurses may be involved in activities at any or all three levels. Whatever the level of prevention undertaken, nurses working with the homeless may be in need of assistance in resolving the problems engendered by homelessness. Selected sources of information and services for the poor and homeless are presented in Table 24–1. For the most part, the agencies and organizations included in the table are national in scope. The community health nurse can also consult the telephone directory for local branches of these organizations. The nurse might also approach local government task forces on homelessness for information and assistance for clients.

As is true in caring for any client, planning care for a homeless client begins with giving priority to the client's health needs. In many instances, for example, the first priority would be obtaining shelter, a secondary preventive measure. Other health needs could then be addressed in terms of their level of priority. For each of the health-care needs identified for the homeless client, the community health nurse would develop specific outcome objectives and design interventions at the primary, secondary, or tertiary level of prevention. Planning efforts should be a joint function of the community health nurse and the homeless client, who best knows his or her situation and the kinds of interventions that are likely to be successful in that situation.

PRIMARY PREVENTION

Primary prevention may be directed either at preventing homelessness or preventing its health consequences. Primary prevention can occur at the individual or family level or at community levels. Community health nurses can help prevent individuals and families from becoming homeless by assisting them to eliminate factors that may contribute to

TABLE 24–1. RESOURCES FOR HOMELESS CLIENTS

Agency or Organization	Services
National Runaway Switchboard 2210 N. Halstead Chicago, IL 60614 (800) 621-4000	Shelter referral for runaways, message to family
Operation Peace of Mind P.O. Box 52896 Houston, TX 78711 (800) 392-3352 or (800) 231-6946	Services to runaways
PUSH (People United to Save Humanity) P.O. Box 5432 Chicago, IL 60680-9919	Advocacy to eliminate poverty, unemployment, drug abuse, political injustice, assistance with community organization to promote employment, provide food, etc.
Runaway Hotline Governor's Office P.O. Box 12428 Austin, TX 78711 (512) 463-1980	Referral for help for runaways, message to parents, statistics
Salvation Army 799 Bloomfield Avenue Verona, NJ 07044 (201) 239-0606	Food, shelter, assistance for the poor and the homeless
Save the Children 54 Wilton Rd. Westport, CT 06880 (203) 226-7271	Self-help education for communities and the poor
United Way of America 701 N. Fairfax St. Alexandria, VA 22314-2045 (703) 836-7100	Coordinates volunteer donations to agencies that may provide assistance for the homeless; information on local services for homeless persons
Women's Equity Action League 1250 I St., NW Washington, DC 20005	Advocacy for the economic advancement of women

homelessness. For example, if a family is threatened with eviction because of a parent's unemployment, the nurse can assist family members to obtain emergency rent funds from local social service agencies. The nurse can also encourage the family to apply for ongoing financial aid programs or assist the parent to find work.

As noted earlier, some people become homeless because of underlying psychiatric illness and an inability to deal with the requirements for maintaining shelter. Severely disturbed people may just wander away from home and take up residence on the streets. Homelessness in this group can be prevented by referrals for psychiatric therapy and counseling. Nurses may also provide support services to families caring for mentally ill members to prevent these persons from becoming part of the homeless population. Placement in a sheltered home might also be an approach to preventing homelessness in the mentally disturbed person when family members either cannot or do not wish to care for the client. In addition, the community health nurse can monitor the effectiveness of therapy and watch for signs of increasing agitation or disorientation that may precede wandering. The nurse can also assist the disturbed person by giving concrete direction in such tasks as paying one's rent.

Runaway children and teenagers are another segment of the homeless population for whom homelessness may be prevented through primary preventive interventions. Efforts of community health nurses to promote effective communication in families and to enhance parenting skills may prevent young people from feeling a need to run away. Similarly, efforts to prevent or deal with child abuse may prevent runaways.

Primary prevention at the community level to reduce the incidence of poverty and homelessness will require major changes in societal structure and thinking. Some suggested avenues for intervention include federal support for low-cost housing, increases in the minimum wage, and providing access to supportive services for the mentally and physically disabled to allow them to function effectively in society.[9] Another suggestion aimed at reducing the incidence of poverty in families with children to prevent their homelessness is to provide child-care assistance and paid parental occupational leaves as needed. Another approach is to offer a supplemental income to all families with children, regardless of need, through programs similar to those in place in other countries.[14]

Creating employment opportunities and programs to train people with employable skills are other possible primary preventive measures for both poverty and homelessness.[15] Another societal intervention could be to provide a guaranteed annual income to all citizens.[13] Such an approach is exemplified in part by social insurance programs such as Social Security and unemployment insurance that are not restricted to the poor but available to all eligible participants.[15]

Community health nursing involvement in such activities will occur primarily through advocacy and political action. As advocates, community health nurses can make policymakers aware of the needs of the homeless and can contribute in efforts to plan programs that will prevent homelessness. Nurses can also engage in political activities such as those described in Chapter 12, The Political Process, to influence policies that will help to eliminate these conditions.

Primary prevention may also be undertaken with respect to specific health problems experienced by homeless persons. Here community health nurses may work with individuals, families, or groups of people. For example, community health nurses working with homeless substance abusers might advocate a program providing clean syringes to intravenous drug users. Failing that, the nurse might provide a simple bleach solution for injection equipment to minimize the risk of blood-borne diseases such as hepatitis and AIDS. Similarly, nurses may provide assistance to families with budgeting and meal planning to provide nutritious meals on limited incomes.

Community-based avenues for preventing homelessness among the mentally ill include providing access to services within the community that will enable these persons to maintain themselves adequately without institutionalization. Efforts may also be needed to ensure hospitalization for those persons who cannot be adequately maintained in the community.[7] Treatment for substance abuse and providing secure places for convalescence after hospital discharge might also serve to prevent homelessness in this subgroup.[9]

Also at the group level, nurses may engage in primary prevention for specific problems by encouraging community groups to provide shelters for homeless individuals. Nurses may also provide basic health care for the homeless, focusing particularly on primary preventive measures such as influenza vaccine and routine immunization for children. They may suggest the use of a bleach solution in the showers of shelters to prevent the spread of fungal infections. Adequate ventilation, reduced crowding, and use of ultraviolet lights in shelters may also help to prevent the spread of communicable disease.[3]

Another area for primary prevention of the health consequences of homelessness is adequate nutrition. Community health nurses can advocate food programs for the needy, including the homeless. They can also serve as consultants to existing food programs to ensure that meals served are nutritionally adequate to meet the needs of the population served. Community health nursing activities in this area may also include attempts to arrange diets for homeless clients with special needs (for example, assisting a diabetic client to select foods from those prepared in a shelter that approximate a diabetic diet as closely as possible).

Community health nurses can also work with other concerned citizens to initiate programs to provide adequate clothing and shoes for homeless clients. Efforts may also be needed to arrange mechanisms for the homeless to bathe and wash their clothing. In some cities, day shelters that do not provide sleeping accommodations often provide homeless individuals an opportunity to shower and wash their clothing. These shelters may also provide a clean change of clothing on a periodic basis.

Another aggregate approach to preventing specific health problems among the homeless is providing universal access to health care through such programs as national health insurance or similar programs at the state level. Nurses can promote such programs through political activity and advocacy and may also be involved in implementing them by providing direct services to the homeless.

One approach to dealing with the many health problems experienced by the homeless would be to separate Medicaid eligibility from eligibility for other forms of public assistance. This is one of the recommendations of a recent Institute of Medicine report on dealing with homelessness.[9] While such action would not prevent homelessness per se, it would certainly mitigate its effects on health and on access to health care.

SECONDARY PREVENTION

Secondary prevention is designed to alleviate existing homelessness and its health effects. At the individual level, secondary interventions may include referral for financial assistance via "means-tested income transfers."[15] ***Means-tested income transfers*** involve the distribution of cash or non-cash assistance to individuals and families on the basis of income. As noted earlier, such programs frequently serve only the poorest of the poor and may necessitate loss of all resources before eligibility can be confirmed. Community health nurses may need to function as advocates to assist clients through the bureaucratic process frequently involved. This is particularly true for elderly clients and those with mental health problems.[5]

At the community level, nurses can advocate a review of eligibility criteria for means-tested income transfer programs so that a greater proportion of the homeless population are served. This type of review was one of the major recommendations of the Institute of Medicine report on strategies needed to alleviate homelessness in the United States.[9]

Shelter is an immediate need for homeless individuals. The community health nurse can assist the homeless client to locate temporary shelter. This may be accomplished by means of referrals to existing shelters. If the nurse is not aware of homeless shelters provided in the community, he or she can contact a local YMCA or YWCA, a Salvation Army service center, or local churches for information on shelter availability. When organized shelter facilities are not available, the nurse may try contacting local houses of worship to see if members of religious congregations can provide shelter for a homeless person on a short-term basis. In making a referral for emergency shelter, the community health nurse would consider the needs of the particular client. Ideally, for example, the elderly and women and children would be referred to shelters where they are protected from victimization. Similarly, homeless persons with chronic health problems should be referred to shelters where health services are available and their conditions can be monitored on an ongoing basis.

At the group level, community health nurses can work with government officials and other concerned citizens to develop shelter programs for homeless individuals or families. Avenues that might be pursued include school gymnasia, churches, or public buildings. Many cities have used these and other buildings as temporary nighttime shelters for the homeless during cold weather. Plans might also be developed for more adequate shelters that provide other services as well as a place to sleep. In designing a shelter program, the community health nurse and other concerned individuals would employ the principles of program planning presented in Chapter 19, Care of the Community or Target Group.

Shelters are an emergency resource, not a solution to the problem of homelessness. Community health nurses should help homeless clients find ways to meet long-term shelter needs. For individual clients, this may mean referrals for employment assistance or other services to eliminate factors that resulted in homelessness. At the community level, nurses can participate in planning long-term solutions to the problems of homelessness. Unfortunately, such planning has not often been the focus of community attempts to deal with the problem. As noted by one observer, "We are, as a society, in danger of creating a shelter system that contains—even warehouses—a deviant and troubling group of people."[7] Community health nurses can advocate and participate in planning efforts to find ways to provide low-cost housing, employment assistance, job training, and other services needed to resolve community problems of homelessness. Initiating these planning activities may require political activity on the part of the community health nurse.

Planning for long-term resolution of the problem of homelessness for runaways will involve a different set of strategies. The community health nurse can explore with the youngster his or her reason for running away from home. Nursing interventions would then be directed toward modifying factors that led the child to run away. For example, if the child was abused, the nurse can institute measures to prevent further abuse if the youngster returns to the home, or foster home placement can be arranged. If problems stem from poor family communication, the nurse can make a referral for family counseling or other therapeutic services. The nurse can also serve as a liaison between the child and his or her family, negotiating for changes that make the child's return possible.

Particular care should be taken to involve the child in planning interventions to resolve his or her situation. If the child is returned to his or her family unwillingly, the youngster will probably run away again. In addition, such actions on the part of the community health nurse may also destroy any faith the child may have had in health-care providers as a source of assistance.

At the aggregate level, community health nurses should alert community policymakers to the need for coordinated services for the homeless offered in a single location to meet the health and social needs of homeless clients. They should also make sure that planning groups in which they participate plan services to address the needs of the homeless for housing, food, clothing, employment, child-care services for working parents, and adequate preventive and therapeutic health-care services. Planning should also include avenues for outreach and follow-up services, particularly for the homeless who may be lost to service. Such comprehensive programs will require changes in health and social systems that may necessitate legislation and public-policy formation that can be guided by nursing input.

Community health nurses can also provide curative services for a variety of health problems experienced by the homeless. For example, they may make referrals for food supplement programs or provide treatment for skin conditions or parasitic infestations. They will also be actively involved in educating clients for self-care. Homeless clients may have difficulty with simple aspects of treatment regimens. For example, if the homeless client does not have access to a clock or watch, it may be difficult to take medications as directed. Nurses can suggest the use of medications that can be taken in conjunction with set activities, such as on arising or at bedtime.

The special needs of homeless children and older persons require particular attention. One suggestion is age-segregated shelters or services specifically designed for older persons and families with children to prevent their victimization by other subgroups within the homeless population. Special attention also needs to be given to meeting the nutritional needs of these vulnerable groups as well as those of pregnant women.

TERTIARY PREVENTION

Tertiary prevention may be aimed at preventing a recurrence of poverty and homelessness for individuals, families, or groups of people affected. Or the emphasis may be placed on preventing the recurrence of health problems that result from conditions of poverty and homelessness.

Community health nursing involvement in tertiary prevention may entail political activity to assure the provision of services to relieve poverty and homelessness on a long-term basis. This will mean involvement by nurses in efforts to raise minimum wages or to design programs to educate the homeless for employment in today's society. Advocacy and political activity may also be needed to ensure the adequacy of community services for the mentally ill to allow them to care for themselves or to support their families as care-givers.

At the individual and family level, community health nurses may be involved in referral for employment assistance or for educational programs that will allow homeless clients to eliminate the underlying factors involved in their homelessness. Moreover, nurses might assist clients to budget their incomes more effectively or engage in cooperative buying efforts to limit family expenses. Community health nurses may also be actively involved in monitoring the status of mentally ill clients in the home and in assisting families of these clients to obtain respite care and other supportive services needed to prevent the mentally ill client from returning to a state of homelessness. In such cases, nurses will also monitor medication use and encourage clients to receive counseling and other rehabilitative services.

IMPLEMENTING CARE FOR HOMELESS CLIENTS

Acceptance of clients and their circumstances is an essential function of community health nurses working with the homeless. Dirty bodies and unwashed clothing are most likely the result of inadequate opportunities for hygiene rather than an indication that the client does not value cleanliness.

Another area in which understanding and acceptance may be required is failure to keep appointments. In the absence of timepieces and calendars, which may not be available to the homeless client, keeping appointments for health care and other services may be difficult. One suggestion is to provide clients with a photocopy of a date book on which they can keep track of days until their next appointment. Providing services on a walk-in basis is another way in which clients can be seen when the need arises, rather than at the convenience of the health-care facility.

EVALUATING CARE FOR HOMELESS CLIENTS

Evaluating the effects of nursing interventions with homeless clients can take place at two levels—the individual level and the group or community level. At the individual level, evaluation of the effectiveness of interventions will reflect the client-care objectives developed by the nurse and client in planning care. For example, if an objective for a homeless family was to provide them with an income sufficient to meet survival needs, the nurse and family would determine whether this objective has been achieved. Does the family now have sufficient income to provide adequate housing, appropriate nutrition, and other needs? If the objective was to find employment for the mother or father, has this been accomplished?

Evaluation of group interventions must also be undertaken. For example, nurses and other concerned individuals will want to determine whether shelter programs are sufficient to meet the needs of the homeless population, or are there still people sleeping under bridges and in doorways? Evaluation of tertiary prevention programs would focus on the extent to which interventions prevent people from returning to poverty and again becoming homeless. Are job training programs effective in increasing the income of participants above the poverty level? Criticism of current welfare programs seems to indicate that such programs do not effectively relieve the problems of the poor and homeless.[16] If current programs are not effectively alleviating the problem, other solutions must be sought; community health nurses will be actively involved in developing those solutions.

CHAPTER HIGHLIGHTS

- Homelessness is a growing problem in all regions of the United States, and groups of homeless individuals are found in both urban and rural areas. The population of the homeless is changing to include a greater number of families, women with children, and elderly persons.
- The homeless may be categorized into four groups: street people, the chronically mentally ill, chronic substance abusers, and the situationally homeless.
- Both young children and the elderly are particularly susceptible to the adverse health effects of homelessness.
- Common physiologic health problems among the homeless population include a variety of communicable diseases, infestations with lice and other parasites, malnutrition, and trauma. Homelessness also complicates control of existing chronic conditions.
- Physical environmental factors such as a lack of available housing units may contribute to homelessness. Physical factors such as exposure to heat and cold may also lead to health problems among the homeless.
- Psychological environmental factors such as mental illness and an inability to cope with everyday life and maintain a place of residence may result in homelessness. Homelessness, in turn, leads to psychological problems of depression and anxiety and may result in suicide.
- Social environmental factors that contribute to homelessness include unemployment, poverty, urban redevelopment, and changes in family structure brought about by population mobility, divorce, separation, or flight from an abusive situation.
- Substance abuse is the primary life-style factor that can lead to homelessness. Homelessness often leads to a life-style that involves prostitution, substance abuse, or both. Homelessness and malnutrition also contribute to a variety of health problems experienced by the homeless population.
- Two health system factors that contribute to homelessness are the deinstitutionalization or non-institutionalization of the mentally ill, and extensive medical bills. Health system factors such as cost and scheduling also make it more difficult for homeless persons to obtain necessary health-care services.
- Primary prevention for homelessness may include referrals for financial assistance, counseling, and therapy for the mentally ill; facilitating family communication; employment assistance; and providing access to low-cost housing for the economically disadvantaged. These measures may be provided at the individual or family level or at the larger societal level.
- Secondary prevention focuses on providing short-term and long-term solutions to the problem of homelessness as well as on the treatment of health problems caused by homelessness.
- Tertiary prevention is aimed at keeping people who have been assisted to find housing from becoming homeless. Again, interventions may involve community health nursing activities at the individual or family level or at the community level in terms of advocacy and program planning.
- To implement primary, secondary, or tertiary preventive measures for homeless clients, community health nurses must accept clients and their circumstances while working to change those circumstances.
- Evaluation of care for homeless clients focuses on the extent to which identified client-care objectives have been met at the individual or family level or at the larger community level.

Review Questions

1. Identify at least three physiologic problems common among homeless individuals. (p. 586)
2. Describe at least three social environmental factors that contribute to homelessness. (p. 587)
3. What are two life-style factors that influence the health of homeless clients? (p. 589)
4. Describe two ways in which health system factors have contributed to homelessness. (p. 589)
5. Describe at least three approaches to primary prevention of homelessness. How might community health nurses be involved in each approach? (p. 591)
6. What are three areas in which secondary preventive activities may be appropriate in the care of homeless clients? What kinds of secondary preventive measures might a community health nurse employ in these areas? (p. 593)
7. Identify at least two strategies for tertiary prevention of homelessness at the aggregate level. How might community health nurses be involved in implementing these strategies? (p. 594)
8. What are two primary considerations in implementing care for homeless clients? (p. 594)
9. What is the primary focus in evaluating care for homeless clients? Is this focus the same for evaluating care for individuals and families and care for groups of homeless people? (p. 595)

APPLICATION AND SYNTHESIS

Jennifer is a 16-year-old girl with a 3-month-old baby boy. She has been referred for community health nursing services by her teacher at a special program for adolescents with children. In this program, the girls attend school while child-care services are provided for the children. During the day, the girls participate in the care of their infants and learn about child care as well as the usual high school subject material. Jennifer has been referred because she has not been coming to school and her teacher is concerned. The school does not have a home address or phone number for Jennifer, but the teacher gives you the phone number of Jennifer's grandmother. After several attempts, you finally contact the grandmother, who agrees to give Jennifer a message to get in touch with you. The grandmother says that Jennifer does not live with her and that she only sees her occasionally.

The following week you receive a call from Jennifer. She is reluctant to give you an address, but agrees to come to the health department with the baby. When she arrives, she tells you that she has not been going to school because the baby was ill and cannot return to the child-care center without a doctor's note that the baby is well. Jennifer says she cannot afford to see a doctor. She has no health insurance and no money for health care. She began the application process for Medicaid but never followed through because it was "too much hassle." She lives with her mother and stepfather in a camper shell at a construction site where her stepfather is temporarily employed. She refuses to give you the location of this construction site, saying that they will probably move to a new site soon. Jennifer says her parents provide her with food and formula for the baby, who appears clean and well nourished. The baby has not begun his immunizations, again because of lack of funds for health services.

Jennifer says she is in good health, but has not had a postpartum checkup. Although not currently sexually active, she has a steady boyfriend and is contemplating sexual intimacy with him. She asks about various types of contraceptives.

The father of her baby is no longer in the area and is not aware that Jennifer had a baby. Jennifer's own father is also removed from the picture and Jennifer does not know where he is. When asked about her grandmother, Jennifer says that they do not get along well and that her grandmother hardly speaks to her since she got pregnant.

Jennifer is anxious to complete high school and go into a program to become a beautician. She tried recently to get a part-time job in a fast-food restaurant, but was told that they wanted someone with experience. She socializes somewhat with the girls at school and goes with several of them to take their babies to the park and similar outings.

1. What are the health problems evident in this situation? What are the human biological, environmental, life-style, and health system factors influencing these problems?
2. What considerations are important in planning care for Jennifer?
3. What primary prevention measures would you undertake with Jennifer and her son?
4. What secondary prevention measures would be warranted to deal with existing health problems? Describe specific actions that you would take to resolve these problems.
5. What could be done in terms of tertiary prevention to prevent further consequences or recurrence of health problems in this situation?
6. How would you evaluate the effectiveness of your interventions with Jennifer? Describe the specific evaluative criteria you would use and how you would obtain the evaluative data needed.

REFERENCES

1. Bowdler, J. E. (1989). Health problems of the homeless in America. *Nurse Practitioner, 14*(7), 44–51.
2. Miller, D. S., & Lin, E. H. B. (1988). Children in sheltered homeless families: Reported health status and use of health services. *Pediatrics, 81*, 668–673.
3. Wlodarczyk, D., & Prentice, R. (1988). Health issues of homeless persons. *Western Journal of Medicine, 148*, 717–719.
4. Robertson, M. J., & Cousineau, M. R. (1986). Health status and access to health services among the urban homeless. *American Journal of Public Health, 76*, 561–563.
5. Damrosch, S., & Strasser, J. A. (1988). The homeless elderly in America. *Journal of Gerontologic Nursing, 14*(10), 26–29.
6. Fischer, P. J., Shapiro, S., Breakey, W. R., Anthony, J. C., & Kramer, M. (1986). Mental health and social characteristics of the homeless: A survey of mission users. *American Journal of Public Health, 76*, 519–524.
7. Chafetz, L. (1988). Perspectives for psychiatric nurses on homelessness. *Issues in Mental Health Nursing, 9*, 325–335.
8. Damrosch, S. P., Sullivan, P. A., Scholler, A., & Gaines, J. (1988). On behalf of homeless families. *MCN, 13*, 259–263.
9. Holden, C. (1988). Health problems of the homeless. *Science, 242*, 188–189.
10. Youssef, F. A., Omokehinde, M., & Garland, I. M. (1988). The homeless and unhealthy: A review and analysis. *Issues in Mental Health Nursing, 9*, 317–324.
11. Belcher, J. R., & McCleese, G. (1988). The process of homelessness among the mentally ill: Rural and urban perspectives. *Human Services in the Rural Environment, 12*(2), 20–25.
12. Danziger, S. (1988). The economy, public policy, and the poor. In H. R. Rodgers (Ed.), *Beyond welfare* (pp. 3–13). Armonk, NY: M. E. Sharpe.
13. Woods, D. W., & Williamson, J. B. (1988). *Think about poverty in the U.S.: Problems and policies.* New York: Walker.
14. Rodgers, H. R. (1988). Reducing poverty through family support. In H. R. Rogers (Ed.), *Beyond Welfare* (pp. 39–65). Armonk, NY: M. E. Sharpe.
15. Meltzer, M. (1986). *Poverty in America.* New York: Morrow.
16. Lewis, G. H., & Morrison, R. J. (1987). *Income transfer analysis.* Brooklyn, NY: Immergut & Siolek.

RECOMMENDED READINGS

Belcher, J. R., & McCleese, G. (1988). The process of homelessness among the mentally ill: Rural and urban perspectives. *Human Services in the Rural Environment, 12*(2), 20–25.

Describes the results of two studies on the needs and response to homeless mentally ill persons in rural and urban communities.

Bowdler, J. E. (1989). Health problems of the homeless in America. *Nurse Practitioner, 14*(7), 44–51.

Discusses the health issues and conditions confronting the homeless in the United States. Also describes a health-care clinic designed to meet the needs of a homeless population.

Chafetz, L. (1988). Perspectives for psychiatric nurses on homelessness. *Issues in Mental Health Nursing, 9*, 325–335.

Addresses the special needs of the homeless mentally ill client and ways to meet those needs.

Damrosch, S., & Strasser, J. A. (1988). The homeless elderly in America. *Journal of Gerontological Nursing, 14*(10), 26–29.

Presents the health problems of homeless elderly persons and nursing interventions designed to meet those needs.

Danis, D. (1987). Bringing nursing care to homeless guests: Barbara McInnis and the Pine Street Inn's nurses' clinic. *Journal of Emergency Nursing, 13*(5), 26A–30A.

Examines the initiation of a nursing clinic for homeless clients in Boston. Addresses the kinds of problems encountered in this population group and nursing interventions designed to resolve those problems.

Francis, M. B. (1987). Long-term approaches to end homelessness. *Public Health Nursing, 4*, 230–235.

Looks at the contributing factors in homelessness from an epidemiologic perspective. Also addresses societal strategies that will be required to solve the problem of homelessness.

Miller, D. S., & Lin, E. H. B. (1988). Children in sheltered homeless families: Reported health status and use of health services. *Pediatrics, 81*, 668–673.

Reports the findings of a study on the health status and needs of homeless children.

Pearson, L. J. (1988). Providing health care to the homeless: Another important role for NPs. *Nurse Practitioner, 13*(4), 38–48.

Describes the work of two nurse practitioners in meeting the health care needs of the homeless population of Atlanta, Georgia.

Woods, D. (1989). Homeless children: Their evaluation and treatment. *Journal of Pediatric Health Care, 3*(4), 194–199.

Addresses the special health needs of homeless children. Describes assessment of homeless children's health status and provides a case study to demonstrate assessment and health-care planning for homeless youngsters.

UNIT FIVE

Care of Clients in Specialized Settings

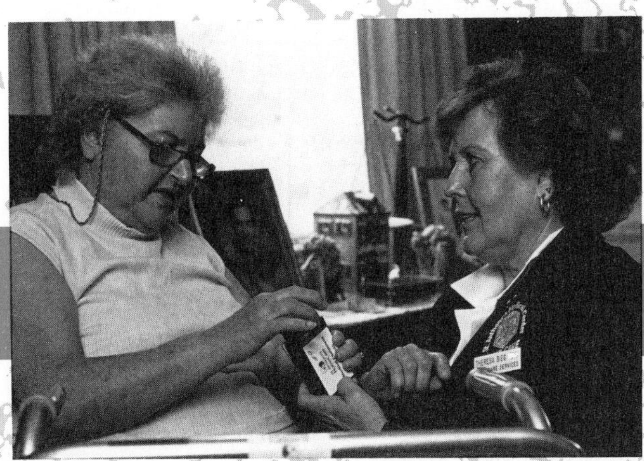

People typically think of community health nursing as nursing care that is provided in public health agencies like state and county health departments. This is, however, a misperception. Community health nursing can take place in any setting in which emphasis is placed on health promotion and illness prevention for groups of people. As noted earlier, community health nursing may even take place in a hospital or other acute-care setting, where community health nurses may engage in roles related to case management and discharge planning.

There are, however, some specialized settings in which community health nursing is likely to take place. Not all nurses who function in these settings may be community health nurses. When community health nurses do work in these settings, though, they incorporate the principles of community health nursing into the care provided to achieve the multiple goals of improving not only the health status of individual clients but also groups of people in the setting and the total population.

The home has been a traditional setting for providing community health nursing services. Because of dwindling resources and changes in the type of clients seen in the home, home visits must be more focused and purposive than was the case in the past. As noted in Chapter 8, The Home Visit Process, community health nursing care provided in the home setting must be well planned and designed specifically to address identified health problems. Not every nurse who provides services in the home setting is a community health nurse. However, nurses who can combine the principles of community health nursing with other nursing skills can contribute more effectively to improving clients' overall health status than can those who do not have a background in community health nursing. Community health nursing and its relevance to home health care are addressed in Chapter 25, Care of Clients in the Home Setting.

School nursing addresses the health-care needs of individual children in the school. When school nurses are also community health nurses, they target their interventions to the school population as a whole, as well as the larger community. This setting is an important one for community health nurses because of the potential for influencing the health and health behaviors of future generations. Community health nursing as practiced in the school setting is addressed in Chapter 26, Care of Clients in the School Setting.

Work settings also afford an opportunity for community health nurses to influence health behaviors and conditions that may contribute to ill health in a large segment of the population. Again, the hallmark of the community health nurse working in this setting is concern for population groups as well as for individual employees. Chapter 27, Care of Clients in the Work Setting, examines the application of community health nursing principles to the care of members of the work force.

Health-care services have often been less accessible or of a lower quality in rural settings than in urban areas. Health-care providers may also be less frequently encountered. In addition to these health system factors, the health status of rural populations is influenced by a variety of environmental factors that make their health-care needs uniquely different from those of their urban counterparts. Community health nurses are important providers of care in rural settings where they may be some of only a few health-care providers available. The unique health-care needs of rural populations and the role of community health nurses in meeting those needs are addressed in Chapter 28, Care of Clients in Rural Settings.

It is common today to hear of natural or man-made disasters that cause tremendous loss of life and property and disrupt the day-to-day routine of those affected. Community health nurses should play a primary role in assisting individuals, families, and communities to prevent such disasters and their aftereffects. They should also be involved in planning, implementing, and evaluating health-care services in the event of an actual disaster. In Chapter 29, Care of Clients in Disaster Settings, the principles of community health nursing are applied to the subject of preventing and resolving the aftermath of disaster situations.

In each of the specialized settings described in this unit, community health nurses use the epidemiologic prevention process model to adapt nursing care to the needs of the individual and the setting. The focus remains on the health care of population groups and the overall society.

From the Community: A Nurse's Voice

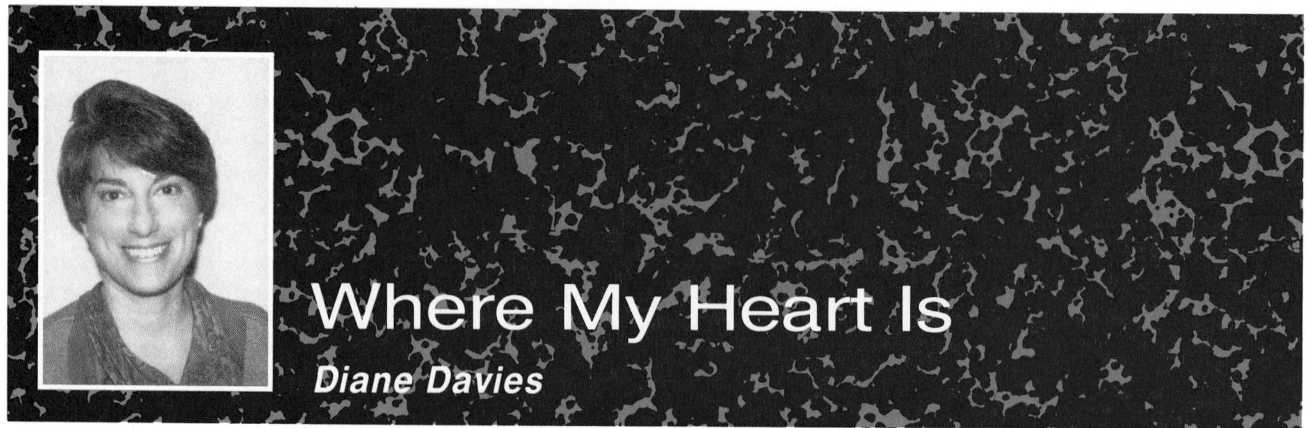

For me, community health nursing has been a daily proving ground for 20 years of nursing practice and education. I work for a community-based, home-care agency in New York's lower Hudson Valley. To accomplish my professional mission I need to assess my clients' needs, plan and implement interventions that work in a home-care environment, and teach clients and their families the process of promoting wellness.

My ability to give priority to and anticipate client needs is exercised each morning as I map out a schedule that maximizes my time spent with clients and minimizes my time spent driving—a difficult goal when I sometimes have to drive up to 500 miles a week! Frequently, I have only a name, diagnosis, and address to guide me. But even at this early stage I've begun to search my knowledge of disease, psychology, family dynamics, growth and development, cultural factors, and local geography to guide my planning.

Client assessment begins even before I've met the client. Driving to the client's home, I note its distance from the nearest health-care facility, pharmacy, grocery store, or neighbor. Approaching the client's house, I take note of its structure, upkeep, and its entrances and exits. I also listen and observe for signs of dogs and other household pets. Once inside, I listen carefully to what the client has to say and, equally important, to what he or she may not be telling me. Indeed, I've learned never to take a conversation at face value. One might say that caring for clients in their homes has trained me to really "see" when I look and "hear" when I listen.

I draw on an array of clinical competencies—some simple, some sophisticated—to provide safe nursing care to clients from infancy to advanced age. For one client, I might only need to teach the safe use of aspirin. For another, I might need to administer chemotherapeutic agents via central or peripheral lines. I am also required to have a working knowledge of the high-tech equipment used in infusion therapy and to know how to develop client-specific drug compatibility lists. For every client, I maintain a clinical record for peer review.

Caring for clients in their homes has taught me to become acutely cost-conscious. Any nursing intervention that requires equipment and supplies is expensive, and outside of the hospital setting many expenses are borne by the client. Working as I do with rural clients who often have limited incomes, developing an effective plan of care requires that I be as sensitive to the cost of a quart of milk as to the cost of a Foley catheter. After all, how would it benefit a client if the cost of my nursing care meant that he or she couldn't afford that week's groceries? Accordingly, I've often shown my clients how to sterilize strips of old sheets in an oven to use for dressings or how to boil salt water to make saline solution. I've even taught a family how to wash a straight catheter in soap and water and reuse it as needed.

Finally, caring for clients in the home setting has made me keenly aware of the client's rights. When I enter a home, I do so only with the expressed permission of the individual client or family. Although I come armed with clinical ability, knowledge of community resources, and a desire to maintain the client at home until he or she recovers or succumbs, I cannot force my services on the client. I can only request that the client allow me to enter and assist, and I must accept it when that permission is denied. To this day, the toughest thing for me to do is to allow a client or family member to refuse help.

If I have been successful as a community health nurse, it has been because I have learned to carry everything I need in my head or in my hand, and I have learned to think on my feet. Although I stand alone at the front door, standing behind me, unseen by the client, is an incredibly complex health-care system. This system, while far from perfect, does recognize that "home is where the heart is." It's where my heart is too.

CHAPTER 25

Care of Clients in the Home Setting

Margaret Myers Sereda

KEY TERMS

certificate of need
fiscal intermediaries
Medicare-certified agency
pre-discharge assessment
pre-process goals
respite care

Community health nursing began with services offered to clients in their homes, and community health nurses continue to care for clients in the home setting. Today, however, the clients who are seen differ in terms of their health problems and the acuity of those problems. In the past, clients were seen at home for purposes of health promotion and health education and to monitor the status of chronic health conditions, or to give technical care such as dressing changes for a short time after hospitalization. Today, clients may receive a variety of health-care services at home including intravenous antibiotic infusions or chemotherapy.

Clients seen in the home today are often sicker than those seen in the past and have a broader range of health-care needs. Reasons for some of the changes in the type of clients seen include the influence of the DRG (diagnosis related group) reimbursement system (discussed in Chapter 13, Economic Influences on Community Health) and the consequent early discharge of more acutely ill clients; a growing recognition of the cost-effectiveness of home care versus hospitalization; and the growing number of elderly clients in the population.

With the advent of DRGs, hospitals are only reimbursed under Medicare for a specific length of stay depending on the client's diagnosis. These restrictions on reimbursement have led many hospitals to encourage physicians to discharge clients earlier. Early discharge frequently means that clients have continuing needs for nursing care that, in the past, were met in the hospital. These clients are usually referred for home-care services. In addition, private insurance carriers are realizing that care in the home is less expensive than hospitalization. Advances in medical technology have made it possible to provide complex therapy in the home setting.

The increase in nursing care in the home setting can also be attributed to the increasing number and proportion of elderly persons in the population.[1] The average age of the population will con-

(*continued*)

LEARNING OBJECTIVES

After reading this chapter you should be able to:

- Identify at least three types of home health-care agencies.
- Describe three general considerations in providing care to clients in the home setting.
- Identify two considerations in assessing the physical environment of the home nursing client.
- Describe at least three organizational considerations in planning nursing care for clients in the home setting.
- Identify two considerations in implementing nursing care in the home setting.
- Describe two aspects of evaluating nursing care of clients in the home setting.

tinue to increase into the next century. Older people have greater needs for health care and use a greater proportion of health-care resources than any other age group. Care-givers of older persons are also frequently elderly and may be chronically ill, thus requiring assistance themselves.[2] In many instances their needs for nursing care can be adequately met in the home setting.

Not all nurses who provide nursing care in the home setting are community health nurses. Many home health nurses focus primarily on providing acute care in the home setting. When community health nurses work in home health agencies, however, they combine acute-care skills with the health-promotion and illness-prevention emphasis of community health nursing, allowing them to deal more effectively with clients' overall health-care needs.

Home health nurses focus on secondary and tertiary levels of care, while community health nurses working in home-care settings provide care at all three levels of prevention. In addition, the community health nurse who provides home care addresses the needs of the population as well as those of the individual client and his or her family. For example, while the community health nurse provides care to the client with AIDS and gives support to the client's significant others, he or she will also engage in health education to prevent the spread of the disease to other members of the community.

HOME HEALTH AGENCIES

Health care in the home setting can be provided by a variety of agencies and organizations. Community health nurses who provide nursing care in the home may be employed by official health departments or by home health agencies. Because home health nursing agencies provide a unique milieu for community health nursing some general information about these agencies, including the types of agencies involved and reimbursement and licensing issues, will be presented here.

TYPES OF HOME HEALTH NURSING AGENCIES

Four basic types of home-care agencies provide skilled nursing services. These include Medicare-certified agencies, private home health agencies, hospice home-care agencies, and public-supported agencies.

MEDICARE-CERTIFIED AGENCIES

Medicare has a great impact on home health care because over half of home health-care expenditures are funded by this federal insurance plan for the elderly and the disabled.[3] A ***Medicare-certified agency*** is a home health-care agency that has been approved by Medicare to provide specific services for which it can be reimbursed under Medicare. As of 1987, there were almost 6000 Medicare-certified home health-care agencies in the United States.[4] To provide home-care services to Medicare recipients, the agency must comply with regulations promulgated under the Social Security Act. These regulations dictate qualifications of personnel, agency structure, restrictions on client eligibility, billing methods, and numerous other facets of agency function.

The Health Care Financing Administration (HCFA) regulates payment for services under Medicare. This agency has designated fiscal intermediaries for each area of the country. ***Fiscal intermediaries*** are organizations that act as reimbursement agents and that deal directly with home-care agencies. For example, in certain sections of Southern California, the Blue Cross-Blue Shield Insurance Company acts as a fiscal intermediary for home health agencies. In other parts of the country, private carriers such as Aetna Life & Casualty and Traveler's Insurance Company serve as intermediaries.

Home health agencies are reviewed periodically by representatives from the fiscal intermediary for adherence to Medicare guidelines related to services, documentation, and billing practices. Medicare-certified agencies must provide a broad spectrum of care including physical therapy, occupational therapy, speech therapy, and social services, in addition to skilled nursing and home health aide services.

The home health-care services billed to Medicare must be intermittent in nature, consisting of skilled services for 8 hours a day or less.[5] Beyond the 8-hour limit, services are considered continuous or extended rather than intermittent. Although the intermittent visit can be up to 8 hours in length, reimbursement by Medicare for one visit is such that a visit of more than 1½ to 2 hours would result in financial loss for the agency. Intermittent services are also episodic, as the nurse may visit the client anywhere from twice a day to once a month.

There are strict regulations regarding the homebound status of clients eligible for home-care services under Medicare. The homebound client must be confined to the home except for visits to the physician's office. The frequency of professional visits must be in accord with the client's documented diagnosis, need for care, and activity restrictions. Many more restrictions exist in the Medicare reimbursement system, some of which will be discussed later in this chapter.

The client must have a demonstrated need for either skilled nursing care or physical or speech therapy in order to be eligible for home health aide or other ancillary services. A physician must certify that the client has a need for skilled home health services and sign a plan of treatment that details the home health-care plan.[5] The home health agency bills Medicare through the fiscal intermediary and is reimbursed for services provided. If Medicare does not cover the total cost of services, the agency *may not* bill the client for outstanding fees.

PRIVATE HOME HEALTH AGENCIES

Major differences between private home health-care and Medicare-certified agencies relate to restrictions on intermittent care, regulation of professional staff qualifications, agency structure, and reimbursement policies. Private agencies may provide services for any individual requesting them, with or without physician orders. The agency may bill the client directly for the amount not reimbursed by the client's private insurance carrier.

Client care may, and frequently does, occur on an extended or continuous basis, for more than 8 hours a day. Private home health agencies may also provide intermittent visits in addition to continuous nursing care, but they are not required to do so. They frequently have a number of services available to the client, such as physical, occupational, and speech therapy, social services, and so on. The availability of these services is not mandatory as in the case of Medicare-certified agencies.

HOSPICE HOME-CARE AGENCIES

There are both private and Medicare-certified hospice organizations. These agencies provide services for terminally ill clients who wish to remain at home. A Medicare hospice client must receive services from a Medicare-certified hospice for the benefits to be covered.[5]

A physician must certify that the Medicare hospice client is terminally ill, and that the client elects to receive hospice care rather than hospitalization. Non-Medicare hospice services may or may not be covered by private health insurance.

Both intermittent and extended or continuous care can be provided by hospice agencies. Hospices may also provide home health aides and other services such as social work assistance as needed. Most hospice agencies have a volunteer component as an adjunct to professional services. Respite services are also provided so family caretakers can carry out responsibilities of everyday life such as shopping and banking.

Community health nurses who work for hospices usually have received special education to prepare them for work with terminally ill clients. This education includes a focus on bereavement issues for the client, family and significant others, and for the nurse.

PUBLICLY FUNDED AGENCIES

Other agencies that are partially funded by public donations may also employ community health nurses (and other nurses) to provide home nursing services. Visiting nurse associations (VNAs) are an example of this type of agency. The client population served by these agencies is similar to that of the Medicare-certified or private home-care agency in addition to indigent persons who have no outside source of funding for services.

Because VNAs have difficulty competing with private agencies for reimbursement, their caseloads include a high proportion of indigent clients for which the agency receives little or no reimbursement for care.[6] This has resulted in the closing of many VNAs or refusal to provide services for clients who cannot pay. The decision of some VNAs not to provide home-care services to the needy population is seen by some as abandonment of clients,[7] creating an ethical dilemma for these agencies.

REIMBURSEMENT FOR HOME NURSING SERVICES

It is clear from the preceding discussion that the organization and operation of home health agencies is intimately bound to reimbursement issues. Reimbursement for home nursing services may occur under both the Medicare and Medicaid programs, private insurance, out-of-pocket payment by clients, and, on occasion, by public donation.

As was the case with Medicare-certified agencies, the types of services that can be provided under the Medicaid program are specifically dictated. Nurses must obtain prior authorization for a specific number of home visits and types of services for Medicaid clients. Reimbursement for these visits is usually so low that agencies lose money serving Medicaid recipients and frequently provide these services only as a favor to physicians who also refer private or Medicare clients.

What are the implications of financial issues in home care for community health nurses? The importance of reimbursement issues has largely been ignored in nursing's traditionally service-oriented philosophy. In home-care agencies, community health nurses must become knowledgeable about reimbursement issues because their documentation of client needs and nursing care given directly influences payment for services. Nurses need to know what services are reimbursable and what criteria clients must meet to be eligible for reimbursable services. Community health nurses, then, need to assess and document the existence of conditions that make clients eligible for services. They also need to be careful to document services provided in such a way that services can be reimbursed. This usually entails becoming intimately familiar with the eligibility and documentation guidelines of each funding agency.

LICENSING OF HOME HEALTH AGENCIES

Licensure of home health-care agencies is state, county, or locally controlled depending upon where the agency is located. In California, for example, licensing is a state regulatory function. Some areas require a "certificate of need" prior to licensing a home nursing agency. A ***certificate of need*** is evidence of the need for home nursing services in that area that are not met by existing agencies. The trend appears to be toward increased legislation regarding licensure of home health agencies; thus the reader is encouraged to seek out licensing requirements for home health agencies in his or her own area.

THE HOME HEALTH CLIENT

There is no "typical" client requiring nursing care in the home. The client profile can include a mother and a 1- or 2-day-old infant born in a short-stay hospital unit or at home who require follow-up care. It can also include the elderly person requiring skilled care and monitoring after surgery for a hip fracture or other medical or health problems. In short, the client can be anyone in need of professionally supervised nursing care in the home.

Some trends are evident, however. With increased frequency, clients requiring nursing care at home are receiving complex therapies or using high-technology equipment that was formerly restricted to acute-care hospital settings. More and more chemotherapy clients, for example, are receiving treatment at home as new technology allows safer infusion of chemotherapeutic agents. Pain management for those with end-stage cancer or chronic disease is also being achieved in the home with good results. Clients on ventilators or who require continuous or intermittent oxygen can also be maintained at home.

Irrespective of the reasons for care, the client is the *primary* recipient of nursing care in the home. But the client's progress in reaching health-related goals can be either greatly facilitated or obstructed by interaction with significant others. Those who interact with the client are potential *secondary* recipients of nursing care. For this reason, community health nurses working in the home setting will often need to use the family assessment skills discussed in Chapter 18, Care of the Family Client.

In addition, because community health nurses are also concerned with the health of groups of people, they may need to employ the principles of community assessment and health program planning discussed in Chapter 19, Care of the Community or Target Group. For example, in the course of providing home care to clients with AIDS, the community health nurse might note that there is little opportunity for family caretakers to obtain relief from the burden of care for their loved one. In such a situation, the nurse might function as an advocate for this population group, initiating activities to plan respite care for the caretakers of clients with AIDS and other terminal illnesses.

GENERAL CONSIDERATIONS IN CARING FOR CLIENTS IN THE HOME SETTING

Before examining the application of the epidemiologic prevention process model in the home health setting, several general considerations should be addressed. These include collaboration, pre-process goals, and continuity.

COLLABORATION

The key to successful use of the epidemiologic prevention process model in home care is collaboration, working jointly with others to ensure successful completion of each stage of the process. Collaboration with the client and the family or care-givers, the home health-care team, the physician, and discharge planner is necessary to provide comprehensive care.

PRE-PROCESS GOALS

Pre-process goals, which are goals identified prior to client assessment and intervention,[8] are needed for the smooth and effective use of the epidemiologic prevention process model. Goals to be accomplished before the nurse can effectively use the model to identify client health needs include establishing trust between the nurse and the client, defining the roles to be played by each during their interaction, providing an opportunity for the client to become comfortable in the relationship, and creating an environment in which the epidemiologic prevention process model can be successfully employed. These pre-process goals are especially important in home-care settings to provide an atmosphere in which client independence, the ultimate goal of community health nursing, can be achieved.

CONTINUITY

Community health nurses need to apply the epidemiologic prevention process model on a continuing basis until the time of problem solution or client discharge from care. The community health nurse uses the model to provide ongoing and cyclic care rather than episodic care. The information garnered in the evaluation of care will be used to restructure further assessment, planning, implementation, and evaluation.

THE EPIDEMIOLOGIC PREVENTION PROCESS MODEL AND CARE OF CLIENTS IN THE HOME SETTING

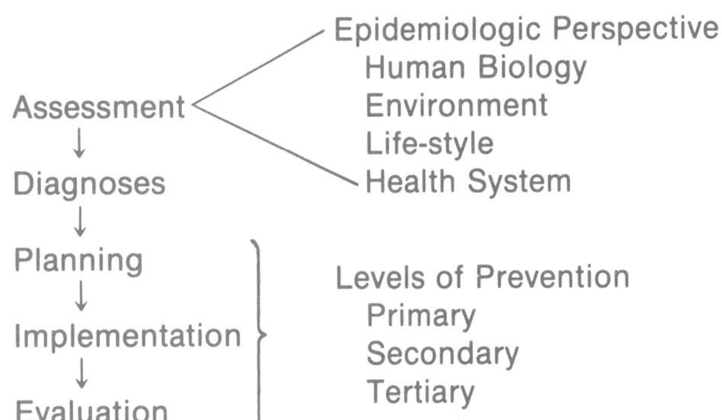

The epidemiologic prevention process model is used to its fullest extent in the community health nurse's interactions with clients and their family and friends. The relatively autonomous nature of community health nursing in the home setting places upon the practitioner the responsibility of ensuring that a total spectrum of care is provided to meet client care goals.

ASSESSING THE CLIENT'S HEALTH NEEDS

REFERRAL

The responsibility of the community health nurse may begin with the referral of the client. In this context, referral is the notification of the community health agency that skilled nursing or other services are required for a client in the home. This notification may come directly from the physician, from a hospital social worker, a discharge planner in the employ of the hospital, or the liaison nurse.

Regrettably, many times requests for home nursing services are nonspecific; for example, "Please go out and see what you can do for this patient. She is in heart failure and refuses hospitalization." Other times, specific procedures and complex treatments are requested, and orders for these treatments must be validated. The client's medications are sometimes listed on the referral, but they must also be validated by a pharmacist if they are to be provided by the nursing agency.

PRE-DISCHARGE ASSESSMENT

Pre-discharge assessment is a desirable first step in the assessment process when caring for clients in the home. ***Pre-discharge assessment*** occurs when the nurse visits the client in the hospital and confers with him or her and, possibly, with the physician and significant others to determine what type of nursing services will be required.

Alternatively, the community health nurse may work in association with a "liaison" nurse, employed either by the hospital or by the community agency, who performs a discharge assessment prior to the client's release. The liaison nurse may recommend home-care services to ease the client's transition to the home setting. Sometimes pre-discharge teaching, such as techniques for intravenous infusion, is provided prior to the client's release from the acute-care institution. This teaching would then be continued and reinforced in the home after discharge.

THE EVALUATION VISIT

An initial evaluation visit to the client's home is made following referral and the pre-discharge assessment, if one is made. During this visit the nurse obtains a health history and determines the client's physical and mental status, need for care, potential for accomplishment of health-related goals, activity level and restrictions, equipment and supplies needed, safety issues, and rehabilitation potential. Some agencies employ nurses whose sole function is to perform evaluation visits and then refer clients to community health nurses who provide the direct care. Other agencies have the community health nurse conduct the evaluation visit as part of the continuous process of care.

It is important to establish a positive working relationship with the client and family members during this initial visit and to obtain their perceptions of goals for care. Emphasizing the partnership aspects of the nurse-client-family relationship will promote client and family independence in assuming responsibility for care.

The community health agency's practices and policies, hours of operation, on-call system, and emergency procedures should be discussed with the client and significant others. The client's rights and responsibilities regarding care should also be discussed. Some agencies endorse the Client Bill of Rights developed by the Community Health Accreditation Program (CHAP), the home health accrediting body of the National League for Nursing, and a copy of this document may be left with the client or with family members. Copies of any agreements for care signed by the client should also be provided.

ASSESSING FACTORS INFLUENCING CLIENT HEALTH

Human Biology

The community health nurse assessing a client's health needs must identify biological factors that may affect the client's condition and care. Several categories of biological factors are genetic inheritance, maturation and aging, and the client's physiologic status. These factors are interdependent in their effect on the client.

Genetic Inheritance. Some genetically influenced diseases are noteworthy in the home-care setting owing to their influence on clients' health status and ability to care for themselves. Diabetes mellitus is an example of this kind of condition; the client with diabetes may have difficulty healing following surgery or injury.

It is imperative that the community health nurse obtain information about genetic diseases through careful questioning of the client or significant others. Neither the client nor his or her family may comprehend the impact of these diseases on the client's condition, prognosis, and care, and may neglect to mention them unless asked.

Maturation and Aging. Maturation and aging affect clients' abilities to carry out self-care techniques and may increase or decrease the need for skilled nursing care. Visual problems associated with aging such as cataracts, glaucoma, or poor vision may prevent elderly clients from providing necessary care for themselves or for others in the home setting.

It may also be the nurse's responsibility to assess an adolescent mother's maturity level and its effect on her ability to care for a sick infant. Skill in assessing maturational factors is valuable and helpful in providing comprehensive nursing care in the home. (See chapters included in Unit 4 for descriptions of client-specific assessment procedures.)

Physiologic Function. Clients are most often referred for home care for treatment of specific health problems. As complete an assessment of biological function as is possible at the time of each visit is critical because the nurse is, at times, the only source of physical assessment the client receives.

A comprehensive system-by-system or head-to-toe approach to assessment should be used. Both clients and family members may forget to mention problems or symptoms or believe them to be inconsequential until the nurse questions them. Sometimes knowing the right question to ask can prevent a minor problem from developing into a dangerous situation.

Environment

Factors in the client's environment may influence the need for nursing care and its provision in the home. These factors can arise out of the client's physical, psychological, or social environment and will be considered by the nurse in assessing the client's health status.

Physical Environment. The client's physical environment is an important factor in providing nursing care in the home. Safety and infection control are two areas of particular concern in the physical environment of the home setting.

Infection Control. Infection control in the home has a dual focus: protecting the client and family and protecting the nurse. The nurse should adhere to the agency's standards of practice and educate the client and family members in infection-control measures.

Nurses perform dressing changes for infected wounds, change intravenous sites, provide central line care and home blood transfusion, and work with clients diagnosed with many communicable diseases. Continuous assessment of the physical environment for established infection-control standards and outcome criteria is a necessary function of the community health nurse in the home setting.

Infection-control procedures are similar to those employed in other health-care settings but may require more creativity on the part of the nurse working in the client's home. For example, a community health nurse made an early morning home visit to change an indwelling urinary catheter in a remote rural area. Because the nurse knew he would be visiting the client before going to the health center, he put the necessary supplies in his car the day before. Unfortunately, the temperature dropped during the night, and when the nurse went to inflate the bulb to keep the catheter in place, the fluid was frozen in the syringe. The nurse could not return 60 miles to the health center to get another catheterization set, so he used the warmth of his sterile-gloved hand to thaw the syringe while maintaining a sterile field and keeping the catheter in place in the client's urethra.

The primary infection-control measure in any setting is adequate handwashing before and after any direct care given to clients. Hands should be thoroughly washed with soap and running water. Again, this may require some creativity on the part of nurses or family members in homes that do not have running water. For example, the nurse may wet his or her hands, apply soap and lather thoroughly, then ask a family member to pour clean water over the hands to rinse off the soap. The nurse can also carry paper towels to avoid using towels that may have been used for other purposes earlier. The nurse should also instruct family members in the importance of handwashing in the care of the client and as a general measure for preventing the spread of disease.

Infection control in the home, as in other settings, also involves the use of sterile precautions in any invasive procedures, appropriate disposal of bodily secretions and excretions, and isolation precautions as warranted by the client's condition. For example, reverse isolation procedures might be needed for the client who is severely immunocompromised. For a visit to a client with active tuberculosis, on the other hand, the nurse does not need to wear a mask, but merely to minimize the time spent in close proximity to the client.

Nurses working in the home with clients who have blood-borne diseases such as AIDS or hepatitis B should use universal blood and body fluid precautions. These precautions apply to any body fluids containing visible blood, semen, vaginal secretions, cerebrospinal fluid, synovial fluid, pleural fluid, peritoneal fluid, pericardial fluid, and amniotic fluid, and any feces, nasal secretions, sputum, sweat, urine, or vomitus that contains visible blood.[9] Universal precautions are summarized in Box 25–1.

Care should also be taken in the disposal of secretions and excretions of clients with other conditions. For example, sputum from clients with active tuberculosis should be handled with care, while the feces of chronic typhoid carriers should be disposed of in a municipal sewer system.

Nurses and significant others caring for clients with certain conditions may need to be immunized. For example, household contacts to chronic typhoid carriers should be immunized against typhoid, and both family members and nurses caring for clients with hepatitis B should be immunized.[10] Careful attention to infection-control measures in the home can minimize risks for clients and their families as well as for the nurse.

Safety. Although safety issues in the home include infection control, other concerns need to be addressed in this area as well. Equipment and preparations that present minimal safety risks in a hospital setting can present considerable, but controllable, risks when used in the client's home. For example, an IV stand becomes a safety hazard when the home has scatter rugs or is particularly crowded. Grounding of electrical outlets is a safety issue for clients requiring infusion pumps. Injectable and other medications can be dangerous in the hands of infants and children.

Continuous chemotherapy infusions are administered in homes with excellent results for clients, but they present unique safety hazards. For example, some of these agents are extremely toxic to skin tissue and can cause severe damage if they come in contact with the skin.[11] Needles and other equipment used to administer these agents also present contamination and injury hazards.

Safety assessment goes beyond factors involved

BOX 25–1

Universal Precautions for Preventing the Spread of Blood-Borne Diseases

1. Use appropriate barrier precautions (for example, gloves) to prevent skin and mucous membrane exposure when contact with human blood or other body fluids is anticipated.
2. Wash hands and other skin surfaces immediately after contamination with blood or other body fluids.
3. Take precautions to prevent injuries stemming from needles and other sharp instruments during or after procedures, when disposing of used equipment, or when cleaning used equipment.
4. Do not recap, bend, or break used needles; place them in a puncture-proof container for disposal.
5. Keep mouthpieces, resuscitation bags, or other ventilation devices at hand when the need for resuscitation is predictable.
6. Refrain from direct care of clients and from handling client-care equipment when you have exudative skin lesions or weeping dermatitis.
7. Implement these precautions with all clients, not just those known to be infected with blood-borne diseases.

(Source: Recommendations for prevention of HIV transmission in health care settings. [1987]. *MMWR, 36* [Suppl 2], 35–185)

in direct provision of care. Bathroom safety equipment, medications, lighting, clothing and shoes, home traffic patterns, and electrical hazards were identified as threats to safety in one study of hazards encountered by nurses working in the home setting.[12] Many of these issues have already been addressed in Chapter 8, The Home Visit Process. (See Appendix C, Home Safety Assessment Guides, as well.) Even if the community health nurse is going into the home to supervise chemotherapy or to change a dressing, this individual should remain alert to safety hazards and intervene to eliminate them.

Psychological Environment. As mentioned in earlier chapters, a stressful environment can appreciably affect a client's health status. This is especially true for the client requiring care at home. A supportive environment is one of the keys to aiding the healing of individual and family clients.

Stress and anxiety may be experienced by the client returning to the home from an acute-care setting. Uncertainty about the client's diagnosis, treatment, and prognosis may create fear and anxiety in both the client and in family members. Interactions between the client and the family or among other family members may also be sources of stress that impair the client's health status.

In assessing the client's health status, the community health nurse would explore the presence of these potential sources of stress. Clients and their significant others should be encouraged to voice fears and anxieties about the client's condition and about its treatment. The client's relationships with others should be assessed as well for situations that may produce additional stress. The interaction patterns observed among family members may provide valuable information if the client appears to be distressed about family pressures. (See Chapter 18, Care of the Family Client.)

Oftentimes families feel inadequate to the demands of meeting the needs of the client as well as their own physical and psychological needs. These feelings may lead to guilt, which can create a whole host of problems. The community health nurse would assess the client's (and others involved with the client) degree of comfort and competence in managing the client's health-care requirements. If the client or family is overly anxious, the community health nurse might assume a negotiated level of responsibility for case management. This might consist of arranging and coordinating care received from other providers, obtaining necessary equipment, or providing assistance in meeting financial needs or obtaining help with housekeeping.

Social Environment. Reinforcement of a client's social environment, usually based on cultural identity, may have a great influence on the client's well-being. For example, the client and significant others are more likely to adhere to folk medicine and culturally based health-care practices and life-styles in the home setting than in the hospital setting. The nurse must develop an awareness of and sensitivity to cultural factors that may influence the client's health. Familiarity with common traditions and practices and careful cultural assessment will aid the nurse in appraising needs and providing appropriate care. Finding a sympathetic resource such as a co-worker or friend with expertise or membership in an unfamiliar culture can be an invaluable asset in establishing a working relationship with the client and family. (See Chapter 15, Cultural Influences on Community Health, for a complete discussion of cultural assessment.)

Life-style

Life-style factors related to employment, consumption patterns, and leisure activities can influence the health of the client in the home setting. Assessment of these factors will give the community health nurse a more accurate picture of the client's needs, assist the nurse to recognize problems, and aid in establishing positive goals for health.

Employment. If the client's condition has interfered with his or her employment or that of family members, the nurse should assess the potential for a return to work. For example, the client may have a need for physical or occupational therapy in order to return to his or her previous occupation. If the client will not be able to return to a former occupation because of consequences of illness or injury, the nurse can assist the client to determine the potential for other avenues of employment. Or, if the client will not be able to work, there may be a need for assistance in filing disability claims.

In a similar vein, the community health nurse would assess factors that may influence the ability of family caretakers to return to work. For example, the mother of a handicapped child may require assistance in making appropriate child-care arrangements so that she can return to work. Or there may be a need for a companion for an elderly client with Alzheimer's disease to free family caretakers for employment.

Consumption Patterns. Assessment of both the client's and family members' consumption patterns and their significance for health can guide the nurse in formulating a realistic plan of care. The client and family will be more likely to revert to traditional eating and drinking practices at home than in the regimented atmosphere of the hospital. Cultural sensitivity in this aspect of life-style is again very valuable.

Clients on a liquid diet might better tolerate it if it has some of the taste, ingredients, or association with their regular diet. Clear instructions about the interaction of the client's medication and alcohol or other substances may also be necessary.

Consumption patterns of family members are also important. If family members smoke, for example, second-hand smoke might further impair the health of a client with a chronic respiratory condition. Smoking by either the client or family members could be a serious safety hazard if the client is receiving oxygen therapy. Substance abuse by family members would be another significant assessment finding because substance abuse can impair family members' abilities to provide adequate care for the client.

Leisure. The atmosphere in the home setting can become so intense and focused on the client and his or her health problems that all parties concerned fail to recognize the need for leisure activities. Assessing the client's and family's normal relaxation habits can help the nurse suggest methods to maintain a healthier, happier period of recuperation from illness or adjustment to chronic disease.

Family members might require respite care so as to have time for leisure pursuits, and the community health nurse should assess both the need for and availability of respite care. ***Respite care*** is the voluntary or paid services of a person to assume on a temporary basis the care responsibilities of a homebound client. This type of service allows family members who have responsibility for the direct care of the client to get some necessary personal time or to meet other responsibilities.

Health System

Health system factors can also influence both the client's health status and the nurse's approach to home care. In assessing this area, the community health nurse would identify the client's usual source of health care and the client's source of health-care funding. The client's usual source of health care will indicate where the nurse may need to go to obtain medical orders for certain interventions that might be needed by the client. For example, if a client has a private physician, the nurse would contact the physician to obtain an order prior to catheterizing the client to relieve a distended bladder.

Information about the client's source of health-care funding may also influence the nurse's ability to provide certain interventions. As noted earlier, reimbursement under Medicare, for example, is only available for those services covered. Both the nurse and the client need to understand what types of nursing services are, or are not, covered by the client's funding source.

DIAGNOSTIC REASONING AND CARE OF CLIENTS IN THE HOME SETTING

Based on client assessment information, the community health nurse will derive nursing diagnoses to direct the care to be given. Nursing diagnoses can be organized in terms of the level of prevention involved. For example, a nursing diagnosis related to primary prevention might be, "Potential for stress-related problems due to lack of knowledge regarding positive effects of exercise on stress reduction," while a diagnosis reflecting secondary prevention might be, "Infection due to inadequate knowledge of care of infusion device." Diagnoses at the tertiary level of prevention would be geared toward preventing the recurrence of problems or complications of existing problems or restoring client function. For example, a nursing diagnosis at this level might be, "Need for education to prevent recurrent episodes of diabetic acidosis." The nursing diagnoses and their implications should be shared with the client and significant others to clarify perceptions prior to presenting and discussing the plan of care.

PLANNING INTERVENTIONS FOR CLIENTS IN THE HOME SETTING

The planning of nursing intervention in the home setting follows the general principles of planning discussed in Chapter 5, The Nursing Process. Because of the setting in which care occurs, special planning considerations exist in providing home-based care. These include organizational considerations and the planning process itself.

ORGANIZATIONAL CONSIDERATIONS

To be effective in providing nursing care in the home, the community health nurse needs to employ a variety of organizational skills. These include skills related to technical competence, time management, cost-effectiveness, and supervision.

Technical Competence

Providing nursing care in the home setting frequently involves maintaining a high level of technical competence to meet the needs of today's more acutely ill client. This can include knowledge of sophisticated treatments of infants with hyperbilirubinemia; monitoring the respiratory condition of ventilator-dependent clients; or home-monitoring of hyperalimentation. Large nursing agencies can employ nursing specialists to perform highly skilled care such as enterostomal therapy or chemotherapy infusion, but the nurse associated with a moderate-size or small agency may need to perform many complex and highly specialized procedures. When planning client care, nurses must honestly examine their competence and expertise in providing the technical care required.

The community health nurse should also consider the competence of the client and significant others in performing tasks required to meet the client's needs. If the client or family members do not have the necessary competencies, the nurse will need to help them develop those competencies. For example, if parents will need to use periodic suction to clear their child's tracheostomy tube, they may need to be taught suctioning techniques. Or, if family members will be administering pain medications for the client with terminal cancer, they may need to learn the associated skills.

Time Management

A common misconception among nurses who do not work in home settings is that home-based care is not a time-intensive mode of nursing. After all, if the nurse must only see five to seven clients a day, what could be the problem? As in any specialty area, community health nurses have their difficulties in managing time. If the nurse could conveniently schedule all of the visits in a geographical sequence and spend precisely 45 minutes with each client, there would be little challenge in time management.

Sequential mapping is ideal and does facilitate efficiency, but there is always the IV dose due across town at a specific time or twice daily dressing changes in a rural area that defeat efforts to schedule visits based on locale. There are also the last-minute referrals of clients who *must be seen* that day.

Time-consuming documentation to meet federal reimbursement regulations constitutes a large portion of a nurse's workload. Conferring with physicians and other team members can also be challenging in a fieldwork situation and must be incorporated into the work schedule.

Cost-effectiveness

Cost-effectiveness is another consideration in planning for care. Traditionally, nursing has used a "whatever-the-client-needs" approach in providing care. This is no longer feasible in today's organizational cost-monitoring systems. As noted earlier, regulations exist for each reimbursement source regarding the types of supplies and services that are reimbursable. By developing an awareness of reimbursement restrictions, the nurse can plan for treatment methods that meet regulations.

Supervision

Nursing supervision of home health aides occurs largely in absentia. This fact underscores the importance of planning for frequent contact between the nurse and the aide and for nursing visits to evaluate the client's status and the quality of care provided by the aide. The aide will usually visit the client more frequently than the nurse and can be a valuable source of information about the client and provide clues to needed areas of assessment. Although the community health nurse does not supervise home care by members of other disciplines such as respiratory therapists, social workers, and so on, the nurse still must maintain close contact with them.

THE PLANNING PROCESS

Once the nurse has determined, through self-examination, that he or she has the background to provide the care required by the client, the planning process begins. Once again, collaboration with the client and significant others is vital.

Designating Goals and Outcome Criteria

As noted in Chapter 5, The Nursing Process, one of the first tasks in planning care is the designation of client care goals and expected outcomes or objectives. Using identified nursing diagnoses as a guideline, the nurse proposes goals designed around client and family needs. Outcome criteria that will indicate goal attainment or successful completion of steps toward the goal are also established.

Some home nursing agencies have strictly imposed outcome criteria for each client problem or diagnosis. These criteria are structured to meet the standards for practice in home health care and will be covered in more detail in the quality assurance section of this chapter.

When planning care with long-term interventions, goal attainment may not occur during the initial period of treatment. This is frequently true at the primary level of prevention. In this situation, goals may be broken down segmentally to provide levels of attainment that can be achieved in a shorter time period. This can have the effect of positive reinforcement for both client and nurse and adds to the success of long-term outcomes.

Planning Interventions

Nursing care in the home setting is likely to involve interventions at the primary, secondary, and tertiary levels of prevention. It is important that the client and family not be overwhelmed with long and complex interventions at the beginning of home care. Often clients and family members become anxious with the responsibility of learning new principles and performing new functions. This anxiety can interfere with the educational process and achievement of goals. For this reason, it may be appropriate to concentrate first on secondary prevention dealing with the client's acute needs and then shift the focus of intervention to primary and tertiary prevention.

Secondary Prevention. Secondary prevention activities will focus on relieving existing health problems identified in the assessment. This may involve planning for activities such as dressing changes, care of central lines, or educating clients and families. Secondary interventions may also involve providing respite care for overburdened caretakers or other nursing interventions designed to meet the immediate needs of the client or significant others.

Other secondary preventive activities might include giving IV medications or other treatments. The community health nurse may also monitor client compliance with taking medications as directed, as well as the therapeutic effects and side effects of medications or treatments.

Primary Prevention. Even though the community health nurse may be going into the home to deal with specific problems related to medical diagnoses, the nurse will not ignore client and family needs for primary preventive actions. For example, the nurse may be involved in the care of a terminally ill grandmother, but can also provide primary preventive assistance to the family in helping to prepare the children for their grandmother's death. Or, the nurse may find that the daughter-in-law in this situation is pregnant and make a referral for prenatal care.

In this example, primary preventive activities may also be warranted for the client herself. For example, the nurse may suggest ways of preventing decubiti when the client becomes bedfast. In this instance, nursing intervention is geared toward preventing the occurrence of a problem, namely decubiti.

Primary preventive interventions required by a particular client will depend upon both the client's current condition and age and developmental status. For example, primary prevention for a handicapped child would include child-proofing a home as described in Chapter 20, Care of Children, while primary preventive measures for an older person might necessitate the installation of a tub rail. Or, as another example of primary prevention tailored to a client's particular needs, primary prevention for the client with AIDS may entail antibiotic prophylaxis for opportunistic infections such as *Pneumocystis carinii* pneumonia.

Tertiary Prevention. The community health nurse may also be involved in tertiary interventions to prevent the recurrence of problems or the development of complications of existing ones. Using the example of the client with decubitus ulcers, the nurse will employ secondary prevention measures to achieve their healing. At the same time, the nurse will educate the client and care-givers regarding the prevention of further decubiti. Again, the type of tertiary preventive measures used will depend upon the client's unique situation and needs.

IMPLEMENTING THE PLAN OF CARE

Two major considerations in implementing nursing interventions in the home setting are decisions regarding the continuation of care and documentation of the care given.

CONTINUATION OF CARE

Adjustment in the implementation phase of home care is an ongoing process. Nurses will design an assessment structure for obtaining needed information at each visit. The period of intervention may need to be lengthened or shortened on the basis of the information obtained during these ongoing assessments.

Experience in providing nursing care in the home setting affords the nurse a background that aids in determining the length of care needed to achieve outcome criteria. There are few absolutes, though, in dealing with acutely ill clients. Their health status may change rapidly because of internal and external factors over which the nurse has little or no control. Use of the epidemiologic prevention process model will facilitate reorganization of care to meet changing needs.

DOCUMENTATION

Written communication and documentation are both very important aspects of implementing nursing care in the home. As noted earlier, agency reimbursement frequently depends upon an accurate portrayal of the client's condition and progress and the nature of services provided.

General Considerations in Documentation

Each agency has its own forms designed to meet the needs of its clientele. There are usually separate forms for initial evaluation visits and progress notes that cover the follow-up period. Most agencies use specific forms to inform the physician of the client's status and to document communications. Each agency has a protocol to be followed with documentation of the plan of care, case conferences, and discharge from home nursing services. Examples of agency forms for documenting nursing assessments and care provided in the home setting are contained in Appendix N, Sample Forms for Documenting Home Nursing Care.

Medicare Documentation

Fiscal intermediaries for payment of Medicare-covered services monitor agency documentation via periodic audits of nursing notes submitted with billing forms and on-site review visits. If inconsistencies or inappropriate statements are found, it is possible for reimbursement for all Medicare services to be denied, even those unrelated to the nursing notes.

Specific information must be obtained and appear on the original certification and plan of treatment form, along with an estimation of the number and frequency of all visits. This information is derived from the initial evaluation form completed by the nurse at the time of the evaluation visit.

Recertification of the client's condition and eligibility for services must occur at specific intervals, usually every 90 days, and the physician must be periodically notified of the client's progress. Copies of both the original Medicare certification form and the recertification form are included in Appendix N, Sample Forms for Documenting Home Nursing Care.

Documenting Nursing Care in Private Home-Care Agencies

Many private reimbursement sources are developing regulations for documentation similar to those for Medicare. They frequently request that copies of the nurse's plan of care and progress notes be forwarded with reimbursement requests.

The old documentation adage "if you haven't documented it, you haven't done it" is applied stringently to home health care. Fortunately, streamlined methods are available for fulfilling documentation requirements. Nurses need to be oriented to the methods and regulations surrounding documentation in a particular agency. Close supervision of the nurse's written communication during a probationary period and thereafter can help to reduce documentation and reimbursement difficulties.

EVALUATING NURSING CARE IN THE HOME SETTING

Evaluating the care of the client in the home setting can be simplified by using the outcome criteria developed in planning care. Success or failure to meet outcome criteria provides a succinct measure of goals that have been achieved and those that need further attention and restructuring of care. For those areas in which goals have not been met, the epidemiologic prevention process model would be used to revise the plan of care.

QUALITY ASSURANCE

In the past two decades there has been increasing recognition of the need to validate the results of service. Quality assurance data serves several functions:

TABLE 25–1. SUPPORT AGENCIES AND SERVICES FOR HOME NURSING CLIENTS

Focus	Agency or Organization	Services
Home care	National Association for Home Care 311 Massachusetts Ave., NE Washington, DC 20002 (202) 547-7424	Advocacy, referral, public information
Hotlines and helplines	Acquired Immune Deficiency Syndrome (AIDS) hotlines (800) 342-AIDS (800) 447-AIDS	Public information, assistance
	Alcoholism Hotline (800) 328-9000	Public information, assistance
	Alzheimer's Disease and Senile Dementia hotline (800) 621-0379	Public information, assistance
	Asthma & Lung Diseases hotline (800) 222-LUNG	Public information, assistance
	Cancer hotline (800) 4-CANCER	Public information, assistance
	Children's Diseases hotline (800) 237-5055	Public information, assistance, Shriner's hospital referrals
	Cystic Fibrosis hotline (800) FIGHT-CF	Public information, assistance
	Diabetes hotline (800) 232-3472	Public information, assistance
	Down's Syndrome hotline (800) 221-4602	Public information, assistance
	Drug Abuse hotlines (800) 662-HELP (800) 554-KIDS	Public information, assistance
	General health information helpline (800) 336-4797	Public information, assistance
	Heart helpline (800) 241-6693	Public information, assistance
	Kidney helpline (800) 638-8299	Public information, assistance
	Lupus hotline (800) 558-0121	Public information, assistance
	Multiple Sclerosis helpline (800) 872-2767	Public information, assistance
	Spinal Cord Injury hotline (800) 526-3456	Public information, assistance
	SIDS (Sudden Infant Death Syndrome) helpline (800) 221-SIDS	Public information, assistance
Hospice	Children's Hospice International 1800 Diagonal Rd., Suite 600 Alexandria, VA 22314 (703) 684-4464	Information
	National Hospice Organization 1901 Fort Myer Dr., Suite 402 Arlington, VA 22209 (703) 243-5900	Information
National support organizations	Alzheimer's Disease and Related Disorders 70 E. Lake St., NW, Suite 600 Chicago, IL 60601 (312) 853-3060	Public information

(*continued*)

TABLE 25–1. (*Continued*)

Focus	Agency or Organization	Services
National support organizations (*continued*)	American Association of Homes for the Aging 1129 20th Street, NW, Suite 400 Washington, DC 20036 (202) 296-5960	Advocacy, information
	American Holistic Medical Association 2727 Fairview Ave., East No. D Seattle, WA 98102 (206) 322-6842	Public information
	American Society of Clinical Hypnosis 2250 E. Devon Ave., Suite 336 Des Plaines, IL 60018 (312) 297-3317	Information
	American Society of Clinical Oncology 435 N. Michigan Ave., Suite 1717 Chicago, IL 60611 (312) 644-0828	Information
	American Society of Plastic and Reconstructive Surgeons 233 N. Michigan Ave., Suite 1900 Chicago, IL 60601 (312) 856-1818	Information
	American Speech-Language-Hearing Association 10801 Rockville Pike Rockville, MD 20852 (301) 897-5700	Information
	Biofeedback Society of America % Francine Butler, Ph.D. 10200 W. 44th Ave., No. 304 Wheat Ridge, CO 80033 (303) 422-8436	Information
	Center for Medical Consumers 237 Thompson St. New York, NY 10012 (212) 674-7105	Information, advocacy
	Office of Consumer and Professional Affairs Food and Drug Administration HFN17 Department of Health and Human Services 5600 Fishers Lane Rockville, MD 20857 (301) 295-8012	Information, advocacy
	Guild for Infant Survival P.O. Box 3841 Davenport, IA 52808 (319) 326-4653	Information
	National Institutes of Health Public Inquiries Building 31, Room 2B-10 9000 Rockville Pike Bethesda, MD 20892 (301) 496-2535	Information
	National Kidney Foundation 2 Park Ave. New York, NY 10016 (212) 889-2210	Information

TABLE 25–1. (*Continued*)

Focus	Agency or Organization	Services
National support organizations (*continued*)	National Sudden Infant Death Syndrome Foundation 8240 Professional Place, Suite 205 Landover, MD 20785 (800) 221-SIDS	Information, support
	United Way Resource Center P.O. Box 23543 San Diego, CA 92123 (619) 492-2115	Information
Pain control	National Chronic Pain Outreach 8222 Wycliffe Court Manassas, VA 22110 (703) 368-7357	Information, support
	National Committee on the Treatment of Intractable Pain P.O. Box 9553, Friendship Station Washington, DC 20016 (301) 983-1710	Information, assistance
	Traditional Acupuncture Institute American City Bldg., Suite 100 Columbia, MD 21044 (301) 596-6006	Information

(1) it identifies the number and scope of problems experienced by clients in the home; (2) it validates the necessity for specialized, skilled nursing for the client in this setting; and (3) it measures the effectiveness of nursing interventions according to client outcomes.

The National League for Nursing[13] has established quality assurance requirements for accrediting home-care agencies that address structure, process, and outcome components of evaluation. Outcome criteria for nursing intervention are also presented in the American Nurses' Association[14] standards for home health nursing. Agencies are responding to the existence of these standards by constructing quality assurance mechanisms that demonstrate the effects of nursing interventions.

DISCHARGE FROM HOME CARE

Discharge from home care begins at the onset of care. At times, there may be a tendency for home-care clients to become dependent upon the nurse. This dependency is the antithesis of the goals of community health nursing, which include promoting client and family independence. Therefore, emphasis on self-care and responsibility at the time of the initial visit, with reinforcement on subsequent visits, will assist home-care recipients to develop this perspective and goal for themselves. The actual decision to terminate home nursing services is made on the basis of evaluative findings regarding the client's health status and needs for further care.

Discharging a client from home nursing services involves providing the client and significant others with appropriate community and professional resources for follow-up care. It takes time for the new community health nurse to develop an awareness of the many agencies available for client support. Strategies for developing this awareness were presented in relation to community assessment in Chapter 19, Care of the Community or Target Group. Typical support agencies and services that may benefit home nursing clients are included in Table 25–1.

CHAPTER HIGHLIGHTS

- Community health nurses combine the skills of the acute-care setting with the principles of community health when providing care to clients in the home setting.
- Four types of home health agencies may employ community health nurses (and others) to do home nursing. These four types are Medicare-certified agencies, private agencies, hospice home-care agencies, and publicly funded agencies.
- Reimbursement for home nursing services may come from Medicare or Medicaid, private insurance coverage, out-of-pocket payment by the client, or public donation.
- Home health agencies may be licensed by state, county, or local jurisdictions depending upon area regulations.
- Home nursing clients today tend to have a broader range of health needs and to be more acutely ill than was true in the past. The client is the primary recipient of nursing care, while family members and significant others may be secondary recipients of care.
- Three general considerations in caring for clients in the home setting include the need for collaboration between the client and the nurse and among health-care personnel providing care for the client, the need for preprocess goals, and the need for continuity in the care provided.
- Responsibility for care of clients in the home begins with a referral for services. If the referral is received before the client is discharged from a hospital, a pre-discharge assessment may be completed by a liaison nurse or the nurse who will provide the client's care.
- Discharge back to the home is followed by an initial evaluation visit to determine the client's health status and care requirements.
- Two primary concerns in assessing the client's physical environment are infection control and safety in the home setting.
- Fear and anxiety about the client's condition on the part of the client or significant others can impair the client's health status. Similarly, interactions among family members may create an unhealthy psychological environment.
- Social environmental factors of particular concern in the care of clients in the home setting reflect the client's culture and culturally based health-related behaviors.
- Life-style factors that might influence the health status of clients in the home setting include employment concerns, consumption patterns, and leisure pursuits. A particular concern with respect to leisure is the need for respite for caretakers.
- Health system factors to be assessed include the client's usual source of health care and means of paying for health-care services including nursing services.
- Special planning considerations in caring for clients in the home setting include the technical competence of those who will implement the plan, time management, cost-effectiveness, and supervision of ancillary personnel.
- Secondary preventive measures will frequently be the initial focus of nursing care in the home setting, but needs for primary and tertiary prevention will be addressed as well.
- Two considerations in implementing care in the home setting are decisions related to continuation of care and documentation. Documentation is particularly important in this setting for reimbursement reasons, and both the need for care and the care given must be adequately documented.
- Two aspects of evaluating care in the home setting include quality assurance regarding the care provided and decisions to discharge the client from home nursing services.

Review Questions

1. Describe at least three types of home health-care agencies. In what ways do they differ? (p. 606)
2. Describe three general considerations in providing care to clients in the home setting. (p. 609)
3. What are the two major considerations in assessing the physical environment of the home nursing client? (p. 611)
4. Describe at least three organizational considerations in planning nursing care for clients in the home setting. Give an example of how each might influence nursing intervention. (p. 614)
5. What are the two major considerations in implementing nursing care in the home setting? (p. 616)
6. What are the two aspects of evaluating nursing care provided in the home setting? (p. 616)

APPLICATION AND SYNTHESIS

Mrs. Santos was scheduled for discharge from the hospital in 2 days when a referral was made to the home nursing agency for which you work. This 67-year-old woman will require antibiotic infusion for 2 weeks following a total hip replacement stemming from advanced rheumatoid arthritis. Physical therapy has also been ordered for Mrs. Santos. Secondary diagnoses in addition to the arthritis include arteriosclerotic heart disease and hypertension.

Information on the referral form indicates that Mrs. Santos lives with her 72-year-old husband, who has some visual problems, and that a granddaughter lives nearby. Mrs. Santos has Medicare coverage for home health services.

During a pre-discharge assessment conducted in the hospital with Mr. and Mrs. Santos and their granddaughter, you learn that the couple live in a small two-story house that is over 50 years old, and the three bedrooms are on the second floor. The lower floor consists of a living room across the front of the house with a small bathroom off to the right. Behind the living room are the kitchen to the right and a dining room off to the left. Doors lead from the living room into both the dining room and the kitchen.

Because of Mr. Santos's poor vision and the crippling resulting from Mrs. Santos's arthritis, it will be difficult for them to administer the antibiotic infusion. Mrs. Santos's granddaughter wants to help as much as possible, but she has three small children, one of whom is in school. The granddaughter's husband works during the day but is home in the evening. The granddaughter thinks she will be able to assist with the infusions but will not have the time to help Mr. Santos with housekeeping chores.

You arrange for an evaluation visit to the home the day after Mrs. Santos is discharged from the hospital. While you are doing a physical examination on Mrs. Santos during the evaluation visit, she shares her fear of her husband's reaction to performing the many "female" types of chores involved in caring for her. She says that her husband was raised in Mexico with very traditional ideas of men's and women's work.

You arrange to visit Mrs. Santos three times a week to monitor her health status. On a subsequent visit, she complains of constipation related to her medications and immobility. Otherwise she progresses well and you feel able to discharge her from home nursing services after 2 weeks.

1. What are the human biological, environmental, life-style, and health system factors operating in this situation?
2. How would collaboration be incorporated into the care of Mrs. Santos?
3. How would you address considerations of competence, time management, cost-effectiveness, and supervision in planning care for Mrs. Santos?
4. What primary, secondary, or tertiary preventive interventions would be appropriate in this situation? Why?
5. On what basis would you make the determination to discharge Mrs. Santos from home nursing services?

REFERENCES

1. Humphrey, C. J. (1988). The home as the setting for care: Clarifying the boundaries of practice. *Nursing Clinics of North America, 23,* 305–314.
2. McCann, J. J. (1988). Long-term home care for the elderly: Perceptions of nurses, physicians, and primary caregivers. *Quality Review Bulletin, 14*(3), 66–74.
3. United States General Accounting Office. (1987). *Medicare: Need to strengthen home health care payments control and address unmet needs.* Report to the Special Committee on Aging, U.S. Senate. December 1986. Washington, DC: GAO.
4. Watkins, V., & Kirby, W. (1987). Health care facilities participating in Medicare and Medicaid programs, 1987. *Health Care Financing Review, 9,* 101–105.
5. Health Care Financing Administration. (1989). *The Medicare handbook.* Publication No. HCFA 10050. Baltimore: Department of Health and Human Services.
6. Kilbane, K., & Blacksin, B. (1988). The demise of free care: The Visiting Nurse Association of Chicago. *Nursing Clinics of North America, 23,* 435–442.
7. Reckling, J. B. (1989). Abandonment of patients by home health nursing agencies: An ethical analysis of the dilemma. *Advances in Nursing Science, 11*(3), 70–81.
8. Yura, H., & Walsh, M. B. (1988). *The nursing process: Assessing, planning, implementing, evaluating* (5th ed.). Norwalk, CT: Appleton & Lange.
9. Update: Universal precautions for prevention of transmission of human immunodeficiency virus, hepatitis B, and other blood-borne pathogens in health care settings. (1988). *MMWR, 37,* 377–382, 387–388.
10. Williamson, K. M., Turner, J. G., Brown, K. C., et al. (1988). Occupational health hazards for nurses: Infection. *Image: The Journal of Nursing Scholarship, 20,* 48–53.
11. Moraca-Sawicki, A. (1991). Antineoplastic chemotherapy. In M. M. Kuhn (Ed.), *Pharmacotherapeutics: A nursing process approach* (2nd ed.) (pp. 1339–1392). Philadelphia: F. A. Davis.
12. Tynan, C., & Cardea, J. M. (1987). Home health hazard assessment. *Journal of Gerontological Nursing, 13,* 25–27.
13. National League for Nursing. (1987). *Accreditation program for home care and community health: Criteria and standards.* New York: National League for Nursing.
14. American Nurses' Association. (1986). *Standards of home health nursing practice.* Kansas City, MO: American Nurses' Association.

RECOMMENDED READINGS

Bedrosian, C. A. (1989). *Home health nursing: Nursing diagnosis and care plans.* Norwalk, CT: Appleton & Lange.

Provides a basic introduction to principles of home health nursing and the use of nursing diagnoses as the basis for care in this setting.

Burbach, C. A., & Brown, B. E. (1988). Community health and home health nursing: Keeping the concepts clear. *Nursing & Health Care, 9*(2), 97–100.

Compares and contrasts community health nursing in the home setting from home health nursing.

Crystal, S., Flemming, C., Beck, P., et al. (1987). *The management of home care services.* New York: Springer.

Offers a practical understanding of reimbursement issues in home health nursing. Discusses approaches to providing cost-effective home care.

Green, J. L., & Driggers, B. (1989). All visiting nurses are not alike: Home health nursing and community health nursing. *Journal of Community Health Nursing, 6*(2), 83–93.

Differentiates home health nursing from community health nursing in the home setting. Presents findings of a study on the activities of home health nurses.

Humphrey, C. J. (1988). The home as a setting for care: Clarifying the boundaries of practice. *Nursing Clinics of North America, 23,* 305–314.

Describes the relationships between community health nursing in the home setting and home health nursing.

Liebermann, C. (1989). *Community and home health nursing.* Phoenixville, PA: Springhouse.

Addresses basic principles of community health and home health nursing.

Marrelli, T. M. (1988). *Handbook of home health standards and documentation guidelines for reimbursement.* St. Louis: C.V. Mosby.

Sets forth standards for care in home health nursing. Also provides documentation guidelines to facilitate reimbursement for home health nursing services.

Schaal, M. G. (1989). Baccalaureate nursing education: The framework for holistic home health nursing practice. *Holistic Nursing Practice, 3*(2), 77–83.

Discusses the need for community health nurses to provide home health nursing care and the educational background needed for practice in the home setting.

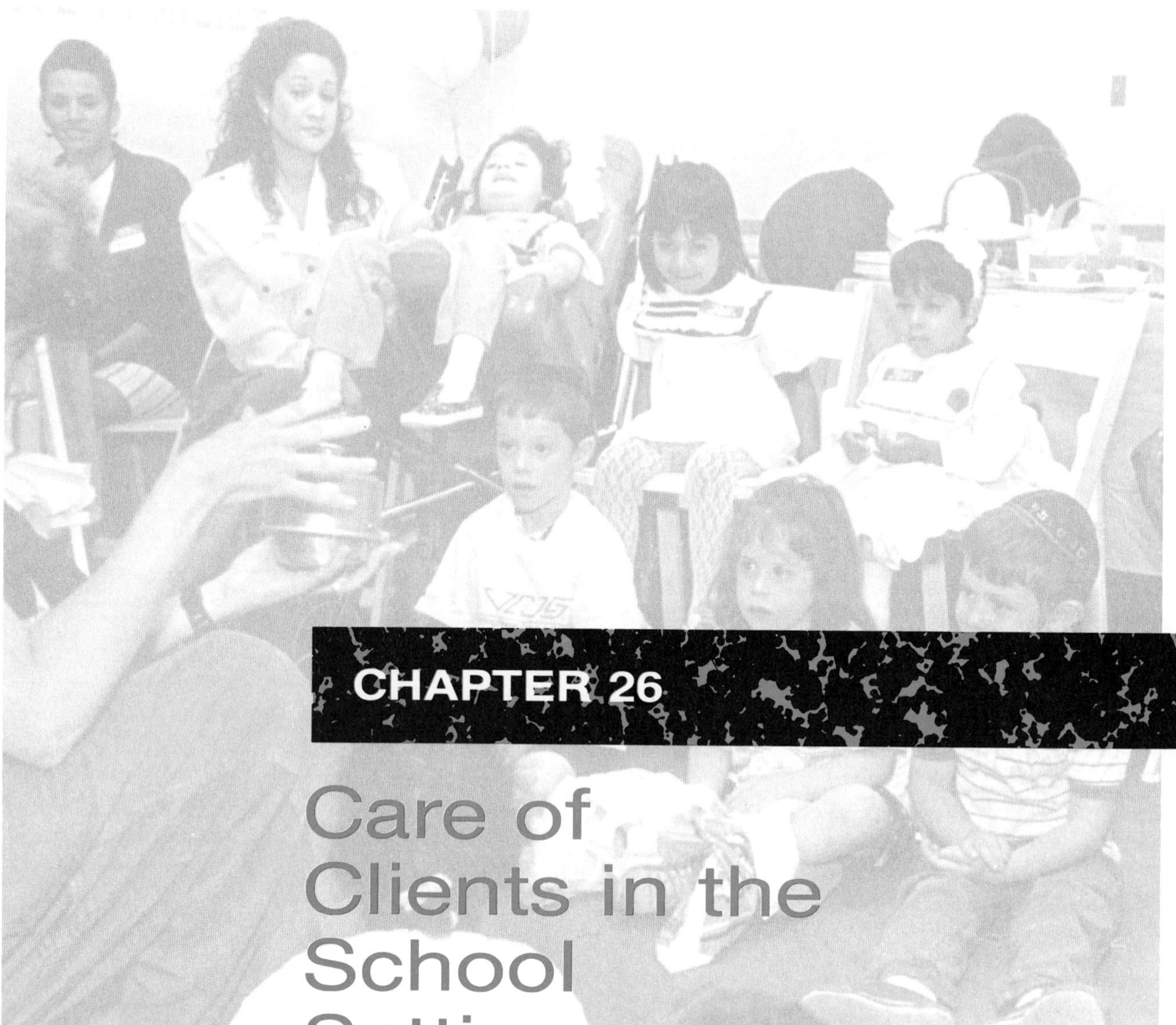

CHAPTER 26

Care of Clients in the School Setting

KEY TERMS

affective learning
cognitive learning
learning disability
school nurse credential program

Education and health have a reciprocal relationship. Health factors influence one's ability to learn. Education affects one's ability to engage in healthful behaviors. This reciprocal relationship makes the school setting an ideal place to provide health care. Most school nurses are community health nurses practicing in a specialized setting. Given their community health preparation, school nurses retain their concern for the health of the community and apply the principles of community health nursing to the needs of the overall community as well as to the needs of the school population.

Community health nurses working in school settings have a threefold concern for the health of school children. First, the health of school children influences the health status of the community at large. Second, health-promotion and illness-prevention efforts directed at youngsters will improve their health status as adults. Finally, healthy children learn better and can take greater advantage of the educational opportunities provided to them.

The importance of the school health program as an avenue for improving the health of the population can be seen in the number of national health objectives for the year 2000 that reflect health measures in schools.[1] These objectives are summarized in Box 26–1.

(*continued*)

LEARNING OBJECTIVES

After reading this chapter you should be able to:

- Identify three goals of a school health program.
- Describe the three components of a school health program.
- Describe at least five roles for community health nurses in school settings.
- Identify three areas of nursing responsibility in school health.
- Describe at least two considerations in assessing physical environmental factors influencing the health of the school population.
- Identify at least four areas to be assessed in relation to the psychological environment in the school setting.
- Describe at least two areas to be addressed in assessing social environmental influences on the health of the school population.
- Identify at least five areas of emphasis in primary prevention in the school setting.
- Describe at least three approaches to secondary prevention in the school setting.
- Describe at least two areas of emphasis in tertiary prevention in the school setting.

HISTORICAL PERSPECTIVES

School nursing is one of several traditional roles for community health nurses and originally arose out of concern for the numbers of children being excluded from school owing to communicable diseases. In New York City in 1902, 15 to 20 children per school were being sent home daily. In response to this problem, Lillian Wald assigned nurses from the Henry Street Settlement to four New York City schools in a pilot project in school nursing. Because of the success of the project, the New York City Board of Health hired additional nurses to continue this type of work.[2]

Early school nursing focused on preventing the spread of communicable disease and treating ailments related to compulsory school attendance. By the 1930s, however, the focus had shifted to preventative and promotive activities including case finding, integration of health concepts into school curricula, and maintenance of a healthful school environment. Treatment of any health problems by the nurse was strongly discouraged to prevent infringe-

BOX 26–1

Summary of National Health Objectives for the Year 2000 Related to School Health

1. Increase to at least 50% the proportion of children in grades 1 through 12 who participate in daily physical education activities at school.
2. Increase to at least 90% the proportion of school lunch and breakfast programs with menus consistent with nutritional principles contained in *Dietary Guidelines for Americans.*
3. Increase to at least 75% the proportion of the nation's schools that provide nutrition education from preschool through 12th grade.
4. Include tobacco use prevention in the curricula of all elementary, middle, and secondary schools.
5. Provide children in all primary and secondary schools with educational programs on alcohol and other drugs.
6. Increase to at least 85% the proportion of people aged 10 through 18 who have discussed human sexuality with their parents or received information from parentally endorsed sources such as schools.
7. Increase to at least 50% the proportion of elementary and secondary schools that teach nonviolent conflict-resolution skills.
8. Provide academic instruction on injury prevention and control in at least 50% of public school systems.
9. Increase to at least 95% the proportion of schools that have age-appropriate HIV education curricula for children in grades 4 through 12.
10. Include in all middle and secondary schools instruction on preventing sexually transmitted diseases.

ment on the private medical sector. School nurse activities at this time consisted of screening for vision, hearing, and orthopedic defects, as well as detecting developmental difficulties and providing minor first aid.[3]

School health nurses, dissatisfied with such a minimal role, continued to provide clandestine diagnostic services and treatment of minor ailments in addition to engaging in classroom teaching related to health. More recently, school nurses have begun to return to activities related to the diagnosis and treatment of health problems. Several factors account for current changes in the school nurse role.[3] Among these are the number of families of school-age children in which both parents work. In these families neither parent may have time to deal with routine health problems of their children. Other factors include the interest of school nurses in expanding their role, the failure of governmental programs (for example, the Early and Periodic Screening, Diagnosis, and Treatment Program, EPSDT) to resolve the health problems of school-age children, the enrollment of handicapped youngsters in regular school programs, and consumer demands for alternative sites for providing health care to children. One other major factor is that approximately one-third of school-age children in the United States have no regular source of health care except for care rendered in emergency rooms.[3] For these children in particular, the school nurse may be the only source of health care.

THE SCHOOL HEALTH PROGRAM

Health care is provided in schools for a number of reasons. The school environment itself may create hazards from which students must be protected. A second reason has already been mentioned: Children need to be healthy in order to learn effectively. Maintaining the health of children today produces healthier adults in years to come. Finally, there is a need to protect and enhance the health of the overall community.[4]

The overall goal of a school health program is enhancing the health of members of the school community.[5] More specific goals of a school health program include promoting health and preventing illness, identifying and resolving existing health problems, and educating students and families for a healthier life-style.

These goals are achieved through the three basic components of a school health program, which include a health services component, a health instruction component, and an environmental component. These components of the school health program are depicted in Figure 26–1.

THE HEALTH SERVICES COMPONENT

School health programs should provide a wide variety of health-care services. Broadly categorized, these services would include teacher observation for health problems, health screening and appraisal, counseling of students and parents regarding appraisal findings, and referral for assistance in resolving health problems. Other categories of health services include preventing and controlling communicable diseases and providing emergency care.[5] In assessing the health of the school population, the nurse would examine the adequacy of services provided in each of these areas. Are services appropriate to the needs of the specific population served? Are they provided in a timely and efficient manner? And, are they adequate to meet the needs of the school population?

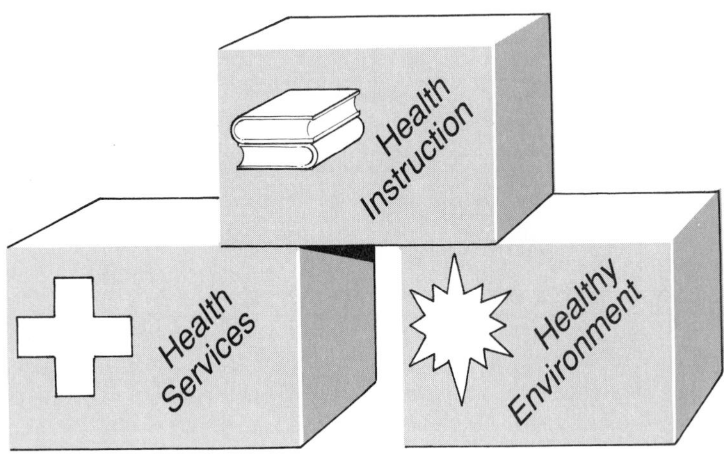

Figure 26–1. Components of the school health program.

THE HEALTH EDUCATION COMPONENT

One of the functions of the school health program is to educate students for health awareness and healthful behavior. This means that the instructional curriculum must include content on health, and instructional strategies must be used that provide information and develop attitudes that foster healthy behavior. Health education in the school setting focuses on both cognitive and affective learning. ***Cognitive learning*** involves learning facts and information related to health and healthful behaviors. ***Affective learning,*** on the other hand, refers to developing attitudes toward health and health behaviors that foster a healthy life-style.

In assessing this component of the health program, the nurse would examine the content of the health curriculum and evaluate its adequacy and appropriateness for the age group involved. For example, nutrition is an area that should be reinforced at each grade level. Basic hygiene is usually introduced at the preschool or early elementary grade levels, while issues related to sexuality are more commonly addressed at upper grade levels. The instructional curriculum, like the health services program, should reflect the needs of the population served and should help to enhance the health status of the overall community.

THE ENVIRONMENTAL COMPONENT

The environmental component of the school health program includes activities directed toward improving the physical, psychological, and social environment of the school and the surrounding community. Later in this chapter each of these aspects of a healthy school environment will be addressed in the use of the epidemiologic prevention process model in the school setting.

EDUCATIONAL PREPARATION FOR SCHOOL HEALTH NURSING

Depending on the requirements of the particular jurisdiction, nurses working in school settings may have varying levels of education. In some parts of the country (for example, the Southeast), a person designated as a "school nurse" may not even be a Registered Nurse. Because of the autonomy of nursing practice in the school setting, ideally the school nurse should be prepared at least at the baccalaureate level. This level of educational preparation guarantees that the nurse has the community health nursing background to deal effectively with the health needs of the school population.

In some states, employment as a school nurse requires advanced preparation beyond a baccalaureate degree in nursing. In California, for example, school nurses must complete a state-approved ***school nurse credential program.***[6] This is a nondegree program offered in an institution of higher learning that meets state requirements for educating school nurses.

Other school nurses may be prepared at the master's level in nursing. These nurses frequently function as nurse practitioners promoting health and diagnosing and treating minor illnesses. Some, however, have advanced preparation in community health nursing and are involved in program planning rather than primary care of minor illnesses.

NURSING ROLES IN SCHOOL HEALTH

Community health nurses may work in various professional capacities within school settings.[7] First, the nurse may serve as a *consultant* to the school system regarding health problems and their solution. In this role the community health nurse would not be an employee of the school system but might be called upon to address special problems encountered by school personnel. For example, a nursing consultant might be asked to help school personnel design a healthy menu for the school lunch program. Second, the nurse may act as a *director,* coordinating the school health program within an entire school system. Third, the nurse may serve as a school health *educator,* teaching theory basic to school nursing and educating those who will practice in this setting. The school nursing *supervisor,* a fourth role, oversees the activities of school nurses within a particular jurisdiction. The *coordinator* of special school health programs is a fifth community health nursing role in the school setting. The school nurse *practitioner* functions in an expanded role, diagnosing and treating health problems as well as performing other aspects of the school nurse role.

A nurse may also work as a *school community nurse.* This individual has had advanced preparation in school and community health nursing but does not function as a nurse practitioner. He or she is usually involved in designing programs at the aggregate level rather than providing direct care at the level of the individual child. A final professional role is that of the *school nurse* who has received basic preparation in community health and school nursing. It is in this capacity that the nurse provides direct services to the children of a specific school or schools. The focus of this chapter is on the community health nurse functioning in the capacity of school nurse.

NURSING RESPONSIBILITIES IN SCHOOL HEALTH

The community health nurse functioning in the school nurse role has a wide variety of responsibilities categorized on the basis of the recipients of school nursing services. Categories of recipients include students and their families, school personnel, and the community.

STUDENTS AND FAMILIES

Health of students is the primary responsibility of the school health program and, therefore, of the school nurse. Responsibilities related to the child and his or her family include case finding, referral, education, counseling, motivation of families to follow through with recommendations, and, occasionally, planning and implementing a treatment plan.

SCHOOL PERSONNEL

The school health nurse also has responsibilities related to other school personnel. Broad areas of responsibility might include direct provision of healthcare services to staff such as screening for tuberculosis, providing counseling and referral for health problems, or providing emergency care in case of illness or injury. Educative and collaborative responsibilities are centered around interpreting student and family needs to school personnel, consulting with school personnel about student health problems, providing information about community health resources, and collaborating with teachers and administrators in planning the health services program and health instruction curriculum. Carrying out educative and collaborative responsibilities involves interactions with teachers, school administrators, and ancillary personnel.

Responsibilities to teachers include consulting with them on matters of health education as well as on health problems of individual children. This may involve assisting a teacher to tailor teaching strategies to a particular child's health status. Other activities might include in-service programs for teachers regarding the health needs of school-age youngsters. For example, school health nurses might educate teachers about how to observe students for signs of health problems and when to refer students to the school nurse. According to one study, when nurses held in-service programs of this sort for teachers, the number of referrals to the school nurse increased significantly, and 84 percent of the referrals were found to be appropriate.[8]

One primary collaborative responsibility of the nurse with respect to school administrators is apprising them of the health needs of the school community (students and personnel). Other areas of nursing responsibility include participation in planning and evaluation—as well as the implementation—of the school health program, delineating and interpreting the role of the school nurse in the overall school health plan, and providing information for budgetary decisions.

The school nurse also has educative and collaborative responsibilities to other school personnel. In addition to monitoring employee health and safety, the nurse may apprise maintenance staff of safety hazards to be remedied, assist clerical personnel with maintenance of student health records, or collaborate with food services staff to plan nutritious meals.

School health nurses might also have supervisory responsibilities for a variety of people. These can include supervising the health-related activities of other school personnel, such as clerical review of children's immunization records and volunteer activities by parents. The nurse might also supervise professional students (for example, nursing students) during learning experiences in the school setting.

THE COMMUNITY

As a community health nurse working in a specialized setting, the school nurse must maintain a concern for the health of the entire community. To achieve this goal, the nurse must strive to build a school health program that addresses both school and community concerns. To accomplish this, the nurse must assess the health status of the community.

To guide health program planning in the school and community, the nurse should examine measures of health status such as morbidity and mortality figures, investigate the extent and adequacy of community health resources, and assess environmental conditions affecting health.[4] The nurse would conduct a community assessment using the principles discussed in Chapter 19, Care of the Community or Target Group.

Based on the results of this assessment, the

school nurse collaborates with other school and community members to plan a school health program addressing identified community problems. For instance, if poor nutrition is identified as a community problem, the school health program might include hot breakfast and/or lunch programs. Similarly, if drug abuse is prevalent in the community, drug education should certainly be included in the health instruction curriculum.

THE SCHOOL HEALTH TEAM

Health problems identified in individual children or in the community served by the school are frequently beyond the capabilities of the community health nurse acting independently. To meet the needs of the school population and the community, the school health nurse will often need to participate as a member of a team.

Because identified health problems may be the consequence of factors beyond the control of health-care professionals, the school health team is often comprised of a variety of individuals, not all of whom have a health or medical background. The team acts to design a school health program that meets the health needs of students and of the larger community.

The school health team should use the strategies discussed in Chapter 11, The Change, Leadership, and Group Processes, to create an effective team that can address the health needs of the population. One of the critical features of group development for the school health team is negotiating member roles. Group members should clarify for themselves the roles that each will play, so that infringement on the professional territory of any one group is avoided.

Specific members of the team will vary with the identified needs of the population, but some of those who may be involved, in addition to the nurse, include parents, teachers, administrators, counselors, psychologists, social workers, physicians and dentists, a health coordinator, food service personnel, janitorial and secretarial staffs, public health officials and other public officials, and students.

Parents, of course, have the primary responsibility for the health of their children. With respect to the school health program, parents have a responsibility to reinforce health teaching at home and to follow up on referrals for assistance with identified health problems in their children. They should also provide input into the planning and evaluation of the school health program. Parents may also provide volunteer services for first aid or "sick room duty" when there is not a nurse employed full-time.

Teachers also have a variety of responsibilities for the health of their students. Among these are the need to motivate students in the development of good health habits, to encourage student responsibility for health, and to observe them for signs of health problems. Teachers have a responsibility to model healthy behavior and to provide health instruction. Other responsibilities include assisting with screening efforts and measures to control the spread of disease and helping to identify factors in the physical, psychological, and social environments that are detrimental to the health status of students and co-workers. In addition, teachers may counsel students with health problems and may make referrals for assistance as appropriate.

School administrators include principals, district superintendents, and school board members. Administrators are responsible for the implementation of the school health program and should provide both material and nonmaterial support. They also function as a liaison between the school and the larger community. In collaboration with other team members, administrators participate in planning and evaluating the school health program. Other administrative responsibilities include the hiring and evaluation of health service employees and fostering collegial relationships among school health team members. Finally, administrators have the ultimate responsibility for the creation of a healthy and safe environment.

Some schools employ counselors, psychologists, or social workers or contract for their services as consultants. Counselors may provide emotional counseling or assistance to students in career decisions. Psychologists may also be involved in counseling for emotional problems. In addition, they may conduct psychological testing on selected youngsters to identify emotional problems or learning disabilities. Or, they may be called upon to administer tests of school readiness to all incoming children. Social workers may likewise counsel students regarding problems and may provide referrals for students and families to assist with socioeconomic problems. When the services of these specialists are not available in a particular school setting, many of these functions may be assumed by the school nurse, if he or she is educationally prepared to carry them out. Or, the nurse might make a referral to an outside source of assistance.

Physicians and dentists usually are not employed by a school system, but they may provide services on a contract or referral basis. Under a contractual arrangement, physicians and dentists may spend a certain amount of time in the school assessing health and dental needs or making treatment recommendations. In other instances, students may be referred to their own physicians or dentists for follow-up treatment on identified health problems.

The school nurse may function as the school's health coordinator, or the school health team may include a health coordinator who is not a nurse. The health coordinator may be a parent, teacher, or other person with some health-related preparation. Responsibilities of the health coordinator include serving as a liaison with families and with the community, arranging in-service education for staff, facilitating team relationships, and coordinating the health instruction program. Other areas of responsibility include planning for speakers on health topics, arranging health-related learning experiences such as field trips or health fairs, and reviewing materials for use in health education.[5]

In schools where meals are provided, food service personnel are responsible for preparing and serving nutritious meals. They may also be responsible for planning menus, depending upon their background and knowledge of the nutritional needs of school-age children.

The janitorial staff is usually responsible for maintenance of the physical environment. Remediation of physical health hazards usually comes under their jurisdiction as well. They also ensure the cleanliness of kitchen and sanitary facilities to prevent the transmission of disease.

Clerical personnel are responsible for maintaining student records and for processing family notification of screening test results and recommendations. They may also be responsible for notifying families in the case of student injury or illness.

Public health officials are not employed by the school but still form part of the school health team in that they are responsible for inspection of school sanitation, cooking facilities, immunization status, and so on. They also act to establish local health policy related to schools and other institutions and to safeguard the health of the overall community. Other public officials may also be involved in planning a school health program to meet the needs of the school's population. Fire or police personnel might be involved, for example, in designing safety education programs for children and their parents.

In older age groups, students within the school may also be part of the school health team. Student responsibilities include helping to maintain a healthful and safe environment and providing input regarding student health needs and planning to meet those needs. Older students should also be involved in evaluating the effectiveness of the school health program.

THE EPIDEMIOLOGIC PREVENTION PROCESS MODEL AND CARE OF CLIENTS IN THE SCHOOL SETTING

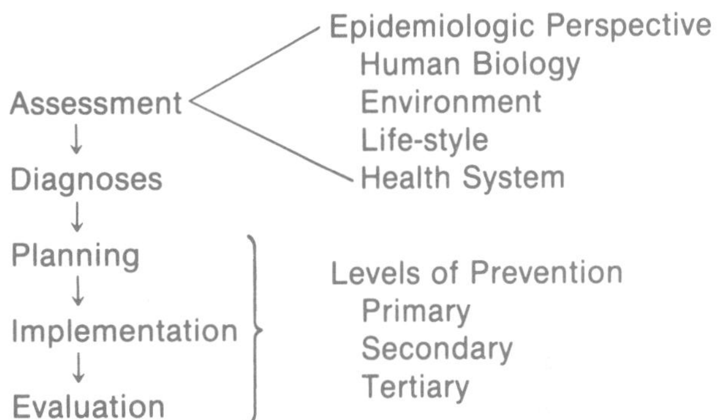

The community health nurse in the school setting will find the epidemiologic prevention process model a useful framework for directing nursing care. Components of the model remain the same as in any other setting and include assessing the school population and setting in terms of the epidemiologic perspective; diagnosing health problems; planning care at primary, secondary, and tertiary levels of prevention; intervening; and evaluating the care given.

ASSESSING HEALTH NEEDS IN THE SCHOOL SETTING

Use of the epidemiologic prevention process model in the school setting begins with assessing the health needs of the school population and identifying the factors influencing those needs. Areas for consideration include human biology, the environment, lifestyle considerations, and the health system.

HUMAN BIOLOGY

Areas for considerations related to human biology include maturation and aging, genetic inheritance, and physiologic function.

Maturation and Aging

School nurses work with students in preschool, elementary school, junior high and high school, and college and university settings. Consequently, the age of the client population will influence the types of health problems that may be present. For example, prevention of communicable disease would receive greater emphasis in the preschool population, while sexuality issues and substance abuse would be of greater concern with adolescent populations. For college students, substance abuse and sexuality issues are also pertinent as are stress-related problems stemming from academic pressures and being away from home.

Client maturation will also influence the content and process of the health instruction component of the school health plan. Basic hygiene conveyed via cartoon films is appropriate to the preschool or early elementary age child; a frank discussion of sexuality and sexually transmitted diseases is appropriate with older groups.

Genetic Inheritance

Aspects of genetic inheritance of particular interest to the school nurse are the sex and racial composition of the population. A predominance of females in an elementary school increases the frequency with which the nurse will encounter students with symptoms of urinary tract infection since these are common in girls in that age bracket. In adolescent girls, on the other hand, there is increased risk of unwanted pregnancy. Boys of all ages tend to have more sports-related injuries with which the nurse must deal.

Racial composition of the school population will also influence the types of health problems encountered. For example, in schools with large black populations, sickle cell screening might be included as a routine part of the school health program. The nurse will also want to be alert to the prevalence of other diseases such as thalassemia and diabetes that exhibit genetic predispositions.

Physiologic Function

An important aspect of the human biological component of the assessment is the physiologic function of the school population. In assessing physiologic function, the community health nurse would look for general indicators of health in elementary and secondary school children. These indicators include:

1. A display of energy and development normal for the child's age group, and the ability to participate regularly in physical education activities;
2. The ability to carry out normal school and home responsibilities without undue fatigue or emotional upset;
3. Normal, progressive gains in weight and height;
4. A clear, smooth skin;
5. Normal experience of illness or accidents expected for the child's age group;
6. Enthusiasm and zest for life;
7. Good social health and peer group interactions; and
8. Emotional control.[9,10]

Many school children may not exhibit these characteristics and suffer from a variety of health problems. These can be categorized as short-lived and self-limiting diseases, environmental and psychological stress, chronic diseases with long-term health and educational implications, chronic diseases and handicaps that interfere with function, and fatal irreversible disease.[4]

Examples of self-limiting conditions include communicable diseases such as the common cold, influenza, or chickenpox and injuries such as a fractured arm or leg. Diabetes, seizure disorders, and minor visual or hearing problems are examples of chronic conditions that may have health and educational implications. Many of these conditions can be controlled if properly diagnosed and treated and do not necessarily interfere with the child's ability to function in school. Other chronic and handicapping conditions do interfere with school function. Examples of such conditions include blindness, deafness, mental retardation, attention deficit hyperactivity disorder, and long-term effects of fetal drug exposure. Conditions related to environmental or psychological stress may or may not affect physiologic function, although they may affect the child's ability to function effectively in the school situation.

The kinds of physical health problems seen by school nurses among students and staff are many and varied. Acute and chronic conditions commonly encountered in the school setting are included in Table 26–1.

The majority of health conditions seen in most school populations are acute respiratory illnesses. One in four school-age children, however, has some type of chronic condition. Most of these (48 percent) are related to asthma, hay fever, or other chronic respiratory conditions. Approximately 12 percent of children in school suffer from paralysis or debilitating orthopedic conditions.[4] An estimated 8 million school children have special education needs due to a handicapping condition. One in five youngsters has some type of vision problem, while approximately 10 percent have hearing difficulties.[9] The school nurse should be conversant with the signs and symptoms of common illnesses and other conditions among children. The nurse should be aware of the prevalence of these and other health conditions among the school population so as to plan health care to meet the needs of children with these conditions.

Immunity is another important consideration re-

TABLE 26–1. ACUTE AND CHRONIC HEALTH PROBLEMS ENCOUNTERED IN THE SCHOOL SETTING

Organ System Affected	Conditions Encountered
Cardiovascular system	Heart murmurs, hypertension
Central nervous system	Mental retardation, blindness, deafness, attention deficit hyperactivity disorder, learning disability, seizure disorder, meningitis, cerebral palsy
Endocrine system	Diabetes mellitus, thyroid disorders
Gastrointestinal system	Encopresis, hepatitis, diarrhea, dental caries, constipation, peptic and duodenal ulcer
Genito-urinary/reproductive system	Sexually transmitted diseases, urinary tract infection, enuresis, dysmenorrhea, pregnancy
Hematopoietic system	Anemia, hemophilia, leukemia, sickle cell disease, lead poisoning
Immunologic system	AIDS and related opportunistic infections
Integumentary system	Acne, eczema, impetigo, lice, scabies, dermatitis, tinea corporis
Musculoskeletal system	Arthritis, sprains, fractures, scoliosis, Legg-Calvé-Perthes disease
Respiratory system	Upper and lower respiratory infections, strep throat, influenza, asthma, hay fever, pertussis, diphtheria, pneumonia
Other diseases	Measles, mumps, rubella, scarlet fever, chickenpox, infectious mononucleosis, otitis media, otitis externa, conjunctivitis

lated to physiologic function in the school population. The community health nurse working in the school setting will monitor the immunization status of students and school employees. For example, maintenance personnel are at risk for tetanus because of the potential for dirty injuries, and their immunization status should also be monitored. For female teachers and other school personnel of childbearing age, the risk of rubella during pregnancy is increased by working with children, and they should also be adequately immunized.

A final health problem frequently encountered in the school population that may have a physiologic basis is learning disability. Approximately 9 to 20 percent of school children experience some form of learning disability. A ***learning disability*** is "a disorder of one or more of the basic psychological processes involved in understanding or in using spoken or written language."[10] This definition does not include inabilities to learn that are the result of hearing or visual problems, emotional difficulties, or mental retardation.

Children with learning disabilities may exhibit any of several characteristics. These include poor visual and/or auditory discrimination or the tendency to confuse shapes, letters, or sounds; poor visual memory in which the child has difficulty remembering what is seen or read; and poor kinesthesia or the inability to discriminate objects by touch. Other characteristics that may be evident are poor eye-hand coordination, poor spatial orientation (for example, the inability to tell right from left), poor figure ground discrimination (inability to pick a specific object from a group), perseverance (the obsessive repetition of a newly learned skill), and poor self-image. Moreover, it is thought that the hyperactivity characteristic of some of these children is due to their bewilderment stemming from the fact that they have not understood what they have seen or heard in their classroom instruction.[10]

ENVIRONMENT

In the school setting, a healthy environment is one that addresses the needs of the total student by providing him or her with health services, food services, opportunities for appropriate physical activity, and satisfactory classroom instruction.[5] Environmental aspects of assessment in the school setting include consideration of the effects of the physical, psychological, and social environments on health.

Physical Environment

The nurse assesses both the internal and external physical environment of the school.[5] The external environment includes the area surrounding the school. Assessment considerations here include traffic patterns, water hazards, use of pesticides, and rodent control in the area. Other environmental concerns include the proximity of hazardous waste dumps or nuclear power plants, industrial hazards, and the presence of various forms of pollution.[4] (See Chapter 16, Environmental Influences on Community Health, for a discussion of environmental health issues.)

Several aspects of the school's internal environment, such as assessing fire hazards and sanitation, are the responsibility of official agencies like the fire department or health department. However, there are other aspects of the physical environment that are rarely adequately assessed.[4] The school health nurse will need to be alert to other hazards to physical safety that may be present in the school setting. Examples of these hazards are toxic art supplies, scientific equipment in labs, kitchen appliances in home economics classrooms, and chemical substances used either in chemistry labs or by maintenance and janitorial staffs. Animals in classrooms may also present safety hazards in terms of the potential for scratches and bites or disease transmission.

Other areas of concern are the safety of industrial arts classrooms, the gymnasium, and play areas. As noted in Chapter 20, Care of Children, the safety of outdoor play equipment should be inspected on a regular basis and repairs made as needed. A similar need exists for periodic assessment of sports equipment and practices. Other hazards associated with play areas include broken glass and other refuse on the playground. Hard surfaces below play equipment increases the potential for injuries stemming from falls.[4]

Other assessment considerations with respect to the school's internal physical environment include noise levels within and outside of classrooms and the adequacy of lighting, ventilation, heating, and cooling. Food sanitation should also be assessed.[5] If hot meals are provided at school, cooking facilities should be inspected regularly. Such inspections are usually the official responsibility of the local health department, but the community health nurse should also assess these facilities periodically. If students bring their lunches, the potential for food poisoning from spoiled foods should be appraised.

Assessing sanitary facilities in the school is another area for consideration. Here the nurse would examine the adequacy of toilet facilities for the size of the school population. The nurse would also periodically inspect sanitary facilities to make sure they are in good working order and do not pose hazards for the transmission of communicable diseases. Again, this is usually an area of responsibility for health department personnel, but official inspections may only occur at lengthy intervals and the nurse should be aware of hazards that might arise in the interim.

Another area of concern with respect to sanitation is the use and cleaning of shower facilities. The nurse should assess that showers are adequately cleaned to prevent transmission of communicable conditions such as tinea pedis (athlete's foot).

Physical facilities for preventing the spread of disease by infected children should also be assessed. Are there places within the school where youngsters with infectious conditions can be isolated? All too often these children are merely kept in the nurse's office until a parent can come for them. This presents opportunities for exposure of all those who visit the nurse while the child is there.

Special consideration should be given to the physical environment as it relates to handicapped children. Many physical barriers may exist, particularly in older schools, that limit the ability of handicapped youngsters to benefit from the educational setting. Areas of concern include the presence of ramps, easily opened doors and windows, nonslip flooring, elevators, and curb modifications to eliminate the need to step up. Another consideration is access to toileting facilities by handicapped children. Are toilets accessible to wheelchairs? Are sinks placed so that a wheelchair can be maneuvered beneath them? Placement and height of mirrors, drinking fountains, and telephones are also of concern. Other considerations with respect to the environment of handicapped children are the adequacy of storage for wheelchairs and other special equipment, wheelchair space in classrooms and auditoria, modification of laboratory and library carrels for wheelchair use, and the adequacy of evacuation plans for the handicapped in case of emergency.[11]

Psychological Environment

The psychological environment of the school can either foster good health or undermine it. Aspects of the psychological environment to be assessed include the organization of the school day, the aesthetic quality of the physical environment, the nature of relationships among students and school staff members, discipline and grading practices, and parent-school relations.[5]

Organization of the School Day. The nurse would determine whether the organization of the school day is conducive to health. Assessment areas to be addressed include the extent to which periods of strenuous physical activity are alternated with periods of quiet study and the extent of opportunities for developing a variety of psychomotor as well as academic skills. The nurse would also assess whether mealtimes are arranged so that students have the energy reserves to handle the tasks of the school day. For younger children, this usually means providing a snack time. Another area for assessment is the scheduling of time for toileting activities. The nurse should determine whether children are given time to go to the lavatory or permitted to go when necessary to prevent chronic constipation or urinary tract infection. There should also be opportunities for children to obtain drinks of water. Such opportunities should increase in frequency with hot weather.

Aesthetic Quality. The appearance of the physical environment is interrelated with the psychological environment, and the nurse would assess the aesthetic quality of the environment. Are the rooms clean, bright, and cheerful and conducive to good psychological health? Or, are they dark, dingy, and depressing?

Peer Relations. The relationships of a student with his or her peers can create a psychological environment that is either conducive or detrimental to mental and physical health. The community health nurse can assess the extent to which students who have difficulties with peer relationships are encouraged to participate in group activities. Is there adequate adult supervision of student activities to moderate unhealthy peer relationships? If school personnel see that particular children are unable to participate or are even victimized, do they act to stop such behaviors? Are opportunities provided within the school setting and the curriculum for values clarification and learning about healthy interpersonal interactions?

Teacher-student Relations. Teacher-student relations also affect the psychological climate of the school. The nurse would assess the quality of student-teacher relationships within the school in general and also between specific teachers and their students. Ideally, teachers are people who listen, reward appropriate behavior, maximize student assets, allow personal expression, and foster responsibility. Teachers who foster good student relationships tend to be enthusiastic and have a way of making learning fun. They exhibit a sincere concern for students and respect, accept, and trust them. They get to know their students well, encourage participation and curiosity, foster healthy competition, and encourage students to perform to their best potential. They also refrain from harsh or sarcastic comments, and they discipline students appropriately.[5]

Unfortunately, not all teachers fit this picture. In assessing teacher-student relationships, the nurse would seek to identify any tendencies on the part of teachers to use undue punishment or to make demands that students are incapable of meeting. Inconsistent demands or conflicting expectations on the part of a teacher can also create stress in students and lead to physical and mental health problems. Nurses might note that certain children are singled out for punishment by a particular teacher and may need to function as advocates. School nurses should also be alert to the potential for emotional, physical, or sexual abuse of students by teachers (and, on occasion, of teachers by students).

Teacher-to-Teacher Relationships. The relationships among teachers in a school and among teachers and other school personnel also influence the psychological environment of students. The nurse should assess the extent to which healthy teacher relationships—those that are supportive, encourage creativity and freedom, and foster cooperation—exist within the school. Effective relationships among teachers foster sharing and self-confidence, recognize achievements, and provide guidance for teacher development. In schools where teacher-to-teacher relationships are strained, students may get caught in the middle between teachers, or student morale may be undermined by the stress created by strife among teachers. For example, if the basketball coach and a particular high school English teacher do not get along well, the coach may demand that basketball players cut English class for an extra practice before a championship game and the English teacher may threaten to fail any player that cuts class. In this instance, the students cannot win. If they cut class, they may fail English. Conversely, if they miss the practice, they may be dropped from the team.

Discipline. In discussing the characteristics of supportive teachers, the issue of discipline was alluded to. In addition to looking at disciplinary measures employed by individual teachers, school nurses should assess the school's philosophy regarding discipline. Discipline should be used for inappropriate behavior and should not be unduly harsh. The nurse would determine whether rules of behavior are clearly communicated to students and whether expectations are realistic. The nurse should also assess whether discipline, when warranted, is administered fairly and in a manner that does not diminish the student's self-respect.[5]

Grading. Likewise, grading policies should be clearly understood and should be fairly implemented. Particular grading practices are usually the province of the individual teacher, but the community health nurse can assess whether grading standards are consistent and grades are communicated to students privately to avoid humiliation. If graded work is displayed, the nurse can examine the extent to which student work is exhibited in such a way that all students are made to feel good about some of their abilities. This is particularly important in elementary grades when children incorporate perceptions of their school performance into either positive or negative self-images.

Parent-school Relationships. Another area for assessment is the quality of relationships between school personnel and parents, which can have a strong influence on the psychological climate of the school setting. When this relationship is cooperative in nature, students do not receive conflicting messages about what is expected of them. On the other hand, when relationships between parents and school personnel are adversarial, students may again be caught in the middle of a power struggle. Or, students may attempt to exploit the situation by manipulating both parents and teachers to their own advantage. Other areas that the nurse might explore in assessing the psychological environment are the quality of students' school performance, and absenteeism and drop-out rates.

Social Environment

The social environment also plays a part in influencing the health status of members of the school community. The nurse needs to assess the community's attitudes toward education because these attitudes will determine, in large part, the degree of support given to the schools and to health care within the schools. Community attitudes will also affect the allocation of funds for both school and health programs.

The extent of crime in the school neighborhood is another aspect of the social environment to be assessed. Is violence a problem for children going to and from school? Is drug dealing going on in the area and will youngsters be exposed to pressure to experiment with drugs?

A social factor that also influences health in the school setting is the prevalence of families in which both parents work. Unfortunately, children are often sent to school when they are ill because there is no one at home to care for them.[6] The nurse should assess the number of students who come to school ill and explore with parents their reasons for sending sick children to school. It may be a lack of awareness on the part of parents of the signs and symptoms of illness or an absence of other options available to parents.

The social environment within the school is also influential. What is the socioeconomic status of students? Of school personnel? What is the racial or ethnic composition of the school population? Are racial tensions present? Do religious beliefs influence the health of the school population? For example, if there are large numbers of children whose parents object to immunization on religious grounds, the nurse needs to be particularly alert to signs of outbreaks of childhood diseases such as measles, rubella, and diphtheria, among others. Another area for consideration is the cultural background of students and school personnel. Are they similar? Do cultural practices influence students' health? Do differences in cultural practices create tension among students or between students and staff?

LIFE-STYLE

Enrollment in school is itself a life-style factor that influences health. School attendance increases one's risk of exposure to a variety of communicable diseases. Children generally experience an increase in the number of acute illnesses during the first few years of school whether this occurs at the day-care/preschool level or with admission to elementary school.

The rigidity of the school day may also affect the health status of students. Attempts to postpone defecation or urination until prescribed times may lead to chronic constipation or to urinary tract infections. Likewise, inability to get a drink of water except at specific times may lead to dehydration, particularly in hot weather. The nurse should assess the effects of these aspects of regimentation on the health of students.

Nutrition is another life-style factor that should be assessed in the school population. The adequacy of lunches brought from home should be examined as well as evidence of poor nutrition of meals eaten at home. For example, the nurse would assess children for evidence of anemia or poor growth and development. In those schools without a dietary consultant, the nurse should appraise the nutritional quality of school lunch and/or breakfast programs. Too often, food for such programs is purchased with an eye toward economy rather than nutritional value.

Recreational activities should also be explored. The need to examine recreational and sports equipment for safety hazards has already been touched upon, but the nurse should also be aware of the types of recreational and competitive activities engaged in by students. Is there ample opportunity for physical activity? Is it adequately supervised? Are sports and recreational programs appropriate to children's ages and developmental levels? For example, contact sports are not appropriate for children in lower elementary grades because of increased risk of injury. Another question is whether recreational activities are suited to children's interests. Are various opportunities available, or must all children engage in the same activity, whether they choose to or not? Is there a sexual bias evident in recreational opportunities provided? For example, is soccer restricted to boys while girls are expected to play hopscotch or jump rope? Attention should also be given to the recreational needs of teachers. Are teachers given a break from classroom and playground duties?

Rest is another component of life-style that is assessed. Nurses and teachers should note whether children appear to be getting sufficient sleep at night. The nurse should also examine the adequacy of rest periods provided for younger children. Are these periods appropriately incorporated into the school day? Are there adequate facilities for rest periods (i.e., cots or mats)? Facilities for rest periods are also an important consideration for handicapped children or those with chronic illnesses who may tire easily.

Other life-style behaviors should also be assessed, particularly among older students. The extent of tobacco use or the use of alcohol or other drugs should be explored as should the extent of sexual activity among preadolescent and adolescent students.

HEALTH SYSTEM

Health system factors that influence the health of the school population occur at both the individual and community level. At the individual level, the community health nurse would assess the usual source of health care for individual children and their families. Do children have a regular source of health care? Do they make use of health-promotive and illness-preventive services as well as curative services? Or is health care for children crisis oriented, focusing only on the treatment of acute conditions? Do children have unmet health needs because their families cannot afford care?

At the community level, the nurse would assess the availability of health-care services to meet the needs of the school-age population. Are health-promotive and illness-preventive services easily accessible in the community? Are there services available for youngsters with special health needs (for example, handicapped children). Are specific pediatric or adolescent services available? Is there access to contraceptive services or treatment of sexually transmitted diseases for the adolescent population? Is community attention to possible child abuse adequate?

The nurse would also assess the relationship between the school and the health-care community. Are private physicians conversant with regulations for excluding children with communicable conditions from school? Do physicians and other health-care providers work cooperatively with school personnel to meet the health-care needs of individual youngsters? Do health-care providers in the community offer services within the school on either a paid or voluntary basis? Appendix O, Special Assessment Consideration in the School Setting, provides guidelines for assessing health needs in schools.

DIAGNOSTIC REASONING AND HEALTH NEEDS IN THE SCHOOL SETTING

The second aspect of the use of the epidemiologic prevention process model in the school setting is deriving nursing diagnoses from assessment data. Diagnoses can be derived at two levels, in relation to individual students and in relation to the school population. Examples of diagnoses related to the population group might be, "Safety hazard due to placement of play equipment on asphalt surface" or "Need for drug abuse education due to high prevalence of drug abuse in the surrounding community." Diagnoses related to an individual student might include, "Inability to participate in vigorous physical exercise due to exercise-induced asthma" or "Need for referral to child protective services due to suspected physical abuse by father."

Again, each of the sample diagnoses provided above contains a statement of the probable underlying cause of the problem. Such a statement provides direction for efforts to resolve the problem. For example, one approach to the playground safety hazard might be to relocate play equipment in a sandy area. With the individual examples, measures might be taken to provide less strenuous forms of exercise for the asthmatic child or to make a referral for child protective services in the abuse situation.

PLANNING TO MEET HEALTH NEEDS IN THE SCHOOL SETTING

Planning to meet health needs identified in the school setting takes place at two levels. The first is the macro level at which the general approach to providing health services in the school is planned. The second is the micro level at which plans are made to meet specific health needs of members of the school population. The community health nurse working in the school setting will participate in planning efforts at both levels.

MACRO-LEVEL PLANNING

Health services are provided in keeping with an overall health services plan. The plan should specify the population to be served and the services to be provided.[4] Typical categories of services include assessment of health status, problem-management services, acute-care services, and other preventative services such as immunizations and safety education. Additional components of the health services plan include specification of the personnel involved and the resources needed to implement the program.

The health services plan should also address the nature of records to be kept. Categories to be addressed include clinical records related to the health of particular children or staff members, administrative records, and evaluative records. Planning for program evaluation should also be included in the plan. Finally, the plan should specify budgetary considerations related to salaries, facilities, and other expenses. Specific elements of the plan in each of these areas are included in Table 26–2. Initial development of a health services plan in the school setting would entail use of the program planning process described in Chapter 19, Care of the Community or Target Group.

TABLE 26–2. ELEMENTS OF THE SCHOOL HEALTH PLAN AND RELATED CONSIDERATIONS

Health Plan Element	Related Considerations
Population served	Ages and grades of students involved Extent of service to be given to staff
Services provided	Assessment/screening services First aid Acute-care services Problem-management services Immunizations Safety education Health education Counseling services
Personnel	Categories of health personnel Qualifications of health personnel Functions and responsibilities Staff development needs
Resources	Facilities Equipment Supplies/postage Health records Telephone
Record system	Clinical records for individuals seen Administrative records Immunization records Absenteeism records Program evaluation records
Program evaluation	Focus of evaluation Data collection procedures Data analysis procedures
Budgetary considerations	Salaries Facility construction and maintenance Equipment and supply costs Record-keeping costs Staff development costs

MICRO-LEVEL PLANNING

The school health program will include planning for activity at all three levels of prevention: primary, secondary, tertiary.

Primary Prevention

Primary prevention in the school setting involves many of the same planning considerations as those used with children in general. Areas of emphasis in planning primary preventative measures in the school setting include immunization, safety, exclusion from school, health education, as well as diet and nutrition.[12] Other concerns in primary prevention include developing a strong self-image, positive coping skills, and good interpersonal skills in students.

Immunization. Young children are at particular risk for a variety of communicable diseases for which immunization is possible. Immunizations against measles, mumps, rubella, diphtheria, pertussis, tetanus, and polio are required for school entry in most states. Immunizations are also available for diseases caused by *Hemophilus influenzae* B and influenza. These diseases are discussed in more detail in Chapter 30, Communicable Disease.

The school nurse may be involved in referring individuals who are not immunized for appropriate services or may be involved in providing immunizations in the school setting. In addition to providing for routine immunizations, school nurses may also suggest other immunizations in the event of exposure to certain diseases, such as hepatitis A.

Safety. Part of the school nurse's responsibility is to identify safety hazards and report them to those responsible for eliminating them. Safety education may also be the responsibility of the school nurse. In addition, the nurse might collaborate with others within and outside the school setting to reduce safety hazards in the surrounding area. Moreover, the nurse and other school personnel might become involved in cooperative efforts with local police to reduce drug traffic in the neighborhood.

Exclusion from School. One of the earliest responsibilities of the school nurse was to determine when children should be excluded from school because they had communicable illnesses. Children were also excluded from school as part of an effort to stop the spread of scabies, lice, and other parasites among a highly susceptible population. Performance of this responsibility still requires the school nurse to be knowledgeable of the signs and symptoms of communicable disease and infestation and to be aware of state and local regulations regarding school exclusion. Several conditions that usually warrant exclusion and guidelines for readmission are included in Table 26–3.

The responsibility of the nurse does not stop with excluding the affected child from school. The nurse should also educate parents and children regarding the need to stay home from school when they are ill and about care during illness. The nurse may also make referrals for medical care as needed. In addition, the nurse will follow up on children excluded from school to make sure that they are receiving appropriate care and that they are able to return to school when there is no longer any danger of exposure to others.

Health Education. Health education in the school setting provides a foundation for healthy behaviors in adulthood. Growing recognition of this is seen in the fact that by 1989 some 25 states had mandated school health education programs and 9 others had recommended implementation of such programs.[1] In addition, 25 states require elementary teachers to have some preparation in health education.[9]

The principles of health education discussed in Chapter 7, The Health Education Process, are particularly relevant to community health nursing in the school setting. The nurse may either serve as a resource for teachers on health content or provide health education classes, or do both. The school nurse will also be involved in the development of the health education curriculum. Activities involved in curriculum development in which the nurse may engage include the assessment of needs and resources, review of health curricula from other school systems, development of goals and objectives, and design of specific learning activities. In addition, the nurse may also be involved in preparing teachers to participate in the health education program. Finally, the nurse

TABLE 26–3. CONDITIONS TYPICALLY WARRANTING EXCLUSION FROM SCHOOL AND GUIDELINES FOR READMISSION

Condition	Readmission Guidelines
Bacterial conjunctivitis	After acute symptoms subside
Chickenpox	Five days after the eruption of the first vesicles or after lesions are dried
Diphtheria	Until negative cultures of nose and throat are obtained at least 24 hours after discontinuing antibiotics
Hepatitis A	One week after the onset of jaundice
Impetigo (staphylococcal)	24 hours after treatment is initiated
Influenza	After acute symptoms subside
Measles	Four days after the onset of the rash
Meningococcal meningitis	24 hours after chemotherapy is initiated or when the child is sufficiently recovered
Mononucleosis, infectious	After acute symptoms subside Delay resumption of strenuous physical activity until spleen is nonpalpable
Mumps	Nine days after the onset of swelling
Pediculosis	24 hours after the application of an effective pediculocide
Pneumonia, pneumococcal, and Mycoplasma	48 hours after the intitiation of antibiotics or when the child is sufficiently recovered
Pertussis	After 5 days of antibiotic therapy or when the child is sufficiently recovered
Respiratory disease (viral) and upper respiratory infection	After acute symptoms subside
Rubella	Seven days after the onset of the rash
Scabies	24 hours after treatment
Streptococcus (strep throat, scarlet fever, impetigo)	24 hours after treatment is initiated or when the child is sufficiently recovered
Tinea corporis	Exclude only from gym, swimming pool, or other activities where exposure of other individuals may occur. Resume activities after treatment is completed.

(Source: Benenson, A. (Ed.). (1990). Control of communicable diseases in man *(15th ed.). Washington, DC: American Public Health Association; Hoekelman, R. A., Blatman, S., & Friedman, S. B., et al. (1987).* Primary Pediatric Care. *St. Louis: C. V. Mosby.*

will participate in the implementation and evaluation of the program.

Food and Nutrition. Nutrition is another important aspect of health promotion with the school population. As noted earlier, when this function is not performed by a dietician or nutritionist, school nurses assess the nutritional status of children and monitor the nutritional value of school lunches. When nutritional offerings are inadequate, the nurse would work with school administrators and food service personnel to improve the nutritional quality of meals served. The nurse may also educate children and their parents regarding nutrition and good dietary habits.

Self-image. Sound mental health is promoted by a strong self-image developed throughout the childhood years. Health promotion in the school setting should focus on the development of a healthy self-image as well as a healthy physical self. School nurses can foster self-image development by serving as role models in their dealings with children. They can also suggest to teachers learning activities that will enhance development of a positive self-image.

On occasion, school nurses may need to function as advocates for children who do not have a strong self-image or for those who may be emotionally (or physically) abused by family members, peers, or even teachers. As noted earlier, the nurse should be aware of disciplinary measures used in the school and be alert to forms of discipline or unfair exercise of authority that are harmful to a child's self-image. When such circumstances are identified, the nurse might discuss his or her observations with teachers or other personnel involved and suggest other avenues for achieving the goals of disciplinary action. When corrective actions do not result from these interactions, the nurse may need to bring the problem to the attention of the appropriate authorities such as the school principal or members of the school board.

Occasionally this will require filing a report of child abuse. In addition to reporting the situation, however, the nurse has a responsibility to provide counseling or referral for assistance to those involved and to serve as a support person for both victim and abuser. In such cases, referrals may also be needed to address socioeconomic problems that may be contributing to the situation.

Coping Skills. Another aspect of primary prevention that should be fostered in schools is the development of coping skills. Students and personnel can be assisted to develop active problem-solving strategies that will promote their abilities to cope with adverse circumstances. School health nurses can serve as role models in this respect and can also provide counseling that assists students and their families or staff to engage in positive problem solving. Nurses can also reinforce evidence of positive coping by making others aware of their abilities to cope. In addition, the nurse can present information on stress, and can offer strategies for dealing with stress that will enhance the development of sound coping skills.

Interpersonal Skills. The ability to interact effectively with others is essential to civilized society. Such abilities are not innate and must be learned. Education for effective interpersonal skills is another aspect of primary prevention with the school population. This is because interpersonal skills enhance mental and social health. Again, the nurse can serve as a role model for effective interpersonal skills and can educate students, parents, and staff regarding interpersonal interactions and the development of communication skills. The nurse can also provide information on group dynamics and communication skills that can enhance interpersonal skills within groups of people. For example, the nurse might promote role-play in a class to which a handicapped child will soon be admitted or help youngsters learn how to express anger at a teacher in an appropriate manner. Aspects of primary prevention in the school setting and related community health nursing responsibilities are summarized in Table 26–4.

Secondary Prevention

Secondary prevention deals with existing problems that require intervention. Generally speaking, secondary prevention involves screening for existing health conditions, referral, counseling, and treatment.

Screening. Screening is a major facet of most school health programs and an important responsibility of the school nurse. The goals of screening programs within the school setting include the obvious goal of detecting disease.[13] Other goals include identifying children with special needs that require adjustment of the educational program, promoting the importance of primary preventative measures, and evaluating the effectiveness of current measures.

Screening can be used to detect health conditions that are amenable to treatment and that can be resolved with appropriate therapy. For example, vision screening is used to identify children with visual problems, the majority of whom can benefit from corrective lenses. Screening may also help to identify children with particular needs that necessitate adjustments in the educational program. For instance, developmental screening may help to identify young-

TABLE 26–4. AREAS OF EMPHASIS IN PRIMARY PREVENTION IN THE SCHOOL SETTING AND RELATED COMMUNITY HEALTH NURSING RESPONSIBILITIES

Area of Emphasis	Community Health Nursing Responsibilities
Immunization	• Refer for immunization services as needed • Provide routine immunizations • Suggest additional immunizations as warranted by circumstances (for example, an epidemic of hepatitis A)
Safety	• Report safety hazards to appropriate authorities • Provide safety education • Collaborate with others to eliminate safety hazards in the community
School exclusion	• Determine need for exclusion from school • Explain need for exclusion to parents • Refer child for treatment of condition if needed • Educate children and parents on preventing the spread of communicable diseases • Follow up on children excluded from school to ensure appropriate care
Health education	• Participate in designing health education curricula • Provide consultation to teachers on health education topics • Provide in-service for teachers related to health education • Teach health education in the classroom • Arrange for other health educational experiences (for example, field trips or guest speakers) • Arrange or provide health education for families
Food and nutrition	• Provide consultation on menu planning • Educate children and families regarding nutrition
Self-image	• Provide a role model for teachers and others in positive interactions with children • Provide consultation to teachers on activities to enhance children's self-esteem • Function as an advocate for children who have poor self-esteem
Coping skills	• Provide a role model for students and staff for effective problem-solving skills • Provide counseling regarding problem-solving skills • Reinforce use of appropriate coping skills • Educate students and staff on stress and coping
Interpersonal skills	• Provide a role model for students and staff for effective interpersonal skills • Educate students, staff, and parents on group dynamics and communication skills

sters with learning disabilities who will benefit from special education programs.

A screening program also provides an opportunity to stress the importance of primary prevention. Dental screening, for example, provides an excellent opportunity to educate students on the need for good dental hygiene. Finally, screening efforts provide one measure of the effectiveness of current preventative efforts. For instance, hematocrit screening can provide evidence of one aspect of the efficacy of a school lunch program or nutrition education program in promoting good nutrition.

Screening is a cost-effective approach to the identification of health problems. Typical costs of a screening program include those of the screening procedure itself and of retesting those with positive results; time spent by the nurse in referral; costs of diagnostic and treatment services; special education costs; and the costs of corrective maintenance (for example, for hearing aids or replacing eyeglasses). These costs tend to be far less than the costs incurred when diagnoses are made later, after problems become more pronounced.[4]

Screening programs typically undertaken in the school setting include screening of vision and hearing, dental screening, developmental screening, school readiness testing, and screening for scoliosis. Other screening tests may also be employed depending upon the needs of the population served by the school. For example, hematocrit testing might be undertaken in populations with high levels of anemia, whereas tuberculin testing would be appropriate in populations with a high incidence of TB. Other tests that might be relevant to particular populations include lead screening, sickle cell testing, and diabetes screening.[9]

The community health nurse in the school setting may perform a variety of roles with respect to screening programs. The nurse might arrange for the screening to be done or might conduct screening tests on one's own. Or, the nurse might train volunteers to perform certain screening procedures. Moreover, the nurse is also responsible for informing students and parents of the results of screening tests and of interpreting those results. The nurse may also need to make referrals for follow-up diagnostic or treatment services. In addition, the nurse will follow up on these referrals to make sure that students are receiving appropriate health-care services.

Referral. School health nurses make a number of referrals. In addition to referrals for following up on positive screening test results, the nurse may make referrals for a variety of other services. For example, the nurse might refer children who are not immunized to the local health department for immunizations. Or, a referral for counseling might be needed for a child with behavior problems. School personnel may also be referred for health problems that require medical attention. In making these and other referrals, the school nurse will use the principles of referral discussed in Chapter 9, The Discharge Planning and Referral Process.

Counseling. Another important role for the school nurse in secondary prevention is that of counseling. As noted in Chapter 4, Community Health Nursing, counseling involves assisting clients to make informed health decisions. Nurses may counsel individual students regarding personal problems, or they may assist students, families, and staff to engage in problem solving.

Treatment. School nurses may also be involved in the actual treatment of existing health conditions. Treatment can involve emergency care in the event of illness or injury. School nurse practitioners might even engage in medical management of minor illnesses such as antibiotic treatment of otitis media and so on.

Nurses may also be involved in providing specific treatments designed to minimize the effects of acute and chronic conditions. For example, the nurse may need to dispense prescribed medications, assist with physical therapy exercises for some children, suction tracheostomies, or perform catheter irrigations. They may also be involved in programs for bowel or bladder training. Community health nurses working with handicapped children in the school setting may also find it necessary to educate other school personnel in procedures required by the child's condition.[6] In addition, the community health nurse will monitor the therapeutic effects and side effects of medications and other treatments. Emphases in secondary prevention in the school setting and related community health nursing responsibilities are summarized in Table 26–5.

Tertiary Prevention

Tertiary prevention is undertaken to prevent the recurrence of a problem or to minimize the effects of an existing one. To a large extent, tertiary preventative measures will depend upon the problems experienced by the student or staff member. Generally speaking, however, there are four aspects of tertiary prevention with which the school nurse is concerned: preventing the recurrence of acute problems, preventing complications, fostering adjustment to chronic illness and handicapping conditions, and dealing with learning disabilities.

TABLE 26–5. AREAS OF EMPHASIS IN SECONDARY PREVENTION IN THE SCHOOL SETTING AND RELATED COMMUNITY HEALTH NURSING RESPONSIBILITIES

Area of Emphasis	Related Community Health Nursing Responsibilities
Screening	• Conduct screening tests or arrange for screening by others • Train volunteers in screening procedures • Interpret screening test results • Notify parents of screening test results • Make referrals for further testing or treatment as needed • Follow up on referrals to determine outcomes and to ensure appropriate care for identified conditions
Referral	• Refer children and families for health-care services and other services as needed • Refer other school personnel for needed services
Counseling	• Assist students, staff, or families to make informed health decisions • Counsel students, staff, or families regarding personal problems • Assist students, staff, or families to engage in problem solving
Treatment	• Provide first aid for illness or injury • Dispense medications prescribed for acute or chronic illnesses • Perform special treatments or procedures warranted by identified conditions • Teach others to perform special treatments or procedures • Monitor therapeutic effects and side effects of medications and other treatments

Acute Conditions. Preventing the recurrence of acute health problems depends upon adequate treatment for existing problems and eliminating conditions that might lead to recurrence. For example, the school nurse might need to educate parents and children regarding the need to complete the course of therapy for otitis media. Or, education might be needed related to toileting hygiene (for example, wiping from front to back) to prevent a recurrent urinary tract infection. The nurse might also engage in efforts to help an abusive parent or unduly harsh teacher find other ways to vent frustrations, or might make a referral to help alleviate financial difficulties that are taxing coping abilities.

Preventing Complications. Tertiary prevention will also be directed toward preventing complications of either acute or chronic health problems. For example, the school nurse might encourage parents of a child with strep throat to complete a course of antibiotics to prevent cardiac and urinary complications. Similarly, the nurse might suggest a cushion and frequent changes of position to prevent pressure sores in a student confined to a wheel chair.

Chronic Illness and Handicapping Conditions. Tertiary prevention for children with chronic or handicapping conditions involves assisting them to adjust to their condition and preventing complications. Specific measures will depend upon the condition involved. For instance, special arrangements for physical education might be needed to prevent recurrent attacks of exercise-induced asthma, while special attention to diet might be required for the diabetic child or staff member.

Major considerations in dealing with children with chronic illness in the school setting involve money, transportation and facilities, and equipment.[14] Additional considerations include nutrition and psychological well-being. The school nurse may need to refer students and parents to sources of financial assistance as a way to deal with the long-term care requirements of chronic and handicapping conditions.

Transportation and facility considerations in the school setting would include issues of physical access to facilities discussed earlier in this chapter. Another area for consideration is that of transportation to and from school and when class members are scheduled for field trips. The nurse will identify barriers to access in the school setting and serve as an advocate for the removal of those barriers. Likewise, the nurse will attempt to arrange transportation and other circumstances so that students with chronic or handicapping conditions can participate in as many regular school activities, including field trips, as possible. Advocacy in this area might also be needed with parents who may have a tendency to overprotect these children.

There may also be a need for special equipment to be used either at home or at school. The school nurse will make referrals to obtain such equipment or attempt to see that necessary equipment is provided by the school itself.

Nutrition may be particularly problematic for school children with chronic diseases or handicapping conditions. Youngsters with diabetes, for example, may need assistance in adapting a school lunch program to a diabetic diet. Severely handicapped children may need assistance with eating or may need to be fed. The school nurse assesses the special nutritional needs of children with these and similar conditions and then assists the child, family, and other school personnel to meet those needs.

The final consideration with children who have chronic illnesses or handicapping conditions is that of psychological well-being. These children should be helped to adjust to their conditions and to participate as normally as possible in the school routine. Parents, teachers, and other children may need to be discouraged from undermining the child's independence by "doing for" them. Values clarification exercises can help other children to understand the problems of the handicapped or chronically ill child rather than to poke fun at them or pity them.

Psychological health may be particularly fragile among those children with AIDS. There is a need to provide emotional support for these children as they deal with a terminal illness that may cause others to withdraw from them in fear.[15] Again, the community health nurse in the school setting may need to function as an advocate to prevent social isolation of these and other children with chronic or handicapping conditions. Another concern about the child with AIDS is the need to protect the child from infection and the use of universal precautions when dealing with blood and body fluids; both of these concerns may heighten the child's sense of isolation and alienation. There is also a need to deal with the child's knowledge of his or her own mortality. Thus the nurse may want to refer the child and family members for counseling. The nurse might also need to help other children, parents, and school personnel deal with their feelings of fear and grief related to AIDS and death.

Learning Disability. Because there does not seem to be any form of primary or secondary prevention available for learning disability, the focus in working with learning-disabled children is on minimizing the effects of their disability.

Some of the interventions that may be planned to assist learning-disabled children include learning by activity; involving multiple senses in learning activities; repetition; providing direction in small steps; and giving directions without irrelevant detail. Teaching at the appropriate level, a level that creates a challenge but does not lead to frustration, may also be helpful. Other useful strategies include avoiding drastic changes in activities, limiting distractions, and creating a climate in which success is ensured and reinforced as often as possible.[10]

The nurse will be involved in the development of an individualized lesson plan that will allow children with learning disabilities, as well as those with other chronic or handicapping conditions, to learn as easily as possible. Again, attention must be given to the psychological effects of being tagged "learning disabled." The nurse may need to function as an advocate with parents, teachers, and other children to avoid the application of labels that undermine the child's self-esteem. The nurse can also function as a role model in providing positive reinforcement for the child's strengths and for his or her accomplishments, however small. Considerations related to tertiary prevention in the school setting and related community health nursing responsibilities are summarized in Table 26–6.

In planning primary, secondary, or tertiary preventative measures in the school setting, the community health nurse may need information or assistance from outside sources. Sources of assistance for specific health problems among children were provided in Chapter 20, Care of Children. Other resources that may be of use in the school setting are presented in Table 26–7.

IMPLEMENTING HEALTH CARE IN THE SCHOOL SETTING

Implementing health care for individuals or groups in the school setting will frequently involve collaboration between the nurse and other members of the school health team. At the individual level, for example, the community health nurse may need to contact the private physician of a child with a chronic illness with information about adverse effects of medications or to request a change in the medical treatment plan based on changes in the child's condition. The nurse will also need to solicit the cooperation of parents in following through on a referral for medical services, testing, counseling, or other services needed by their child.

Implementing care for groups within the school setting will also require collaboration between the nurse and others. For example, the nurse may invite local police personnel to participate in a drug education program to be presented in the school. Or, the nurse might work with teachers, media specialists, food service personnel, and others to implement an educational program on basic nutrition for elementary school children. Parental permission may be re-

TABLE 26–6. AREAS OF EMPHASIS IN TERTIARY PREVENTION IN THE SCHOOL SETTING AND RELATED COMMUNITY HEALTH NURSING RESPONSIBILITIES

Area of Emphasis	Related Community Health Nursing Responsibilities
Prevention recurrence of acute conditions	• Eliminate risk factors for the condition • Teach students, staff, or parents how to prevent recurrence of problems • Make referrals that can assist in eliminating risk factors
Preventing complications of and promoting adjustment to chronic and handicapping conditions	• Assist parents with finding sources of financial aid to deal with chronic and handicapping conditions • Facilitate meeting special nutritional needs • Assist with meeting special needs for transportation and facilities • Provide for special equipment needs • Promote psychological well-being • Assist students, families, and staff to deal with the eventuality of death in terminal illnesses • Refer for counseling as needed • Function as an advocate as needed
Preventing adverse effects of learning disabilities	• Provide consultation for teachers in dealing with children's learning disabilities • Participte in the design of individualized learning programs for children with learning disabilities • Function as an advocate for the learning-disabled child as needed • Serve as a role model in positively reinforcing the child's accomplishments

TABLE 26–7. RESOURCES FOR COMMUNITY HEALTH NURSES WORKING IN SCHOOL SETTINGS

Area of Focus	Agency or Organization	Services
Health education	Abbott Laboratories Abbott Park, D-383 North Chicago, IL 60064	Health education material
	Aetna Life and Casualty Companies Public Relations and Advertising 151 Farmington Ave., DA06 Hartford, CT 06115	Health education material
	Allstate Corporate Relations Dept. Allstate Plaza Northbrook, IL 60062	Health education material
	American Alliance for Health, Physical Education, Recreation and Dance 1900 Association Dr. Reston, VA 22091	Health education material
	American Automobile Association Traffic Safety Dept. 8111 Gatehouse Rd. Falls Church, VA 22047	Health education material on automobile safety
	American Dental Association Bureau of Health Education and Audiovisual Services 211 Chicago Ave. Chicago, IL 60611	Educational material on dental health
	American Health Foundation 320 E. 43rd St. New York, NY 10017 (212) 953-1900	Health education material
	American Medical Association Department of Health Education 535 N. Dearborn St. Chicago, IL 60610	Health education material
	Charles E. Merrill Publishing Company 1300 Alum Creek Dr. Columbus, OH 43216	Health textbooks for elementary and secondary schools
	Chicago Heart Health Curriculum Project Chicago Heart Association 20 N. Wacker Dr. Chicago, IL 60606 (312) 346-4675	Educational material on preventing heart disease
	Department of Medicine School of Medicine University of California Los Angeles, CA 90024 (213) 825-6709	Health education materials
	Darte: Drug Abuse Reduction Through Education 33500 Van Borm Rd. Wayne, MI 48184 (313) 326-9300	Educational materials on drug abuse
	Distilled Spirits Council of the United States 1300 Pennsylvania Bldg. Washington, DC 20004	Health education material on alcohol abuse
	Environmental Protection Agency 401 M. St., SW Washington, DC 10460	Educational materials on environmental health

(*continued*)

TABLE 26–7. (*Continued*)

Area of Focus	Agency or Organization	Services
Health education (*continued*)	Epilepsy Foundation of America 4351 Garden City Dr. Landover, MD 20785 (301) 638-5229	Materials on epilepsy in the school
	Harcourt Brace Jovanovich 757 Third Ave. New York, NY 10017	Health textbooks for elementary and secondary schools
	Hogg Foundation for Mental Health University of Texas, Austin P.O. Box 7998, University Station Austin, TX 78712	Health education material on mental health
	Institute for Experimentation in Teacher Education SUNY, College at Cortland Cortland, NY 13045 (607) 753-4705	Health education material on heart disease
	Institute of Makers of Explosives 1575 Wye St., NW, Suite 550 Washington, DC 20005	Health education material on gun safety
	Laidlaw Brothers Thatcher and Madison River Forest, IL 60305	Health textbooks for elementary and secondary schools
	Mental Health Materials Center 30 E. 29th St. New York, NY 10016	Health education material on mental health
	National Center for Education Materials and Media for the Handicapped Ohio State University Faculty for Exceptional Children Columbus, OH 43210 (614) 422-7596	Bibliographies of education aids for the handicapped
	National Center for Health Education 30 E. 29th St. New York, NY 10016	Health education material for primary and secondary schools
	National Congress of Parents and Teachers 700 N. Rush St. Chicago, IL 60611 (312) 787-0977	Health education, advocacy
	National Fire Protection Association Batterymarch Park Quincy, MA 02269	Educational material on fire safety
	Office on Smoking and Health 5600 Fishers Lane Room 1-10 Park Building Rockville, MD 20857	Health education material on smoking
	Planned Parenthood Association of Humboldt County 2316 Harrison Ave. Eureka, CA 95501 (707) 442-2961	Family life sex education curriculum guide
	President's Council on Physical Fitness and Health 400 Sixth St., SW Washington, DC 20202	Health education material on exercise and fitness
	Rutgers Center of Alcohol Studies Smith Hall New Brunswick, NJ 08903	Health education material on alcohol abuse

TABLE 26–7. (*Continued*)

Area of Focus	Agency or Organization	Services
Health education (*continued*)	School Health Curriculum Project Center for Health Promotion and Education Centers for Disease Control Atlanta, GA 30333 (404) 329-3115	Curriculum for health education
	School Health Curriculum Project Primary Grades Curriculum Project National Center for Health Education 1130 Burnette Ave., Suite G Concord, CA 94520	Materials on school health curricula
	Scott, Foresman & Co. 1900 East Lake Ave. Glenview, IL 60025	Health textbooks for elementary and secondary schools
	Sex Information and Education Council of the United States 80 Fifth Ave., Suite 801 New York, NY 10011	Materials for sex education
	Stech-Vaughn Company Box 2028 Austin, TX 78768	Health textbooks for elementary and secondary schools
	The Travelers Film Library One Tower Square Hartford, CT 06115	Health education films
	United Way Health Foundation 618 Second St., NW Canton, OH 44703 (216) 455-0378	Health education curriculum
Nutrition	American Dry Milk Institute 130 N. Franklin St. Chicago, IL 60606	Health education material
	American Institute of Baking Communications Dept. 1213 Bakers Way Manhattan, KS 66502	Health education material
	Consumer Nutrition Center Human Nutrition Information Service U.S. Department of Agriculture Hyattsville, MD 20782	Health education material on nutrition
	National Dairy Council 6300 North River Rd. Rosemont, IL 60018	Educational material on nutrition
	National Livestock and Meat Board Nutritional Department 444 N. Michigan Ave. Chicago, IL 60611	Health education material on nutrition
	U.S. Department of Agriculture Food and Nutrition Service National School Lunch Program National School Breakfast Program Park Office Bldg., Room 512 3101 Park Center Dr. Alexandria, VA 22302 (703) 756-3590	Administers funds for school lunch and breakfast programs
	Utah State University Foundation UMC 93 Logan, UT 84322 (801) 750-2603	Nutrition education curriculum

(*continued*)

TABLE 26–7. (*Continued*)

Area of Focus	Agency or Organization	Services
School health	American School Health Association P.O. Box 708 Kent, OH 44240 (216) 678-1601	Standards for school health programs, help in establishing a school health program, publications related to school health, health education material
School nursing	National Association of School Nurses P.O. Box 1300 Scarboro, ME 04074 (207) 883-2117	Advocacy, assistance with school health program implementation

quired in certain school-based health programs. For example, parents will need to grant permission for screening procedures such as hematocrit testing. The nurse may also need to recruit parent or community volunteers to assist with screening programs or with other health-related programs such as a health fair.

EVALUATING HEALTH CARE IN THE SCHOOL SETTING

Evaluating the effectiveness of care in the school setting focuses on the outcomes of that care. Evaluation can occur at two levels, that of the individual child or the total school health program. Evaluative criteria for the care of the individual child will reflect the effects of nursing care on the youngster's health status. For example, if a child is no longer abused by his parent, or no longer has recurrent ear infections, or is now able to interact effectively with peers, the interventions of the nurse have probably been effective.

Evaluation of the overall school health program will focus on indicators of the health status of the total population. For instance, absentee rates might indicate how effective the program has been in preventing disease. Student screening test results may also provide information on the effectiveness of primary preventative efforts.

Changes in the prevalence of certain health problems within the school population may also indicate the efficacy of secondary preventative measures. For example, if alcohol abuse has been a problem among the student population, a declining prevalence of alcohol abuse would indicate that secondary measures are having an effect. Similarly, a decline in the teenage pregnancy rate would indicate that a sex education program is effective. Guidelines for evaluating the effectiveness of school health programs have been developed by a coalition of organizations concerned with school health (see the Recommended Readings at the end of this chapter) and can be used by the community health nurse to evaluate the health program in a particular school.

The processes used in evaluating the school health program are those discussed in Chapter 19, Care of the Community or Target Group. The school nurse will collaborate with other members of the school health team in designing and implementing an evaluation of the program. Moreover, the nurse may also be involved in data collection related to the evaluation and in interpreting that data. Finally, the nurse should be actively involved in decisions made on the basis of evaluative data.

CHAPTER HIGHLIGHTS

- Health care in the school setting provides community health nurses with an opportunity to improve the health status of the entire population.
- Goals of a school health program include promoting health and preventing illness, identifying and resolving existing health problems, and educating students and families for healthier life-styles.
- The school health program is comprised of three components: a health services component, a health education component, and an environmental component.
- School nurses should be educated at least at

the baccalaureate level in nursing. In some areas, school nursing requires a credential beyond the baccalaureate level. Some community health nurses working in school settings are prepared at the master's level in nursing.

- Community health nurses may perform a variety of roles in the school setting. These roles include consultant, director, educator, supervisor, coordinator, school nurse practitioner, and the roles of the school community nurse and the school nurse.
- Community health nurses working in school settings have responsibilities to three types of clientele: students and their families, school personnel, and the community.
- In addition to the community health nurse, potential members of the school health team include parents, teachers, administrators, counselors, social workers, physicians and dentists, health coordinators, food service personnel, janitorial and secretarial staff, public health and other public officials, and students.
- Human biological factors influencing the health of the school population may be related to the age and maturation of the students, genetic inheritance including race and sex composition of the population, and physiologic function.
- Considerations in assessing physiologic function include the characteristics of healthy children, the presence of existing physical health problems, and immunization levels among students and staff.
- Assessment considerations related to the physical environment reflect the influence of both the internal and external environment on the health of the school population.
- Areas to be addressed in assessing the psychological environment include the organization of the school day, the aesthetic atmosphere of the school, peer relations, teacher-student relations, teacher-to-teacher relations, discipline and grading practices, and parent-school relationships.
- Social environmental factors to be considered in assessing the health of the school population include community attitudes to education and school health, crime in the school neighborhood, the prevalence of working parents, the socioeconomic status of students and staff, and the influence of cultural and religious beliefs on health.
- Health system factors that influence the health of the school population include the source and use of health-care services by the population and the availability and accessibility of services needed within the community. The nurse would also assess the quality of relationships between the school and the health-care community.
- Planning to meet health needs in the school setting occurs at both macro and micro levels. Macro-level planning involves developing the overall plan for health services in the school. Micro-level planning involves planning for primary, secondary, and tertiary preventative measures to address the identified health needs of the population.
- Areas for emphasis in primary prevention in the school setting include immunization, safety, exclusion of students with communicable diseases from school, health education, food and nutrition, developing healthy self-images in students, developing student's coping skills, and fostering effective interpersonal skills.
- Secondary prevention foci in planning health care in the school setting include screening, referral, counseling, and treatment of existing conditions.
- Emphases in tertiary prevention in the school setting include preventing recurrence of acute health conditions, preventing consequences of and facilitating adjustment to chronic illnesses and handicapping conditions, and dealing with learning disabilities.
- Implementing health-care plans in the school setting requires collaboration between the community health nurse and a variety of others including parents, school personnel, other health-care providers, and community residents.
- Evaluation in the school setting addresses the effectiveness of the overall health-care program as well as the extent to which the health needs of individual children have been met.

Review Questions

1. What are the three goals of a school health program? (p. 627)
2. What are the three components of a school health program? (p. 627)
3. Describe at least five roles for community health nurses in school settings. (p. 628)
4. Describe three areas of nursing responsibility in school health. (p. 629)
5. Describe at least two considerations in assessing physical environmental factors influencing the health of the school population. Give an example of the health effects of factors in each area. (p. 633)
6. Identify at least four areas to be assessed in relation to the psychological environment in the school setting. Describe the influence of factors in each area on the health of the school population. (p. 634)
7. Describe at least two areas to be addressed in assessing social environmental influences on the health of the school population. Give an example of the health effects of factors in each area. (p. 636)
8. Identify at least five areas of emphasis in primary prevention in the school setting. Describe at least two activities that might be performed by community health nurses in school settings promoting health in each area. (p. 638)
9. Describe at least three approaches to secondary prevention in the school setting. Identify at least two community health nursing responsibilities related to each approach. (p. 640)
10. Describe at least two areas of emphasis in tertiary prevention in the school setting. How might the community health nurse be involved in each of these areas? (p. 642)

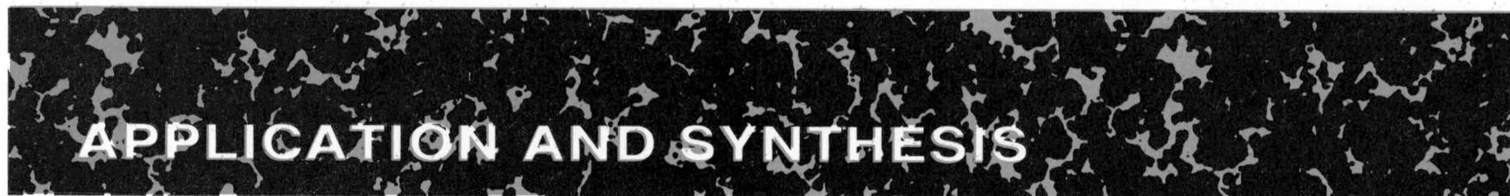

APPLICATION AND SYNTHESIS

Jimmy is a third grader in the school where you work as a school nurse. He comes to see you because he "has a stomachache." This is his third visit to your office in as many days. Each day you have seen him for a similar complaint but have found no physical evidence of illness. According to his teacher, his appetite has been good at lunch, although his lunches are large and not particularly nutritious. Jimmy says he is not constipated and has not had any diarrhea or vomiting. His abdominal pain usually disappears after lying down in your office for about 20 minutes.

When you talk to the teacher, she tells you that lately the other children have been making fun of Jimmy because he always comes in last in running games and can't run very fast during PE. Jimmy is about 35 pounds overweight for his height and becomes short of breath with strenuous physical exercise. Jimmy has two younger brothers who are both slender and have no difficulties with physical activity.

The teacher also mentions that Jimmy has been talking during class and disturbing the other children. She has tried to take him aside and explain why he should not talk in class, but he continues. His grades are not the best in the world (they're not the worst either), but he has been discouraged lately because he is having trouble mastering long division.

1. What human biological, environmental, life-style, and health system factors are operating in this situation?
2. What nursing diagnoses would you derive from the information provided above? How would you prioritize Jimmy's problems? Why?
3. Write at least two client-care objectives for Jimmy.
4. What primary, secondary, and tertiary prevention measures would be appropriate in this case?
5. How would you evaluate the effectiveness of your interventions with Jimmy? Be specific.

REFERENCES

1. United States Department of Health and Human Services. (1991). *Healthy people 2000: National health promotion and disease prevention objectives.* Washington, DC: Government Printing Office.
2. Buhler-Wilkerson, K. (1985). Public health nursing: In sickness or in health. *American Journal of Public Health, 75,* 1155–1161.
3. Igoe, J. B. (1980). Changing patterns in school health and school health nursing. *Nursing Outlook, 28,* 486–492.
4. Lynch, A. (1983). *Redesigning school health services.* New York: Human Services Press.
5. Redican, K., Olsen, L. K., & Baffi, C. R. (1986). *Organization of school health programs.* New York: Macmillan.
6. Young-Cureton, V. (1991). Its more than Band-Aids for kids. *California Nursing, 13*(2), 20–22.
7. Bryan, D. S. (1973). *School nursing in transition.* St. Louis: C. V. Mosby.
8. Chen, S. C., Rose, D. A., & Chen, E. H. (1987). A health-awareness program for elementary school teachers. *Public Health Nursing, 4,* 105–110.
9. Cornacchia, H. J., Olsen, L. K., & Nickerson, C. J. (1984). *Health in elementary schools.* St. Louis: Times Mirror/Mosby.
10. Rhodes, R. L., Hafen, B. Q., Karren, K. J., & Rollins, L. M. (1981). *Elementary school health: Education and service.* Boston: Allyn & Bacon.
11. Albanese, M. K. (1986). A barrier-free school environment. In G. Larson (Ed.), *Managing the school age child with a chronic health condition* (pp. 51–57). Falls Church, VA: DGI Publishing.
12. Dagg, N. V. (1981). Primary prevention: Health promotion and specific protection. In S. J. Wold (Ed.), *School nursing: A framework for practice* (pp. 39–48). St. Louis: C. V. Mosby.
13. Wold, S. J. (1981). Secondary prevention: Theoretical and ethical issues. In S. J. Wold (Ed.), *School nursing: A framework for practice* (pp. 49–60). St. Louis: C. V. Mosby.
14. Kern, N. (1986). Using community resources. In G. Larson (Ed.), *Managing the school age child with a chronic health condition* (pp. 59–62). Falls Church, VA: DGI Publishing.
15. Leuhr, R. E. (1986). Helping the student with AIDS virus infection. In G. Larson (Ed.), *Managing the school age child with a chronic health condition* (pp. 123–136). Falls Church, VA: DGI Publishing.

RECOMMENDED READINGS

American School Health Association. (1985). *An evaluation guide for school nursing practice designed for self and peer review.* Kent, OH: American School Health Association.

Provides guidelines for evaluating the effectiveness of school health nursing programs.

Lovato, C. Y., Allensworth, D. D., & Chen, M. (1989). *School health in America: An analysis of state requirements for school health programs* (5th ed.). Kent, OH: American School Health Association.

Addresses state mandates in areas of instruction, environment, services, physical education, guidance and counseling, food services, and school psychology. Describes certification requirements for health professionals in schools and provides guidelines for the ideal school health program.

Nelson, S. (1986). *How healthy is your school? Guidelines for evaluating school health promotion.* Kent, OH: American School Health Association.

Sets forth guidelines for assessing, planning, implementing, and evaluating each of the three components of a school health program.

Rudman, J. (1989). *School nurse practitioner.* Washington, DC: National Learning.

Describes the role of the nurse practitioner in the school setting.

Task Force on Standards of School Nursing Practice. (1983). *Standards of school nursing practice.* Kent, OH: American School Health Association.

Examines standards for school health nursing and outcome criteria for measuring achievement of the standards.

United States Department of Agriculture and United States Department of Health and Human Services. (1990). *Dietary guidelines for Americans.* Washington, DC: United States Department of Agriculture and United States Department of Health and Human Services.

Presents guidelines for basic nutrition that can be used to plan the nutritional content of school lunch and breakfast programs.

CHAPTER 27

Care of Clients in the Work Setting

KEY TERMS

employee assistance program
ergonomics
occupational health nursing
paraoccupational exposure
risk factor

Because most American adults are employed, the work setting is an important place for promoting the health of the general population. Although the work environment contributes to a wide variety of health problems, it also provides opportunities to influence a major segment of the population regarding personal health behaviors.

Over the years, employers have come to appreciate that healthy employees are more productive and that it is in the employer's interest to promote and maintain employee health. Moreover, the escalating cost of health insurance, accounting for almost half of all corporations' total operating costs in 1988,[1] makes health promotion increasingly cost-effective. One way that some companies have chosen to decrease health-related costs is to provide on-site health care for employees.

The importance of health care in the occupational setting can be seen in the national objectives related specifically to this setting. In fact, one entire section of the national objectives for the year 2000 deals with health in the occupational setting.[2] These objectives are summarized in Box 27–1.

LEARNING OBJECTIVES

After reading this chapter you should be able to:

- Describe at least three advantages in providing health care in the work setting.
- Identify at least six of the ten leading causes of health problems encountered in the work setting.
- Identify at least five types of health and safety hazards encountered in work settings.
- Describe four spheres of social influence on the health of employees.
- Describe four potential types of health-care programs in the work setting.
- Describe the three main areas of emphasis in primary prevention in the work setting.
- Describe three major considerations in secondary prevention in the work setting.
- Describe three emphases in tertiary prevention in the work setting.

BOX 27–1

National Objectives for the Year 2000 Related to Occupational Health

1. Reduce deaths from work-related injuries to no more than 4 per 100,000 full-time workers.
2. Reduce work-related injuries resulting in medical treatment, lost work time, or restricted work activity to no more than 6 cases per 100 full-time workers.
3. Reduce the incidence of cumulative trauma disorders to no more than 60 cases per 100,000 full-time workers.
4. Reduce the incidence of skin occupational disorders to no more than 55 cases per 100,000 full-time workers.
5. Reduce the number of hepatitis B infections due to occupational exposure to no more than 1250 cases per year.
6. Increase to at least 75% the proportion of work sites with 50 or more workers that mandate employee use of occupant protection systems for work-related motor vehicle travel.
7. Reduce to no more than 15% the proportion of workers exposed to average daily noise levels exceeding 85 dB.
8. Eliminate exposures that result in blood lead levels greater than 25 μg/dL.
9. Increase hepatitis B immunization levels to 90% of occupationally exposed workers.
10. Implement occupational safety plans in all 50 states to identify, manage, and prevent leading work-related diseases and injuries.
11. Establish in all 50 states exposure standards adequate to prevent the major occupational lung diseases.
12. Increase to at least 50% the proportion of work sites with 50 or more employees that have implemented programs for employee health and safety.
13. Increase to at least 50% the proportion of work sites with 50 or more employees that offer back-injury prevention and rehabilitation programs.
14. Establish in all 50 states programs that provide consultation and assistance to small businesses to implement health and safety programs for employees.
15. Increase to at least 75% the proportion of primary care providers who routinely elicit occupational exposures as part of a client history and who provide relevant counseling.

ADVANTAGES OF PROVIDING HEALTH CARE IN THE WORK SETTING

From a community health nursing perspective, there are a number of advantages to providing health care in the work setting.[3] These include the amount of time that people spend in this setting and the fact that this time is spent on a regular basis. In addition, when employees are present, they are essentially a "captive audience" subject to powerful pressures from peers and from employers to engage in healthy behaviors. For example, nonsmoking peers may object to smoking in their work or recreation areas, or employers may provide financial or nonfinancial incentives for healthy behavior. Another advantage is that the work force frequently consists of people who may be at risk for a variety of health problems or who may be motivated to maintain their health to ensure their continued ability to work. Because there are frequently health-care personnel present in the setting and mechanisms are already in place for communicating health messages, health promotion in the work setting is efficient and cost-effective.

More and more companies are acknowledging the advantages of providing health care in the occupational setting. Studies of representative employers and employees indicate that the number of companies with established on-site health-care units rose from 14 percent during the 1970s to 24 percent after 1980. Similarly, the percentage of companies employing at least one nurse rose from 8 percent to 17 percent during the same period. Although this percentage may seem low it represents a majority of working Americans, so that today approximately 80 percent of the American work force is now employed in businesses where there is access to the services of at least one nurse (compared to less than 60 percent in previous years). These figures indicate the growing recognition of occupational health concerns and of the role of nurses in dealing with those concerns.

OCCUPATIONAL HEALTH NURSING

Not all nurses who practice in occupational settings are community health nurses. However, the community health nurse is uniquely prepared to meet the health needs of the working population because of his or her knowledge of community health principles. Occupational health nursing is not a new role for the community health nurse. As noted in Unit One, nurses were employed in the work setting as early as 1895. Since that time, the role of the occupational health nurse has been expanded along with other nursing roles. Several years ago, the United States Department of Labor defined ***occupational health nursing*** as "giving nursing service under general medical direction to ill or injured employees or other persons who become ill or suffer an accident on the premises of a factory or other establishment."[4]

This definition does not, however, fully describe today's community health nursing role in the work setting. It concentrates on the treatment aspects of care and the nurse's dependent functions and does not acknowledge the promotional and preventive aspects that are of paramount importance in this practice setting. Occupational health nursing, then, is nursing practice directed toward promoting health, preventing illness, and restoring function for the working population.

NURSING ROLES IN THE WORK SETTING

Nursing roles in occupational health are based on the standards for practice in this setting developed by the American Association of Occupational Health Nurses (AAOHN).[5] These standards are summarized in Box 27–2.

The roles of the community health nurse in an occupational setting are many and varied. These roles include promoting the health of the employee population, preventing illness and injury, providing preemployment assessment of prospective employees, conducting periodic screening tests, and monitoring the work environment for health hazards. Other roles include providing first aid for injuries and treating existing health problems. In addition, the community health nurse working in the occupational setting should be a participant in planning the occupational health program and in evaluating its effectiveness.

Employers' expectations of nurses in the work setting are changing to incorporate more community

BOX 27–2

Standards for Occupational Health Nursing

1. The nurse collaborates with management in developing objectives for employee health services.
2. The nurse administers the employee health service.
3. The nurse defines nursing authority and responsibility and collaborates with management in determining the nurse's position in the organization.
4. The nurse administers nursing care and develops procedures and protocols with specific goals and interventions related to employee health needs.
5. The nurse coordinates responsibilities in health assessment, and promotes health maintenance and prevention of illness and injury.
6. The nurse collaborates with other on-site members of the occupational health team to evaluate the work environment and uses outside resources as needed.
7. The nurse establishes and promotes working relationships with appropriate community agencies.

(Source: American Association of Occupational Health Nurses[5])

health nursing functions aimed at improving the health of working people. In one study, for example, the five most frequently reported current activities of occupational health nurses were care of illnesses and emergencies, health risk counseling, follow-up on employee compensation claims, periodic health assessment, and evaluation of employees' readiness to return to work. Future roles envisioned by corporate executives for occupational health nurses included analysis of health promotion and risk-reduction trends and expenditures, development of health programs, planning efficient and cost-effective health operations, research, and collaboration with other disciplines to solve health problems.[6] Each of these future roles demands the community health background possessed by the community health nurse and highlights the importance of community health nurses functioning in occupational settings.

NURSING RESPONSIBILITIES IN THE WORK SETTING

As was true in the school setting, community health nurses working in the occupational health setting have responsibilities to several constituencies: the employee, the employer, and the community.

With respect to the employee, the community health nurse has responsibilities for safeguarding and promoting health and preventing illness, as well as identifying and dealing with existing health conditions. In some settings, responsibilities to employees may also be extended to care of the employee's family.

Nursing responsibilities to the employer include ensuring that employees are able to function effectively in their job. The nurse may also need to make recommendations for employee removal from certain positions when their continued presence in a particular job might jeopardize their safety or that of others. On occasion, conflicting responsibilities to employees and employers may pose ethical dilemmas for the nurse. These dilemmas should be resolved using the ethical principles discussed in Chapter 14, Ethical Influences on Community Health. The nurse is also responsible for providing a cost-effective health-care program that is not a financial drain on the employer.

Finally, the community health nurse, because of this individual's concern with the health of the total population, has responsibilities to the larger community. These responsibilities may entail assessing the effects of the business or industry on the community and working with company executives to minimize adverse effects on community health. The nurse will also assess the effects of the community environment on the health of company employees.

EDUCATIONAL PREPARATION FOR OCCUPATIONAL HEALTH NURSING

Several types of nursing personnel may be found in occupational settings including Registered Nurses prepared in associate degree and diploma programs in nursing as well as in baccaluareate degree programs; Licensed Practical Nurses; and nurses prepared at the master's level. Because of the need to apply principles of community health nursing, nurses who engage in the full scope of the occupational health nurse's role should be prepared at least at the baccaluareate level in nursing. Advanced preparation in occupational health nursing may result in certification by the American Association of Occupational Health Nurses (AAOHN). Nurses working in occupational settings might also hold master's degrees in nursing. Educational preparation at this level might be in occupational health nursing, in community health nursing, or as a nurse practitioner.

THE OCCUPATIONAL HEALTH TEAM

Community health nurses working in occupational health settings may be part of an occupational health team. In some small companies, the nurse is the only health professional employed by the company. In such instances, other health professionals interact with the nurse on a consultant basis. For example, the community health nurse might collaborate with an employee's private physician to plan for the employee's return to work after an illness or injury. In other instances, the company may contract with outside physicians for consultation services related to employee health needs.

Other companies have a well-developed occupational health team present within the facility. In addition to the community health nurse, such teams may include physicians, safety engineers, industrial hygienists, counselors, ancillary nursing personnel (for example, Licensed Practical Nurses), toxicologists, emergency medical technicians, physicians' assistants, epidemiologists, laboratory and X-ray technicians, safety coordinators, and nurse practitioners.[6] The functions and roles of most of these individuals will already be familiar to the reader. A few, however, may be unfamiliar. A safety engineer, for example, is responsible for monitoring the safety of the physical environment in the work setting, while the industrial hygienist has similar responsibilities for identifying and controlling physical, biological, and chemical hazards in the work setting.[7] Toxicologists may be involved in research on the toxic effects of chemical exposures in the work setting as well as contributing to plans for the control and treatment of such exposures.

THE EPIDEMIOLOGIC PREVENTION PROCESS MODEL AND CARE OF CLIENTS IN THE WORK SETTING

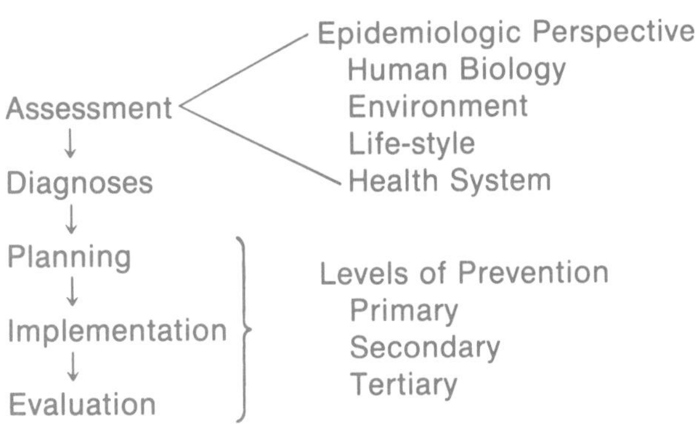

ASSESSING HEALTH NEEDS IN THE WORK SETTING

Assessment of employee health status and health needs is undertaken from the epidemiologic perspective of the epidemiologic prevention process model. Factors related to human biology, environment, life-style, and the health system are explored in light of their contribution to health or illness in the working population.

HUMAN BIOLOGY

Human biological factors to be addressed in assessing employee health status include those related to maturation and aging, genetic inheritance, and physiologic function.

Maturation and Aging

The age composition of a firm's work force will affect its health status. If employees are primarily young adults or adolescents, health conditions that may be noted with some frequency include sexually transmitted diseases, hepatitis, and pregnancy. If, on the other hand, the workers are middle-aged, problems such as heart attack and cancer are more likely to be common.

Genetic Inheritance

Genetic inheritance factors likely to be of greatest importance in the work force are those related to race and sex. For example, in a largely black labor force, problems of sickle cell disease and hypertension may be prevalent. In an Asian population, particularly if large numbers are refugees, communicable diseases such as tuberculosis and parasitic diseases may be common.

The sex composition of the employee population will also affect the types of health conditions seen. For instance, if large numbers of employees are women of childbearing age, there may be a need to provide prenatal or contraceptive services. There is also a need with this population to monitor more closely environmental conditions that may cause genetic changes or damage to an embryo.

Physiologic Function

The community health nurse in an occupational setting must be prepared to recognize and deal with the multitude of illnesses and injuries likely to be encountered in the workplace. While these will vary with the occupational setting, the National Institute for Occupational Safety and Health (NIOSH) has established a list of the 10 leading causes of work-related diseases and injuries in the United States (see Box 27–3). The list was derived from data related to the frequency of occurrence of problems, their severity, and their amenability to preventative efforts.

Community health nurses working in any occupational setting should be aware of the prevalence of these conditions and of the factors that influence the development of these problems. These contributing factors may be related to the work environment itself or to the personal behaviors of employees within and outside the workplace.

Of the common occupation-related conditions reviewed by NIOSH, 52 involve some form of occupational lung disease and include illnesses such as

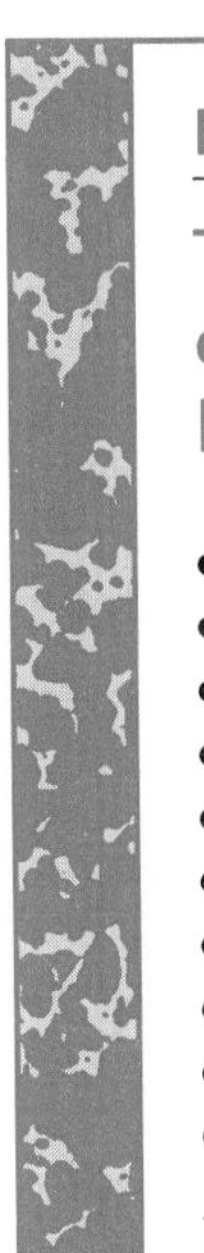

BOX 27–3

Ten Leading Causes of Occupational Illness and Injury

- Occupational lung diseases
- Musculoskeletal injuries
- Occupational cancers
- Severe traumatic injuries
- Cardiovascular disease
- Disorders of reproduction
- Neurotoxic disorders
- Noise-induced hearing loss
- Dermatologic conditions
- Psychological disorders

(Source: Monson[10])

silicosis, byssinosis (due to inhalation of cotton dust), asbestosis, and coal worker's pneumoconiosis. The effects of these conditions range from mild respiratory irritation to lung cancer and asphyxia.

Musculoskeletal injuries are the leading cause of lost workdays among American employees and include injuries due to the cumulative trauma of repetitive activities as well as acute trauma. Musculoskeletal injuries accounted for 57 percent of the total occupational injuries and illnesses reported in 1985.[8] One particular condition related to cumulative musculoskeletal injury that is of growing concern is carpal tunnel syndrome. This condition, characterized by pain, numbness, and tingling in the hand, is caused by compression of the median nerve where it passes under the carpal ligament as a result of swelling of tissues in the wrist. It is estimated that 47 percent of carpal tunnel syndrome cases are work-related and the proportion of employees affected has been reported as high as 15 percent in some types of occupations (for example, food processing, carpentry and other jobs that involve repetitive wrist movements).[9]

Several types of cancers are attributable to occupational influences.[10] Cancers that may result from occupational exposures include those of the bladder, blood, bone, larynx, liver, lung, nasal cavity and sinuses, peritoneum, pharynx, pleura, and skin (including scrotal malignancies). Occupational cancers may result from any of 61 substances and conditions currently identified by NIOSH.[11]

Serious traumatic injuries are those in which multiple injuries occur as a result of trauma, where musculoskeletal injuries are usually confined to localized areas. In 1987, 10 of every 100,000 workers were killed in occupational accidents and 1800 persons experienced severe disabling injuries.[12]

For the most part cardiovascular diseases (CVD) are influenced by personal risk factors of employees. However, evidence suggests that occupational factors may also contribute to the incidence of CVD.[13] Ten such factors have been identified in NIOSH recommendations for occupational health and safety and are included in Box 27–4.

With greater numbers of women working today, there is growing concern for the reproductive and social effects of working conditions. Thus far, 15 potentially hazardous substances or conditions have been identified by NIOSH as having effects on the reproductive system. While the primary concern is with the impact on the female reproductive system, evidence indicates that exposure to some of these conditions (for example, heat) can also affect the reproductive capabilities of men. Reproductive effects related to occupational conditions include infertility, spontaneous abortion, low birth weight, prematurity and postmaturity, birth defects, chromosomal abnormalities, childhood cancers such as leukemia and central nervous system tumors, and preeclampsia.[10]

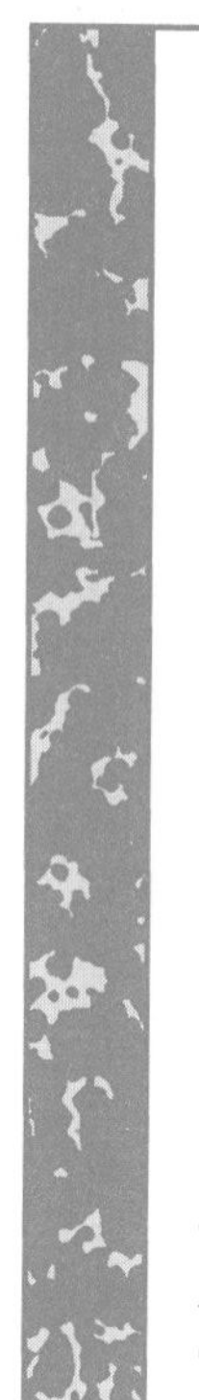

BOX 27–4

Occupational Factors Contributing to Cardiovascular Disease

- Exposure to metals
- Dust exposure
- Chemical inhalants (for example, carbon monoxide)
- Exposure to carbon disulfide
- Exposure to ethylene compounds
- Halogenated hydrocarbon exposures
- Exposure to nitroglycerin
- Exposure to nitrates
- Noise exposures
- Psychosocial stress

(Source: Leading work-related diseases and injuries[13])

Neurotoxic conditions are another of the 10 leading concerns in occupational health. Some of the conditions encountered include heavy metal poisonings, behavior changes related to chemical exposures, and difficulty concentrating and performing one's job. An estimated 850 substances found in various work settings are potentially neurotoxic.[14]

Noise-induced hearing loss is a serious problem both within and outside the occupational setting. According to the Occupational Safety and Health Administration (OSHA) over 9 million people in the United States have worked in areas where continuous noise-exposure levels exceed those at which hearing loss is possible. Approximately one-fourth of those exposed to high noise levels develop noticeable hearing impairment. During the years from 1978 to 1987, workers' compensation claims for this problem alone approached $835 million.[15]

With respect to dermatologic conditions arising from occupational factors, the nurse is again in a position to assess the health status of employees. As with other types of health problems, the nurse should be aware of outbreaks of dermatologic conditions that indicate the presence of hazards in the environment and a need for control measures. Conditions encountered include a variety of rashes, pruritus, chemical burns, and desquamation. NIOSH recommendations are available for 31 substances and conditions that result in dermatologic problems, and such problems account for more than 40 percent of reported work-related conditions. The annual cost to business and individual employees for medical care and lost work time resulting from these dermatologic problems is estimated at nearly $10 million.[16]

The occupational health problems discussed here are only a few of the many physical health problems likely to be encountered by the community health nurse working in an occupational setting. The occurrence of psychological health problems will be addressed in relation to the psychological environment. Each occupational setting will contain factors unique to that setting and that influence the health of employees. The nurse should be congnizant of the factors operating in any given place, their effects, and the appropriate measures of control.

Immunization is the final physiologic consideration in assessing health needs in the workplace. The nurse would assess the immunization status of employees, with special emphasis on groups of employees who may be at increased risk for certain diseases preventable by immunization. For example, employees who may be at risk for dirty injuries should be assessed for immunity to tetanus, while immunity to rubella should be assessed in women of childbearing age. Health-care workers, on the other hand, should be particularly assessed for immunity to hepatitis B.

ENVIRONMENT

Physical Environment

Physical environmental factors contribute to a variety of health problems encountered in the work setting. Categories of health hazards in the physical environment include chemical hazards, physical hazards (radiation, noise, vibration, and exposure to heat and cold), electrical hazards, fire, heavy lifting and uncomfortable working positions, and potential for falls.[17]

Poor lighting or high noise levels may adversely affect vision and hearing, respectively. Heavy objects that must be moved may cause musculoskeletal injuries. In addition, there is the potential for falls or exposure to excessive heat or cold in many workplaces.

The use of toxic substances in work performance is another source of possible health problems related to the physical environment. As noted earlier, a great number of toxic substances are present in the work environment that may result in respiratory, dermatologic, and other health problems. Of particular concern in this area is exposure to heavy metals (Table 27–1). The adverse effects of occupational exposure to lead, for example, have been known for over 2000 years.[18] Despite this knowledge and efforts to minimize occupational exposure to lead and other heavy metals, approximately 827,000 workers in the United States have the potential for work-related lead exposure,[19] and in many industries no mechanism is in place for biological monitoring of lead levels in employees with potential for exposure.[18] Other metals of concern include mercury, arsenic, and cadmium.[20] Exposure to lead and other metals occurs in a variety of occupations including those presented in Table 27–1.

Equipment may also constitute an occupational

TABLE 27–1. OCCUPATIONAL SOURCES AND HEALTH EFFECTS OF HEAVY METAL EXPOSURES

Metal	Occupational Sources	Health Effects
Antimony	Iron works, red dye manufacture	Irritation, cardiovascular and lung effects
Arsenic	Photographic equipment and supplies	Lung and lymphatic cancer, dermatitis
Cadmium	Soldering, battery manufacture, fuses, paint manufacture and painting, nuclear reactors	Lung cancer, prostatic cancer, renal system effects
Chromium	Steel manufacture, chrome plating, dye and paint manufacture, leather tanning	Lung cancer, skin ulcers, lung irradiation
Lead	Soldering, dispensing leaded gas, cable cutting and splicing; painting, casting or melting lead; radiator repair; welding, grinding, or sanding lead-painted surfaces; battery manufacture, construction, paper hanging, foundries, plumbing	Kidney, blood, and nervous system effects
Mercury	Metal foil and leaf application, industrial measurement instruments, gold and silver refining	Central nervous system and mental effects
Nickel	Nickel plating, steel manufacture, heating coils, hydrogenation processes	Lung and nasal cancer, skin effects
Tungsten	Steel manufacture, X-ray tubes	Lung and skin effects
Zinc oxide	White paint manufacture	Metal fume fever

health hazard. The use of heavy equipment or sharp tools can result in injury. There is also the potential for hand-arm vibration syndrome in the use of tools that vibrate or visual disturbance related to the use of computer display terminals. Another relatively recent physical hazard generated by widespread computer use is the potential for tendonitis and other similar conditions stemming from the use of word processors.

The nurse in the occupational setting will identify the presence of any hazards in the physical environment that contribute to health problems. In addition, the nurse will monitor the status of known hazards and their effects on the health of employees.

BOX 27–5

Indicators of Psychological Problems in Employees

- Increased absenteeism (especially on Mondays, Fridays, and the day after being paid)
- Mood changes or changes in relationships with others (especially health-care providers)
- Increased incidence of minor accidents on and off the job
- Fatigue, weakness, or a general decrease in energy
- Sudden weight loss or gain
- Increased blood pressure
- Frequent stress-related illnesses (for example, stomach distress, sore throat, chronic gastritis, headache, or other vaguely defined illnesses)
- Bloodshot or bleary eyes
- Facial petechiae (especially over the nose)
- Ulcer

(Adapted from Csiernik[22])

Psychological Environment

In assessing psychological environmental factors influencing the health of clients in the work setting the community health nurse would identify psychological health problems prevalent in the population and assess factors contributing to psychological problems. While compensation claims for other work-related disorders were decreasing, claims for "work-related neuroses" doubled during the years between 1980–1982 and account for approximately 11 percent of all occupational disease claims.[21] Psychological health problems may manifest in substance abuse, violence, psychiatric disorders such as psychoses and neuroses; somatic complaints such as ulcers or fatigue; or a general inability to cope. Some of the indicators of psychological health problems that the nurse might assess include increased absenteeism, poor interpersonal relationships, increased accident rates, complaints of fatigue, sudden weight loss or gain, or frequent illnesses.[22] Additional indicators of psychological problems are included in Box 27–5.

Occupational health nurses also need to be able to identify sources of stress in and out of the work setting that may contribute to the development of psychological health problems. Psychological stress is the tenth leading occupational disease. Employees particularly prone to work-related psychological stress include health-care and other service personnel, blue-collar workers, and those who work nights or who rotate shifts. Nurses who work with these groups should be particularly aware of the potential for stress-related illnesses.

Other sources of stress in the work setting include work overload, the organizational structure of the company, job insecurity, and interpersonal relationships with co-workers or supervisors.[17] Stress may also be created by sexist or racist attitudes of others in the workplace. Perceptions of the source of occupational stress may differ greatly between employees and employers. Sources of stress most frequently identified by workers include, for example, lack of control over the content, process and pace of one's work; unrealistic demands and lack of understanding by supervisors; lack of predictability and security regarding one's job future; and the cumulative effects of occupational and family stressors. Employers, on the other hand, most often perceive employees' life-styles and health habits as the primary contributors to stress.[23]

Social Environment

The social environment of the work setting can influence employee health status either positively or negatively. The quality of social interactions among employees, attitudes to work and health, and the presence or absence of racial or other tensions can all affect health status as well as employee productivity.

Four spheres of influence in the workplace social environment may affect the health status of individual employees, and the effects of each sphere on health should be assessed by the community health nurse in the occupational health setting. The first sphere of influence involves the health-related behaviors of employees themselves and will be addressed in the discussion of life-style factors affecting health. The other three spheres are more directly part of the social environment of the work setting.

The second sphere of influence on health in the workplace occurs among groups of co-workers, and the community health nurse should assess the influence of co-worker groups on the health of individual employees and on the group as a whole. A group of co-workers may decide, for example, that they do not wish to be exposed to smoke in their work area. This decision can lead to formal or informal bans on smoking in certain areas. Formal bans may occur when groups of employees request no-smoking policies from company management. When this is not the case, work groups may enforce the decision informally by exerting peer pressure on the smokers in the group. In other words, they can make life unpleasant for those who wish to smoke by ostracizing them or using other social sanctions.

The third sphere of influence is the management sphere. The nurse would assess management's attitudes to health and health-related policies and the effects of these policies (or the lack of them) on employee health. For example, management may decide on and enforce a no-smoking policy throughout the company, whether or not employees favor such a policy. Management makes other kinds of policy decisions that affect employee health. For instance, the type of health-care coverage provided to employees is a management decision. Or, a policy that provides "well leave" or extra vacation for those who have not taken sick leave may prompt employee efforts to promote health and prevent illness.

The last sphere of influence involves legal, social, and political action that influences the health of employees. A prime example of this is the regulation of conditions in the work setting by agencies such as the Occupational Safety and Health Administration (OSHA). Through legislation, society can mandate that business and industry create specific conditions that enhance the health of employees. Another example of such a mandate is legislation that companies over a certain size must offer employees a health maintenance organization (HMO) as one option for health insurance coverage. In assessing health needs in the work setting, the community health nurse would examine the extent to which the employer adheres to legislative and regulatory standards and the effect of these standards in promoting employee health.

Unfortunately, regulations promulgated by OSHA are not as effective in promoting and protecting employee health as one might wish. One reason for this lack of efficacy is the fact that OSHA tends to focus on the industrial sector while attention is also needed in other occupational sectors.[7] Other difficulties in realizing the aims of OSHA include exclusion of certain types of industries from complying with industry standards; and changes in OSHA exposure levels once considered safe but with further research have been shown to exceed levels now known to cause adverse health effects.

In addition, regulations are not uniformly enforced.[18] For example, in one study in California, less than 3 percent of facilities with potential for employee exposure to lead had instituted environmental monitoring systems and less than 2 percent had initiated biological monitoring of employees at risk for exposure.[24] In another study, only 18 percent of companies in the manufacturing sector with reported cases of elevated blood lead levels in employees were investigated by OSHA and about 1 percent of companies outside of the manufacturing sector were investigated.[20] Finally, regulatory policies within OSHA are frequently inconsistent. For example, four OSHA policies related to carcinogens in the work setting display marked inconsistencies with each other.[25]

LIFE-STYLE

As noted above, life-style factors exemplified in individual decisions about health-related behaviors comprise the first sphere of social influence on employee health. Life-style factors to be considered here include the type of work performed, consumption patterns, patterns of rest and exercise, and use of safety devices.

Type of Work Performed

The type of work performed by an individual within a company can significantly influence the employee's health. The type of work performed will determine the risk of exposure to various physical hazards and level of stress experienced. For example, factory workers in industries using lead may run the risk of lead poisoning, while executives in the same companies may be exposed to more stress.

The type of work done will also influence the extent of exercise that employees obtain. Construction workers, for example, have ample opportunities for physical activity but also risk serious injury in the use of heavy equipment. Bank tellers, on the other hand, are at risk for cardiovascular and other diseases related to a sedentary life-style.

The community health nurse in an occupational setting will be conversant with the variety of jobs performed in that setting. The nurse will also be aware of the health hazards posed by each type of work performed and will be alert to signs of health problems deriving from the work itself.

Another aspect of the type of work performed is that of ***ergonomics,*** the degree of fit between the employee and the job performed. The nurse should assess the degree to which employees are qualified to perform their particular job function and their interest in that job. Employees who work at jobs that do not interest them, that are beyond their capabilities, or that do not provide sufficient challenge may be at greater risk for both emotional and physical health problems than those who are better suited to their jobs.

Consumption Patterns

Consumption patterns of interest to the occupational health nurse include those related to food and nutrition, smoking, and drug and alcohol use. The influence of nutrition on health is well established, and the occupational health nurse will assess the nutritional patterns of employees with whom he or she works. In addition, the nurse will assess how the work environment affects eating habits. For example, there may not be sufficient opportunity provided for employees to eat despite OSHA regulations regarding time and place for breaks and meals.

The nurse would also determine whether there is food service available to employees. If there is an employee cafeteria, the nurse may need to assess the nutritional quality of the food provided. If there are no food services available in the workplace, the nurse would determine whether they are available nearby, or whether adequate storage facilities exist for employees who bring meals from home.

Smoking is another consumption pattern of concern to the occupational health nurse. Smoking is harmful to health in and of itself. In addition, smoking may increase the adverse effects of other environmental hazards in the work setting, particularly those that affect respiration. Many employers have recently begun to prohibit smoking except in carefully controlled areas in the workplace and have been active in promoting programs to help employees quit smoking. The nurse would assess the extent of smoking in the employee population as well as the specific implications of smoking in that particular environment.

As noted earlier, employees may have problems with substance abuse. The prevalence of these problems should be monitored and the nurse should be alert to signs and symptoms of substance abuse in the employee population. Overindulgence in other substances, such as caffeine, may also pose a health hazard to employees.

Rest and Exercise

Work puts many physical and psychological demands on people. Sometimes these demands result in inadequate rest and recreation as with the executive who works constantly, or the blue-collar worker who holds two jobs in an attempt to make ends meet. Conversely, work may also lead to too much sitting and too little exercise.

The nurse in the work setting will assess the amount of activity engaged in by employees and the balance between rest and exercise. This individual will also obtain information on the types of recreation used by employees and any potential health hazards posed by recreational choices.

Many companies are recognizing the benefits of exercise in terms of both the physical and psychological health of employees. These companies are promoting physical exercise and may even provide facilities for exercise and recreation in the workplace. If this is the case, the nurse should be alert to potential health hazards and the potential for too much exercise. For example, if there is a company pool, the epileptic employee who swims to relieve tension should be cautioned against swimming alone. Similarly, the overweight executive should engage in physical activity cautiously to lessen the risk of heart attack or injury.

Use of Safety Devices

A last life-style factor that is particularly relevant to health in the occupational setting is the use or nonuse of safety devices. Physical hazards present in the workplace frequently can be mitigated by the use of appropriate safety devices. However, this can only occur if employees use these devices consistently and appropriately. Emphasis on the use of safety devices in the work setting is more pronounced today than in the past. For example, as of 1985, some 85 percent of American businesses required or recommended the use of some type of protective device compared to only 74 percent in previous years.[16]

The community health nurse would identify the need for safety devices and would also monitor the extent to which they are used. For example, do individuals working in high noise areas wear earplugs? Are those earplugs correctly fitted? Do people involved in heavy lifting wear weight belts or do they ignore the potential for injury? Are heavy shoes or gloves worn in areas with dangerous equipment?

HEALTH SYSTEM

Health system factors influencing employee health relate to both external and internal health-care systems. The external system reflects the availability and accessibility of health-care services outside the workplace, whereas the internal system is comprised of those services offered within the workplace.

The External System

In assessing employee health status, the community health nurse in the occupational setting will gather information about the use of health services in the community at large. The nurse will examine the type of services used and the reasons for and appropriateness of their use. The nurse will also assess the availability of services needed by company employees in the external health-care system.

One of the work-related factors influencing use of outside health services is the availability of insurance coverage. Health insurance is an employment benefit for many, but large segments of the working population still do not have health insurance coverage. Many of these uninsured workers do not have sufficient income to afford health insurance themselves or out-of-pocket health-care expenses. The occupational health nurse will become familiar with the insurance status of employees in his or hei company and with the kinds of benefits covered under group policies where they exist.

The Internal System

The internal health-care system is comprised of those health services and programs provided to employees in the work setting. Four general types of occupational health programs can be found in business and industry.[26] These include programs aimed at controlling exposure to toxic substances; those emphasizing health-promotion policies in the workplace; those focusing on limited health-promotion efforts; and comprehensive programs that attempt to meet a variety of employee health needs.

Programs to Control Toxic Exposures. Programs to control or eliminate toxic substances and other hazardous conditions in the workplace usually occur in response to Occupational Safety and Health Administration (OSHA) regulations. Control programs may involve engineering controls, use of safety equipment or devices, or elimination of toxic substances from the work environment. In industries with this type of program, the community health nurse should assess the efficacy of these control measures and the extent to which they are adhered to in the setting.

Health-Promotion Policies. The second type of program involves policies that are initiated by employers to keep health-care expenditures to a minimum. These policies seek to limit hospitalization and expenses for acute-care services by promoting the health of the employee population and by encouraging a less expensive approach to providing services. For example, employers may have policies related to the need for a second opinion before covering employee expenses for elective surgery or encouraging home care rather than hospitalization whenever possible. In this type of an occupational health program, the community health nurse would assess the effect of these and similar policies on the health of the employee population.

Limited Health-Promotion Programs. The third type of program provides a limited approach to health promotion. Generally, these programs focus on one aspect of health care and may make use of prepackaged health-promotion and education programs that do not meet the specific needs of the employee group. These programs also tend to be illness-oriented rather than to focus on the promotion of overall health. For example, there may be emphasis on education for good body mechanics to prevent injuries or first aid for injuries, but little attention to overall health promotion. These programs also focus on the individual employee's responsibility for his or her health and may neglect conditions within the work setting that create health problems. In this type of a system, the community health nurse would identify the type of health-promotion programs provided and the extent to which they meet employees' identified health needs.

Comprehensive Programs. The fourth type of occupational health program is a comprehensive approach to health care. These programs educate employees so as to promote health and prevent illness, but they also emphasize organizational programs, policies, and environmental changes that are conducive to health. For example, a company with a comprehensive health-care approach might provide educational sessions on stress management *and* engage in organizational changes aimed at reducing the amount of stress engendered by the work setting. Again, the nurse assessing the influence of health system factors on employees' health would determine the extent to which the designated program meets employees' health needs.

Family Care. In some work settings, comprehensive health-care programs go beyond the provision of care to employees to include some form of direct care for family members. Employees who are concerned about their families may be less productive than they would be were their family situation less stressful. As more and more families are supported by two wage earners, employment of both husband and wife has implications for the life of the family and the well-being of children. Community health nurses who care for clients in the work setting should be aware of the stresses involved in dual-career (or single-parent) families and how work schedules and conditions may affect the health of the family. Work schedules that allow for outside responsibilities and family life are very helpful, and the nurse may be able to influence management in the creation of flexible scheduling systems. The nurse may also be of assistance in helping employees deal with the stress of role overload.

Some companies are becoming more aware of the interplay of family influences and occupational factors in employee performance and are establishing systems designed to assist families. One recent effort is the establishment of child-care centers in company premises. Some centers provide care whether the child is well or ill. In such cases, the community health nurse working in this setting may assume responsibilities relative to the health of the children in the centers. These nurses will need to be versed in pediatric as well as adult health care.

Even in occupational settings where there are no child-care facilities, nurses are asked for assistance in dealing with health problems of family members. The nurse may counsel the employee regarding resolution of family problems or may provide referrals to outside sources of assistance that can be found in Chapter 20, Care of Children.

The last aspect of the occupational health nurse's role in the care of employees' families deals with the concept of paraoccupational exposures to hazardous substances. ***Paraoccupational exposure*** occurs when employees are exposed to hazardous substances and in turn expose their families (usually via contaminated clothing). For example, in one industry a man involved in making lead belt buckles was found to have blood lead levels five times the normal. When family members were examined, all three of his children were found to have elevated blood lead levels.[27] Because lead poisoning has even more serious consequences for children than for adults, paraoccupational exposure to lead can be very harmful.

Nurses who have knowledge of problems experienced by members of employees' families are in a position to recognize paraoccupational exposure and to take action to correct such exposure. Nurses should be aware of the potential for such exposures and should make it a practice to ask employees questions designed to elicit information about family exposure to hazardous substances.

Factors related to human biology, environment, life-style, and internal and external health systems can influence the health status of clients in the work setting. These epidemiologic factors are summarized in Box 27–6.

DIAGNOSTIC REASONING AND HEALTH NEEDS IN THE WORK SETTING

Community health nurses working in occupational settings derive nursing diagnoses from assessment information related to individuals or groups of employees. For example, the nurse might make a diagnosis of "inability to sleep due to work pressures" for a company executive or diagnose "poor employee morale due to increased tension and stress in the work setting." Other nursing diagnoses related to individual employees might include a "need for referral for counseling due to heavy drinking" or "moderate hearing loss due to failure to use hearing protection in high-noise areas." Additional nursing diagnoses at the group level might include a "potential for exposure to hepatitis B due to frequent contact with blood" for a group of laboratory technicians in a hospital or the "potential for falls due to work in elevated areas" for a group of construction workers.

PLANNING NURSING INTERVENTIONS IN THE WORK SETTING

Interventions may be developed by the occupational health nurse alone or in conjunction with others in the work setting to address the health needs identified. In the case of individual clients, interventions would be tailored to individual needs and circumstances. When identified health problems affect groups of employees, planned interventions are likely to be more involved. Planning to meet the needs of groups in the workplace will employ the principles of health programming discussed in Chapter 19, Care of the Community or Target Group.

Whether the client is an individual, a group of employees, or the total population in the work setting, interventions may be planned at primary, secondary, and tertiary levels of prevention.

PRIMARY PREVENTION

As in other settings, primary prevention in the occupational setting is directed toward preventing the occurrence of health problems. This is accomplished

BOX 27–6

Epidemiologic Factors Influencing Employee Health

Human Biology
- Age, race, and sex composition of employee population
- Presence or absence of other health conditions
- Immunization status

Environment

Physical environment
- Presence of safety hazards in equipment and tools
- Potential for exposure to toxic substances
- Potential for exposure to vibration
- Potential for exposure to temperature extremes
- Potential for exposure to radiation
- Potential for exposure to noise
- Poor lighting or ventilation
- Potential for falls

Psychological environment
- Evidence of psychological problems in employees
- Stress levels in the work setting and outside
- Relationships among employees and with management

Social environment
- Influence of co-worker group on health behavior
- Influence of management on health behavior
- Influence of society on working conditions
- Attitudes to work and health
- Presence of intergroup or intragroup tensions

Life-style
- Type of work performed
- Consumption patterns related to food, alcohol, and drugs
- Rest and exercise patterns
- Use of safety devices

Health System

External system
- Availability of health-care services
- Extent of health insurance coverage

Internal system
- Type of health services provided in the work setting
- Availability of family care

through planning activities related to health promotion, illness prevention, and prevention of injury.

Health Promotion

Community health nurses in occupational settings educate employees to lead healthier lives. Planned interventions might include education on healthy nutrition, stress management, or exercise. Occupational health nurses may also work to influence the types of food provided in employee dining areas or to initiate no-smoking policies throughout the company.

Nurses also work with clients on a one-to-one basis to promote health. Development of exercise regimens for employees and education on coping strategies are two examples of the occupational health nurse's health-promotion efforts directed at individual clients.

Another avenue for health promotion is providing prenatal care to pregnant workers. This could involve referral for prenatal care if this service is not provided by the company health facility. The nurse might also monitor the employee for signs and symptoms of complications of pregnancy. The nurse may find it necessary to function as an advocate for the employee who needs to be relieved of some of her duties as the pregnancy progresses. For example, it may be necessary to move the employee to another position that does not require heavy lifting. The nurse may also be involved in childbirth education for pregnant employees or male employees and their spouses.

Illness Prevention

Preventing illness is the second aspect of primary prevention in the workplace. Illness prevention can involve either employee education or prevention of specific illness through immunization. For example, some industries routinely offer employees influenza immunization to cut down on illness-related absenteeism.

Another aspect of illness prevention involves modifying risk factors. **Risk factors** are personal or group characteristics that predispose one to develop a specific health problem. For example, it is well known that smoking increases one's risk of developing heart disease and lung cancer, so smoking is a risk factor for both of these problems.

Some risk factors can be modified or eliminated, thus decreasing one's chances of developing specific health problems. Again, using smoking as an example, people who quit smoking lower their risk of developing lung cancer. Occupational health nurses can be instrumental in assisting employees to modify risk factors, helping them to prevent health problems. Some risk factors that receive particular attention in the occupational setting are smoking, elevated blood pressure, sedentary life-style, stress, and being overweight.

Occupational health nurses can work on risk-factor modification with individuals or groups of employees. They can also engage in risk-factor modification efforts at the company level. One example of this would be efforts to convince company policymakers that a no-smoking policy should be instituted and enforced within the workplace. Nurses can also develop weight standards for job categories in which being overweight is particularly hazardous.

At the individual level, the nurse can counsel employees regarding the hazards of smoking, particularly in conjunction with occupational exposure to respiratory irritants. They can also provide assistance to individuals who wish to quit smoking.

Restructuring the work environment can help in minimizing occupational stress as a risk factor for health problems. Efforts in this direction include developing flexible scheduling plans to minimize conflicts with employees' outside responsibilities. The nurse can also facilitate employee input into work-related decisions and strive to minimize role overload and role ambiguity. The nurse can also promote opportunity for social interaction, job security, and career development.

As is obvious, most of these efforts must be undertaken by management, but the nurse can provide management with evidence of related research and can provide the impetus for change in these areas. At the individual level, the occupational health nurse can be aware of the stressors experienced by employees in various jobs in the work setting. The nurse is also in a position to monitor the effects of stress on the individual employee and to counsel employees in stress management.

Injury Prevention

Injury prevention may again entail employee education in a variety of areas. Employees will need to be acquainted with safety procedures to prevent accidents. There may also be a need to educate employees in the correct use of safety equipment. For example, individuals working in some areas should wear protective clothing or use breathing apparatus. The nurse should explain the need for safety equipment and be responsible for monitoring its use. This may entail planning periodic visits to certain areas of the workplace to determine whether employees are indeed using safety equipment as directed.

Employees may also be in need of education in other areas related to injury prevention. Handling of hazardous substances, proper use of machinery, need for fluid replacement in high heat areas, and good body mechanics are all educational topics that may be appropriate in certain industrial settings. Nurses may also provide education on first aid and cardiopulmonary resuscitation.

One aspect of injury prevention in which the nurse may be involved is monitoring hazardous conditions in the workplace. The nurse should be aware of potential hazards and their appropriate management. In the absence of an industrial hygienist, the nurse may plan and conduct environmental testing to detect hazardous levels of chemicals, heat, or noise.

The nurse may need to acquaint management regarding the occurrence of injuries due to hazardous conditions and advocate changes designed to protect employees from injuries. Recommendations for dealing with the problem of noise-induced hearing loss include engineering efforts to minimize noise production, use of properly fitted hearing-protection devices, education of employees and managers in the use of protective devices and their importance, and periodic audiometric screening. The occupational health nurse may be actively involved in planning and executing the majority of these recommended activities particularly in screening for hearing loss, fitting protective devices, and educating employees and supervisors. Control of noise-related hearing loss requires commitment on the part of employees and management to the proper use of protective devices. Motivating employees to use these devices and monitoring their use are crucial functions of the occupational health nurse.

Primary prevention in the occupational health setting focuses on health promotion, illness preven-

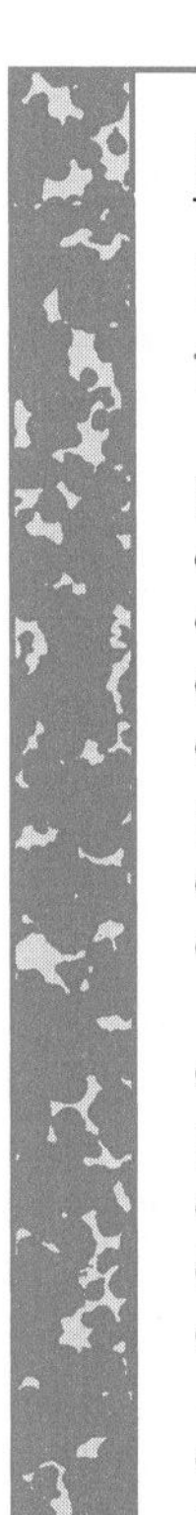

BOX 27–7

Primary Prevention in the Work Setting

Health promotion
- Health education
- Good nutrition
- Rest and exercise
- Prenatal care for pregnant employees

Illness prevention
- Immunization
- Modification or elimination of risk factors
- Stress reduction and management

Injury prevention
- Safety education
- Use of safety devices
- Safe handling of hazardous substances
- Elimination of safety hazards
- Good body mechanics

tion, and prevention of injury. Various aspects of these three foci are summarized in Box 27–7.

SECONDARY PREVENTION

Secondary prevention in the work setting is aimed at recognizing and resolving existing health problems. General areas of involvement for occupational health nurses include screening, treatment for existing conditions, and emergency care.

Screening

Screening activities can take any of three directions. Screening efforts begin with pre-employment assessment of potential employees. Screening may also be conducted at periodic intervals to monitor employee health status. Finally, the work environment may be screened periodically for the presence or absence of hazardous conditions. The community health nurse would be involved in planning and implementing screening efforts at all three of these levels.

Pre-employment Screening. For many employees, their first interaction with an occupational health nurse is the pre-employment screening examination. The purpose of this initial screening is to facilitate employee selection and placement. Hiring an employee for a particular job is in part dependent on his or her physical, mental, and emotional capabilities for performing that job. These capabilities can be determined in an initial screening exam. At this time the nurse will usually obtain a complete health history from the employee and conduct a battery of routine screening tests. Nurse practitioners in the occupational setting may also conduct the physical examination.

Based on the information derived from the screening, the nurse may make determinations regarding the person's employability in a particular capacity. To make such determinations, the nurse must be familiar with the type of activities involved and stressors encountered in a particular job. The pre-employment screening also provides baseline data for determining the effects of working conditions on the health of employees.

Periodic Screening. The nurse in the occupational setting would also plan periodic screening activities to monitor employees' continuing health status. This is particularly true of employees working under hazardous conditions. For example, monitoring devices are used by personnel working with radiation and are periodically checked for exposure limits. Likewise, blood chemistries may be done at periodic intervals to test for exposure to toxic substances. Periodic blood pressure screenings and pulmonary function tests may also be warranted. In some occupational groups such as the armed forces, employees are routinely screened for overweight and for physical capacity.

The types of screening done will depend on the type of job performed, the risks involved, and the capabilities required. Some screenings are routinely performed on all employees in a particular setting. For example, employees may receive a routine physical examination at periodic intervals. Other screening tests are performed only on specific employees. For instance, lead screening may be done routinely on individuals who work in the company plant, but not on clerical personnel.

Occupational health nurses are frequently responsible for conducting these and other screening tests on employees. They may also interpret test results, explain them to employees, and take action when warranted by positive test results.

Environmental Screening. Periodic screening of the environment may also be warranted and, in the absence of industrial hygienists or safety engineers, the nurse may be responsible for planning and conducting environmental screenings. For example, the nurse may plan to measure noise levels in various work areas at specific intervals to determine areas in which hearing protection is required. Similarly, measurements of volatile chemicals or radiation might be done in high-risk areas.

Treating Existing Conditions

The second aspect of secondary prevention is the diagnosis and treatment of existing health problems. Community health nurses will be actively involved in planning health interventions for individual employees and should also participate in planning health programs to meet the needs of groups of clients.

Many industries go beyond treating only job-related illness and conditions to treating a variety of major and minor conditions. The rationale for the extension of services to non-job-related conditions is that any health problem, physical or emotional, can serve to impair the employee's performance. Also, treatment of these conditions within the work setting itself limits time lost in pursuing outside treatment, saving the company money in the long run.

Depending upon the capabilities of the occupational health unit, employees with existing health problems may be referred to the external health-care system for problem resolution. Or, treatment may be provided within the workplace itself. Those occupational health nurses who are nurse practitioners may treat illness in the work setting. Even those nurses who are not nurse practitioners may treat minor conditions on the basis of protocols established in conjunction with medical consultation.

Occupational health nurses will also need to plan to monitor the effectiveness of therapy, whether or not that therapy is provided by the occupational health unit. For example, an employee with hypertension might be followed by his or her private physician, but the occupational health nurse will monitor medication compliance and effects on the employee's blood pressure. In addition, the nurse will educate the employee regarding the condition and its treatment.

In the case of employees with problems related to substance abuse or stress, the community health nurse would usually plan a referral to an appropriate source of assistance. The nurse may also need to function as an advocate for impaired employees, encouraging employers to provide coverage for treatment for psychological as well as physical illness. Nurses may also find it necessary to report conditions of abuse to supervisory personnel when either the health or the safety of other employees is threatened.

Community health nurses in occupational settings may also be involved in planning and implementing employee assistance programs (EAPs) for employees with psychological problems. An ***employee assistance program*** is a program within the occupational setting designed to counsel employees with psychological problems and assist them in dealing with those problems. Employee assistance programs usually focus on motivating individuals to seek help and on referring the person for needed services.

The nurse can plan to motivate the employee to get help through seven feedback steps performed in sequence until the employee (client) is willing to seek assistance.[22] In the first step, the nurse discusses with the client (employee) his or her observations of the client's behavior or appearance that indicate the existence of a problem. In the second step, the nurse would comment on several instances of the client's behavior that suggest a psychological problem, making connections between discrete behavioral events to show the employee a definite pattern in his or her behavior. In the third step, the nurse would ask the employee to explain the causes for the observed signs and symptoms. Interpreting possible causes for behavior is the fourth feedback step in motivating employees with psychological problems to take action. The fifth step is to provide suggestions for change that would eliminate or modify factors contributing to the problem. If the employee has not decided to take action by this point, the nurse may need to provide a warning on the progressive nature of most psychological problems and on possible consequences if no action is taken. Finally, the nurse may strongly recommend action to correct the problem. The choice of whether or not to take action, however, remains with the employee (client).

Once the individual is motivated to seek help for the problem, the nurse can make a referral to counselors within the organization or on the outside. In addition to planning the referral, the nurse should plan activities to support and encourage the employee and to monitor his or her progress in resolving problems. Finally, the community health nurse should plan interventions that will help reintegrate the employee into the work setting if an extended absence has been necessary.

Emergency Response

Another aspect of secondary prevention in the work setting is response to emergency situations. Nurses may find themselves dealing with both physical and psychological emergencies and should have a basic plan for dealing with various types of emergencies that may arise. Physical emergencies may result from serious accidents or from physical conditions such as heart attack, stroke, seizure disorder, or insulin reaction. Traumatic injuries in the occupational setting are often fatal. The period between 1980 and 1984 saw a crude death rate for occupational trauma fatalities of 8.8 per 100,000 employees. Approximately 7000 fatalities occurred annually in each of the 50 states and the District of Columbia.[28] Again, appropriate treatment for such emergencies will usually be based on established protocols.

With respect to emergencies due to illnesses, it is helpful if the nurse has prior information related to the employee's condition. For example, if the nurse has prior knowledge that the client is diabetic, the diagnosis of hypoglycemic reaction will be reached and treatment initiated more rapidly than would otherwise be the case. For this reason, occupational health nurses should be well acquainted with employees' health histories.

Psychological emergencies may result in homocide, suicide, or both. Of the occupational fatalities occurring each year, 13 percent are classified as occupational homicide and almost 3 percent constitute occupational suicides.[28] While businesses may have generalized protocols for dealing with such emergencies as threatened homocide or suicide, the nurse faced with such situations will probably need to exercise a great deal of creativity in planning to address a psychological emergency. General considerations include remaining calm and removing others from the immediate vicinity. The nurse *should not* plan any heroic measures that may endanger oneself, the employee, or others. Additional interventions will need to be dictated by the situation. Again, prior identification of employees under excessive stress may help to prevent psychiatric emergencies.

One further type of emergency that requires an occupational health nursing response is the emergency that affects large numbers of people. Examples of mass emergencies include fires or explosions, radiation exposure, or hazardous substance leaks. In addition to providing treatment for those injured in such emergencies, the nurse may be responsible for assisting in evaluating affected areas and in organizing to provide needed care. Occupational health nurses should be involved in planning for the overall company response to such situations as well as planning for health care in such an eventuality. The role of the nurse in disaster preparedness will be discussed in greater detail in Chapter 29, Care of Clients in Disaster Settings. Considerations in secondary prevention in the work setting are summarized in Box 27–8.

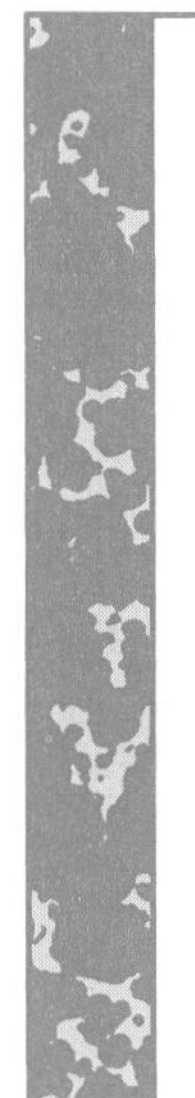

BOX 27–8

Secondary Prevention in the Work Setting

Screening
- Pre-employment screening
- Periodic screening of employees at risk for health problems
- Environmental screening

Treatment of existing conditions

Emergency response
- Physical emergencies
- Psychological emergencies
- Occupational disasters

TERTIARY PREVENTION

Tertiary prevention in the work setting is directed toward preventing a recurrence of health problems and limiting their consequences. The type of tertiary intervention measures employed will depend on the problems to be prevented. In many instances, primary prevention measures, which would be used to prevent a problem from occurring in the first place, can also be used as tertiary prevention to prevent its recurrence. For example, engineering measures may be used to prevent leakage of a toxic chemical or to prevent subsequent leaks if one has already occurred.

Generally speaking, tertiary prevention will be geared toward preventing the spread of communicable diseases, preventing recurrence of other acute conditions, and preventing complications of chronic conditions. Sick-leave policies and employee immunization are examples of tertiary preventative measures that might be taken to stop the spread of influenza in the employee population. By encouraging employees to take advantage of sick-leave benefits when they or family members are ill, the nurse can minimize exposure of others in the occupational set-

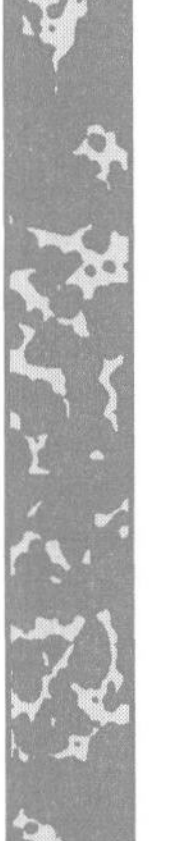

BOX 27–9

Tertiary Prevention in the Work Setting

Preventing the spread of communicable diseases
- Immunization
- Sick leave for ill employees

Preventing the recurrence of other acute conditions

Preventing complications of chronic conditions

TABLE 27–2. RESOURCES FOR NURSES IN OCCUPATIONAL HEALTH SETTINGS

Focus	Agency or Organization	Services
Disease prevention	National High Blood Pressure Education Program 120/80 National Institutes of Health Bethesda, MD 20014	Literature on control of high blood pressure in work settings
Health promotion	American Association of Fitness Directors in Business and Industry 400 6th St., SW Washington, DC 20201	Information on health promotion and fitness
	American College of Preventive Medicine 1015 15th St. NW, Suite 403 Washington, DC 20005	Information on health-promotion programs
	American Physical Fitness Research Institute 654 N. Sepulveda Blvd. Los Angeles, CA 90049 (213) 476-6241	Public education on fitness and health promotion
	Health Education Foundation 600 New Hampshire Ave, NW Suite 425 Washington, DC 20037 (202) 338-3501	Health-education programs for business and industry
	National Center for Health Education 30 E. 29th St. New York, NY 10016	Health-promotion programs in the workplace
	National Health Information Clearinghouse P.O. Box 1133 Washington, DC 20013	Information on federal resources on health issues
	Occupational Health Institute 2340 S. Arlington Heights Rd. Arlington Heights, IL 60005 (312) 228-6850	Assistance in developing and maintaining occupational health programs
	President's Council on Fitness and Sports 400 6th St., SW, Room 3030 Washington, DC 20201	Public information
	U.S. Department of Health and Human Services Office of Health Information and Health Promotion Washington, DC 20203	Health-promotion information
Mental health	American Institute of Stress 124 Park Ave. Yonkers, NY 10703 (914) 963-1200	Information
	National Clearinghouse for Mental Health National Institute of Mental Health Room 11A33 Parklawn Bldg. 5600 Fisher's Lane Rockville, MD 20857	Video series on stress management in the workplace
	The Other Victims of Alcoholism P.O. Box 921 Radio City Station New York, NY 10101 (212) 247-8087	Information on the effect of alcoholism on families and industry, advocacy
	Western Center for Behavioral and Preventive Medicine 208-125 East 13th St. North Vancouver, BC V7L2L3 Canada	Literature on stress management

TABLE 27–2. (*Continued*)

Focus	Agency or Organization	Services
Safety	American Industrial Health Council 1330 Connecticut Ave., NW Washington, DC 20036 (202) 659-0060	Advocacy, identification of industrial carcinogens
	National Institute of Occupational Health and Safety Division of Technical Services Public Dissemination 4676 Columbia Parkway Cincinnati, OH 45226	Technical information on toxins and safety hazards
	Public Citizen's, Inc. Health Research Group 2000 P St., NW, Suite 708 Washington, DC 20036 (202) 872-0320	Information on toxic substances, food, drugs, and occupational safety
	Toxic Project Clearinghouse Environmental Action Foundation 724 Dupont Circle Bldg. Washington, DC 20036	Information on toxic substances and exposure
	National Safety Council 444 N. Michigan Ave. Chicago, IL 60611	Public information on occupational safety
Other	American Association of Occupational Health Nurses 50 Lennox Pointe Atlanta, GA 30324 (404) 262-1162	Information on occupational health nursing and certification
	International Commission on Occupational Health 10, Avenue Jules Crosnier CH 1206 Geneva, Switzerland	Public education
	Just One Break 373 Park Avenue South New York, NY 10016 (212) 725-2500	Consultation to industry in job placement for the disabled
	National Institute for Occupational Safety and Health 1600 Clifton Rd. Atlanta, GA 30333 (404) 329-3771	Research
	U.S. Department of Labor Occupational Safety and Health Administration Publications, Room N-3423 200 Constitution Ave., NW Washington, DC 20210 (202) 523-7162	Employee complaints, establish standards, public information
	U.S. House of Representatives Committee on Education and Labor Subcommittee on Health and Safety B 345-A Rayburn House Office Bldg. Washington, DC 20515	Policy formation
	U.S. Senate Committee on Appropriations Subcommittee on Labor, Health and Human Services, Education and Related Agencies SD-186 Dirksen Senate Office Bldg. Washington, DC 20510 (202) 224-7283	Policy formation
	Women's Occupational Health Resource Center 117 St. John's Place Brooklyn, NY 11217 (718) 230-8822	Education on occupational hazards for women, advocacy

ting to communicable diseases and can control the spread of disease. Safety education might prevent a recurrence of accidental injuries due to hazardous equipment, and use of hearing protection might prevent further deterioration of an employee's hearing after noise exposure has already caused some damage. Similarly, treatment of an employee's hypertension can prevent further health problems. These three foci of tertiary prevention in the work setting are summarized in Box 27–9.

Community health nursing involvement in occupational health may entail primary, secondary, or tertiary prevention activities. Whatever the level of prevention, the nurse may experience a need for assistance with information or other services. Some sources of assistance for nurses working in occupational health settings are presented in Table 27–2.

IMPLEMENTING HEALTH CARE IN THE WORK SETTING

Implementing nursing interventions in the work setting frequently involves collaboration with others. Most often, collaboration occurs between the nurse and the employee. In other instances, the nurse may collaborate with health-care providers and others within or outside of the occupational setting. For example, the nurse might collaborate with a pregnant employee's private physician to monitor her progress throughout the pregnancy. Implementing the plan of care for an employee with carpal tunnel syndrome might involve collaboration with the physician and with a supervisor to facilitate movement to a job that does not necessitate repetitive wrist movements.

When health problems affect groups of employees, implementing the plan of care might involve collaboration with other health-care providers and with company management and other personnel. For example, the nurse who has documented an increased incidence of respiratory conditions due to aerosol exposures will advocate plans to resolve the problem. These plans will need to be approved by management and implemented by engineering personnel, if engineering controls are required, or by company purchasing agents if special respiratory protective devices are needed. In the latter instance, the nurse may be involved in determining the type of protective devices needed and recommending their purchase to management.

EVALUATING HEALTH CARE IN THE WORK SETTING

As in all other settings for nursing practice, the effectiveness of health care in the work setting must be evaluated. Evaluation can focus either on the outcomes of care for the individual employee or for the total employee population. Evaluation will be conducted on the basis of principles discussed in Chapter 5, The Nursing Process, and Chapter 19, Care of the Community or Target Group, and will focus on the achievement of expected outcomes and the processes used to achieve those outcomes. For example, the occupational health nurse may evaluate the effectiveness of body mechanics education in decreasing the incidence of back injuries. At the individual level, evaluation might focus on the impact of no-smoking education on an individual employee's smoking behavior.

CHAPTER HIGHLIGHTS

- Community health nurses have been providing health care in American occupational settings for almost a century.
- Advantages of providing health care in occupational settings include access to a large segment of the population—who may be at risk for a variety of health problems—as a "captive audience"; pressures in the work setting for healthier behavior; motivation to stay well in order to continue working; efficiency; and cost-effectiveness.
- Occupational health nursing is nursing practice directed toward promoting health, preventing illness, and restoring function in the working population.
- Human biological factors to be assessed in the work setting include the composition of the work force in terms of age, race, and sex; the presence or absence of a variety of acute and chronic conditions; and immunization status.
- Health and safety hazards present in the physical environment of the work setting include chemical hazards, physical hazards, electrical hazards, fire, heavy lifting and uncomfortable working positions, and potential for falls.
- Four spheres of social influence on health operating in the work setting include the sphere of personal behaviors, the co-worker sphere, the management sphere, and the societal sphere.
- Life-style factors to be assessed in the work setting include types of work performed, consumption patterns, patterns of rest and exercise, and use of safety devices.
- Four types of internal health-care systems that may be present in the work setting are programs to control toxic wastes, health-promotion policies, limited health-promotion programs, and comprehensive programs. In some comprehensive programs, care may also be provided to family members.
- Areas of emphasis for primary prevention in the work setting include health promotion, illness prevention, and injury prevention.
- Secondary prevention foci in the work setting include screening, treating existing disease, and emergency response. Screening may involve pre-employment examinations, periodic screening of employees at risk for certain problems, and environmental screening to detect health hazards in the workplace.
- Emphases in tertiary prevention in the work setting include preventing the spread of communicable diseases, preventing the recurrence of other acute conditions, and preventing consequences of chronic conditions.

Review Questions

1. Describe at least three advantages in providing health care in the work setting. (p. 654)
2. Identify at least six of the ten leading causes of health problems encountered in the work setting. Give at least one example of how a community health nurse working in an occupational setting might be involved in preventing conditions in each category. (p. 657)
3. Identify at least five types of health and safety hazards encountered in work settings. Describe at least one potential control measure for hazards in each category. (p. 659)
4. Describe four spheres of social influence on the health of employees. (p. 661)
5. Describe four potential types of health-care programs in the work setting and the community health nurse's focus in assessing each. (p. 663)
6. What are the three main areas of emphasis in primary prevention in the work setting? Give an example of a community health nursing intervention related to each area. (p. 664)
7. Describe three major considerations in secondary prevention in the work setting. What activities might a community health nurse be involved in with respect to each? (p. 667)
8. Describe three emphases in tertiary prevention in the work setting. Describe at least one community health nursing responsibility related to each area of emphasis. (p. 669)

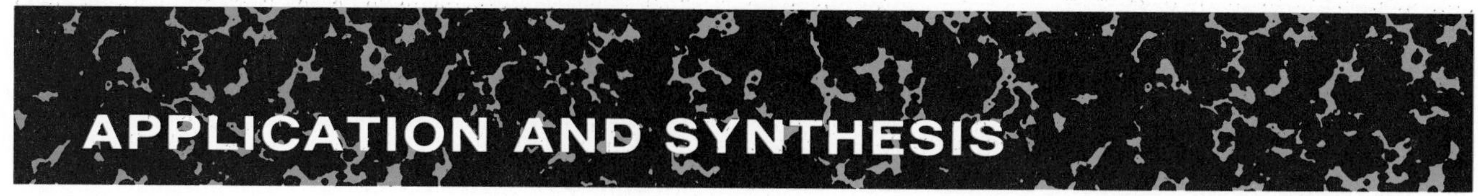

APPLICATION AND SYNTHESIS

You are a community health nurse employed by a large manufacturing plant. On Wednesday you see several employees complaining of abdominal cramping and diarrhea. They all state that their symptoms started at home during the night. You get word from one of the plant supervisors that several of her employees called in sick this morning because of similar symptoms. In checking with other departments, you find that there are a number of absences throughout the plant. Two of the older employees and one whom you know has AIDS have been hospitalized with severe dehydration. All of the people with cramps and diarrhea eat regularly in the cafeteria.

1. What are the human biological, environmental, life-style, and health system factors operating in this situation?
2. What are your nursing diagnoses?
3. What are you client-care objectives?
4. What secondary prevention measures will you employ in relation to your diagnoses? Why? What primary preventive measures might have prevented the occurrence of these problems? What tertiary prevention measures are warranted to prevent the recurrence of problems or complications?
5. How will you evaluate the effectiveness of your interventions?

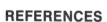

REFERENCES

1. Heier, R. (1989, June 26). Workers can expect big changes in health-care benefits. *San Diego Union*, A-11.
2. United States Department of Health and Human Services. (1991). *Healthy people 2000: National objectives for health promotion and disease prevention*. Washington, DC: Government Printing Office.
3. Warner, K. E. (1987). Selling health promotion to corporate America: Uses and abuses of the economic argument. *Health Education Quarterly, 14*(1), 39–55.
4. Hughes, H. V. (1979). A view from the top: Today's needs in occupational health service. *Occupational Health Nurse, 27*(2), 13–15.
5. American Association of Occupational Health Nurses. (1988). *Standards for occupational health nursing practice*. Atlanta, GA: American Association of Occupational Health Nurses.
6. Lusk, S. L. (1990). Corporate expectations for occupational health nurses' activities. *AAOHN Journal, 38*, 368–374.
7. Marbury, M. (1987). Workers' health. In M. R. Greenberg (Ed.), *Public health and the environment* (pp. 76–104). New York: Guilford Press.
8. Work-related injuries and illnesses in an automotive parts manufacturing company—Chicago. (1989). *MMWR, 38*, 413–416.
9. Franklin, G. M., Haug, J., Heyer, N., et al. (1991). Occupational carpal tunnel syndrome in Washington State, 1984–1988. *American Journal of Public Health, 81*, 741–746.
10. Monson, R. R. (1990). *Occupational epidemiology* (2nd ed.). Boca Raton, FL: CRC Press.
11. Centers for Disease Control. (1986). NIOSH recommendations for occupational safety and health standards. *MMWR, 35*(Suppl. 1), 1S–33S.
12. United States Department of Commerce. (1990). *Statistical abstract of the United States, 1989*. Washington, DC: Government Printing Office.
13. Leading work-related diseases and injuries—United States. (1985). *MMWR, 34*, 219–222, 227.

14. Leading work-related diseases and injuries—United States. (1986a). *MMWR, 35,* 113–116, 121–123.
15. Leading work-related diseases and injuries—United States. (1986b). *MMWR, 35,* 185–188.
16. Centers for Disease Control. (1985). Trends of a decade—A perspective on occupational hazard surveillance, 1970–1983. *CDC Surveillance Summaries, MMWR, 34*(Suppl. 2), 15SS–24SS.
17. Stellman, J. M. (1986). Occupational safety and health hazards. In M. F. Cataldo & T. J. Coates (Eds.), *Health and industry* (pp. 270–284). New York: Wiley.
18. Landrigan, P. J. (1990). Lead in the modern workplace. *American Journal of Public Health, 80,* 907–908.
19. Control of excessive lead exposure in radiator repair workers. (1991). *MMWR, 40,* 139–141.
20. Baser, M. E., & Marion, D. (1990). A statewide registry for surveillance of occupational heavy metals absorption. *American Journal of Public Health, 80,* 162–164.
21. Leading work-related diseases and injuries—United States. (1986c). *MMWR, 35,* 613–614, 619–621.
22. Csiernik, R. P. (1990). An EAP intervention protocol for occupational health nurses. *AAOHN Journal, 38,* 381–384.
23. Singer, J. A., Neale, M. S., Schwartz, G. E., et al. (1986). Conflicting perspectives on stress reduction in occupational settings. In M. F. Cataldo & T. J. Coates (Eds.), *Health and industry* (pp. 162–180). New York: Wiley.
24. Rudolph, L., Sharp, D. S., Samuels, S., et al. (1990). Environmental and biological monitoring for lead exposure in California workplaces. *American Journal of Public Health, 80,* 921–925.
25. Annas, G. J. (1991). Public health and the law: OSHA's four inconsistent carcinogen policies. *American Journal of Public Health, 81,* 775–780.
26. Pelletier, K. R. (1984). *Healthy people in unhealthy places: Stress and fitness at work.* New York: Delta/Seymour Lawrence.
27. Occupational and paraoccupational exposure to lead—Colorado. (1989). *MMWR, 38,* 338–340, 345.
28. Traumatic occupational fatalities—United States, 1980–1984. (1987). *MMWR, 36,* 461–464, 469–470.

RECOMMENDED READINGS

Csiernik, R. P. (1990). An EAP intervention protocol for occupational health nurses. *AAOHN Journal, 38,* 381–384.

Describes the role of the occupational health nurse in an employee assistance program for employees with psychological problems. Presents a seven-step feedback protocol for motivating employees to seek help.

Frazier, F. (1988). *Principles and practice of occupational health nursing.* New York: Delmar.

Provides an overview of occupational health nursing.

Lusk, S. L. (1990). Corporate expectations for occupational health nurses' activities. *AAOHN Journal, 38,* 368–374.

Sets forth findings of a study of the perceptions of corporate executives regarding the role and responsibilities of occupational health nurses.

Manchester, J., Summers, V., Newell, J., et al. (1991). Development of an assessment guide for occupational health nurses. *AAOHN Journal, 39,* 13–19.

Reports the development of a tool for assessing an occupational health nursing program in light of the standards for occupational health nursing. Includes a copy of the tool.

Monson, R. R. (1990). *Occupational epidemiology* (2nd ed.). Boca Raton, FL: CRC Press.

Reviews findings of epidemiologic research in occupational health. Provides an overview of studies on major occupational health problems.

CHAPTER 28

Care of Clients in Rural Settings

Charlene M. Hanson

KEY TERMS

frontier
nurse generalist
rural
stroke belt
urban

Although rural community health nursing requires high levels of skill and competence and may offer less opportunity for interchange with colleagues, there are many rewards to rural nursing practice. Nurses who practice in small rural communities form close relationships with clients and their families. They also tend to exhibit higher levels of autonomy and job satisfaction than do their urban counterparts.[1] The unique relationship with client and family includes "knowing" the family well, understanding some of the strengths and weaknesses of the family structure, and sensitivity to family support systems. Community activities related to helping families prevent illness can be one of the most rewarding aspects of rural community health nursing. Rural community health nursing, with its commitment to health promotion and holistic family-centered primary care, plays a central role in improving the health of rural Americans.

Rural community health nursing offers the nurse unique opportunities to care for clients within a broad practice environment with high potential for autonomy and job satisfaction. The focus of this chapter is to identify the many ways in which community health nurses can provide health care to rural-based people within the context of rural culture and ethnicity. Differences in life-style and in the health problems rural populations experience are explored using the epidemiologic prevention process model.

(*continued*)

LEARNING OBJECTIVES

After reading this chapter you should be able to:

- Identify five differences between rural and urban communities.
- Describe three roles for community health nurses in rural areas.
- Identify at least three work environments for community health nurses in rural settings.
- Describe at least four barriers to effective health care in rural areas.
- Identify two age groups at particular risk for health problems in rural settings.
- Describe at least five environmental concerns unique to rural settings.
- Identify four major occupational and safety risk factors for rural populations.
- Discuss two aspects of the impact of health policy on rural community health care.
- Identify three aspects of primary prevention in rural settings.
- Describe four approaches to secondary prevention in rural settings.

WHAT IS URBAN? WHAT IS RURAL?

"Rural" is often defined as anything that is not urban. According to the U.S. Census Bureau, "urban" and "rural" are "type of area" concepts rather than specific areas outlined on maps. The term ***urban,*** when used to define a population, includes persons living in metropolitan areas and in places with 2500 or more residents, whereas the term ***rural,*** used to define populations, includes all other persons. The rural population is further divided into farm and nonfarm populations. The Census Bureau definition of rural as places with fewer than 2500 residents is the most specific measure used.[2] "Frontier" is another term used in relation to rural areas. A ***frontier*** is an area with a population density of six or fewer persons per square mile. Frontier areas are common in the western half of the United States. Figure 28–1 indicates the distribution of frontier counties throughout the nation.

The Far West, the Midwest, and the rural South are often designated as known rural areas although there are rural populations scattered throughout all regions of the country. About 25 percent of the nation's population lives in rural areas, and this number is growing. The areas of greatest rural growth include rural counties of the Southwest, Florida, and the Southeastern coast, southern Texas, the Ozarks, the southern Appalachian area, and the mountains of New England.

New census data (available in 1992–1993) will help community health nurses and others to more clearly estimate the extent of rural populations in the United States. In addition, statisticians who work with national health-related data are breaking morbidity and mortality statistics into urban and rural components. This information will help to identify rural and high-risk urban areas that need health-care resources and technology.

THE RURAL POPULATION

There are some misconceptions about who makes up the rural population. The rural population of America is a diverse group of people who are born to or choose to live and work within a rural environment. The notion that rural people are predominantly farmers is no longer true and is becoming less so over time. It is important to remember that only about one-third of rural families live and work on farms. The majority of the rural population are not agricultural workers, although they live in rural communities.

Over the past few years, large companies have seen the tax advantage of moving their production facilities to rural areas. This factor has not only facilitated the movement of rural communities away from agriculture but has also contributed to some of the health problems experienced by people in rural areas. For example, increased industry has contributed to pollution of water sources with manufacturing residues.

Other factors that contribute to the changing face of the rural population include work in nearby cities and movement of young people away from rural areas. A growing number of people who live in small rural communities work in nearby cities and commute to work each day. Researchers also note the tendency of young people to move out of rural areas, leaving behind the elderly and high-risk needy.

RURAL COMMUNITY HEALTH NURSING

Peggye Lassiter,[3] a rural nurse educator credited with developing early concepts of rural nursing, believed that the demands of rural nursing are different from community health nursing demands in the urban setting. The rural community health nurse is a nurse generalist rather than a nurse specialist. The ***nurse generalist*** possesses a broad base of knowledge and skills rather than in-depth knowledge in a specialized field. Being a generalist requires an ability to be flexible and innovative and to possess broad-based assessment skills.

Rural nursing is interdisciplinary with the community health nurse working closely with other members of the health-care team such as physicians, pharmacists, psychologists, and others who strive to bring

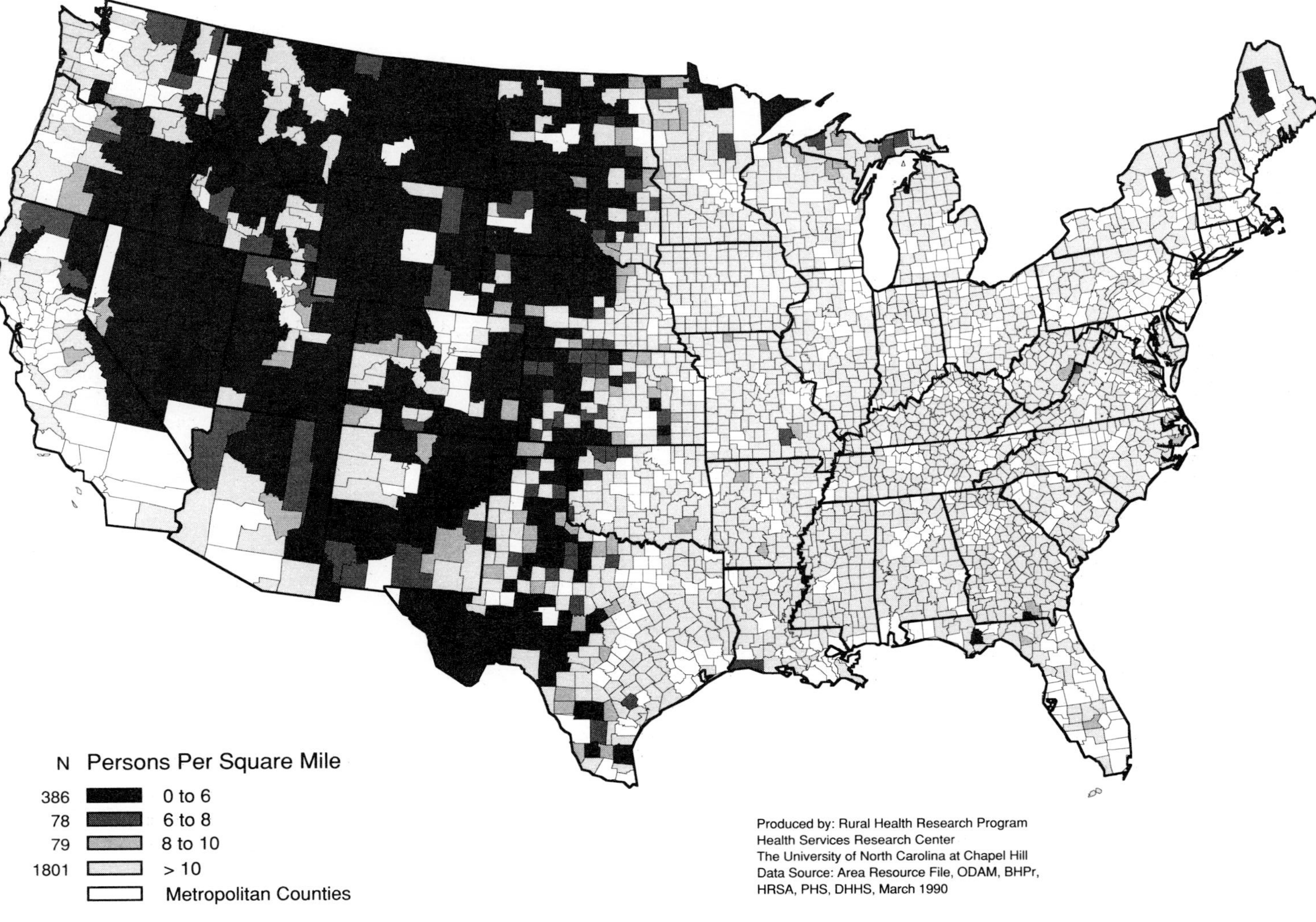

Figure 28–1. Map of frontier counties, 1987. Shading indicates frontier regions of the United States where distance to health care is a major factor. (*Courtesy Health Services Research Center, The University of North Carolina at Chapel Hill*)

comprehensive health care to rural families. Because of the scarcity of other health-care providers, the community health nurse often moves into other roles as needed to provide care for clients. The need to rely frequently on nonprofessional persons to provide care, such as family members, nursing assistants, and emergency medical technicians (EMTs), requires strong leadership and management skills on the part of the rural community health nurse.

Rural community health nursing also frequently involves working within tight financial constraints and with fewer resources than may be found in urban settings. These factors require innovative care strategies on the part of the community health nurse.

It is important to remember that rural settings can cover large territories where distance and communication are major influencing factors in the delivery of health care. In the past, factors related to travel time and difficulty finding coverage while away from the job have limited the ability of rural community health nurses to attend continuing education programs or pursue advanced education. New incentives for education in rural areas and innovative telecommunication systems, however, are beginning to alter this situation.

Rural nurses usually do not change jobs as frequently as their urban counterparts. Initial recruitment of nurses to work in rural communities, however, is a major national concern. Federal and state incentives for rural practice may facilitate recruitment in the future. These incentives should improve access to health care by encouraging rural practice by many health disciplines, including nursing.

SETTINGS FOR RURAL COMMUNITY HEALTH NURSES

Employment opportunities for community health nurses in rural settings are diverse and challenging. The local health department is very often the mainstay of health care in the rural community, and the community health nurse is the key care-giver within this agency. Community health nurses in health departments are frequently involved in well-child care, prenatal care, care of migrant workers, and screening and immunization programs. In many states, public health agencies employ community health nurses to provide both preventative care and primary care for episodic illnesses.

Another rural community health nursing role is in the area of occupational health, working in small businesses and plants to meet the preventative and primary health-care needs of employees. Small rural industries often cannot afford full-time occupational health nurses and rely on community health nurses in the local health department to do pre-employment physical examinations and blood and urine screening as well as vision and hearing checks. In addition, testing may be provided for lunch-room workers and cooks to rule out hepatitis and gastrointestinal parasites.

There is also a great need for the community health nurse in rural home health care. Coordinating the care of chronically ill and elderly clients has been identified as a critical role for community health nurses throughout the 1990s. This role is even more important in communities lacking human resources, where the community health nurse may need to function as nutritionist, epidemiologist, and social worker, as well as nurse.

Federal and community-funded rural primary-care clinics and private office settings afford opportunities for community health nurses to function as primary-care providers or as liaisons with community resources. Indian health and migrant health settings also employ community health nurses as primary care-givers. In addition, there is a widespread need for preschool and school-based community health nurses in rural areas.

The lack of qualified EMTs and ambulance networks in isolated rural areas, small rural hospitals without the technological capabilities for complicated neurological and vascular procedures, and extended distances to major trauma centers place the rural community health nurse in a situation that requires constant readiness to assess and make decisions accurately regarding emergency care. In this capacity, the rural community health nurse may function as a paid or volunteer ambulance service professional.

HEALTH-RELATED PROBLEMS IN RURAL AREAS

Preventing illness presents a challenge to the rural community health nurse. Both the young and the aged are in need of special immunization efforts. AIDS and other sexually transmitted diseases, tuberculosis, and childhood communicable diseases are cited as some of the current national concerns for illness prevention. Health-promotion programs are severely lacking in many rural areas. This fact is, in large part, attributable to the lack of funding for wellness activities in the current U.S. health-care system.

Nursing management of chronic health problems such as high-risk diabetes, alcoholism, cancer, and cardiovascular disease is an important facet of rural nursing. Risk factors such as high-fat and high-carbohydrate diet, obesity, and smoking remain prevalent among rural people. Rural-based Native Americans, for example, have some of the highest rates for diabetes and alcoholism in the country. In addition, the rural South is often referred to as the ***stroke belt,*** an area of particularly high morbidity and mortality due to hypertension and cardiovascular disease, especially among rural southern blacks.

Farm workers are at risk for serious work-related disease, particularly lung disease such as occupational asthma, hypersensitivity reactions, leukemia, non-Hodgkin's lymphoma, and hearing loss. Farm accidents and motor vehicle accidents remain continuing sources of injury and death in rural areas, especially among the young. Both farm safety and emergency medical services (EMS) are eliciting strong national and state concern and support.

Often thought to be safe from serious substance abuse problems, rural communities are experiencing the same severe increases in crack-cocaine use and other substance abuse as their urban counterparts. Mental illness and chronic stress are serious health problems facing rural communities in all regions of the country.

Teenage pregnancy, with a subsequent high rate of infant mortality and morbidity, ranks as one of the most serious rural health concerns facing the nation. Moreover, the incidence of AIDS and sexually transmitted diseases continues to rise alarmingly in rural counties. Figure 28–2, for example, shows the increase in the incidence of syphilis in rural southern Georgia in recent years.[4]

BARRIERS TO EFFECTIVE HEALTH CARE IN RURAL AREAS

Health problems in rural areas are intensified by several major barriers to effective health care. These barriers include poverty; distance and lack of transportation; the presence of several high-risk aggregates in the population; health policy inequities; and lack of health-care providers.

POVERTY

One of every four poor Americans (about 9 million people) lives outside of urban areas. Poverty rates are higher in rural areas than in metropolitan areas. The poverty rates for whites, blacks, and Hispanics are as high or higher in nonmetropolitan areas than they are in inner or central cities.[5] Figure 28–3 depicts the distribution of rural poverty in the southern, northeastern, midwestern, and western regions of the country.

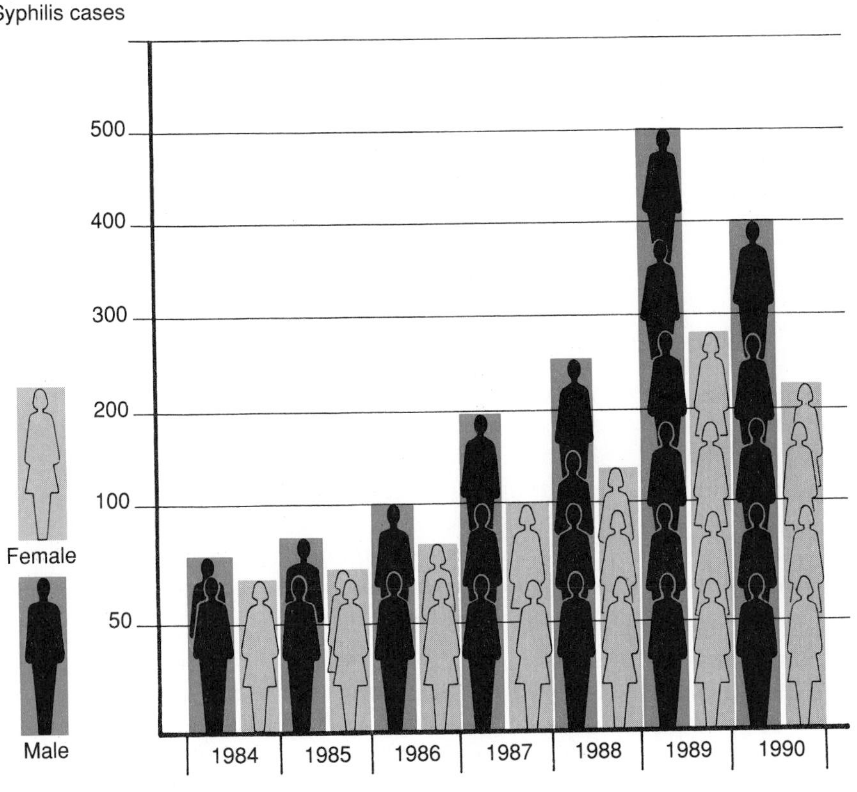

Figure 28–2. Syphilis cases reported in southeast Georgia from 1984 to 1990. Note the sharp increase in cases for 1989. (*Source: Fortney, M. A., & Holloway, T. [1990]. Crack, syphilis, and AIDS: The triple threat to rural Georgia. GAPF, 12[2], 6.*)

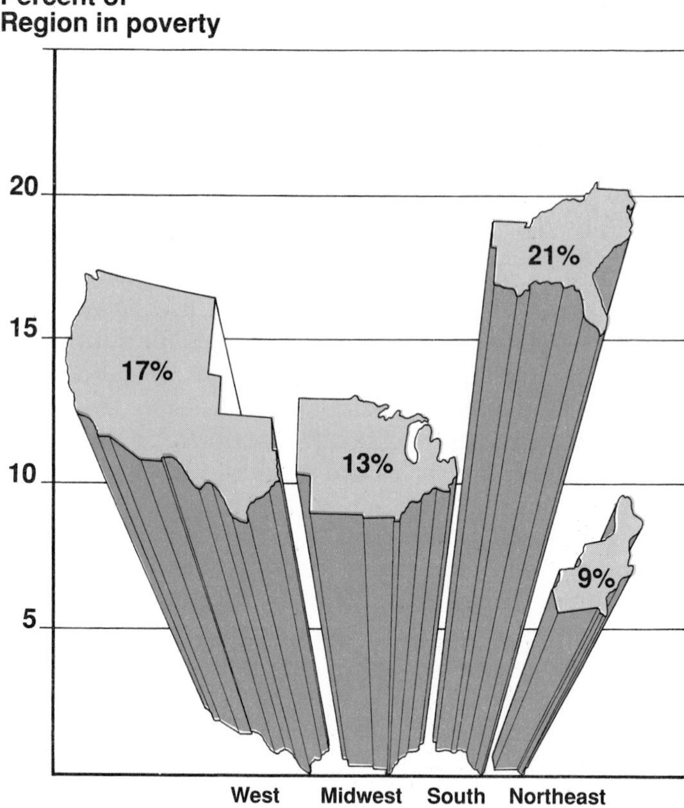

Figure 28–3. Rural poverty rates in the United States by region, 1986. (*Courtesy Center on Budget and Policy Priorities, Washington, DC*)

Poverty rates for the elderly are also higher in rural areas. This problem is compounded by the migration of the rural young to the city, in many instances leaving the aged without strong family support.

DISTANCE AND LACK OF TRANSPORTATION

It may take an hour or more for residents of remote, isolated frontier areas to reach health-care providers and facilities. Health services may be difficult to come by in these diverse and sparsely populated regions. The distance to health-care services is one of the factors in increased mortality from myocardial infarction and motor vehicle accidents in rural areas. Distance to health care is one of the major barriers to health care in the frontier West in contrast to the more populated rural areas of the South where poverty is the major barrier to rural health care.

HIGH-RISK RURAL AGGREGATES

Aggregates of migrant farm workers, Asian immigrants, Native Americans, elderly persons, and those with mental illness compound the rural community health nurse's illness-prevention and primary-care tasks. These groups may comprise a significant portion of the rural population in some areas. Members of these groups are at high risk for a variety of health problems and frequently have more limited resources to deal with them than do their urban counterparts.

Migrant farm workers are usually poor and may experience language barriers that limit their access to health care. Because of their mobile life-style, it is hard to provide consistent health-care services to meet their needs. The health needs of Native Americans, addressed in Chapter 15, Cultural Influences on Community Health, are compounded by rural residence and associated life-styles. Asian immigrants are frequently refugees from countries torn by war and famine and are at high risk for a variety of communicable diseases as well as the psychological problems attendant on physical and emotional trauma. Similarly, older rural residents with multiple chronic health concerns find that they are disadvantaged with respect to housing, income, education, transportation, and access to health care.[6]

HEALTH POLICY INEQUITIES

Two health policy factors tend to worsen the health status of rural Americans. First, health policy formulations treat the problems of the rural poor as though they were the same as those of the urban inner-city poor. Second, when policies are designed specifically for rural areas, they falsely assume that all rural residents are farmers. These two policy factors result in inequities in appropriation of funds and often cause financial barriers to rural health care.

LACK OF HEALTH-CARE PROVIDERS

To make matters worse, there is a severe lack of qualified health-care personnel, especially minority personnel, in many poor rural areas. The absence of technological support for health-care practice and the meager economic status of many rural clients deter many health-care providers from practicing in rural areas. This lack of qualified personnel, coupled with the paucity of technological resources, has created serious health problems for rural residents.

THE EPIDEMIOLOGIC PREVENTION PROCESS MODEL AND CARE OF CLIENTS IN RURAL SETTINGS

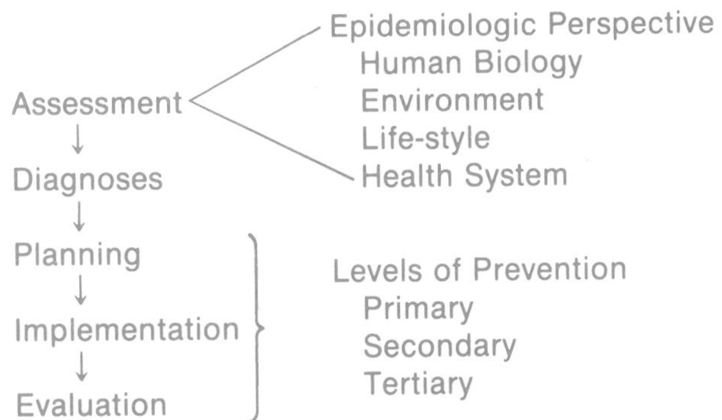

The epidemiologic prevention process model lends itself to the assessment of health needs and planning for primary, secondary, and tertiary care in several types of rural community settings. Using this model, the community health nurse can identify the health needs of rural residents and explore ways to improve their access to care.

ASSESSING HEALTH STATUS

Assessing the health status of rural populations is carried out using the four components of Dever's epidemiologic model (human biology, environment, life-style, and health system). These factors are assessed within the context of rural culture and rural living patterns.

HUMAN BIOLOGY

Genetic Inheritance

Genetic factors most prevalent within the rural setting are those associated with rural-based minority aggregates. For example, the genetic predisposition to diabetes mellitus and chronic alcoholism among Native Americans is a well-known and serious health problem. Rural black families may have unusually strong histories of hypertension, stroke, or sickle cell anemia. Moreover, black women have a higher risk for breast cancer. As America's rural Asian population continues to increase, genetic disorders related to these ethnic groups will become statistically more evident in the rural population mix of the United States.

These and other genetic factors influencing the health of rural people can be found within most geographic sections of the country, and the community health nurse would assess their incidence and prevalence in one's own area. Information on the incidence and prevalence of selected conditions can be obtained for rural counties from state health departments. Health professionals and local health-care facilities are also sources of information on the extent of genetically determined diseases in the population.

Physiologic Function

People living in rural settings are prone to the same illnesses and accidents that afflict urban residents. Large numbers of high-risk infants and elderly, however, and fewer hospital and community resources mean that community health nurses working in rural settings must assess and manage their clients more thoroughly, often relying on family members to help provide care.

Physiologic illnesses vary somewhat by rural regions of the United States. As noted earlier, the rural South has a high incidence of essential hypertension and stroke, particularly among blacks. Coal miners in rural Appalachia, on the other hand, tend to have more respiratory diseases. Again, the community health nurse might obtain information on health problems common to one's own area by studying data collected by state offices or by reviewing the records of local health providers and agencies.

Maturation and Aging

The age composition of the rural population is another factor to be assessed by community health nurses. Two client subpopulations merit special attention. In both children and elderly populations, physical and psychosocial developmental factors can seriously affect client health, and the nurse should determine the size of both subgroups in his or her jurisdiction.

Like youngsters everywhere, rural children of all ages require several assessments over time to evaluate appropriate physical and mental growth and development. The rural community health nurse plays a key role in this assessment process within the child health component of health department services and the school-based health system. Types of assessments that may be conducted on a regular basis include the Denver Developmental Screening Test (DDST) for young children, scoliosis checks for preteens, vision testing and tests for amblyopia in preschoolers, and breast examinations for adolescents.

The rural elderly also require assessment on a regular basis for both the prevention of new changes or problems related to the aging process and to monitor ongoing health problems such as diabetes, hypertension, COPD, or depression. Chapter 20, Care of Children, and Chapter 23, Care of Older Clients, provide generic protocols that the rural community health nurse can use to assess these groups of clients.

ENVIRONMENT

Physical Environment

The rural environment is often thought to be a healthy, stress-free place to live. However, weather-related, chemical, and occupational hazards may constitute risks for a variety of health and safety-related problems.

Threats from the Natural Environment. Hazards of nature, such as tornadoes, drought, wind, and rain clearly affect rural families, especially those who depend on the land for their livelihood. Fire is a major risk factor for rural families because of the extended response time for volunteer fire companies. Rarely a day goes by without media coverage documenting adverse weather conditions or fire with associated health risk or morbidity. The role of the community health nurse, as a member of the rural community disaster team, is to help citizens and community leaders assess areas at risk for weather-related hazards and to plan for disaster response. This role is addressed in more detail in Chapter 29, Care of Clients in Disaster Settings.

Rural living also places clients at higher risk for problems caused by animal and insect vectors. An awareness of the need to assess for stings and bites from insects and snakes and wild animal bites (especially those of animals that may have rabies) falls within the day-to-day assessment tasks of the rural community-based nurse. The nurse should also obtain information on the kind of wildlife present in the area and the frequency of bites and stings as well as the prevalence of rabies and other diseases that can be transmitted to humans. This information can be obtained from wildlife personnel, veterinarians, or vector-control personnel in local health departments.

Rural Public Health and Sanitation. Most rural homes are not connected to public water and sewage lines. Drinking water obtained from natural springs and wells is common. Septic tanks and outdoor toilets placed too close to wells can cause water contamination. Local industry may also serve as a source of contamination for groundwater that eventually finds its way into wells used for drinking purposes. Often, evidence of polluted drinking water is found while the community health nurse is assessing for other health-related problems in rural families. The community health nurse assists rural sanitation directors to identify homes that have contaminated wells, a lack of indoor plumbing, or septic systems that are improperly maintained. Use of reclaimed water from sewage for crop irrigation in areas with low rainfall may also pose health hazards should groundwater become contaminated.

Families living in farm communities are also at risk for pollution from insecticides and sprays used for crops and animals. A common source of respiratory ailments is repeated exposure to poisons in farm chemicals. Chemical and pesticide exposure was listed as the second most important farm safety concern of parents in a recent CDC report.[7]

Psychological Environment

Many people think of rural areas as places to get away from the stress of urban life. Persistent economic problems experienced by farmers in the last decade, however, have brought the stress faced by rural farming families to national attention. Crop failures triggered by severe weather conditions, coupled with a declining economy, have caused excessive emotional and physiological stress for farm families nationwide. These factors have contributed to mental and physical disabilities among rural clients as well as to substance abuse and family violence. Increased cases of suicide, situational depression, gastrointestinal diseases, and eating disorders are only a few of the rural health problems arising from economic stress.

Another area needing assessment from a psychological standpoint is that of family violence and neglect. Research indicates that isolation and lack of day care and other support services for the young and the aged are contributing factors in child abuse, wife and elder battering, and neglect. The close contact that community health nurses have with rural families offers an opportunity for early identification of all kinds of family violence. The lack of resources for early referral for mental health problems increases the prevalence of these problems for both individual clients and family members.

In assessing the psychological environment, the community health nurse would examine the effects of the economic climate of the area on residents' psychological health as well as the incidence of indicators of emotional distress such as substance abuse, violence, and depression. In addition, the nurse would assess individual clients and families for evidence of psychological distress.

Social Environment

Each rural community is unique and needs to be considered separately from others. Because of the special flavor of the social environment in rural communities, researchers have found that urban models of health-care delivery superimposed on rural communities frequently do not work. For this reason the community health nurse needs to know the internal workings of the community in order to design health-care programs that will best meet the needs of rural people.

The social isolation of these communities and the importance placed by rural families on religious beliefs and church attendance foster close kinship networks. Family and friends are relied on, and self-help and self-reliance are important factors to assess. The church family is often an important social resource for rural community living. Phenomena such as culture, distances, work demands, and family values (for example, early sexual activity leading to high-risk pregnancy) all need to be considered before health-care services can be tailored to suit the preferences of these rural families and communities. Chapter 15, Cultural Influences on Community Health, offers a more general discussion of the role that culture plays in healthy or unhealthy life-styles.

The assessment of social supports and resources within the rural community is an important role for the community health nurse. Specific assessment considerations in this area are included in Box 28–1.

LIFE-STYLE

Life-style assessment considerations in rural settings relate to patterns of occupational risks, leisure activity, and daily consumption.

Occupational Risks

Occupational risks vary for persons living in a rural environment and fall into farming and nonfarming categories. The risks of farming and ranching, which include working with heavy machinery, pesticides, and large animals, present opportunities for physical injury. Child safety, within the context of the farm setting, is of serious concern.[7] Farm accidents are one

BOX 28–1

Social Environmental Assessment Considerations in Rural Settings

- What is the economic status of the community? What are the mean and median salaries of community residents?
- What are the transportation needs of community members? How are they met?
- What educational facilities are available to community residents? Are they adequate to meet the educational needs of community members?
- What social support services are available within the community? How accessible are these services to the needy? Are services adequate to meet the needs of community members?
- How cohesive is the community? Is there conflict between groups within the community?
- What are the attitudes of community members to health and healthy behaviors?
- What cultural groups are represented in the community? To what extent does culture influence the health and healthy practices of community members?
- What religious groups are represented in the community? What is the influence of religion on the health of community members?
- What values are held by members of the community? How do values influence health and health care?
- Who can be relied on to help with finances, transportation, meals, and other needs?
- What child-care services are available in the community? Are they adequate to meet community member's needs?

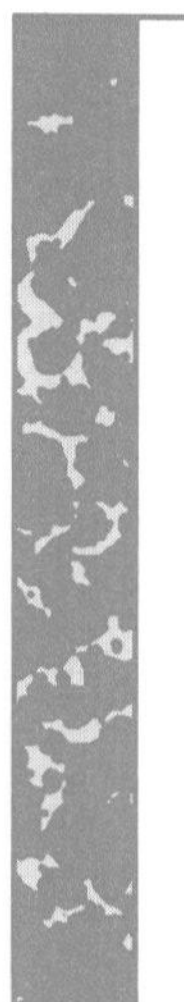

BOX 28–2

Safety Concerns of Farm Families

Farm machinery accidents
Chemical/pesticide exposure
Breathing problems
Skin cancer
Hearing loss
Injury by animals
Stress

(Adapted from Hawk, Gay, & Donham[7])

source of parental safety concerns presented in Box 28–2.

The persistent economic downturn in farming has caused many women to seek employment outside the home, while the farmer-father combines farm chores with child care. This practice increases the risk of child-related farm accidents as children are playing in close proximity to large machinery and toxic substances.

An added concern is that many rural elderly people work beyond the years that they should safely undertake hard physical labor so they can keep their land and maintain their family. These farm-related risk factors require careful assessment and education in order for the nurse to engage in injury prevention.

Nonfarming occupational considerations are becoming more and more important as rural communities become more diversified. The same types of occupational hazards described for urban occupations are present in rural factories and businesses; however, both emergency care and trauma surveillance related to occupational injury are less available. In addition, the necessity for traveling to and from work on two-lane highways adds to the potential for injury for rural dwellers. The considerable risks of working in mining and lumbering industries or near nuclear plants and dumping grounds, which are often located in rural areas, also need assessment by the community health nurse.

Leisure Activity Risks

Some rural families tend to be "tied down" by the need to care for crops and animals. The majority, however, go to work each day in structured nonfarm work settings. Getting together for family outings and church programs is common, and food-oriented activities are prevalent. Obesity, diabetes, and high cholesterol levels are common health problems related to leisure-time activities in rural areas.

Organized recreational activities are carried out primarily in either the schools or churches. There are few job-related or free-standing "health clubs" with professional personnel to oversee exercise programs. Community-sponsored recreation centers and state parks offer other avenues for leisure-time activities.

The one outstanding health risk is motor vehicle accidents on two-lane roads. Head-on collisions produce extremely high morbidity and mortality and are the leading cause of death for young males. Children riding in the back of pickup trucks and drivers who drive while intoxicated represent a serious toll of lives each year. Hunting accidents also account for many injuries, mostly related to improper training and poor gun-safety practices.

Consumption Patterns

Major health-related consumption patterns of rural people include those related to smoking, diet and nutrition, and substance abuse (with alcohol being a most serious problem). Table 28–1 offers a comparison of the prevalence of selected preventive and high-risk behaviors for rural and urban areas.

Community health nurses should assess the nutritional patterns of clients in rural settings. This can be done by exploring dietary patterns, food preferences, and modes of preparation with families in the community. The nurse may also examine the types of restaurants and foods served in the area to determine general food preferences. Observations of foods available and purchased in area grocery stores can also provide a picture of dietary practices in the area. The prevalence of obesity in the population is another indicator or food consumption patterns.

Nurses would also assess other consumption patterns including the extent of smoking behaviors and the use of alcohol and other drugs. The nurse might obtain information on tobacco and alcohol sales from local merchants or determine the extent of arrests related to drug and alcohol abuse. Information on hospitalizations for substance abuse will enable the nurse to determine the extent of these problems.

HEALTH SYSTEM

Both the external and internal health-care systems influence health and illness within rural communities. The goal for successful access to rural health care is to coordinate the efforts of the external federal and state programs with the internal community-based health-care system to create a strong collaborative partnership.

TABLE 28–1. SELECTED PREVENTIVE BEHAVIORS AND RISK EXPOSURES OF METROPOLITAN AND NONMETROPOLITAN RESIDENTS, 1985

Behavior	Percent of Adult Population Engaging in Particular Behavior	
	Metropolitan Area	*Nonmetropolitan Area*
Use seat belts all or most of the time	38.9	25.2
Exercise regularly	41.5	35.2
Had Pap smear in last year (women only)	46.8	41.8
Had breast exam in past year (women only)	51.8	45.4
Had blood pressure check in past year	85.3	83.7
Have been told they have high blood pressure at least twice	16.8	19.4
Those with high blood pressure who take medication	64.9	67.9
20% or more above desirable body weight	23.1	26.9
Currently smoke cigarettes	30.3	29.4
Of smokers, smoke 25 or more cigarettes a day	26.0	28.7
Of women aged 18 to 44 years giving birth in past 5 years:		
Smoked in 12 months before giving birth	31.7	31.9
Quit smoking when pregnant	22.0	18.8
Reduced smoking when pregnant	35.4	38.0
Of drinkers, in the past year:		
Consumed 5 or more drinks in one day on at least 5 occasions	24.5	26.0
Had driven a vehicle after having had too much to drink	16.6	17.9
Exposed to at least one job-related hazard in current job	59.5	68.7

(*Source: Office of Technology Assessment. [1990].* Health care in rural America. *[GPO publication No. 052-003-01205-7]. Washington, DC: Government Printing Office.)*

The formal health-care system in rural settings needs to fit into the informal rural helping system. The use of old and trusted resources rather than "outsider" influence is often the key to success in health-care programming in rural areas. It is important to recognize that rural people comprise a large segment of the population who have little or no health insurance coverage. Rural residents without insurance often "fall through the cracks" of the health-care system and are in need of health-care services. Fixing the health-care system from outside the community often does not have lasting effects because of environmental constraints related to distance, poor transportation, and few economic resources.

The External System: National and State Programs

The heightened awareness of health concerns in rural areas has strengthened federal support for rural health care. Figure 28–4 depicts the organizational structure of the newly formed Office of Rural Health and the Office of Rural Mental Health designed to advise the Secretary of Health and Human Services on matters related to health, health-care provision, and health-care financing in rural areas.

Federally funded rural health clinics and community health clinics offer primary health care to local residents. In these clinics, nurse practitioners, supported by collaborative physician backup, assess clients and manage care for a variety of health problems. Mental health clinics, detoxification units, and substance abuse follow-up programs receive funding priorities at both the state and national level. In addition, new programs for addicted pregnant women are springing up throughout the nation. These federal and state initiatives provide community health nurses with much needed resources to assist high-risk rural clients.

Both Medicare and Medicaid programs provide health-care coverage for members of rural population groups. Programs for high-risk maternal and infant care, elder care, mental health services, and dental care are most often cited as key areas of rural need. Implementing federal and state initiatives for migrant health care often becomes the responsibility of community health nurses as well. New grant-supported incentives through CDC are supporting case finding, fieldwork, and epidemiologic follow-up by community health nurses as a way to track rural health accidents and illness.[8]

State rural health associations and state offices of rural health are two relatively new health-care provider groups that are proving to be strong support systems for rural health professionals and consumers.

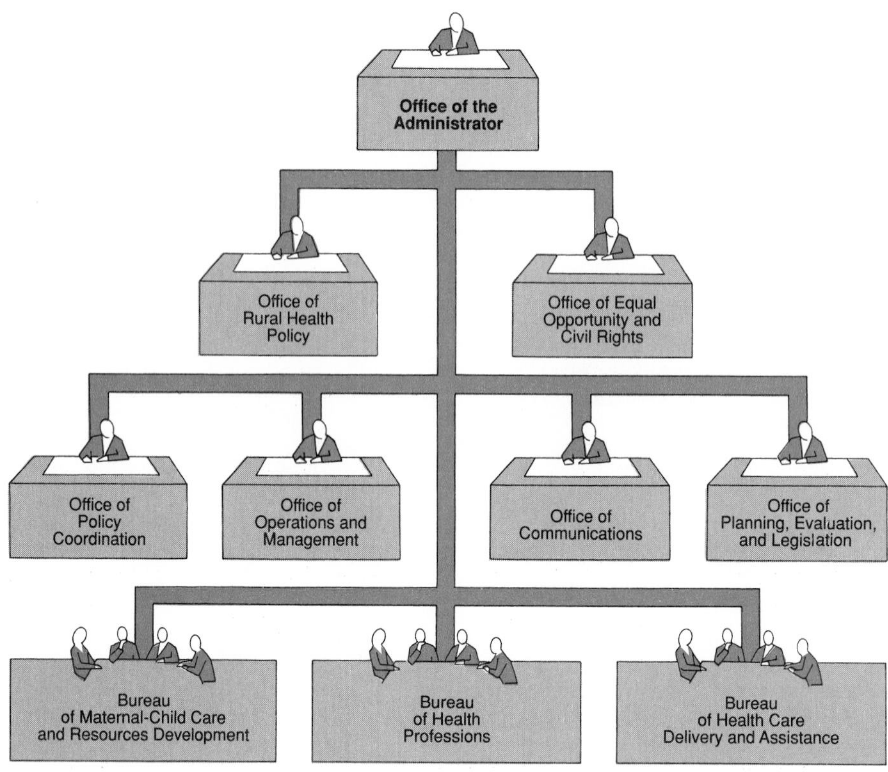

Figure 28–4. Organizational chart of the U.S. Health Resources and Services Administration showing placement of the Office of Rural Health policy.

The nurse in a rural setting would assess the availability and influence of these and other groups and programs in their jurisdictions.

The Internal System: Local Community Care and Family-centered Care

Health-care services for many rural residents are less accessible, more costly to deliver, narrower in range and scope, and fewer in number than those available to their urban counterparts. This is true for most professional services including those of physicians, dentists, nurses, and social workers and is particularly true of services for the elderly in rural areas.[6]

Informal care-giving by relatives and friends in rural communities is an essential component of a rural community's internal health-care system[9] and should be a major focus of efforts for assessing care-giving activities. This informal care is often provided to frail and immobile elderly persons who have limited resources.[10] Assisting relatives and friends in their capacity as care-givers helps individuals and families better control health problems that affect their lives. This is important for rural people who value independence and control over their lives.

Folk beliefs and alternative methods of care other than those provided by health professionals are common in rural areas of the United States. Herbalists, witch doctors, and healers are viewed by some rural clients as very acceptable sources of care. Assessment of these alternative providers and practices is essential to understanding the rural health-care system.

In rural areas, the Church, regardless of denomination, is seen as a stronghold for local community care to high-risk groups, especially for the elderly and for the rural homeless. The rural pastor is often a key player in finding monies or other resources for members of the congregation. Rural health nurses may look to clients' churches for resources in emergency situations. Volunteerism and charitable acts to members of the community are part of the rural way of life.

The emergency medical system within the rural community is a critical component of the health-care system. Because the rural community health nurse may rely heavily on the stability and quality of the EMS program to provide client care, it is an important assessment consideration, and the nurse would assess the type of services available and the expertise of those providing them.

The loss of large numbers of obstetricians from rural communities, due to prohibitive malpractice costs and lack of professional support, places pregnant women and infants in rural settings at risk for complications. This outflow of physicians from rural America places responsibility for much of the assessment of healthy prenatal women and infants on the community health nurse, leaving delivery and high-risk care to the overburdened rural obstetrician.

DIAGNOSTIC REASONING AND CARE OF CLIENTS IN RURAL SETTINGS

In rural areas, the etiology of nursing diagnoses is frequently related to a lack of resources and limited access to health care in the community. A nursing diagnosis of "potential for poor infant outcome due to 3-hour travel time to nearest maternity delivery service" is common in today's rural health system and requires that the rural nurse providing prenatal care be most astute in assessing this client during her pregnancy. A second nursing diagnosis might be, "Increased suicide risk due to lack of access to mental health services." Again, this diagnosis is attributable to limited access to health care.

The financial pressures of farming in rural America have caused rural mothers to seek outside employment and leave the farm father to care for the children while he is attending to farm chores. This change in child care might suggest a nursing diagnosis of "increased potential for farm accidents due to lack of day-care services for rural preschoolers during the absence of working mothers." Rural nurses are often the care-givers who can identify the potential safety problems in this situation and help the family work toward solutions.

PLANNING CLIENT CARE IN RURAL SETTINGS

Planning primary, secondary, and tertiary levels of prevention can be directed toward meeting the needs of individual clients, families, or the community itself. The community health nurse plays a pivotal role in planning preventative strategies for rural communities.

PRIMARY PREVENTION

In rural settings, primary prevention focuses on preventing high-risk health problems endemic to rural communities. Prevention is achieved through health-promotion activities, preventing common illnesses, and preventing accidents and injuries related to work and leisure activities.

Health Promotion

Planning for health-promotive activities in selected community agencies is a rewarding task for the community health nurse. One of the items of the national school agenda for the next decade is to introduce health-promotion practices to children beginning in kindergarten. Rural school nurses and community health nurses can play major roles in this endeavor. Community health nurses can also plan to teach principles of good nutrition to pregnant women and to cafeteria workers and cooks who plan and serve meals in schools and other institutions.

The lack of access to healthy foods is sometimes apparent in rural communities where elderly persons must shop at "convenience" stores that sell high-cholesterol, high-fat, sodium-laden foods. To alleviate problems of this sort, the community health nurse can help to plan community support for transportation for communal shopping trips to the nearest supermarket to allow the elderly to maintain healthy eating habits.

A strong emphasis on organized athletics in junior and senior high schools provides another opportunity for health promotion. Nurses can also emphasize healthy activities and use of appropriate safety equipment in organized summer camps sponsored by churches and other organizations.

There is a pressing need for school-based clinics for adolescents for both family planning and prenatal care, and community health nurses can be actively involved in planning and implementing care in such clinics. These clinics offer the rural nurse prime opportunities for teaching women's self-care practices, including breast self-examination, encouraging Pap smears, and explaining safe sexual practices. Community health nurses in rural areas play a critical role in sex education and in helping both girls and boys to develop prudent sexual practices.

In rural communities, there are often few formal programs for cardiovascular fitness, and community health nurses can be instrumental in designing programs of this type. Public health and church-based aerobics classes and diet programs are other ways for nurses to lend their professional expertise to health promotion in the rural community.

Illness Prevention

Rural community health nurses can plan nursing interventions aimed at modifying risk factors among aggregates of rural clients in several ways. Booths at yearly country fairs offer excellent opportunities for children and adults to present projects related to health promotion and illness prevention. The nurse is a resource person in these types of activities. Planning hypertension, cholesterol, breast self-exam, or glaucoma screening opportunities through the auspices of a local church or other community organization is another way to assist the community to focus on the need to lower health risks.

Sitting on school, public health, or mental health boards affords the rural community health nurse an opportunity to help the community set the "health agenda" around illness prevention. Rural community leaders are often not well advised on how to carry out these matters. Speaking at Rotary or Lion's Club meetings, Jaycees, or the local garden club are other ways that the rural nurse can encourage clients to assume a role in illness prevention. Many resources are available from national and state groups to support these efforts. Table 28–2 identifies state and national resources to which rural community health nurses can turn for help.

Injury Prevention

Planning to prevent accidents within the rural community is a major role for the rural community health nurse. Farm and motor vehicle accidents rank as the number-one cause of morbidity and mortality for young people in rural America. Moreover, the fatality rate for agricultural industries is 2.6 times greater than the national average for all other industries.[8] Farm accidents, especially those involving children, are receiving national emphasis. Children operating farm equipment, hearing and eye protection, machine safety education, and preventing childhood poisonings are all areas requiring education and preventative strategies. The rural community health nurse serves as both formal and informal educator as well as community planner for accident-prevention strategies.

SECONDARY PREVENTION

As in other nursing settings, planning for secondary prevention is geared toward resolving health problems identified during assessment. Rural nurses focus on screening for health problems; treating clients with ongoing problems and providing episodic care; performing triage and referring clients in emergency situations; and monitoring clients' health status.

Screening

Major screening activities of rural community health nurses may be carried out in one of two settings—the local school system or the public health department. Children, for example, typically are screened for scoliosis, hearing and vision problems, and immunization status. Community health nurses also routinely monitor children's growth patterns and test for anemia. Adults are screened for hypertension and tuberculosis, and screening examinations for breast, cervical, and colon cancer may also be performed.

Funding for most of the monitoring and screening activities that nurses provide is derived from state and federal sources. Therefore, it is crucial that rural community health nurses take an active part in the assessment, planning, and decision-making process to allocate program funds. Coalition-building and political activity for a rural health-care platform are professional activities of rural community health nurses.

Environmental Screening

Rural community health nurses frequently assist environmentalists to plan for community improvement based on environmental health problems identified during assessment. This includes concerns about indoor plumbing, lack of heat for the elderly, poor or contaminated water supplies, unacceptable care of animals, reporting of animal bites, and outbreaks of infectious illness—for example, gastrointestinal infections due to giardiasis or salmonella.

Treating Existing Conditions

Community health nurses working in rural settings will spend a major portion of their time caring for clients with existing health problems and providing episodic health care. New legislation that will allow rural hospitals to expand into primary-care centers to provide care management for clients across a continuum of health states will further increase this component of rural nursing care.

In rural areas, where mental health services are severely lacking, it is most often the nurse who assists client and family to deal with the burden of emotional stress and chronic mental illness. Homeless mental health patients are part of the rural extended family, and their health-care needs are part of the rural nursing repertoire.

Management of chronic illness is a family affair in rural settings, with the community health nurse acting as a resource person and facilitator. The nurse may plan several strategies to assist family-centered services.[11] For example, encouraging Congress and state legislatures to continue to target health-care programs to rural areas, offering reimbursement to families in the planning and delivery of this care, encouraging neighbors and friends to help, and recognizing the diversity that exists among communities and families are some strategies that would assist families in these situations.

Emergency Care, Triage, and Referral

Another important area of rural community health nursing is that of emergency care. Research has

TABLE 28–2. RESOURCES FOR NURSES IN RURAL HEALTH SETTINGS

Focus	Agency or Organization	Services
Education	Rural Clearinghouse for Education and Development Division of Continuing Education College Court Bldg. Kansas State University Manhattan, KS 66506 (913) 532-5560	Information on rural education
Health promotion	Cooperative Extension Service Local chapter in each state	Client education
	National Health Information Clearinghouse P.O. Box 1133 Washington, DC 20013	Health resources
Rural elderly	Center on Rural Elderly University of Missouri 5245 Rockhill Kansas City, MO 64110 (816) 276-2180	Information on rural aged
Rural health	National Mental Health Association 1021 Prince St. Alexandria, VA 22314	Rural mental health issues
	National Rural Health Association 301 East Armour Blvd. Suite 420 Kansas City, MO 64111 (816) 756-3140	Information on rural health care
	Office of Rural Health Policy U.S. Dept. of Health and Human Services 5600 Fisher's Lane, Room 14-22 Rockville, MD 20857 (303) 443-0835	Rural health clinics, information about rural health policy
	U.S. Department of Agriculture Rural Information Center National Agricultural Library Room 304 Beltsville, MD 20705 (301) 344-2547	Resources on rural health
	U.S. House of Representatives Rural Health Care Coalition 2244 Rayburn House Office Bldg. Washington, DC 20515 (202) 225-2911	Federal rural health issues
	U.S. Senate Rural Health Caucus 511 Hart Senate Office Bldg. Washington, DC 20510 (202) 224-2551	Federal rural health issues
Rural issues	State Rural Health Association State Offices of Rural Health (contact local state government)	Information
Rural nursing	American Nurses' Association 2420 Pershing Road Kansas City, MO 64108 (816) 474-5720	Nursing incentives to improve rural health care
Safety	National Institute for Occupational Safety and Health 1600 Clifton Rd. Atlanta, GA 30333 (404) 329-3771	Farm safety and rural accident prevention

shown that the early hours of care are critical to successful outcomes for emergency situations. New telecommunications networks such as telemetry and Fax capabilities put the rural nurse in close contact with medical and nursing expertise. Simulations and protocols assist the nurse to implement emergency care until support arrives. Careful planning and coordination of members of the emergency team is essential to successful emergency care services.

Monitoring Health Status

The last focus for community health nurses involved in secondary prevention in rural settings is monitoring the health status of clients with chronic health problems. For example, monitoring elderly clients with the triad of diabetes mellitus, hypertension, and renal disease is a common activity in rural care. Patients with chronic illnesses are treated during the acute phase of their illness in tertiary urban settings and then discharged to convalesce at home. Planning to monitor their status may include plans to continue chemotherapy and observe for treatment effects for clients with cancer; monitoring cardiac status after coronary bypass surgery; or monitoring clients on respirators or home dialysis.

TERTIARY PREVENTION

Tertiary preventive efforts of community health nurses who work in rural practice settings are directed toward preventing complications of chronic illness and preventing recurrences of acute health problems. These nursing care measures are carried out primarily by community-based home health nurses who care for elderly and chronically homebound clients who are monitored closely to assure stability of their disease process. Case-management activities to coordinate care and resources can be quite effective in preventing complications.

Community health nurses carefully monitor the nation's health through the administration of immunizations to both children and adults. Pneumonia and influenza vaccines are available for the rural elderly. Rural communities are just seeing the tip of the iceberg with regard to AIDS, and community health nurses are the mainstay of AIDS care both as counselors for HIV-infected individuals and as providers of nursing care for clients with full-blown AIDS.

A great deal of the follow-up care in rural communities is carried out through "being neighborly." The local nurse is viewed as the person to contact before making the return visit to the city physician. In both the school and community setting in rural communities, education about safety and high-risk health behaviors is a key strategy of rural nurses involved in tertiary prevention.

IMPLEMENTING HEALTH CARE IN RURAL SETTINGS

Nursing interventions in rural settings usually involve the client and family and any other available resources. The case-management approach within the context of continuity of care for the entire family is the desired outcome. The plan of care should be implemented locally whenever possible because distant services are not only expensive but also difficult for clients to manage. A broad understanding of what health services are available and how to obtain these services is critical. Good communication skills and building strong interprofessional networks are vital to successful nursing intervention in the rural practice setting.

EVALUATING HEALTH CARE IN RURAL SETTINGS

Evaluating health care in the rural setting is done by focusing on outcomes for rural clients and for the rural community. One way that community health nurses can evaluate outcomes is by carrying out clinical research projects within the community. For example, are nursing interventions lowering the teen pregnancy rate in the local high school? Are the infants who receive milk through the rural health department progressing satisfactorily in terms of their growth and development? Is the overweight elderly population in a community-based hypertension clinic losing weight? These and other issues are of concern to community health nurses in rural areas.

CHAPTER HIGHLIGHTS

- Barriers to effective rural health care include poverty, distance from health-care services, the presence of high-risk aggregates, health policy inequities, and lack of personnel.
- The hallmark of rural community health nursing is generalist, family-centered care.
- Rural communities are made up of diverse populations.
- A major reward of rural community health nursing is the close interaction with local families.
- Rural community health nurses are found in a myriad of community settings including public health and home health agencies; rural community primary-care clinics; occupational and environmental health settings; and schools.
- The rural elderly, and infants and children are two population aggregates that require special consideration by community health nurses.
- In rural communities, the etiology of a nursing diagnosis is often related to a lack of health-care resources and limited access to care.
- Informal care-giving by family and neighbors is essential to planning health-care interventions.
- Rural community health nurses assist environmentalists to plan for improved environmental health in rural communities.
- Education about safety and high-risk lifestyles is a key role for community health nurses in rural settings.

Review Questions

1. Describe five differences between rural and urban communities. (p. 678)
2. Describe three roles for community health nurses in rural areas. (p. 678)
3. What are three work environments where community health nurses might be found in rural settings? (p. 680)
4. Describe at least four barriers to effective health care in rural areas. What might community health nurses do to eliminate these barriers? (p. 681)
5. What two age groups in rural settings are at particular risk for health problems? Why? (p. 683)
6. Describe at least five environmental concerns unique to rural settings. What influence might they have on the health of rural residents? (p. 684)
7. Identify four major occupational and safety risk factors for rural populations. (p. 685)
8. In what two ways do inequities in health policy create barriers to health care in rural settings? (p. 682)
9. Identify three aspects of primary prevention in rural settings. How might community health nurses be involved in each? (p. 689)
10. Describe four approaches to secondary prevention in rural settings. What interventions might community health nurses employ with respect to each? (p. 690)

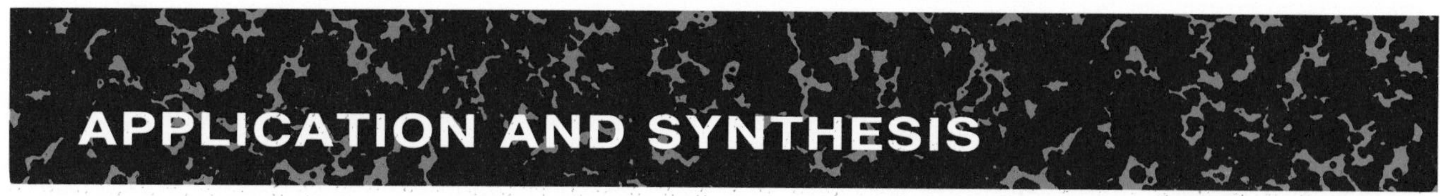

APPLICATION AND SYNTHESIS

You are a rural community health nurse assigned to the county health department mobile van visiting a large migrant community at a local farm. Mr. Robert Kelbert is a 64-year-old black migrant worker who comes into the mobile unit to have his blood pressure medication refilled. He will be in the county for the next 3 to 4 weeks to harvest the soybean crop. He usually attends a rural health clinic in the northern part of the state where he has been receiving his care and medications free.

Today his blood pressure is 154/98; his pulse is 88; height is 69 inches, and weight 198 pounds. He states he is "worn out" from the heat. He chews tobacco and drinks alcohol "some." He travels and stays with his son and family. His daughter-in-law does the cooking. During your interview, Mr. Kelbert tells you he is worried because two of the migrant workers have been given medicine for lung congestion and one of them has been coughing up blood.

1. What are some of the human biological, environmental, life-style, and health system factors operating in this situation?
2. List three nursing diagnoses that you would identify for Mr. Kelbert.
3. What are your objectives for today's client visit?
4. How might your care for Mr. Kelbert differ from that provided to a client you see regularly at the rural health department?
5. What primary, secondary, and tertiary prevention measures are appropriate for Mr. Kelbert?
6. How will you follow up on this visit?

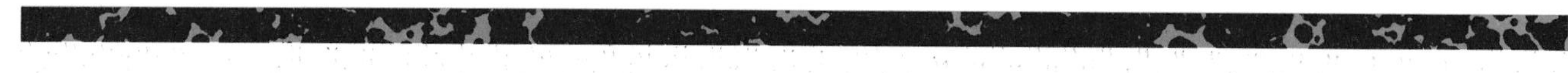

REFERENCES

1. Hanson, C. M., Ryan, R., & Jenkins, S. (1990). Job satisfaction and autonomy as correlates of retention in rural hospital nurses. *The Journal of Rural Health, 6*(7), 302–316.
2. Office of Technology Assessment. (1989). *Defining "rural" areas: Impact on health care policy and research.* (GPO publication No. 052-003-01156-5). Washington, DC: Government Printing Office.
3. Lassiter, P. G. (1985). Rural practice: How do we prepare providers?—Nurses. *The Journal of Rural Health, 1*(1), 23–26.
4. Holloway, T. (1989). *Syphilis, crack, and AIDS: Rural Georgia's new epidemic.* Waycross, GA: Southeast Health Unit.
5. Porter, K. H. (1989). *Poverty in rural America: A national overview.* Washington, DC: Center on Budget and Policy Priorities.
6. Coward, R. T., & Lee, G. R. (Eds.). (1985). *The elderly in rural society: Every fourth elder.* New York: Springer.
7. Hawk, C., Gay, J., & Donham, K. J. (1991). Rural youth disability prevention survey: Results from 169 Iowa farm families. *The Journal of Rural Health, 7*(2), 170–175.
8. National Institute for Occupational Safety and Health (NIOSH). (1990). *Announcement 031, Program Guidance.* Atlanta: Centers for Disease Control.
9. Weinert, C., & Long, K. A. (1988). Understanding the health care needs of rural families. In R. Marotz-Baden, C. B. Hennon, & T. H. Brubaker (Eds.), *Families in rural America* (pp. 225–232). St. Paul, MN: National Council on Family Relations.
10. Newhouse, J. K., & McAuley, W. J. (1988). Understanding the health care needs of rural families. In R. Marotz-Baden, C. B. Hennon, & T. H. Brubaker (Eds.), *Families in rural America* (pp. 238). St. Paul, MN: National Council on Family Relations.
11. Mertensmeyer, C., & Coleman, M. (1988). Correlates

of inter-role conflict. In R. Marotz-Baden, C. B. Hennon, & T. H. Brubaker (Eds.), *Families in rural America* (pp. 142–148). St. Paul, MN: National Council on Family Relations.

RECOMMENDED READINGS

Bushey, A. (Ed.). (1991). *Rural nursing, Vols. 1 & 2.* Newbury Park, CA: Sage.

Both volumes present an excellent overview of the many facets of rural life and rural health care and describe the nature and scope of rural nursing practice. Authors are drawn from rural areas in all parts of the nation to share their views, their research, and their expertise about the role of nursing in rural families and communities.

U. S. Congress, Office of Technology Assessment. (1991). *Rural America at the crossroads: Networking for the future.* (S/N 052-003-01228). Washington, DC: Government Printing Office.

Outlines the changing infrastructure of rural America. Proposes new models for orchestrating cooperation and change within rural communities.

Barger, S. E. (1991). The nursing center: A model for rural nursing practice. *Nursing and Health Care, 12*(6), 290–294.

Identifies the unique health-care delivery issues of rural populations and describes how nursing centers have addressed these issues. The role of the community health nurse is explored. Characteristics of nursing centers are clearly defined and methods of implementation by rural nurses are suggested.

Lindseth, G. (1990). Evaluating rural nurses for preparation in implementing nutrition interventions. *The Journal of Rural Health,* 6(3), 231–245.

Examines nursing interventions—specifically nutrition education practices—based on nutrition knowledge that is used in health promotion. Provides information on the nutrition education information that is most frequently sought by rural clients.

Marotz-Baden, R., Hennon, C. B., & Brubaker, T. H. (Eds.). (1988). *Families in rural America.* St. Paul, MN: National Council on Family Relations.

An interdisciplinary look at the dimensions of culture, married life, parenting, aging, and other phenomena that affect rural nursing and health care. The readings help one to understand rural life and especially the family issues surrounding the farm crisis.

Reinhardt, A. M. & Quinn, M. D. (1980). *Family centered community nursing, A socio-cultural framework.* St. Louis: C. V. Mosby.

Proposes that community health nurses must understand the totality of health factors influencing rural health in order to nurse rural clients successfully. The community and its many community health-care settings are explored. Various emerging community health nursing roles are described in depth. The community health nurse is viewed as a catalyst for rural community change.

CHAPTER 29

Care of Clients in Disaster Settings

KEY TERMS

adaptive capacity
direct victims
disaster
emergency consensus
immediate care
indirect victims
inventory
logistical coordination
mitigation
normative context
post-event response
pre-event response
pre-impact mobilization
reconstitution
remediation
restoration
triage

Throughout history, people have been subjected to unexpected events that cause massive destruction, death, and injury. Almost any day of the week, the news media cover some kind of disaster somewhere in the world. Preparation for disasters and effective response when a disaster occurs can help minimize the long-term effects of these events. This chapter will explore the role of the community health nurse with respect to disaster care before, during, and after the event.

(*continued*)

LEARNING OBJECTIVES

After reading this chapter you should be able to:

- Describe four ways in which disaster events may vary.
- Describe three factors that influence a community's response to disaster.
- Describe the three dimensions of a disaster.
- Identify at least three benefits of disaster planning.
- Identify at least two human biological, two environmental, two life-style, and two health system factors to be assessed in relation to a disaster.
- Discuss at least six principles of community disaster planning.
- Describe four characteristics of a successful disaster plan.
- Discuss at least five elements of an effective disaster plan.
- Describe the role of the community health nurse in primary, secondary, and tertiary prevention related to disaster situations.

DISASTERS

Disasters are overwhelming events that exceed the ability of those affected to respond adequately. Disasters test the adaptational responses of communities or individuals beyond their capabilities and lead to at least a temporary disruption of function.[1] In characterizing disasters, one observer spoke of the "sudden and massive *disproportion* between hostile elements of any kind and the survival resources which can be brought into action in the shortest possible time."[2]

Individuals, families, and groups or communities all experience disasters. Most people experience "personal disasters" in their own lives, events with which they are unable to cope using the resources at hand and that require assistance from the outside. In this chapter, however, the focus is on both natural and manmade disasters that affect relatively large numbers of people at once rather than isolated individuals or families.

TYPES OF DISASTERS

Disasters can be categorized as either natural or manmade. Manmade disasters can occur as a result of technology gone awry or acts of aggression such as war. Natural disasters are those produced by epidemics, famine, and forces of nature such as storms, floods, and earthquakes. Whether they are natural or manmade, disasters vary considerably in terms of their frequency, predictability, preventability, imminence, and destructive potential.

Some disasters occur relatively frequently in certain parts of the world. Consequently, people in those areas have some knowledge of what to expect and what can be done to minimize the effects of the event. For example, earthquakes occur periodically in California, and residents in earthquake-prone areas are encouraged to be prepared in the event of a large quake. Similarly, hurricanes and other severe storms are frequently experienced during certain seasons in other parts of the country.

Some disaster events are predictable. The probability of destructive tornadoes increases from April through July.[3] Similarly, many rivers are known to flood periodically with heavy spring rains. Other events, such as a plane crash or fire in a chemical plant, are not predictable.

Similarly, some types of disasters are more easily prevented than others. For example, periodic flooding can be prevented by rerouting waterways or by building dams. Others, such as earthquakes, cannot be controlled or prevented.

Disasters also vary with respect to their imminence in terms of their speed of onset, extent of forewarning, and duration. Some disasters provide evidence of their imminent occurrence and allow time for forewarning and preparation prior to impact. For example, hurricanes can be tracked and their probable path determined. People along that path usually have sufficient warning to take preventive actions that minimize the potential for death and destruction. Other disasters such as fires or explosions occur instantaneously, with no prior warning. In some cases, the disaster event itself is of short duration, as in the case of an earthquake or a transportation disaster. At other times, the disaster event lasts for some time. Examples of prolonged disasters are epidemics, famine, and war.

Finally, disasters vary in terms of their impact and their destructive potential. Some disasters are fairly limited in scope, affecting a small geographic area or a relatively small number of people. For example, the effects of a mine cave-in are generally restricted to the area where the mine is located. The effects of war or famine, on the other hand, may be more far-reaching. Disasters also vary in terms of the severity of their effects. Some disasters cause moderate loss of life or property and result in only temporary inability to function, while others are devastating in their destruction. The destructive potential of a nuclear explosion, for example, is far greater than that of a plane crash.

FACTORS AFFECTING DISASTER RESPONSE

Three factors influence the adequacy of a community's response to a disaster event: (1) the event's magnitude, (2) the community's adaptive capacity, and (3) the normative context in which the event occurs.[4] The magnitude of the disaster event can be measured in terms of the number of fatalities and serious injuries it produces, the extent of property loss, and the degree to which it disrupts the community's ability to function. The community's ***adaptive capacity*** is its ability to respond to the disaster event and its effects with minimal disruption of everyday life. A community that is prepared for a variety of emergency situations has greater adaptive capacity than one that is not, influencing the effectiveness of disaster response. The ***normative context*** in which the disaster event occurs is the extent to which the community has developed norms for responding to a disaster. For example, when a catastrophe occurs in a community that has developed norms for responding to disasters, the community is better able to respond effectively than if no such norms existed.

DIMENSIONS OF A DISASTER

In order to plan, with other members of the community, for an effective response to a disaster, community health nurses need to understand the three dimensions of a disaster: the temporal dimension, the spatial dimension, and the role dimension.

THE TEMPORAL DIMENSION: STAGES OF DISASTER RESPONSE

Several stages occur in a community's response to a disaster. These include the pre-event response, the post-event response, and the recovery response.

Pre-event Response

The ***pre-event response*** of a community involves activities that take place prior to the occurrence of a disaster. The pre-event response can be divided into three distinct stages: planning, warning, and pre-impact mobilization. The planning stage should occur before there is any indication that a disaster is about to occur, while the warning and pre-impact mobilization stages occur when there is evidence that a disaster is likely to occur or when the disaster is imminent.

The Planning Stage. Disaster planning within a community takes place at individual, group, and aggregate levels, and planning at each of these three levels should be coordinated. Community health nurses would assist individuals, families, and other groups (for example, personnel in a health-care facility) to plan for their response in the event of a disaster, but the focus of the discussion here will be on planning for disaster response at the aggregate level. Actual activities involved in disaster planning will be discussed in greater detail later in this chapter.

It is hoped that communities will engage in comprehensive disaster planning, and community health nurses should advocate this type of comprehensive planning. Communities, however, may also react by denying the threat of possible disasters and the need for planning.

The Warning Stage. The warning phase of a disaster event occurs when the disaster is an imminent possibility,[1] and members of the community are apprised of the danger. People are encouraged to be on the alert and to plan for the possibility of evacuation or other action. For example, storm warnings are broadcast when there is potential for a severe storm, but people do not immediately go to a storm cellar or leave the area, because the possibility remains that the storm will bypass the area.

Just as communities may accept or deny the need for disaster planning, members of the community may respond positively or negatively to warnings of possible disasters. Several factors can influence a person's response to warnings of imminent disaster.[5] These factors include the content of the warning message, individual perceptions, warning confirmation, and belief. Warning messages that are clear, practical, and relevant are more likely to be acted upon than those that are vague or impractical. Warnings need to specify the exact nature of the threat and provide specific recommendations for action. Warnings should also contain sufficient information to allow people to decide on an appropriate course of action. It is sometimes erroneously believed that detailed information about a disaster will cause panic. In effect, failure to provide information usually leads to failure to act on warnings; providing information does not seem to contribute to panic among individual citizens.

Response to a warning will also be affected by each individual's perceptions about the possibility of disaster. These perceptions arise from past experiences with disaster, one's psychological traits, and sociocultural factors. For example, if people have previously only been on the fringes of a hurricane path, they may not perceive a hurricane as a very frightening event, and they may ignore storm warnings. Or, if the individual has a fatalistic attitude that one's own actions will not make much difference in the outcome of an event, he or she might not act in response to warnings. Such an attitude may be the result of an individual personality trait or a sociocultural norm in the group.

Warning confirmation also influences the way people respond. Warnings tend to be believed if the source of the warning is an official one, if the probability of the event is increasing, and if one is in close geographic proximity to the area where the disaster is likely to occur. For example, people who live on a recognized geological fault line are more likely to take warnings about potential earthquakes seriously than those who do not live on a fault.

Finally, belief influences action with respect to warnings. Again, belief in the potential for disaster is enhanced if the source of the warning is an official agency and if that agency has credibility. For example, if there have been numerous false alarms in the past, people are less likely to pay attention to warnings. Belief is also enhanced if the medium of the warning is personal rather than impersonal. People are more likely to evacuate their homes if someone comes to their door to warn them than if they hear a warning on the radio. Previous experience also influences the likelihood of belief. If one has experienced the full force of a hurricane before, one is more likely to believe and act on a hurricane warning than would otherwise be the case.

The frequency with which the warning is received also influences belief, as do observable changes in the situation. For instance, if people see evidence of flames on a nearby hill, they are more likely to believe in the danger posed by a brush fire. Perceived behavior of others can influence belief either positively or negatively. When others are acting in response to the warning, belief is enhanced. If, however, others appear to be ignoring the warning, belief is less likely. People are also more likely to believe warnings if they are with family members than if they are with other groups of people. In fact, the group environment may reinforce disbelief rather than belief. Finally, men and older people tend to place less credence in warnings than do women and younger individuals.

People's beliefs about warnings can be represented as a hierarchical series of decisions[6] (Fig. 29–1). The first decision involves determining whether a serious risk exists if no action is taken. If no serious risk is perceived, no action is taken. The second decision involves determining whether protective action poses any risk. If there is little or no risk involved, action will be undertaken.

At the third decision point, the individual determines whether action increases one's hope of escape. If the answer is no, the person is likely to engage in defensive avoidance rather than positive action. Defensive avoidance can involve buck-passing, ignoring the warning, and/or rationalizing the decision not to take action. The final decision is whether there is time

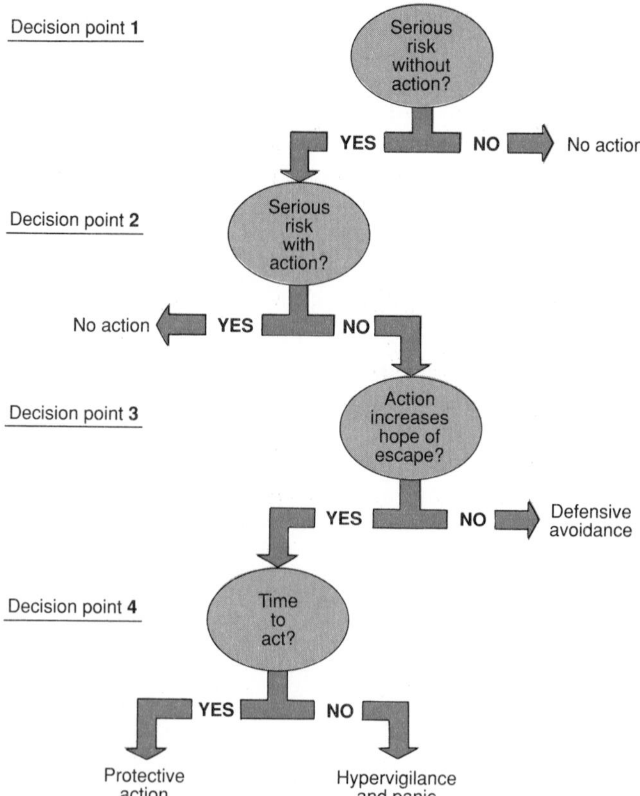

Figure 29–1. Decision points and action following warning of disaster.

BOX 29–1

Factors Influencing Response to Disaster Warnings

Factors related to the warning message
- Clarity
- Practicality
- Relevance
- Informativeness

Factors related to individual perceptions
- Past experience with disasters
- Psychological traits
- Sociocultural attitudes

Factors related to warning confirmation
- Official source for the warning
- Increasing probability of the disaster event
- Geographic proximity to the expected disaster location

Factors related to beliefs
- Credibility of the warning source
- Personal, rather than impersonal, contact
- Previous experience of disaster
- Frequency of warning
- Observable changes in the situation
- Belief and action by others

to take action that will enhance one's chances of escape. When the answer is yes, vigilance and effective coping are likely to occur, resulting in protective action. If the answer is no, the result may be hypervigilance and panic with ineffective action. Factors influencing individual responses to disaster warnings are summarized in Box 29–1.

The Pre-impact Mobilization Stage. ***Pre-impact mobilization*** is action aimed at averting the disaster or minimizing its effects. Categories of activity involved in this stage might include efforts to prevent the disaster or its effects, seeking shelter from the effects of the disaster, evacuating people from areas threatened by the disaster, and implementing plans to deal with the effects of a disaster. For example, in the threat of a flood, people may sandbag river banks to divert floodwaters from a town, or board up windows and tie down equipment when a hurricane is forecast. People may seek shelter from tornadoes or other storms by moving to a basement, a storm cellar, or an interior room of a house. Pre-impact mobilization might also involve evacuating people from an area threatened by fire, radiation, or chemical leakage. Finally, the initial phases of a disaster response plan may be implemented. For example, health-care personnel may be recalled to health facilities in preparation for treating anticipated casualties.

The Post-event Response

The ***post-event response*** consists of actions taken during and immediately following a disaster. This response involves three types of activity: inventory, rescue, and remediation.[1]

An inventory of the extent of damage and injury wrought by the disaster is the first component of the post-event response. ***Inventory*** involves a rapid assessment of the damage to buildings and the type and extent of injuries suffered. This information will be used to determine actions needed in carrying out other aspects of the immediate response. For example, if the local hospital is badly damaged, other arrangements will need to be made for handling casualties.

The second type of activity in the post-event response of a community to disaster involves rescuing victims and providing immediate care. The degree of difficulty in rescuing victims will depend on the nature of the event and the type of hazards involved in extricating them. It is also necessary that the appropriate types of equipment and personnel be available for the job. For example, if the disaster is due to a toxic gas leak, rescue workers must use appropriate breathing apparatus, and health-care providers must be prepared to deal with the physical effects of the gas. If, on the other hand, victims are trapped in rubble from collapsed buildings following an earthquake or explosion, heavy construction equipment and personnel will be needed for rescue operations, and health-care personnel will need to be prepared to deal with crushing injuries and broken bones.

The third activity in the post-event response is remedying the immediate effects of the disaster. ***Remediation*** includes providing more involved health care and meeting needs of victims for shelter, food, and clothing. Post-event remediation activities also include providing necessities for disaster workers.

The Recovery Response

The recovery stage of a community's response to a disaster consists of a return to normal equilibrium. This stage is divided into the substages of restoration, reconstitution, and mitigation.

Restoration is the reestablishment of a basic way of life and occurs within the first 6 months following

BOX 29–2

Stages of Community Disaster Response

Pre-event response
- The planning stage
- The warning stage
- The pre-impact mobilization stage

Post-event response
- Inventory
- Rescue
- Remediation

Recovery response
- Restoration
- Reconstitution
- Mitigation

a disaster. Activities of this stage include returning to or rebuilding homes, replacing lost or damaged property, and continuing life without those who were killed in the catastrophe. At the community level, restoration involves reestablishing community services that may have been disrupted by the disaster. After a flood, for example, people may return to their homes, clean up the mud, and replace water-damaged furniture. Schools will reopen, and residents will return to work. If a prominent community official was killed in the flood, someone will be appointed to fill that post until an election can be held.

Reconstitution occurs when the life of the community has returned, as far as possible, to normal. This return to normal may take from several months to several years depending upon the degree of damage sustained in the disaster. It may take several years after a flood, for example, to restore the landscape of the community to its former self or to replenish the city treasury after disaster costs have depleted it. It may also take some time for individuals to adjust to the loss of loved ones or for the community government to be reconstituted.

The final stage of recovery after a disaster is ***mitigation,*** which involves future-oriented activities to prevent subsequent disasters or to minimize their effects. For example, a community that has experienced a flood may take engineering action to prevent the likelihood of subsequent floods. Or, a community that was unprepared for disaster may develop a disaster response plan. The stages of community response to a disaster are summarized in Box 29–2.

THE SPATIAL DIMENSION

The spatial dimensions of a disaster refer to the extent of its effects on specific geographic regions. These regions include the area of total impact, the area of partial impact, and outside areas (Fig. 29–2).[1]

The area of total impact is the zone where the most severe effects of the disaster are found. In an earthquake, for example, this would include the area where the greatest damage to buildings has occurred and where the greatest number of injuries were sustained.

In the area of partial impact, evidence of the disaster can be seen but the effects are not of the magnitude of those in the total impact area. Using the earthquake example, there may be broken windows or objects shaken from shelves in the partial impact area, but buildings are intact and injuries, if any, are infrequent and relatively minor. Or, only telephone and electrical services might be disrupted in the partial impact area.

The outside area is not directly affected but may be a source of assistance in response to the disaster. Areas immediately adjacent to the disaster area will be called upon first to provide assistance, with further outlying areas being involved later as needed.

Spatial dimensions of a disaster vary greatly from event to event. For example, the total and partial impact areas affected by a nuclear accident would be far larger than those affected by a fire at an industrial chemicals plant. The area from which assistance might be requested will also be larger given the greater magnitude of the problem, the number of victims involved, and the damage sustained.

THE ROLE DIMENSION

The final dimension of a disaster is its role dimension. Two basic roles for people involved in a disaster are *victim* and *helper* roles.[1]

People may be direct or indirect victims of a disaster. ***Direct victims*** are those who experience maximum exposure to and effects of the event. ***Indirect victims*** are friends and family of direct victims. Direct victims may require medical or psychological assistance or help with basic survival necessities. Indirect victims need reassurance and may require help in locating family members affected by the disaster.

Helpers include designated rescue and recovery personnel as well as community members who help provide care or who assist in the provision of necessities such as food, shelter, and clothing. It is important to remember that victim and helper roles may overlap and that rescue and recovery personnel or other community helpers may themselves have suffered injury or loss as a result of the disaster.

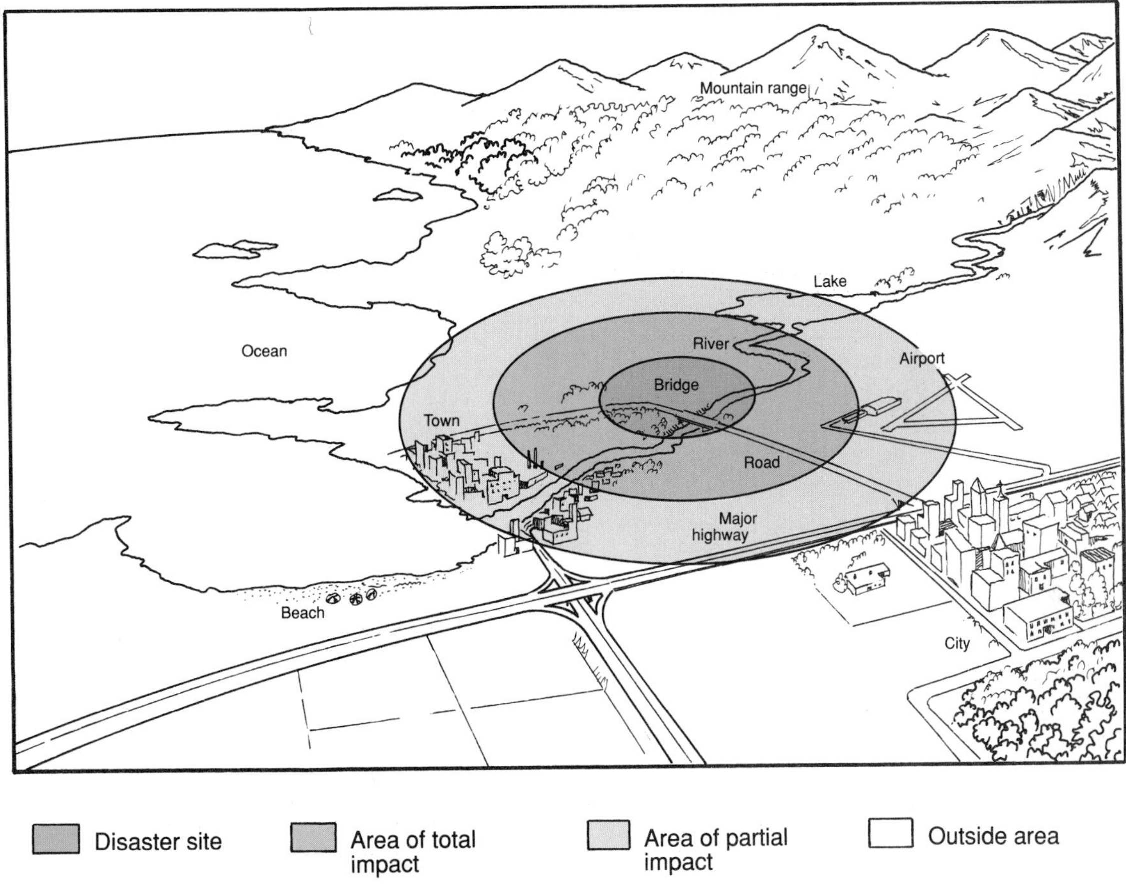

Figure 29–2. Areas of disaster impact.

Both victims and helpers are under stress as a result of the disaster. Stressors for victims may be quite obvious and include injury and the loss of loved ones or property. Stressors for helpers during the rescue and recovery periods include encounters with multiple deaths that are frequently of a shocking nature; experiencing the suffering of others; and role stress. Frequently the overwhelming nature of role demands or needs for assistance by victims leads to feelings of helplessness and depression. Other sources of role stress include communication difficulties, inadequacies in terms of resources or staff, lack of access to people needing assistance or resources to help them, bureaucratic difficulties, exhaustion, uncertainties regarding role or authority, and intragroup or intergroup conflicts. Stress may also arise from conflicts between demands of the helper's family members and the needs of victims, and between demands of one's regular job and the disaster role.

DISASTER PLANNING

As noted earlier, it is to be hoped that the earlier stages of a community's response to a disaster involve planning for a disaster event. For this to occur, community health nurses and others in the community must have an understanding of the concepts and principles of disaster planning.

BENEFITS OF DISASTER PLANNING

The need for disaster preparation and plans for disaster response is greater today than at any time in history. Increased population density throughout the world has heightened the potential for widespread effects of disasters. Technologies such as nuclear reactors and dams to provide water and electricity have also contributed to increased potential for disastrous events, as has man's increased capacity to wage destructive warfare.

The costs of all types of disasters are staggering in terms of death and human suffering as well as dollars. Economic costs for natural disasters in the United States alone could reach as high as $18 billion annually by the year 2000. With adequate preparation and timely response, it is estimated that the monetary costs of disaster could be reduced by as much as 20 percent to 40 percent.[1] The savings in human lives that could result are another strong motivation for concerted community efforts in disaster planning.

The need for disaster planning is reinforced by observations that there is less confusion regarding responsibilities and communications when specific agencies have been assigned specific functions in keeping with an overall disaster response plan. In addition, the development of interagency linkages that take place in disaster planning increases the smoothness of response in an actual disaster situation. A final reason for concerted disaster planning is that well-developed existing plans can be used in the event of other unforeseen events.[4]

Disaster planning can modify, to some degree, the three factors influencing a community's response to a disaster event discussed earlier, thus increasing the effectiveness of the community's response to a disaster and limiting its damaging effects. In some instances, disaster planning can limit the magnitude of the catastrophe. For example, if there is a response plan in the event of a major fire, the fire may be contained before extensive damage has been done or lives have been lost. Similarly, community preparedness in the event of a hurricane can minimize damage and loss of life.

Disaster planning can also increase the adaptive capacity of the community. Planning for a disaster event heightens the community's ability to respond effectively to the aftermath of the disaster. For instance, if there is a plan for emergency food and shelter that can be put into operation in the event of a disaster, the number of lives that are disrupted can be minimized. Or, if contingency plans exist for different situations, performance of critical functions will be less disrupted than they would otherwise be. For example, plans may call for casualties to be brought to a certain hospital during a disaster. If that hospital is affected by the disaster and there is no alternative planned, the community will be less able to adapt to the situation, care of victims will suffer, and more lives may be lost.

Finally, disaster planning creates a normative context that enhances the effectiveness of community response to the disaster. For example, if there is community awareness that, in the event of a disaster, the local police will take over a coordination function, there will be less confusion in dealing with the exigencies of the disaster than if there is no norm for the situation.

PURPOSES OF DISASTER PLANNING

Disaster planning has two major purposes.[1] The first is to reduce the community's vulnerability to the disaster and to prevent it, if possible. For example, when the threat of flood is imminent, work crews may sandbag river banks in an attempt to prevent flooding of homes and businesses. Or, in an area where flooding occurs periodically, a dam might be built to control water flow and prevent flooding. A community's vulnerability to the effects of flooding may also be reduced by locating vital community services on high ground to prevent their disruption by floodwaters.

The second purpose of disaster planning is to ensure that resources are available for effective post-event response in the event of a disaster. This aspect of planning involves determining procedures that will be employed in response to a disaster event and obtaining material and personnel that will be required to implement the disaster plan.

PRINCIPLES OF DISASTER PLANNING

Disaster planning should be based on several general principles.[4] The first principle is that measures used for everyday emergencies typically are not useful for major disasters. Disasters and everyday emergencies differ in their degree of uncertainty, urgency, and "emergency consensus." They also differ in terms of the role played by private citizens and the emphasis placed on contractual and interpersonal relationships. Disasters typically present a greater degree of uncertainty than do everyday emergencies in that the latter tend to be more predictable. For example, the types of activities needed to respond to the usual residential fire are well known and predictable. The precise needs in a disaster situation are largely dependent on the type and extent of the disaster and, while some of this can be predicted, the exact extent of needs is uncertain until the event occurs.

Disasters are also attended by a greater degree of urgency than everyday emergencies. Traffic accidents, for example, occur frequently and pose a need for action. People may be trapped in damaged vehicles, and there is a need to get them out. In a large-scale plane crash or train wreck, there is less knowledge of what the status of those trapped may be than in the case of the individual trapped in a single vehicle. There may also be greater urgency if the train was carrying hazardous materials that may cause further damage.

In a disaster there is also less of an ***emergency consensus*** or agreement on what must be done and how to do it than is usually true of an everyday emergency. In addition, private citizens may play a very active role in rescue and response activities in a disaster situation, but have little or no role in responding to everyday emergencies. In the case of a residential fire, for example, once fire department personnel have arrived, private citizens are expected to stay out of the way rather than assist in fighting the blaze. However, when a lengthy section of a major highway collapsed during an earthquake in San Francisco, residents in the area began immediately to help rescue people trapped in their cars and continued to help with rescue operations even after emergency personnel arrived.

Finally, in a disaster there often is less emphasis on contractual relationships than there is in an everyday emergency. For example, a supermarket might provide food to people regardless of their ability to pay, which is not the usual contractual relationship. Similarly, the rules that typically govern interpersonal relationships may be suspended during a disaster. For example, people may offer shelter to perfect strangers in a disaster, whereas they would be more likely to limit assistance to family and friends in the event of an everyday emergency.

The second principle in disaster planning is that plans need to be adjusted to people's needs and not vice versa. If a large portion of the population is non-English-speaking, for example, it is unreasonable to issue disaster warnings only in English in the hope that someone will be available to translate the message. The third principle is that disaster planning does not stop at the development of a written plan. Rather, disaster planning is a continuing process that changes as community circumstances change.

Fourth, the greater the incorporation of disaster "myths" into the plan, the less effective the plan will be. For example, some individuals believe that disasters inevitably trigger widespread looting and theft when this is not usually the case. If disaster planning focuses on such myths, supplies and personnel will be diverted from necessary activities and directed instead toward preventing events that are unlikely to occur.[4]

The need for information about a disaster is reflected in the fifth principle. All too frequently, some planners believe that providing the public with detailed information about the disaster and its effects will lead to panic. For this reason, vital information may be withheld, actually leading to a lack of response or to an inappropriate response on the part of the public.

The sixth principle is that, in the event of a disaster, people are likely to respond without direction, in the absence of a specific disaster plan. The typical response of most community members will be to do what seems best in the circumstances, sometimes even with heroic action. While such efforts are commendable, they may result in duplication of effort, inefficient use of resources, and confusion.

Another principle is that the disaster plan should enlist the support and coordinate the efforts of the entire community. To achieve this end, major components of the community that would be involved in a disaster response should be involved in developing the response plan. Some of those that might be involved include police and fire departments, local governing bodies, major health-care facilities, and large corporations. Pre-disaster incorporation of these various segments of the community limits confusion with respect to authority and direction for disaster-related activities and enhances the smooth operation of a disaster effort.

An eighth principle is that there is a need to link the disaster plan for one area with those of surrounding areas to allow coordination of efforts in the face of widespread catastrophe. Conversely, when help is needed from surrounding areas, that help will better complement local efforts if plans are coordinated.

The ninth principle is that there is a need for a general plan that addresses all potential types of disasters in the community. When there are several separate plans for different types of disasters, there is potential for confusion regarding roles and responsibilities in any particular situation. If, for example, fire personnel are supposed to have primary authority in disasters involving fires and military personnel in disasters related to destruction of property (say, an earthquake), there may be confusion about authority in any disaster involving both. Conversely, in an unanticipated disaster, neither group may take responsibility for decision making, and the response will be hampered by lack of leadership.

In addition, disaster plans should be based as much as possible on everyday working methods and procedures. If one approach to communication is used in dealing with everyday emergencies, the same approach should be used in the event of a major disaster. This eliminates the need for personnel to learn new procedures and prevents confusion over which procedure is applicable in a given situation.

The eleventh principle is that a disaster plan should be flexible enough to fit the specific situation.

If the disaster event has eliminated usual means of communication, there should be a contingency plan to adapt to that circumstance. Similarly, if injured victims were to be taken to a specific hospital for treatment after stabilization and that hospital is damaged in an earthquake, there is a need to change the plan to adapt to this situation.

The twelfth and final principle of disaster planning is that the plan should not specify responsible persons by name but by position or title. This prevents a need to revise the plan whenever one person leaves and another takes over the position. For example, the plan may specify that the chief of police will be notified of the emergency situation and will put the disaster plan into effect. Then, whoever happens to be chief of police will know that it is his or her responsibility to mobilize personnel in the event of a disaster. The principles of disaster planning at the community level are summarized in Box 29–3.

PARTICIPANTS IN DISASTER PLANNING

Planning for community response in the event of a disaster should involve a broad cross section of the community. Categories of people who should be involved in developing a disaster response plan are those discussed in Chapter 19, Care of the Community or Target Group, and include individuals who have the authority to sanction the plan, those who will implement the plan, beneficiaries of the plan, experts in the area, and those who are likely to resist the plan.

In disaster planning, the people who have authority to sanction a disaster plan are usually local government officials, so local governing bodies should be represented in the planning group. Representatives of those who will implement the plan might include health-care professionals (including community health nurses) and personnel from local health-care facilities; fire department and police department spokespersons; personnel from major industries in the area; and others who have special capabilities that might be needed in a disaster (for example, representatives of local radio and TV stations). Beneficiaries of the disaster plan are community residents, so members of concerned citizen's groups might be asked to participate in developing a disaster response plan. Consultants in disaster planning may also be invited to participate and to share their expertise. Finally, those who might object to the plan could include people who are concerned with the cost of mounting disaster planning efforts. They should be included in the planning group because they might be able to envision less expensive ways of achieving the ends of disaster planning.

BOX 29–3

Principles of Community Disaster Planning

- Measures used for everyday emergencies are not sufficient for major disasters
- Disaster plans should be adjusted to people's needs and not vice versa
- Disaster planning does not stop with the development of a written plan, but is a continuous process changing with community circumstances
- The greater the incorporation of disaster myths, the less effective the disaster plan will be
- Lack of information, rather than too much information, causes inappropriate response by community members
- People will respond to a disaster situation with or without direction
- The disaster plan should coordinate the efforts of the entire community so that large segments of the citizenry should be involved in its development
- The community's disaster plan should be linked to those of surrounding areas
- Plans should be general enough to cover all potential disaster events
- As much as possible, plans should be based on everyday work methods and procedures
- Plans should be flexible enough to be used in a variety of situations
- Plans should specify persons responsible for implementing segments of the plan by position or title rather than by name

CHARACTERISTICS OF SUCCESSFUL DISASTER PLANS

Disaster plans can be either more or less effective. An effective plan has four basic qualities.[4] First, an effective plan typically is based on realistic expectations of the effects and needs a disaster will generate. Sec-

BOX 29–4

Characteristics of Successful Disaster Plans

- The plan is based on realistic expectations of effects and needs
- The plan is brief and concise
- The plan unfolds and expands by stages
- The plan possesses an official stamp of authority

ond, a sound disaster plan is brief and concise. A lengthy or complicated plan is unlikely to be properly implemented. Third, an effective plan unfolds by stages. The plan designates activities that must be carried out first and establishes priorities and time lines appropriate to the situation. Finally, a good disaster plan possesses an official stamp of authority. When a plan is officially sanctioned by all of the participating agencies and governing bodies, those agencies are more likely to cooperate in implementing the plan. The characteristics of successful disaster plans are summarized in Box 29–4.

If these qualities are the hallmarks of an effective disaster plan, what are the indicators of an ineffective plan? A plan may be ineffective if it does not adequately deal with large-scale disasters that produce large numbers of casualties.[4] An ineffective disaster plan may fail to specify resources available in the community. Some plans fail because of undue intrusion of political machinations. Finally, many inadequate disaster plans lack review mechanisms that allow planners to correct past mistakes.

GENERAL CONSIDERATIONS IN DISASTER PLANNING

General considerations in planning the response to a disaster event include designating authority, developing communication mechanisms, providing transportation, and developing a record-keeping system.

AUTHORITY

An effective disaster response plan designates a central authority figure and lays out the responsibilities that are delegated to specific persons and organizations. For example, if it is clear that evacuation decisions are made by the mayor and implemented by members of a local military installation, while police have the responsibility for keeping roads open, there will be less confusion and evacuation efforts will be carried out more smoothly. Central authority may be assigned to several people in a hierarchical order so that in the absence of the first person designated, the second person has authority to implement the plan. In his or her absence, a third person would assume that authority, and so on.

COMMUNICATION

Communication is critical to the effective implementation of a disaster response plan. Modes of communication should be established, and disaster personnel and the general public should be familiarized with them. Specific considerations in this area include how warnings of an imminent disaster will be communicated; how communication between various emergency teams and facilities will be handled; and how communication with the outside world will be facilitated. It is important to remember that normal means of communication may be disrupted during an emergency. There should also be some consideration given to facilitating communication among members of the community. For example, there may be a central bulletin board where messages can be left or a specific agency that is responsible for handling personal communications that permit family members separated by a disaster to locate each other.

TRANSPORTATION

General plans for the provision of necessary transportation must also be considered. There will be a need to transport personnel and equipment to the disaster site as well as to transport victims away from the site. There will also be a need to move personnel to areas where they are most needed. Another consideration with respect to transportation is keeping access roads open so that emergency vehicles can pass.

RECORDS

Records will be needed prior to a disaster regarding the availability of supplies and equipment and areas where they are stored. This information should be updated on a regular basis and a systematic process for its updating should be established. Local institutions such as schools and businesses should be encouraged to keep records of all those present at any given time to allow everyone to be accounted for and to permit the identification of those missing as early as possible.

During the disaster itself, there is a need for a variety of other types of records. Victims need to be identified and their condition and treatment documented. Deaths should also be recorded. Records will also be needed of the use of supplies and equipment so that additional materials can be obtained if required. Records of the deployment of rescue personnel will also be needed to ensure the most effective use of personnel. It would be difficult to develop systematic record-keeping systems during an actual disaster, so it is important that such systems be in place before a disaster occurs.

ELEMENTS OF A TYPICAL DISASTER PLAN

A thorough disaster plan should address notification, warning, control, coordination, evacuation, and rescue. Additional elements of the plan should specify protocols for immediate care, supportive care, recovery, and evaluation.

NOTIFICATION

A disaster plan specifies in a systematic fashion the means of notifying the person or persons who can set the plan in motion. Persons who might be in a position to have advance warning of a disaster (local weather service personnel, for example) should have a clear understanding of who should be apprised of the potential for disaster. There must also be specific plans for notifying personnel and organizations involved in the disaster response. Notification should always include the fact of occurrence of a disaster, the type of disaster involved, and the extent of damage as far as it is known at the time. Notification should also convey any other relevant information that is known about the situation.

WARNING

The disaster plan should also spell out the procedures for disseminating disaster warnings to the general public. Procedures should specify the content of warnings, who will issue the warnings, and the manner in which warnings will be communicated. For example, the plan might specify that warnings should include the type of disaster involved, the area affected, and specific directions on actions to be taken by community members. Warnings may be issued by local radio and TV stations and by police vehicles with loudspeakers. Or, sirens may be used to alert people if they have been informed beforehand of the meaning of the siren and where to turn for more information. If warnings are to be communicated by media personnel, the plan should specify contact persons at radio and TV stations.

CONTROL

A disaster plan will also specify how the effects of a disaster are to be controlled. Different control efforts will be required for different types of disasters, and a community should be prepared to implement a variety of control activities. In the case of an earthquake, for example, control measures are directed at preventing and extinguishing fires before further damage is caused. Again, the procedures, materials, and personnel needed to carry out control measures must be specified in the plan.

LOGISTICAL COORDINATION

Another element of a community disaster plan deals with logistical coordination. ***Logistical coordination*** is the coordination of attempts to procure, maintain, and transport needed materials. The disaster plan will specify where and how supplies and equipment will be obtained, where these will be stored, and how they will be transported to the disaster site.

Traffic control is another aspect of logistical coordination. The disaster plan should specify personnel and procedures for controlling access to the disaster site. Traffic control procedures should also specify means by which access to the disaster site is ensured for rescue vehicles and vehicles carrying personnel, supplies, and equipment.

EVACUATION

A disaster plan also specifies evacuation procedures. The plan should indicate how those to be evacuated will be notified, what they can take with them, and how the evacuation will be accomplished. The plan may need to specify several contingency evacuation procedures depending upon the type of disaster.

The disaster response plan also would provide for the logistics of evacuation. This would include specifying the personnel needed to carry out the evacuation, how they are to be recruited and assigned, and how they will be notified. The plan would also specify the forms of transportation to be used during evacuation, where appropriate vehicles can be obtained, and how they will be refueled.

RESCUE

The response plan should specify the process to be used to assess rescue needs and who is responsible for carrying out the assessment. Once the assessment is made, there should be procedures in place for obtaining the appropriate personnel and equipment. For example, in the event of an earthquake, heavy construction equipment and operators will be needed, whereas fire department personnel are needed in a fire-related disaster.

The rescue operation should focus on removing

victims from hazardous conditions and providing first aid as needed. Rescue personnel should refrain from providing other forms of care as much as possible. This care can be provided by others, thus freeing rescue personnel to carry out the rescue operation.

IMMEDIATE CARE

Provision of immediate care is another consideration detailed in a disaster response plan. ***Immediate care*** is care required on the spot to ensure a disaster victim's survival or a disaster worker's continued ability to function. Plans for providing immediate care in four areas in the vicinity of the disaster site (Fig. 29–3) should be detailed in the disaster response plan.[2] Immediate care begins at the actual site of the disaster with a rapid initial assessment of all victims by the first health-care provider on the scene. This phase of immediate care is geared to correcting any life-threatening problems.

The second area of immediate care is the triage area. ***Triage*** is the process of sorting casualities on the basis of urgency and their potential for survival to determine priorities for treatment, evacuation, and transportation. Triage decisions are intended to maximize the number of survivors of a disaster event.[2] In a disaster in which victims are easily accessible, triage can take place right at the site. Victims are then removed to treatment areas based on their triage priority. In a disaster occurring in an enclosed environment (for example, in a mine or in a building), victims may not be easily accessible and will probably need to be removed to a more distant triage area as they are found.

The triage process usually involves placing color-coded tags on victims. Typically, black tags are attached to victims who are already dead. Red tags indicate top priority and are attached to victims who have life-threatening injuries but who can be stabilized and who have a high probability of survival. Priority is automatically given to injured rescue workers, their family members, hysterical persons, and children.[2] Yellow tags, indicating second priority, are assigned to victims with injuries with systemic complications that are not yet life-threatening and who are able to withstand a wait of 45 to 60 minutes for medical attention. Yellow tags are also assigned to victims with severe injuries who have a poor chance of survival. Green tags indicate victims with local injuries without immediate systemic complications who can wait several hours for treatment.

The third area of immediate care at the disaster site is the treatment area to which victims are removed after triage. In this area medical stabilization, temporary care, and emergency surgical stabilization are provided as needed. There may also be a need for psychological first aid at this point. The final area at the site of the disaster is the staging area. It is here that immediate-care operations are coordinated and vehicles and personnel are directed to areas of greatest need. The disaster plan should specify the procedures for setting up and operating each of the four areas of intermediate care. The plan should also address the supplies, equipment, and personnel needed in each area, how they will be obtained, and how they will be transported to the area.

Another area related to immediate care that

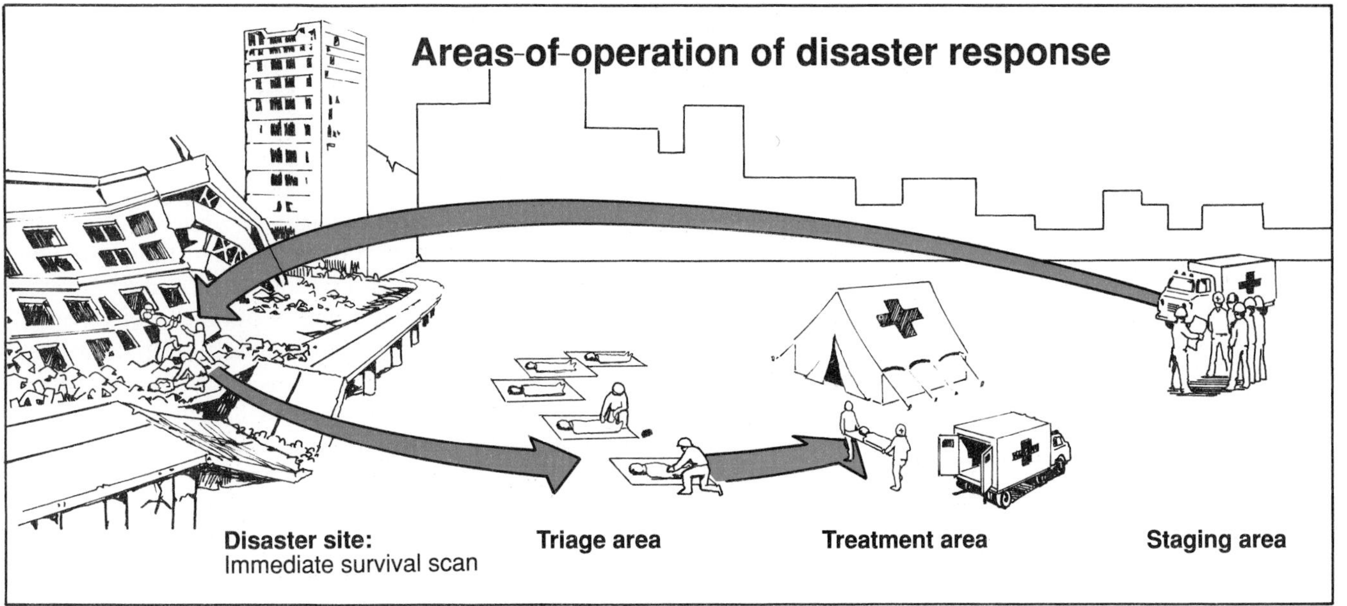

Figure 29–3. Areas of operation in the rescue phase of disaster response.

should be addressed in the disaster plan is care of the dead. Plans should be included for procedures to identify bodies and transport them to a morgue of some sort. Records of deaths should be kept, and procedures for rapid disposal of bodies should be specified should contagion be a problem. Plans should also include where and how body bags and identification tags will be obtained.

SUPPORTIVE CARE

Supportive care must also be addressed in an effective disaster response plan. Supportive care includes providing food, water, and shelter for victims and disaster relief workers. Other considerations in this area are sanitation and waste disposal; providing medications and routine health care; and reuniting families separated by the disaster.

Shelter will be required for those who are evacuated from their homes or whose homes are damaged in the disaster. The disaster response plan should specify which community buildings can be used to shelter victims and how victims will be transported to shelters. There may also be a need to use the homes of private citizens to shelter victims if public shelters are insufficient. When such is the case, the plan should specify how to notify concerned citizens of the need to place victims in their homes and how placement will be handled. It will be helpful to have a prepared list of people willing to provide shelter to others should a disaster occur.

Within the shelter, there is also a need for supplies to sustain daily living. Shelters should have adequate sanitation and sleeping facilities. There should also be plans for heating shelters and cooking food if area gas and electrical power systems are disrupted. Mechanisms should also be specified for governance and security within the shelter, particularly if the shelter will be in use for some time. Shelter leaders can be appointed or elected, and persons within the shelter should have a means of providing input into governance in long-term shelter situations.

Food supplies should be planned and obtained prior to a disaster. There should also be a mechanism for obtaining more food and other supplies from outside the community in the event of damage to stores and stockpiled supplies. A source of clean water will be needed, and the disaster plan should identify how and where water will be supplied. Equipment for water purification should be stored in case of need. There is also a need to plan for adequate sanitation and waste disposal at shelters and throughout the community following a disaster.

Victims may have other health-care needs unrelated to the disaster that will need to be met, so plans for providing basic health care in shelters should also be specified. These plans should include stores of medications most likely to be needed by the general public and critical to survival. For example, diabetics will continue to need insulin or oral hypoglycemics, whereas individuals with heart conditions may need a variety of medications. Priority should be given to medications required for serious illnesses rather than for minor conditions. Because communicable diseases spread more rapidly in a debilitated population following a disaster, antibiotics and vaccines should also be stored in case of need.

Supportive care also includes psychological counseling for those who are not coping adequately with the situation. Counseling may be required by both victims and disaster workers, and plans should be made to provide crisis intervention services during the response stage of the disaster. Psychological support can be provided through comforting and consoling those in distress and by protecting them from the ongoing disaster threat.[1] The disaster plan should include mechanisms for identifying those in need of counseling and for providing them with the services required.

Disaster victims may require goal orientation and guidance, and they can be directed to perform specific tasks that will help them achieve a sense of control. Support will also be needed for those who must identify loved ones among the dead. Expression of feelings should be fostered, and victims should be encouraged to make use of available support networks. Immediate referral to mental health personnel may be required in some instances. Structuring the environment and regularizing schedules, particularly in shelters, can also help to reestablish a sense of security.

Some relief from psychological stress can frequently be obtained if victims can be assured that family members are safe. Disaster plans should therefore include mechanisms for locating people and reuniting families. Names of persons admitted to shelters or health-care facilities should be recorded and communicated to a central location where others can check for word of loved ones. Deaths should also be reported if the dead can be identified, and information should be kept on the assignment of disaster workers to specific areas. It is helpful if institutions, such as schools and businesses, compile the names of those who were present prior to a disaster so that they can be accounted for afterwards.

RECOVERY

Another component of the disaster plan is mechanisms for supporting community rehabilitation. There may be a need to rebuild or repair damaged structures, and plans should be made for obtaining

TABLE 29–1. RESOURCES IN DISASTER PLANNING

Agency or Organization	Services
Agency for International Development Office of Planning and Budget Bureau for Program and Policy Coordination Washington, DC 20010 (202) 647-6483	Provides support and relief in international disasters
Agricultural Stabilization and Conservation Service Department of Agriculture P.O. Box 2415 Washington, DC 20013 (202) 447-5237	Provides emergency assistance to farmers after a disaster
American National Red Cross 17th & D Streets Washington, DC 20006 (202) 737-8300	Information and literature on disaster preparedness Assists with supportive care in the event of a disaster
Doctors for Disaster Preparedness P.O. Box 1057 Stark, FL 32091 (904) 964-5397	Professional education for disaster preparedness
Emergency Shelter Grants Program Office of Block Grant Assistance Department of Housing and Urban Development 451 7th St. SW Washington, DC 20410 (202) 755-5977	Provides funds for conversion of buildings for emergency shelter and for operating costs
Farmers' Home Administration Department of Agriculture Washington, DC 20250 (202) 447-4323	Provides funds to rebuild farms and homes after a disaster Also provides loans for watershed development and flood prevention
Federal Crop Insurance Corporation Department of Agriculture Washington, DC 20250 (202) 447-6795	Insures farm crops against storm damage, fire, flood, earthquake, etc.
Federal Emergency Management Agency 500 C Street SW Washington, DC 20472 (202) 646-4600	Information and literature Development of national preparedness policy; 24-hr dissemination of emergency information
National Flood Insurance Program Federal Insurance Administration Washington, DC 20472 (202) 646-2774	Provides insurance against flood damage and assists with floodplain management
Office of Emergency Transportation Department of Transportation 400 7th St. SW Washington, DC 20590 (202) 366-5270	Provides transportation in emergencies related to national defense and other disasters and crisis events
Office of U.S. Foreign Disaster Assistance Washington, DC 20011 (202) 647-8924	Assistance with disaster relief in other countries
Small Business Administration Imperial Bldg. 1441 L St. NW Washington, DC 20416 (202) 368-5855 (800) 653-7561	Provides loans to small businesses to rebuild or replace homes or businesses after floods, riots, or civil disorder
U.S. Fire Administration Washington, DC 20010 (202) 646-2449	Provides assistance with fire and arson prevention and firefighter health and safety.

financial and material assistance in these endeavors. Mechanisms should be developed that will help victims to process insurance claims as rapidly as possible. There may also be a need for outside assistance in rebuilding, and plans should be made for obtaining that assistance. Several sources of such assistance are presented in Table 29–1.

There will also be a need for psychological counseling in the aftermath of a disaster, and mechanisms should be developed for identifying and referring those in need of counseling. Post-disaster counseling may be delegated to specific mental health agencies that would plan how post-event counseling will be handled, who will be eligible for care, and procedures for obtaining care. Particular attention should be given to the counseling needs of both disaster workers and victims, because research has indicated the potential for psychological trauma to both as a result of a disaster experience.

EVALUATION

Plans should also be made prior to the disaster for evaluating the effectiveness of the disaster plan and its implementation. Again, consideration should be given to procedures, personnel, and materials needed to carry out the evaluation. Records will be needed that permit evaluation of the efficiency and effectiveness of the plan, and procedures should be developed for obtaining and storing data. Plans should also be made for follow-up meetings with disaster workers to provide input into the evaluation process. The focus of these meetings would be on what worked and what did not work and what could be done to improve the plan and its implementation in subsequent disasters. Elements of a comprehensive disaster plan are summarized in Box 29–5.

BOX 29–5

Elements of a Typical Disaster Plan

- Mechanisms exist for notifying individuals responsible for authorizing disaster plan implementation
- Mechanisms exist for warning individuals likely to be affected by the disaster
- Mechanisms exist for controlling damage due to disaster
- Procedures are specified for logistical coordination in traffic control, tranportation of equipment, supplies, and personnel to the disaster site
- Procedures are specified for evacuating individuals in the potential disaster area
- Plans are in place for rescue operations to remove victims from hazardous situations
- Plans and procedures have been designed to meet immediate-care needs of disaster victims related to:
  - Triage
  - First aid
  - Transportation to other facilities
  - Care of the dead
- Plans and procedures have been designed to provide supportive care to meet ongoing needs of disaster victims and relief workers related to:
  - Emergency shelter
  - Food and water
  - Sanitation and waste disposal
  - Health care, medications, etc.
  - Reuniting families
- Mechanisms are in place to provide assistance to victims during the recovery period
- Mechanisms exist for evaluating the adequacy of the disaster plan in meeting the community's needs

NURSING RESPONSIBILITIES IN DISASTER PLANNING

Community health nurses are well suited to assist in the actual development of a disaster plan. Because of their background in program planning and group dynamics, they can help ensure that planning is a systematic rather than a haphazard process. Community health nurses also have knowledge of what the health-related needs of the population would be in a disaster and can provide input regarding needs as well as potential resources for meeting needs.

Another role for community health nurses in disaster preparation is to train rescue workers in triage techniques and basic first aid. Nurses might also help educate personnel who will staff shelters regarding the needs of disaster victims and considerations related to group interactions that will make shelter operations run more smoothly. A final responsibility of community health nurses in the disaster planning stage is educating the public regarding the disaster plan and the need for personal preparation for a disaster.

THE EPIDEMIOLOGIC PREVENTION PROCESS MODEL AND CARE OF CLIENTS IN DISASTER SETTINGS

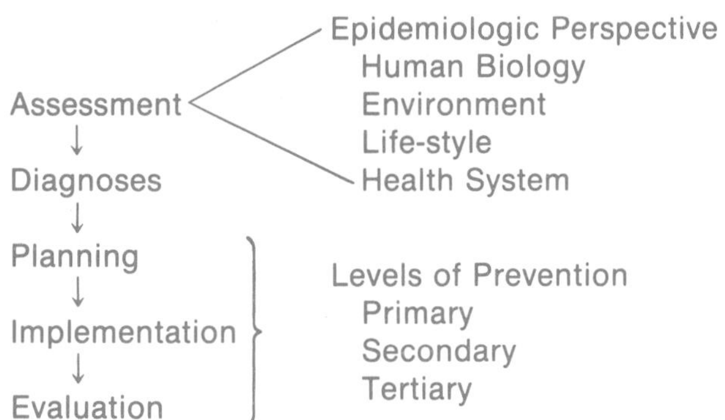

The epidemiologic prevention process model can be used by community health nurses and others involved in disaster response planning to guide the development, implementation, and evaluation of the disaster plan.

ASSESSING THE POTENTIAL FOR, AND THE EFFECTS OF, DISASTERS

There are two aspects of assessment in providing disaster care. These include assessing the potential for disaster and assessing possible effects of a disaster. Identifying the potential for disaster in a particular community involves forecasting the types of disasters possible and the likelihood of their occurrence. The possible types of disasters will, of course, vary from community to community. Disaster potential and the probable effects can be systematically assessed by examining factors related to each of the four components of the epidemiologic perspective of the model. The epidemiologic perspective can also be used to assess the effects of an actual disaster.

HUMAN BIOLOGY

One determinant in forecasting regarding potential disasters is that of human biology. Certain groups of people are more likely than others to be affected by a disaster. For example, if the anticipated disaster is an epidemic of influenza, those most likely to be severely affected are the very young and the elderly. However, there also will be illness among the work force that may impede efforts to halt the spread of disease. On the other hand, if there is potential for an explosion in a local chemical plant, those affected are likely to be company employees and persons in surrounding buildings that might be damaged as well. Again, this might include children if there is a school nearby.

Human biology is also a factor in predicting the effects expected as a result of the disaster. In the case of an influenza epidemic, illness potentially accompanied by dehydration and electrolyte imbalance may be expected. In an explosion, expected injuries may consist of burns and trauma, whereas a flood will result primarily in drownings.

The overall health status of the community will also influence disaster planning requirements. For example, if hypertension is prevalent in the community, provisions will need to be made in a disaster plan for ongoing treatment of hypertension or other prevalent diseases. Human biological considerations related to several types of disasters are presented in Table 29–2.

In the event of an actual disaster, the community health nurse will also be involved in assessing the physiological effects of the event on human biology. The nurse will appraise the extent of injuries incurred by victims and relief workers and may also assess other needs for health care. For example, the nurse might need to assess the health status of a disaster relief worker with diabetes or of a child with a fever. The nurse will also assist in assessing the health status of groups of people. For example, the nurse may note an increased incidence of diarrhea among evacuees in a shelter or identify nutritional needs in war refugees.

ENVIRONMENT

Elements of the physical, psychological, and social environments influence the types of disasters that may occur and their effects on the community. Examples of specific considerations related to each type of environment are presented in Table 29–3.

Physical Environment

Many disasters arise out of features of the physical environment. For example, the presence of a river near the community and the likelihood of heavy rainfall both contribute to the potential for flooding, as does the construction of homes and businesses on floodplains. The existence of a geological fault, a nuclear reactor, or a chemical plant are other examples of factors in the physical environment that may increase the potential for a disaster.

Elements of the physical environment can either help or hinder efforts to control the effects of a disaster. For example, limited traffic access to the part of town where an explosives plant is located could

TABLE 29–2. HUMAN BIOLOGICAL CONSIDERATIONS RELATED TO SELECTED TYPES OF DISASTERS

Type of Disaster	Considerations Related to Human Biology
All disasters	• Greater loss of life and injury will occur among the elderly, young children, and chronically ill and disabled persons
Avalanches	• May result in asphyxiation • May result in frostbite and other effects of exposure to cold • May result in fractures or other forms of trauma
Chemical spills	• May result in chemical burns of the skin • May result in respiratory irritation and illness • May result in poisoning with a variety of symptoms depending on the chemical involved • May result in eye irritation
Earthquake	• May result in crushing injuries and fractures from falling bricks, masonry, and other objects • May result in burns suffered in fires and explosions due to ruptured natural gas mains • May result in waterborne diseases because of ruptured water mains and lack of safe drinking water • May result in electrocutions from fallen power lines
Epidemics	• May result in communicable diseases with a variety of symptoms depending upon the disease involved
Explosions	• May result in burns due to associated fires • May result in fractures or crushing injuries due to explosion impact or falling masonry, bricks, other debris
Famine	• May result in developmental delay in young children • May result in failure to thrive in nursing infants because of inadequate lactation by mothers
Fire	• May result in minor to severe burns • May result in respiratory problems due to inhalation of smoke and hazardous fumes from burning objects
Floods	• May result in drownings • May result in waterborne and insectborne diseases from contaminated water supplies and insect breeding grounds
Radiation leakage	• May result in radiation burns or radiation sickness • May result in later cancer • May result in later infertility, spontaneous abortion, or fetal defects
Storms	• May result in crushing injuries due to windblown objects and debris • May result in minor to severe lacerations due to flying glass from broken windows
Transportation disasters	• May result in crushing injuries and other trauma • May result in burns with associated vehicle fires • May result in drownings or asphyxiation if disasters occur over water or in tunnels • May result in exposure to the elements if disaster occurs in a remote area

hinder movement of emergency vehicles in the event of a fire or explosion. Similarly, the physical isolation of a mountain community may impede rescue efforts in the event of a forest fire or flood. On the other hand, such isolation might spare the community from the effects of an epidemic in the surrounding area.

In conducting a community assessment, the community health nurse would identify physical environmental factors that might contribute to the occurrence of a disaster. The nurse would also determine whether the community is prepared for potential disasters that might occur. When the community is not prepared, the nurse would advocate the planning activities described earlier in this chapter.

The nurse would also identify factors that might impede the community's response in the event of a disaster. The nurse can then share these observations with others involved in disaster planning, and interventions to modify or circumvent these factors can be incorporated into the community's disaster response plan.

Psychological Environment

Components of the psychological environment can also influence the effects of a disaster on health. As noted earlier, a number of psychological factors can affect the way people respond to a warning of disaster. Similarly, psychological factors can influence

TABLE 29–3. ASSESSING ENVIRONMENTAL FACTORS IN RELATION TO DISASTER

Type of Environment	Assessment Considerations
Physical environment	• Is there potential for flooding in the community? • Are homes constructed in areas subject to flooding? • Are vital community services located in areas subject to flooding? • Is there potential for forest or brush fires? • Are residences and other buildings constructed of fire-retardant materials and in keeping with fire safety codes? • Are public buildings (and others) equipped with sprinkler systems and alarms in the event of fire? • Is the community located on a geological fault? • Are buildings constructed to withstand the stress of an earthquake? • Are bookcases and cabinets securely bolted to walls? • Are there features of the community that may impede access to disaster victims or transportation of supplies and personnel to disaster sites (for example, limited highway access to certain areas)?
Psychological environment	• What prior experience with disaster have community members had? • How do community members perceive disaster warnings? • What is the level of coping ability among members of the community? • What are the psychological effects of a disaster event on victims? On disaster relief workers?
Social environment	• Is there a potential for intergroup violence within the community? • Is there potential for involvement in war? Are battles likely to occur in the immediate area? • Does the economic status of most community members permit them to prepare adequately for a potential disaster? • Is the community economically able to engage in disaster preparedness? • What languages are spoken in the community? Will language barriers hamper disaster response efforts? • To what extent do groups within the community work together to solve common problems? • What is the extent of community support for disaster preparedness? • What community agencies are responsible for disaster planning? • Is there a communitywide disaster response plan? Is the plan coordinated with existing disaster plans of subgroups in the population? Or, do plans conflict? • What are the attitudes of community members to disaster preparedness? • To what extent are community members prepared for a disaster? • Is there evidence of friction between groups of disaster victims in shelters? • Do disaster relief activities enhance social cohesion or detract from it? • What buildings are available in the community to serve as potential shelters for disaster victims?

responses once a disaster has occurred. For example, familiarity with earthquakes may limit panic in some people, while those new to the area, who have never before experienced an earthquake, may panic and respond inappropriately. Communities and persons with good coping skills will usually respond more effectively in a disaster situation than those who have poor coping skills.

The community health nurse should assess the attitudes of community members to disaster preparedness. To what extent are individuals and families in the area prepared for potential disasters? Have families in an earthquake-prone region, for example, gathered supplies that will be needed in the event of an earthquake and placed them in an accessible location? Have emergency escape routes from homes, schools, and other buildings been identified? Have families discussed an emergency contact person who can relay messages for and about family members separated in a disaster? Or, are these types of preparation largely ignored?

In the event of an actual disaster, the community health nurse will assess the psychological effects of the disaster event. As noted earlier, both victims and relief workers may experience stress related to a disaster, and the nurse should be alert to signs of emotional distress in both groups. Signs of psychological distress might include confusion, inability to make decisions, excessive crying, aggressive behavior, restlessness, inability to sleep, and nightmares.

Social Environment

The social environment can also influence the way people respond to a disaster and may even give rise to one. For example, the presence of racial tensions could trigger outbreaks of violence in some communities. War is another disaster arising out of social environmental conditions. In assessing a community, the nurse would attempt to identify social factors that might contribute to disasters and to the way people respond to them.

Elements of the social environment also may increase or limit the effects of a disaster on a community. For example, the economic status of community members and of the community at large may limit the ability of people to prepare for potential disasters or to recover after a disaster event. Language barriers may hamper evacuation or rescue efforts. Strong social networks in the community that can be tied into disaster planning will aid in effective disaster response, whereas intragroup friction will hamper response effectiveness. The nurse would identify social factors present within the community that may decrease the effectiveness of the community's response to a disaster and participate in planning efforts to modify these factors. The nurse would also identify social factors that will enhance the community's ability to respond effectively in the event of a disaster. Planning groups could then capitalize on these factors in designing an effective disaster plan. For example, well-established cooperative relationships between groups and agencies in the community are an asset in designing and implementing a disaster plan.

Another aspect of the social environment that should be assessed is the extent of existing community preparation for possible disasters. The first consideration in this area is the community structure related to disaster preparedness. Is there a community agency responsible for coordinating overall disaster preparedness? In some communities, this may be a function of local government, while in others it might be a local chapter of the American Red Cross or civil defense unit.

The nurse and others concerned with disaster preparedness would also determine whether there is a communitywide disaster plan and whether an existing plan incorporates the elements discussed earlier. It is also important to examine the disaster plans of various organizations and agencies in the community and their congruence with the community disaster response plan (if one exists). For example, is the plan of a local chemical plant for dealing with an explosion and fire congruent with the community's plan for dealing with such a disaster, or do provisions of the two plans contradict each other?

Finally, those responsible for planning a disaster response should assess community attitudes to, and participation in, disaster planning. Are local governmental agencies supportive of planning efforts? Do community members exhibit concern for disaster planning and do they follow through on recommendations for disaster preparedness?

In the event of an actual disaster, the nurse might also assess social factors influencing the community's disaster response. For example, the nurse might identify growing intergroup tensions in shelters for disaster victims or disorganization in efforts to reunite families separated by the disaster. Other areas for consideration include the degree of cooperation among groups providing disaster relief and, following the disaster, the availability of recovery assistance to individuals and families.

LIFE-STYLE

Life-style factors related to consumption patterns, occupation, and even leisure pursuits can also influence the occurrence of disasters and their effects on the health of community members.

Consumption Patterns

Consumption patterns such as smoking, drinking, and drug use can contribute to disasters. Smoking, for example, is often the cause of residential fires and forest and brush fires that result in loss of life as well as extensive property damage. Drinking and drug abuse have both been known to contribute to transportation disasters, and they may also contribute to industrial disasters when the abuser is working in a setting with disaster potential. For example, if a person responsible for monitoring the safety of a nuclear reactor is drunk, he or she is unlikely to recognize or respond appropriately to signs of danger. The community health nurse will assess the extent of smoking and substance abuse in the community in relation to the potential for disaster. The nurse may also want to assess (or encourage others to assess) the effectiveness of substance-abuse policies in transportation services and industries where there is potential for disaster. Another area for assessment is the extent of safety education in regard to smoking (for example, not smoking in bed) that occurs in the community.

Consumption patterns may also intensify the effects of a disaster on the health of a population. A community whose members are poorly nourished, for example, will be at greater risk for consequences of disaster such as communicable diseases. Substance abuse may limit one's potential for appropriate behavior in an emergency and lead to injury and even death due to failure to respond appropriately. For example, intoxication may prevent someone from fleeing a burning building.

TABLE 29–4. LIFE-STYLE CONSIDERATIONS RELATED TO DISASTER ASSESSMENT

Consumption patterns	• What is the general nutritional status of the population? Does the population's nutritional status place residents at risk for adverse health effects in the event of a disaster? • What provisions should be made to meet special nutritional needs in the population (for example, low-sodium foods for those with hypertension)? • What is the extent of drug and alcohol use or abuse in the community? Will the prevalence of drug or alcohol abuse impede disaster response in the community? • Are there policies related to drug and alcohol use in settings with the potential for disaster events? • Are these policies enforced? • What is the extent of smoking in the community? To what extent do smokers engage in unsafe smoking practices (for example, smoking in bed)? • To what extent do members of the population engage in regular physical activity? Will lack of physical activity impede disaster response capabilities?
Occupation	• What industries are present in the community? Do any of these industries pose disaster hazards related to fire, explosion, radiation, chemical leaks, or transportation disasters? • To what extent do local industries adhere to safety procedures that would prevent disasters from occurring? • Is adherence to safety procedures by local industries adequately monitored by regulatory bodies? • What occupational groups in the community could enhance the effectiveness of the community's response to a disaster (for example, construction workers, media companies, military units)? • Is the number of rescue personnel (for example, police and fire personnel) adequate to meet community needs in the event of a disaster? • Do rescue personnel have the equipment that might be needed in the event of a disaster?
Leisure pursuits	• Do community members engage in leisure pursuits that pose a disaster hazard (for example, use of off-road vehicles or campfires in fire-prone areas)? • To what extent do community members engage in recreational safety practices that may serve to prevent disasters? • How are recreational safety practices enforced? • What leisure pursuits by community members would enhance the community's response to a disaster?

Lack of exercise in the population can limit their ability to engage in strenuous labor that might be demanded in a disaster situation. Unaccustomed activity may result in exhaustion or heart attack. The nurse would assess the levels of exercise engaged in by the general population. Community health nurses in occupational settings may also be responsible for determining the physical fitness of personnel who would be involved in rescue operations in the event of a disaster (for example, firefighters).

Occupation

Occupational factors can contribute to the potential for disaster in a community and should be assessed by the nurse. For example, the community health nurse should be aware of industries in the area that pose hazards related to fire or explosion. The potential for radiation exposure or leakage of toxic chemicals in the community should also be determined. The nurse may also want to appraise the extent to which local industries adhere to safety regulations related to hazardous conditions. Community health nurses working in industrial settings would be particularly likely to have access to this type of information. Other community health nurses may need to advocate regular inspection of industrial conditions by the appropriate authorities.

The community health nurse will also identify occupational factors that may enhance a community's abilities to respond effectively in the event of a disaster. The nurse and others involved in disaster planning would explore the adequacy of rescue services and personnel for dealing with potential disasters. Is the number of firefighters in the community, for example, adequate to deal with an explosion and fire in a local chemical plant? Do firefighting units possess the equipment needed to deal with such an event? Planners would also assess the existence of other occupational groups that may assist with disaster response. For example, are there construction companies in the community that could supply heavy equipment that might be needed for rescue operations?

Leisure Pursuits

The leisure pursuits of community members may, on occasion, contribute to the occurrence of a disaster event. Careless campers, for example, could ignite a forest fire, or skiers might trigger an avalanche. Fires can also be started by sparks from recreational vehicles. The community health nurse and others involved in disaster planning will assess the extent of such leisure pursuits in the community, the existence of safety regulations related to these pursuits, and the degree of adherence to safety regulations. Do campers, for example, refrain from lighting fires in fire-prone areas, or do skiers avoid restricted areas where avalanches are possible?

Leisure pursuits can also enhance the community's response to a disaster event, and the nurse would assess the presence of leisure pursuits that may have this effect. For example, the existence of a group with an interest in wilderness survival may be an advantage in the event of an avalanche or a plane crash in a remote area. Or, people with citizen-band radios may assist with communications in the event of an emergency. Assessment considerations related to life-style and its influences in a disaster setting are summarized in Table 29–4.

HEALTH SYSTEM

The adequacy of the health system's response capability in the event of a disaster will influence the extent to which a disaster effects a community and the health of its members. Assessing the ability of the health system to respond to a disaster would include examining facilities and personnel as well as the organizational framework in which they operate. A community that has a variety of health-care facilities joined in a cooperative network can respond more effectively to the health-care demands of a disaster situation than can a community with limited facilities or where there is no existing system for coordinating joint efforts.

The nurse and other disaster response planners would identify the types of health-care facilities available in the community and the number and type of health-care personnel that could be called upon in the event of a disaster. Planners might also determine the existence and adequacy of disaster plans developed by health-care facilities. For example, has a local hospital developed a plan for evacuating patients if the hospital is involved in the disaster? Or, is there a plan for handling mass casualties of various types in the event of a disaster? Assessment of potential avenues for obtaining health-care personnel is also important. For example, local professional organizations might serve as a means of contacting and organizing health-care providers. Or, area educational programs for health professionals may provide a source of manpower. Health system considerations related to disaster settings are summarized in Box 29–6.

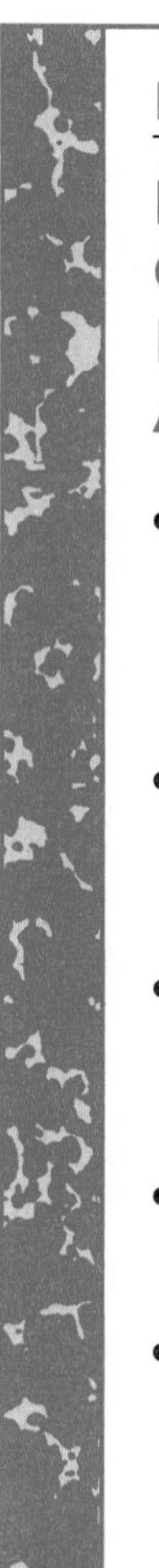

BOX 29–6

Health System Considerations Related to Disaster Assessment

- What health-care facilities are available in the community? Are the facilities in danger of being affected by potential disasters? To what extent?
- Have health-care facilities developed disaster response plans? Are they congruent with the community's disaster response plan?
- How many hospitals are there in the community? What is their total bed capacity? What specialty services are available at each?
- What facilities are available to care for trauma victims? What is their capacity?
- How many and what types of health-care providers are available in the community? How can they be contacted most efficiently in the event of a disaster?
- What is the extent of first-aid knowledge in the general population?

DIAGNOSTIC REASONING AND CARE OF CLIENTS IN DISASTER SETTINGS

Based on the assessment of human biological, environmental, life-style, and health system factors, the nurse derives nursing diagnoses related to disaster care. These diagnoses may reflect the potential for disaster occurrence, the adequacy of disaster preparation, or the extent of effects in an actual disaster. A diagnosis related to forecasting might be "potential for major earthquake damage and injury due to community location on a geological fault." A diagnosis of "inadequate disaster planning due to fragmentation of planning efforts among community agencies" is a possible nursing diagnosis related to disaster preparedness. A diagnosis derived from information about the effects of an actual disaster might be "need for additional shelter sites due to destruction of planned shelters by fire."

In the event of an actual disaster, nursing diagnoses might relate to individual clients as well as to the status of the overall community. For example, individual diagnoses might include "grief due to loss of husband" or "pain due to leg fracture suffered in the collapse of a wall." Nurses may derive diagnoses related to both helpers and victims, such as "role overload due to need to rescue disaster victims and care for own family" or "stress related to constant exposure to death."

PLANNING CARE OF CLIENTS IN DISASTER SETTINGS

Activities related to disaster care take place in several areas.[7] Two of these areas, prevention and education, involve primary prevention. The third area of activity, the actual emergency response, reflects secondary prevention, whereas recovery, the fourth area of activity, involves tertiary prevention.

PRIMARY PREVENTION

Primary prevention is geared toward preventing the occurrence of a disaster or limiting consequences when the event itself cannot be prevented. Activities to prevent or minimize the effects of a disaster take place during the pre-impact mobilization stage of the disaster. Community health nurses may be involved in eliminating factors that may contribute to disasters to the extent that they identify these factors and report their existence to the appropriate authorities. For example, the community health nurse working in an occupational setting may note that an employee who is responsible for monitoring pressure levels in a boiler may be drinking heavily. This employee's drinking problem may lead to lack of attention to rising pressures and an explosion and fire in the plant. In such a case, the nurse would call the employee's drinking behavior to the attention of a supervisor.

Community health nurses may also become politically active in order to assure that risk factors for potential disasters present in the community are eliminated or modified. For example, the nurse might campaign for stricter safety regulations for nuclear power plants or stricter building safety codes or serve as a mediator in an attempt to defuse social unrest in the community.

Community health nurses are more often involved in educating the public about how to prevent disasters and minimize their consequences. This may involve planning education to help individuals, families, or groups of clients on home safety practices to prevent fires and explosions, how to prepare for a possible community disaster, and what to do in the event of a disaster situation.

The nurse would plan to acquaint clients with whom he or she works with the types of disasters possible in their community and about actions they can take to minimize the consequences should an emergency arise. The nurse can also guide clients to resources that will help them prepare for the possibility of a disaster. A variety of government agencies publish literature containing guidelines for emergency preparation by individual citizens. One such guideline, entitled "In Time of Emergency: A Citizen's Handbook," is published by the Federal Emergency Management Agency. The American Red Cross also publishes a guideline entitled "Family Disaster Plan and Personal Survival Guide." These and similar publications offer general guidelines for emergency preparation as well as more specific recommendations for certain common types of disasters. Some areas for client education related to disaster are presented in Box 29–7.

SECONDARY PREVENTION

Secondary prevention involves the response to a disaster occurrence. Implementing the community's disaster plan is a secondary preventative measure. Secondary prevention is geared toward halting the disaster and resolving problems caused by it. Secondary prevention may take place at the community level or at the level of individual victims. For example, efforts to provide food and shelter are secondary preventative measures taken at the group level, whereas treatment of burns and other injuries is secondary prevention related to specific individuals.

Community health nurses are actively involved in the response to an actual disaster event. Areas for involvement include triage, treatment of injuries and other health conditions, and shelter supervision. Community health nurses may be some of several health-care providers who perform triage activities described earlier and who determine priorities for treatment, evacuation, and transportation of disaster victims. In planning for triage responsibilities, community health nurses would familiarize themselves with criteria for assigning priority.

Community health nurses may also be involved in treating injuries or other health conditions. This may occur in "definitive care sites" (hospitals or other health-care facilities removed from the disaster site itself)[8] or in shelters. Nurses involved in first aid for victims should plan to update their skills in basic first aid on a periodic basis. Community health nurses,

BOX 29–7

Areas for Client Education Related to Disaster Preparedness

- Install and maintain smoke detectors in homes.
- Bolt bookcases and cabinets to walls in areas with earthquake potential.
- Seek shelter in a reinforced area (for example, a doorway) during an earthquake and face away from windows. Stay indoors.
- Seek shelter from hurricanes or tornadoes in basements or inner rooms without windows.
- Seek high ground in the event of a flood.
- Drop to the ground and roll about to extinguish flaming clothing, or smother flames with a rug.
- Close doors and windows to prevent the spread of a fire, and place wadded fabric beneath doors to prevent smoke inhalation.
- Determine avenues of escape from the home or other buildings.
- Install fire escape ladders as needed at upper windows.
- Keep stairways and doors free of obstacles to permit easy egress.
- Identify a place for family members to meet after escape from the home.
- Designate a person living outside the area as a family contact if family members are separated during a disaster.
- Learn community disaster warning signals and their meaning.
- Keep a battery-operated radio and extra batteries available (replace batteries periodically).
- Collect and store, in an accessible location, sufficient emergency supplies for one week, including:
  - Nonperishable foods (including pet foods)
  - Drinking water
  - Warm clothing
  - Bedding (blankets or sleeping bags)
  - A tent or other type of shelter
  - A source of light (flashlights or lanterns)
  - Chlorine bleach for treating suspect water supplies to prevent infection
  - First-aid supplies and a first-aid manual
  - Medications needed by family members.
- Replace stored food, water, and medications periodically.
- Know where natural gas and water valves are located and how to turn them off. Attach a wrench close to valves.
- Determine what valuables are to be taken if evacuation is required.
- Assign activities related to evacuation (for example, designate the person responsible for taking the baby or family pets).
- Know the general plan for evacuating the community.
- Know where proposed shelters will be located.
- Know what actions should be taken when warning is given.
- Know where to seek additional information.

particularly those working in shelters, will need to plan to deal not only with existing health conditions, such as hypertension or diabetes, but also with acute conditions that may arise. For example, the nurse may encounter a child with a middle ear infection that requires treatment, or a woman in labor. In planning for these and similar activities, the nurse should be familiar with procedures included in the disaster plan for care of minor illnesses and dispensing medications for clients with chronic diseases. The nurse will need to know to whom to refer those in need of services and how to arrange for transportation or other needs. The disaster plan may call for nurses to treat minor illnesses on the basis of protocols developed in conjunction with medical personnel. If such is the case, the nurse should become familiar with those treatment protocols. Finally, the nurse will need to plan for activities to monitor client's health status. For example, the nurse might schedule periodic blood pressure measurements for a disaster relief worker with hypertension.

Community health nurses may also be respon-

TABLE 29–5. SECONDARY PREVENTIVE ACTIVITIES BY COMMUNITY HEALTH NURSES IN DISASTER SETTINGS

Secondary Prevention Focus	Related Nursing Activities
Triage	• Assess disaster victims for extent of injuries • Determine priority for treatment, evacuation, and transportation • Place appropriate colored tag on victim depending on priority
Treatment of injuries	• Render first aid for injuries • Provide additional treatment as needed in definitive-care areas
Treatment of other conditions	• Determine health needs other than injury • Refer for medical treatment as required • Provide treatment for other conditions based on medically approved protocols
Shelter supervision	• Coordinate activities of shelter workers • Oversee records of those admitted and discharged from the shelter • Promote effective interpersonal and group interactions among those housed in the shelter • Promote independence and involvement of those housed in the shelter

sible for supervising and coordinating shelter activities. Responsibilities involved might include supervising the meeting of health-care and other needs by other disaster relief workers; supervising record-keeping related to people brought to and released from the shelter; assisting people housed in shelters on a long-term basis to develop some form of governance; and using interpersonal skills to keep the shelter running smoothly. Secondary preventative activities by community health nurses in a disaster setting are summarized in Table 29–5.

TERTIARY PREVENTION

Tertiary prevention with respect to a disaster has two major goals. The first of these is recovery of the community and its members from the effects of the disaster and return to normal. The second aspect of tertiary prevention is preventing a recurrence of the disaster.

Community health nurses have responsibilities in both of these areas after the disaster is over. Community health nurses may be called upon to provide sustained care to both victims and disaster workers following the disaster. They may also be involved in identifying health and psychosocial problems that require further assistance. Community health nurses should plan to provide counseling or referral for persons with psychological problems stemming from their experiences during the disaster. There may also be a need to refer disaster victims to continuing sources of medical care. Community health nurses may also need to plan referrals for clients in need of social and financial assistance. For example, disaster victims may require help in finding housing or in getting financial aid to rebuild homes or businesses.

Community health nurses may also provide input into interventions designed to prevent future disasters or to minimize their effects. For example, if the disaster involved rioting by minority groups, the community health nurse might advocate measures to meet the needs of minority group members prevent further rioting. Or, community health nurses might campaign for stronger building codes to prevent the collapse of buildings in subsequent earthquakes. Community health nurses can also help to educate the public on disaster preparedness to minimize the effects of subsequent disasters. Tertiary prevention foci in disaster settings and related community health nursing activities are summarized in Table 29–6.

IMPLEMENTING DISASTER CARE

Prior to the occurrence of a disaster, the community health nurse may be involved in activities preliminary to implementing a disaster plan, particularly in disseminating the plan to others. Dissemination needs to occur among persons and agencies who will have designated responsibilities during a disaster. The community health nurse participating in disaster planning will be responsible for communicating elements of the plan to members of the nurse's employing agency. They may also ensure that the plan is disseminated to nursing organizations in the area (for example, to members of a district nurses' association). The nurse who assumes this responsibility should be sure that the general plan is understood, as well as the specific part to be played by members of the agency or organization.

The essential features of the community's disaster response plan should also be communicated to the general public so residents will be prepared to follow the plan in the event of a disaster. The community health nurse may be involved in helping to communicate the plan to the public by apprising clients with whom he or she works of relevant aspects

TABLE 29–6. TERTIARY PREVENTIVE ACTIVITIES BY COMMUNITY HEALTH NURSES IN DISASTER SETTINGS

Tertiary Prevention Focus	Related Nursing Activities
Follow-up care for injuries	• Provide continued care for people injured as a result of the disaster or during rescue operations • Monitor response to treatment
Follow-up care for psychological problems resulting from the disaster	• Provide counseling for those with psychological problems resulting from the disaster • Refer clients for counseling as needed • Monitor progress in resolving psychological problems
Recovery assistance	• Refer clients for financial assistance • Provide assistance in finding housing
Prevention of future disasters and their consequences	• Advocate measures to prevent future disasters • Educate the public about disaster preparation to minimize the effects of subsequent disasters

of the plan. The public should be informed of mechanisms that will be used to inform them of a disaster and where to go for additional information. Community members should also know the general procedures to be followed in terms of caring for disaster victims and setting up shelters. They should also be informed of the locations of proposed shelters. Finally, community members should be told of specific disaster preparations that should be undertaken by individuals and families.

EVALUATING DISASTER CARE

The final responsibility of community health nurses with respect to disaster care is evaluating that care. Nurses and others involved in the disaster will participate in evaluative activities outlined in the disaster plan. The focus for the evaluation will be on the adequacy of the plan for curtailing the disaster and meeting the needs of those involved in it.

In this effort it may be helpful to examine the disaster response in light of the four components of the epidemiologic perspective. Did the plan adequately provide for the needs of the people affected and the kinds of health problems that resulted? Were there physical, psychological, or social environmental factors that impeded implementation of the plan or that limited its effectiveness? What influence did lifestyle factors have on plan implementation, if any? Were health-care services adequate to meet the health needs posed by the disaster itself as well as those encountered in the period after the disaster? Data obtained in the evaluative process will be used to assess the adequacy of the community disaster plan and to guide revisions of the plan to better deal with future disasters.

The effectiveness of care provided to individual disaster victims should also be assessed. Evaluation in this area will focus on the degree to which individual needs were met and the extent to which problems resulting from the disaster were resolved.

CHAPTER HIGHLIGHTS

- A disaster is an overwhelming event that exceeds the ability of those affected to respond effectively.
- Effective community response to a disaster requires planning and preparation.
- Disasters vary in terms of their frequency, their predictability, and their preventability. Disasters also vary with respect to their speed of onset, extent of forewarning, duration, and destructive potential.
- Three factors affecting a community's response to a disaster are the magnitude of the disaster event, the adaptive capacity of the community, and the normative context in which the disaster occurs.
- There are three dimensions of a disaster: the temporal dimension, the spatial dimension, and the role dimension.
- The temporal dimension of a disaster refers to the stages of a community's response to a disaster event. These include the pre-event response, the post-event response, and the recovery response.
- The three stages of the pre-event response to a disaster are the planning stage, the warning stage, and the pre-impact mobilization stage.
- The spatial dimension of a disaster involves three areas. The area of total impact is the zone where the most severe effects of the disaster are found. In the area of partial impact, there is evidence of the disaster but the effects are of a lower magnitude than in the area of total impact. The outside area is not directly affected by the disaster, but may be a source of assistance in dealing with the consequences of the disaster.
- The role dimension of a disaster encompasses the roles of the disaster victim and the helper. These roles frequently overlap, and both involve high levels of stress.
- The potential benefits of disaster planning include decreased economic costs related to damage, reduced loss of life, less confusion regarding roles in the disaster response, and utility for responding to unforeseen disasters.
- The purposes of disaster planning are to reduce the community's vulnerability to disaster and to prevent its occurrence.
- Planning a community disaster response is based on several principles related to the differences between a disaster and an everyday emergency: the need to fit the plan to people's needs; the continuous nature of disaster planning; the need to eliminate myths from the plan; the need for information about the disaster; and the tendency of people to respond, in the absence of a plan, in the way they see fit. Additional principles reflect the need to involve large segments of the community in planning; the need to coordinate with the disaster plans of surrounding areas; the need for a general plan that addresses all types of disaster; the need to base the plan, as much as possible, on everyday working methods and procedures; the need for flexibility; and the need to specify responsible individuals by position title rather than by name.
- Participants in disaster planning should include those with authority to sanction the plan, those who will implement the plan, beneficiaries of the plan, experts in disaster planning, and those who are likely to resist the plan.
- A successful disaster plan is characterized by realistic expectations of the effects of a disaster and the needs generated, brevity and conciseness, expansion in stages, and official sanction by community authorities.
- General considerations in disaster planning include designation of authority, plans for communication during and after the disaster, plans for transportation, and plans for recordkeeping.
- Elements of a typical disaster plan include mechanisms and procedures for notification, warning, control, logistical coordination, evacuation, rescue, immediate care, supportive care, recovery, and evaluation.
- Data derived from assessing a potential or actual disaster situation give rise to nursing diagnoses that may reflect the potential for a disaster, the adequacy or inadequacy of disaster planning, or the effects of an actual disaster. Nursing diagnoses may be derived in relation to groups of people or to individuals involved in the disaster.
- Nursing involvement in planning for disaster care occurs at primary, secondary, and tertiary levels of prevention.
- Implementing a plan for disaster response involves communicating it to those who will be responsible for implementation and to members of the general public.
- Evaluation in a disaster setting will focus on the effectiveness of the disaster plan in dealing with a disaster event and on the effectiveness of care provided to individual disaster victims.

Review Questions

1. Describe four ways in which disaster events can vary. (p. 698)
2. Describe three factors that influence a community's response to a disaster. Give an example of the influence of each factor. (p. 699)
3. Describe the three dimensions of a disaster. (p. 699)
4. Identify at least three benefits of disaster planning. (p. 703)
5. Identify at least two human biological, two environmental, two life-style, and two health system factors to be assessed in relation to a disaster. Describe how each of the factors identified might influence a disaster or a community's response to a disaster. (p. 713)
6. Discuss at least six of the twelve principles of community disaster planning. (p. 704)
7. Describe four characteristics of a successful disaster plan. (p. 706)
8. Discuss at least five elements of an effective disaster plan. (p. 708)
9. Describe the role of the community health nurse in primary, secondary, and tertiary prevention related to disaster situations. (p. 719)

APPLICATION AND SYNTHESIS

Two commuter trains have collided in a tunnel at rush hour. Both trains derailed and one of them struck the side of the tunnel causing it to collapse on two of the derailed cars. Approximately 300 people were passengers on the two trains, with 50 or more people trapped in the two buried cars. The accident occurred approximately one-quarter mile from the west end of the tunnel and 2 miles from the east end. Most of both trains lie on the west side of the collapsed portion of the tunnel.

One of the passengers is a community health nurse. The nurse was not injured in the accident and was able to get out of the wreckage to the west end of the tunnel where most of the survivors are gathered.

1. What are the human biological, environmental, life-style, and health system factors that may be influencing this disaster situation?
2. What role functions might the community health nurse carry out in this situation?
3. What primary, secondary, and tertiary preventative activities might be appropriate in this situation? Why?

REFERENCES

1. Raphael, B. (1986). *When disaster strikes.* New York: Basic Books.
2. Dixon, M. (1986). Disaster planning, medical response: Organization and preparation. *AAOHN Journal, 34,* 580–584.
3. Tornado disaster—Illinois, 1990. (1991). *MMWR, 40,* 33–36.
4. Drabek, T. E. (1986). *Human systems responses to disaster.* New York: Springer/Verlag.
5. Mileti, D. S., Drabek, T. E., & Haas, J. E. (1975). *Human systems in extreme environments: A sociological perspective.* Boulder: University of Colorado Institute of Behavioral Sciences.
6. Janis, I. L., & Mann, L. (1977). Emergency decision-making: A theoretical analysis of responses to disaster warnings. *Journal of Human Stress, 3*(6), 35–45.
7. Merchant, J. A. (1986). Preparing for disaster. *American Journal of Public Health, 76,* 233–235.
8. Brandt, E. N., Mayer, W. N., Mason, J. O., et al. (1985). Designing a national disaster medical system. *Public Health Reports, 100,* 455–461.

RECOMMENDED READINGS

Drabek, T. E. (1986). *Human systems responses to disaster.* New York: Springer/Verlag.

Provides an introduction to disaster preparation at the individual, family, organizational, and community levels.

Garcia, L. M. (1985). *Disaster nursing: Planning, assessment, and intervention.* Rockville, MD: Aspen.

Describes nursing involvement in planning for and responding to a disaster event.

Raphael, B. (1986). *When disaster strikes.* New York: Basic Books.

Presents information related to disaster response and planning for disaster.

Vance, M. (1989). *Disaster preparedness: A bibliography.* Mansfield, OH: Vance Biblios.

Offers a selection of additional readings related to disaster preparation.

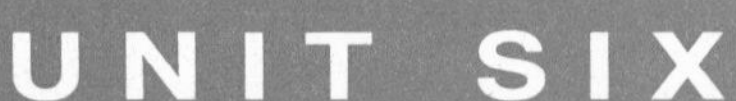

UNIT SIX

Common Community Health Problems

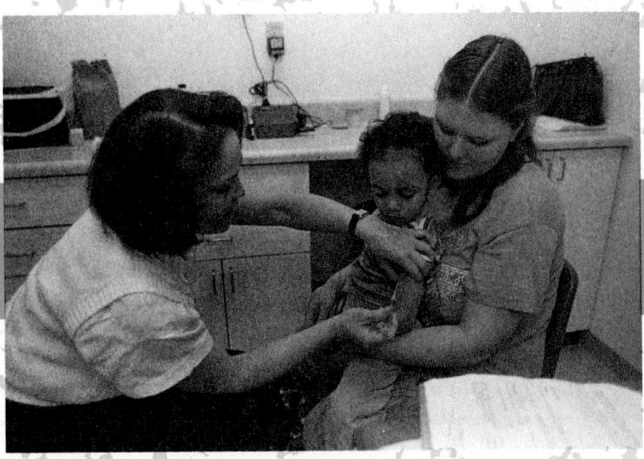

Community health nurses care for a variety of clients in a variety of settings. Although the needs of each client are unique, there are several categories of health problems that community health nurses encounter relatively frequently. These problems not only impair the health of the individual clients and families affected but also pose serious health risks for society as a whole. Because the primary focus of community health nursing is the health of the total population, these problems are of serious concern to community health nurses. In order to be in a position to deal with these problems, however, community health nurses need to have knowledge of the factors contributing to them and of strategies that can be used to control them.

For centuries, communicable diseases were the bane of human existence, and epidemics periodically eliminated large segments of the population. In fact, the plagues of the fourteenth century killed nearly one-fourth of the total population of Europe. Modern medical science and improved sanitation have allowed humankind to limit to some extent the death and suffering wrought by communicable diseases. However, diseases like acquired immunodeficiency syndrome (AIDS) and other sexually transmitted diseases continue to take their toll. Preventable childhood diseases still contribute to human morbidity and mortality. Chapter 30, Communicable Disease, addresses the epidemiology of childhood diseases, AIDS and other sexually transmitted diseases, viral hepatitis, tuberculosis, and influenza as well as the community health nurse's role in measures to control these diseases.

Despite the attention given to AIDS and its control in today's society, chronic illnesses have become the primary focus of epidemiologic research and control effects. Although medical science has helped to prolong the life of many Americans, it has been less successful in improving the quality of life, and many people suffer the debilitating consequences of chronic health problems. With the exception of heart disease and stroke, control strategies for chronic diseases have not been particularly successful. Chronic physical illnesses contribute to increased morbidity and mortality throughout the world and account for a large portion of health-care expenditures in the United States. In Chapter 31, Chronic Physical Health Problems, epidemiologic factors and control strategies are presented for chronic conditions such as trauma due to accidents, diabetes, cancer, heart disease, and obesity.

Chronic mental health problems are also of growing concern today, and clients with emotional disorders are encountered relatively frequently by community health nurses. Problems such as schizophrenia and depression may create tremendous difficulties for the individuals and families affected and for society as a whole. The epidemiology and control of these and other chronic mental health problems are presented in Chapter 32, Chronic Mental Health Problems.

Mental distress can also be manifested in substance abuse and violence. Abuse of alcohol and other drugs is a growing concern for community health nurses and for the general public. Alcohol and drug abuse not only affect the individuals experiencing these problems but may also profoundly affect their families. In addition, there is a growing number of children with a variety of health problems resulting from fetal exposure to alcohol and other drugs. Society, too, suffers from the effects of addictive behaviors involved in alcohol and drug abuse. Epidemiologic factors contributing to these problems and the community health nurse's role in dealing with them are the focus of Chapter 33, Substance Abuse.

But substance abuse is only one of several contributing factors in the growing problem of violence enacted against others or against oneself. Violence against others can manifest in family violence such as child abuse, spouse abuse, or elder abuse, or in homicide. Violence against oneself can culminate in suicide. More and more frequently, community health nurses encounter families with problems of violence. These nurses need a working knowledge of contributing factors and of interventions that may prevent violence. Chapter 34, Violence, presents information needed by community health nurses in dealing with these problems.

Communicable disease, chronic physical and mental health problems, substance abuse, and violence are the major deterrents to health encountered in contemporary society. Action to resolve these problems is needed at the individual, family, group, and societal levels, and community health nurses should be actively involved in interventions at each of these levels.

From the Community: A Nurse's Voice

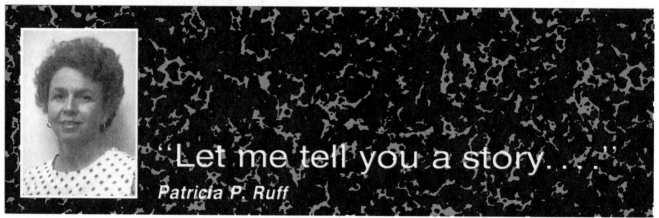

More likely than not, stories and tales have been used to teach ever since the time of the earliest human societies. Aesop had his fables, and Jesus Christ taught using simple parables. I too use stories in my work as a community health nurse to teach and to motivate my clients to overcome health-related problems. I have found that the more a story touches a client personally, the greater its power to produce positive change.

Accordingly, I draw on my personal experiences and those of my clients. First, I take time to get to know my clients and what is important in their lives. I often recall the words of the author of *Desiderata*, who penned, "Listen to others, even the dull and ignorant; they too have their own story." I then draw on their story to motivate them. Two major teaching foci, medication compliance and safety, illustrate how this process works.

Letitia Thompson, the beloved 84-year-old matriarch of an extended black family, had consistently refused to take her medication to help prevent another CVA. Questioning her, I learned that she had decided it was time to die and that another stroke would be "a blessing." Mrs. Thompson had few cognitive deficits and enjoyed the support of a nurturing family. I explained that in the event of her death her family would bury her as she wished. If she survived another stroke, however, she could become aphasic, bedfast, and incontinent, thus increasing the burden of care for her family. If placement in an extended-care facility became necessary, it would increase the financial burden to the taxpayer. Mrs. Thompson was not moved.

I pulled my chair closer, held her hand, and looked around the room at the proudly displayed pictures of her dozen grandchildren. Mrs. Thompson had raised her own family during a time when budgeting meant that every penny had to be stretched twice as far, and still her children often got less than they needed. I explained that the tax budget is the same as her family's household budget. Should limited tax monies be spent to care for a woman who was in a nursing home because she wouldn't take her pills, I asked, or should the money go to build playgrounds and provide college educations for her grandchildren? Aha! She saw that by keeping well she could continue her lifelong effort of furthering the welfare of her family. Mrs. Thompson started taking her medication.

Another client, Mrs. Bertini, who had arthritis and severely deformed hands, used wooden kitchen matches to light the burners on her gas stove. She refused to have the automatic pilot activated because it would cost her an extra dollar a month in gas. Mrs. Bertini seldom dressed for the day, and the sleeves of her loose-fitting housecoat offered ample opportunity for catching fire each time a match was struck and the burner ignited. Many family members and other health-care providers had failed to convince her to make a change.

I told her a story from my childhood about Mrs. Graham, a neighbor lady who would invite my friends and me into her home for singing, games, and cookies. All of us loved Mrs. Graham. One day her clothing caught fire while she was cooking and she died of the burns. I was heartbroken and cried for days. On my next visit, Mrs. Bertini was beaming and couldn't wait to turn on the gas stove. The automatic pilot was working! She still doesn't share my depth of concern in this situation, but she was touched by the depth of my feelings over my childhood recollection and realized that I had her well-being in mind.

My job is to effect positive change in the lives of my clients. For Mrs. Thompson and Mrs. Bertini, some simple stories helped me do my job.

CHAPTER 30

Communicable Disease

KEY TERMS

attack rates
case fatality rates
chain of infection
chemoprophylaxis
communicable diseases
contact notification
droplet nuclei
incubation period
mode of transmission
opportunistic infection
prodromal period
sensitive occupations

Communicable disease was the scourge of the Middle Ages when epidemics wiped out huge segments of the population in a short period of time. By and large, epidemics of this magnitude do not occur today. With the advent of antibiotics and immunization, the morbidity and mortality associated with communicable diseases have decreased significantly. Despite this progress, however, communicable disease continues to be a serious concern in community health practice.

Acquired immunodeficiency syndrome (AIDS) is probably the primary communicable disease of concern in today's society. By September 1990, more than 150,000 cases of AIDS had been diagnosed in the United States, accounting for more than 92,000 deaths.[1] By March of that same year, more than 35,000 cases had been diagnosed in Europe.[2] Sexually transmitted diseases such as gonorrhea, syphilis, and hepatitis continue to occur with alarming frequency. Finally, despite the availability of vaccines, cases of preventable diseases such as measles, pertussis, and influenza still occur.

Community health nurses are actively involved in preventing, identifying, and controlling communicable disease. For this reason, they must have a firm understanding of general concepts related to communicable diseases as well as knowledge of specific disease entities. General concepts and control measures related to communicable disease are addressed in this chapter. Community health nursing roles and responsibilities with respect to communicable disease are also discussed; information related to childhood diseases, along with information on AIDS and other sexually transmitted diseases, hepatitis A and non-A, non-B hepatitis, tuberculosis, and influenza, is presented to give the nurse a strong foundation for dealing with the problems posed by communicable disease.

(continued)

LEARNING OBJECTIVES

After reading this chapter you should be able to:

- Describe trends in the incidence of at least five major communicable diseases.
- Identify six major modes by which communicable diseases are transmitted.
- Identify at least four roles for community health nurses in controlling communicable diseases.
- Identify the two major approaches used to control communicable diseases.
- Discuss the influence of at least two factors in each component of the epidemiologic perspective on childhood diseases.
- Describe at least two nursing interventions for controlling childhood diseases related to each level of prevention.
- Compare and contrast the epidemiologic factors contributing to the development of HIV infection and other major sexually transmitted diseases.
- Describe at least two nursing interventions for controlling HIV infection and other sexually transmitted diseases related to each level of prevention.

(*continued*)

- Discuss the influence of at least two factors in each of the components of the epidemiologic perspective on the development of hepatitis A and non-A, non-B hepatitis.
- Describe at least two nursing interventions for controlling hepatitis A and non-A, non-B hepatitis related to each level of prevention.
- Discuss the influence of at least two factors in each of the components of the epidemiologic perspective on the development of tuberculosis.
- Describe at least two nursing interventions for controlling tuberculosis related to each level of prevention.
- Discuss the influence of at least two factors in each of the components of the epidemiologic perspective on the development of influenza.
- Describe at least two nursing interventions for controlling influenza related to each level of prevention.

GENERAL CONCEPTS OF COMMUNICABLE DISEASE

Communicable diseases are those diseases spread by direct contact with an infectious agent. Communicable diseases affecting humans arise from both human and animal sources. In some instances, however, there is an extended period of time between the excretion of the organism by the *reservoir* and infection of a new *host*. (For a complete discussion of these terms, see Chapter 6, The Epidemiologic Process.) Thus, it may sometimes be difficult to identify the immediate source of infection in a particular person.

Several communicable disease concepts must be understood prior to examining specific diseases. These include concepts related to the "chain of infection" such as modes of transmission and portals of entry and exit, concepts of incubation and prodromal periods, and the concept of "sensitive occupations."

CHAIN OF INFECTION

In communicable diseases, epidemiologic factors related to human biology, environment, life-style, and health system create what may be termed a "chain of infection." A *chain of infection* is a series of events or conditions that lead to the development of a particular communicable disease. The "links" in the chain are the infected person or source of the infectious agent, the reservoir, the agent itself, the mode of transmission of the disease, the agent's portals of entry and exit, and a susceptible new host. The concepts of reservoir, agent, and host were introduced in Chapter 6. This discussion will focus on the remaining links in the chain: modes of transmission and portals of entry and exit.

MODES OF TRANSMISSION

The *mode of transmission* of a particular disease is the means by which the infectious agent that causes the disease is transferred from an infected person to an uninfected one. Communicable diseases may be spread by any of several modes of transmission: airborne transmission, fecal-oral (gastrointestinal) transmission, direct contact, sexual contact, direct inoculation, insect or animal bite, or via inanimate objects or soil.

Airborne Transmission

Airborne transmission occurs when the infectious organism is present in the air and is inspired (inhaled) by a susceptible host during respiration. Diseases transmitted by the airborne route include the exanthems (diseases characterized by a rash, such as measles and chickenpox), infections of the mouth and throat (such as streptococcal infections), and infections of the lower respiratory system (such as tuberculosis, pneumonia, and influenza). Certain systemic infections are also products of airborne transmission. Examples of these are meningococcal meningitis and pneumococcal pneumonias.

Fecal-oral Transmission

Fecal-oral transmission of an infectious agent may be either direct or indirect. Direct transmission occurs when the hands or other objects (fomites) are contaminated with organisms from human feces and then put into the mouth. Indirect transmission occurs via contaminated food or water. For example, a person with hepatitis A may defecate, fail to wash his or her hands properly, and then prepare a sandwich for someone else. The second person would ingest the virus with the sandwich and, if susceptible, might develop hepatitis A.

Direct Contact

Direct contact transmission involves skin-to-skin contact or direct contact with mucous membrane discharges between the infected person and another person. Diseases typically spread by this route include infectious mononucleosis, impetigo, scabies, and lice. Scabies, lice, and other parasitic diseases also may be transmitted through contact with clothing and other items containing the eggs of the parasites.

Sexual Transmission

Transmission of diseases via sexual contact is a special instance of direct contact transmission. Diseases spread by this mode of transmission are usually referred to as sexually transmitted diseases (STDs). Diseases spread during sexual intercourse include (but are not limited to) AIDS, gonorrhea, syphilis, genital herpes, hepatitis B, and delta hepatitis. These diseases may also be spread by other modes of transmission. For example, both hepatitis B and AIDS may be spread by direct inoculation.

Transmission by Direct Inoculation

Direct inoculation occurs when the infectious agent is introduced directly into the bloodstream of the new host. Direct inoculation can occur transplacentally from an infected mother to a fetus, via transfusion with infected blood or blood products, or through the use of contaminated hypodermic equipment. Health-care workers are particularly at risk for several communicable diseases owing to the likelihood of needle sticks or puncture injuries from objects contaminated with blood and other body fluids. Diseases commonly spread by direct inoculation include AIDS, hepatitis B, and delta hepatitis. Some evidence suggests that hepatitis A can also be spread by intravenous drug use with contaminated needles.

Transmission by Insect or Animal Bite

Insect and animal bites can also transmit infectious agents. For example, the bite of the Anopheles mosquito is the mode of transmission for malaria. Similarly, rabies frequently is transmitted via a bite from infected, warm-blooded animals such as dogs, skunks, and raccoons. Another disease transmitted by an insect bite is Lyme disease, which is transmitted by the bite of an infected tick.

Transmission by Other Means

Some communicable diseases are transmitted through contact with spores present in the soil or with inanimate objects. For example, exposure to the bacillus that causes tetanus frequently occurs through a dirty puncture wound. Modes of transmission and typical diseases most often transmitted by each mode are summarized in Table 30–1.

TABLE 30–1. MODES OF DISEASE TRANSMISSION AND TYPICAL DISEASES

Mode of Transmission	Diseases Transmitted
Airborne	Measles, mumps, rubella, poliomyelitis *Hemophilus influenzae* type B (HiB) infection, tuberculosis, influenza, scarlet fever, diphtheria, pertussis
Fecal-oral	Hepatitis A, non-A, non-B hepatitis, salmonellosis, shigellosis, typhoid, polio (in poor sanitary conditions)
Direct contact	Impetigo, scabies, lice
Sexual contact	Chlamydia, gonorrhea, hepatitis B, delta hepatitis, human immunodeficiency virus (HIV) infection, herpes simplex virus (HSV) infection, syphilis
Direct inoculation	Syphilis, hepatitis A and B, non-A, non-B and delta hepatitis, human immunodeficiency virus (HIV) infection
Insect or animal bite	Malaria, plague, rabies
Other means of transmission	Tetanus, hookworm

TABLE 30–2. PORTALS OF ENTRY AND EXIT FOR EACH MODE OF DISEASE TRANSMISSION

Mode of Transmission	Portal of Entry	Portal of Exit
Airborne	Respiratory system	Respiratory system
Fecal-oral	Mouth	Feces
Direct contact	Skin, mucous membrane	Skin, mucous membrane
Sexual contact	Skin, mouth, urethra, vagina, rectum	Skin lesions, vaginal or urethral secretion
Direct inoculation	Across placenta, bloodstream	Blood
Animal or insect bite	Wound in skin	Blood, saliva
Other means of transmission	Wound in skin, intact skin	Animal feces, soil

PORTALS OF ENTRY AND EXIT

Communicable diseases also differ in terms of the portals through which the infectious agent causing the disease enters and leaves an infected host. Portals of entry include the respiratory system, the gastrointestinal tract, and the skin and mucous membrane.

Portals of exit also differ among communicable diseases. Infectious agents may leave an infected host through the respiratory system or through feces passed from the gastrointestinal tract. Blood and other body fluids such as semen, vaginal secretion, and saliva are the portals of exit for infectious agents causing diseases such as AIDS, gonorrhea, and hepatitis B. The skin acts as a portal of exit as well as a portal of entry for conditions such as impetigo and syphilis. Portals of entry and exit and related modes of disease transmission are summarized in Table 30–2.

INCUBATION AND PRODROMAL PERIODS

The *incubation period* of a communicable disease is the interval from the time one is exposed to an infectious organism until one develops the symptoms of the disease. The length of the incubation period for a particular disease may influence the success of efforts to halt the spread of the disease. Some diseases, such as influenza and scarlet fever, have incubation periods of less than a week. Others typically require incubation periods of 1 to 2 weeks (gonorrhea, measles, pertussis, and polio), 2 to 3 weeks (rubella, chickenpox, and mumps), or months (viral hepatitis, syphilis). In some diseases, such as AIDS, the incubation period can be years.

The *prodromal period* of a communicable disease is the period between the first symptoms and the appearance of the symptoms that typify the disease. For example, prior to the appearance of the jaundice that is characteristic of viral hepatitis, the client may experience prodromal symptoms of nausea, fatigue, and malaise. Similarly, a runny nose and watery eyes are prodromal symptoms for measles.

SENSITIVE OCCUPATIONS

Sensitive occupations are those that foster the spread of disease by virtue of contact with susceptible individuals, which occurs because of the type of work performed. The types of occupations considered sensitive for specific diseases vary with the mode of transmission of the disease. For example, people who are chronic carriers of typhoid, a disease communicated by fecal-oral transmission, are not allowed to work as food handlers. For airborne diseases, sensitive occupations are those where transmission of respiratory secretions would be likely to occur.

In some jurisdictions, persons in sensitive occupations who are even exposed to certain diseases may be removed from work until they are deemed incapable of giving the disease to others. This judgment may occur when the incubation period has passed without the onset of symptoms, or when direct evidence of noncommunicability is available. For example, a negative throat culture for streptococci or prophylactic treatment for scarlet fever would allow a nurse whose child has this disease to return to work.

COMMUNITY HEALTH NURSING ROLES IN CONTROLLING COMMUNICABLE DISEASES

Community health nurses have a variety of roles and responsibilities in efforts to control communicable diseases. These roles generally fall into the categories of contact notification, providing chemoprophylaxis, education, immunization, case finding, referral, treatment, supportive care, and political activity. The roles of the nurse in notifying contacts and providing chemoprophylaxis will be addressed later in the chapter.

The nurse's educational role involves educating the general public about means to prevent communicable diseases, signs and symptoms of existing diseases, and where to seek help for possible communicable diseases. The nurse may also be involved in educating other health-care providers on the appropriate diagnostic and screening procedures for certain communicable diseases, particularly sexually transmitted ones. It is the responsibility of community health nurses in some public health agencies, for example, to contact private physicians who report cases of gonorrhea and syphilis to educate them regarding appropriate treatment measures.

Community health nurses also educate the public regarding the need for immunizations. They would also be involved in planning, implementing, and evaluating immunization campaigns and in giving the actual immunizations to susceptible individuals.

Community health nurses are also actively involved in case finding with respect to communicable diseases. Because they service large segments of the population who may not receive care from other health-care providers, community health nurses are in a unique position to identify possible cases of communicable diseases. Once a person with a potential communicable disease has been identified, the community health nurse may make a referral for further diagnosis and treatment. Or, in some cases, the nurse may be involved in diagnosing and treating communicable diseases on the basis of medically approved protocols. Community health nurses may also either refer contacts (those exposed) to communicable diseases for chemoprophylaxis as appropriate, or they may provide chemoprophylaxis themselves.

Another role for community health nurses related to communicable diseases is providing supportive care for clients with these conditions. Supportive care can include educating clients and families on measures for reducing fever or enhancing comfort until the disease has run its course, or providing emotional support and assistance in adjusting to the long-term consequences of some communicable diseases. Supportive care might also involve helping clients and their families to deal with the psychological implications of incurable diseases such as genital herpes and AIDS.

Finally, the role of the nurse in the control of communicable diseases may involve political activity and advocacy. For example, the nurse might be actively engaged in efforts to ensure access to health care for persons with AIDS or in promoting legislation to make immunization for *Hemophilus influenzae* type B infections mandatory for day-care admission.

PRINCIPLES OF COMMUNICABLE DISEASE CONTROL

The interventions of community health nurses and other health-care providers in the control of specific communicable diseases are determined by the nature of the disease. Two basic approaches are used to control communicable disease. The first is preventing the spread of the disease. The second is to increase the resistance of the host.

PREVENTING THE SPREAD OF INFECTION

Preventing the spread of infection may be accomplished through measures aimed at the agent or at the source of the infection. For example, the use of ultraviolet light and adequate ventilation in areas where *Mycobacterium tuberculosis* is found is an attempt to control or kill the infectious agent that causes tuberculosis. Interventions aimed at the source of infection might include measures such as eradicating the mosquito that spreads malaria or isolating persons with disease to prevent infection of others. Other specific methods of preventing the spread of infection to others are "contact notification" and "chemoprophylaxis."

CONTACT NOTIFICATION

Contact notification is the process of identifying persons who have been exposed to a communicable disease, informing them of exposure, testing them for the particular disease, and, in some cases (for example, syphilis, gonorrhea, tuberculosis, and hepatitis), offering treatment to prevent them from becoming symptomatic and exposing others to the disease. Who is considered a contact to a particular disease depends of the mode of transmission of that disease. For AIDS and hepatitis B, for example, contacts would include past and present sexual partners, persons who shared needles in IV drug use, and young children born to women with AIDS. For tuberculosis and hepatitis A, people living with the infected person are considered contacts.

Contact notification is usually handled in such a way that individuals notified of their potential exposure to a communicable disease are not told the source of that exposure, thereby protecting the anonymity of the infected person. In fact, in many jurisdictions, legislation prohibits subpoenaing client records of communicable disease treatment so as to ensure confidentiality.[3]

Contact notification can be carried out in one of two ways: client referral and provider referral. In client referral, individuals who are known to have a communicable disease notify their contacts themselves and refer them for testing and possible treatment. In provider referral, designated health-care personnel solicit names of contacts from infected persons and notify the contacts of potential exposure. When given the option, many people with communicable diseases select provider referral as the preferred mechanism of contact notification. For example, in some studies, up to 59 percent of those with human immunodeficiency virus (HIV) infection (the virus that causes AIDS) preferred provider referral as a means of notifying their contacts.[4]

Community health nurses are frequently involved in the provider referral approach to contact notification. The process used is a systematic one and begins with an interview of the client with a communicable disease. In this interview, the community health nurse explains the need for notification, testing, and possible treatment of contacts, and then elicits names, addresses, and other information that will allow contacts to be located and informed of their exposure. Depending on how the notification system is organized, this same nurse may follow up on contacts whose names were elicited or communicate this information to another health-care provider (frequently another community health nurse) who will get in touch with the individuals named. The identity of the client with the communicable disease from whom the names were elicited is not included in the information communicated.

Nurses involved in contact follow-up can either make home visits or approach contacts at work or any other place where they can be located. When contacts are approached, nurses should speak to them in a setting that ensures privacy and inform them that they have been exposed to a communicable disease. Nurses frequently need to exercise creativity to prevent others from knowing why the person is being contacted by a nurse.

The nurse who approaches the contact never divulges information about the source of the exposure, but explains that the person has potentially been exposed to a communicable disease. In addition to notifying the contact regarding the exposure, the nurse will educate the client about the potential for developing the disease and for spreading it to others and make a referral for testing and treatment for the condition as needed.

CHEMOPROPHYLAXIS

Chemoprophylaxis is the use of medications to prevent the onset of disease in exposed individuals. When individuals are prevented from developing symptomatic disease, they are usually also prevented from spreading the disease to others. Chemoprophylaxis is used for a variety of communicable disease including tuberculosis, gonorrhea, syphilis, hepatitis A and B, *Hemophilus influenzae* type B (HiB) infection, diphtheria, and tetanus. Chemoprophylaxis has also been shown to be effective in slowing the development of AIDS in persons with human immunodeficiency virus (HIV) infection[5] and in preventing some of the opportunistic infections that occur in people with AIDS, but its effectiveness in preventing the spread of the disease has not been demonstrated.

INCREASING HOST RESISTANCE

The second approach to the control of communicable disease is to increase the resistance of the host. Means of achieving this include promoting general health, producing immunity, and preventing complications of communicable diseases, all of which involve nursing action. Chapter 6, The Epidemiologic Process, addressed measures that can be used to promote health. Measures to prevent complications of communicable diseases will be addressed for each of the diseases presented later in this chapter. Here, the focus is on developing host immunity to disease.

Immunity to communicable diseases can occur in three ways: transplacental transfer of maternal antibodies, having the disease, or immunization. Transplacental transfer provides short-term immunity in young infants, but depends on the mother having antibodies to a particular infectious agent. If the mother is immune, the newborn will have some degree of short-term immunity to the same diseases.

Having the disease is an effective, though sometimes dangerous, means of developing immunity to some diseases. Immunity seems to be conferred in such diseases as measles, diphtheria, pertussis, mumps, chickenpox, and hepatitis A and B. Having other diseases such as gonorrhea and early stages of syphilis, however, does not appear to protect one from being infected again.

Immunization is available for many communicable diseases including polio, measles, mumps, rubella, diphtheria, pertussis, tetanus, hepatitis B, diseases caused by *Hemophilus influenzae* type B, and pneumococcal pneumonia. In the United States, routine immunization of all persons (preferably in childhood) is recommended for measles, mumps, rubella, diphtheria, pertussis, tetanus, and polio. Immunization of children, especially those in day-care centers, against *Hemophilus influenzae* type B is also recommended. In developing countries, BCG immunization for tuberculosis is also suggested. Immunization for other diseases is recommended for certain groups at higher risk of developing them (discussed later in sections dealing with each disease). Recommendations for routine immunization are summarized in Table 30–3.

TABLE 30–3. RECOMMENDATIONS FOR ROUTINE IMMUNIZATION

Immunizing Agent	Recommendations for Administration
Diphtheria, Tetanus, Pertussis vaccine (DTP)	Children aged 2, 4, 6 months, 18 months, and school entry
Tetanus, diphtheria (Td)	Children over 8 and adults: booster every 10 years
Trivalent Oral Polio vaccine (OPV)	Children aged 2 and 4 months (third dose at 6 months in areas of high incidence), 18 months, and school entry
Measles, Mumps, Rubella vaccine (MMR)	Children 15 months of age; measles booster at junior high entry
Hemophilus influenzae type B (HiB)	Children 2, 4, 6, months of age (or 2 and 4 months of age) and a booster at 15 months of age
Hepatitis B vaccine	Health-care workers, prostitutes and others with multiple sex partners, IV drug users
Influenza vaccine	Annually for persons over 65 years of age and those with debilitating physical illness
Pneumonia vaccine	Persons at risk for pneumococcal pneumonia

(Source: MMUR[81]; State of California, Department of Health Services[22])

OTHER CONTROL MEASURES

Other measures that aid in the control of communicable diseases include legislation requiring screening for specific diseases in high-risk groups and mandatory reporting of cases of communicable disease. Additional control measures include compulsory immunization prior to school entry, compulsory examination of contacts and treatment of infected persons, and regulation of vehicles of transmission such as second-hand mattresses and pillows. Use of these and related measures will be addressed in more detail later in this chapter.

THE EPIDEMIOLOGIC PREVENTION PROCESS MODEL AND CONTROL OF COMMUNICABLE DISEASE

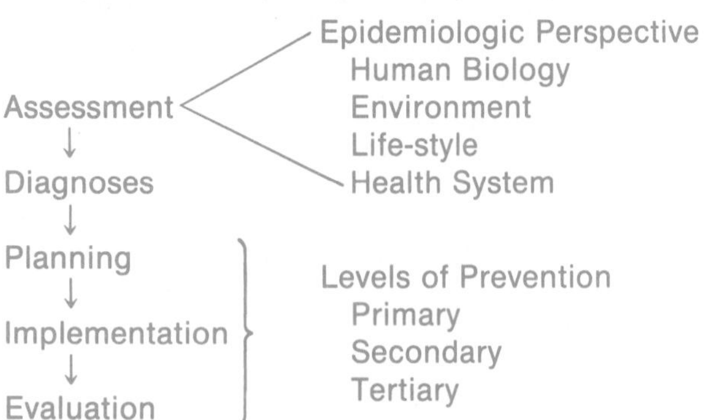

The epidemiologic prevention process model can be used to enhance the control of communicable disease. In the remainder of this chapter, the model will be applied to childhood illnesses, AIDS and other sexually transmitted diseases, hepatitis, tuberculosis, and influenza.

CHILDHOOD DISEASES

Childhood diseases are so named because, in the past, the incidence of these diseases was higher among children than adults. These diseases were also the major source of mortality among children. They are not, however, experienced exclusively by children. A growing number of young adults are susceptible to measles, while older adults are frequently unprotected against tetanus. Although adults develop these diseases relatively infrequently, consequences of infection in adults are frequently more severe than in children. The childhood diseases to be discussed here include measles, mumps, rubella, diphtheria, pertussis (whooping cough), tetanus, poliomyelitis, and diseases caused by *Hemophilus influenzae* type B (HiB) virus. Unless otherwise specified, incidence rates reflect the total population, not just cases of disease among children.

The importance of community health efforts to deal with the problems posed by the continued incidence of childhood diseases is reflected in the national objectives for the year 2000 related to control of these conditions. These objectives are summarized in Box 30–1.

TRENDS IN CHILDHOOD DISEASES

Measles is a relatively mild viral disease that used to be common in childhood in the United States and still is in developing countries. Ever since the develop-

BOX 30–1

Summary of National Objectives for the Year 2000 Related to Childhood Diseases

1. Reduce the number of cases of diphtheria and tetanus in persons aged 25 and younger to zero cases annually.
2. Reduce the number of cases of wild-virus polio, measles, rubella, and congenital rubella syndrome to zero cases per year.
3. Reduce the number of cases of mumps to 500 cases per year.
4. Reduce the number of cases of pertussis to 1000 per year.
5. Reduce bacterial meningitis (usually due to HiB) to no more than 4.7 cases per 100,000 population.
6. Complete the basic immunization series in 90% of children under age 2.
7. Complete the basic immunization series in 95% of children in licensed child-care facilities and kindergarten through postsecondary education.
8. Expand immunization laws for schools, preschools, and day-care settings to all states for all antigens.
9. Increase to at least 90% the proportion of primary-care providers who provide information and immunizations for their clients as appropriate.
10. Ensure that virtually no American child experiences a financial barrier to immunization services.
11. Increase to at least 90% the proportion of public health departments that provide adult immunization for tetanus and diphtheria.

(Source: U.S. Department of Health and Human Services[87])

ment of a vaccine, there has been a 98 percent decline in the incidence of measles in the United States,[6] reaching a low of 0.64 per 100,000 population in 1983. After 1983, however, a slight rise in incidence was noted for several years. Incidence for 1988 was 1.38 cases per 100,000 population, approximately double the rate for 1983,[7] and the number of cases occurring in 1989 increased 300 percent over those of 1988.[8] In recent measles outbreaks in Chicago and Los Angeles, 75 percent to 80 percent of the cases reported occurred in individuals who had not been immunized.[9–10]

Rubella is a relatively mild disease in itself but poses serious consequences to children who are exposed in utero. The number of cases of rubella declined 99 percent from the initiation of rubella immunization in 1969 to 1988. There was a concomitant 96 percent decrease in the incidence of congenital rubella syndrome (CRS) from 1970 to 1988.[11] In 1988, the incidence rate for rubella was 0.09 per 100,000 population, while that for CRS was zero per 1000 live births.[7] In 1989, however, the number of cases of rubella increased twofold and jumped another threefold in 1990 to reach an incidence rate of 0.4 cases per 100,000 population, the highest rate since 1982. Despite the recent increase in the number of cases of rubella, however, the incidence of this disease remains 98 percent lower than pre-immunization rates.[12]

Mumps, also called infectious parotitis, is an acute viral disease characterized by swelling and tenderness of salivary glands, especially the parotid gland. The incidence of mumps decreased significantly following the development of a vaccine. This decline continued until 1985, when incidence rates reached a low of 1.3 cases per 100,000 population. Since that time, rates have begun to increase slightly to 2.3 cases per 100,000 population by 1989.[13]

Deaths due to mumps are rare, but approximately 15 percent to 25 percent of adult males infected develop orchitis (inflammation of the testes) with subsequent potential for infertility. Other complications include oophoritis (inflammation of the ovaries) in females, pancreatitis, nephritis, arthritis, mastitis, thyroiditis, and pericarditis. Meningitis may also occur.[14]

Diphtheria, pertussis, and *tetanus* are three more childhood diseases for which the availability of vaccines has resulted in a marked decline in incidence. Since 1980, the incidence rate for diphtheria has been negligible with only an occasional case occurring throughout the population. The decline in the incidence of pertussis is not quite so dramatic, and cases continue to occur at a rate of 1.9 per 100,000 persons, a rate that has been relatively stable over the last few years. Tetanus incidence declined from 0.28 cases per 100,000 population in 1955 to 0.02 per 100,000 population in 1990.[13]

Despite the dramatic decline in the incidence of these three diseases, there has been recent concern over the fact that approximately 18.5 percent of inner-city women have inadequate immunity levels for both diphtheria and tetanus.[15] Because protection against disease in newborns is dependent upon maternal antibody levels, lack of immunity in these women increases the risk of disease among their children.

Incidence rates for *poliomyelitis* have been stable at zero per 100,000 population each year since 1979 except during 1983 when there was a temporary increase to 0.01 cases per 100,000 population. Approximately one in every 200 children will experience an illness caused by *Hemophilus influenzae* type B (HiB) before the age of 5.[16] HiB is suspected of causing 60 percent of cases of meningitis in children and is the most common cause of epiglottitis, another life-threatening disease. Other diseases caused by HiB include septic arthritis, pneumonia, and cellulitis. Because HiB-related diseases are not reportable as a class, specific incidence rates are not available.

ASSESSING CONTRIBUTING FACTORS IN CHILDHOOD DISEASES

Human Biology

Human biological factors can increase one's risk of developing childhood diseases. Biological factors to be assessed by the community health nurse include the age and sex composition and physical health status of the population.

The nurse would assess the age of population groups in a community to determine their susceptibility to childhood diseases. Young children tend to be more susceptible to childhood diseases and their effects than are older children. Many of these cases in recent outbreaks of measles have occurred in children too young to have received routine immunization.[17] Mumps, too, is most often seen in young children. Pertussis is rarely seen in children above 8 to 10 years of age; and although diphtheria can affect all age groups, the risk of fatality due to diphtheria is highest for infants and young children. Among susceptible populations, in fact, fatality rates of 5 percent to 10 percent continue to occur despite treatment with diphtheria antitoxin.[14] Newborns delivered in less than sterile conditions (especially in developing nations) are at risk for tetanus neonatorum, particularly if their mothers are unimmunized. Diseases caused by *Hemophilus influenzae* type B are found almost exclusively in children under age 5,[14] and younger children seem to be at greater risk for complications of these diseases. Polio tends to occur primarily in children and adolescents in developed countries and infants and young children in the developing world.

Older children and adults may also be at risk for childhood diseases and their consequences. For example, evidence suggests that some children who have been immunized against measles have decreasing levels of immunity over time. These "secondary vaccine failures" contribute to outbreaks of measles, particularly in schools and in college-age students.[18] Rubella in adults is also a cause for concern in that an estimated 10 percent to 20 percent of women 15 to 29 years of age may not be adequately immunized. Because these women are of childbearing age, their lack of immunity increases the potential for congenital rubella syndrome in their children. Further evidence of low immunity levels to rubella in young adults can be seen in recent outbreaks of rubella on college campuses.[11]

Complications of mumps, especially those of the reproductive tract, are more common in adults than in children. Measles is another disease that tends to be more severe in adults than in children. Older persons tend to be at slightly greater risk than younger ones for developing tetanus. This is primarily because they grew up in an era before DPT immunizations and because immunization of adults has not been pursued as actively as that of young children. Currently, about 60 percent of cases of tetanus occur in people over age 60.[14] Older persons are at a somewhat lower risk for diphtheria, however, if they were exposed to the disease and developed immunity during their youth when the disease occurred far more frequently.

Sex may also be an influencing factor in the development of childhood diseases and their consequences, so the nurse would determine the sex composition of the population to determine the extent of risk for specific childhood diseases. Complications of mumps, for instance, are more common in adult males than females. Morbidity and mortality for pertussis, on the other hand, are higher among females than among males of all ages. Males, however, more frequently develop tetanus, probably due to occupational exposure.

Physical health factors can increase both susceptibility to disease and complications of childhood illnesses, and the community health nurse would assess the community for the prevalence of conditions that increase susceptibility to childhood diseases. For example, malnutrition places young children at higher risk of death and complications from measles. Malnutrition in children with measles may contribute to diarrhea and dehydration, severe skin infections, and vitamin A deficiency, resulting in blindness. Tonsillectomy predisposes one to bulbar involvement and motor center-mediated paralysis due to polio. In addition, increased susceptibility to polio is noted in pregnancy.[14] The presence of certain physical conditions including asplenia, sickle cell disease (which occurs primarily in blacks), and immunodeficiency also contributes to the incidence of HiB-related diseases. In addition, immunodeficient children may not develop adequate immunity in response to HiB immunization.

Environment

Factors related to both the physical and social environments influence the development of childhood diseases and should be assessed by the community health nurse. Crowded living conditions, particularly in inner-city areas, enhance the spread of airborne diseases such as measles, mumps, rubella, pertussis, polio, and HiB infection.[8,14] College campuses and military installations experience frequent outbreaks of measles among young adults in close quarters who are not immunized, or whose immunity levels have declined over time.

Sanitation and disposal of both human and animal feces are other factors in the physical environment that affect the development of childhood diseases, particularly tetanus and polio. The organism causing tetanus is found on a variety of surfaces and is more common in areas where there is animal excrement. In addition, home delivery births and poor hygiene on the part of untrained midwives in developing countries and some parts of the United States contribute to the development of tetanus in neonates and, occasionally, in postpartum women. Poor sanitation also fosters the spread of polio in underdeveloped countries. The polio virus is excreted in the feces of an infected person and then contaminates food and water supplies ingested by others, spreading the disease.

Social environmental factors that influence the incidence and consequences of childhood diseases include poverty, unemployment, lower educational levels, and religion. Poverty and unemployment, with consequent loss of health insurance, may limit the ability of parents to have their children immunized or to provide prompt medical care when illness does occur, resulting in more serious consequences of disease. For example, the number of children adequately immunized against measles in inner-city areas ranges from only 49 percent to 65 percent,[8] far lower than in more affluent communities. Pregnant women with low incomes might not receive prenatal care, thus denying them the opportunity to obtain screening and counseling for congenital rubella syndrome.

Racial and ethnic group differences are factors in the incidence of childhood illnesses. The incidence of childhood illnesses is higher, for example, among minority group children than their Caucasian counterparts, although these findings probably reflect access to health care rather than increased susceptibility among these minority groups. American Indians and Alaskan Natives have higher rates of HiB infection than do their white counterparts and, in recent measles outbreaks, incidence was highest among black and Hispanic children.

Language barriers and lower educational levels among some ethnic and socioeconomic groups may impede awareness of the need for immunization against childhood diseases. In addition, the religious beliefs of some religious sects prohibit immunizations, thus increasing the size of the susceptible population among members of these sects and the community at large. Because of reduced herd immunity (see in Chapter 6, The Epidemiologic Process, for a discussion of herd immunity), the presence of these unimmunized individuals increases the potential for the spread of disease throughout the community.

Other social factors that can increase the incidence of childhood diseases include media communications and homelessness. Media reports of adverse reactions to immunization have led some parents to put off immunizing their children, while the fatigue, malnutrition, exposure to cold and crowding, and general debilitation associated with homelessness have contributed to increased incidence of pertussis in the homeless population.

Life-style

The community health nurse will also assess the presence of life-style factors that might increase the susceptibility of a population to childhood diseases. Individuals and families in lower socioeconomic groups tend to engage in a "present-oriented" life-style in which energies are focused on dealing with current problems. Consequently, immunization of young children may not be assigned a high priority in light of other needs. Moreover, inattention to routine health-care needs and poor nutrition also contribute to increased susceptibility to childhood diseases. Overexertion and fatigue are also risk factors for childhood diseases, particularly polio.

Intravenous drug use is another life-style factor that contributes, on occasion, to the development of childhood diseases. Intravenous use of drugs contaminated with tetanus bacilli has been implicated in some cases of tetanus.[14]

Occupation is also a life-style factor that plays a part in the development of some childhood diseases. Tetanus occurs more frequently among people who work outdoors, particularly among those working around animals or in outdoor occupations in which there is a high potential for puncture wounds such as trash collection or construction work. Pertussis occurs with some frequency among health-care workers who have low immunity levels.

Children of working parents who are placed in day care are at higher risk for HiB infection than children cared for at home.[16] Social and economic conditions that require both parents to work or that limit support networks, particularly for single parent families, contribute to the incidence of HiB-related illness.

Health System

The community health nurse will assess the effects of health system factors on the incidence of childhood diseases in the population. Health system factors have contributed in several ways to the continued incidence of childhood diseases. Some of the contributing factors related to the health-care system include errors in recommendations for routine immunizations and predictions of their efficacy; limiting access to immunizations; failure to educate the public adequately on the need for immunization; and failure to plan effective immunization strategies for groups at risk for disease.

Because of incomplete knowledge of the efficacy of various vaccines, health-care providers have sometimes failed to give routine immunizations at appropriate times and have erroneously assured the general public of protection from disease when such may not have been the case. In the past, for example, measles immunization was given to many children prior to the first birthday. These children frequently did not develop adequate levels of immunity, leaving them susceptible to measles. Even when the first dose of measles vaccine is delayed to 15 months of age (the current recommendation), it appears that immunity may not be lifelong and that a booster dose is required.

The health-care system also may have contributed to the rise in the incidence of some childhood illnesses by limiting the availability of immunization services. The increasing practice in the public health-care system of charging fees for immunization services that were formerly free deters economically disadvantaged clients from seeking immunizations for young children, thus limiting their ability to protect their youngsters from disease. In addition, health-care providers in some areas have, in the past, been reluctant to provide rubella immunization to women of childbearing age, this despite evidence that no harm has come to children of women inadvertently immunized during pregnancy.[11] Furthermore, failure to monitor immunization rates among school children in some areas may also contribute to increased incidence of disease.

Failure of health-care providers to educate the public in the appropriate treatment of wounds and failure to stress the need for immunization are contributing factors in the occurrence of tetanus. There has also been relatively little attention given to educating the general public regarding the need for and availability of a vaccine for diseases caused by HiB virus (particularly compared to educational campaigns related to both the Salk and Sabin polio vaccines).

Finally, failure to mount intensive immunization campaigns directed toward populations at risk has resulted in the continuing incidence of many childhood diseases. Inattention to booster immunization for persons beyond childhood and the lack of initiation of tetanus immunization for older persons, for example, have both resulted in a pool of susceptible adults. Similarly, failure to target immunization campaigns to members of minority groups and those of lower socioeconomic levels and to design an intensive campaign for HiB immunization for children in daycare centers have contributed to the extent of preventable morbidity and mortality related to childhood diseases.

Factors related to human biology, environment, life-style, and the health system influence the incidence and consequences of childhood diseases. These epidemiologic factors are summarized in Box 30–2. Additional information related to each of the diseases discussed here is presented in Appendix P, Additional Information Related to Selected Communicable Diseases.

DIAGNOSTIC REASONING IN CHILDHOOD DISEASES

The community health nurse may derive a variety of nursing diagnoses related to the problem of childhood diseases. These diagnoses may reflect the health needs of individuals, families, or population groups. For example, the nurse working with a family may make a diagnosis of "inadequate immunization status due to poor knowledge of children's immunization needs." A nursing diagnosis related to an individual client might be "potential for infection with tetanus due to increased risk of occupational injury." Or, "failure to obtain routine immunizations due to lack of transportation."

Other nursing diagnoses may reflect the health needs of groups of people. For example, the community health nurse might diagnose "poor immunization levels among minority children due to limited access to immunization services." Another community-related diagnosis might be "potential for measles outbreak due to large number of unimmunized children and young adults with declining immunity levels." Still another nursing diagnosis might be "increased incidence of congenital rubella syndrome due to low rubella immunity levels among women of child-bearing age."

PLANNING AND IMPLEMENTING CONTROL STRATEGIES FOR CHILDHOOD DISEASES

Efforts to control childhood illnesses and their effects can occur at the primary, secondary, or tertiary levels of prevention. Planning of control strategies at each level is based on the general principles of program planning discussed in Chapter 19, Care of the Community or Target Group.

Primary Prevention

Primary prevention for childhood disease will include planning for immunization, chemoprophylaxis, and other measures as appropriate.

Immunization. The major primary preventative measure for reducing the incidence of childhood diseases is, of course, immunization. The community health nurse should plan to ensure that all susceptible individuals, particularly children, receive immunizations as appropriate.

The usual recommended schedule for measles immunization is an initial dose at 15 months of age with a booster either at school entry or entry into junior high.[19] The initial dose of measles vaccine may be given earlier (at a few months of age) in areas of high incidence, but should be repeated after the child's first birthday. Measles immunization can also be given to susceptible adults, but should not be given to pregnant women because of the theoretical risk of harm to the fetus.[20] Immunization is also contraindicated for those who are immunosuppressed.[21]

Immunization for rubella should be planned for all susceptible persons except pregnant women,[20] particularly women of childbearing age. Planned immunization sites targeting women of childbearing age might include postpartum and family planning clinics, college health services, and WIC clinics.

Planning for mumps immunization should include all youngsters over the age of 1 and susceptible adults, especially males. Immunity appears to be lifelong with no need for booster doses. Immunization is contraindicated in immunosuppressed clients, and live-virus vaccines should not be given to pregnant women.

Immunization with DTP vaccine in childhood with continued boosters for tetanus and diphtheria (TD) every 10 years throughout life is the major pri-

BOX 30–2

Factors in the Epidemiology of Childhood Diseases

Human Biology

Genetic inheritance

- Many women of childbearing age are unimmunized for rubella
- Complications of mumps are more frequent in males

Maturation and aging

- Measles may occur in children too young for immunization
- Children under 2 years of age are at greater risk for HiB infection and complications of measles
- Complications of mumps more frequent in adults than in children
- Polio occurs in young children and adolescents in developed nations and in infants and young children in developing nations

Physiologic function

- Presence of asplenia, sickle cell, or immunodeficiency increases susceptibility to HiB infection
- Immunodeficiency may inhibit immunization response
- Tonsillectomy may predispose one to bulbar involvement and paralysis in polio
- Malnutrition increases the risk of complications in measles

Environment

Physical environment

- Overcrowding increases spread of airborne diseases
- Incidence of measles, mumps, rubella, pertussis, polio, and HiB infection is high in inner-city areas
- Poor sanitation leads to fecal-oral polio spread in developing nations

Social environment

- Poverty impedes access to immunization services for all age groups and to prenatal care for pregnant women
- Media coverage of adverse reactions to immunization results in fear of immunization
- Increased incidence of pertussis occurs in the homeless
- Social factors necessitating employment of both parents and day care for children increases risk of HiB infection
- Poverty impedes access to care when disease occurs

Life-style

Consumption patterns

- Poor nutrition is a contributing factor
- Lack of attention to immunization needs contributes to disease
- Lack of rest may increase susceptibility to polio

Occupation/employment

- Working parents increase potential for exposing child to communicable diseases in day-care settings

Health system

Inaccurate knowledge of immunization needs has led to

- Giving immunizations at inappropriate times
- Assuming adequate immunity to measles following initial immunization

Access to immunization services has been impeded by

- Fees for immunization services
- Refusal of some agencies to immunize women of childbearing age against rubella

Failure to educate public about need for immunization and failure to mount intensive immunization campaigns have lowered immunity levels

mary preventative strategy for diphtheria, tetanus, and pertussis. Immunization for diphtheria and pertussis are particularly recommended for health-care personnel, whereas tetanus should be of particular concern in occupational groups prone to injury. Older persons should be evaluated for their diphtheria and tetanus immunization status, and an initial series of immunization should be planned and initiated as needed. Immunization of unimmunized travelers to areas with high incidence rates for these diseases is also recommended, especially for young children.

Oral polio vaccine (OPV) should be given to infants beginning at 2 months of age. Persons who are immunodeficient and their family members should be given inactivated polio vaccine (IPV) rather than OPV. Immunization is not generally recommended for adults unless they are working with infectious clients during a polio outbreak, in which case IPV should be given.

Planning for primary prevention for HiB-caused illnesses involves immunizing children under 6 years of age. Immunization may consist of three doses at 2, 4, and 6 months of age with a booster at 15 months (HibTITER) or two doses at 2 and 4 months of age, followed by a booster at 15 months (PedvaxHiB). Because HiB vaccines are not interchangeable, the nurse should make careful note on both the agency record and the client's personal immunization record of the type of vaccine used so the appropriate series of immunizations can be given.[22] Overall vaccine efficacy of 62 percent to 90 percent has been demonstrated for these vaccines.[23]

Chemoprophylaxis. Chemoprophylaxis may be used as a primary preventative measure for those childhood diseases for which prophylactic medications are available. Chemoprophylaxis is given when an unimmunized person has already been exposed to the infectious agent causing a particular disease. In most cases, routine immunization for the disease should be initiated once the immediate danger has been averted. The community health nurse would use the following guidelines in planning chemoprophylaxis:

- **Measles.** Live vaccine given within 72 hours of exposure may provide protection. Measles immune serum globulin may be given to household contacts and those at particular risk for complications within 6 days of exposure.[14]
- **Rubella.** Chemoprophylaxis is not recommended.[14]
- **Mumps.** It is not known whether post-exposure immunization for mumps is effective, but it is not contraindicated.[14]
- **Diphtheria.** Previously immunized contacts should receive a booster. Antibiotic prophylaxis should be given to immunized contacts with positive nose and throat culture and to unimmunized contacts.[14]
- **Pertussis.** Close contacts under age 7 who have not received four doses of DPT or one dose in the last 3 years should be given a booster. All close contacts should be given a 14-day course of erythromycin regardless of immunization status.
- **Tetanus.** Previously immunized persons should be given a booster dose of TD vaccine if 10 years or more have elapsed since the last dose (5 years for major or contaminated wounds). Unimmunized persons should receive a dose of tetanus toxoid. If the wound is major or contaminated, unimmunized persons should receive tetanus immune globulin (TIG).[14]
- **Poliomyelitis.** Chemoprophylaxis is not recommended.[14]
- **HiB infection.** Chemoprophylaxis using rifampin, an antituberculin drug, may be given to all household contacts in homes with children under age 4 and to children under age 2 exposed in day-care settings.[24]

Other Primary Prevention Measures. In some cases, other primary prevention measures may be planned and implemented to prevent childhood diseases. These measures would include public education regarding control of these diseases and advocacy.

Education of clients would include the use of protective clothing in certain occupational groups to prevent injuries and the need for adequate cleansing of wounds with soap and water to prevent tetanus when injuries do occur. Education of individual clients and the general public regarding the need for immunization is another community health nursing activity directed toward primary prevention. At present there is also a need to inform previously immunized persons of the need for a booster dose of measles vaccine and periodic boosters for tetanus and diphtheria after school entry.

Interventions related to advocacy might entail ensuring access to immunization services for those most in need of them. Eliminating fees for primary immunization of children would be one means of ensuring access to services. The community health nurse might also advocate the enactment and enforcement of immunization policies designed to protect the general public. For example, community health nurses might advocate requirements that college entrants provide evidence of measles immunity; college students are one of the groups at risk for this disease.[21] Community health nurses can also advocate HiB immunization prior to day-care admission, and may be involved in efforts to promote legislation to this effect.

Secondary Prevention

Generally speaking, secondary preventive measures usually include screening efforts and activities designed to diagnose and treat existing illness. However, with the exception of screening pregnant women for susceptibility to rubella and screening contacts to diphtheria for carrier status, screening is not an effective control measure for childhood illnesses because of the relatively short incubation periods involved. Consequently, this discussion will focus on planning other categories of secondary prevention: diagnosis and treatment.

Diagnosis. Secondary prevention of childhood diseases, as well as other communicable diseases, involves prompt identification and care of persons with the disease. Diagnosis of childhood diseases is usually made on the basis of the clinical symptomatology and immunization history, but may be confirmed by laboratory procedures in some instances. The community health nurse would plan to refer suspected cases of childhood diseases for diagnostic confirmation. The nurse also would inform clients of the type of diagnostic procedures likely to be used, based on the following guidelines:

- **Measles.** Diagnosis may be confirmed by isolation of the virus from blood, conjunctivae, nasopharynx, or urine, or by a rise in measles antibody titre.
- **Rubella.** Presumptive diagnosis made on the basis of history and physical findings should be confirmed by rising rubella antibody titres. Diagnosis may also be made on the basis of viral cultures of the pharynx, blood, urine, or stool within 1 to 2 weeks after the onset of rash.
- **Mumps.** Diagnosis is usually made on the basis of physical findings but may be confirmed by serologic tests or isolation of the virus from saliva, blood, urine, or cerebrospinal fluid.
- **Diphtheria.** Diagnosis is made on the basis of the characteristic lesion in the throat and is confirmed by bacteriologic examination of lesions.
- **Pertussis.** Diagnosis is based on identifying the causative organism on nasopharyngeal swabs during the early stages of disease. In the whooping stage, a very high white blood cell count assists diagnosis.
- **Tetanus.** Diagnosis is made on the basis of clinical symptoms.
- **Polio.** Diagnosis is based on clinical signs and confirmed by isolating the virus from feces or oropharyngeal secretions.
- **HiB infections.** Diagnosis is based on clinical signs and may be confirmed by isolating the virus from a variety of locations.[14]

Treatment. Community health nursing involvement in the treatment of childhood diseases includes referring clients with suspected diseases for diagnosis and for medical supervision. The community health nurse will also plan to educate parents or clients regarding the disease and its treatment. Community health nurses can educate parents or clients on measures to reduce fever and promote comfort for all childhood diseases, until the particular disease runs its course. Nurses also should plan to educate caretakers on the symptoms of potential complications. Families whose members have rubella should be specifically cautioned by the community health nurse about the risks of exposing pregnant women. In the event the exposure does occur during pregnancy, the nurse can counsel the family on options available and aid them in decisions about the pregnancy. Specific education about treatment measures for childhood illnesses should be planned to include the following information.

- **Measles, rubella, mumps,** and **polio.** Treatment is symptomatic in nature and focuses on fever control and maintaining hydration and nutrition.
- **Diphtheria.** Treatment includes administering diphtheria antitoxin and antibiotics such as penicillin or erythromycin.
- **Pertussis.** Treatment may include antibiotics such as erythromycin to limit the period of communicability although they do little to speed recovery. Attention to rest is important. Rest may be facilitated by the use of cough suppressants.
- **Tetanus.** Treatment involves the use of tetanus immune globulin (TIG) or tetanus antitoxin accompanied by intravenous penicillin. Other treatment measures might include excision of the wound, airway maintenance, sedation or muscle relaxants, or use of ventilators.[14]
- **HiB infections.** Treatment usually involves giving ampicillin or other antimicrobials.[16]

Tertiary Prevention

Tertiary prevention for the individual client with a childhood disease involves planning to prevent complications and long-term sequelae. For population groups, tertiary prevention is aimed at curtailing the spread of infection and preventing a recurrence of an outbreak. Preventing recurrent infection is not relevant for individual clients with most childhood diseases because infection usually confers lifelong immunity. In planning for tertiary prevention of childhood illnesses, the community health nurse would consider the following interventions.

- **Measles.** People who have suffered complications of measles may need help in adjusting to handicaps such as blindness or mental retardation. Families can be referred to sources of assistance and can be given emotional support in caring for handicapped members.

Recurrent outbreaks of measles can be prevented by immunizing children as young as 6 months of age with measles vaccine alone[17] and the regular measles, mumps, and rubella (MMR) immunization at 15 months of age.[21] Using door-to-door immunization teams and giving immunizations in emergency rooms can also curtail the spread of an epidemic.

- **Rubella, mumps, diphtheria,** and **pertussis.** Tertiary prevention is not usually required for individuals who recover from these diseases. Recurrent outbreaks of disease in the community can be prevented by immunizing susceptible individuals.
- **Tetanus.** Tertiary prevention is not usually required for individuals who recover from tetanus. Control of animal feces in the environment can prevent the spread of disease. Hygienic midwifery practices in developing countries and immunizing susceptible persons can prevent recurrent epidemics.
- **Polio.** Rehabilitation may be required to strengthen affected muscles or to promote individual and family adjustment to permanent disabilities. Active and passive range of motion may help restore muscle strength and prevent contractures. Maintaining skin integrity for clients with braces or those confined to bed or wheelchair is also important. Observation for recurrent disease is also needed. Families may also require assistance in financing rehabilitative care and procuring needed equipment and appliances. Mass immunization campaigns can curtail the spread of polio in the community and prevent recurrent epidemics.
- **HiB infections.** Rehabilitation may be required for lasting consequences of HiB infections in individuals. Developmental levels should be carefully monitored and referrals made for assistance as needed. Parents should also be discouraged from becoming overprotective.

Immunization of household contacts and children in day-care centers can curtail the spread of infection; immunization of all children under the age of 5 can prevent recurrent epidemics in the community.

TABLE 30–4. PRIMARY, SECONDARY, AND TERTIARY PREVENTION MEASURES AND COMMUNITY HEALTH NURSE FUNCTIONS IN CONTROL OF CHILDHOOD DISEASES

Level of Prevention	Community Health Nurse Function
Primary Prevention	
Immunization	Identify persons in need and refer for immunization; provide immunizations
Prophylaxis (diphtheria, pertussis, measles, rubella, polio, HiB infection)	Identify persons in need and refer for prophylaxis; monitor use of prophylactics
Secondary Prevention	
Diagnosis and symptomatic treatment for most diseases	Case finding and referral for diagnosis and treatment
	Assistance with supportive measures
	Observe for complications
Antibiotics/antitoxins (pertussis, diphtheria, tetanus, HiB infection)	Educate regarding medications
Tertiary Prevention	
Prevention of complications	Observation for complications
Mass immunization to prevent spread of disease	Plan and implement immunization programs
Rehabilitation (poliomyelitis, HIB infection, complications of measles)	Monitor and promote development; promote client and family adjustment

Primary, secondary, and tertiary preventive activities are very similar for all of the diseases discussed thus far. Interventions at each level of prevention are summarized in Table 30–4.

EVALUATING CONTROL STRATEGIES FOR CHILDHOOD DISEASES

A number of the health-related statistics discussed in Chapter 6 can be used to evaluate the effects of primary prevention of childhood illnesses at the community level. Incidence rates for each of the childhood diseases provide information on the efficacy of primary preventive measures. Immunization levels in the population also indicate whether immunization programs, a primary preventative measure, are reaching high-risk populations. Evidence of primary prevention for the individual client is reflected in whether the client gets immunized or develops a particular disease.

Another approach in evaluating control measures is examining the extent to which the 1990 objectives for childhood diseases have been met (Table 30–5). For the most part, these objectives have not been achieved, with the exception of those related to rubella, diphtheria, and polio and for immunization of school-age children and those in day-care centers. The objective for tetanus had been met in 1987 (48

TABLE 30–5. STATUS OF 1990 OBJECTIVES FOR CHILDHOOD DISEASES

Objective	Evaluative Data	Status
1. Reduce measles incidence to under 500 total cases per year	3396 cases in 1988	Objective unmet
2. Reduce mumps incidence to under 1000 total cases per year	4866 cases in 1988	Objective unmet
3. Reduce rubella incidence to under 1000 total cases per year	225 cases in 1988	Objective met
4. Reduce incidence of congenital rubella syndrome to under 10 cases per year	6 cases in 1988	Objective met
5. Reduce diphtheria incidence to under 50 total cases per year	2 cases in 1988	Objective met
6. Reduce pertussis incidence to under 1000 total cases per year	3450 cases in 1988	Objective unmet (cases doubled since 1979)
7. Reduce tetanus incidence to under 50 total cases per year	53 cases in 1988	Objective unmet (48 cases in 1987, but incidence rose again)
8. Reduce polio incidence to under 10 total cases per year	9 cases in 1988	Objective met
9. Reduce incidence of bacterial meningitis (due to HiB) to 2 per 100,000 population	3 per 100,000 population in 1987	Objective unmet
10. Completion of basic immunization series by age 2 in 90% of all children	76%–85% of children immunized depending on disease	Objective unmet
11. Complete immunization of 95% of children in day-care facilities	97%–98% of children immunized depending on disease	Objective met
12. Annual immunization of 60% of persons in high-risk groups for influenza	18% immunized in 1985	Objective unmet

(Source: U.S. Department of Health and Human Services[25])

cases), but the number of cases rose again in 1988 beyond the target of 50 cases.[25]

Rates of death due to childhood illnesses are indicators of the success or failure of secondary and tertiary interventions. Another evaluative criterion for secondary and tertiary prevention is the incidence of complications resulting from these conditions. For example, if there are fewer instances of measles encephalitis among persons who get measles, secondary and tertiary preventive measures are probably effective.

HUMAN IMMUNODEFICIENCY VIRUS INFECTION AND AIDS

Human immunodeficiency virus (HIV) infection, which results in AIDS in its most extreme manifestation, may well go down in the history of the twentieth century as a disease comparable in terms of human devastation to the plagues of the Middle Ages. The growing concern about HIV infection and AIDS prompted the inclusion of several objectives related to control of this disease in the national health objectives for the year 2000. The relevant objectives are summarized in Box 30–3.

HIV infection occurs on a continuum of related conditions[26] characterized by inadequate immune system function. Soon after exposure to the virus (probably within 14 days)[27] the new host may develop mild symptoms similar to those of infectious mononucleosis including fever, splenomegaly, enlarged lymph nodes, fatigue, and, possibly, a rash. (Negative mono-spot and heterophile tests help to rule out mononucleosis.) Symptoms generally subside to be followed by a variable period of asymptomatic HIV infection.

At some point, as yet undetermined, infected individuals begin to develop symptomatic HIV infections. In the past, these conditions were designated as AIDS-related complex (ARC) or generalized lymphadenopathy syndrome (GLS). Some of those infected with HIV will go on to develop one of a group of opportunistic infections that are diagnostic of AIDS, the end-stage of HIV infection.[26] *Opportunistic infections* are diseases caused by organisms that either do not usually cause illness in humans or that usually cause only mild disease. Opportunistic infections that serve as diagnostic indicators of AIDS are included in Box 30–4.

Additional data presently known about AIDS, such as incubation period, transmission, and com-

BOX 30–3

National Objectives for the Year 2000 Related to HIV Infection and AIDS

1. Confine the annual incidence of diagnosed cases of AIDS to no more than 98,000 cases.
2. Confine the prevalence of HIV infection to no more than 800 per 100,000 population.
3. Increase to at least 50% the proportion of sexually active, unmarried people who used a condom at last sexual intercourse.
4. Increase to at least 50% the proportion of estimated intravenous drug users who are in drug-treatment programs.
5. Increase to at least 50% the proportion of estimated intravenous drug users who use only uncontaminated drug paraphernalia.
6. Reduce the risk of transfusion-transmitted HIV infection to no more than 1 per 250,000 units of blood and blood components.
7. Increase to at least 80% the proportion of HIV-infected people who have been tested for HIV infection.
8. Increase to at least 75% the proportion of primary-care and mental-health-care providers who counsel clients on preventing HIV infection and other STDs.
9. Increase to at least 95%, the proportion of schools that have age-appropriate HIV education curricula in grades 4 through 12.
10. Provide HIV education for students and staff in at least 90% of colleges and universities.
11. Increase to at least 50% the proportion of family planning, maternal and child, STD, and tuberculosis clinics, drug-treatment centers, and primary-care clinics that provide screening, diagnosis, treatment, counseling, and partner notification services for HIV infection, gonorrhea, syphilis, and chlamydia.
12. Extend to all facilities where workers are at risk for occupational exposure to HIV infection regulations to protect workers from blood-borne infections, including HIV.

(Source: U.S. Department of Health and Human Services[87])

municability, are presented in Appendix P, Additional Information Related to Selected Communicable Diseases. It should be particularly noted that the modes of transmission for HIV infection are relatively limited. Despite widespread fear of casual transmission, actual transmission of HIV infection has been found to be limited to sexual contact; inoculation by contaminated needles and syringes; exposure to infected blood, blood products, or tissue; and transplacental or perinatal transmission from mother to infant.[26] Specific behaviors that contribute to transmission of the disease include IV drug use (particularly using contaminated needles and syringes) and anal intercourse as practiced by male homosexuals and bisexuals and by some heterosexuals.

TRENDS IN HIV INFECTION AND AIDS

The incidence of AIDS has risen alarmingly since general reporting began in 1984. At that time the annual incidence of new cases was 1.88 per 100,000 population. For the period from October 1989 through September 1990, the incidence of new cases AIDS in the United States was 17.1 per 100,000 population.[1]

The prevalence of HIV infection, of course, greatly exceeds the number of persons with actual cases of AIDS. Incidences of both HIV infection and AIDS are expected to continue to rise in the next few years. Currently, AIDS is believed to be uniformly fatal. Many authorities predict an overall *case fatality rate* (the number of persons who have a disease who will die as a result of it) of 100 percent within 5 to 13 years of exposure.[28]

The economic costs of AIDS are also of concern. With the possibility of the use of zidovudine (AZT) and other substances as preventative and therapeutic measures for those with HIV infection, the demand for therapy will undoubtedly increase. At present,

BOX 30–4

Indicator Diseases for Diagnosing AIDS

Section 1: Indicator diseases diagnosed definitively
- Candidiasis of esophagus, trachea, bronchi, or lungs
- Extrapulmonary cryptococcosis
- Cryptosporidiosis with diarrhea for longer than 1 month
- Cytomegalovirus disease of an organ other than liver, spleen, or lymph nodes in a client over 1 month of age
- Herpes simplex virus infection with lesions for over 1 month or causing bronchitis, pneumonitis, or esophagitis in a client over 1 month of age
- Kaposi's sarcoma in a client under 60 years of age
- Primary lymphoma of the brain in clients under 60 years of age
- Lymphoid interstitial pneumonia or pulmonary lymphoid hyperplasia in a child under 13 years of age
- Disseminated disease caused by *Mycobacterium avium* or *M. kansasii*
- *Pneumocystis carinii* pneumonia
- Progressive multifocal leukoencephalopathy
- Toxoplasmosis of the brain in a client over 1 month of age

Section 2: Indicator diseases diagnosed definitively
- Multiple or recurrent infections with septicemia, pneumonia, bone or joint infection, meningitis, or abscess of an internal organ (except otitis media or skin abscess) due to *Hemophilus*, *Streptococcus*, or other pyogenic bacteria in a child under 13 years of age
- Disseminated coccidioidomycosis
- HIV encephalopathy
- Disseminated histoplasmosis
- Isosporiasis with diarrhea for longer than 1 month
- Disseminated mycobacterial disease caused by any agent other than *M. tuberculosis*
- Extrapulmonary disease due to *M. tuberculosis*
- Recurrent salmonella septicemia
- HIV wasting syndrome

Section 3: Indicator diseases diagnosed presumptively
- Candidiasis of the esophagus
- Cytomegalovirus retinitis with loss of vision
- Lymphoid interstitial pneumonia or pulmonary lymphoid hyperplasia in a child under 13 years of age
- Kaposi's sarcoma
- Disseminated mycobacterial disease
- *Pneumocystis carinii* pneumonia
- Toxoplasmosis of the brain in a client over 1 month of age

(Source: Centers for Disease Control[32])

use of zidovudine temporarily delays the onset of AIDS, but the addition of newer therapies may actually prevent disease in those infected.[29] It is unclear at present whether the use of zidovudine and other agents will increase or decrease the economic cost of AIDS to society. On one hand, currently available therapies could potentially decrease the cost of the AIDS epidemic by keeping those infected healthier. On the other hand, they could also increase the overall cost by allowing HIV-infected individuals to live longer.[30] Because outpatient care costs for clients with ARC and GLS have been found to average $489 per person per year[31] and because outpatient costs for those with AIDS vary from $2300 to $6500 per person annually, it would appear that keeping those infected with HIV healthier would be the less expensive alternative. Additional data on the incidence and prevalence of AIDS and HIV infection, AIDS mortality, and the economic costs of AIDS and HIV infection can be found in Box 30–5.

ASSESSING CONTRIBUTING FACTORS AND EFFECTS OF HIV INFECTION AND AIDS

Factors in all four areas of the epidemiologic prevention process model influence the development and effects of HIV infection and AIDS.

BOX 30–5

Facts and Figures Regarding AIDS Incidence and Prevalence, Mortality, and Economic Costs

Incidence and Prevalence

- By September 1990, a total of 152,126 cases of AIDS had been diagnosed in the United States. (*Centers for Disease Control*[1])
- Approximately 2% of cases of AIDS have occurred in children. (*Centers for Disease Control*[1])
- Eighty-five percent of cases of AIDS among women occurred in women of childbearing age. (*Aids in Women*[33])
- An estimated 15 per 1000 American women giving birth in 1989 were infected with HIV. (*Gwinn, M., Pappaioanou, M., George, J.R., et al.* [*1990*]. *Prevalence of HIV infection in childbearing women in the United States.* JAMA, 265, *1074–1078.*)
- The incidence of HIV infection among blood donors in 1989 ranged from 0.014% to 0.021%. (*Human T-lymphotropic virus type 1 screening in blood donors—United States, 1989.* [*1990*]. MMWR, 39, *915, 921–924.*)
- An estimated 1 million people in the United States are currently infected with HIV. (*HIV prevalence estimates and AIDS case projections for the United States. [1990].* MMWR, 39 [*No. RR-16*], *1–31.*)
- Anywhere from 61,000 to 98,000 new cases of AIDS are projected for 1993. (*HIV prevalence estimates and AIDS case projections for the United States.* [*1990*]. MMWR, 39 [*No. RR-16*], *1–31.*)
- In 1993, some 53,000 to 76,000 deaths due to AIDS are expected. (*HIV prevalence estimates and AIDS case projections for the United States.* [*1990*]. MMWR, 39 [*No. RR-16*], *1–31.*)

Mortality

- Since the start of the epidemic, AIDS has resulted in more than 92,000 deaths. (*Centers for Disease Control*[1])
- Nearly 62% of all people diagnosed with AIDS before September 1990 have died. (*Centers for Disease Control*[1])
- By September 1990, AIDS has resulted in 1374 deaths in children under 13 years of age. (*Centers for Disease Control*[1])

Economic Costs

- From 1984 to 1988, Public Health Service expenditures related to AIDS amounted to more than $1.6 billion. (*United States Department of Commerce.* [*1990*]. Statistical Abstract of the United States, 1989. *Washington, DC: Government Printing Office.*)
- State expenditures for AIDS from 1984 to 1988 exceeded $269 million (California, $113 million). (*United States Department of Commerce.* [*1990*]. Statistical Abstract of the United States, 1989. *Washington, DC: Government Printing Office.*)
- Economic costs of AIDS in the year 1992 may be as high as $5 billion to $16 billion. (*Koop, C.E., & Samuels, M.E.* [*1988*]. *Surgeon General's report on AIDS. In I.B. Corless & M. Pittman-Lindeman* [*Eds.*], AIDS: Principles, practices and policies [*pp. 5–18*]. *New York: Hemisphere. Quarterly report to the Domestic Policy Council on the prevalence and rate of spread of HIV and AIDS—United States.* [*1988*]. MMWR, 37, *551–559.*)
- Economic costs of research for 1991 are projected at $2.3 billion. (*Scitovsky, A.A., & Rice, D.P.* [*1987*]. *Estimates of the direct and indirect costs of acquired immunodeficiency syndrome in the United States, 1985, 1986, and 1991.* Public Health Reports, 102, *5–17.*)
- Lost productivity due to AIDS in 1991 may amount to $55.6 billion. (*Scitovsky, A.A., & Rice, D.P.* [*1987*]. *Estimates of the direct and indirect costs of acquired immunodeficiency syndrome in the United States, 1985, 1986, and 1991.* Public Health Reports, 102, *5–17.*)

Human Biology

Knowledge of the epidemiology of HIV infection has been growing ever since the condition was first identified. Human biological factors, particularly age and health status, are known to influence the incidence of HIV infection and AIDS. An individual's race and sex also influence the disease's incidence, probably through differential risk of exposure. In conducting an assessment related to AIDS and HIV infection, the community health nurse would identify factors related to the community or to individuals that will foster the spread of disease. The nurse also assesses the effects of the disease on the individual, his or her family, and the community.

Maturation and Aging. The nurse would begin by assessing the client or community for factors related to age that may increase susceptibility to HIV infection. AIDS is currently primarily a disease of young adults because of behaviors that put them at risk. There is, however, a growing number of young children who have developed AIDS. In 1989, the incidence of AIDS in youngsters under 13 years of age was 1.1 per 100,000 children.[13] The relative age distribution of all pediatric cases of AIDS diagnosed through September 1990 is presented in Figure 30–1. Infants appear to be more susceptible to HIV infection,[32] and up to 30 percent of infants born to HIV-infected mothers are themselves infected. Sources of pediatric HIV infection and their relative magnitude are presented in Figure 30–2.

Sex and Race. Far more men than women have AIDS, again probably because men are more likely to engage in high-risk behaviors such as anal intercourse and IV drug use. However, more and more women are becoming infected, either through these risk behaviors or through sexual intercourse with someone who engages in high-risk behaviors. Based on recent trends in AIDS incidence among females, AIDS will be among the five leading causes of death for women aged 15 to 44 years for 1991. Because the majority of females with AIDS are of childbearing age, there is increasing potential for pediatric infection.[33] In addition, there seems to be greater potential for transmission of HIV infection from infected males to female sexual partners than from infected females to male sexual partners.[26]

Racial and ethnic group differences are noted as well in the incidence of AIDS. While the majority of cases to date have occurred among Caucasians, the incidence of AIDS is disproportionately high for blacks and hispanics. Relative incidence rates for AIDS among whites, blacks, Hispanics, Asians and Pacific Islanders, and Native Americans and Alaskan Natives are depicted in Figure 30–3. Racial and ethnic group differences in the incidence of pediatric AIDS are even more marked, as indicated in Figure 30–4.

There are also racial and ethnic group differences in the prevalence of HIV antibodies in the population. Blood tests indicating that the presence of HIV antibodies are seropositive are almost nine times more often in black women as in their Caucasian counterparts and 14 times more often than in Hispanic women. Black and Hispanic prostitutes also are more than twice as likely to test seropositive for HIV antibodies than other prostitutes.[34] Similar differences in rates of seropositivity are noted among black, Caucasian, and Hispanic military recruits.[35]

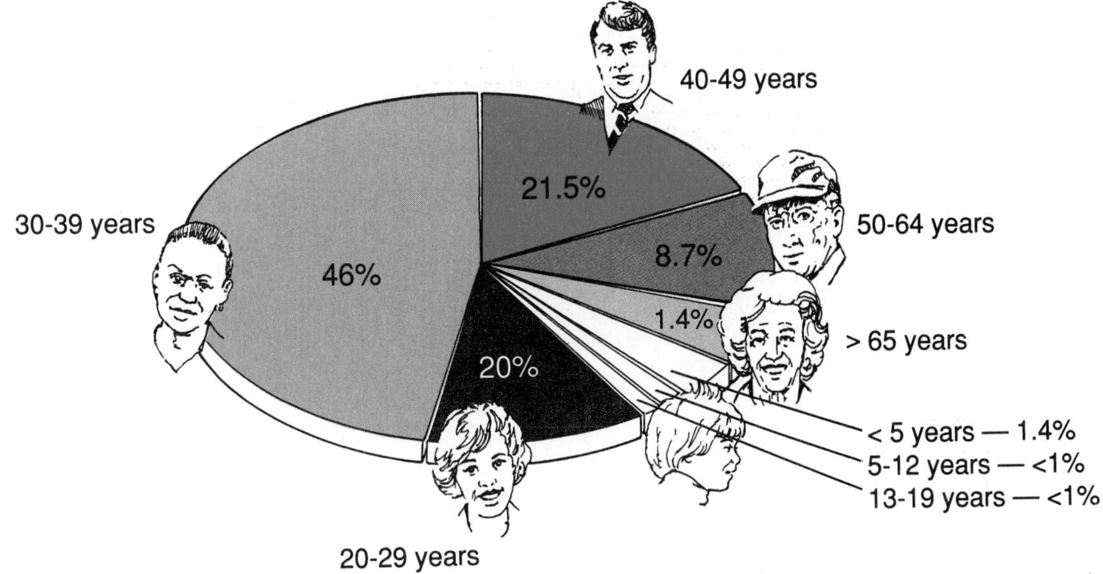

Figure 30–1. Age distribution of AIDS cases diagnosed prior to October 1990. (*Source: Centers for Disease Control*[1])

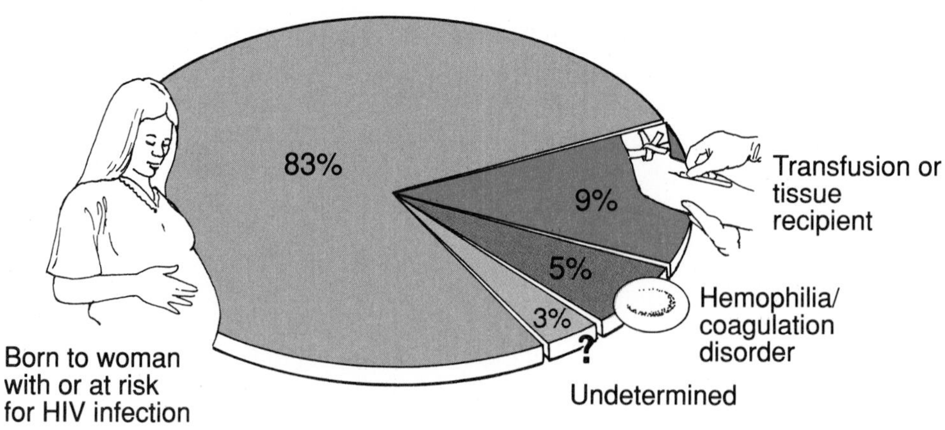

Figure 30–2. Sources of exposure in pediatric AIDS cases diagnosed prior to October 1990. (*Source: Centers for Disease Control*[1])

Physiologic Function. The presence or absence of other health conditions can influence the transmission of HIV infection as well as the development of AIDS. In assessing the potential for AIDS in the community, the community health nurse would determine the prevalence of these conditions and their relationship to other risk factors. To determine an individual client's risk of AIDS, the nurse would assess the presence or absence of these conditions in the client.

Health conditions requiring transfusion or organ transplantation provide the potential for HIV transmission. The potential for transfusion-related HIV transmission has been greatly reduced by screening of potential donors for HIV antibodies. Only a few transfusion-related cases of AIDS have been diagnosed since 1985 when donor screening and blood testing began. However, HIV seropositivity occurs in almost 100 percent of those persons who were transfused with infected blood prior to donor screening.[36]

Pregnancy is a risk factor in the development of AIDS for both mother and baby. As noted earlier, the majority of pediatric AIDS cases are due to perinatal transmission. Thirty to 50 percent of babies born to HIV-positive mothers will be infected as well. The potential for infection of the infant appears to increase if the mother is actually symptomatic for AIDS.[26,36] Transmission can also occur, however, if the mother is asymptomatic.[3] Perinatal transmission may occur in utero with transplacental transfer of the virus, by contact with maternal blood and vaginal secretions during delivery, or through breast feeding.[36] Mothers

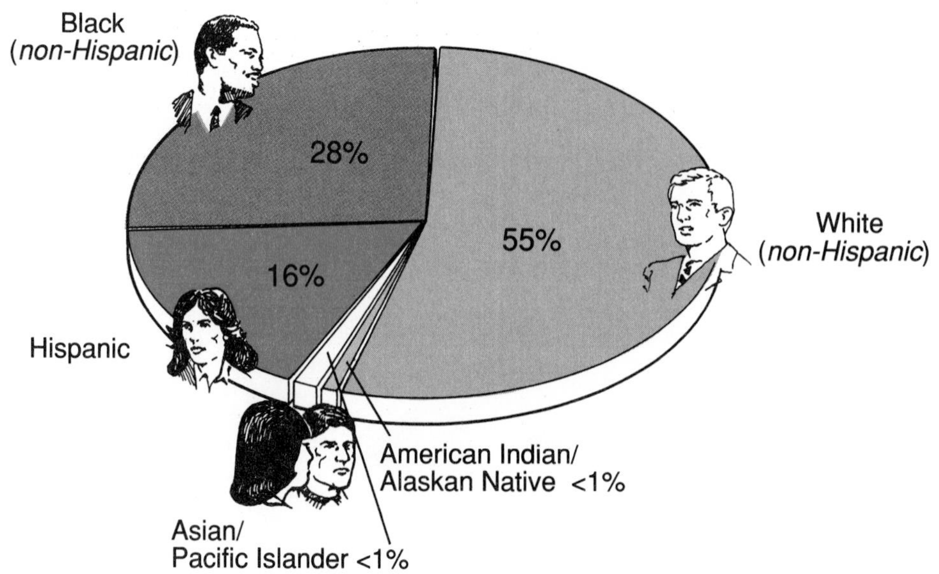

Figure 30–3. Racial distribution of cases of AIDS diagnosed prior to October 1990. (*Source: Centers for Disease Control*[1])

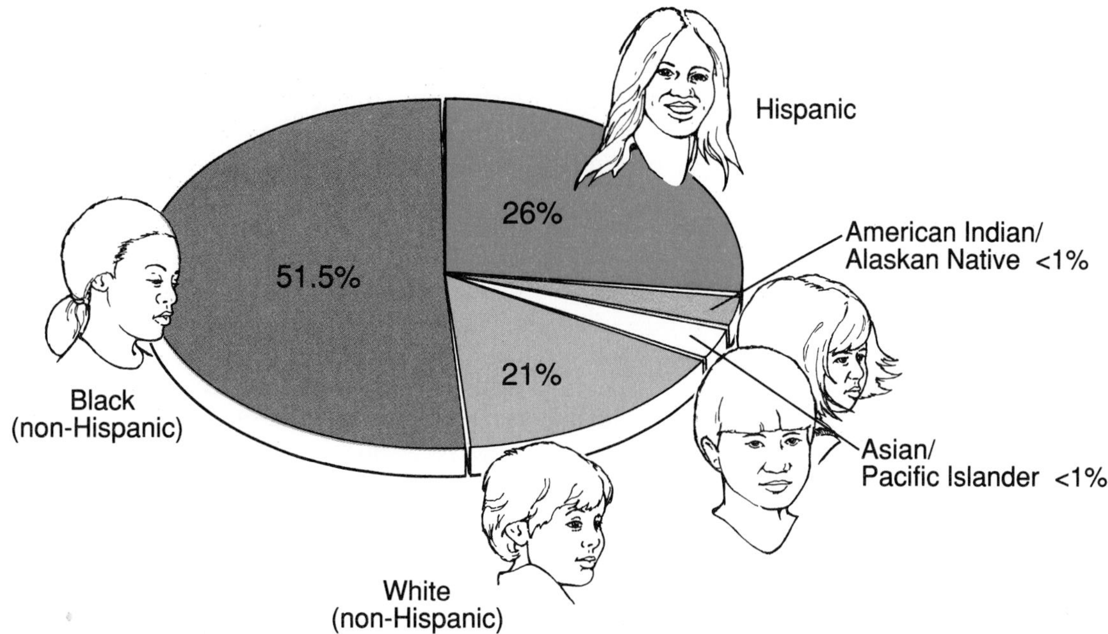

Figure 30–4. Racial distribution of pediatric AIDS cases diagnosed prior to October 1990. (*Source: Centers for Disease Control*[1])

are also at risk during pregnancy. Pregnant women with HIV infection have a greater probability of developing AIDS than those who are not pregnant.[3]

Several other physical conditions appear to increase an individual's susceptibility to HIV infection. Women experiencing cervicitis or vaginitis or who are menstruating are at greater risk of infection during intercourse with an infected partner.[36] For both men and women, the presence of genital ulcers from diseases such as syphilis or genital herpes also increases the potential for HIV infection.

Because HIV compromises and eventually destroys the immune system, persons with AIDS are highly susceptible to a variety of other infections, and the community health nurse would assess the person with AIDS or HIV infection for signs and symptoms of opportunistic infections. Persons with AIDS, for example, have approximately one hundred times the risk of developing tuberculosis as those in the general public.[37] The physiologic effects of AIDS can also be seen in the increased levels of mortality due to pneumonia and influenza among individuals with AIDS. In New York City, for example, 80 percent of deaths due to pneumonia of individuals between the ages of 25 and 45 occurred in those with risk factors for HIV infection. Mortality for pneumonia and influenza together has doubled in those cities with the highest incidence of AIDS.[38] Symptoms of common opportunistic infections for which the community health nurse should assess the client with AIDS are presented in Table 30–6.

Environment

The community health nurse would also assess both the community and the individual for environmental

TABLE 30–6. SYMPTOMS OF SELECTED OPPORTUNISTIC INFECTIONS IN HIV-INFECTED INDIVIDUALS

Opportunistic Infection	Typical Symptoms in HIV-infected Individuals
Bacterial gastroenteritis	Diarrhea, abdominal cramping, dehydration
Bacterial pneumonia	Cough, fever, malaise, dyspnea, chest pain
Cerebral toxoplasmosis	Altered mental state, convulsive seizures
Esophagitis (candida, herpes, cytomegalovirus)	Difficulty swallowing, or a burning sensation on swallowing
Oral candidiasis	Oropharyngeal white patches, sore mouth
Oral herpes simplex	Painful, ulcerative perioral lesions
Meningitis (cryptococcal, cytomegalovirus, herpes tubercular, aseptic)	Fever, headache, stiff neck
Pneumocystis carinii pneumonia	Shortness of breath, exertional dyspnea, cough, chest tightness, fever, malaise
Tuberculosis, pulmonary	Fatigue, night sweats, weight loss, hemoptysis

factors that may contribute to HIV infection and its effects on health. The primary social environmental factors related to becoming infected with HIV are the prevalence of HIV infection within a particular population and the extent to which individuals within that population engage in high-risk practices. The prevalence of HIV seropositivity varies across the country as does the incidence of full-blown cases of AIDS. AIDS has been diagnosed in all 50 states, Washington, DC, and U.S. territories. Figure 30–5 presents AIDS incidence rates by state for the period from October 1989 through September 1990.

AIDS tends to occur at higher rates in cities with population over 1 million. However, incidence rates are beginning to rise in areas with less than 500,000 population.[39] Table 30–7 presents data on the cities with the highest incidence rates for AIDS from October 1989 through September 1990.

Specific risk behaviors prevalent in areas with high AIDS incidence rates account for those high rates. In New York City, for example, the highest incidence of HIV infection occurs among intravenous drug users. In other cities, such as San Francisco, the highest incidence of HIV infection occurs among homosexual men. The nurse in a particular community would assess the prevalence of these risk behaviors in the population to determine community risk for problems related to AIDS.

Residential facilities for the developmentally disabled offer opportunities for the spread of HIV infection among residents through sexual exploitation of the mentally retarded, and 45 cases of AIDS are known to have occurred in such environments. Despite this potential, however, only 21 states have policies related to control of AIDS in these institutions. Six of the states without such policies are those with diagnosed cases of AIDS in these populations.[40] The nurse would determine the presence of residential facilities for the developmentally disabled in the community and would also assess the policies of these institutions related to AIDS control.

Some of the differences between racial and ethnic groups in the incidence of AIDS and the prevalence of HIV infection may be due to the social environmental factor of lack of knowledge regarding the transmission of AIDS. Knowledge differences related to AIDS and HIV infection have been noted among members of different racial and ethnic groups. In at least one study, white adolescents had greater knowledge regarding the transmission of AIDS than did black adolescents, who, in turn, were more knowledgeable than Hispanic youths. In addition to less overall knowledge, black and Hispanic adolescents were twice as likely as whites to hold misconceptions about casual transmission of AIDS.[41]

Community attitudes toward AIDS can often influence the effect of having AIDS on individual clients. The social stigma attached to a diagnosis of AIDS may deter people with possible infection from being tested or from seeking treatment. The social stigma and fear attendant on a diagnosis of HIV infection may also prevent those who know that they are infected with HIV from notifying their contacts or limiting their sexual or needle sharing drug-use behaviors.

In communities with high anxiety levels and fear of casual exposure to HIV infection, individuals with AIDS are unlikely to seek assistance until they are desperate. Such attitudes by community members may also limit the availability of services for persons with AIDS. In assessing individual and community risk of health problems related to AIDS, the com-

TABLE 30–7. CUMULATIVE CASES OF AIDS THROUGH SEPTEMBER 1990 AND AIDS INCIDENCE FROM OCTOBER 1989 THROUGH SEPTEMBER 1990 IN MAJOR U.S. METROPOLITAN AREAS

City	Total AIDS Cases Diagnosed	Percent of National Total	Oct. 1989–Sept. 1990 Incidence of AIDS Per 100,000 Population
New York	28,595	19	80.3
Los Angeles	10,106	7	27.1
San Francisco	8,933	6	129.3
Houston	4,481	3	40.3
Washington, DC	4,323	3	31.5
Newark, NJ	4,136	3	53.0
Miami	4,049	3	61.8
Chicago	3,722	2	16.6
Philadelphia	3,156	2	16.9
Atlanta	3,075	2	33.0

(Source: Centers for Disease Control[1])

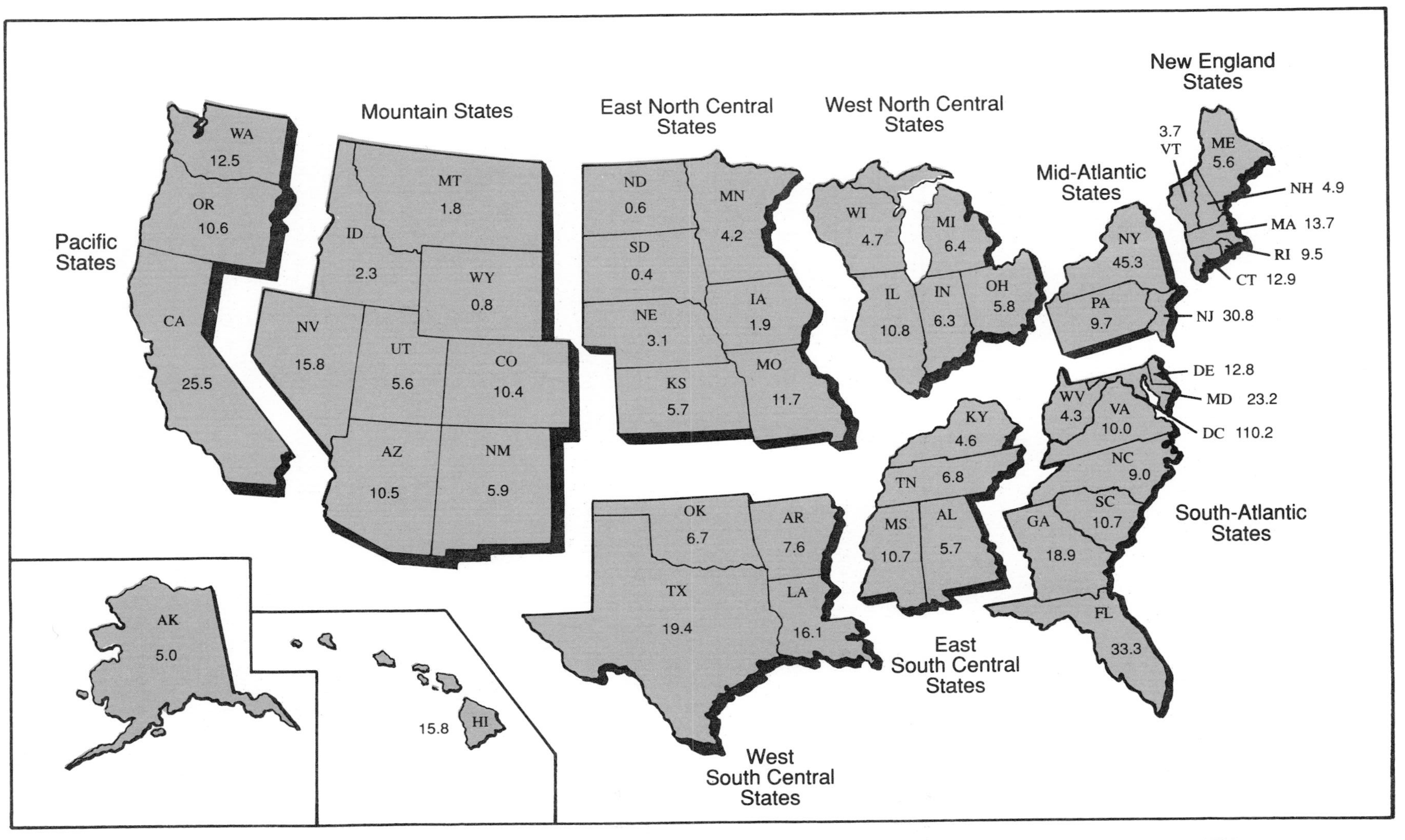

Figure 30–5. Incidence of AIDS per 100,000 persons by state for cases reported October 1989 through September 1990. (*Source: Centers for Disease Control*[1])

munity health nurse would explore community members' knowledge, beliefs, and attitudes to AIDS as well as the sources of their knowledge, beliefs, and attitudes.

Social norms that contribute to high-risk behaviors also foster the spread of HIV infection. For example, relaxed sexual mores have led to greater sexual promiscuity and increased risk of exposure to HIV infection. Similarly, a social environment in which it is relatively easy to obtain drugs for IV drug use promotes the spread of infection.

One aspect of the social and physical environment is *not* considered to influence the transmission of HIV infection. Casual social or physical contact with persons who have AIDS or who are infected with HIV has not been implicated in transmission of the infection. In studies of over 400 families with AIDS, household contact with infected persons has not led to seroconversion in any other members of the household.[36] This has also been true of health-care workers caring for clients with AIDS; casual contact has not been a source of infection. Beliefs by community residents that casual contact does transmit infection, however, can impede efforts to provide care for people with AIDS and should be identified by the community health nurse.

The nurse working with individuals with AIDS should assess the extent of their social support networks. Clients with AIDS may have diminished social networks due to social isolation resulting from other people's reactions to their diagnosis or to the death of significant others from AIDS. In addition, abstinence from sexual contact to prevent the spread of disease may limit the client's social contacts. Loss of occupational and financial resources may also occur as a result of reaction to the diagnosis or as a result of diminishing health.[42] The nurse should determine the people who comprise the client's social support network and the types of support available from each. Gaps in social support available and additional avenues for obtaining support from the social network can also be determined.

Elements of the psychological environment can also present problems related to AIDS that should be assessed by the community health nurse. Psychological factors such as poor self-esteem and poor interpersonal skills may lead individuals to engage in behaviors such as sexual promiscuity and IV drug use, thus increasing their risk of exposure to HIV infection. In addition, fear of a diagnosis of AIDS may cause individuals to delay seeking treatment for suspected illness.

For clients who have been diagnosed as having HIV infection or AIDS, there are tremendous psychological implications. These clients may face guilt related to past high-risk behaviors that contributed to their diagnoses and to possibly infecting loved ones with HIV. In addition, they face the possibility of rejection by significant others and of their own untimely death. Suicide is a serious problem among persons with HIV infection and AIDS, and the community health nurse should assess these clients for depression, withdrawal, and suicidal ideation or gestures. The nurse should also assess family members for signs of emotional stress, fear and anxiety, or grief regarding the client's possible death.

The final psychological factor to be assessed is confusion or disorientation in the client with AIDS. HIV infection has central nervous system effects that may result in loss of memory, and confusion, or, as noted earlier, in aggressive or combative behavior. The community health nurse would assess the client's level of orientation using the mental status examination described in Chapter 17, Care of the Individual Client.

Life-style

Life-style factors play a greater role in the development of AIDS than any other epidemiologic factor. The primary life-style factors involved in the development of HIV infection and AIDS are sexual activity and intravenous drug use (IVDU). One other less prominent risk factor is occupation. In assessing the risk of HIV infection and its effects in a community or for an individual client, the community health nurse would determine the presence of factors in each of these areas.

Sexual Activity. Three-fourths of all cases of AIDS are related to sexual transmission. Most cases of sexually transmitted AIDS early in the epidemic (approximately 95 percent) occurred among homosexual men. More recently, however, heterosexual transmission of AIDS has increased.[36] As of September 1990, some 5 percent of all AIDS cases among adults were the result of heterosexual transmission.[1] Heterosexual transmission usually only occurs among persons engaging in high-risk behavior.[43] For example, 28 percent of women with AIDS report a history of intercourse with partners in high-risk groups.[1]

Among men, certain forms of homosexual or bisexual activity remain the primary risk factor in HIV transmission, accounting for 66 percent of AIDS in males.[1] HIV infection among homosexual men varies throughout the country, being as low as 14 percent in some places and as high as 50 percent in cities such as San Francisco.[28] Homosexuals who engage in receptive anogenital intercourse (RAI) are at greater risk than those who engage in insertive anogenital intercourse.[26,44] Oral sex without contact with blood or semen appears to be safer than vaginal or anal intercourse.[45]

An individual's risk of HIV infection increases as the number of his or her sexual partners increase. This is true whether one engages in homosexual or heterosexual activities.[43–46] Recent figures indicate that a significant number of people aged 18 to 44 engage in sexual activity with multiple partners, thus increasing their risk of AIDS and other sexually transmitted diseases.

One final factor related to sexual activity that influences the incidence of HIV infection and AIDS is the use of condoms. In a 1987 study, 45 percent of homosexual men reported that condoms had never been used by their partners when the subjects engaged in receptive anogenital intercourse, and half reported never using condoms for insertive anogenital intercourse.[47] In another study, prostitutes who reported consistent use of condoms with every partner had no incidence of seropositivity to HIV antibodies, whereas in those who did not use condoms, the rate of seropositivity was 11 percent.[34] The use of a spermicide in conjunction with condom use is even more effective in preventing HIV infection than the use of condoms alone.[48]

Intravenous Drug Use. Intravenous drug use (IVDU) is another life-style factor implicated in the transmission of HIV infection. Intravenous drug use accounted for 22 percent of all AIDS cases in adults diagnosed through September 1990. Women are more likely than men to acquire AIDS through IVDU. For example, IVDU accounted for 48 percent of all cases of AIDS diagnosed in American women from October 1989 through September 1990 but accounted for only 20 percent of men diagnosed during the same time period.[1]

The prevalence of HIV infection among intravenous drug users varies widely across the country. From 10 percent to 70 percent of IVDUs in a given locale may be HIV positive.[36] Incidence rates for diagnosed cases of AIDS among intravenous drug users also vary geographically. Areas with particularly high rates of AIDS related to IVDU are presented in Box 30–6. The very low prevalence of HIV infection occurring among drug users in Los Angeles (1.8 percent) may be due to environmental factors that limit the potential for spread of the infection. These include the widespread nature of metropolitan Los Angeles and the absence of large "shooting galleries," where multiple patrons share needles and syringes, common on the East Coast. Because of relatively great distances between small groups of IVDUs in the Los Angeles area and the lack of a mass transportation system, there is little interaction between groups of drug users. Hence, HIV infection is confined to the small local group of IVDUs rather than being spread to drug users throughout the city.[49]

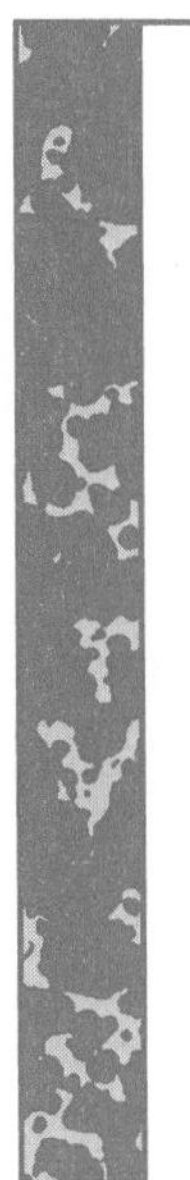

BOX 30–6

Areas with High AIDS Incidence Attributable to IV Drug Use, 1988

Puerto Rico—31.6 cases per 100,000 population
New Jersey—21.4 cases per 100,000 population
New York—19.2 cases per 100,000 population
Washington, DC—15.1 cases per 100,000 population

(Source: MMWR[39])

Some of the differences in AIDS incidence and the prevalence of HIV infection among racial and ethnic groups may be explained by differences in the prevalence of IVDU within groups.[50] Black and Hispanic clients are 20 times more likely to develop AIDS as a consequence of IVDU than their white counterparts.[51]

Specific behaviors among drug users increase the risk of HIV infection. The primary risk behavior in this group is needle sharing (this includes sharing any drug-related paraphernalia such as needles and syringes that may be contaminated with blood). Several studies have indicated widespread needle sharing among IVDUs. In one study, more than 20 percent of males arrested for crimes unrelated to drug use in 11 cities reported needle sharing at some time in their lives. Because study subjects were arrested for crimes unrelated to drug use, these findings probably considerably underrepresent the extent of needle sharing behaviors.[52] In Los Angeles, 95 percent of IVDU subjects reported sharing needles, usually within a small group of friends, but occasionally with strangers.[49] In another study conducted in New York, 40 percent of drug users reported sharing needles, again primarily with friends, although one quarter of the subjects reported sharing in shooting galleries.[53]

Needle sharing among IVDUs appears to be influenced by peer group behavior, financial considerations, not owning personal injection equipment, and a sense of fatalism regarding AIDS.[53] Drug users whose sexual partners and close friends also used drugs frequently reported needle sharing because of a wish not to offend friends by refusing to share. Most of those sharing needles rarely sterilize their equipment after use by friends. Financial inability to purchase personal injection equipment and fears of being found by police with equipment on one's person were other factors related to needle sharing. Finally, individuals who believed that they would get AIDS whether they shared needles or not engaged in more sharing than did others. Knowledge about the risk of acquiring AIDS by sharing needles did not seem to be associated with this practice. Needle sharers appeared to be well acquainted with the risks involved, but chose to share anyway.[53]

In assessing the risk of AIDS in the community and for the individual client, the community health nurse would explore the extent of intravenous drug use (if any). The nurse would also determine the extent to which unsafe practices such as needle sharing are prevalent.

Drugs and Sexual Activity. The nurse would also assess the extent to which sexual and drug-use behaviors are combined by members of the community, because the combination of risk behaviors associated with intravenous drug use and sexual activity is particularly significant in the transmission of HIV infection. Eight percent of all American males with AIDS engaged in both drug use and homosexual activity.[39] Increased prevalence of HIV infection is also noted among males who combine drug use with bisexual behavior.[51] HIV seropositivity for heterosexuals is higher for those whose partners are drug users than for those whose partners are not.[26] Other findings that link combined sexual and drug use behaviors with HIV infection include the fact that three-fourths of prostitutes who are seropositive for HIV antibodies are intravenous drug users.[34] Moreover, an increased incidence of AIDS is linked to sexual contact with multiple partners from urban areas with high rates of IVDU, prostitution, and other sexually transmitted diseases.[26]

Condom use by IVDUs engaging in sexual activity could significantly reduce the risk of HIV infection. However, several studies indicate that condoms are rather infrequently used by intravenous drug users. In one study, 68 percent of drug users in New York City did not use condoms regularly.[54] Other investigators have reported decreased use of condoms in sexual encounters by gay men in which alcohol or drug use were involved.[47] Condom use among drug users has been found to be associated with personal acceptance of condoms, partner receptivity to use, and recent entry into a methadone treatment program.[54]

Occupational Risk. Health-care workers are at a slightly higher risk for HIV infection than the general population because of the potential for contact with blood and other contaminated body fluids. As of 1988, the incidence rate for AIDS in health-care workers was only 5.4 per 100,000 persons. The majority of these persons (95 percent) were members of other high-risk groups (primarily homosexual men rather than intravenous drug users). Among health-care personnel reporting needle-stick injuries while working with HIV-infected clients, 0.5 percent (4 persons) eventually tested seropositive for HIV. However, one of these individuals also had a history of other risk factors for HIV infection. The conclusion reached as a result of these findings is that the risk of infection following needle-stick exposures to blood from HIV-infected clients is less than 1 percent.[55] Another recent study found that military medical personnel had higher rates of HIV seropositivity than other groups of military personnel. In-depth analysis of these cases, however, indicated that these increases were generally attributable to risk factors other than occupational exposure.[56]

Although the risk of transmission of HIV infection to health-care workers is small, the possibility exists. For this reason, the Centers for Disease Control recommends the application of universal blood and body fluid precautions by all health-care workers working with clients with AIDS and other blood-borne diseases. Under these recommendations, blood and other body fluids of all patients are to be treated as though HIV infection were present. Potentially infectious bodily fluids include blood, semen, vaginal secretions, cerebrospinal fluid, pleural fluid, pericardial fluid, and amniotic fluid. Universal precautions *do not* apply to feces, nasal secretions, sputum, sweat, tears, urine, or vomitus. Special precautions for dental professionals are suggested for contact with saliva, more because of the likelihood of transmission of hepatitis B than concern for HIV infection.[57] Observance of universal precautions will provide protection against hepatitis and other blood-borne diseases, as well as AIDS.

Health System

As noted earlier, blood transfusions were a source of HIV infection prior to the institution of donor screening. HIV transmission has also occurred in organ transplants from infected donors; HIV screening of organ donors was instituted in 1985.[58] However, recently a bone-transplant recipient developed AIDS as a result of transplantation from a donor who tested antibody negative. The donor had been screened following multiple transfusions that decreased the sensitivity of the HIV screening test.[59]

Additionally, HIV transmission via infected semen used in artificial insemination has also been documented. At present, no known mechanism exists for processing human semen that can prevent transmission of HIV infection.[60] The Centers for Disease Control also recently released a report that, in a few cases, HIV infection was transmitted from infected health-care workers to their patients.

The reimbursement policies of Medicaid and private insurers also influence the effects of AIDS on individuals and on the community at large. In 1988, Medicaid programs in 46 states provided coverage for zidovudine (AZT) to persons with AIDS, but only 13 provided coverage for hospice care.[61] Health insurance is sometimes a problem for persons with AIDS as it has been the practice of many insurance companies to deny coverage to those with HIV infection. There has been political activity in some areas to guard against this type of discrimination. As of 1988, six of the 10 states with the most diagnosed cases of AIDS had legislation prohibiting the denial of insurance coverage because of HIV seropositivity.[62]

Refusal of some health-care workers to provide care to persons with AIDS is another health system factor influencing the impact of this disease. Both the American Medical Association and the American Nurses' Association have issued statements relative to the responsibility of health professionals to care for those with communicable diseases, including AIDS. As stated by the report of the Institute of Medicine and the National Academy of Sciences, "The health professions have a compact with society to treat all forms of illness including HIV infection and AIDS" (p. 99).[26] The ethical implications of this statement and refusal to care for clients with AIDS were addressed in Chapter 14, Ethical Influences on Community Health.

Finally, the lack of facilities for the care of persons with AIDS may lead to an increased burden of suffering for the individual and his or her family. This is particularly true for clients with central nervous system effects of the disease that cause aggressive behavior. In many instances, these clients are not able to be placed in nursing homes, hospices, or other facilities for the terminally ill because of their combativeness. This may either place the entire burden of care for the client on significant others or create a situation in which the person with AIDS becomes part of the homeless population discussed in Chapter 24, Care of Homeless Clients.

Human biological, environmental, life-style, and health system factors contributing to HIV infection are summarized in Box 30–7.

DIAGNOSTIC REASONING, HIV INFECTION, AND AIDS

A number of nursing diagnoses are related to HIV infection and AIDS that may be derived relative to population groups and individual clients and their families. Diagnoses at the community level may reflect the current incidence of disease or the potential for spread of infection. Examples of such diagnoses might be "increased incidence of AIDS due to intravenous drug use" or "potential for increased transmission of HIV infection due to widespread use of unsafe sexual practices by a large homosexual population."

Diagnoses related to individual clients and families may also reflect potential for infection or active disease. A possible diagnosis for a sexually active adolescent might be "potential for HIV infection due to multiple sexual partners and failure to use condoms." Nursing diagnoses for a client who has AIDS and his or her significant others may be many and varied. Examples of nursing diagnoses for the client with AIDS are presented in Box 30–8.

PLANNING AND IMPLEMENTING CONTROL STRATEGIES FOR HIV INFECTION AND AIDS

Planning and implementation of control strategies for HIV infection and AIDS occur at the primary, secondary, and tertiary levels of prevention.

Primary Prevention

Efforts to control the incidence of HIV infection and AIDS are hampered by several factors. The first of these is the disease's prolonged incubation period, during which infected persons are communicable but asymptomatic and thus difficult to identify. Second, based on current knowledge and owing to a lack of effective therapy, HIV-infected individuals are likely to remain communicable for the remainder of their lives. Finally, AIDS is largely spread by private behaviors that are associated with some degree of social stigma, making it difficult to identify individuals at greatest risk for the disease.[26]

Currently, there is no vaccine for AIDS, although human testing of a potential vaccine has been initiated.[63] Progress in developing an AIDS vaccine has been hampered by the ease with which the virus mutates, creating new strains. Zidovudine (formerly AZT) has proven effective in slowing the course of infection among many individuals, but whether it will

BOX 30–7

Factors in the Epidemiology of HIV Infection

Human Biology

Genetic inheritance:

- Males more often affected than females

Maturation and aging:

- Infants in utero particularly susceptible
- Highest incidence in young adults

Physiologic function:

- Conditions requiring transfusion or organ transplantation slightly increase risk of HIV infection
- Pregnancy increases maternal susceptibility and potential for infant exposure in utero
- Presence of cervicitis, vaginitis, or menstruation increases suceptibility to HIV infection
- Presence of genital ulcer disease increases susceptibility

Environment

Physical environment:

- Prevalence of HIV infection in population affects risk of exposure
- Increased prevalence noted in large metropolitan areas
- Increased potential for spread in institutions for mentally disabled
- Casual contact *does not* transmit HIV infection

Psychological environment:

- Psychological factors that increase high-risk behaviors increase the potential for exposure
- Fear associated with diagnosis of HIV infection may prevent infected individuals from seeking screening
- Persons with HIV infection may experience fear, guilt, anxiety

Social environment:

- Social stigma attached to HIV infection impedes control efforts
- Social norms that contribute to high-risk behaviors lead to increased incidence
- Lack of knowledge about HIV transmission may lead to high-risk behaviors
- Social support networks of persons with AIDS may be diminished

Life-style

Sexual activity:

- Increased number of sexual partners increases risk of exposure
- Receptive anal intercourse increases risk of infection
- Homosexual and bisexual behavior increases risk of exposure
- Use of condoms and spermicides decreases risk of infection

Intravenous drug use:

- Drug use and needle-sharing practices increase risk of exposure
- Prostitution to support a drug habit increases risk of exposure

Occupation:

- Use of universal precautions for blood and body fluids limits chances of health-care worker exposure

Health system

- Screening of blood and organ donors limits potential for exposure
- Failure to provide health insurance for persons with HIV infection leads to decreased access to care
- Refusal of health-care workers to care for infected persons leads to poor care
- Lack of facilities for care leads to increased suffering and societal burden

render these individuals noncommunicable is not known.

At present the most effective method of decreasing the incidence of HIV infection and AIDS is eliminating high-risk behaviors. Two approaches can be taken to achieve this end. The first is to change behaviors among those who are uninfected so as to prevent or minimize exposure to HIV infection. The second is to promote behavioral changes in those who are infected to prevent transmission to others.

BOX 30–8

Potential Nursing Diagnoses for the Client with AIDS

Diagnoses related to physical health

- Fever due to opportunistic infection
- Cough due to opportunistic infections of the respiratory system
- Dyspnea due to lung congestion related to opportunistic pulmonary infection
- Skin lesions related to opportunistic infection
- Weakness due to debilitation from recurrent opportunistic infections
- Fluid and electrolyte loss due to diarrhea from opportunistic gastrointestinal infection
- Poor nutritional status due to loss of appetite, nausea, and vomiting related to opportunistic infections
- Increased susceptibility to infection due to immune deficiency

Diagnoses related to psychological health

- Confusion/disorientation due to CNS effects of AIDS
- Fear of impending death due to diagnosis of AIDS
- Grief of individual and/or family due to impending death
- Impaired self-image due to diagnosis of AIDS
- Guilt related to past high-risk behavior and possible exposure of loved ones

Diagnoses related to socioeconomic health

- Potential for spread of disease due to communicability of HIV infection
- Social isolation due to stigma of AIDS diagnosis
- Financial problems resulting from loss of job, medical bills
- Lack of source of care due to inadequacy of facilities for caring for clients with AIDS

Several approaches have been suggested for decreasing the risk of exposure for persons who are currently uninfected. These include avoiding unsafe sexual practices and high-risk drug behaviors, continued screening of blood and organ donors, the use of universal precautions in the handling of blood and body fluids, and premarital/preconceptual HIV testing and counseling.

Optimal risk reduction relative to sexually transmitted HIV infection would result from abstinence or lifelong monogamy. Serial monogamy (only one partner at a time) is less effective than lifelong monogamy, but less risky than having multiple partners. It has been suggested that legitimizing homosexual relationships in terms of the rights and privileges accorded to married people might contribute to greater lifelong monogamy among homosexuals, thus reducing the incidence of AIDS in this group.[64] Community health nurses can educate the public on the advantages of monogamous relationships, or they can use political activity to legitimize homosexual unions.

In the absence of monogamy or abstinence, the use of barrier methods such as condoms and spermicidal preparations limit exposure to HIV infection as well as to other sexually transmitted diseases and pregnancy. Education about condom use alone does not seem to affect use appreciably. However, education coupled with easy access to condoms does seem to increase use of this barrier method.[65] Limiting the number of sexual partners and refraining from anogenital intercourse are other ways to limit sexual transmission of HIV infection. Community health nursing activities in this area might include planning to educate individual clients and the general public about safe sexual practices and advocacy to ensure easy availability of condoms. For example, community health nurses might participate in programs to provide free condoms to sexually active young people.

For drug users, preventative measures might include increased availability of drug-treatment centers and methadone programs. Failing elimination of drug use, clients can be educated regarding "safe shooting" practices such as not sharing needles or disinfecting them after use. Again, education along with ready access to bleach as a disinfectant has resulted in some behavioral changes among intravenous drug users.[66]

Another strategy suggested for use with drug users is to provide assertiveness training and support groups that might improve users' abilities to resist peer pressure to share needles or avoid condom use during intercourse.[53] Community health nurses can plan to refer willing drug users to drug-treatment centers. They might also be involved in advocating access to drug-treatment centers and in planning educational programs for IVDUs related to safe shooting practices, avoiding needle sharing, and the use of bleach to disinfect equipment. Nurses might also plan and implement needle exchange programs for IVDUs to reduce needle-sharing behaviors.

Another approach to reducing high-risk sexual activity and drug use is to provide alternatives to prostitution and drug abuse. This might be accomplished in part by providing for employment and other social needs.[64] Other approaches to the primary prevention of drug abuse are discussed in Chapter 33, Substance Abuse.

Education is one approach to bring about some of the behavioral changes suggested. First, there is a need to educate health-care providers about risks for HIV infection and the kinds of interventions that can prevent transmission of disease. When health professionals are knowledgeable, they can more effectively educate clients on safe and unsafe behaviors. As noted earlier, community health nurses may play a role in educational programs for health professionals related to AIDS and other sexually transmitted diseases. They may be involved in planning and implementing formal educational programs for other health-care providers, or they may educate other providers more informally on a one-to-one basis.

Educating the general public and members of high-risk groups about AIDS has had some impact, and community health nurses can be actively involved in educational endeavors. Increases in knowledge of AIDS and its transmission have been noted both among adolescents[67] and the general public.[68] In neither group, however, did knowledge of the risk of transmission lead to greater use of condoms. In addition to providing information about HIV infection and its transmission, community health nurses should plan educational campaigns that motivate clients to change their behavior. Motivational techniques were reviewed in Chapter 7, The Health Education Process.

Among high-risk groups, education and counseling have been somewhat more effective. Homosexuals have demonstrated rather profound decreases in numbers of sexual partners and unsafe sexual practices.[44] In fact, the decreasing incidence of AIDS among homosexuals is attributed to changes in behavior made in response to knowledge of the risks of transmission through certain specific practices. Among some groups of drug users as well there has been evidence of a decrease in high-risk behaviors as a result of education and counseling.[66] Community health nurses should plan to reinforce positive behavior changes among clients that diminish potential for exposure to HIV infection.

Measures can also be taken to prevent the spread of HIV infection from infected individuals to others in the community. By and large, these should be voluntary measures. Research indicates that voluntary changes in behavior to reduce the risk of transmission to others have occurred in groups of homosexual men.[44,69]

Some people, however, have called for isolation of those with AIDS and HIV carriers as a means of preventing the spread of the epidemic. Because casual contact is not a means of transmission for HIV infection, isolation measures would be unwarranted. There may occasionally be a need to restrict persons who knowingly continue to infect others. Authority to do so should be provided to the states as is the case in other communicable diseases, but this should only be exercised as a last resort and only in instances in which the individual is definitely infected, continues to put others at risk, and refuses to control his or her behavior. Control in such cases should be exercised using the least restrictive method possible.[26] Community health nurses should be active in assuring that punitive measures not be enacted against persons with AIDS. They might also need to plan and implement political campaigns to promote legislation against broad-based measures to isolate individuals with AIDS and to monitor isolation proceedings when they occur to be sure that they are warranted.

Prenatal or even preconceptual screening for HIV infection in high-risk groups could serve as a primary prevention measure in the control of pediatric AIDS. Community health nurses could be active in planning and implementing screening programs for high-risk women in STD and family planning clinics and drug-treatment centers so as to facilitate counseling those with seropositive results regarding the risks of pregnancy. Any counseling should be coupled with opportunities to receive contraceptive services. Women who are HIV positive and who are already pregnant can be counseled regarding the potential for infection of the infant and options available to them. Community health nurses can also plan to refer women of childbearing age in high-risk groups for HIV infection to screening and counseling services.

Secondary Prevention

Secondary prevention of AIDS involves identifying HIV-infected persons and those with AIDS and appropriately treating their infection. The first step is screening those at risk. Other secondary prevention measures involve diagnosis and treatment of AIDS and related opportunistic infections.

Screening. For screening programs to be effective in controlling the incidence of AIDS, health-care professionals should be adequately educated regarding those who need screening, the interpretation of screening tests, and the need for counseling after testing.[3] Community health nurses can be active in planning and implementing this education. Initial screening is done using an enzyme immunoassay test (EIA), the most common of which is the enzyme-linked immunosorbent assay (ELISA). Reactive (positive) tests should be repeated until there have been more than two reactive tests on the same sample. They should then be confirmed by means of the Western blot (WB) test.[70]

Screening results are reported as positive, indeterminate, or negative. A positive test is one in which more than two positive reactions were obtained on an EIA test subsequently confirmed with a Western blot. Indeterminate tests necessitate further observation of the client and retesting, as he or she may be in the process of seroconverting (changing from a negative to a positive test). Generally, seroconversion occurs within 3 months of exposure.[70] Health-care providers, including community health nurses, who are interpreting screening tests for HIV should be aware that false-positive results may be obtained due to pregnancy, immune globulin derived from infected persons, and circulating maternal antibodies in young infants.[71–73] Test results should be assessed in the light of client history and questionable results confirmed with subsequent blood tests before clients are informed that they are infected with HIV.

HIV screening has been suggested for a number of groups. These include blood and tissue donors, persons with other sexually transmitted diseases, prisoners, hospitalized persons, intravenous drug users, women of childbearing age, pregnant women, men and women contemplating impregnation, children of infected women, those who have been transfused, those with tuberculosis and other signs of opportunistic infection, prostitutes, persons applying for marriage licenses, military recruits, and the general public.[74]

Screening of the general public is unwarranted at this time. Because of the slow spread of HIV infection in populations without identified risk factors, the cost of screening and post-test counseling would outweigh the benefits in terms of cases of HIV infection identified.[71] Premarital screening for HIV infection in the general population has also been suggested. Because the incidence of HIV seropositivity in the general population is relatively low, screening has not been cost-effective in this group either. Premarital screening for HIV infection has been mandated in two states, Louisiana and Illinois. Screening was never implemented in Louisiana, and the Illinois law mandating screening was repealed. Studies during its implementation indicated that the law, rather than promoting HIV screening, caused increasing numbers of couples to be married in adjoining states rather than be tested for HIV infection.[75]

Mandatory testing of prisoners has been advocated by some because of the increased prevalence of both drug abuse and homosexual activity within correctional settings. Current recommendations are for the provision of voluntary testing for inmates, with emphasis on those in high-risk groups or who have symptoms suggestive of AIDS. Federal prisons have received directives to test all inmates on admission and at release.[74] Screening for HIV infection is mandatory for sex offenders, prostitutes, and drug users arrested in some states.

Routine HIV screening is advisable among some population groups. HIV screening for clients seen in STD clinics and drug-treatment centers, for example, is warranted because of the prevalence of risk behaviors among these groups. Routine screening of pregnant women or women of childbearing age is not recommended at present, but screening should be offered to those who are intravenous drug users; those who have had sexual contact with people in high-risk groups; prostitutes; those who have had multiple partners; or those who reside in areas with a high prevalence of HIV seroprevalence. Screening is also warranted for individuals in high-risk groups who are contemplating pregnancy or those who feel themselves to be at risk for AIDS. In addition, screening is recommended for all people who were transfused between 1978 and 1985.[74]

It has been suggested that all hospital admissions be screened for HIV infection. The advantages of this practice include identifying the need for infection control precautions and alerting health-care providers to the presence of a condition that may affect the client's prognosis and clinical course. Disadvantages include the high costs of testing and counseling in view of limited returns, the problem of false-positive and false-negative tests, and the risk of disclosure of confidential information. An additional disadvantage of testing all clients is the delay in implementing potentially necessary control measures while waiting for test results.[27] Current Public Health Service recommendations are for screening of hospital admissions in age groups with a high incidence of HIV infection (for example, young adults) and the use of universal precautions with all clients admitted.[74]

Screening for HIV, even in groups in which screening is recommended, should be a voluntary activity, with adequate provision for the protection of confidentiality. Positive screening results were reportable to the state department of health in 28 states as of July 1989 with legislation pending in 10 additional states. Eighteen of these states require reporting by name.[76] Reporting of positive test results facilitates determination of the incidence of HIV infection, allows for follow-up of infected individuals for medical care, and permits contact notification.[77] Screening also permits earlier diagnosis and promotes better medical management and efforts to prevent opportunistic infections.[26]

The only generally accepted exception to voluntary HIV screening is screening of blood and tissue donors. The costs of screening in these instances are outweighed by the benefits of identifying infected donors. Also, calculations of the relative costs and benefits per case of AIDS prevented are comparable to those for other screening programs.[78]

Community health nurses are often actively involved in planning and implementing HIV screening programs. They educate clients at risk for HIV infection of the need for testing and may either refer them to screening clinics or conduct screening tests in those clinics. Community health nurses working in HIV-screening clinics will also plan to interpret test results for clients and counsel them on avoiding high-risk behaviors that may lead to HIV exposure. For clients with positive tests, nurses will plan referrals for further diagnosis and treatment as needed and provide counseling to prevent the spread of disease to others. Community health nurses may also make referrals for counseling related to the psychological effects of positive test results.

Diagnosis. Community health nurses will plan to refer clients with positive HIV screening results and others with conditions suggestive of AIDS for further diagnostic evaluation. Diagnosis of AIDS is based on diagnostic criteria developed by the Centers for Disease Control.[32] In the presence of serologic evidence of HIV infection, the presence of any of the diseases listed in Sections 1, 2, or 3 of Box 30–4 constitutes a case of AIDS. In the absence of serologic evidence of HIV infection and in the absence of other reasons for immunodeficiency (for example, steroid or other immunosuppressive therapy, lymphocytic leukemia, or cancers of lymphoreticular or histiocytic tissue), a definitive diagnosis of one of the indicator diseases in Section 1 of Box 30–4 is diagnostic of AIDS. When HIV serologies are negative, a diagnosis of AIDS is not considered unless there is no other reason for immunodeficiency *and* the client has either definitively diagnosed *Pneumocystis carinii* pneumonia (PCP) or any of the diseases listed in Section 1 of Box 30–4 and a T-helper/inducer (CD4) lymphocyte count greater than 400/mm^3.[32] A diagnosis of AIDS is a reportable condition in every state.[76]

Treatment. At present, treatment for AIDS and HIV infection is limited. Zidovudine is currently being used to treat those with symptomatic AIDS and those with asymptomatic HIV infection. The efficacy of zidovudine (AZT) and other therapies is not completely known; zidovudine provides some hope for prolonging the life of AIDS patients.[5] The drug has been shown to improve neurodevelopmental abnormalities, increase appetite and weight, decrease lymphadenopathy and hepatosplenomegaly, and decrease immunoglobulin and increase CD4 cell levels. Effects were most noticeable in children with encephalopathy.[79] Other drugs that may have potential for treating AIDS are under investigation.

Treatment of clients with AIDS is primarily supportive in nature. Treatment for current opportunistic infections is provided as needed as a secondary prevention measure. Community health nurses working with clients with AIDS can plan to educate them regarding treatment with zidovudine or other primary drugs for AIDS and treatment for opportunistic infections. Areas to be addressed in planning include the client's need to know the effects and side effects of the medications and how to take medications as prescribed. Community health nurses should also plan interventions related to maintaining nutritional status, oral and personal hygiene, observation for effects and side effects of medications, and advocacy. At the community level, secondary prevention by community health nurses may include political action to ensure the availability of funding and adequate diagnostic and treatment facilities for those with HIV infection and AIDS.

Tertiary Prevention

Tertiary prevention in AIDS may be directed toward the individual client or to population groups.

The Individual Client. Tertiary prevention measures for HIV-infected clients is aimed at limiting the debilitating effects of infection, preventing the occurrence of opportunistic infections, and normalizing the client's life as much as possible. Prophylaxis may be given to prevent certain opportunistic infections such as *Pneumocystis carinii* pneumonia (PCP) and tuberculosis. Tuberculosis chemoprophylaxis is given to persons with HIV infection who have a reactive tuberculin skin test and no evidence of active disease. Isoniazid (INH) is the drug most often used. In the presence of HIV infection, INH is given for at least a year compared to the usual prophylactic regimen of 6 months.

Trimethoprim-sulfamethoxazole is sometimes used for prophylaxis of PCP, especially in client's with multiple episodes.[73] PCP prophylaxis may also be achieved by aerosolized pentamidine, which ensures delivery of drug to the alveolar site of infection. Dapsone has also been demonstrated to prevent PCP in small comparative studies with HIV-infected adults. Both trimethoprim-sulfamethoxazole and aerosolized pentamidine may also be used for PCP prophylaxis in children, although the effectiveness of pentamidine is influenced by the child's ability to use the nebulizer.[80]

The community health nurse working with HIV-infected clients receiving prophylaxis for tuberculosis, PCP, or other opportunistic infections will plan to educate clients regarding the medication used, its therapeutic effects, and its side effects. In addition, the nurse will plan to monitor the effectiveness of medication and the occurrence of side effects.

Community health nurses will also plan to modify routine preventative health-care measures to prevent untoward reactions in HIV-infected clients. For instance, inactivated polio vaccine (IPV) should be substituted for oral polio vaccine (OPV) for immunosuppressed persons and their family members. Despite the caution against the use of live vaccines in the presence of AIDS, giving measles, mumps, and rubella vaccine (MMR) may be considered because measles infection in persons with AIDS is extremely serious and outweighs the risks of immunization. Routine immunization with HiB and DPT should be given. Immunization for pneumococcal infection and for influenza should also be provided for persons with HIV infection and AIDS.[81] BCG vaccine (a preventive for tuberculosis) should not be used in the presence of HIV infection.[82]

Community health nurses can plan referrals for clients with AIDS and HIV infection to health-care sources that provide both prevention for opportunistic infection and routine health care. Nurses may also be involved in educating health-care providers regarding the special health needs of those with AIDS or HIV infection.

The community health nurse working with clients with AIDS and HIV infection should plan to monitor them closely for signs of opportunistic infection. When signs or symptoms of opportunistic infections are noted, the nurse would make a referral for treatment. The nurse would also monitor the effectiveness of treatment for opportunistic infections.

Community health nurses may also need to function as advocates to prevent AIDS-related discrimination and to foster a client's integration into the community to the extent permitted by the client's health status. To achieve this, the nurse may need to plan to educate those who interact with the client about how HIV infection is and is not transmitted. When working with children with AIDS, advocacy by the community health nurse may necessitate planning activities that foster normal growth and development in each child. Owing to fear of infection, for example, teachers and schoolmates and their parents may be reluctant to let the child with AIDS participate in group activities. Or, parents of the child with AIDS may become overprotective and prevent the child from engaging in activities that would promote growth and development.

Another role for the community health nurse in tertiary prevention to limit the impact of AIDS on the individual client and his or her family lies in planning to provide emotional support. Clients will probably need assistance in working through their feelings about having the disease and their guilt at possibly having infected others (especially their children). Clients and family members may need the help of the community health nurse in adjusting to the debilitating effects of the disease and in dealing with the possibility of death. If referral is needed for additional counseling, the community health nurse should be prepared to make such referrals and to act as a liaison in linking the client and family with appropriate resources.

Assistance may also be needed in dealing with the financial impact of AIDS. The community health nurse can help in this respect by referring the client and his or her family to sources of financial assistance. Advocacy by community health nurses may be required to ensure client eligibility for financial assistance programs. At the level of public policy, community health nurses may need to plan for political activity to ensure necessary funding for AIDS-related assistance programs.

The Community Client. Tertiary prevention with population groups is directed primarily toward preventing the spread of infection. In the absence of a cure for AIDS, the most significant approach to tertiary prevention at the community level is contact notification.

Contact notification for AIDS and HIV infection has been a controversial issue because of fear about loss of confidentiality and discrimination against HIV-infected individuals. Other arguments against contact notification for HIV are based on concerns over cost and the lack of a definitive treatment.[83] These concerns are largely unfounded. The history of contact notification in other sexually transmitted diseases and the precautions taken against loss of confidentiality have been very effective,[83] and similar precautions would be taken in notifying contacts to HIV infection.

The cost of contact notification is a consideration. Estimated annual costs based on projected incidence figures for HIV infection amount to $13.5 million.[83] Although this may seem like a large sum, it is actually less than the current cost of contact notification for diseases like gonorrhea and syphilis, for which contact notification has proved to be an effective control measure.

Some argue that contact notification is of no benefit in the absence of a cure for HIV infection. It is argued that knowledge of exposure only creates anxiety on the part of contacts. However, with the advent of zidovudine and drugs used to prevent opportunistic infections, HIV infection is closer to becoming a manageable chronic illness than it was heretofore.

Even in the absence of effective treatment for HIV infection, contact notification can help control the spread of this disease, particularly in view of the fact that 11 percent to 19 percent of contacts tested prove seropositive and are in danger of infecting others.[4] Contact notification and subsequent testing for HIV infection counteracts the tendency of many high-risk individuals to avoid testing. Contact notification also permits several avenues for action that would be unavailable without this measure. If contacts are seronegative on examination, they can be counseled regarding measures that may limit their chances of subsequent exposure (for example, condom use, not sharing needles, discontinuing receptive anogenital intercourse). If contacts are seropositive, they can be encouraged to take precautions to avoid infecting others. Studies have shown that contacts tend to change high-risk behaviors whether they test positive or negative for HIV infection.[44,69,84,85]

Furthermore, earlier identification of HIV-infected persons through contact notification and testing permits preventative measures for opportunistic infections. For example, seropositive contacts can be screened for tuberculosis and given chemoprophylaxis to prevent development of active disease. Female contacts who are HIV positive can be assisted to make informed decisions regarding pregnancy. Contact notification also provides opportunities to offer other needed services such as treatment for other sexually transmitted diseases, immunization, contraceptive services, and psychological support services.[4,86]

In some jurisdictions community health nurses are involved in notifying contacts to HIV infection. In carrying out contact notification, community health nurses need to keep in mind that individuals might be emotionally devastated by news of possible HIV infection. Fear of AIDS can cause contacts to react with anger, depression, or anxiety. Consequently, the nurse should plan for interventions to assist the contact to deal with his or her emotional reaction. The nurse can be an effective support person in helping the contact deal with these feelings. The nurse can

TABLE 30–8. PRIMARY, SECONDARY, AND TERTIARY PREVENTION MEASURES TO CONTROL HIV INFECTION

Level of Prevention	Community Health Nurse Function	Goal
Primary prevention	• Educate clients and public on preventive measures	• Decrease number of sex partners
	• Educate on "safe sex"	• Increased use of condoms and spermicides • Decreased receptive anal intercourse
	• Refer drug abusers for treatment	• Decreased IV drug use
	• Educate drug users on "safe shooting" practices	• Decreased needle sharing
	• Political activity	• Ensure funding for education and prevention
Secondary prevention	• Identify and refer those in need of screening	• Screening of members of high-risk groups
	• Provide screening and counseling	
	• Monitor treatment for HIV infection	• Compliance with treatment
	• Monitor treatment for opportunistic infections	• Adequate treatment of opportunistic infections
	• Political activity	• Ensure funding for facilities and treatment
Tertiary prevention	• Counsel HIV-infected women	• Prevent fetal HIV infection
	• Counsel and screen blood and tissue donors	• Safe blood and tissue supply
	• Educate infected persons on means of preventing transmission	• Prevent spread of infection
	• Interview cases and notify contacts	• Prevent spread of infection
	• Provide prophylaxis for opportunistic infections	• Prevent opportunistic infection
	• Assist clients and families with grieving	• Acceptance of death
	• Political activity	• Ensure funds to care for terminally ill (including hospice care)

explain that not everyone becomes seropositive after exposure to HIV and that testing can help determine whether the contact is indeed infected. The nurse can also use the opportunity to educate the client regarding high-risk practices and can suggest changes in behavior to minimize risk of disease transmission. Nurses who are engaged in contact notification also have the opportunity to refer contacts for other needed services. For example, an intravenous drug user can be referred to a treatment program if desired. Or, the nurse may discuss the potential effects of HIV infection in pregnancy with a female contact of childbearing age and refer her for contraceptive services (or high-risk prenatal services if she is already pregnant).

Contacts should be reassured as to the confidential nature of screening. The nurse should emphasize that information about the need for screening and test results will not be shared with others (employers, for example). Reassurance should also be provided that illegal behaviors will not be reported to the authorities and that, while information about high-risk behaviors will be requested at the time of screening, this information is strictly confidential and will not be used in criminal proceedings.

When contacts arrive for screening tests, they might encounter the same nurse or other community health nurses. These nurses will plan to reinforce information about the screening test and about high-risk behaviors and how these behaviors can be modified. When the client returns to obtain test results, the community health nurse has another opportunity to inform the client about measures to prevent the transmission of AIDS. Clients who have positive test results will need a great deal of emotional support from the nurse. They may need assistance in dealing with feelings and fears regarding AIDS and HIV infection. The nurse can provide information about the need for medical supervision and make referrals for these services as well as for psychological counseling. Referrals may also be needed for other services such as drug abuse treatment, prenatal or contraceptive services, or financial aid.

Numerous primary, secondary, and tertiary prevention measures can be employed to control HIV infection. Community health nurses are actively involved in controlling this disease at all three levels. Table 30–8 summarizes primary, secondary, and tertiary prevention activities for HIV infection and AIDS.

EVALUATING CONTROL STRATEGIES FOR HIV INFECTION AND AIDS

The effects of control strategies for HIV infection and AIDS for various population groups can be evaluated in terms of trends in HIV incidence and HIV-related mortality as well as indicators of the extent of risk behaviors in the population. For example, the nurse could examine the extent to which members of a community or target group engage in unsafe sexual practices or needle sharing during drug use. Because the problems of HIV infection and AIDS had not yet been recognized when the national objectives for 1990 were formulated, there were no stated goals to aid evaluation in this area. These problems are addressed, however, in the objectives for the year 2000, and these objectives can provide criteria for future evaluation of the effectiveness of control measures in preventing HIV infection.

Evaluation of care for individuals with HIV infection and AIDS focuses on the extent of disruption of clients' lives caused by their condition. Evaluative questions might include: How effective is zidovudine therapy in preventing the development of AIDS? Has the person with HIV infection refrained from practices that enhance the spread of infection? Have further opportunistic infections been prevented or resolved in the client with AIDS? Have the social and economic effects of his or her condition been minimized?

OTHER SEXUALLY TRANSMITTED DISEASES

Several other diseases are also transmitted via sexual intercourse. This section will examine trends, epidemiologic factors, nursing diagnoses, control strategies, and evaluation related to syphilis, gonorrhea, herpes simplex virus (HSV) infection, *Chlamydia trachomatis*, and hepatitis B. Epidemiologic and treatment information about each of these diseases is summarized in Appendix P, Information Related to Selected Communicable Diseases.

TRENDS IN SEXUALLY TRANSMITTED DISEASES

Overall, the incidence of most sexually transmitted diseases (STDs) has risen in recent years. Because of the sometimes devastating consequences of these diseases (for example, blindness in infants exposed to syphilis, gonorrhea, or herpes), their increasing incidence is of concern to community health practitioners and the general public. Evidence of this concern can be seen in the fact that 15 of the national health objectives for the year 2000 are specifically related to sexually transmitted diseases other than AIDS.[87] These objectives are summarized in Box 30–9.

Syphilis

Through the use of antibiotics and the contact-notification strategies discussed earlier, the incidence of

BOX 30–9

National Objectives for the Year 2000 Related to Sexually Transmitted Diseases

1. Reduce gonorrhea incidence to no more than 225 cases per 100,000 population.
2. Reduce nongonococcal urethritis (usually due to *Chlamydia trachomatis* infection) to no more than 170 cases per 100,000 population.
3. Reduce the incidence of primary and secondary syphilis to no more than 10 cases per 100,000 population.
4. Reduce the incidence of congenital syphilis to no more than 50 cases per 100,000 live births.
5. Reduce the annual number of first-time physician consultations for genital herpes to 142,000.
6. Reduce hospitalizations for pelvic inflammatory disease to no more than 250 per 100,000 women aged 15 through 44.
7. Reduce the annual number of cases of sexually transmitted hepatitis B to no more than 30,500.
8. Reduce the rate of repeat gonorrhea infection within 1 year to no more than 15%.
9. Reduce the proportion of adolescents who have engaged in sexual activity by age 15 to no more than 15% and by age 17 to no more than 40%.
10. Increase to at least 50% the proportion of unmarried, sexually active people who used a condom at last sexual intercourse.
11. Increase to at least 50% the proportion of family planning, maternal and child health, STD, tuberculosis, and primary-care clinics and drug-treatment centers that provide screening, diagnosis, treatment, counseling, and partner notification services for STD.
12. Include instruction in grades 6 through 12 on preventing STDs.
13. Increase to at least 90% the proportion of primary care-givers who correctly manage cases of STD.
14. Increase to at least 75% the proportion of primary-care and mental-health-care providers who do age-appropriate counseling on preventing STD.
15. Increase to at least 50% the proportion of clients with gonorrhea, syphilis, and chlamydia who are offered provider referral services.
16. Reduce hepatitis B incidence among occupationally exposed workers to no more than 1250 cases.
17. Increase hepatitis B immunization levels to 90% among persons with potential for occupational exposure.
18. Reduce overall incidence of hepatitis B to 40 cases per 100,000 population.
19. Increase hepatitis B immunization to at least 90% of infants of seropositive mothers and at least 50% of IV drug users and male homosexuals.
20. Increase to at least 90% the proportion of local health departments that offer hepatitis B immunization.

(Source: U.S. Department of Health and Human Services[87])

syphilis seemed to be well controlled for several years. Recently, however, there has been an increase in both early syphilis among adults and congenital syphilis in young children. In 1979, the overall rate of incidence for primary and secondary syphilis (two early stages of the disease) was 11.1 cases per 100,000 population.[7] By 1990, incidence had risen to 20 cases per 100,000 population.[88]

One baby in every 10,000 live births in 1986 had congenital syphilis.[89] But, from 1986 to 1988, the number of cases of congenital syphilis in New York City, already a high incidence area, increased by more than 500 percent.[90] Congenital syphilis causes fetal or perinatal death in approximately 40 percent of cases,[89] and those infants who survive typically have a variety of mental and physical health problems.

Gonorrhea

Adequate treatment for gonorrhea has been available since the 1940s. Nevertheless, attempts to control gonorrhea have not been as successful as attempts to control syphilis. Incidence rates for gonorrhea have declined somewhat in the last decade, but the incidence remains at epidemic proportions. The 1979 incidence rate for gonorrhea was 450 cases per 100,000 population. By 1988, the rate, while lower, was still 298 cases for very 100,000 people in the United States.[7] To make matters worse, there is some evidence that these figures actually underrepresent the incidence of gonorrhea in the United States. Although private clinics and physicians' offices treat one-third to two-thirds of all cases of gonorrhea, they report only a portion of these cases[91] despite legal requirements for reporting all cases of gonorrhea.

Further complicating the situation, the incidence of antibiotic resistant strains of *Neisseria gonorrhoeae*, the causative organism in gonorrhea, has risen steadily in the last few years. Most antibiotic resistance is related to penicillinase-producing *Neisseria gonorrhoeae* (PPNG). However, other strains such as chromosomally mediated resistant *Neisseria gonorrhoeae* (CMRNG) and tetracycline-resistant *Neisseria gonorrhoeae* (TRNG) have been reported. Not only is CMRNG resistant to penicillin therapy but also to tetracycline, spectinomycin, and cephalosporin treatment.[92]

Herpes Simplex Virus Infection

Unlike the sexually transmitted diseases discussed so far, reporting of herpes simplex virus (HSV) infection, or genital herpes, is not required by law. Consequently, precise incidence figures are not available. It is estimated that 200,000 to 500,000 new cases occur each year and that the overall prevalence of HSV infection in the United States is 20 million people.[24] Based on figures for the number of first physician visits, the incidence of symptomatic HSV infection increased almost ninefold from 1966 to 1984,[93] and estimates from the Centers for Disease Control place the incidence of HSV infections at 10 times the incidence of syphilis in the United States.[94]

Chlamydia Trachomatis

Chlamydial infection is the most prevalent of all sexually transmitted diseases, with a possible incidence of 3 million to 4 million cases annually. This is more than two and a half times the incidence of gonorrhea. Like HSV infection, chlamydia is not a reportable disease in most places, so its precise incidence is unknown.

Chlamydia is suspected as the causative agent in 50 percent of nongonococcal urethritis (NGU) and epididymitis, and is implicated as well in the development of pelvic inflammatory disease (PID), ectopic pregnancy and infertility, increased perinatal mortality, postpartum endometritis, ophthalmia neonatorum, and pneumonia in the neonate. It is estimated that direct and indirect costs of chlamydial infection amount to $1 billion a year.[24]

Hepatitis B

Hepatitis B is a viral infection transmitted by sexual intercourse or direct inoculation. Just prior to the availability of an effective vaccine, the incidence of hepatitis B increased 30 percent between 1978 and 1981.[95] A vaccine became available in 1982, but the incidence of hepatitis B continued to climb from 7 cases per 100,000 population in 1979 to 11.5 per 100,000 in 1985. A slight decline in incidence has been noted since then with a 1988 rate of 9.4 per 100,000 population.[7]

Among high-risk groups (prostitutes, intravenous drug users, and Alaskan Natives), the lifetime risk of developing hepatitis B approaches 100 percent compared to a 5 percent risk for the general U.S. population.[96]

ASSESSING FACTORS CONTRIBUTING TO SEXUALLY TRANSMITTED DISEASES

Factors in each of the four areas of Dever's epidemiologic perspective contribute to the growing problem of STDs.

Human Biology

Human biological factors to be assessed in relation to STDs are age, race, sex, and physiologic function.

Age. The incidence of all sexually transmitted diseases is higher among adolescents and young adults than in other age groups. But this is primarily a function of life-style factors rather than biological susceptibility because of one's age. Infants are, however, more susceptible to the effects of STD exposure, particularly in utero or during birth.

Women of childbearing age constitute 90 percent of all women with syphilis,[97] increasing the potential for congenital syphilis in babies born to these women. Syphilis does not cross the placental barrier until some time after the 12th week of gestation, so gestational age does influence the infant's susceptibility to infection. Congenital syphilis may result in fetal death, blindness, mental retardation, or cardiovascular disease.

Children exposed to other sexually transmitted diseases are also at higher risk of complications than are adults. Infants exposed to gonorrhea during passage through the birth canal, for example, may develop a gonorrheal conjunctivitis called ophthalmia neonatorum. In addition, as many as 400 to 1000 babies with neonatal herpes simplex virus infection are born each year in the United States. Transmission of HSV infection to infants rarely occurs transplacentally, but is usually due to perinatal exposure as the infant passes through the birth canal of an infected mother.[98] HSV-infected infants have a high incidence of visceral and central nervous system complications. Sixty-five percent of infants with untreated HSV infection die, while fewer than 10 percent of those with CNS complications have normal development.[24]

Although hepatitis B occurs relatively rarely in children, those children who do develop the disease have a greater probability than do infected adults of developing liver cancer later in life.[99] Hepatitis B infection of the infant can occur in utero, and fetal infection contributes to the development of a chronic carrier state. Seventy to 90 percent of infants born to mothers seropositive for the hepatitis B "e" antigen (one of the serologic markers indicative of active infection and a high degree of infectivity) become infected perinatally. Eighty-five to 90 percent of hepatitis B-infected babies become chronic carriers, and approximately 25 percent of these children will die of cirrhosis or liver cancer before age 50.[24]

Community health nurses should assess both the extent of these pediatric effects of STDs in the community and the factors contributing to them. The extent of disease in other age groups should also be assessed.

Sex. Gender also plays a part in the incidence and effects of some STDs, and the nurse assessing the potential for cases of STD in the community would determine the community's sex composition and the relative incidence of STD in males and females in the community. For example, women are more likely than men to be seropositive for HSV antibodies,[94] and women account for more physician visits for symptomatic herpes than men.[100] Men, on the other hand, account for more cases of gonorrhea than women. This is probably due, however, to difficulty in obtaining reliable diagnostic test results in women. Women seem to have a greater risk of gonorrhea infection after exposure to an infected male than males do after exposure to an infected female.[91]

Males and females may also differ somewhat in the symptoms associated with STDs. Males with gonorrhea, for example, may experience a penile discharge with burning on urination, while females may have an increased vaginal discharge that may have a foul odor. In addition, females are more likely than males to be asymptomatic, with gonococcal infection creating a large reservoir of untreated persons capable of spreading disease.

Race. Generally speaking, members of minority groups have higher incidence rates for STDs than do whites. This is primarily a function of socioeconomic factors rather than innate racial susceptibility. Blacks, however, may be more susceptible to gonorrhea than other racial groups. Some evidence indicates that having ABO blood group type B, which is prevalent among blacks, may increase one's susceptibility to gonorrhea.

Race as a biological factor may also account for differences in the risk of developing a chronic carrier state. For example, the prevalence of a chronic carrier state is 1.9 cases per 1000 population for whites and 8.5 per 1000 for blacks.[101]

Physiologic Function Physiologic factors also influence the incidence and course of several STDs, and the community health nurse would assess the presence of specific factors in an individual client as well as their prevalence in the community in assessing the risk of STDs. For example, concurrent HIV infection influences the diagnosis, treatment, and consequences of syphilis. The presence of HIV infection may cause false-negative results on screening and confirmatory tests for syphilis. HIV-infected individuals also have a greater risk of developing neurosyphilis (deterioration of the central nervous system in the late stages of syphilis). In addition, treatment for syphilis may be ineffective when HIV infection is present.[102]

Certain physiologic conditions are also associated with increased incidence of hepatitis B. These include Down's syndrome and lymphoproliferative disorders such as lymphocytic leukemia and malignant lymphoma. Clients in need of hemodialysis are also at greater risk for the development of hepatitis B.

The presence of nicks or abrasions of the skin or mucosa also increase the potential for infection in the event of exposure to an infected individual.[99] Concurrent infection with syphilis is another biological condition related to increased incidence of hepatitis B.[101]

Environment

Environmental factors also contribute to the growing incidence of STDs in the United States. The nurse would assess factors present in the psychological and social environments of both the individual client and the community that may increase the risk of STD.

Psychological Environment. The psychological environment contributes to the incidence of STDs to the extent that it creates an emotional climate conducive to exposure to infection, usually through sexual activity or intravenous drug use. Individuals with low self-esteem or poor interpersonal skills may use sexual activity as a means of interacting with others. In a similar vein, those with poor coping skills or those confronting feelings of hopelessness may turn to illicit drug use as an escape.

Among teenagers, the sense of invulnerability characteristic of this age group may lead to experimentation with sex or drugs in the belief that adverse consequences are unlikely. In addition, the need for peer acceptance and for conformity to peer group norms may lead the adolescent to engage in sexual activity or drug use in an effort to be accepted by peers.

Social Environment. One of the major social factors in the incidence of sexually transmitted diseases to be assessed is the prevalence of the disease in the community. In areas where the incidence of disease is high, large reservoirs of infected individuals increase the risk of exposure to disease. Generally speaking, the incidence of STDs is higher in urban than in rural areas. Incidence rates for gonorrhea, for example, are twice as high in cities with populations over 200,000 than in smaller cities and rural areas.[91] Variations in incidence rates for gonorrhea by state for 1989 are depicted in Figure 30–6. Incidence of syphilis and hepatitis B also vary from place to place. State-by state-variations in annual incidence rates for syphilis and hepatitis B are shown in Figures 30–7 and 30–8, respectively.

Incidence rates for gonorrhea and syphilis also seem to rise during the summer and at certain holidays (particularly Labor Day and Memorial Day). It is unclear whether this increase is due to increased sexual activity at these times or because antibiotics used to treat wintertime infections may treat incubating gonorrhea and syphilis, thus reducing their incidence during the winter months.[91]

Other social environmental factors that contribute to STDs include poverty, lack of access to health care, and social attitudes condoning behaviors that foster exposure to these diseases. For example, higher incidence rates for congenital syphilis among blacks may be a function of lack of prenatal care and associated opportunities for early diagnosis and treatment of pregnant women with syphilis.[103] Similar factors may be operating in recent outbreaks of syphilis among Native Americans.[97]

Changes in behavioral norms in the society at large, with greater acceptance of sexual activity outside of marriage, have led to increases in sexual activity and subsequent increases in the incidence of STDs. At the same time, social constraints on discussing sexuality have limited the ability of public health officials and school personnel to provide sex education to young people at high-risk for STD.

Media presentations of sexual activity as desirable behavior have also contributed to the incidence of STD. Portrayals of popular heroes and heroines as "sexy" and sexually active have fostered imitative behavior, particularly among adolescents.

Life-style

Life-style factors to be assessed by the nurse in determining the risk of STDs in the community or for the individual client include sexual activity, intravenous drug use, and occupational risks.

Sexual Activity. The primary life-style factor associated with sexually transmitted diseases is, of course, sexual activity itself. Increased sexuality, failure to use protective devices, and homosexuality are some of the specific factors that contribute to STDs.

As noted earlier, changes in social mores have led to increased sexual activity by large numbers of Americans. Increased sexual activity, particularly with multiple partners, increases one's risk of exposure to STDs. In one study, almost 5 percent of people aged 18 to 29 reported having intercourse with more than 10 people in a 12-month period,[46] thereby increasing their risk of exposure to disease. Widespread use of oral contraceptives over the last few decades has led to more sexual activity among women as fear of pregnancy diminished. In addition to prompting an increased level of sexual activity, use of oral contraceptives may actually increase one's susceptibility to STD. For example, oral contraceptive use has been found to increase susceptibility to HSV infection.[98] Another effect of increased use of oral contraceptives is a concomitant decline in the use of barrier methods

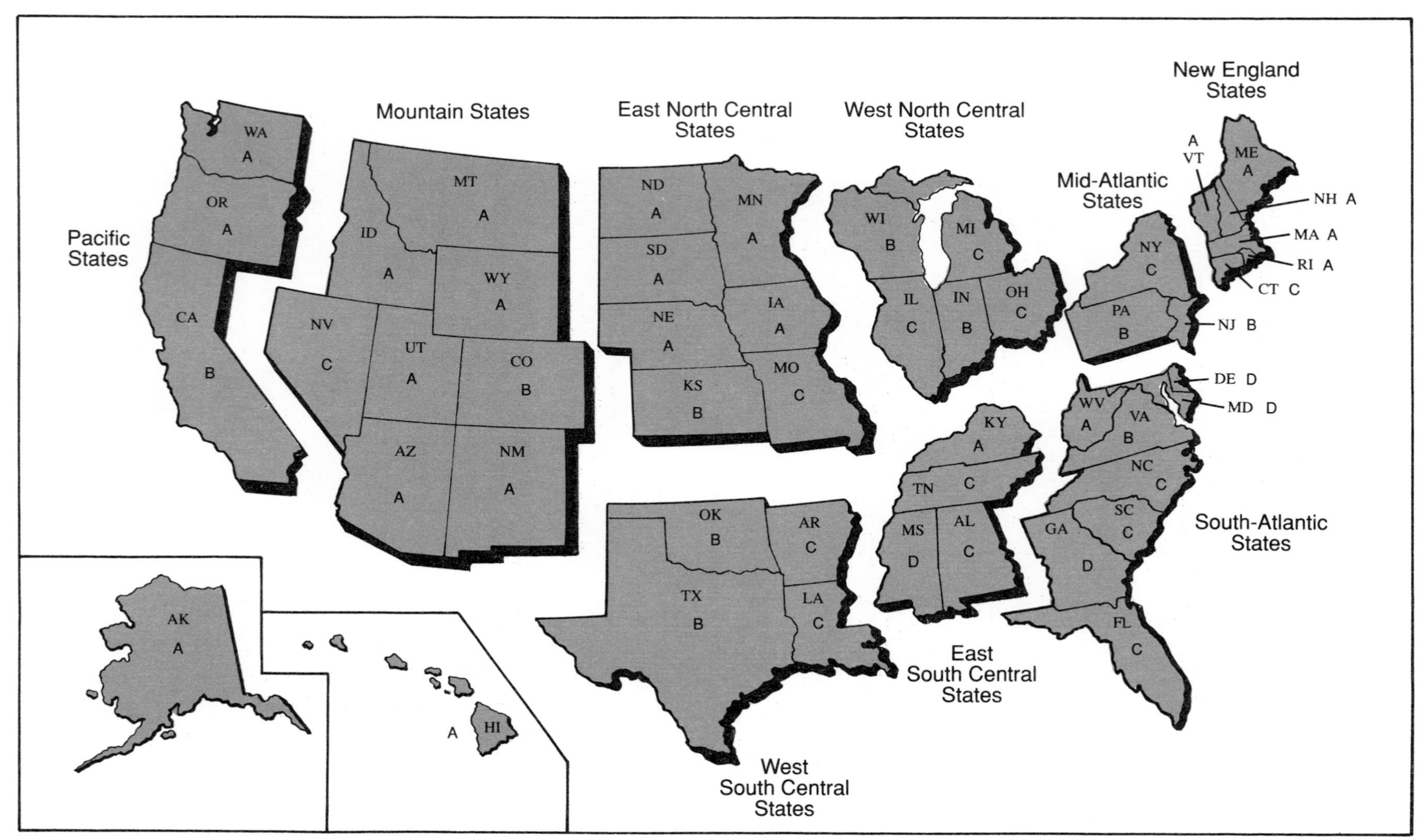

Figure 30–6. 1989 gonorrhea incidence per 100,000 population, by state. Legend: A = < 200 cases per 100,000 population; B = 200–299 cases per 100,000 population; C = 300–499 cases per 100,000 population; D = > 500 cases per 100,000 population. (*Source: Summary of notifiable diseases*[13])

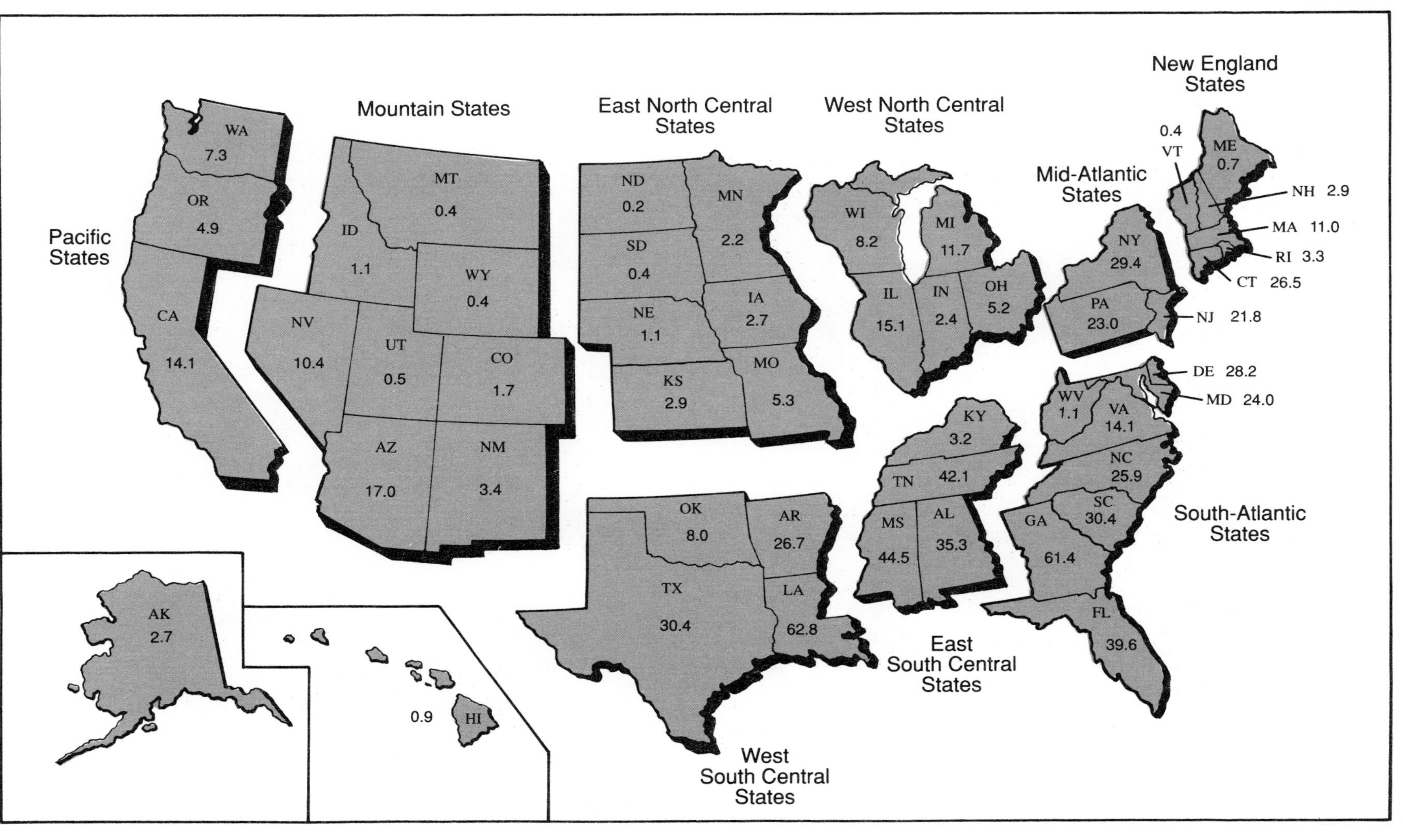

Figure 30–7. 1990 incidence of primary and secondary syphilis per 100,000 population, by state. (*Source: MMWR*[88])

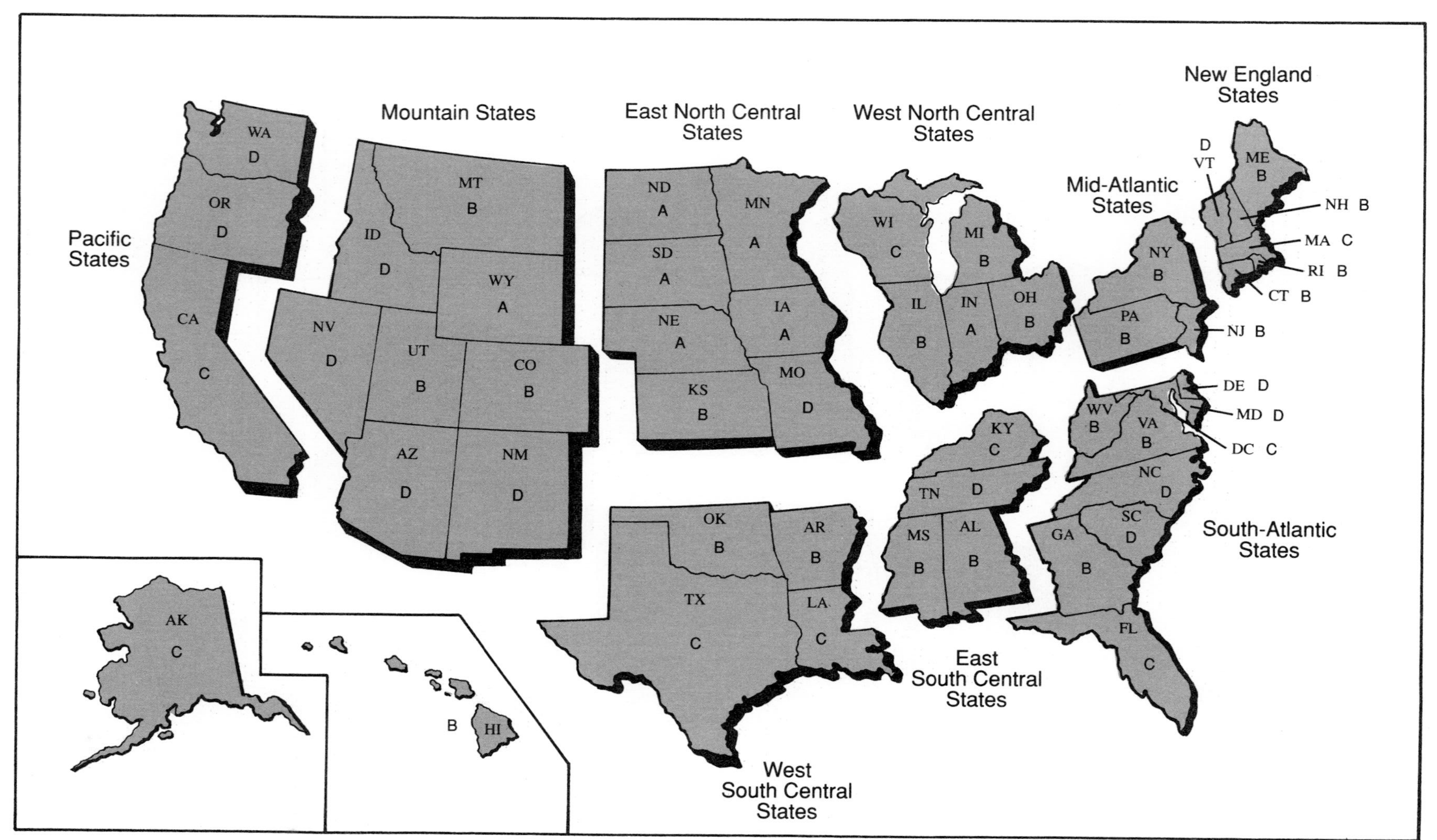

Figure 30–8. 1989 hepatitis B incidence per 100,000 population, by state. Legend: A = 0–3.9 cases per 100,000 population; B = 4.0–7.9 cases per 100,000 population; C = 8.0–11.9 cases per 100,000 population; D = >11.9 cases per 100,000 population. (*Source: Summary of notifiable diseases*[13])

of contraception that also provided protection against sexually transmitted diseases.

A homosexual life-style has also been associated with increased incidence of some STDs. Both gonorrhea and syphilis have been more prevalent among male homosexuals than among the general population. However, the incidence of both these diseases and the incidence of hepatitis B among homosexuals have recently begun to decline, probably in response to behavioral changes occurring as a result of efforts to prevent the spread of HIV infection in this population.[101,104,105] Homosexuality does not seem to be a significant risk factor for chlamydia since the incidence rate among gays is only one-third that among heterosexuals. However, homosexuals are more likely to develop chlamydial proctitis than other forms of the disease.[106]

Intravenous Drug Use. Intravenous drug use is a life-style factor implicated in the development of some STDs. Both syphilis and hepatitis B may be transmitted via contaminated drug paraphernalia.[14] Drug-related prostitution is another life-style factor that increases the incidence of STDs. Some drug users, particularly those who use crack cocaine, trade sex directly for drugs or engage in prostitution to obtain money to support their drug habits.

Occupation. Occupation is a life-style factor contributing to some STDs. Prostitutes and their customers are at risk for a variety of sexually transmitted diseases. A recent outbreak of gonorrhea among Colorado prostitutes is one indicator of increased risk in this population group.[107]

Military duty and occupations involving frequent travel away from home can pose increased risk of exposure to STDs through intercourse with prostitutes. It is believed that initial cases of antibiotic-resistant strains of gonorrhea were brought to the United States by military personnel returning from Southeast Asia. Surveillance of gonorrhea, syphilis, and HIV incidence among military personnel is used as a barometer of the prevalence of disease in the civilian population.

Occupation is also a life-style factor contributing to hepatitis B incidence. Health-care providers have a relatively high rate of infection. Dental professionals are at particularly high risk because of frequent exposure to blood and saliva.[108]

Health System

Health system factors have also contributed to the rise of STDs. Health system factors that influence the occurrence of STDs include lack of adequate attention to the problem on the part of many health-care providers, failure of health-care providers to educate individuals and the general public about STDs, inappropriate use of antibiotics, and failure to provide diagnostic and treatment facilities. In some instances, health-care providers may even be the source of STDs in their clients. Community health nurses would assess the extent to which factors in each of these areas contribute to problems related to STD in the community.

Unless clients specifically request services for signs and symptoms that may be related to sexually transmitted diseases, many health-care providers do not address sexuality issues with their clients. Despite recommendations for obtaining a sexual history on all adolescent and adult clients,[24] only 10 percent of primary-care providers regularly do so.[87] By and large, health-care providers have also failed to educate their clients regarding high-risk sexual behaviors and means of preventing STDs.

Health-care providers often use antibiotics inappropriately both in treating STDs or in treating other conditions. For example, a sizable proportion of primary-care providers do not prescribe the appropriate drugs for treating STDs.[87] In addition, many providers fail to recognize the fact that clients with one sexually transmitted disease may have been exposed to others and thus fail to provide treatment with broad-spectrum antimicrobials that will treat both incubating and symptomatic disease. For example, the use of spectinomycin to treat gonorrhea is not effective in treating incubating syphilis and may contribute to an otherwise preventable case of syphilis.[109] Finally, health professionals may prescribe antibiotics inappropriately for other conditions (for instance, a viral respiratory infection). If the client is exposed to a sexually transmitted disease, the amount of antibiotic prescribed may not be sufficient to treat the STD, but may present the infecting organism with an opportunity to develop resistance to the antibiotic, creating antibiotic-resistant strains of microorganisms.

Failure to provide adequate preventative, diagnostic, and treatment services to clients with STDs is another way in which the health-care system has contributed to the rising incidence of these diseases. For example, not targeting hepatitis B immunization campaigns to groups at risk for hepatitis B (prostitutes, intravenous drug users, and health-care workers) has contributed to the failure of efforts to control this disease.[108] Lack of affordable prenatal care for pregnant women at risk for STDs has added to an increased incidence of STDs such as gonorrhea, syphilis, hepatitis, and HSV infection in newborns. In addition, concern for the rising incidence of AIDS has led to diversion of funds from control programs for other

BOX 30–10

Factors in the Epidemiology of Other Sexually Transmitted Diseases

Human Biology

Genetic inheritance:

- Increased incidence of syphilis in women of childbearing age leads to increased congenital syphilis
- Type B blood may increase susceptibility to gonorrhea
- More women than men are asymptomatic for gonorrhea
- Women are more likely than men to be seropositive for HSV infection
- Blacks more often develop chronic hepatitis B carrier states than do Caucasians

Maturation and aging:

- STD incidence is highest among adolescents and young adults
- Infants in utero are at risk for infection with syphilis after about the 12th week of gestation
- Children have greater risk of cancer after hepatitis B than do adults
- Infants are at risk of ophthalmia neonatorum due to gonorrhea and chlamydia infection

Physiologic function:

- Concurrent HIV infection may invalidate tests for syphilis
- Presence of Down's syndrome, leukemia, and lymphoma increase susceptibility to hepatitis B
- Conditions requiring hemodialysis increase risk of exposure to hepatitis B
- Skin abrasions increase risk of being infected with syphilis and hepatitis B
- Syphilitic infection is associated with hepatitis B risk
- Passage through birth canal may infect infant with HSV, gonorrhea, or chlamydia
- Presence of one sexually transmitted disease increases potential for others

Environment

Physical environment:

- Higher incidence of some STDs is noted in summer than winter
- Use of articles contaminated by blood increase the risk of syphilis and hepatitis B

Psychological environment:

- Psychological factors that lead to increased sexual activity increase risk of exposure
- Psychological factors that contribute to drug use increase risk of exposure to syphilis and hepatitis B

Social environment:

- STD incidence is higher in large urban areas
- Incidence of hepatitis B is higher on both coasts than in the Midwest
- Changes in social norms and increased use of contraceptives have led to greater sexual activity and risk of exposure
- Media presentations of sexual activity as desirable have led to increases in risk behaviors
- Peer pressure for IV drug use increases the risk of exposure to syphilis and hepatitis B

Life-style

- Sexual activity with multiple partners increases risk of infection
- Homosexual activity increases risk of exposure to some STDs
- Failure to use condoms or other barrier methods increases risk of exposure to STDs
- Intravenous drug use and needle sharing increase risk of exposure to syphilis and hepatitis B

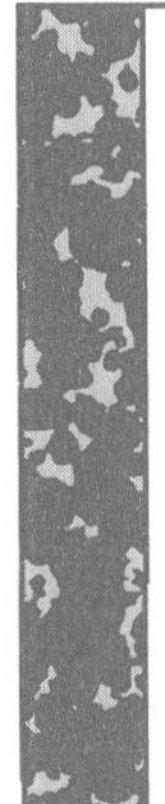

BOX 30–10 (*continued*)

Health system
- Failure to educate public regarding STDs impedes control
- Inappropriate use of antibiotics leads to ineffective control of STDs
- Reduced funding impedes adequate control of STDs
- Lack of access to prenatal care contributes to congenital infections
- Failure to provide immunization to persons at risk for hepatitis B contributes to increased incidence
- Failure to use precautions with blood and body fluids may cause spread of hepatitis B to health workers
- Use of contaminated injector guns contributes to spread of hepatitis B

STDs and has resulted in a shortage of diagnostic and treatment services for these diseases.[109]

Finally, health-care providers have, on occasion, transmitted STDs to their clients. Dental procedures (especially extractions and oral surgery) and hemodialysis, for example, are facile modes of transmission from infected health-care providers to clients. In fact, dental professionals have a higher prevalence of chronic carriers of hepatitis B than many other occupational groups. Despite the increased risk of disease in this population, studies indicate that only 15 percent of dentists and oral surgeons routinely use gloves, and in 1986 only 44 percent had been immunized for hepatitis B.[108]

Transmission of hepatitis B via jet-gun injector has also been reported. Tests indicate that jet-guns are relatively hard to contaminate, but, once contaminated, are very hard to disinfect.[110] Transmission via transfusion is also possible but has declined with the advent of donor screening.

Factors related to human biology, environment, life-style, and the health system influence the development of sexually transmitted diseases in communities and in individual clients. Factors in each of these areas are summarized in Box 30–10.

DIAGNOSTIC REASONING AND SEXUALLY TRANSMITTED DISEASES

Nursing diagnoses related to other STDs, like those for HIV infection, may be related to individual clients or population groups. Examples of diagnoses for the individual might be "potential for exposure to hepatitis B due to intravenous drug use and needle sharing" or "pain on urination due to gonococcal urethritis." At the group level, nursing diagnoses might reflect an "increased incidence of *Chlamydia trachomatis* infection in adolescent girls due to sexual activity with multiple partners" or "potential for increased incidence of congenital syphilis due to lack of prenatal care for women in high-risk groups."

PLANNING AND IMPLEMENTING CONTROL STRATEGIES FOR SEXUALLY TRANSMITTED DISEASES

Planning control strategies for STDs may occur at the primary, secondary, or tertiary levels of prevention.

Primary Prevention

Primary prevention strategies for sexually transmitted diseases consist of immunization, prophylaxis, and other general prevention measures.

Immunization. Unfortunately, the only sexually transmitted disease for which immunizing agents are available is hepatitis B. Pre-exposure immunization for hepatitis B is recommended for sexually active homosexual men and heterosexuals of both sexes, intravenous drug users, recipients of certain blood products, and health-care workers.[24] Other candidates for immunization include contacts to infected persons, prostitutes, persons with multiple episodes of other STDs, clients on hemodialysis, inmates of long-term prison facilities, and members of ethnic groups with high incidence rates such as Alaskan Natives and refugees from Indochina and Haiti. Americans traveling abroad to areas where hepatitis B is endemic should be immunized for hepatitis B as should the residents and staff of institutions for the developmentally disabled.[111] Community health nurses can be active in planning to publicize the need for immunization among these high-risk groups and may also be involved in providing immunizations.

Chemoprophylaxis. Prophylactic treatment of those exposed to an STD can not only prevent the spread of STDs to others but also prevent development in the exposed individual. Prophylaxis is available for several STDs including syphilis, gonorrhea, chlamydia, and hepatitis B. Community health nurses can plan to notify contacts who are candidates for chemoprophylaxis of their exposure to one of these diseases and inform them of the availability of prophylactic treatment. Community health nurses might refer clients to other sources of prophylactic services or provide prophylactic treatment themselves on the basis of medically approved protocols. In either case, the nurse would plan to educate the client about the medications used, how to take them, and potential side effects.

Prophylactic treatment of those exposed to syphilis is usually accomplished with a long-acting form of penicillin in a dose similar to that used for treatment of confirmed cases of early syphilis. Early treatment of pregnant women with syphilis is also prophylactic for congenital syphilis in the infant.

Prophylaxis is also available for ophthalmia neonatorum due to gonorrhea or chlamydia in the newborn. Prophylaxis for gonorrhea is accomplished with the instillation of a 1 percent silver nitrate solution or tetracycline or erythromycin ointment in both eyes immediately after birth.[112] Prevention of ophthalmia neonatorum due to chlamydia involves the application of erythromycin ointment in the eyes of the newborn immediately after delivery. Tetracycline can also be an effective prophylactic for this condition. Silver nitrate solution has not been found to be effective in preventing chlamydial conjunctivitis in the newborn.[24] Treatment of pregnant women who have chlamydial infection provides primary prevention for other forms of the disease in the neonate.

Cesarean section can be performed on pregnant women with active HSV infection at the time of delivery to prevent transmission of infection to the newborn. Another alternative is prophylactic use of acyclovir in infected mothers. This is not routinely used, however, due to lack of knowledge regarding the effects of acyclovir on the fetus. Community health nurses would refer pregnant women with possible HSV infection for appropriate diagnostic and treatment services to prevent infection of their infants.

Prophylaxis for unimmunized persons exposed to hepatitis B infection is also available and involves providing hepatitis B immune globulin (HBIG) and hepatitis vaccine (three doses). This combination of chemoprophylactic agents provides both long-term and short-term protection against hepatitis B.[111]

Other Measures. Several other measures may also be used in the primary prevention of sexually transmitted diseases. Primary prevention of all STDs relies heavily on achieving change in high-risk behaviors such as limiting the number of sexual partners (preferrably to a monogamous relationship), using barrier forms of contraception such as condoms and spermicides that may also prevent exposure to sexually transmitted diseases, and refraining from drug use.

Primary prevention for congenital syphilis, neonatal herpes infection, and ophthalmia neonatorum involves early identification and treatment of pregnant women with early syphilis, HSV infection, gonorrhea, and chylamydia. This may be accomplished by screening pregnant women in the first trimester of pregnancy and again early in the third trimester. An alternative approach is to screen women for pregnancy if they have STDs or are sexual contacts to men who have STDs. Pregnant women living in neighborhoods with a high incidence of STDs also can be screened for these conditions as well as referred for prenatal care and treatment if necessary. Women diagnosed as having an STD might also need counseling regarding the risks associated with pregnancy and the need for prenatal care for current or future pregnancies.

Women who are intravenous drug users are at high risk for pregnancy, hepatitis, and syphilis and should be asked about their menstrual history and referred for pregnancy testing as needed. Screening for STDs in WIC clinics, family planning clinics, and drug-treatment centers and among female prisoners can also identify pregnant women for whom treatment would constitute primary prevention of sexually transmitted diseases in their babies.[89]

Pregnant women with genital lesions can be tested for HSV infection. Those with positive tests or those who have a history of prior episodes of symptomatic herpes or contact with an infected person can be closely monitored for symptoms near term. If lesions are present at delivery, a cesarean section can be performed.

Community health nurses may also plan to educate and motivate clients to modify life-style factors that contribute to STDs. Limiting sexual activity and using condoms are primary preventive measures aimed at the population of sexually active individuals at risk for infection. Limiting needle sharing and treatment for drug abuse may reduce transmission of STDs in intravenous drug users.

Primary prevention aimed at health system factors related to STDs can also be undertaken. Care and training in the use of jet-guns, as well as technological redesign to limit potential for contamination and increase ease of disinfection, may also prevent infection with hepatitis B. Similarly continued donor screening will limit transfusion-related infection. Finally, use of universal precautions for blood and body fluids will help protect health-care workers against infection.

Community health nurses are actively involved in primary prevention of STDs. They are frequently involved in educating the public, particularly young people regarding the risks of indiscriminate sexual activity and the use of preventative measures such as condoms to reduce the risk of infection.

Nurses also make frequent referrals for prenatal

care and follow women throughout their pregnancy. During this prenatal period they can continue to educate clients regarding the risks of STD and identify women whose babies are at risk for congenital syphilis. Women with identified risk factors can then be referred for diagnosis and treatment to prevent disease in their babies.

At the aggregate level, primary prevention of STDs entails the allocation of adequate funds for STD control efforts. Community health nurses can plan to influence policymakers using the processes described in Chapter 12, The Political Process, to ensure that monies will be made available for education regarding STDs and for prenatal care for women at risk.

Nurses can also campaign for adequate sex education for young people that includes information on the prevention of STDs. In addition, they can plan to educate intravenous drug users regarding "safe shooting practices" or to refer clients desiring assistance with drug abuse problems. Nurses can also monitor legislative and regulatory activities related to blood-donor screening and use of jet-guns.

Secondary Prevention

Several strategies are used in secondary prevention of sexually transmitted diseases. These include screening, diagnostic, and treatment activities, each of which will be discussed briefly.

Screening. Screening procedures are available for syphilis, gonorrhea, HSV infection, chlamydia, and hepatitis B. Community health nurses will plan to educate individual clients and the public about the need for and availability of screening for STDs. Areas to be addressed in educational programs include groups at high risk for disease who should be screened and the signs and symptoms of these STDs that indicate a need for screening. Information about symptoms of the STDs discussed here is presented in Appendix P. Nurses can also make referrals for screening or actually conduct screening programs. In addition, they will explain screening results to those tested and educate them regarding the meaning of the tests. When screening tests are positive, they will refer clients for further diagnosis or treatment as needed.

Screening for STDs should be routinely performed on persons seen for other sexually transmitted diseases; those in family planning clinics who are at risk because of multiple sexual partners; prostitutes; male homosexuals; and intravenous drug users.[24] Screening for selected STDs may also be done on a routine basis for arrestees, hospital admissions involving persons in high-risk groups such as young adults or drug users, and persons with identified high-risk behaviors or sexually active persons who live in areas with a high incidence of sexually transmitted diseases. Premarital screening for syphilis is required to obtain a marriage license in most states. However, this approach to screening has not been shown to be cost-effective because of the low prevalence of the disease in the general population.[71,113]

Screening for reactive serology is usually the initial step in identifying persons with syphilis. Screening for syphilis is generally done with a non-treponemal test such as that developed by the Venereal Disease Research Laboratory (VDRL), or the Rapid Plasma Reagin test (RPR). These tests are relatively inexpensive and easy to perform. They are not, however, specific for syphilis because they react to a variety of other conditions and circumstances in addition to the presence of syphilis. For example, pregnancy or intravenous drug use, as well as several other diseases, may cause a biological false-positive (BFP) reaction. Positive screening tests are followed by specific diagnostic tests discussed later in this chapter.

Screening for gonorrhea is accomplished by culture of vaginal secretions in women or urine culture in men. Vaginal cultures are not foolproof in women, and a negative test should not be interpreted as conclusive evidence of the absence of infection.

Screening for HSV infection using Papanicolaou smears, immunoperoxidase tests, immunofluorescence, or enzyme assay has been suggested. However, the sensitivity of such tests is too low and the yield of positive cases too few to warrant routine screening except in the case of pregnant women at high risk as noted earlier.[24]

It is possible to screen for chlamydial infection with urethral or endocervical cultures, but this is not cost-effective in the general population. There is potential for rapid, low-cost screening using direct antigen testing, but these methods are not readily available at present.[24]

Routine screening of the general public for hepatitis B is not recommended. However, screening is suggested for all pregnant women at the first prenatal visit, and those in high-risk groups should be retested in the third trimester. Screening should also be done for sexual contacts of infected persons to determine susceptibility to infection before administration of HBIG. The usual screening test is for the presence of hepatitis B surface antigen (HBsAg) in the blood. A chronic carrier state may also be determined via screening. Presence of HBsAg in two blood samples taken 6 months apart indicates a chronic carrier state for hepatitis B.[24]

Diagnosis. Diagnoses of sexually transmitted diseases are made using a variety of laboratory procedures as well as physical signs and symptoms and history of risk behaviors or actual exposure to disease. Community health nurses might plan to refer clients with suspected STDs for diagnostic evaluation or obtain specimens for diagnostic tests themselves based on medically approved protocols.

Laboratory diagnosis of syphilis is made on the basis of confirmatory treponemal antibody tests such as the Fluorescent Treponemal Antibody test (FTA) and the Treponema Pallidum Immobilizing test (TPI), or actual identification of treponemes on darkfield examination of material taken from primary or secondary lesions. Diagnosis of gonorrhea and chlamydia may be confirmed through urine, vaginal, or rectal cultures.

Symptomatic HSV infection is diagnosed on the basis of clinical findings and the result of viral cultures of lesions. However, it is estimated that as many as two-thirds of infected persons are asymptomatic. The typical lesion in genital herpes is vesicular in nature and very painful. Lesions tend to occur in anogenital and oral-facial areas depending upon the site of exposure. Viral culture of lesions is an effective method of identifying HSV infection in an initial episode of symptomatic genital herpes. Cultures of lesions are less sensitive during recurrent episodes. Immunofluorescent and enzyme assay tests for HSV antibodies indicate the presence of infection, but they do not predict the likelihood of infecting others.

Diagnosis of hepatitis B is based on the presence of clinical signs and the presence of viral antigens such as HBsAg or HBeAg. Presence of appreciable amounts of Anti-HBe in serum usually indicates a resolving infection and declining communicability.[99]

Treatment. Antibiotic therapy is available for syphilis, gonorrhea, and chlamydia. Medications used to treat these diseases are presented in Appendix P. Community health nurses can plan to refer clients with suspected STDs for medical management, or they might plan to provide treatment themselves when there are established protocols for doing so. Community health nurses are also responsible for educating clients about medications used, how to take them if they are self-administered, and about potential side effects. Nurses will also monitor the effectiveness of treatment. To prevent the spread of infection, community health nurses should also plan to caution clients to refrain from sexual activity until they have returned for follow-up testing and cure has been demonstrated.

At the community level, community health nurses can be active in educating the public, especially those at risk, regarding the signs and symptoms of STDs and the availability of treatment. Nurses may also need to educate health-care professionals, particularly those in the private sector, regarding the appropriate diagnostic and treatment measures for STDs. Political activity by nurses might also be needed to ensure the adequacy of facilities for the diagnosis and treatment of STDs.

The treatment of choice for syphilis is still penicillin. Gonorrhea can be treated with a variety of antibiotics, although a regimen of ceftriaxone and doxycycline is recommended because of its effectiveness in treating strains of gonorrhea resistant to other antibiotics as well as incubating syphilis.

Systemic acyclovir can be used to treat asymptomatic HSV infection. Treatment appears to control symptoms and speed healing of lesions but does not cure the client or prevent subsequent recurrences.[112] Other therapy is symptomatic in nature and includes warm soaks of affected areas. Application of a tea bag soaked in water as hot as the client can tolerate may help relieve the pain of herpetic lesions as well.

Treatment for chylamydia may be provided routinely in conjunction with gonococcal therapy because the two infections often occur together. Both doxycycline and tetracycline have been found to be effective in treating chlamydia. Treatment for hepatitis B is symptomatic in nature and includes a diet relatively low in fat to minimize nausea. Pruritis related to jaundice can be minimized by the use of lotions.

Tertiary Prevention

Tertiary prevention of STDs in the individual client involves follow-up to determine the efficacy of treatment and education to prevent reinfection. Community health nurses should plan to emphasize to all clients the necessity for returning for follow-up to determine the effectiveness of treatment. This is particularly true of syphilis, in which the VDRL is used to monitor treatment effects.

Community health nurses should also plan to inform clients with syphilis that blood tests for syphilis usually continue to be positive even after adequate treatment. For this reason, these clients should be encouraged to inform subsequent health-care providers that they have been treated for syphilis in the past. Records of initial and posttreatment VDRLs can then be obtained from the Centers for Disease Control and compared to current test results to determine whether reinfection has occurred and treatment is required.

Babies with STDs may have a variety of subsequent health problems, even though they have been adequately treated and the progression of the disease halted. For this reason, community health nurses will continue to monitor these children over extended periods to provide for early identification of developmental delays and other problems.

Preventing reinfection, another aspect of tertiary prevention with the individual client, requires limiting exposure to the causative organism. Community health nurses can plan to educate clients on the need to limit their sexual activity and the number of sexual partners and on the efficacy of condoms and other barrier methods in preventing sexually transmitted diseases.

Another means of preventing reinfection with syphilis among drug users is discontinuing needle sharing. When an infected person shares equipment contaminated with his or her blood, the infection is transmitted to the new host. Community health nurses should plan to educate intravenous drug users regarding the risks of needle sharing and refer those who desire treatment to available treatment centers.

There is no need for intervention to prevent reinfection with hepatitis B, because hepatitis B infection confers lifelong immunity. However, community health nurses should caution clients with hepatitis against activities that could further damage their liver such as the use of alcohol and other drugs metabolized or detoxified by the liver.

Tertiary prevention at the community level involves preventing the spread of STDs. The primary mode of preventing the spread of many STDs is contact notification. Contrary to the situation with HIV infection, contacts to syphilis, gonorrhea, chlamydia, and hepatitis B, if identified and treated soon after exposure, can be prevented from developing the disease and transmitting it to others.

When STDs in children are the result of child abuse, the nurse will be involved in referrals and counseling to prevent subsequent abuse and reinfection. The involvement of community health nurses in cases of child abuse is dealt with in more detail in Chapter 34, Violence.

Tertiary prevention may also require planning for political activity on the part of nurses. As noted earlier, monies previously allocated to contact notification and STD prevention programs have been shifted to HIV infection control. Community health nurses can help to acquaint policymakers with the need to continue to fund control programs for syphilis as well as for other communicable diseases. Primary, secondary, and tertiary control measures for sexually transmitted diseases are summarized in Table 30–9.

TABLE 30–9. PRIMARY, SECONDARY, AND TERTIARY PREVENTION MEASURES TO CONTROL OTHER SEXUALLY TRANSMITTED DISEASES

Level of Prevention	Community Health Nurse Function	Goal
Primary prevention	• Referral for chemoprophylaxis	• Prophylaxis for persons exposed to STD
	• Use of antibiotics that not only treat gonorrhea but also treat incubating syphilis and chlamydia	• Prevent developing infection
	• Educate on condom use	• Increased condom use
	• Educate persons at risk	• Decrease number of sexual partners
	• Refer pregnant women for prenatal care and STD screening	• Identification and treatment of women with STD to prevent fetal infection
	• Refer drug users for treatment	• Decreased drug use and potential for exposure
	• Educate on "safe shooting" practices	• Decreased needle sharing
	• Correct use and cleaning of jet-guns	• Reduced potential for exposure
Secondary prevention	• Refer for screening persons at risk for STD	• Screening of groups at risk
	• Refer persons with symptoms for diagnosis and treatment	• Adequate diagnosis and effective treatment of STD
	• Educate clients on relief of symptoms of STD	• Relief of symptoms of STD
	• Educate clients on use of medications	• Effective treatment of STD
	• Political activity	• Ensure funds and facilities for treatment
Tertiary prevention	• Monitor effects of treatment	• Client compliance and effective treatment of STD
	• Educate clients about risk behaviors	• Prevent reinfection
	• Educate drug abusers on "safe shooting" practices	• Prevent reinfection
	• Interview cases and notify contacts	• Prevent communicability and spread of infection
	• Observe for signs of complications and refer for care as needed	• Prevent long-term consequences of infection
	• Refer children with STDs for child protective services	• Investigate possible sexual abuse and prevent recurrence

TABLE 30–10. STATUS OF 1990 OBJECTIVES FOR SEXUALLY TRANSMITTED DISEASES

Objective	Evaluative Data	Status
1. Reduce gonorrhea incidence to fewer than 280 cases per 100,000 population per year	305.5 cases per 100,000 population in 1988	Objective unmet
2. Reduce incidence of gonococcal pelvic inflammatory disease to 60 cases per 100,000 females per year	595.7 cases per 100,000 in 1988	Objective unmet
3. Reduce incidence of primary and secondary syphilis to 7 cases per 100,000 population per year	16.8 cases per 100,000 in 1988	Objective unmet
4. Reduce incidence of congenital syphilis to 1.5 cases per 100,000 population per year	16.9 cases per 100, 000 in 1988	Objective unmet
5. Reduce hepatitis B incidence to 20 cases per 100,000 population per year	Estimated 64 cases per 100,000 in 1987	Objective unmet
6. Educate all junior and senior high school students regarding sexually transmitted diseases	95% of high schools offer at least one class on STD as of 1988, but only 77% of students report STD education and overall knowledge is low	Objective unmet

(Source: U.S. Department of Health and Human Services[25])

EVALUATING CONTROL STRATEGIES FOR SEXUALLY TRANSMITTED DISEASES

For individual clients, evaluation of the effectiveness of control strategies focuses on whether clients develop STDs (evaluation of primary prevention), whether they are adequately treated for existing STDs (secondary prevention), and whether they develop complications or become reinfected (tertiary prevention). At the aggregate level, criteria for evaluation can be derived from the 1990 objectives for control of communicable diseases. Objectives for syphilis, gonorrhea, hepatitis B, and herpes, as well as knowledge of STD, have not yet been met, while no objectives were developed relative to chlamydia.[25] Evaluative data and the status of sexually transmitted disease objectives are presented in Table 30–10.

HEPATITIS A AND NON-A, NON-B HEPATITIS

There are other forms of viral hepatitis that, unlike hepatitis B, are not usually transmitted sexually. These include hepatitis A and non-A, non-B hepatitis (NANB). In addition, there is another form of sexually transmitted viral hepatitis called delta hepatitis, or hepatitis D. Delta hepatitis is caused by a dependent virus (hepatitis D virus, or HDV) that can only cause infection in the presence of hepatitis B.[114] Transmission occurs via perinatal, sexual, or parenteral exposure, and risk factors and prevention are similar to those for hepatitis B. Consequently, this discussion will be limited to a consideration of hepatitis A and NANB.

TRENDS IN HEPATITIS A AND NON-A, NON-B HEPATITIS

Hepatitis A is caused by the hepatitis A virus (HAV) and is primarily transmitted fecal-orally. The incidence of hepatitis A had been declining over the last several years, dropping from 13.8 cases per 100,000 population in 1979 to 11.6 per 100,000 in 1988.[7] However, during 1989, hepatitis A incidence increased to 14.4 per 100,000 population.[13] Serologic evidence of hepatitis A is found in approximately 45 percent of adults and 20 percent to 25 percent of children in urban areas in the United States.[115]

There are apparently two forms of non-A, non-B hepatitis, an enteric form transmitted fecal-orally and another transmitted parenterally. The enteric form may also be transmitted via contaminated food and water and occurs primarily in underdeveloped nations.

Parenterally transmitted NANB hepatitis accounts for 20 percent to 40 percent of cases of acute viral hepatitis in the United States. The incidence of this form of the disease has remained rather stable over the last few years, ranging from 1.8 cases per 100,000 population in 1985,[7] to 1 per 100,000 in 1989.[13]

ASSESSING FACTORS CONTRIBUTING TO HEPATITIS A AND NON-A, NON-B HEPATITIS

Factors related to human biology, environment, lifestyle, and the health system influence the incidence of both hepatitis A and NANB hepatitis. The community health nurse would assess for factors present in each area to determine the risk of these diseases for an individual client or for a community.

Human Biology

Although hepatitis A occurs in all ages, the severity of the disease tends to increase with age. Children usually remain asymptomatic.[111] Males and females are equally affected and all racial and ethnic groups are equally susceptible.

Enteric NANB hepatitis occurs most often in adults demonstrating ***attack rates*** (the proportion of persons exposed who actually develop the disease) of 10 percent for persons over 15 years of age and 1 percent for those under age 15.[116] The presence of health conditions necessitating multiple transfusions or hemodialysis increases the risk of parenterally transmitted NANB infection.[117]

Environment

Poor sanitation, inadequate plumbing, and overcrowding are environmental conditions that contribute to the incidence of hepatitis A. Contamination of food or water supplies is frequently implicated in common-source outbreaks. Incidence rates for hepatitis A vary from state to state. Relative incidence in 1989 is indicted for each state in Figure 30–9.

Incidence of enteric NANB hepatitis is also increased in conditions of poor sanitation and water control. Health-care providers need to be aware of the potential for NANB hepatitis in individuals from areas outside the United States.

Life-style

Poor personal hygiene, particularly lack of handwashing after toileting, is a life-style factor associated with hepatitis A. Recently, outbreaks of hepatitis A have been reported in conjunction with marijuana use and intravenous use of methamphetamines, heroin, and cocaine. It is unclear whether the contributing factor in theses outbreaks is contamination of drug supplies with fecal material during production of parenteral inoculation due to needle sharing.[118,119] The frequency of HAV seropositivity in intravenous drug users in Denmark has been found to be four times that of the general population,[119] suggesting that parenteral transmission is a possibility. Intimate household or sexual contact with infected persons has also been associated with increased risk of infection.[111]

From 23 percent to 42 percent of NANB hepatitis is related to intravenous drug use and 8 percent to 11 percent is transfusion-related. Another 4 percent to 8 percent of cases occur as a result of occupational exposure in health-care workers. Regretably, in up to 57 percent of cases no specific source of infection can be identified, although it is known that increased numbers of sexual partners and sexual or household contact with diagnosed cases are associated with increased risk.

Health System

Hepatitis A has, on rare occasions, been linked to blood transfusion.[96,118] These cases provide further support for the possibility of parenteral transmission of the disease during intravenous drug use. Factors associated with the incidence of hepatitis A and NANB hepatitis are summarized in Box 30–11.

DIAGNOSTIC REASONING AND HEPATITIS A AND NON-A, NON-B HEPATITIS

Nursing diagnoses related to hepatitis A and NANB hepatitis in the individual may reflect either the potential for developing either disease or health problems associated with them. Typical nursing diagnoses might be "potential for exposure to hepatitis A due to poor sanitary conditions" or "nausea and vomiting

BOX 30–11

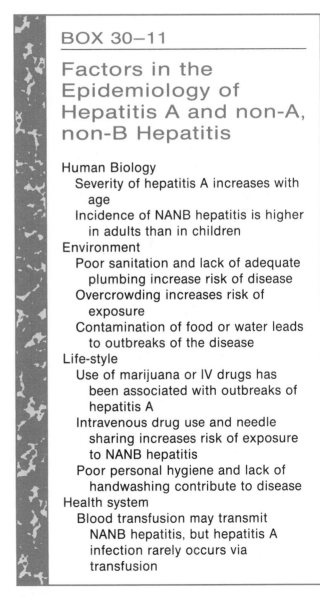

Factors in the Epidemiology of Hepatitis A and non-A, non-B Hepatitis

Human Biology
- Severity of hepatitis A increases with age
- Incidence of NANB hepatitis is higher in adults than in children

Environment
- Poor sanitation and lack of adequate plumbing increase risk of disease
- Overcrowding increases risk of exposure
- Contamination of food or water leads to outbreaks of the disease

Life-style
- Use of marijuana or IV drugs has been associated with outbreaks of hepatitis A
- Intravenous drug use and needle sharing increases risk of exposure to NANB hepatitis
- Poor personal hygiene and lack of handwashing contribute to disease

Health system
- Blood transfusion may transmit NANB hepatitis, but hepatitis A infection rarely occurs via transfusion

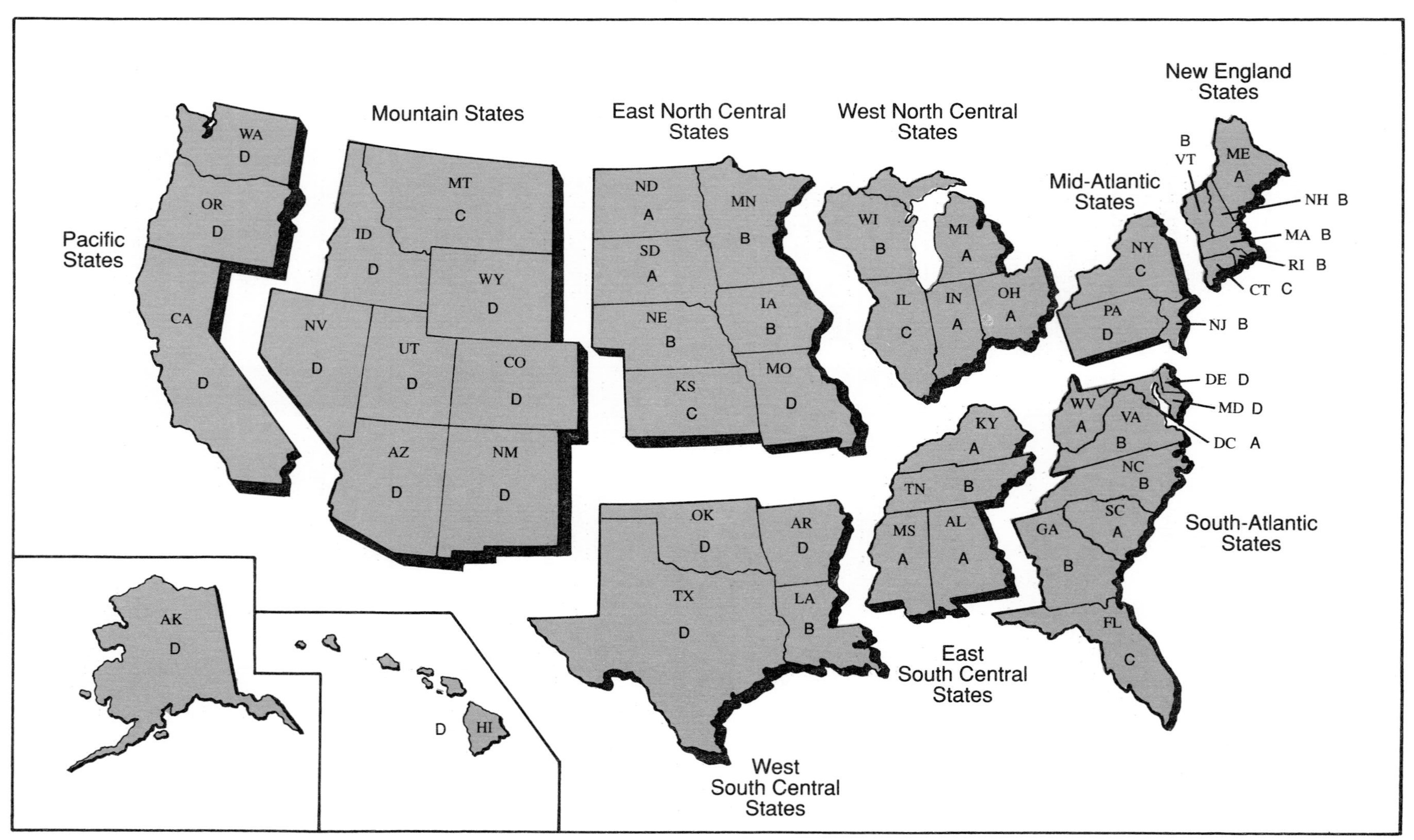

Figure 30–9. 1989 hepatitis A incidence per 100,000 population, by state. Legend: A = 0–3.9 cases per 100,000 population; B = 4.0–7.9 cases per 100,000 population; C = 8.0–11.9 cases per 100,000 population; D = > 11.9 cases per 100,000 population. (*Source: Summary of notifiable diseases*[13])

due to inability to digest fatty foods." Nursing diagnoses for population groups might reflect increased incidence of these diseases or the existence of conditions contributing to them. Examples of community diagnoses might be "increased incidence of NANB hepatitis due to contaminated blood supplies" or "potential for outbreak of hepatitis A due to broken sewer lines following earthquake."

PLANNING AND IMPLEMENTING CONTROL STRATEGIES FOR HEPATITIS A AND NON-A, NON-B HEPATITIS

Primary, secondary, and tertiary prevention measures may be planned to control the incidence and consequences of hepatitis A and NANB hepatitis.

Primary Prevention

Primary prevention of hepatitis A focuses on both chemoprophylaxis and general control measures. For NANB hepatitis, only general primary preventive measures are available.

Chemoprophylaxis. Pre-exposure chemoprophylaxis for hepatitis A is recommended for international travelers to developing countries. Chemoprophylaxis with immune globulin (IG) is particularly warranted for travelers who live in or visit rural areas, eat or drink in areas with poor sanitation, or engage in close contact with persons (especially children) in areas with poor sanitation.[111]

Primary prevention of hepatitis A can also involve prophylaxis following exposure to HAV infection. Immune globulin (IG) should be given within 2 weeks of exposure to a definitively diagnosed case of hepatitis A.[99] Prophylaxis can also be given to household and sexual contacts of cases, day-care staff and children exposed to the disease, and staff and residents of institutions for the developmentally disabled. Routine prophylaxis is no longer recommended for health-care personnel or persons exposed at work.[111] Community health nurses will frequently be involved in identifying contacts and in educating them regarding the need for prophylaxis. Nurses may then either plan to refer contacts to appropriate health-care services or administer IG directly under appropriate protocols.

General Measures. Currently, primary preventive measures for hepatitis A and enteric NANB hepatitis are aimed at improving sanitation, protecting food and water from contamination, and promoting adequate handwashing. Washing of fruits and vegetables before eating, boiling contaminated water, and discouraging use of human waste as fertilizer may also serve to prevent both hepatitis A and the enteric form of NANB hepatitis. There is some potential for a vaccine for hepatitis A in the near future.[118] Use of such a vaccine would be indicated for persons living in conditions of poor sanitation or for intravenous drug users if parenteral transmission is confirmed. For the parenteral form of NANB hepatitis, education of intravenous drug users regarding needle sharing and discouraging infected persons from donating blood may prevent infection.

Community health nurses should plan to educate the public in the primary prevention of hepatitis A and NANB hepatitis. Thorough handwashing after toileting and before preparing food should be encouraged. Persons traveling to areas where incidence of hepatitis is high should be cautioned by community health nurses against using unboiled water or eating foods that have not been cooked or peeled. Uncooked shellfish should also be avoided.

Community health nurses in developing countries where sanitation is a problem can plan to discourage the use of human fecal material as fertilizer. Clients can also be encouraged to wash fruits and vegetables thoroughly before eating them. Similar precautions are advisable in the United States especially if there is potential for infection via crop irrigation with water reclaimed from inadequately treated sewage.

Secondary Prevention

Secondary preventive measures for hepatitis A and NANB hepatitis include diagnostic and treatment measures. Screening for hepatitis A susceptibility is possible prior to administering IG to contacts, but this is not recommended because screening costs outweigh the expense of IG administration. Nor is screening for the disease itself suggested as a general approach to secondary prevention.

Diagnosis of hepatitis A is based on the presence of the clinical symptoms described in Appendix P, Information Related to Selected Communicable Diseases, and the presence of IgM anti-HAV antibodies, which indicate acute infection with HAV.[99] Community health nurses may need to identify persons with symptoms of hepatitis A and then refer them to appropriate health-care facilities for diagnosis.

Unfortunately, no serologic test for NANB hepatitis exists at present, so screening of donated blood is not possible. Diagnosis of NANB hepatitis is based on the presence of one or more diagnostic criteria including a history of exposure, travel to an endemic area, transfusion, intravenous drug use, or clinical symptoms of hepatitis in the presence of negative tests for hepatitis A and B. Treatment for hepatitis A and NANB hepatitis, as is the case in all forms of viral hepatitis, is symptomatic and is similar to that employed in hepatitis B.

Tertiary Prevention

Tertiary prevention of a recurrence of hepatitis A for individual clients is unnecessary because the disease confers lifelong immunity. Community health nurses should, however, plan to caution clients against the use of alcohol and other substances detoxified by the liver so as to prevent further liver damage.

Nurses should also instruct clients with hepatitis A on adequate handwashing to prevent transmission of the disease to others. Another tertiary prevention measure that curtails the spread of disease is removal of food handlers from work until they are considered noncommunicable. Other sensitive occupations for hepatitis A are health-care providers and child-care workers.

Tertiary prevention of NANB hepatitis involves preventing the spread of the disease through behavior changes related to hygiene, sexual activity, and drug use similar to interventions discussed for hepatitis A and B. Primary, secondary, and tertiary prevention strategies for hepatitis A and non-A, non-B hepatitis are summarized in Table 30–11.

EVALUATING CONTROL STRATEGIES FOR HEPATITIS A AND NON-A, NON-B HEPATITIS

Evaluation of control strategies for hepatitis A and NANB hepatitis involves monitoring the incidence and prevalence of both diseases in the population. Other indicators of successful control include declining mortality figures for these diseases. Incidence rates for hepatitis A have declined steadily in recent years, while NANB hepatitis incidence has remained stable. Mortality rates for both conditions are also relatively low. National objectives for the year 2000 for hepatitis A include reducing the overall annual incidence of hepatitis A to 23 cases per 100,000 population and reducing the annual incidence of hepatitis A among international travelers to 640 cases per 100,000 population. In the future, these objectives can be used as criteria for evaluating the effectiveness of primary preventive measures related to hepatitis A. The national objectives do not address non-A, non-B hepatitis.[87]

TUBERCULOSIS

Tuberculosis (TB) in the United States is primarily a disease of the lungs. In developing countries, however, tuberculosis occurs in a variety of extrapulmonary sites including bone, kidneys, pericardium, joints, and the lymphatic system. There is also a disseminated form of the disease that manifests in multiple organ systems. Tuberculosis is transmitted by the airborne route as ***droplet nuclei*** (small droplets of respiratory secretions propelled into the air by coughing, sneezing, or talking) that are inhaled by the host.

TABLE 30–11. PRIMARY, SECONDARY, AND TERTIARY PREVENTION MEASURES TO CONTROL HEPATITIS A AND NON-A, NON-B HEPATITIS

Level of Prevention	Community Health Nurse Function	Goal
Primary prevention	• Monitor community sanitation	• Prevent spread of disease
	• Monitor food and water supplies	• Ensure safe food and water supplies
	• Discourage use of human waste as fertilizer	• Prevent contamination of food and water supplies
	• Educate clients and public	• Handwashing and hygiene to prevent the spread of infection
	• Contact notification and referral for chemoprophylaxis	• Prophylactic treatment of contacts
	• Refer drug users for treatment	• Decreased drug use and potential for exposure
	• Educate drug users on "safe shooting" practices	• Decreased needle sharing
	• Political activity	• Ensure adequate sanitation and safe food and water supplies
Secondary prevention	• Educate clients about relief of symptoms	• Relief of symptoms
Tertiary prevention	• Educate infected persons to prevent spread to others	• Behavior changes to prevent the spread of infection
	• Interview individuals and notify contacts	• Chemoprophylaxis for exposed persons
	• Educate clients about alcohol effects on inflamed liver	• Prevent complications

Several strains of related bacteria produce tuberculosis, but the primary cause of pulmonary tuberculosis in humans is *Mycobacterium tuberculosis*. Basic information about tuberculosis is presented in Appendix P.

TRENDS IN TUBERCULOSIS INCIDENCE

With the advent of anti-tuberculin drugs, both morbidity and mortality due to tuberculosis have declined precipitously. In fact, chemotherapy is credited with a 94 percent drop in TB-related mortality since 1953. Prior to the availability of treatment, approximately half of those with tuberculosis died. The 1987 mortality rate for TB was 0.7 deaths per 100,000 population.[120]

Despite the remarkable decline in mortality, new cases of tuberculosis continue to occur, and incidence rates have increased somewhat in recent years (9.4 cases per 100,000 population in 1988).[13] The rise in TB is due in part to the influx of refugees from regions of the world with high TB rates. Tuberculosis might also be rising because of larger numbers of homeless persons living in shelters, especially in urban areas. The disease also occurs as an opportunistic infection among those with HIV infection and AIDS.

ASSESSING FACTORS ASSOCIATED WITH TUBERCULOSIS

The incidence and consequences of TB are influenced by factors in each of the four areas of epidemiologic perspective. The community health nurse would assess factors related to human biology, environment, life-style, and the health system that may place individual clients or communities at risk for TB. Factors that may affect the course of the disease for the individual or the community would also be identified.

Human Biology

Both the very young and the very old are at particular risk for tuberculosis. Currently, the highest rates of incidence occur among the elderly, whereas rates for children under 5 have declined.[121] Approximately 16 percent of older persons with TB die of the disease compared with approximately 1 percent to 2 percent of adolescents. However, children under age 15 are more likely to have extrapulmonary disease.

Differences in TB incidence rates also are noted in relation to gender. Men develop TB almost twice as often as women.

The presence of other physiological conditions can also contribute to the incidence of TB, and the community health nurse would identify physical conditions that increase the susceptibility of disease in the individual. The nurse would also assess the prevalence of these conditions in the population to determine the aggregate risk for TB. Leanness and diabetes are both risk factors for tuberculosis, as in immunosuppression due to any cause. Persons with HIV infection have approximately 100 times the risk of developing TB as noninfected persons.[37] Pregnancy or any other condition that puts undue stress on the body may also increase one's susceptibility to tuberculosis. Poor nutrition, particularly that experienced by alcohol and drug abusers, also increases the risk of TB. The presence of these conditions also heightens the severity of tuberculosis.

Environment

Stress is an element of the psychological environment that may lead to the development of active TB in persons who have been exposed. Other environmental factors influencing TB incidence and outcomes arise from the physical and social environments.

Physical Environment. Exposure to infected individuals in one's environment increases the risk of disease. This is particularly true in conditions of overcrowding. Approximately 29 percent of all close contacts to individuals with tuberculosis are found to be infected.[120] The more crowded the living conditions, and the more frequent and prolonged the contact with an infected person, the greater the risk of infection. Areas of the country in which exposure to TB is most likely to occur owing to the widespread nature of the disease are presented in Figure 30–10.

Social Environment. Social environmental stressors can contribute to increases in cases of TB. War and social upheaval cause TB rates to rise. The recent influx of refugees from parts of the world with high incidence rates for TB has contributed to the rising incidence in the United States.

Differences in TB incidence and mortality are noted among members of different racial or ethnic groups, probably as a result of poverty and its effects. In 1988, 65 percent of tuberculosis occurred among minority group members. Blacks accounted for nearly one-third of reported cases, while Hispanics accounted for 14 percent, Asians and Pacific Islanders 11 percent, and American Indians and Alaskan Natives 2 percent.[24] Statistics indicate that morbidity rates for blacks are four to nine times higher in various age groups than those for whites, while TB mortality rates are four to 16 times higher.[122] Incidence rates for Asians and Pacific Islanders are more than eight times those for whites,[123] while those for American Indians and Alaskan Natives are more than four times higher than rates for whites.[124]

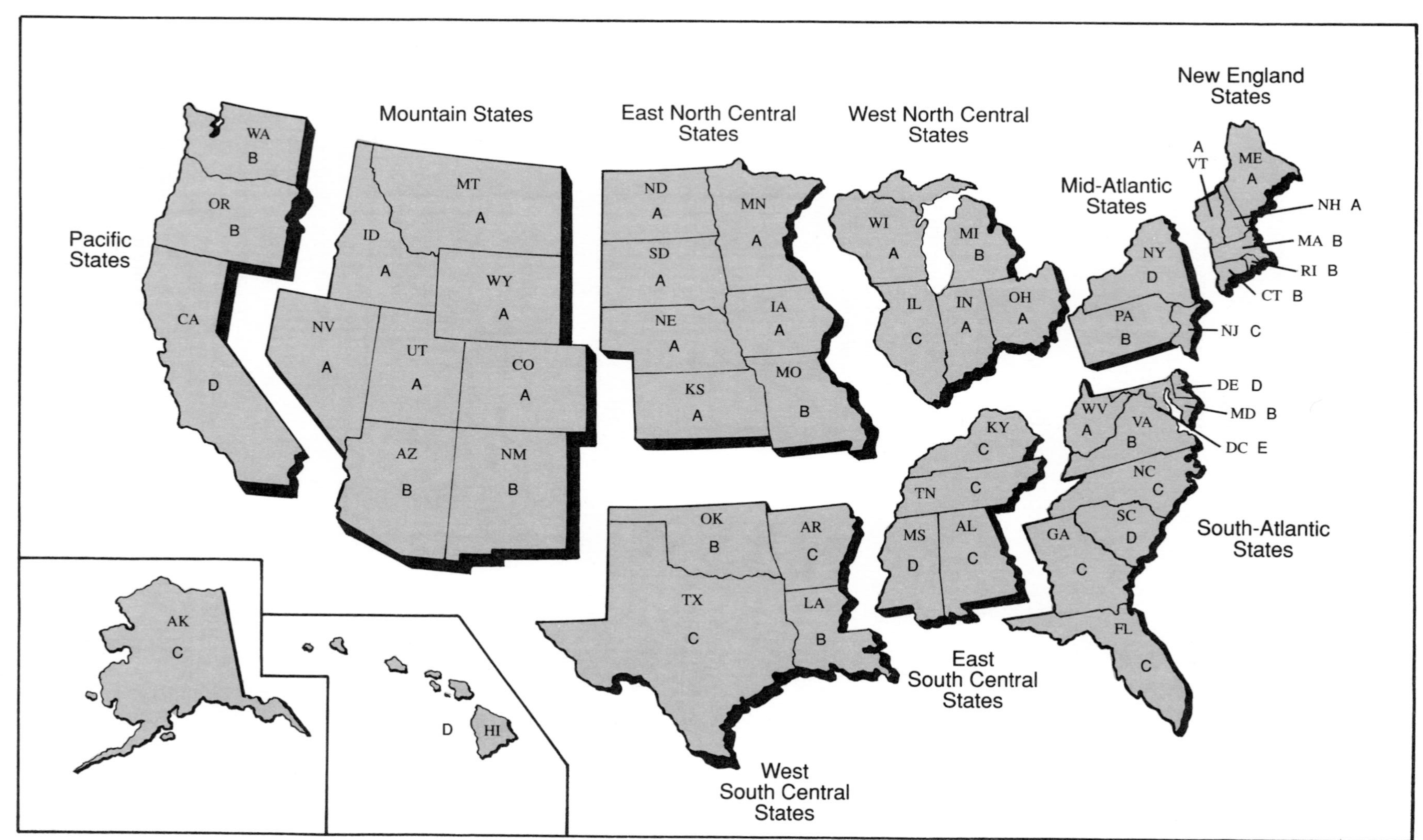

Figure 30–10. 1989 tuberculosis incidence per 100,000 population, by state. Legend: A = 0–4.7 cases per 100,000 population; B = 4.8–9.4 cases per 100,000 population; C = 9.5–14.1 cases per 100,000 population; D = 14.2–18.8 cases per 100,000 population; E = > 18.8 cases per 100,000 population. (*Source: Summary of notifiable diseases*[13])

Life-style

The life-style associated with homelessness has been implicated in the increased incidence of TB. From 2 percent to 7 percent of homeless persons have active tubercular disease, and 22 percent to 50 percent show evidence of infection.[24] Poor nutrition and other consumption patterns related to substance abuse and smoking also increase susceptibility to TB.

Occupation is another life-style factor that poses a risk for health-care providers caring for persons with communicable tuberculosis. The risk of infection is probably less, however, in working with persons diagnosed as having TB than in working with those in high-risk groups who are undiagnosed. This is so because, when a definitive diagnosis of TB has been made, precautions can be taken to prevent transmission to health-care providers. Any person providing services to people in high-risk groups is at increased risk for infection. These include those working with immigrants and refugees, and persons who work in shelters for the homeless.

Health System

Health system factors contribute to the incidence of TB in that many health-care providers are not aware of the growing magnitude of the problem and fail to consider TB as a potential diagnosis. Health-care professionals also may be unfamiliar with appropriate treatment regimens and, therefore, provide inadequate therapy to clients with TB, thus promoting disease recurrence. In addition, based on the number of cases of TB occurring in people under 35 years of age who should have received chemoprophylaxis, prophylactic services are not being provided to those in need of them.[124] Another health system factor contributing to tuberculosis incidence is the relaxation in many parts of the country of requirements for routine tuberculin testing for children, teachers, and others who work with susceptible populations. Factors in the epidemiology of tuberculosis are summarized in Box 30–12.

DIAGNOSTIC REASONING IN TUBERCULOSIS

Nursing diagnoses related to tuberculosis in the individual may be related to the potential for exposure to disease or to problems arising from existing disease. Examples of individual diagnoses might be "need for chemoprophylaxis due to close contact with family member with TB" or "visual disturbances due to ethambutol therapy for TB." At the aggregate level, nursing diagnoses may reflect increased incidence of TB or the existence of conditions that increase the risk of infection. Typical diagnoses at this level might be "increased incidence of TB among homeless persons" or "increased incidence of TB due to recent settlement of Southeast Asian refugees."

PLANNING AND IMPLEMENTING CONTROL STRATEGIES FOR TUBERCULOSIS

Planning control strategies for tuberculosis is based on general principles of program planning presented in Chapter 19, Care of the Community or Target Group. Control efforts may be planned and implemented at primary, secondary, and tertiary levels of prevention.

Primary Prevention

Primary prevention for tuberculosis includes basic health promotion to limit susceptibility to disease. Prevention of HIV infection by measures described earlier in this chapter can also limit susceptibility to tuberculosis in the population. Improvement in living conditions, promotion of good nutrition, and efforts to relieve conditions of poverty will also increase the resistance of the population to developing TB.

Immunization. There is a vaccine available for tuberculosis—bacille Calmette-Guérin (BCG) vaccine. Its efficacy is somewhat unpredictable, however. For this reason, and because it causes conversion of tuberculin skin tests to be positive, BCG is not widely used in the United States, where the prevalence of tuberculosis is relatively low and tuberculin screening is widely used as a control measure.[24] However, BCG is recommended for children who experience continuous exposure to persons with active TB but who cannot be given routine chemoprophylaxis. The vaccine should also be administered to those individuals exposed to persons who have TB that is resistant to the usual forms of therapy. Additionally, BCG should not be given to individuals who are immunocompromised and should be administered only with caution to those at risk for HIV infection. No longer is BCG recommended for health-care workers, who should rely instead on respiratory isolation precautions to prevent exposure.[120]

Finally, BCG vaccine is routinely used in a number of developing countries where the incidence of TB is high. Because BCG causes a positive reaction to tuberculin skin tests, community health nurses should ask about BCG vaccination before skin-testing persons from other countries. If BCG has been given, X-ray, rather than skin testing, is used for screening purposes.

Chemoprophylaxis. Chemoprophylaxis is used for primary prevention of tuberculosis in the United States. Persons who are at risk for TB or who have reactive tuberculin skin tests without evidence of cur-

BOX 30–12

Factors in the Epidemiology of Tuberculosis

Human Biology

Genetic inheritance:

Men are more often affected than women

Maturation and aging:

The very young and elderly are at greater risk of infection than other age groups

Risk of death is greater for the elderly than other age groups

Physiologic function:

Presence of leanness or diabetes increases susceptibility to infection

Pregnancy increases susceptibility

Immunosuppression or immunodeficiency increases susceptibility

Environment

Physical environment:

Overcrowding increases risk of exposure

Psychological environment:

Increased psychological stress heightens potential for developing active disease

Social environment:

Times of social disruption such as war and famine increase incidence

Immigration from countries with a high incidence of TB contributes to increased prevalence and incidence of disease in the United States

Members of minority groups account for a large portion of TB incidence in the United States

Life-style

Persons caring for those with active TB are at increased risk of exposure

Homelessness contributes to increased risk of disease

Substance abuse contributes to physical debilitation leading to increased susceptibility to disease

Poor nutrition increases susceptibility to TB

Smoking increases susceptibility to TB

Health system

Failure to diagnose and adequately treat TB contributes to spread of infection and recurrence of active disease

Relaxation of tuberculin screening requirements for certain groups of people has contributed to the spread of disease

Failure to provide chemoprophylaxis to persons under age 35 with positive TB skin tests contributes to the incidence of active TB

rent disease are offered antibiotic treatment to prevent its development. The most frequently used form of prophylaxis is administration of isoniazid (INH), an anti-tuberculin medication. Chemoprophylaxis is recommended for individuals who are in close contact to an infected person, those under 35 years of age whose tuberculin skin test has converted from negative to positive, persons with diabetes with positive skin tests, persons with HIV infection or silicosis, those of less than ideal body weight, postgastrectomy clients, and people on immunosuppressive therapy.[125]

Other Measures. Other primary prevention measures include the use of adequate ventilation and ultraviolet light in areas that increase the risk of TB transmission.[125] For example, areas in which aerosol sputum specimens are collected provide an environment conducive to the spread of disease that can be modified using these measures. Providing appropriate facilities for isolating infectious clients in hospitals will also minimize the risk of transmission to healthcare personnel.

Community health nurses are often involved in primary preventive efforts for control of tuberculosis. In a few cases, they may identify persons in need of BCG vaccine and assist them to obtain needed services. It is more likely, however, that they will supervise chemoprophylaxis for clients at risk for developing TB. Prophylaxis has been shown to be 90 percent effective in preventing the development of TB if the regimen is completed. For this reason, community health nurses should carefully educate clients regarding the need for preventive therapy and should monitor their compliance. When clients are judged to be unreliable, it is suggested that they be given directly observed therapy twice a week.[125] (In directly observed therapy, the nurse actually watches the client take the medication.) Another means of assessing compliance is periodic spot-testing of urine for INH metabolites.

Community health nurses should plan to educate clients regarding medication dosage and potential side effects. They also monitor clients on chemoprophylaxis for evidence of side effects.

Nurses are also involved in efforts to alleviate social conditions that contribute to tuberculosis incidence. They can help to influence policymakers to provide for the needs of the homeless and to improve the conditions of others in poverty. They can also intervene directly with these clients to refer them to sources of housing and financial assistance.

Secondary Prevention

Secondary preventive efforts for tuberculosis center around screening, diagnosis, and treatment of existing disease.

Screening. Secondary prevention of TB begins with screening members of high-risk groups. Persons who should be screened include those in contact with someone with active TB (especially household contacts) and others at risk for close contact with infected persons such as staff in tuberculosis clinics, shelters for the homeless, nursing homes, substance abuse programs, and prisons. Other high-risk groups that should be screened include recent immigrants from areas of high TB incidence, migrant workers, prisoners, nursing home residents, the homeless, and persons with HIV infection and other debilitating conditions.

The screening test of choice is the Mantoux skin test, an intradermal injection of tuberculin purified protein derivative (PPD). Health-care providers evaluation persons with HIV infection for evidence of TB should bear in mind that these clients may have a false-negative PPD and that a negative test result should not exclude a diagnosis of TB.[82]

A positive tuberculin skin test indicates that the person has at some time been exposed to TB and has developed circulating antibodies to infection. It does not, however, indicate whether the person has active disease. Unlike HIV infection, TB infection is not *necessarily* communicable. Individuals with what is termed a "primary" infection have been exposed to the causative agent, but bodily defense mechanisms have successfully combatted the invading organism. Usually the organism is walled off in an encapsulated area within the lung. During this process, antibody formation is stimulated and the tuberculin skin test becomes reactive.

Persons with primary infection cannot transmit the disease to others. However, when any of a variety of physical or psychological stressors undermine the body's ability to confine the invading organism, active disease can occur. Clients with active disease can transmit the disease to others. Preventing the development of active disease is the aim of chemoprophylactic therapy discussed earlier.

Community health nurses are frequently involved in referring clients for screening. They may also give and interpret the TB test. The nurse should be sure to plan to inform clients of the need to return to have the TB skin test read in 48 to 72 hours. When the test results are positive, the nurse would plan a referral for further diagnostic studies and treatment as needed.

Diagnosis. When a person has a reactive TB skin test, there is a need for further diagnostic testing to determine whether the individual does or does not have active tuberculosis. Diagnosis of active pulmonary disease is based on sputum cultures positive for acid-fast bacilli. In the absence of positive cultures, diagnosis is made in the presence of any two of the following: symptoms suggestive of TB (see Appendix P), X-ray findings consistent with TB, and a positive PPD.[120] Diagnosis of TB in persons with HIV infection may be complicated by the fact that symptoms may not reflect the typical clinical picture of TB and by differences from characteristic X-ray findings. In addition, 40 percent to 75 percent of TB in those with concurrent HIV infection is extrapulmonary in nature.[82]

Treatment. Treatment with anti-tuberculin drugs is highly effective in most clients, resulting in return to negative sputum cultures in 54 percent of clients within 3 months and 100 percent of clients within 6 months when the infecting organism is sensitive to the drugs of choice and the client is consistent in taking the medication.[126] Treatment for tuberculosis usually involves at least two drugs, and occasionally three, to minimize the potential for developing antibiotic resistance. The usual drugs of choice are isoniazid (INH) and rifampin (RIF). Streptomycin occasionally may be added as a third drug. When bacteria are resistant to INH or RIF, ethambutol (EMB) or para-aminosalicylate (PAS) may be substituted.

Community health nurses working with clients with active TB will most likely be monitoring clients' compliance with the treatment regimen and observing them for side effects. It is important that the nurse plan to emphasize to clients the need to complete therapy and to take the medications as directed because sporadic therapy frequently results in the development of drug-resistant bacteria. Again, directly observed therapy or periodic spot-testing of urine for INH metabolites might be warranted in client whose compliance is in doubt.

Community health nurses should plan to educate clients on anti-tuberculin therapy regarding potential side effects of medications and measures that can be taken to minimize them. They should also ensure that periodic testing of vision, liver function, hearing, and kidney function is done to identify adverse effects of chemotherapy.

Tertiary Prevention

Tertiary preventive efforts for tuberculosis focus on three areas: preventing recurrence of the disease in the individual; notifying and treating contacts to cases of tuberculosis; isolating infected persons as needed.

Prevention of Recurrence. Tertiary prevention of TB takes place at both the individual client level and the community level. With the individual client, there is the potential for reactivation of disease following treatment, particularly if treatment has been inadequate. In one study of clients who experienced recurrent episodes of active tuberculosis, 20 percent had never received any treatment for their disease, and an additional 20 percent had received inadequate or inappropriate therapy. Inadequate treatment tended to occur more frequently among clients receiving treatment from private health-care providers than among those receiving care in public clinics. Finally, 33 percent of the recurrent TB was related to poor compliance with treatment.[127]

Community health nurses can prevent all of these situations that lead to recurrence of TB. Case finding and referral of clients for treatment can eliminate lack of therapy as a cause of recurrent disease. Community health nurses are frequently involved in educating other health-care providers regarding the appropriate treatment for tuberculosis as well as other communicable diseases. Community health nurses can also help to ensure that clients take their medications as directed and complete their therapy.

Some of the actions that can be taken to achieve this have already been discussed and include directly observed therapy, periodic spot-testing of urine, and, most importantly, education to promote client understanding of the need to complete an adequate course of therapy. In addition, community health nurses can monitor clients after treatment for signs of recurrent disease and may be involved in obtaining follow-up sputum cultures or arranging for follow-up X-rays to determine the adequacy of treatment.

Contact Notification. At the community level, tertiary prevention of TB focuses on preventing the spread of disease within the community. Contact notification is the major activity in this area. The strategic plan for tuberculosis control developed by the Centers for Disease Control calls for interviews of clients with diagnosed cases of TB within 3 days of

TABLE 30–12. PRIMARY, SECONDARY, AND TERTIARY PREVENTION MEASURES TO CONTROL TUBERCULOSIS

Level of Prevention	Community Health Nurse Function	Goal
Primary prevention	• Educate public regarding health promotion and good nutrition	• Increased resistance to disease
	• Identify and refer those in need of BCG immunization	• Increased resistance to disease
	• Identify and refer those in need of chemoprophylaxis	• Prevent developing active disease
Secondary prevention	• Provide screening and counseling services	• Screening for persons at risk
	• Case finding and referral for treatment	• Diagnosis and treatment with appropriate antituberculin agents
	• Educate regarding medications	• Ensure client compliance and effective treatment of disease
	• Monitor and treat medication side effects	• Prevent adverse reactions
Tertiary prevention	• Interview cases and notify contacts	• Prevent spread of infection
	• Monitor effects of treatment	• Ensure effective treatment
	• Educate health-care providers on appropriate treatment	• Prevent inadequate treatment
	• Identify need for and initiate isolation procedures for noncompliant clients with active disease	• Prevent spread of infection

diagnosis and examination of close contacts within 7 days, at which time contacts would be offered prophylactic chemotherapy.[125]

Isolation. A final tertiary preventive measure for TB is involuntary isolation of persons with active disease; this is designed to prevent the spread of disease. This intervention has the potential for use in the control of several communicable diseases, but is most frequently invoked in tuberculosis control. What is involved is the involuntary isolation or quarantine of an infected person who refuses to discontinue behaviors that expose others to infection. Such measures are a last resort and are used only when all other efforts to control the spread of infection fail.[125] A summary of primary, secondary, and tertiary preventive measures for tuberculosis is presented in Table 30–12.

EVALUATING CONTROL STRATEGIES FOR TUBERCULOSIS

Evaluating primary preventive measures for TB control involves monitoring the incidence and prevalence of the disease as well as the effectiveness of measures to prevent active disease. Secondary and tertiary prevention can be evaluated on the basis of mortality rates for TB and adequacy of therapy in individual cases.

One of the national objectives for the year 1990 was a reduction in the incidence of tuberculosis from 13.1 cases per 100,000 population in 1978 to 8 cases per 100,000 population in 1990. Progress has been made toward this objective, but, as of 1988, when the incidence of TB was 9.1 per 100,000 population, the objective had not been met.[7] Future evaluation of measures for controlling tuberculosis at the community level will be based on the national objectives for the year 2000 related to tuberculosis. These objectives are summarized in Box 30–13.

BOX 30–13

National Objectives for the Year 2000 Related to Tuberculosis

1. Reduce the incidence of tuberculosis to no more than 3.5 cases per 100,000 population.
2. Increase to at least 90% the proportion of local health departments that have ongoing programs for identifying cases of tuberculosis and latent infection in populations at risk.
3. Increase to at least 85% the proportion of people found to have tuberculosis infection who completed courses of preventive therapy.

(Source: U.S. Department of Health and Human Services[87])

INFLUENZA

Influenza is a viral disease caused by three types of influenza viruses (influenza A, B, and C). Type A influenza virus has three subtypes, and both type A and type B viruses undergo frequent genetic mutations that cause periodic development of variant strains for which prior immunization is ineffective. Thus, despite the presence of vaccines for influenza, this disease continues to occur throughout the world. It is usually type A and type B viruses that cause major epidemics of influenza, whereas type C influenza appears only sporadically throughout the world.[14] For most people, influenza is a short-lived illness producing moderate discomfort. For others, however, influenza is a far more serious illness.

TRENDS IN INFLUENZA INCIDENCE

Thousands of people are exposed to influenza and develop active disease each year. From 1982 to 1986, mortality due to influenza and resultant pneumonia rose by 40 percent. From 1980 to 1987, the average rate for epidemic-related pneumonia and influenza deaths among persons 65 years of age and older was 9.1 per 100,000 population.[87] While this represents a decline from the 1970 rate of 22.1 deaths per 100,000 population, it is still far higher than it need be. Basic information on influenza is presented in Appendix P.

ASSESSING FACTORS ASSOCIATED WITH INFLUENZA

Human biological, environmental, life-style, and health system factors contribute to the development of influenza and affect its outcome.

Human Biology

Human biological factors influence susceptibility to and consequences of influenza infection, and the nurse should identify factors present in individual clients or in communities that may place them at risk for influenza or its complications. Influenza occurs in all age groups, but mortality rates are highest among the very young and the very old. Males are more often affected than females, and all racial groups are susceptible.

Persons with other debilitating physical conditions, particularly chronic pulmonary diseases, diabetes, stroke, and heart disease, are at higher risk for death due to influenza.[128] Other illnesses that increase susceptibility include renal dysfunction, hemoglobinopathies, and diseases or treatment regimens that result in immunosuppression. Persons with HIV infection are at particular risk for influenza and, as noted earlier, the death rate among persons with both diseases is much higher than that for the general public. Children who are on long-term aspirin therapy are of particular concern because of the potential for developing Reye's syndrome following viral infections such as influenza.[129]

In working with clients with influenza, the nurse would also assess the extent of the disease. Clients' complaints generally include fever, headache, muscle aches, coryza, sore throat, and cough. The cough, in particular, may linger for some time after other symptoms have resolved. Gastrointestinal symptoms such as nausea, vomiting, and diarrhea can also occur, particularly in children, so the nurse should assess clients for signs of dehydration resulting from these symptoms. The nurse would also assess clients for signs of croup, pneumonia, and other respiratory complications of influenza.

Environment

The community health nurse would also assess environmental factors that may contribute to the development of influenza and affect its outcome in an individual client or result in an influenza epidemic in a community. For the most part, these factors are found in the physical and social environments, although psychological stress can also lower the individual's resistance to influenza.

Like other diseases spread by airborne transmission, influenza occurs more frequently when people congregate in close quarters. This would explain the increased incidence of influenza in temperate areas in the winter months[14] because people are gathered indoors, making the spread of disease from an infected individual to others more likely. Similarly, epidemics typically occur in the rainy season in tropical areas—again, a time when people tend to spend more time indoors.[14] Transmission of influenza is particularly likely in conditions of overcrowding. On rare occasions, animal strains of influenza virus may be transmitted to humans. Animals that can serve as reservoirs for disease include swine, horses, mink, and seals, as well as many domestic and wild birds.[14]

A variety of social factors also contribute to the spread of influenza and to the severity of its effects. For example, poverty can prevent people at risk for influenza from obtaining immunizations or prevent infected persons from seeking medical assistance, thereby increasing their chances for complications from the disease.

Homelessness may also contribute to the onset of influenza. Exposure to cold, poor nutrition, and other conditions related to homelessness can increase the homeless individual's susceptibility to disease. In addition, crowded conditions in shelters or in other areas where the homeless sleep can increase the spread of disease from infected individuals.

Life-style

Any life-style factor that contributes to a generally poor state of health increases one's susceptibility to influenza, so the community health nurse should be alert to life-style factors that may contribute to the development of influenza. Consumption patterns such as poor nutrition and substance abuse lower one's general state of health, while smoking impairs respiratory function and increases susceptibility to infection. Overexertion and fatigue can decrease one's resistance to disease in general, including influenza.

Occupational factors also play a part in increased susceptibility to infection or increased exposure to influenza virus. Occupations that result in exposure to high levels of dust and other particulate matter or chemical vapors that may damage lung tissue can increase susceptibility to disease. Health-care workers are at particular risk of exposure to influenza because of the many clients with influenza for whom they provide services. School teachers are also frequently exposed to infected children in their classrooms.

Health System

The nurse would also assess health system factors that may influence the risk of influenza in an individual or in a community. For example, the nurse might explore the extent to which immunization programs are targeted to members of high-risk groups. In some areas, influenza vaccine is available primarily to those who can pay for it, so many who are in need of protection do not obtain it. In addition, health-care providers may not recognize the need for supportive services in persons with influenza who are at greatest risk for complications such as pneumonia. Factors in the epidemiology of influenza are summarized in Box 30–14.

BOX 30–14

Factors in the Epidemiology of Influenza

Human Biology

Maturation and aging:

- The elderly are at increased risk for influenza and death due to complications of influenza

Physiologic function:

- Presence of conditions such as COPD, diabetes, stroke, and heart disease increase susceptibility to disease
- Renal dysfunction, hemoglobinopathies, and immunosuppression increase susceptibility and risk of complications
- Children on long-term aspirin therapy are at risk for Reye's syndrome as an influenza-related complication
- Persons with HIV infection are more susceptible to influenza infection and complications

Environment

Physical environment:

- Overcrowding contributes to spread of disease
- Influenza incidence increases during weather that keeps people indoors
- Animal strains of influenza may occasionally be transmitted to humans

Psychological environment:

- Presence of psychological stress increases susceptibility

Social environment:

- Poverty may prevent people at risk from seeking immunization or disease-treatment services
- Conditions associated with homelessness can contribute to increased susceptibility to influenza

Life-style

Occupation/employment:

- Care providers in residential and health-care facilities are at increased risk of exposure
- Persons with occupational exposure to dust, fumes, etc., may be at increased risk of influenza infection

Consumption patterns:

- Poor nutrition increases susceptibility to influenza
- Substance abuse increases susceptibility to influenza
- Failure to get adequate rest increases susceptibility to influenza
- Smoking increases susceptibility to influenza infection

Health system

- Failure to provide immunization to persons at risk impedes control of influenza

DIAGNOSTIC REASONING AND INFLUENZA

Nursing diagnoses for the individual client will probably be related to the potential for exposure to, or problems resulting from, influenza. Examples of individual diagnoses might be "need for influenza immunization due to chronic respiratory disease" or "impaired oxygen exchange due to respiratory effects of influenza." Other diagnoses at the individual level might include "electrolyte imbalance from diarrhea due to influenza" or "dehydration due to vomiting and diarrhea."

Nursing diagnoses at the community level may reflect the incidence or consequences of influenza or the potential for an outbreak in the population. Examples of population-oriented diagnoses are "increased mortality from influenza in minority group members due to lack of access to medical care" or "potential for increased influenza incidence due to poor immunization levels in high-risk groups."

PLANNING AND IMPLEMENTING CONTROL STRATEGIES FOR INFLUENZA

Primary, secondary, and tertiary preventive efforts are warranted in the control of influenza. Primary measures are geared toward preventing outbreaks or individual cases of disease, while secondary measures focus on resolving existing problems. Tertiary prevention is directed toward preventing complications or recurrence of disease.

Primary Prevention

Primary preventive measures center on immunizing susceptible individuals. Other primary strategies include chemoprophylaxis and general hygiene and health promotion.

Immunization. The major emphasis in primary prevention of influenza is immunization. Because of the tendency of the influenza virus to produce new strains, a vaccine is developed each year to provide protection against the viral strains identified in early cases of the disease and expected to cause most of that year's cases of influenza. For this reason, community health nurses should plan to educate those persons at greatest risk (for example, the elderly or those with debilitating illnesses) about the need to be reimmunized annually. Routine yearly influenza immunization is recommended for health-care workers, the elderly, and persons with chronic diseases including chronic pulmonary or cardiovascular diseases, asthma, chronic metabolic diseases such as diabetes, renal dysfunction, hemoglobinopathies, or immunosuppression.[130]

Immunization should also be provided to household contacts of persons in high-risk groups to minimize the risk of exposing high-risk individuals to influenza. Other candidates for immunization include travelers to areas of high incidence, children 6 months to 18 years of age who are on long-term aspirin therapy (immunization is to prevent the development of Reye's syndrome), and persons with HIV infection. Influenza vaccine is made from inactivated viruses and cannot cause influenza in the person immunized. For this reason, it is safe to administer influenza vaccine to persons with immunosuppression due to AIDS, and immunization is recommended. However, these individuals may not develop adequate immunity in response to the vaccine and should be protected from exposure to the virus whenever possible. Immunization can also be safely given to pregnant women who demonstrate risk factors for influenza. Immunization is most effective in preventing disease when it is administered before the onset of the influenza season in late fall. Immunization is not recommended for those who have experienced an anaphylactic reaction to egg protein or to persons with febrile illness. The latter may be immunized after their symptoms have abated.[130]

Community health nurses will identify persons at risk for influenza and plan to refer them for immunization services. Nurses may also plan and implement immunization programs, targeting groups at high risk for influenza. In addition to referring clients for or providing immunizations, the community health nurse would plan to educate clients about potential side effects of immunization (soreness at injection site, fever, and myalgia) and their control.

Chemoprophylaxis. Chemoprophylaxis is not routinely used as a primary preventative measure for persons exposed to influenza. However, prophylaxis with an antiviral agent such as amantadine is recommended for individuals involved in outbreaks of influenza A in closed populations. For example, if an outbreak of influenza has taken place in a nursing home or institution for the developmentally disabled, all residents and staff who do not already have the disease might be given amantadine to prevent illness. Chemoprophylaxis is also recommended for persons at high risk for influenza who cannot be immunized (for example, those having severe allergic reactions to eggs). Amantadine is not effective in the prevention of influenza B.[130]

Other Measures. Public education regarding personal hygiene, particularly respiratory hygiene, is another primary prevention measure for influenza. Community health nurses can be instrumental in such education as well as in identifying persons at risk for influenza. The nurse can then acquaint those at risk with the need for immunization and refer them to the appropriate source of care. Oftentimes community health nurses are also involved in the implementation of influenza immunization programs.

Secondary Prevention

No routine screening test exists for influenza. Even if there were a test available, it would not be widely used because the incubation period for influenza is not long enough for action to be taken to prevent development of symptomatic disease in those infected. Persons who had reactive tests would more than likely already be exhibiting symptoms of the disease.

Diagnosis of influenza is based on the presence of characteristic respiratory or gastrointestinal symptoms and the absence of indicators that these symptoms are due to some other cause. Diagnosis also depends on the potential for exposure at any given time. Because influenza in temperate zones is a cold-weather disease, influenza-like symptoms experienced in the summer months are probably not due to influenza but to some other disease process. Likewise, if jaundice accompanies gastrointestinal upset, a more likely cause is hepatitis rather than influenza.

Treatment for influenza is generally symptomatic, although early administration of amantadine in influenza A infection may reduce symptoms. Unimmunized clients who are at particular risk for influenza or its complications may be referred for amantadine therapy in areas where viral cultures of infected persons demonstrate the presence of influenza A strains.

The community health nurse working with individuals with influenza should give particular attention to planning to maintain hydration and conserve energy. If gastrointestinal symptoms are severe, antiemetics or antidiarrheal agents may be given. Antipyretics can be given for fever and analgesics for the headache and myalgia frequently associated with influenza. Nonsalicylate analgesics and antipyretics (for example, acetaminophen) are recommended for influenza-related fever and discomfort in children because of the risk of Reye's syndrome.

Community health nurses are frequently involved in educating the public regarding the symptoms of influenza and elements of self-care. They may also be instrumental in identifying clients who need professional care for severe infection. In such cases, community health nurses would plan to make a referral for medical care. If clients are seriously ill or markedly dehydrated, hospitalization may be necessary, and the nurse may need to plan an emergency referral.

BOX 30–15

National Objectives for the Year 2000 Related to Influenza

1. Reduce epidemic-related pneumonia and influenza deaths among people aged 65 and older to no more than 7.3 per 100,000.
2. Increase pneumococcal pneumonia and influenza immunization among institutionalized chronically ill or older people to at least 80%.
3. Increase pneumococcal pneumonia and influenza immunization among noninstitutionalized, high-risk populations to at least 60%.
4. Increase to at least 90% the proportion of public health departments that provide adult immunization for influenza and pneumococcal disease.

(Source: U.S. Department of Health and Human Services[87])

Tertiary Prevention

Tertiary prevention for the individual client involves preventing complications due to influenza. Clients who are infected should be cautioned by community health nurses not to overexert themselves. Particularly debilitating strains of influenza may require a relatively prolonged period of convalescence before the client is able to return to normal activity levels. Community health nurses may need to help clients give priority to their activities until they are fully recovered. For example, a mother with influenza may need to continue feeding her children if no other help is available, but she can suspend other activities until she is recuperated. Resuming one's former activity level before fully recuperating from influenza frequently leads to relapse or the onset of complications.

Another aspect of tertiary prevention with the individual is dealing with complications that do arise. Antibiotic therapy is warranted for persons with bacterial infections secondary to influenza. Again, community health nurses would plan to monitor the health status of persons with influenza, identifying those who have developed disease complications and referring them for appropriate treatment.

TABLE 30–13. PRIMARY, SECONDARY, AND TERTIARY PREVENTION MEASURES TO CONTROL INFLUENZA

Level of Prevention	Community Health Nurse Function	Goal
Primary prevention	• Educate clients on nutrition and health promotion	• General health promotion
	• Identify and refer persons at risk; provide immunizations	• Immunization of persons at risk
Secondary prevention	• Educate clients in symptom control	• Relief of symptoms
Tertiary prevention	• Educate clients for self-care and about signs of complications	• Prevent complications
	• Monitor for signs of complications and refer for treatment	• Prevent long-term consequences
	• Plan and implement mass immunization campaigns	• Prevent spread of disease through immunization

TABLE 30–14. RESOURCES FOR COMMUNICABLE DISEASE CONTROL

Agency or Organization	Focus
American Council for Healthful Living 439 Main St. Orange, NJ 07050 (201) 674-7476	Public education on sexually transmitted diseases
American Foundation for AIDS Research 40 W. 57th St. New York, NY 10019 (212) 333-3118	Research, public education
American Foundation for Prevention of Venereal Disease, Inc. 799 Broadway, Suite 638 New York, NY 10003 (212) 759-2069	Public education on sexually transmitted diseases
American Hepatitis Association 208 W. 13th St. New York, NY 10011 (212) 340-8986	Low-cost screening and vaccine, education, support groups, research
American Medical Association Order Department, OP-383 P.O. Box 821 Monroe, WI 53566	Educational materials on sexually transmitted diseases
American Social Health Association P.O. Box 13827 Research Triangle Park, NC 27709 (919) 361-2742	Research, information, education on sexually transmitted diseases; resources to assist in local control efforts
American Venereal Disease Association P.O. Box 22349 San Diego, CA 92122 (619) 453-3238	Assistance in efforts to decrease prevalence of sexually transmitted diseases
Center for Health Information P.O. Box 4636 Foster City, CA 94404 (415) 6669	Information on sexually transmitted diseases
Centers for Disease Control Center for Infectious Diseases 1600 Clifton Rd. Atlanta, GA 30333 (404) 329-3401 (404) 377-9563	Public information, research, policy formation Infoline, computerized AIDS information telephone service
Citizens' Alliance for VD Awareness 222 W. Adams St. Chicago, IL 60606 (312) 236-6339	Public information on sexually transmitted diseases
Herpes Resource Center/ASHA 260 Sheridan Ave., #307 Palo Alto, CA 94306 (415) 328-7710	Public information on herpes virus infection; support groups
Kaposi's Sarcoma Research and Education 470 Castro St., #207 P.O. Box 3360 San Francisco, CA 94114 (415) 864-4376	Research, education in Kaposi's sarcoma
March of Dimes Birth Defects Foundation 1275 Mamaroneck Ave. White Plains, NY 10605 (914) 428-7100	Public education on sexually transmitted diseases

TABLE 30–14. (*Continued*)

Agency or Organization	Focus
National AIDS Information Clearinghouse P.O. Box 6003 Rockville, MD 20850 (800) 342-AIDS (800) 344-SIDA	Information materials on AIDS AIDS information hotline—English AIDS information hotline—Spanish
National Institute of Allergy and Infectious Diseases Office of Communications Building 31, Room 7A32 9000 Rockville Pike Bethesda, MD 20892 (301) 496-5717	Research, public information
Operation Venus 1213 Clover St. Philadelphia, PA 19107 (215) 567-6969	Toll-free hot line for STD services in Pennsylvania; assistance to groups in other areas to start similar service
Pacific Financial Companies Products Information Office—4 P.O. Box 9000 Newport Beach, CA 92658-9952 (800) 544-3600	Material on AIDS education in the workplace
People with AIDS Coalition 236A W. 19th St. #125 New York, NY 10011 (212) 627-1810	Support for clients with AIDS, research, public education
San Francisco AIDS Foundation 333 Valencia St., 4th Floor P.O. Box 6182 San Francisco, CA 94101-6182 (415) 864-4376	Public education on AIDS prevention; assistance to those with AIDS for housing, Social Scurity, medical, and legal referrals
Shanti Project 890 Hayes St. San Francisco, CA 94117 (415) 558-9644	Counseling and support for those with AIDS and loved ones; assistance with hospice, housing; public information and education on AIDS
State AIDS Policy Center Intergovernmental Health Policy Center 2011 I Street, NW, Suite 200 Washington, DC 20006	Information on AIDS, policy formation
VD National Hotline 260 Sheridan Ave. Palo Alto, CA 94306 (415) 327-6465	Information on sexually transmitted diseases, referral for services
World Health Organization Collaborating Center on AIDS ℅ Centers for Disease Control 1600 Clifton Rd., NE Atlanta, GA 30333 (404) 239-3311	Coordinates international efforts for AIDS control
World Health Organization Publications Centre USA ℅ Lloyd Publications 49 Sheridan Ave. Albany, NY 12210 (518) 436-9686	Educational materials on sexually transmitted diseases

Tertiary prevention measures used with other diseases to prevent spread are not routinely employed for influenza. Contact notification is not useful because of the short incubation period of the disease. Contacts at high risk for fatality may be provided with chemoprophylaxis and immunization provided for those not yet exposed. Both of these measures may limit the spread of disease within the population. Community health nurses are likely to be involved in immunization as a tertiary as well as a primary preventive measure. Isolating persons with influenza is usually not practical because of the short incubation of the disease.[14] Occasionally, schools and other institutions may be closed in major epidemics to limit the spread of disease to any persons who are not already infected, but more often because there are too few teachers, students, or employees well enough to make it practical to keep the institution operating. Primary, secondary, and tertiary measures for control of influenza are presented in Table 30–13. Resources for information related to the control of influenza and other communicable diseases discussed in this chapter are presented in Table 30–14.

EVALUATING CONTROL STRATEGIES FOR INFLUENZA

Evaluating the extent to which the 1990 objective for influenza immunization has been achieved is one way of assessing the effectiveness of primary prevention strategies in the control of influenza in a community. The objective was for 60 percent of people in high-risk groups to receive annual immunization for influenza. At the national level, the percentage of those in these groups who have been immunized has not changed appreciably since 1979, with less than 20 percent of high-risk persons immunized by 1985.[25] Approximately 62 percent of nursing home residents in six states had been immunized.[87] The community health nurse would examine the extent to which immunization coverage had been achieved in his or her community. In the future, national objectives related to influenza for the year 2000 may serve as evaluative criteria for the effectiveness of intervention. These objectives are summarized in Box 30–15. Other criteria for evaluating the effectiveness of control measures for influenza include the annual incidence of the disease and complications and mortality attributable to influenza.

CHAPTER HIGHLIGHTS

- Despite the use of antibiotics and improved sanitation measures, several communicable diseases continue to contribute to the morbidity and mortality experienced by human beings.
- Epidemiologic factors contributing to communicable diseases create what is sometimes referred to as a chain of infection consisting of an infected person, the infectious agent, the reservoir in which the agent is found, the mode by which the agent is transmitted, the agent's portals of entry and exit, and the new host.
- Communicable diseases can be spread by several modes of transmission, including airborne, fecal-oral, direct contact, and sexual transmission, as well as transmission by direct inoculation, by animal or insect bite, or by contact with soil or inanimate objects containing the agent.
- An agent's portal of entry is its means of infecting the host and may include the respiratory tract, gastrointestinal tract, skin and mucous membrane, the circulatory system, and across the placental barrier from mother to fetus.
- An agent's portal of exit is the means by which it leaves the infected person. Portals of exit include the respiratory tract, feces, the skin and mucous membrane, blood, and saliva.
- The incubation period of a communicable disease is the time from exposure to the agent to the development of symptoms of the disease.
- The prodromal period associated with some communicable diseases is the time from the appearance of early symptoms of the disease to the development of symptoms that typify the disease.
- Community health nursing roles related to the control of communicable diseases include contact notification, providing chemoprophylaxis, education, immunization, case finding, referral, treatment, supportive care, and political activity.
- Two major approaches to the control of communicable diseases are preventing the spread of the disease and increasing host resistance to the disease. Preventing the spread of disease may be accomplished by eliminating the infectious agent or preventing its transmission to others through contact notification and chemoprophylaxis. General health promotion and immunization are the two major means of increasing host resistance.
- Childhood diseases of particular concern to community health nurses include measles, rubella, mumps, diphtheria, pertussis, tetanus, poliomyelitis, and diseases caused by HiB.
- Children are generally more susceptible than adults to childhood diseases, but adults more

often experience severe cases and complications.

- Crowded living conditions, poverty, unemployment, lower educational levels, and religion are environmental factors that may influence development of childhood diseases.
- Intravenous drug use and occupation as well as a present-oriented life-style that does not emphasize prevention of disease may contribute to the incidence of childhood diseases.
- Health system factors contributing to childhood diseases include lack of access to health-care services and failure to educate the public about immunization for childhood diseases.
- Primary prevention for childhood diseases includes immunization for measles, rubella, mumps, diphtheria, pertussis, tetanus, poliomyelitis, and HiB infection. Chemoprophylaxis is available for persons exposed to measles, diphtheria, pertussis, tetanus, and HiB infection.
- Secondary prevention for all communicable diseases involves diagnosis and treatment, although treatment for measles, rubella, mumps, and poliomyelitis is symptomatic and supportive rather than curative in nature. Screening is not usually employed as a secondary prevention measure for childhood diseases.
- Tertiary prevention in childhood diseases entails preventing or dealing with complications of disease in individuals and preventing the spread of disease in the community. Preventing the recurrence of disease is not usually necessary because of antibody development following most of these diseases.
- Young adults and males are most at risk for HIV infection of AIDS, although incidence of disease in children and women is increasing.
- Susceptibility to HIV infection and its consequences is enhanced by conditions requiring blood transfusion or organ transplantation, pregnancy, cervicitis or vaginitis, menstruation, and the presence of genital ulcers. HIV infection also increases one's susceptibility to a variety of diseases.
- Environmental factors that contribute to HIV infection and its effects include social mores that foster high-risk behaviors, fear and anxiety related to HIV infection and AIDS, lack of knowledge of risk factors, the presence of residential facilities for the mentally incapaicitated, and the extent of social support available to persons with AIDS.
- Life-style factors influencing the development of HIV infection include sexual activity, intravenous drug use, and occupations that lead to exposure to infected persons. Combined sexual activity and drug use is particularly significant in developing HIV infection.
- Health system factors influencing HIV infection include the use of contaminated blood and other bodily tissues, health-care costs for persons with AIDS, lack of adequate care facilities, and transmission of infection from infected health-care providers to their clients.
- Primary prevention in HIV infection currently focuses on preventing the spread of infection by avoiding high-risk sexual and drug-use behaviors, screening of blood and organ donors, and preventing opportunistic infections in persons who are already infected.
- Secondary prevention of HIV infection may include measures aimed at screening, diagnosis, and treatment. Treatment of HIV infection with zidovudine (formerly AZT) may slow the progression of disease. Treatment of opportunistic infection is also necessary.
- Tertiary prevention in HIV infection involves preventing the spread of infection through contact notification, preventing recurrent opportunistic infections, modifying routine health-care measures as needed, and providing assistance in dealing with the social and psychological implications of infection.
- Epidemiologic factors in other sexually transmitted diseases are similar to those for HIV infection except that gonorrhea, chlamydia, and herpes simplex virus (HSV) infection are not spread via direct inoculation.
- Curative treatment is available for gonorrhea, syphilis, and chlamydial infection, but not for hepatitis B or HSV infection.
- Poor sanitation and hygiene are the major contributing factors in the epidemiology of hepatitis A and enterically transmitted NANB hepatitis, while intravenous drug use is the primary contributor to parenterally transmitted NANB hepatitis.
- Adequate sanitation and good hygiene are the major primary preventative measures for hepatitis A and enterically transmitted NANB hepatitis, while avoiding unsafe drug-use practices will prevent parenterally transmitted NANB hepatitis. Treatment for both forms of hepatitis is symptomatic.

(*continued*)

- The very young and the elderly are at greatest risk for both influenza and tuberculosis, and conditions of poverty and overcrowding, poor nutrition, and fatigue increase one's susceptibility to both diseases.
- Control of tuberculosis involves general health promotion, screening, contact notification and chemoprophylaxis, and treatment of active cases. BCG immunization is not generally used in the United States because it invalidates the TB skin test as a screening tool.
- Control of influenza involves annual immunization of those at risk, symptomatic treatment of persons with disease, and preventing complications of disease.
- National health objectives for 1990 and the year 2000 may be used to evaluate the effectiveness of control measures for communicable diseases.

Review Questions

1. Describe the trends in at least five major communicable diseases. Identify at least one factor contributing to each of these trends. (pp. 738, 748, 767, 782, 787, 793)
2. What are the six major modes of transmission for communicable diseases? Describe a preventative strategy that would be appropriate to each mode of transmission. (p. 733)
3. Identify at least four roles for community health nurses in controlling communicable diseases. Give an example of a nursing activity that might be performed by a nurse in fulfilling each role. (p. 735)
4. Name the two major approaches to the control of communicable diseases. Give an example of how each approach might be implemented. (p. 735)
5. Discuss the influences of at least two factors in each component of the epidemiologic perspective dealing with childhood diseases. (p. 739)
6. Describe at least two nursing interventions for controlling childhood diseases at each level of prevention. (p. 742)
7. Compare and contrast the epidemiologic factors contributing the HIV infection and other sexually transmitted diseases. (pp. 751, 769)
8. Describe at least two nursing interventions for controlling HIV infection and other sexually transmitted diseases related to each level of prevention. (p. 759)
9. Discuss the influence of at least two factors in each of the components of the epidemiologic perspective on the development of hepatitis A and NANB hepatitis. (p. 782)
10. Describe at least two nursing interventions for controlling hepatitis A and NANB hepatitis related to each level of prevention. (p. 785)
11. Discuss the influence of at least two factors in each of the components of the epidemiologic perspective on the development of tuberculosis. (p. 787)
12. Describe at least two nursing interventions for controlling tuberculosis related to each level of prevention. (p. 789)
13. Discuss the influence of at least two factors in each of the components of the epidemiologic perspective on the development of influenza. (p. 793)
14. Describe at least two nursing interventions for controlling influenza related to each level of prevention. (p. 796)

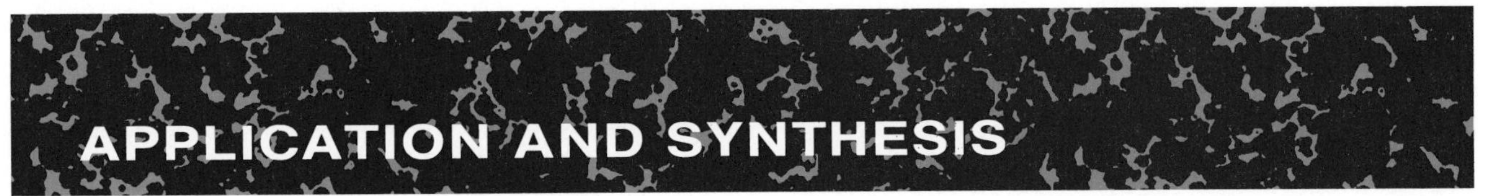

APPLICATION AND SYNTHESIS

Jane is an 18-year-old college student. She lives in the dorm with her roommate, Sally. Shortly after Jane returned from Christmas vacation, she developed a fever and a rash. She didn't feel too bad, but Sally persuaded her to see a doctor. Because it was Saturday, Jane went to the emergency room of the local hospital. The physician there made a diagnosis of rubella. Later that night he and the nurses in the ER became very busy with victims of a multi-car accident. As a result no one completed the health department form reporting Jane's rubella until 2 days later.

By the time a community health nurse contacted Jane to complete a rubella case report, Sally and several other girls in Jane's dorm also developed rubella. Sally gave it to her boy friend, who exposed those in his classes. One of the women in his English class is pregnant.

1. What primary preventive measures could have been employed to prevent this situation? What primary prevention measures are appropriate at this point?
2. What secondary and tertiary measures by the community health nurse are appropriate at this time?
3. What roles will the community health nurse perform in dealing with this situation.

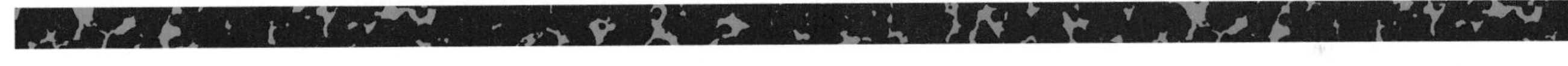

REFERENCES

1. Centers for Disease Control. (1990, October). *HIV/AIDS Surveillance*. Atlanta: Centers for Disease Control.
2. Update: Acquired immunodeficiency syndrome—Europe. (1990). *MMWR, 39*, 850–853.
3. Murphy, J. S. (1988). Women with AIDS. In I. B. Corless & M. Pittman-Lindeman (Eds.), *AIDS: Principles, practices and policies* (pp. 65–79). New York: Hemisphere.
4. Partner notification for preventing human immunodeficiency virus (HIV) infection—Colorado, Idaho, South Carolina, Virginia. (1988). *MMWR, 37*, 393–402.
5. Broder, S., & Fauci, A. S. (1988). Progress in drug therapies for HIV infection. *Public Health Reports, 103*, 224–229.
6. Measles—United States, 1986. (1987). *MMWR, 36*, 301–305.
7. Summary of notifiable diseases, United States—1988. (1989). *MMWR, 37*(54), 1–57.
8. American Academy of Pediatrics, Committee on Infectious Diseases. (1989b). Measles: Reassessment of the current immunization policy. *Pediatrics, 84*, 1110–1113.
9. Update: Measles outbreak—Chicago, 1989. (1990). *MMWR, 39*, 317–319, 325–326.
10. Measles—Los Angeles County, California, 1988. (1989). *MMWR, 38*, 49–57.
11. Rubella and congenital rubella syndrome—United States, 1985–1988. (1989) *MMWR, 38*, 173–182.
12. Increase in rubella and congenital rubella syndrome—United States, 1988–1990. (1991). *MMWR, 40*, 93–99.
13. Summary of notifiable diseases, United States—1989. (1990). *MMWR, 38*(54), 1–59.
14. Benenson, A. S. (Ed.). (1990). *Control of communicable diseases in man* (15th ed.). Washington, DC: American Public Health Association.
15. Koblin, B., & Townsend, T. (1989). Immunity to diphtheria and tetanus in inner-city women of child-bearing age. *American Journal of Public Health, 79*, 1297–1298.
16. Haemophilus influenzae type B. (1985). Evansville, IN: Mead Johnson.
17. Measles outbreak—Chicago, 1989. (1989). *MMWR, 38*, 591–596.
18. Mathias, R., Meekison, W., Arcand, T., & Schechter, M. (1989). The role of secondary vaccine failures in measles outbreaks. *American Journal of Public Health, 79*, 475–478.

19. Measles—United States, 1988. (1989). *MMWR, 38,* 601–605.
20. Immunization recommendations for health care workers. (1989). Atlanta: U.S. Department of Health and Human Services.
21. American Academy of Pediatrics, Committee on Infectious Diseases. (1989a). *Haemophilus influenza Type b Conjugate vaccines: Update. 84,* 386–387.
22. State of California, Department of Health Services. (1991). *Haemophilus influenzae type B immunization guidelines.* Sacremento: State of California, Department of Health Services.
23. Harrison, L. H., Broome, C. V., Hightower, A. W., & Haemophilus Vaccine Efficacy Study Group. (1989). Haemophilus influenzae type b polysaccharide vaccine: An efficacy study. *Pediatrics, 84,* 225–261.
24. United States Preventive Services Task Force. (1989). *Guide to clinical preventive services.* Baltimore: Williams & Wilkins.
25. United States Department of Health and Human Services. (1990). *Health—United States, 1989.* Hyattsville, MD: Public Health Service.
26. Institute of Medicine, National Academy of Sciences. (1988). *Confronting AIDS: Update 88.* Washington DC: National Academy Press.
27. Hughes, J. P. (1989). Report on a symposium: Occupational HIV infection: Risk and risk reduction. *Health Hazards, 1*(3), 1–6.
28. AIDS and human immunodeficiency virus infection in the United States: 1988 update. (1989). *MMWR, 38*(S-4), 1–38.
29. Estimates of HIV prevalence and projected AIDS cases. (1990). *MMWR, 39,* 110–112, 117–119.
30. Dentzer, S. (1988, January). Why AIDS won't bankrupt us. *U. S. News & World Report,* pp. 20–22.
31. Seage, G., Landers, S., Mayer, K. H., et al. (1988). Medical costs of ambulatory patients with AIDS-related complex. *American Journal of Public Health, 78,* 969–970.
32. Centers for Disease Control. (1987). Revision of the CDC surveillance case definition for acquired immunodeficiency syndrome. *MMWR, 36*(1S), 1S–15S.
33. AIDS in women—United States. (1990). *MMWR, 39,* 845–846.
34. Antibody to human immunodeficiency virus in female prostitutes. (1987). *MMWR, 36,* 157–161.
35. Prevalence of human immunodeficiency virus antibody in U.S. active-duty military personnel, April, 1988. (1988). *MMWR, 37,* 461–463.
36. Rogers, M. F. (1987). Transmission of human immunodeficiency virus infection. In B. K. Silverman & A. Waddell (Eds.), *Report of the Surgeon General's Workshop.* Washington, DC: U.S. Department of Health and Human Services.
37. Tuberculosis and AIDS—Connecticut. (1987). *MMWR, 36,* 133–135.
38. Increase in pneumonia mortality among young adults in the HIV epidemic—New York City, United States. (1988). *MMWR, 38,* 593–596.
39. Update: Acquired immunodeficiency syndrome—United States, 1981–1988. (1989). *MMWR, 38,* 229–235.
40. Marchetti, A., Nathanson, R., Kastner, T., & Owens, R. (1990). AIDS and state developmental disability agencies: A national survey. *American Journal of Public Health, 80,* 54–56.
41. DeClemente, R., Boyer, C., & Morales, E. (1988). Minorities and AIDS: Knowledge, attitudes, and misconceptions among black and Latino adolescents. *American Journal of Public Health, 78,* 55–57.
42. McGough, K. N. (1990). Assessing social support of people with AIDS. *Oncology Nursing Forum, 17*(1), 31–35.
43. Update: Heterosexual transmission of AIDS and HIV infection—U.S. (1989). *MMWR, 38,* 423–434.
44. McCusker, J., Stoddard, A., Mayer, K., et al. (1988), Effects of HIB antibody test knowledge on subsequent sexual behaviors in a cohort of homosexually active men. *American Journal of Public Health, 78,* 462–467.
45. Paalman, M. E. (1988, November). Safer sex. *World Health,* pp. 14–15.
46. Number of sex partners and potential risk of sexual exposure to HIV. (1988). *MMWR, 37,* 565–568.
47. Valdiserri, R., Lyter, D., Leviton, L., et al. (1988). Variables influencing condom use in a cohort of gay and bisexual men. *American Journal of Public Health, 88,* 801–805.
48. Feldblum, P. J., & Fortney, J. A. (1988). Condoms, spermicides, and transmission of human immunodeficiency virus: A review of the literature. *American Journal of Public Health, 78,* 52–54.
49. Mascola, L., Lieb, L., Iwskoshi, K., et al. (1989). HIV seroprevalence in intravenous drug users. *American Journal of Public Health, 79,* 81–82.
50. Distribution of AIDS cases, by racial/ethnic group and exposure category, United States, June 1, 1981–July 4, 1988. (1988). *MMWR, 37,* 1–10.
51. Selik, R. M., Castro, K. G., & Pappaioanou, M. (1988). Racial/ethnic differences in the risk of AIDS in the United States. *American Journal of Public Health, 78,* 1539–1545.
52. Urine testing for drug use among male arrestees—United States, 1989. (1989). *MMWR, 38,* 780–783.
53. Magura, S., Grossman, J., Lipton, D., et al. (1989). Determinants of needle sharing among intravenous drug users. *American Journal of Public Health, 79,* 459–462.
54. Magura, S., Shapiro, J., Siddiqi, Q., & Lipton, D. (1990). Variables influencing condom use among intravenous drug users. *American Journal of Public Health, 80,* 82–84.
55. Update: Acquired immunodeficiency syndrome and human immunodeficiency virus infection among health-care workers. (1988). *MMWR, 37,* 229–239.
56. Kelley, P. W., Miller, R., N., Pomerantz, R., et al. (1990). Human immunodeficiency virus seropositivity among members of the active duty U.S. Army, 1985–1989. *American Journal of Public Health, 80,* 405–410.

57. Update: Universal precautions for prevention of transmission of human immunodeficiency virus, hepatitis virus and other bloodborne pathogens in health-care settings. (1988). *MMWR, 37,* 377–388.
58. Human immunodeficiency virus infection transmitted from an organ donor screened for HIV antibody—North Carolina. (1987). *MMWR, 36,* 306–313.
59. Transmission of HIV through bone transplantation: Case report and public health recommendations. (1988). *MMWR, 37,* 597–599.
60. HIV-1 infection and artificial insemination with processed semen. (1990). *MMWR, 39,* 249, 255–256.
61. Buchanan, R. J. (1988). State Medicaid coverage of AZT and AIDS-related policies. *American Journal of Public Health, 78,* 437–438.
62. Faden, R. R., & Kass, N. E. (1988). Health insurance and AIDS: The status of state regulatory activity. *American Journal of Public Health, 78,* 437–438.
63. Human tests starting on possible AIDS vaccine. (1990). *Legislative Network for Nurses, 7*(22), 172.
64. Bateson, M. C., & Goldsby, R. (1988). *Thinking AIDS: The social response to the biological threat.* Reading, MA: Addison-Wesley.
65. Solomon, M., & DeJong, W. (1989). Preventing AIDS and other STDs through condom promotion: A patient education intervention. *American Journal of Public Health, 79,* 453–458.
66. Coordinated community programs for HIV prevention among intravenous-drug users—California, Massachusetts. (1989). *MMWR, 38,* 369–378.
67. Kegeles, S. M., Adler, N. E., & Irwin, C. E., Jr. (1988). Sexually active adolescents and condoms: Changes over one year in knowledge, attitudes and use. *American Journal of Public Health, 78,* 460–461.
68. HIV epidemic and AIDS: Trends in knowledge—United States, 1987 and 1988. (1989). *MMWR, 38,* 353–363.
69. Van Griensven, G., de Vroome, E., Tielman, R., et al. (1988). Impact of HIV antibody testing on changes in sexual behavior among homosexual men in the Netherlands. *American Journal of Public Health, 78,* 1575–1576.
70. Interpretation and use of the Western blot assay for serodiagnosis of human immunodeficiency virus type 1 infections. (1989). *MMWR, 38*(S-7), 1–7.
71. Brandt, A. (1988). AIDS in historical perspective: Four lessons from the history of sexually transmitted diseases. *American Journal of Public Health, 78,* 367–371.
72. Novello, A. (1989). Final report of the United States Department of Health and Human Services Secretary's Work Group on Pediatric Human Immunodeficiency Virus infection and disease. *Pediatrics, 84,* 547–555.
73. Rutherford, G. W., Oliva, G. E., & Grossman, M. (1987). Guidelines for the control of perinatally transmitted human immunodeficiency virus infection and care of infected mothers, infants and children. *Western Journal of Medicine, 147,* 104–108.
74. PHS guidelines for counseling and antibody testing to prevent HIV infection and AIDS. (1987). *MMWR, 36,* 509–515.
75. McKillip, J. (1991). Public health and the law: The effect of mandatory premarital HIV testing on marriage: The case of Illinois. *American Journal of Public Health, 81,* 650–653.
76. HIV infection reporting—United States. (1989). *MMWR, 38,* 496–499.
77. Judson, F. (1989). What do we really know about AIDS control? *American Journal of Public Health, 79,* 878–882.
78. Eisenstaedt, R. S., & Getzen, T. E. (1988). Screening blood donors for human immunodeficiency virus antibody: Cost-benefit analysis. *American Journal of Public Health, 78,* 450–454.
79. Pizzo, P. A., Eddy, J., & Falloon, J. (1988). Effect of continuous intravenous infusion of zidovudine (AZT) in children with symptomatic HIV infection. *The New England Journal of Medicine, 319,* 888–896.
80. Centers for Disease Control. (1991). Guidelines for prophylaxis against *Pneumocystis carinii* pneumonia for children infected with human immunodeficiency virus. *MMWR, 40*(no. RR-2), 1–13.
81. ACIP: General recommendations on immunization. (1989). *MMWR, 38,* 205–227.
82. Tuberculosis and human immunodeficiency virus infection. (1989). *MMWR, 38,* 850–854.
83. Potterat, J., Spencer, N., Woodhouse, D., & Muth, J. (1989). Partner notification in the control of human immunodeficiency virus infection. *American Journal of Public Health, 79,* 874–875.
84. Coates, W., Jr., & Handsfield, H. H., (1988). HIV counseling and testing: Does it work? *American Journal of Public Health, 78,* 1533–1534.
85. Schechter, M., Craib, K., Willoughby, B., et al. (1988). Patterns of sexual behavior and condom use in a cohort of homosexual men. *American Journal of Public Health, 78,* 1539–1545.
86. Howe, E. G. (1988). Ethical aspects of military physicians treating service persons with HIV. Part three: The duty to protect third parties. *Military Medicine, 153,* 140–144.
87. United States Department of Health and Human Services. (1991). *Healthy people 2000: National health promotion and disease prevention objectives.* Washington, DC: Government Printing Office.
88. Primary and secondary syphilis—United States, 1981–1990. (1991). *MMWR, 40,* 314–315, 321–323.
89. Guidelines for the prevention and control of congenital syphilis. (1988). *MMWR, 37*(S-1), 1–13.
90. Congenital syphilis—New York City, 1986–1988. (1989). *MMWR, 38,* 825–829.
91. Barnes, R. C., & Holmes, K. K. (1984). Epidemiology of gonorrhea: Current perspectives. *Epidemiologic Reviews, 6,* 1–30.
92. Antibiotic-resistant strains of *Neisseria gonorrhoeae.* (1987). *MMWR, 36*(5S), 1S-18S.
93. Becker, T. M., Stone, K. M., & Cates, W., Jr. (1986). Epidemiology of genital herpes infections in the United States: The current situation. *The Journal of Reproductive Medicine, 31,* 359–362.
94. CDC's director for STDs gives an overview. (1989, May-June). *The Nation's Health,* p. 16–17.

95. ACIP: Update on hepatitis B prevention. (1987). *MMWR, 36,* 353–366.
96. ACIP: Recommendation for protection against viral hepatitis. (1985). *MMWR, 34,* 313–335.
97. Gerber, A., King, L., Dunleavy, G., & Novick, L. (1989). An outbreak of syphilis on an Indian reservation: Descriptive epidemiology and disease-control measures. *American Journal of Public Health, 79,* 83–85.
98. Guinan, M. E., Wolinsky, S. M., & Reichman, R. C. (1985). Epidemiology of genital herpes simplex virus infection. *Epidemiologic Reviews, 7,* 127–146.
99. Schreeder, M. (1988). Viral hepatitis. *Primary Care, 15,* 157–173.
100. Becker, T. M., Blount, J. H., & Guinan, M. E. (1985). Genital herpes infections in private practice in the United States, 1966 to 1981. *JAMA, 253,* 1601–1603.
101. Racial differences in rates of hepatitis B virus infection—United States, 1976–1980. (1989). *MMWR, 38,* 818–821.
102. Pariser, H. (1989). Syphilis. *Primary Care, 16,* 603–619.
103. Syphilis and congenital syphilis—United States, 1985–1988. (1988). *MMWR, 37,* 486–489.
104. Changing patterns of groups at high risk for hepatitis B in the United States. (1988). *MMWR, 37,* 429–437.
105. Landrum, S., Beck-Sague, C., & Kraus, S. (1988). Racial trends in syphilis among men with same-sex partners in Atlanta, Georgia. *American Journal of Public Health, 78,* 66–77.
106. Chlamydia trachomatis infections. (1985). *MMWR, 34*(3S), 53S–74S.
107. Multiple strain outbreak of PPNG—Denver, Colorado, 1986. (1987). *MMWR, 36,* 534–543.
108. Outbreak of hepatitis B associated with an oral surgeon—New Hampshire. (1987). *MMWR, 36,* 132–133.
109. Continuing increase in infectious syphilis—United States. (1988). *MMWR, 37,* 35–47.
110. Hepatitis B associated with jet-gun injection—California. (1986). *MMWR, 35,* 373–376.
111. Protection against viral hepatitis: Recommendations of the Immunization Practices Advisory Committee. (1990). *MMWR, 39*(No. RR-2), 1–26.
112. Sexually transmitted diseases treatment guidelines. (1989). *MMWR, 38*(S-8), 1–43.
113. Haskell, R. J. (1984). A cost-benefit analysis of California's mandatory premarital screening program for syphilis. *The Western Journal of Medicine, 141,* 538–541.
114. Poss, J. (1989). Hepatitis D virus infection. *Nurse Practitioner, 14,* 12–18.
115. Williams. R. (1986). Prevalence of hepatitis A virus antibody among Navajo school children. *American Journal of Public Health, 76,* 282–283.
116. Enterically transmitted non-A, non-B hepatitis—Mexico. (1987). *MMWR, 36,* 597–601.
117. Non-A, non-B hepatitis—Illinois. (1989). *MMWR, 38,* 529–531.
118. Harkness, J., Gildon, B., & Istre, G. (1989). Outbreaks of hepatitis A among illicit drug users, Oklahoma, 1984–1987. *American Journal of Public Health, 79,* 463–466.
119. Hepatitis A among drug abusers. (1988). *MMWR, 37,* 297–305.
120. ACIP: Use of BCG vaccines in the control of tuberculosis: A joint statement by the ACIP and the Advisory Committee for Elimination of Tuberculosis. (1988). *MMWR, 37,* 663–675.
121. Tuberculosis, final data—United States, 1986. (1988). *MMWR, 36,* 817–820.
122. Tuberculosis in blacks—United States, (1987). *MMWR, 36,* 212–220.
123. Tuberculosis among Asians/Pacific Islanders—United States, 1985. (1987). *MMWR, 36,* 331–334.
124. Tuberculosis among American Indian and Alaskan natives—United States, 1985. (1987). *MMWR, 36,* 493–495.
125. A strategic plan for the elimination of tuberculosis in the United States. (1989). *MMWR, 38*(S-3), 1–25.
126. Bacteriologic conversion of sputum among tuberculosis patients—United States. (1985). *MMWR, 34,* 747–750.
127. Kopanoff, D., Snider, D., & Johnson, M. (1988). Recurrent tuberculosis: Why do patients develop disease again? A United States Public Health Service cooperative survey. *American Journal of Public Health, 78,* 30–33.
128. Pneumonia and influenza mortality on the increase. (1987, April-June). *Statistical Bulletin,* 10–16.
129. ACIP: Prevention and control of influenza: Part 1. Vaccines. (1989). *MMWR, 38,* 297–311.
130. Prevention and control of influenza: Recommendations of the Immunization Practices Advisory Committee. (1990). *MMWR, 39*(no. RR-7), 1–15.

RECOMMENDED READINGS

Benenson, A. S. (Ed.). (1990). *Control of communicable diseases in man* (15th ed.). Washington, DC: American Public Health Association.

Presents an overview of the epidemiology and control of communicable diseases affecting humankind.

Centers for Disease Control. *HIV/AIDS Surveillance*

A quarterly publication by the Centers for Disease Control that provides the most up-to-date figures on the incidence of HIV infection and AIDS. Also contains information on sources of exposure, mortality, and incidence among specific age, sex, and racial/ethnic groups in the United States.

Centers for Disease Control. *Morbidity and Mortality Weekly Report* (MMWR).

A weekly publication based on data from the Centers for Disease Control. Addresses recent trends in the incidence of a variety of communicable and noncommunicable conditions and on the epidemiologic factors contributing to them.

Cummings, D. (1988). Caring for the HIV-infected adult. *Nurse Practitioner, 13* (11), 28–47.

Describes the clinical manifestations of HIV infection and management plans for common health problems in HIV-infected clients.

Durham, J., & Cohen, F. L. (1991). *The person with AIDS: Nursing perspectives* (2nd ed.). New York: Springer.

Examines the nursing care of persons with AIDS as well as the epidemiology of AIDS. Also deals with ethical issues in the care of people with AIDS.

Grimes, D.E. (1991). *Infectious diseases.* St. Louis: Mosby-Yearbook.

Presents the epidemiology, clinical presentation, pathophysiology, complications, diagnosis, treatment, and nursing care related to communicable diseases. Addresses assessment of clients with communicable diseases as well as relevant nursing diagnoses and interventions.

Gibbons, W. (1991). Cluing in on chlamydia: Microbial stealth leads to reproductive ravages. *Science News, 139*(16), 205–252.

Discusses the role of Chlamydia trachomatis *in PID (pelvic inflammatory disease) and infertility in women.*

Huber, J., & Schneider, B. E. (1991). *The social context of AIDS.* Newbury Park, CA: Sage.

Addresses social issues in the prevention of AIDS and high-risk behaviors contributing to HIV infection.

Mays, V. M., Albee, G. W., & Schneider, S. F. (Eds.). (1989). *Primary prevention of AIDS: Psychological approaches.* Newbury Park, CA: Sage.

Sets forth findings of research on preventing high-risk behaviors related to HIV infection. Discusses the implications of research findings for controlling the AIDS epidemic.

McGough, K. N. (1990). Assessing social support of people with AIDS. *Oncology Nursing Forum, 17*(1), 31–35.

Presents a tool for systematically assessing the social support available to persons with AIDS.

Ungvarski, P. (1988). Assessment: The key to nursing an AIDS patient. *RN, 51*(9), 28–33.

Describes approaches for obtaining a sexual history from clients at risk for HIV infection and nursing interventions to prevent or deal with HIV infection.

CHAPTER 31

Chronic Physical Health Problems

KEY TERMS

chronic health problems
disability
years of potential life lost (YPLL)

Because of the effectiveness of control measures developed for many previously fatal communicable diseases, chronic health problems have largely replaced communicable disease as the leading causes of death and disability in the United States. Each year millions of people experience the suffering and the economic costs associated with chronic conditions, and many die as a result of these health problems. Coronary heart disease, for example, kills more than 500,000 Americans and costs the U.S. economy over $50 billion annually.[1]

Chronic health problems are those that are present for extended periods of time and that are characterized by one or more distinctive features. These features may include nonreversible pathological changes, a need for life-style adjustment, or a prolonged period of supervision and care by health professionals.[2] Chronic conditions are also frequently characterized by ***disability***, or an inability to perform one or more functions of everyday life satisfactorily.

Chronic health problems may be either physical or emotional in nature, and both types of chronic conditions are addressed in the national health objectives developed for the year 2000. The focus of this chapter, however, is chronic physical health problems, and relevant national objectives are summarized in Box 31–1. Chronic conditions of an emotional nature are addressed in Chapter 32, Chronic Mental Health Problems.

LEARNING OBJECTIVES

After reading this chapter you should be able to:

- Identify at least three major roles for community health nurses in controlling chronic physical health problems.
- Describe at least three personal effects and four population effects of chronic physical health problems.
- Identify at least three human biological factors that influence the development of chronic physical health problems.
- Describe at least two factors related to the physical, psychological, and social environments that influence chronic physical health problems and their consequences.
- Identify at least five life-style factors that contribute to the development of chronic physical health problems.
- Describe three health system factors that impede efforts to control chronic physical health problems.
- Describe at least four general approaches to primary prevention of chronic physical health problems.
- Identify at least three aspects to the treatment of chronic physical health problems.
- Describe five considerations in tertiary prevention of chronic physical health problems.

BOX 31–1

Summary of Selected National Health Objectives for the Year 2000 Related to Chronic Physical Health Problems

- Increase length of healthy life to at least 65 years.
- Reduce to no more than 8% the proportion of people who experience a major activity limitation due to chronic conditions.
- Reduce coronary heart disease deaths to no more than 100 per 100,000 people.
- Reduce stroke deaths to no more than 20 per 100,000 people.
- Increase the proportion of people with high blood pressure whose blood pressure is under control to at least 50%.
- Reduce the mean serum cholesterol level among adults to no more than 200 mg/dL.
- Reduce dietary fat intake to an average of 30% of calories and saturated fat intake to less than 10% of calories.
- Increase foods with complex carbohydrates and fiber to 5 or more servings of vegetables and fruits and 6 or more servings of grain products per day for adults.
- Reduce the prevalence of overweight to no more than 20% among people aged 20 and older.
- Increase to at least 30% the proportion of people aged 6 and older who engage in regular exercise.
- Reduce cigarette smoking to no more than 15% of people aged 20 and older.
- Establish tobacco-free environments and include tobacco-use prevention in the curricula of all elementary, middle, and secondary schools.
- Enact laws in all 50 states prohibiting or strictly limiting smoking in the workplace and enclosed public places.
- Reverse the rise in cancer deaths to no more than 130 per 100,000 population.
- Reduce cancer deaths to:
  a. 42 per 100,000 population for lung cancer
  b. 20.6 per 100,000 women for breast cancer
  c. 1.3 per 100,000 women for cervical cancer
  d. 13.2 per 100,000 population for colorectal cancer
- Increase to at least 60% the proportion of people who limit sun exposure or use sun screen or protective clothing.
- Increase to at least 80% the proportion of women aged 40 and older who have ever had a clinical breast examination and a mammogram.
- Increase to at least 95% the proportion of women aged 18 and older who have ever had a Pap test.
- Reduce diabetes-related deaths to no more than 34 per 100,000 population.
- Reduce diabetes incidence to no more than 2.5 per 1000 population.
- Slow the rise in deaths due to chronic obstructive pulmonary disease (COPD) to a rate of no more than 25 per 100,000 people.
- Reduce hospitalizations from nonfatal accidental injuries to no more than 754 per 100,000 population.
- Reduce the incidence of secondary disabilities due to injuries of the head and spinal cord to no more than 16 and 2.6 per 100,000 people, respectively.
- Increase use of occupant protection systems (seat belts, child safety seats) to at least 85% of motor vehicle occupants.
- Increase use of helmets to at least 80% of motorcyclists and 50% of bicylists.
- Extend to all 50 states laws requiring safety belt and motorcycle helmet use for all ages.
- Reduce work-related injuries requiring medical treatment, lost time from work, or restricted work activity to no more than 6 cases per 100 full-time workers.

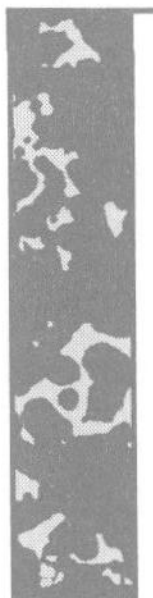

- Increase the proportion of primary health-care providers who routinely
  a. counsel clients about tobacco use cessation to 75%.
  b. provide age-appropriate safety education to 50%.
  c. counsel clients about physical activity needs to 50%.
  d. assess and counsel clients about nutritional needs to 75%.

(Source: U.S. Department of Health and Human Services[48])

COMMUNITY HEALTH NURSING AND CHRONIC HEALTH PROBLEMS

Community health nurses are actively involved in several aspects of efforts to control the effects of chronic health problems for both individuals and their families and for the population at large. They identify factors that place individuals or communities at risk for problems related to chronic conditions and take action to modify those factors. Additionally, they might identify persons with existing chronic conditions and assist them to deal with consequent problems.

The community health nurse should also function as a role model displaying appropriate health behaviors that prevent or control chronic conditions. A nurse weighing 300 pounds, for example, will have limited credibility when he or she talks to clients about the need to lose weight. Similarly, nurses who smoke will probably not be very effective in encouraging clients with COPD to quit smoking or persuading high school students of the hazards of smoking.

Finally, community health nurses can become politically active to promote access to health-promotive services or to control risk factors for chronic health problems. For example, nurses may lobby for legislation prohibiting smoking in public buildings in states that do not already have them or for legislation to require seat-belt use to prevent serious disability resulting from motor vehicle accidents.

THE EFFECTS OF CHRONIC HEALTH PROBLEMS

Chronic health problems can arise from a variety of sources. For example, a person might develop a chronic disability as a result of a serious accident or because of arthritis. Other chronic conditions arise out of other disease processes such as cardiovascular disease, chronic respiratory diseases, or cancer. Some chronic conditions, such as some cancers or other diseases, may result in death. Others, while not fatal cause persistent pain and disability.

The effects of chronic health conditions are experienced not only by individuals. Population groups and society at large are also affected by the consequences of chronic health problems.

PERSONAL EFFECTS

The advent of a chronic condition has many personal effects for individual clients. Among these effects are disability, changes in life-style, social isolation, and financial burdens. Disability due to chronic conditions contributes to some limitation of activity in approximately 14 percent of adult men and women in the United States, and more than 9 percent of the U.S. population experiences major activity limitations.[3]

Activity restrictions often require a change in life-style. Individuals with arthritis, for example, may need to adjust to their inability to do some things that they have done in the past or may need to learn to use special implements to accomplish everyday tasks like closing a zipper or buttoning a shirt. Similarly, clients with chronic respiratory conditions may find that they are less able to engage in vigorous activity than in the past and may require more frequent rest periods, while the client seriously injured in an automobile accident may need to adjust to using a wheelchair. Frequently, physical limitations such as these make it necessary to rely on others to perform routine tasks of daily living. This enforced dependence on others may, in turn, adversely affect an individual's self-image.

Even when activities are not restricted, the presence of a chronic health problem usually requires life-style adjustments. For the person with diabetes or a heart condition, for example, changes in diet are required. The person with diabetes may also need to make changes in eating patterns. This might mean not skipping meals or not eating on the run.

Pain also accompanies a number of chronic conditions and is often unremitting. The client with arthritis or cancer, for example, may have to endure a long period of pain despite the continued use of analgesics. The constant battle with chronic pain can be disheartening and can lead to depression and possible suicide.

The pain, life-style changes, decreased activity levels, and impaired mobility associated with chronic conditions can contribute to social isolation. The chronically ill individual may be less able to interact with others in familiar patterns or be unable to engage in activities that friends and family enjoy. Consequently, this person may feel left out unless concerted efforts are made to incorporate him or her into family and community life.

Finally, chronic health problems often entail considerable financial burdens. Most chronic conditions will require the individual to take prescribed medications for the rest of his or her life. For those taking medications for several chronic conditions, the cost can escalate rapidly. Add to this the cost of frequent visits to health-care providers to monitor the condition and the effects of therapy. Moreover, many individuals with chronic conditions require expensive special equipment or services.

POPULATION EFFECTS

Chronic conditions also affect the general population. These effects are reflected in financial costs, mortality and morbidity, and years of life lost.

FINANCIAL COSTS

Chronic health problems cost society millions of dollars each year. As noted earlier, the costs of coronary heart disease amount to $50 billion annually, while asthma costs more than $4 billion a year.[4] In 1988, the economic cost of diabetes in one state was approximately $301 million. These costs are the result of lost productivity due to work absenteeism and disability, as well as medical care.[5]

MORBIDITY

Societal costs of chronic health conditions are measured not only in dollars but also in terms of the extent of morbidity resulting from these conditions. While some progress has been made in preventing mortality due to chronic conditions, their prevalence has been increasing over the years. Because the reporting of chronic health conditions is not mandatory, however, prevalence figures probably grossly underrepresent the extent of these conditions in the population.

For example, the prevalence of hypertension in the general population was less than 100 per 100,000 persons in 1960, but had climbed to 122 per 100,000 by 1986.[3] Lung cancer incidence has also increased from 52 per 100,000 population in 1980 to 55.5 per 100,000 in 1986. According to the National Health Interview Survey, more than 14 percent of the U.S. population in 1987 was affected by arthritic conditions such as arthritis, bursitis, gout, and rheumatism.[6] In that same year, 6.8 million Americans were affected by diabetes, more than 27 in every 1000 people.[7]

Some of the increase in incidence and prevalence figures for chronic health problems is attributable to better diagnosis as well as to the ability to prevent deaths due to these conditions. However, these and similar figures for other chronic conditions also indicate that Americans are making little progress in the primary prevention of chronic health problems.

MORTALITY

Many chronic health conditions contribute to increased mortality and loss of productive years of life among the population. As with morbidity figures, mortality figures also provide only a partial picture of the extent of chronic health problems within the population; however, they can provide information on patterns and trends in chronic conditions over time.

Despite a marked decline in mortality, cardiovascular disease remains the leading cause of death in industrialized nations. Provisional data for 1988 indicated a mortality rate for heart disease in the United States of 314 deaths per 100,000 population.[8] This figure compares unfavorably with a mortality rate of 167 deaths per 100,000 for heart disease in 1900.[9] Some progress has been made in preventing deaths due to heart conditions, however. From 1979 to 1986, for example, a 20 percent decline in mortality due to coronary heart disease was noted in the United States.[10]

Mortality due to stroke is also declining. At the turn of the century the mortality attributable to stroke was 134 deaths per 100,000 population, while the age-adjusted stroke mortality for 1980 was only 41.5 per 100,000.[9] From 1968 to 1985 the United States saw a 50 percent decline in mortality due to stroke,[11] indicating that some progress has been made in controlling the effects of cerebrovascular disease. Much of this progress, however, has been in preventing deaths due to stroke rather than in preventing the occurrence of stroke.

Mortality figures for malignant neoplasms are more disheartening. Age-adjusted death rates for all forms of malignancy increased from 130 per 100,000 in 1970[3] to 200 per 100,000 in 1989.[12] In 1983, malignant neoplasms accounted for nearly 443,000 deaths, 36 percent of which occurred among persons under 65 years of age.[13] Because of the recent and projected future increases in the incidence of most cancers and overall cancer mortality, it is estimated that approximately one-third of children born in 1985 will develop cancer at some time in their lives and 20 percent of them will die of cancer.[13]

Some forms of cancer are greater contributors to increased cancer mortality than others. Deaths due to lung cancer, for example, increased by 15 percent between 1979 and 1986,[10] a figure alarming enough in itself. However, lung cancer mortality among women has shown the most alarming increase, rising 127 percent from 1968 to 1980, while breast cancer deaths increased by 8.5 percent during the same time period[14] and rose a further 5 percent from 1979 to 1986.[10] Deaths from colorectal cancer have also increased in recent years with a 7 percent increase in mortality noted from 1979 to 1986.[10] Cervical cancer, on the other hand, showed a decline of 18 percent in the same time period.

Other chronic conditions also contribute to mortality figures for the nation. Diabetes mellitus, for example, accounted for almost 19 deaths per 100,000 population in 1989.[12] This figure somewhat underrepresents the extent of the problem since diabetes may contribute to death without being reported on death certificates. Chronic obstructive pulmonary diseases (COPD) and allied conditions have also shown marked increases in mortality rates in recent years and were the fifth leading cause of death in the United States in 1988. For the general population, age-adjusted COPD mortality has increased from 12 deaths per 100,000 in 1970[15] to 34 deaths per 100,000 in 1989.[12]

YEARS OF POTENTIAL LIFE LOST

Another indicator of the effect of chronic health problems on society is the number of years of potentially productive life lost as a result of premature death. ***Years of potential life lost*** (YPLL) is a measure of the number of years that a person might have continued to live given the average life expectancy. For example, the average life expectancy for a male is approximately 71 years. If a man dies of a heart attack at age 50, he has lost 21 potential years of life. The YPLL is a measure of premature mortality and highlights the effects of chronic health problems on younger people, where crude mortality rates weigh all deaths equally. Table 31–1 presents the relative ranking of causes of death in terms of years of potential life lost. From this perspective, of chronic health conditions, malignant neoplasms and cardiovascular diseases have the greatest impact on society, followed by cerebrovascular disease, chronic liver disease, diabetes, and chronic obstructive pulmonary disease.[12]

TABLE 31–1. YEARS OF POTENTIAL LIFE LOST (YPLL) BEFORE AGE 65 DUE TO SELECTED CHRONIC CONDITIONS, 1989

Chronic Condition	YPLL in 1989
Malignant neoplasms	1,876,515
Diseases of the heart	1,383,355
Cerebrovascular disease	234,832
Chronic liver disease and cirrhosis	223,389
Diabetes mellitus	143,659
Chronic obstructive pulmonary diseases	140,683

(Source: MMWR[12])

THE EPIDEMIOLOGIC PREVENTION PROCESS MODEL AND CONTROL OF CHRONIC PHYSICAL HEALTH PROBLEMS

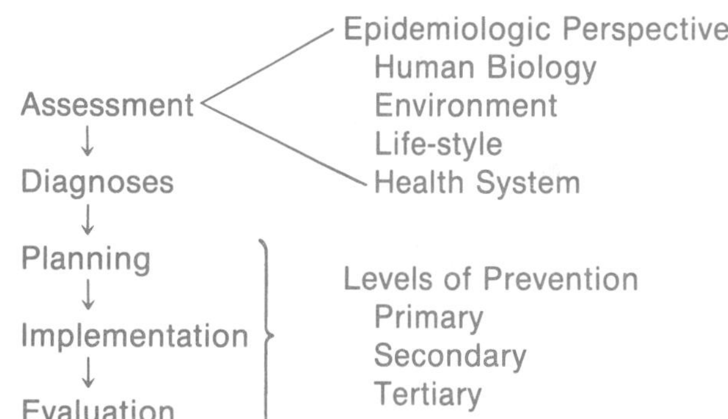

The epidemiologic prevention process model can be used to direct community health nursing actions to control chronic physical health problems experienced by individual clients or by population groups.

ASSESSMENT OF HEALTH STATUS

Community health nurses would use their assessment skills to assess for risk factors that contribute to chronic health problems and for existing chronic conditions and their effects. Factors related to human biology, environment, life-style, and the health system can increase the risk of the individual or a population group with respect to a particular chronic condition. Conversely, the presence of a chronic health problem might affect factors in each of these four areas.

HUMAN BIOLOGY

Human biological factors related to age, sex, race, specific genetic inheritance, and physiologic function can increase one's risk of developing several chronic health problems.

Maturation and Aging

Many people think of chronic health problems as occurring primarily among the elderly, despite the fact that chronic conditions can occur in any age group. Both the young and the elderly, for example, are at higher risk for accidental injuries and resulting disabilities. In part, this increased risk is due to maturational events of childhood. The inability of a young infant to roll over or support his or her head contributes to suffocation as the leading cause of accidental death and disability in this age group.[16] Similarly, normal toddler development involves a great deal of experimentation that may lead to accidental injury and disability if close supervision and safety precautions are not employed. The risk-taking and feelings of invulnerability characteristic of preadolescent and adolescent development places young people at risk for motor vehicle and firearms accidents. In one study, for example, 31 percent of those injured in firearms accidents were under 15 years of age.[17] Among the elderly, death and disabilities due to fires and falls are of the greatest concern.[16] Typical causes of accidental injury and disability for selected age groups are presented in Table 31–2.

Some chronic conditions and their effects are more prevalent in adult age groups. For example, despite the popular belief that people with arthritis are elderly, most cases of arthritis have their onset in the fourth decade of life. Older persons do, however, tend to experience greater disability as a result of this condition.[18] The prevalence of chronic obstructive pulmonary disease (COPD) tends to increase dramatically in the fifth through the seventh decades of life. The incidence of malignant neoplasms in general also increases with advancing age, particularly after midlife.[11,19,20]

TABLE 31–2. TYPICAL CAUSES OF INJURY AND DISABILITY

Age Group	Typical Causes of Injury and Disability
Infants (birth to 1 year)	Suffocation, aspiration of food and other objects, fire, drowning
One to 9 years	Motor vehicle accidents, drowning, poisoning, fires
Ten to 14 years	Motor vehicle accidents, drowning, firearms, fires
15 to 64 years	Motor vehicle accidents, occupational injury, falls, fires
Over 65 years	Falls, fires

Sex

One's gender can also influence the risk of developing a variety of chronic health conditions. Women, for example, less frequently develop colon cancer than do men.[19] Women who do develop forms of cancer other than bladder also have survival rates and lower mortality rates than do men.[11,20,21] Women also have lower mortality rates for cardiovascular and cerebrovascular disease than do men[22] and a lower risk of development emphysema.[23] On the other hand, women appear to be three times more likely than men to develop arthritic conditions.[6] Gender differences in arthritis prevalence, however, tend to diminish with age until elderly men and women seem to be equally affected.[18]

Race

Distance differences exist in the incidence and prevalence of some chronic conditions among different racial and ethnic groups. These may, in part, be due to environmental factors and access to health care, but some differences may be the result of genetic factors. For example, there are differences in cancer survival rates among racial and ethnic groups that are not totally explained by stage of the neoplasm at diagnosis and the quality of care received. Persons of Japanese ancestory have the highest cancer survival rates followed by Hispanics, Chinese, and Caucasians. Survival rates for blacks and Filipinos are less encouraging, and Native Americans experience the worst survival rates for cancer in general.[21]

The incidence and prevalence of other chronic health problems also differs among racial and ethnic groups. Blacks, for instance, tend to have higher diabetes prevalence rates than do whites.[24] Among some Native American tribes, the prevalence of diabetes is as high 10 percent of the population.[25] Race may also play a part in the propensity to develop arthritis, as the incidence of this disease is low in Asian and Native American populations, and whites are more likely to report being affected by arthritis than blacks.[6]

Genetic Inheritance

Some chronic diseases seem to be associated with genetic predisposition. Thus, community health nurses should obtain a family history of chronic disease to help determine the individual client's risk for these conditions. Genetic inheritance is thought to be a major contributing factor for some cancers, for diabetes, and for cardiovascular disease. Evidence also suggests that there is a genetic component to arthritic conditions.[6]

Breast and colon cancers, in particular, seem to have a hereditary component. In one study of people belonging to 24,000 "family trees" nearly 2 percent of the families were designated as "cancer prone" with multiple instances of cancer within these family groups. In the same study, 7.5 percent of the families were found to be "coronary prone," and young adults in these families had a sixfold to tenfold increase in risk for coronary disease. Similarly, nearly 4 percent of the families studied were at high risk for stroke.[26] The genetic component of coronary disease is further supported by findings that about 5 percent of the families in the general American population account for approximately 50 percent of early coronary deaths (those occurring before age 55). A family history of diabetes is also a strong indicator that an individual client may be at risk for diabetes, while a possible genetic disposition to rheumatoid arthritis is suggested by the presence of a specific histocompatibility antigen in 59 percent of persons with rheumatoid arthritis compared to only 16 percent of the general population.[6]

In assessing the potential for chronic health problems in individual clients, the nurse would obtain a family history and construct a genogram as described in Chapter 17, Care of the Individual Client. Positive findings related to chronic conditions with a genetic component would direct the assessment to possible signs and symptoms of existing chronic health problems discussed later in this chapter.

Physiologic Function

Assessment of physiologic factors related to chronic conditions focuses on three areas. These three foci are the presence of physiologic risk factors, physiologic evidence of existing chronic health problems, and evidence of physiologic consequences of chronic conditions.

Certain physiologic conditions may predispose one to develop some chronic health problems. Activity limitations and impaired balance and mobility, for instance, may contribute to injuries with long-term consequences, particularly in elderly individuals, whereas hypertension, elevated serum cholesterol, and diabetes are all physiologic factors in the development of cardiovascular disease.[9] The contribution of diabetes to heart disease appears to be greater for women than for men and for younger than for older persons. Among males, diabetes tends to increase the risk of stroke.[27]

Obesity is a physiologic factor that can contribute to diabetes, and coexistent hypertension may increase the risk of diabetic complications such as blindness.[27] Obesity also places greater strain on joints and may exacerbate the effects of arthritis on affected joints.

Past infection may also be implicated in the development of some chronic conditions. For example, viral infection is suspected as a contributing factor in both cancer and diabetes, particularly in children. As noted in Chapter 30, Communicable Disease, genital herpes simplex virus may contribute to later development of cervical cancer. A history of recurrent respiratory infections, particularly a history of severe viral pneumonias early in life, has been found to be associated with COPD. Respiratory allergy and asthma may also be predisposing physiologic factors in COPD.[23]

In addition to assessing individual clients for the presence of physiologic risk factors for chronic health problems, the community health nurse would examine the incidence and prevalence of these risk factors in the general population to determine the potential for chronic health problems in the community. The nurse would also assess individual clients and groups of people for indications of existing chronic health problems. Finally, the nurse would assess clients with existing chronic conditions for evidence of related physical effects. Assessment considerations related to physiologic risk factors, signs and symptoms of existing chronic conditions, and evidence of physical problems related to selected conditions are summarized in Table 31–3.

ENVIRONMENT

The nurse would assess environmental factors that might contribute to the development of chronic health problems and those that influence the effects of chronic conditions on clients' lives.

Physical Environment

Physical environmental factors contribute to chronic health problems such as long-term sequelae of accidents, cancer, and COPD. Road conditions, weather, dangerous conditions for swimming, and other physical safety hazards can contribute to accidents that result in permanent physical disability, and the nurse would assess the existence of these types of hazardous conditions in the community.

The community health nurse would also assess the environment for pollutants that may be carcinogenic. Air pollution, in particular, also contributes to COPD. Both incidence and mortality rates for this disease are elevated in highly industrialized urban areas, with increased levels of sulfur dioxide (SO_2) and particulates.[23] The effects of environmental pollution on health were addressed in more detail in Chapter 16, Environmental Influences on Community Health.

TABLE 31–3. ASSESSMENT CONSIDERATIONS RELATED TO SELECTED CHRONIC PHYSICAL HEALTH PROBLEMS

Condition	Physiologic Risk Factors	Signs and Symptoms	Potential Effects
Arthritis	Previous injury	Painful, swollen joints, limited range of motion	Contractures, limited mobility, inability to perform ADL
Cancer	Cervical dysplasia, viral infection	Weight loss, change in bowel or bladder habits, change in voice quality, pain, skin changes, palpable lumps or growths, persistent cough, rectal bleeding or blood in stool	Debility
Cardiovascular disease	Hypertension, hypercholesterolemia, diabetes, atherosclerosis, obesity	Chest pain, shortness of breath on exertion, fatigue, arrhythmias, elevated blood pressure, cardiac enlargement, edema	Debility, myocardial infarction
Cerebrovascular disease	Hypertension, atherosclerosis, congenital anomaly, heart disease, diabetes, polycythemia	Headaches, confusion, vertigo, diplopia, parasthesia of extremities, transient ischemic attacks (TIAs), slurred speech, weakness	Paralysis, aphasia, incontinence
Chronic obstructive pulmonary disease (COPD)	Asthma, respiratory allergy, frequent respiratory infections	Shortness of breath on exertion, cough, weakness, weight loss, diminished libido	Debility, inability to perform ADL, heart failure
Diabetes mellitus	Obesity	Polyuria, polydipsia, polyphagia, weight loss, frequent infections (especially monilia)	Ketoacidosis with nausea, anorexia, vomiting, air hunger, and coma; diabetic retinopathy, poor wound healing and infection, sensory loss, postural hypotension, male impotence, nocturnal diarrhea
Hypertension	Atherosclerosis	Headache, blurred vision, dizziness, flushed face, fatigue, epistaxis, elevated blood pressure	Heart disease, stroke

The other aspect of the physical environment related to chronic health problems is its effect on the functional abilities of persons with existing chronic conditions. From this perspective, the nurse would assess the need to adapt the environment to accommodate the needs of the client with a chronic condition. For example, does the home have a shower to make personal hygiene easier for the person with arthritis who may have difficulty getting in and out of a bathtub? Or does the home of the person with cardiovascular disease or COPD have numerous stairs that cause the individual to become short of breath? Similarly, the nurse would assess for potential barriers that limit community services for persons with chronic disabilities.

Psychological Environment

The major psychological environmental factor contributing to chronic health problems is stress. Stress can result in carelessness and contribute to accidents that lead to chronic disability. Similarly, stress has been implicated as a contributing factor in the development of cancer and cardiovascular disease. Stress may also lead to poor compliance with control measures in persons with diabetes, resulting in diabetic complications.

In addition to assessing individual clients for levels and sources of stress experienced and the adequacy of mechanisms for coping with stress, the community health nurse would assess the psychological effects of chronic health problems on persons experiencing them. In assessing this area, the nurse would examine the client's emotional response to his or her condition and its treatment, the effects of the condition on the client's self-image, and any effects of the condition on the client's ability to interact effectively with others. The psychological consequences of pain should also be assessed and evidence of depression and potential for suicide sought. Considerations in assessing clients for depression are addressed in Chapter 32, Chronic Mental Health Problems.

Social Environment

The social environment contributes to the development of chronic health problems primarily in terms of social support for unhealthful behaviors and factors that enhance or impede access to health care. Social norms that condone or promote life-style behaviors such as smoking, drinking alcohol, and a sedentary life-style contribute to the development of a variety of chronic health problems.

Social environmental factors may also promote health and healthy behaviors and impede the development of chronic health problems. For example, social pressures to quit smoking may motivate many smokers to abandon their habit. Similarly, no-smoking policies in work settings have led to an overall decrease in smoking behavior in many instances. Similarly, the existence of strong social support networks have been shown to reduce the risk of cardiovascular disease.[28]

Social environmental factors such as low income, low educational levels, and unemployment may prevent access to health care for persons who have existing chronic conditions. Lack of care leads to the development of complications that might be averted if those with chronic conditions received adequate treatment and monitoring. These types of socioeconomic factors explain some of the differences in survival rates for members of different ethnic groups who have cancer, and particularly explain the poor survival rates of blacks with cancer.[21,29] Such factors also explain the sharp increase in cardiovascular mortality among Native Americans and the fact that blacks account for 28 percent of the years of potential life lost as a result of cerebrovascular diseases.[22] Blacks are also more likely than whites to develop hypertension at an early age and to have more severe disease because of the lack of adequate care.[9]

The community health nurse would also assess the social effects of chronic health problems on those clients experiencing them. For example, the nurse might note that the physical effects of arthritis or COPD may prevent clients from engaging in activities that provided them with opportunities for social interaction in the past, thus resulting in social isolation.

In addition, the nurse should assess the adequacy of client's social support networks for dealing with the problems posed by chronic health problems. Areas to be considered include those who make up a client's social support network, the assistance provided by each, the adequacy of the network for meeting the client's needs, and the extent to which the network is appropriately utilized. For example, the nurse might note that the client's support network is not sufficiently broad to meet his or her needs or that the client is not using the existing network as fully as possible.

LIFE-STYLE

Life-style factors are the major contributors in the development of most chronic health problems. Life-style considerations to be assessed by the nurse include consumption patterns, occupational factors, exercise, and other behaviors.

Consumption Patterns

Consumption patterns that play a role in the development and course of chronic health problems include diet, and the use of tobacco and alcohol. Poor dietary patterns contribute to chronic diseases such as diabetes and cardiovascular disease and to obesity, which is a risk factor for both of these conditions. Individuals who are 50 percent over their optimal weight have a fivefold increase in their risk of diabetes when compared with those who are near their optimal weight.[24]

Cholesterol consumption patterns are well-known correlates of cardiovascular disease, and excess blood cholesterol is a prevalent problem throughout the United States. It is estimated that 80 percent of Americans consume excess fats,[30] and the average daily per capita caloric intake in the United States in 1987 was 3500 calories.[3] Approximately 60 percent of the fat consumed by Americans comes from animal sources known to be high in cholesterol.[31]

Diet has also been implicated in the development of some forms of cancer. For example, rates of colon cancer have been shown to increase in immigrants from countries with low rates of colon cancer when they adopt a Western life-style including a diet higher in fat and lower in fiber than their traditional diet.[19] One study of the dietary patterns of Americans indicated that 43 percent to 55 percent of people in this country consumed foods that increase cancer risks, whereas only 16 percent to 33 percent ate foods consistent with cancer prevention guidelines.[32]

Use of tobacco is another consumption pattern highly correlated with the development of a variety of chronic health problems. In fact, smoking is estimated to be the underlying cause of 390,000 deaths annually in the United States. These smoking-related deaths are due to heart disease, various forms of cancer, COPD, stroke, and other conditions caused by smoking.[33]

Tobacco use remains one of the primary life-style factors contributing to lung, bladder, and other cancers.[34] In fact, tobacco consumption patterns are thought to explain some of the regional variation in cancer incidence. For example, higher rates of oral cancer in the rural South are related to the use of snuff, whereas "unusually intense" cigarette smoking is associated with high lung cancer rates in Louisiana.[35] Pipe smoking on the other hand is associated with cancers of the oral cavity and lips.

Smoking has also been found to influence the incidence of cardiovascular disease and complications of diabetes and COPD. The association between smoking and cardiovascular disease is supported by findings that people who quit smoking reduce their risk of coronary heart disease by about half after a year of abstinence from tobacco. Smoking cessation also markedly reduces the risk of premature death in persons with existing cardiovascular disease.[33] Smoking has been found to interact with diabetes to result in greater risk of heart disease, blindness, and stroke.[27] Smoking is also the primary contributing factor in the development of COPD. In addition to being the single most significant factor in the development of this disease, smoking interacts with all other contributing factors to increase the potential for COPD.[23]

Despite a 45 percent decline in the number of smokers in the United States prior to 1986,[36] the 1988 findings of the Behavioral Risk Factor Surveillance System (BRFSS) indicated that the roughly 15 percent to 34 percent of people in states surveyed continue to smoke.[37] These figures indicate that smoking will continue to be a contributing factor in the incidence of cancer and cardiovascular disease and complications of diabetes and COPD.

Alcohol use also contributes to the development of certain chronic health problems and their consequences. For example, alcohol is implicated in motor vehicle accidents, bicycling accidents, fires, falls, and boating accidents, many of which result in chronic disability. In one study, for instance, half of those individuals who sustained brain injuries in bicycling accidents were found to be legally intoxicated,[38] attesting to the contribution of alcohol to their chronic disability. Alcohol use also contributes to mortality due to diabetes.[39]

In assessing the influence of consumption patterns on chronic health problems, the community health nurse would identify consumption patterns that place individuals at risk for chronic conditions. The nurse would also determine the prevalence of high-risk consumption patterns in the community. In addition, the nurse would explore unhealthful consumption patterns with clients who have existing chronic diseases and determine their effects on the course of the condition. For example, the nurse would want to determine whether a client with diabetes is adhering to a diabetic diet or how well a client with hypertension is complying with a low-sodium diet. The nurse would also assess for factors related to food preferences and modes of preparation that may impede adherence to special diets.

Occupational Factors

Occupational factors can also contribute to the development of chronic health problems. As noted in Chapter 27, Care of Clients in the Work Setting, safety hazards in the work environment can result in accidents that lead to chronic disability. Clients' occupations may also increase their potential for exposure to various carcinogens found in the workplace. Repetitive movements involved in some jobs can lead to joint injuries and subsequent arthritis; research has indicated that increased job demands, loss of control over one's work, and low levels of social support from co-workers are associated with higher prevalence of cardiovascular disease.[28] Reduced cardiovascular mortality has also been found to be associated with white-collar versus blue-collar occupations.[40] Occupations involving exposure to organic and inorganic dusts or noxious gases increase the probability of COPD. Employment in plastics factories and in cotton mills is particularly associated with increased incidence of COPD.[23]

The community health nurse will assess the jobs performed by individual clients and identify any risk factors for chronic health problems posed by the work environment or the work performed. The nurse would also assess the community for potential occupational risk factors related to chronic health problems by determining the major employers and occupations present in the community, the types of products, services, and processes involved.

Exercise and Leisure Activity

Exercise, or the lack of it, can also influence the development and course of some chronic conditions. Exercise may enhance the control of diabetes or contribute to hypoglycemic reactions. In one study, a community-based exercise program for persons with diabetes resulted in weight loss, reduced blood glucose levels, and decreased needs for insulin.[41] The community health nurse should be sure to assess, however, the extent of the diabetic client's exercise in relation to his or her dietary intake and the amount of insulin used to determine the potential for hypoglycemic reaction related to exercise.

Physical activity has also been shown to be directly related to the incidence of heart disease. In one study, those adults with active life-styles had a 30 percent lower risk of developing heart disease than their less-active contemporaries.[42] A sedentary life-style, on the other hand, is closely associated with obesity, a risk factor for cardiovascular disease. The association of lack of exercise and obesity holds true for children as well as for adults.[43]

Television viewing is frequently a component of a sedentary life-style and has been shown to be associated with obesity. Watching television is the third most time-consuming activity in the United States, and the typical adult watches TV an average of 4 hours each day. As viewing time increases, physical fitness declines and, in one study, persons who watched TV more than 3 hours a day were twice as likely to be obese as those who watched less than 1 hour.[44]

Despite the strong association between a sedentary life-style and cardiovascular diseases, many people fail to get sufficient exercise to promote their health. In the 1988 Behavioral Risk Factor Surveillance System, 45 percent to 73 percent of persons responding in the states surveyed reported a sedentary life-style. In fact, the majority of people in all age groups over 18 years were sedentary.[37] The nurse assessing an individual client or a community for risk factors related to exercise or its lack would determine the extent of regular exercise obtained by the individual or the proportion of sedentary individuals who make up the population.

Other Behaviors

Other life-style behaviors that might influence the development and course of chronic diseases include the practice of self-assessment behaviors for breast and testicular cancers and use of safety devices and precautions.

Despite the advantages of early detection of breast cancer through breast self-examination, only 48 percent of women in one study engaged in this practice on a regular basis[45] and even fewer men engage in regular testicular examinations. In assessing this aspect of life-style and its effects on chronic health problems, the nurse would ascertain how often individual clients engage in breast or testicular self-examination. The nurse would also assess the extent to which these practices are employed within the community to determine the community's potential for increased mortality due to breast and testicular cancer.

The use of safety devices and safety precautions can prevent accidents that may result in chronic disability, and the nurse should determine the extent to which individual clients and their families practice safety measures. Do family members consistently use seat belts? Are there smoke detectors in the home? Are hazardous items, such as sharp objects and poisons, stored appropriately? Is there potential for falls owing to multiple obstacles in the homes of elderly persons?

The community health nurse would appraise the extent to which these and similar safety conditions and practices are found in the general population or in the work setting. For example, are there smoke detectors and sprinkler systems present in public buildings or in business and industries? Is seat-belt use mandatory in the jurisdiction and, if so, is it enforced? Are appropriate safety equipment and safety precautions employed in work settings?

HEALTH SYSTEM

Health system factors may contribute to the development of chronic health problems or influence their course and consequences. The failure of health-care professionals to educate their clients and the general public on the effects of diet, exercise, smoking, alcohol, and other factors in the development of chronic health problems may contribute to increased incidence of these conditions.

The extent of screening services for existing chronic conditions may influence their course and effects. It is estimated that diabetic screening programs, for example, detect only about half of the population affected by this disease.[5]

The extent to which screening procedures for various forms of cancer are used also varies considerably. In 1987, 33 state health agencies provided screening services for cervical cancer and 30 screened for breast cancer. Routine screening exams for other forms of cancer are performed even less often. Only 19 state agencies provide screening for colon cancer, 12 for oral cancer, 9 for testicular cancer, and 7 for skin cancer.[46] While screening services may often be obtained from private health-care providers, they are often costly and many low-income people are prevented from taking advantage of them.

Even in those states where screening services are provided, they may not be utilized effectively. In 1987, for example, only 81 percent of adult women included in the National Health Interview Survey reported ever having had a Pap smear for screening purposes, while manual breast examination by a health professional was reported by only 44 percent of the women. Older women were less apt to receive either screening test than were younger women.[47]

Health system factors also influence the availability and quality of treatment available for persons with chronic conditions. In 1987, only 10 states reported state-sponsored programs related to arthritis control, and 14 states reported activities related to COPD.[46]

The aggressiveness of treatment received also affects the outcome of chronic health conditions. Some studies suggest, for example, that poorer cancer survival rates among blacks may be related to less aggressive (primarily nonsurgical) therapy than that provided to their white counterparts.[29] The quality of treatment received for diabetes may also vary widely and affect the consequences of this disease. In one study of individuals under 65 years of age who died as a result of diabetes, only 80 percent had received a fundoscopic examination in the year prior to death despite knowledge of the relationship between diabetes and retinopathy, while 10 percent had not had a blood pressure check or a urinalysis in the year prior to death.[39]

Medical technology, on the other hand, has greatly reduced mortality from cardiovascular and cerebrovascular diseases. This is largely due to a concerted effort to control hypertension, smoking, and diet. In 1987, 42 state health agencies provided hypertension screening services and 39 states provided hypertension control programs. Thirty-two states engaged in smoking cessation or prevention activities and 19 had programs related to dietary modifications.[46]

In assessing individual and community risk for chronic health problems, the community health nurse would determine the extent of preventative, diagnostic, and treatment services offered to community residents as well as their cost and accessibility. The nurse would also assess the extent to which available services are used and possible reasons for nonuse if appropriate.

Risk factors related to human biology, environment, life-style, and the health systems all influence the development and outcomes of chronic physical health problems. Risk factors for selected chronic conditions are summarized in Appendix Q, Factors in the Epidemiology of Selected Chronic Physical Health Problems.

DIAGNOSTIC REASONING AND CHRONIC HEALTH PROBLEMS

Nursing diagnoses are derived from information collected relative to the incidence and prevalence of chronic health problems in the population and the factors contributing to these conditions. These diagnoses may relate to individual clients or to the general population. Examples of nursing diagnoses related to an individual client might be "potential for cardiovascular disease due to smoking and sedentary life-style" or "uncontrolled diabetes due to failure to adhere to diabetic diet." At the group level, the nurse might derive diagnoses such as "increased prevalence of lung cancer due to smoking and occupational exposure to carcinogens." In each case, the nursing diagnosis contains a statement of the probable cause or etiology of the problem that directs interventions designed to resolve it.

PLANNING AND IMPLEMENTING INTERVENTIONS FOR CHRONIC HEALTH PROBLEMS

Planning interventions related to chronic health problems is based on the understanding of contributing factors derived from the assessment. When the client is an individual with a chronic health problem, the nurse plans care in keeping with the principles discussed in Chapter 17, Care of the Individual Client.

It is particularly important to involve the client and his or her family in planning for solutions to chronic health problems because the client or a significant other will probably be responsible for implementing the plan. By involving the client and members of the client's family, the plan of care can be tailored to the client's circumstances. It is important to remember that the presence of a chronic health problem affects many facets of life for the client and his or her family. Effective planning accounts for these effects and minimizes the consequences of chronic illness for client and family alike.

When chronic health problems exist at the community or group level, the nurse collaborates with other members of the community to plan health programs that address the problems identified. For example, if the prevalence of cardiovascular disease is particularly high in the community, programs to prevent and control cardiovascular disease might be developed. In planning these programs, the nurse and other health planners would employ the general principles of health programming discussed in Chapter 19, Care of the Community or Target Group.

Control strategies for chronic health problems can be undertaken at the primary, secondary, or tertiary level of prevention. To date, the major emphasis has been on secondary prevention with only recent attention to primary and tertiary levels.

PRIMARY PREVENTION

Nursing strategies for primary prevention of chronic conditions focus on two major areas—health promotion and risk-factor modification. Both aspects of primary prevention can be applied to individual clients or to population groups.

Health Promotion

General health promotion is aimed at making people healthier and reducing their chances of developing a variety of health problems including chronic conditions. Health promotion at both the individual and group levels involves education for a healthier lifestyle and political activity to create conditions that promote health.

Health Education. Health education efforts in primary prevention of chronic health problems would focus on diet, exercise, and coping skills. The nurse would employ the principles of health education discussed in Chapter 7, The Health Education Process, to educate both individual clients and the general public on basic nutrition and specific nutritional requirements based on a person's age and activity level. For example, the nurse would plan to prevent obesity by teaching parents about the nutritional needs of infants and young children and by encouraging a well-balanced diet with minimal amounts of junk food. Similarly, the nurse would plan to teach a pregnant woman, a nursing mother, or a physically active person about their specific nutritional needs. The nurse would also engage in efforts to inform the general public about proper nutrition.

Exercise is another area in which health education may be required, and nurses would plan to inform both individual clients and the general public about the need for regular exercise. The nurse might also assist clients to plan ways of incorporating exercise into their daily routine, or develop plans for exercise programs in the community or for employees of local businesses.

Teaching general coping skills is another way for community health nurses to promote health and prevent chronic health problems that are influenced by stress. In this respect, the nurse might plan to assist a harried mother of several small children to develop ways of coping with stress, or the nurse might assist school personnel to develop a program to teach basic coping skills as part of elementary and secondary school curricula. Another approach might be to plan a program to foster adequate coping among employees of local businesses.

Political Activity. Political activity related to primary prevention would focus on measures to promote access to preventative health services and to create a healthful environment. Nursing involvement in efforts at this level would include planning strategies to influence health policymaking discussed in Chapter 12, The Political Process. For example, community health nurses might plan to campaign for better access to prenatal care for pregnant women or legislation to prevent or reduce pollution so as to prevent its contribution to chronic respiratory conditions and other chronic health problems.

Risk-Factor Modification

Activities designed to eliminate or modify risk factors include quitting smoking, weight reduction, control of hypertension, the use of safety and protective devices, and the creation of environments free of safety hazards. Again, educational efforts by community health nurses are an important aspect of risk-factor modification, and nurses would plan to educate both individual clients and the general public about the elimination or modification of identified risk factors for chronic health problems.

Smoking. Some progress has been made in eliminating smoking as a risk factor for chronic health problems. Two general approaches have been used in this area—personal efforts and public activity. Personal efforts are designed to keep people from ever starting to smoke and encouraging smokers to quit. Among adults, these efforts have been relatively successful, and, as of 1987, only 29 percent of the adult population in the United States were smokers.[48] Roughly one-fourth of the American population is comprised of former smokers[49] and almost half of those now living who have ever smoked have quit.[50]

In 1985 there were approximately 56 million smokers in the United States. Estimates suggest that without the recent antismoking campaigns this number would have approached 91 million. Such campaigns are also credited with preventing or postponing 3 million deaths between 1964 and the year 2000.[50] However, 50 million Americans continue to smoke, although many have attempted to quit owing to smoking-related illness, medical advice, and social support or pressure to quit.[51]

Community health nurses can plan to educate smokers regarding the hazards of smoking and to direct them to sources of assistance to quit smoking. In addition, the community health nurse can provide support and encourage family members to support the smoker's efforts to quit. Nurses can also plan to educate young people regarding the hazards of smoking and develop programs that discourage them from initiating the habit. Finally, nurses can educate individual clients and groups of people to eliminate other forms of tobacco use such as snuff and chewing tobacco.

Community health nurses may also be involved in planning political activity to limit smoking. Legislative and regulatory activities to control smoking can be of two types—legislation controlling smoking in public places and taxation of tobacco sales. In Great Britain, for example, prohibitively high taxes on cigarettes and other forms of tobacco have greatly reduced tobacco use.

Legislation has also been effective in controlling smoking behavior by limiting smoking in public places. As of 1986, 41 states and the District of Columbia had passed laws restricting smoking in various places, and 80 percent of the American population now resides in states with such restrictions. Most of the states without laws limiting smoking in public places are heavy tobacco growers with strong lobbies opposed to any such legislation.[52] It is in these states, in particular, that community health nurses should employ the political strategies outlined in Chapter 12, The Political Process, to promote legislation to control smoking.

Another area of the public effort to reduce smoking lies in workplace restrictions, and community health nurses can be active in promoting no-smoking policies in business and industry. The recent increase in workplace smoking restrictions has been attributed to four basic factors: public support, state and local workplace smoking legislation, company costs related to smoking, and scientific evidence of the risks of smoking for all employees.[52] Public support for smoke-free workplaces is widely demonstrated. In 1985, 79 percent of adults and 76 percent of smokers favored on-the-job smoking in restricted areas only. Smoking-associated costs to employers include employee absences, medical care and insurance costs, lost productivity, and maintenance costs (for example, more frequent cleaning of drapes). Community health nurses can apprise policymakers in business and industry of the advantages of no-smoking policies and encourage development and enforcement of such policies in the work setting.

Obesity. Control efforts for obesity have been less extensive than those for smoking. Health education related to caloric intake and fat consumption, particularly saturated fats, is required, and community health nurses should plan to educate individual clients about the need for fewer calories and to reduce fat consumption. A recent National Research Council report recommended reducing fat intake to less than 30 percent and saturated fat to less than 10 percent of total caloric intake.[53] Community health nurses can educate clients about reading package labels to determine the fat and caloric content of various foods. They can also inform clients about foods that are low in saturated fats and about food preparation methods that minimize fat consumption.

Development of modified food products will also assist in controlling fat intake. Community health nurses can plan to support campaigns to encourage the food industry to pursue research on food modification. They can also campaign for legislation to require accurate labeling of food packages and disclosure of food contents.

Regular exercise can also be emphasized as a control strategy for obesity, as well as a means of counteracting the effects of a sedentary life-style, itself a risk factor in many chronic conditions. Community health nurses can encourage overweight or sedentary clients to incorporate more exercise into their daily routine. Nurses may also be involved in planning exercise programs for groups of overweight or sedentary clients in the community or in work settings.

Hypertension Control. In addition to being a chronic condition itself, hypertension is a risk factor for several other chronic health problems and their complications. For this reason, efforts to control hypertension constitute primary prevention for cardiovascular and cerebrovascular diseases as well as for complications of diabetes. The two primary aspects of hypertension control are increasing public knowledge related to hypertension and encouraging behaviors conducive to control.[54]

Public awareness of hypertension has increased in recent years. In 1974, for example, only 51 percent of people with hypertension were aware of their condition compared to 85 percent in 1984. Control of hypertension also seems to have improved. Only 36 percent of those with hypertension in 1974 were under treatment and 16 percent had their blood pressure under control. Ten years later, 74 percent of people with hypertension were under treatment and 24 percent had their blood pressure under control.[55]

Public knowledge of the effects of hypertension has also increased, and the general public is engaged in more healthful behaviors designed to control blood pressure. For example, from 1972 to 1985 food-grade salt sales decreased by 36 percent, indicating an overall reduction in sodium consumption. Recently, many more low-salt products can be found on supermarket shelves.

Community health nurses should plan to educate individual clients and the general public regarding the effects and signs and symptoms of hypertension. They can also identify people with hypertension and be involved in planning hypertension screening programs or in referring clients with elevated blood pressures for further evaluation and treatment.

The second aspect of hypertension control is encouraging behaviors that promote control of existing hypertension. Community health nurses can educate hypertensive clients regarding the need for reduced sodium in their diets and about foods that are high and low in sodium content. They should also plan to instruct clients on the appropriate use of antihypertensive medications and potential side effects. In addition, nurses should convey to clients the need to continue with therapy and to report any adverse effects of treatment to their primary-care providers.

Safety Precautions. The use of safety devices and other safety precautions can modify risk factors for accidents that may lead to chronic disability. Community health nurses can plan to encourage clients to install smoke detectors in residences, provide adequate supervision for small children, store hazardous items appropriately, and remove hazards that promote falls for the elderly. They can also plan to promote the use of seat belts in vehicles and campaign for legislation that makes seat-belt use mandatory in all vehicles. Finally, community health nurses can promote use of safety devices and safety precautions in the work setting to prevent accidental injury. Primary prevention goals in the control of chronic physical health problems and related community health nursing activities are summarized in Table 31–4.

SECONDARY PREVENTION

Secondary prevention activities in the control of chronic illness are aimed at dealing with chronic health problems once they have occurred. The three major foci at this level of prevention are screening for existing chronic conditions, early diagnosis, and prompt treatment of these conditions.

Screening

Screening tests are available for several chronic health problems. Pap smears, for example, are used to

TABLE 31–4. GOALS FOR PRIMARY PREVENTION AND RELATED COMMUNITY HEALTH NURSING INTERVENTIONS IN THE CONTROL OF CHRONIC PHYSICAL HEALTH PROBLEMS

Primary Prevention Goal

1. Promote general health
   a. Provide prenatal care
   b. Maintain appropriate body weight through adequate nutrition
      i. Breast-feed infants
      ii. Delay introduction of solid foods
      iii. Avoid use of food as pacifier or reward
      iv. Establish healthy food habits from childhood
   c. Engage in graduated program of exercise
2. Control risk factors
   a. Quit smoking and prevent initiation of smoking
   b. Decrease dietary intake of saturated fats, cholesterol, sodium, alcohol, etc.
   c. Identify and treat existing health problems that are risk factors for chronic illness (hypertension, obesity)
   d. Eliminate environmental pollutants contributing to chronic disease
   e. Decrease exposure to sources of radiation (X-ray, sunlight)
   f. Eliminate occupational exposure to hazardous substances
   g. Eliminate or modify effects of emotional stress
      i. Avoid stressful situations when possible
      ii. Develop sound coping skills

Nursing Intervention

1. Promote client health
   a. Educate clients and public on the need for prenatal care
      Refer to or provide prenatal care
   b. Educate clients and public on adequate nutrition
      Obtain diet history and identify poor food habits
      Assist with breast-feeding
      Assist with menu planning and budgeting
      Refer for food-supplement plans as needed
      Encourage use of nonfood reward systems
   c. Educate public on need for exercise
      Assist clients to plan appropriate exercise program
2. Screen for risk factors
   Educate public regarding risk factors
   a. Foster self-help groups for smokers, overeaters, etc.
      Educate nonsmokers on the hazards of smoking
      Promote no-smoking policies in public places and in the workplace
   b. Educate and help clients plan adequate nutritional intake
   c. Screen for and refer clients with existing conditions
      Educate clients regarding therapy for existing conditions
      Adjust therapy to client's situation when possible
      Monitor for compliance, therapeutic effects, and side effects
   d. Public education on pollution
      Political action on environmental legislation
   e. Public education on risks of radiation
      Discourage sunbathing
      Encourage use of sunscreen, protective clothing, etc.
   f. Monitor occupational safety conditions
   g. Assist clients to identify stressful situations
      i. Explore with clients ways of decreasing stress
      ii. Assist clients to develop positive coping skills

screen women for cervical cancer, while breast self-exam and mammography assist in early detection of breast cancer. Testicular self-exam is an equally important screening procedure for men. Early detection of colorectal cancers is assisted with regular stool examination for occult blood and an annual rectal exam. Dermatologic screening for skin cancers and hypertension and diabetes screenings are readily available and easily accessible in most areas.

Community health nurses play an important role in screening for chronic illness. They are conversant with the prevalence of various risk factors in the community and can plan screening programs needed to detect conditions related to those risk factors that are most prevalent. They may also plan to motivate client participation in screening by educating the public regarding the need for screening. Interpretation of test results and referrals for further diagnosis and treatment of suspected conditions are also functions of community health nurses in secondary prevention of chronic health problems.

Early Diagnosis

The effects of many chronic health conditions can be minimized when they are diagnosed and treated early in the course of the disease. As noted earlier, positive screening test results are always an indication of a need for further diagnostic testing. Persons with obvious symptoms associated with chronic diseases should also be referred for diagnostic evaluation.

Because of their exposure to community members, community health nurses frequently engage in case finding with respect to chronic diseases, identifying those with possible symptoms of disease and referring them for diagnosis and treatment as appropriate. Community health nurses are also actively involved in efforts to educate clients and the general public regarding signs and symptoms of chronic diseases and the need for medical intervention. Community health nurses functioning as nurse practitioners may also be involved in making medical diagnoses of chronic illness.

Prompt Treatment

The third aspect of secondary prevention in the control of chronic health problems is the treatment of existing conditions. Treatment considerations in chronic conditions include stabilizing the client's condition as rapidly as possible, establishing a medical treatment regimen, and preventing progression of the disease by monitoring treatment effectiveness.

Stabilizing the Client's Condition. Community health nurses may need to provide emergency care to stabilize clients who are experiencing some chronic conditions. For example, the client having a heart attack may need CPR, while emergency care will also be required for the client in diabetic coma. Community health nurses may actually provide emergency care in situations of this type, or may educate clients and the public in emergency-care procedures. Once the client has been stabilized, the nurse would refer the client to an appropriate source of medical care.

Establishing a Treatment Regimen. The medical treatment regimen for a chronic health problem can involve medication, radiation, chemotherapy, surgery, or other types of therapy. While nurse practitioners may be involved in providing some of these forms of care, most community health nurses will not. They will, however, be involved in preparing clients for treatments both physically and psychologically, and they will plan to provide supportive measures as needed during therapy. For example, the nurse may administer intravenous pain medication to clients in the terminal stages of cancer, or help clients deal with the side effects of radiation or chemotherapy.

Nurses will also educate clients about their treatment and motivate them to comply with treatment recommendations. For example, community health nurses can educate clients with hypertension about antihypertensive medications and their effects and side effects as well as about diet, weight loss, and the need for continued medical supervision.

At the community level, community health nurses may be politically involved in efforts to assure the presence and accessibility of prompt treatment for chronic conditions. They may also be involved in planning health-care programs for the treatment of a variety of chronic health problems using the principles of health program planning discussed in Chapter 19, Care of the Community or Target Group.

Motivating Compliance. An estimated 30 percent to 50 percent of persons with chronic conditions are noncompliant in following prescribed recommendations.[56] Reasons for noncompliance include inability to understand recommendations, inconvenience of required actions, disruption of life-style, financial or situational constraints, and lack of belief in the severity of the problem or the efficacy of treatment.

Monitoring client compliance with therapy for chronic conditions is an important community health nursing function. Identifying and eliminating factors in a client situation that promote noncompliance may foster compliance instead. Clients may be physically or mentally unable to comply with recommendations. Clients who cannot remove the child-proof cap, cannot get into the tub for a sitz bath, or cannot remember to take their medication will not be compliant because of sheer inability. These are some of the considerations the nurse must make when planning to enhance client compliance with the recommended treatment plan. This is also further reason for incorporating the client and/or family members in the design of the treatment plan.

Other clients may be noncompliant because treatment requires too great an alteration in life-style. In this case the nurse can plan adjustments in the treatment plan to more closely fit the client's life-style. For example, the nurse can assist the client who has diabetes to incorporate culturally preferred foods into a diabetic diet.

Situational constraints can also lead to noncompliance. Clients who cannot afford to purchase their medication will not take it. Lack of running water may make warm soaks difficult for the arthritic. The effort of bringing water from a well and heating it on the stove may be more detrimental to inflamed joints than doing nothing. The nurse will plan measures to eliminate situational barriers to clients' compliance with treatment plans. For example, the nurse may plan a referral to assist a client to obtain Medicaid coverage to help pay for medical expenses, or help the client plan for other ways to provide moist heat to arthritic joints.

Noncompliance can also result when the client has a vested interest in being ill. Clients who use illness as a means of getting attention or qualifying for disability benefits are unlikely to comply fully with a treatment program. In such cases, community health nurses must identify the goal of the client's noncompliance. They may then be able to help the client plan for other means of achieving that goal and motivate greater compliance.

Finally, lack of motivation can contribute to noncompliance. Clients may lack motivation owing to a poor self-concept or because of discouragement. The nurse, as well as family members and friends, can help to improve the client's self-concept. This can be done by encouraging independence, enhancing successful accomplishment of short-term goals, and positive reinforcement of accomplishments. Above all, the client must be accepted by those around him as a unique individual worthy of respect.

Discouragement can be abated through realistic goal setting and achievement of short-term goals. Emotional support by the nurse, provided through opportunities on the part of the client to express feelings of fear and frustration, as well as positive reinforcement of accomplishments, can help to alleviate discouragement and foster compliance. Another way to deal with this type of noncompliance is referral to an appropriate self-help group.

Monitoring Treatment Effects. The nurse involved in secondary prevention for chronic health problems will also plan to monitor clients for the presence of side effects related to treatment. For example, the nurse may note that a client is experiencing postural hypotension due to antihypertensives and will then educate the client about the need to change position gradually and will continue to monitor blood pressure levels to be sure that they do not drop too low.

At the same time, the nurse monitors the therapeutic effects of treatment. For instance, the nurse may plan to obtain periodic blood pressure measurements for the client with hypertension. In the event that the nurse determines that antihypertensive therapy has not noticeably affected the client's blood pressure, the nurse would make sure that the client is taking the medication appropriately and refer the client to his or her physician for further follow-up. Goals for secondary prevention of chronic physical health problems and related community health nursing interventions are summarized in Table 31–5.

TERTIARY PREVENTION

In tertiary prevention the aim is to promote the client's optimal level of function in spite of the presence of a chronic health problem. This entails preventing further loss of function in affected and unaffected systems, restoring function, monitoring health status, and assisting the client to adjust to the presence of a chronic condition.

Preventing Loss of Function in Affected Systems

Chronic health problems frequently result in some loss of function in organ systems affected by the condition, and tertiary prevention activities should be planned to prevent further loss of function in these systems. Activities may be planned to minimize losses or to eliminate risk factors that might lead to adverse consequences of the condition. Such activities on the part of the community health nurse might include motivating client compliance with treatment recommendations and assisting clients to identify and change risk factors that may lead to further loss of function. For example, the client with arthritis may be assisted to identify safety factors in the home that might contribute to falls, leading to further mobility limitation. Or, the client who has had a myocardial infarction may be assisted to plan a regimen of diet and exercise that will prevent future infarcts.

Preventing Loss of Function in Unaffected Systems

Chronic health problems may also result in loss of function in other physical and nonphysical systems

TABLE 31–5. GOALS FOR SECONDARY PREVENTION AND RELATED COMMUNITY HEALTH NURSING INTERVENTIONS IN THE CONTROL OF CHRONIC PHYSICAL HEALTH PROBLEMS

Secondary Prevention Goal	Nursing Intervention
1. Screening a. Periodic health exams b. Periodic screening for chronic disease	1. Screen for existing chronic diseases a. Educate public on need for health exams Provide periodic exams b. Educate public on need for periodic screening Plan and implement screening programs of high-risk groups
2. Early diagnosis	2. Educate public on warning signs and symptoms of chronic disease Engage in case finding and refer for diagnosis as appropriate Prepare client for diagnostic procedures (physically and emotionally) Conduct diagnostic tests as appropriate
3. Prompt treatment a. Stabilize condition as soon as possible b. Establish treatment regimen i. Medication ii. Radiation iii. Chemotherapy iv. Surgery c. Prevent disease progression	3. Assist with management of chronic disease a. Provide emergency care as needed Educate public to provide emergency care (CPR) Refer for further treatment b. Prepare client for treatment procedures (physically and emotionally) Carry out treatment regimen Provide supportive measures during treatment (relief of pain) Educate clients on medications: dosage, side effects, etc. Encourage client compliance with treatment c. Monitor therapeutic effects of treatment Monitor side effects Refer for follow-up as needed

that are not directly affected by the condition. For instance, the client with arthritis may develop skin lesions due to limited mobility, or the client with COPD may become malnourished because meal preparation is too exhausting.

Nursing interventions will be directed toward preventing both physical and social disability. Physical complications of chronic conditions may be prevented by activities such as teaching breathing exercises to clients with COPD, providing good skin care for the client with arthritis, and teaching foot care for clients with diabetes.

Nurses can also help prevent social disability by encouraging the client to interact with others, assisting clients to maintain their independence as much as possible, assisting with necessary role changes within the family, and referring the client to appropriate self-help groups. At the group level, community health nurses can work to prevent social isolation of those with chronic illnesses by advocacy and political activities to ensure access to services. They can also work to educate the public and to develop positive attitudes to persons with chronic or disabling conditions.

Restoring Function

The restoration aspect of tertiary prevention focuses on regaining as much lost function as is possible given the client's situation. Particular areas of function to be considered include bed activities, positioning, range of motion, transfer abilities, dressing, bowel and bladder control, hygiene, locomotion, and eating. Other functional considerations include vision, hearing, speech, mental ability, and capacity for social interaction. The nurse, together with the client and his or her significant others, can plan to foster renewed abilities to perform these functions. For example, the nurse may develop a plan and teach the client and family how to reestablish bowel control following a stroke, or the nurse might assist the client with passive and active range-of-motion exercises to restore function after a broken arm has healed.

Monitoring Health Status

Another aspect of tertiary prevention in the control of chronic health problems is monitoring the client's health status. The nurse would be actively involved in periodic reassessment of a client's situation, being particularly alert to changes in circumstances that may affect health. For example, the nurse may note that cessation of unemployment benefits will limit the client's capacity to pay for health care. In this case, a referral might be made for additional financial assistance.

The nurse monitors the client's overall health status as well as the status of the chronic condition. When warranted, the nurse will refer the client for medical follow-up. For example, the nurse may note that a client disabled by a serious accident is developing pressure sores due to long periods in a wheelchair. In this case, the nurse would suggest interventions to heal the pressure sores and prevent their recurrence or refer the client for medical assistance for severe lesions.

Promoting Adjustment

Adjustments to the presence of a chronic disease need to be both functional and psychological. Functional adjustments reflect changes in life-style that are necessitated by the illness. Such changes may involve diet, activity patterns, restrictions (for example, limiting alcohol use or caloric intake), and the need to take medications. Some diseases necessitate learning of special skills. For instance, insulin-dependent diabetic clients will need to learn to give themselves insulin injections, while the hypertensive client may need to learn how to take a blood pressure. In other chronic conditions, such as arthritis, there may be a need for special apparatus to assist in performing routine activities. The need for medication may also necessitate budgetary changes that the client must adjust to.

Psychological adjustments are also necessary. There are five general areas in which psychological adjustment to a chronic condition may be required.[57] First, the client must learn to trust health-care providers to assist in prolonging life and in dealing with the symptoms arising from the chronic condition. Trust that providers and family members will not abandon the client must also be cultivated. Others may withdraw from the person with chronic condition, leading to isolation and loneliness. Community health nurses can foster trust in health-care providers and can assist families to deal with the chronic condition of a family member without withdrawing.

Self-esteem is the second area that may require adjustment. The presence of a chronic disease may make a client more dependent on others and less able to engage in activities that promote a positive self-image. For example, the client may need to stop working or begin to rely on others for assistance with basic functions such as eating or toileting. This dependence may be demeaning to one who has been independent and self-reliant. The nurse can encourage the client to maintain as many previous functions as possible and can help families to see the client's need for independence.

Third, the loss of independence also necessitates adjustments in one's sense of control. Clients may not feel they are in control of events when the food they eat or the activities they perform are dictated in part by the presence of a chronic health problem. For some clients, noncompliance with recommendations might be an attempt to regain control over their own lives. Nurses can help prevent noncompliance by providing the client with other avenues for exercising control. Ways of doing this include involving the client in planning interventions and providing, whenever possible, choices in which the client can exercise control over actions and outcomes.

Guilt may also require adjustments in the way clients think about themselves. Since life-style factors are widely known to make a significant contribution to the majority of chronic conditions, clients may feel guilty about behaviors that may have contributed to their current health problems. The nurse can help clients explore their feelings and assist them to turn from an irredeemable past to present behaviors that minimize the effects of health problems.

The fifth and final area that may require adjustment for clients with chronic conditions is that of intimacy. For males, some chronic conditions or their treatments may result in impotence, for example. In other cases, pain or changes in self-image may limit a client's ability to maintain intimate relationships with others. Another potential problem may be the withdrawal of significant others noted above. Clients and their families can be encouraged to discuss intimacy issues openly, and significant others can be assisted to find ways of fulfilling intimacy needs that are congruent with the presence of a chronic health problem.

In dealing with clients with chronic illness, the nurse must plan to assist the client in returning to a normal level of function as far as this is possible. In addition to the assistance of the nurse, it may be appropriate to refer the client to a relevant self-help group. Self-help groups can be particularly helpful in dealing with the psychosocial adjustments required by a chronic condition.[58] Clients may be able to relate better to persons experiencing similar problems than to the authority figures represented by health professionals.

Self-help groups have been shown to be quite effective in dealing with many health problems. The effectiveness of these groups stems from several assumptions. First, the emotional support of others with similar problems reduces the social isolation experienced by many clients with chronic conditions. Second, a collective self-identity emerges through group participation, allowing group members to develop new personal self-concepts. The third assumption is that group participation permits sharing of experiential knowledge and practical suggestions for coping with problems encountered. Finally, group participation fosters a more active orientation to health, greater reliance on individual and group support systems, and less dependence on health-care providers.[58]

Community health nurses may be involved in the

TABLE 31–6. RESOURCES FOR DEALING WITH CHRONIC PHYSICAL HEALTH PROBLEMS

Problem Area	Agency or Organization	Services
Accident prevention	American Association of Poison Control Centers Regional Poison Center 225 Dickinson St. San Diego, CA 92103 (619) 294-6000	Information on household poisons
	American National Red Cross 17th & D Sts. Washington, DC 20006 (202) 639-3563	Water safety education
	American Trauma Society 875 N. Michigan Ave., Suite 3010 Chicago, IL 60611 (312) 649-1810	Information on trauma
	National Safety Council 444 N. Michigan Ave. Chicago, IL 60611 (312) 527-4800	Assistance with accident prevention programs; information
	National Spinal Cord Injury Association 369 Elliot St. Newton Upper Falls, MA 02164 (617) 964-0521	Research, information on prevention of spinal cord injury
Airway disease	American Lung Association 1740 Broadway New York, NY 10019 (212) 245-8000	Research, information, antismoking programs
	Asthma and Allergy Foundation of America 1701 N. St., NW Washington, DC 20036 (202) 293-1260	Research, information
	Children's Lung Association of America 150 N. Pond Way Roswell, GA 30076 (404) 993-5859	Research, education, legislation
	Emphysema Anonymous, Inc. P.O. Box 66 Ft. Myers, FL 33902 (813) 334-4226	Self-help group
	National Asthma Center 875 Avenue of the Americas New York, NY 10001	Information
	National Foundation for Asthma, Inc. P.O. Box 50304 Tucson, AZ 85703 (602) 624-7481	Outpatient treatment
Arthritis	Arthritis Foundation 1314 Spring St., NW Atlanta, GA 30309 (404) 872-7100	Information
	Arthritis Rehabilitation Center 1234 19th St., NW Washington, DC 20036 (202) 223-5320	Diagnostic and treatment services
	Arthritis Society 920 Young St., Suite 420 Toronto, Canada M4W 3J7 (416) 967-1414	Professional training, research, information

TABLE 31–6. (*Continued*)

Problem Area	Agency or Organization	Services
Cancer	American Cancer Society 90 Park Ave. New York, NY, 10016 (212) 599-8200	Research, information, rehabilitation
	Cancer Care, Inc. and The National Cancer Foundation, Inc. 1180 Avenue of the Americas New York, NY 10036 (212) 221-3300	Social work assistance, counseling, home management, financial assistance, bereavement counseling
	Cancer Connection H & R Block Bldg. 4410 Main St. Kansas City, MO 64111 (816) 932-8453	Support group, referral for second opinion
	Cancer Coordinating Council for Metropolitan Washington Howard University Cancer Ctr. 2041 George Ave., NW Washington, DC 20006 (202) 659-5136	Information
	National Cancer Cytology Center 88 Sunnyside Blvd., Suite 204 Plainview, NY 11803 (516) 349-0610	Information on cancer screening
	Reach to Recovery 90 Park Ave. New York, NY 10016 (212) 973-8759	Support group for breast-cancer victims
	United Cancer Council, Inc. 1803 N. Meridian St., Room 202 Indianapolis, IN 46202 (317) 923-6490	Research, information
	United Ostomy Association 1111 Wilshire Blvd. Los Angeles, CA 90017 (213) 255-4681	Mutual aid and support, information
Diabetes	American Diabetes Association National Service Center P.O. Box 25757 1660 Duke St. Alexandria, VA 22313 (703) 549-1500	Research, information
	Becton Dickinson Consumer Products Franklin Lakes, NJ 07417 (800) 627-1579	Materials for client education on diabetes
	Joslin Diabetes Center One Joslin Place Boston, MA 02215 (617) 732-2415	Curriculum materials for children with diabetes
	Juvenile Diabetes Association 23 E. 26th St. New York, NY (212) 889-7575	Research, information
	National Diabetes Information Clearinghouse Box NDIC Bethesda, MD 20892 (301) 468-2162	Information on diabetes care and education

(*continued*)

TABLE 31–6. (*Continued*)

Problem Area	Agency or Organization	Services
Heart disease	American Heart Association 7320 Greenville Ave. Dallas, TX 75231 (214) 373-6300	Research, information
	Council on Arteriosclerosis of American Heart Association 7320 Greenville Ave. Dallas, TX 75231 (214) 750-5300	Coordinate research on artersclerosis, provide information
	Mended Hearts, Inc. 7320 Greenville Ave. Dallas, TX 75231 (214) 750-5442	Assistance to persons having heart surgery
Hypertension	National High Blood Pressure Education Program 120/80 National Institutes of Health Bethesda, MD 20014	Literature for blood pressure control in the workplace
	National Hypertension Association 324 E. 30th St. New York, NY 10016 (212) 889-3557	Referral, public and professional education
Obesity	Overeaters Anonymous World Service Office 2190 190th St. Torrance, CA 90504	Self-help group for weight loss, literature
	TOPS Club P.O. Box 07360 4575 S. 5th St. Milwaukee, WI 53207 (414) 482-4620	Self-help for weight reduction
	Weight Watchers International 800 Community Dr. Manhassett, NY 11030	Support group for weight loss, food plan, exercise, behavior modification
Smoking	American Cancer Society (see entry under *Cancer*)	Stop-smoking programs, information
	American Heart Association (see entry under *Heart disease*)	Stop-smoking programs, information
	American Lung Association (see entry under *Airway disease*)	Stop-smoking programs, information
	Action on Smoking and Health 2013 H St., NW, Suite 302 Washington, DC 20006 (202) 659-4310	
	The Non-smokers Club of Gasp 8928 Bradmoor Dr. Bethesda, MD 20817 (301) 530-1664	Arrange smoke-free travel for nonsmokers
Other	U.S. Senate Committee on Labor and Human Resources Subcommittee on the Handicapped SH-639 Hart Building Washington, DC 20510 (202) 224-5630	Policy formation
	Medic Alert Foundation International 2323 Colorado Turlock, CA 95381 (209) 668-3333	Identification and information file on persons with life-threatening conditions, membership fee (waived for the needy)
	National Chronic Pain Outreach Association 4922 Hampden Lane Bethesda, MD 20814 (301) 652-4948	Emotional support, self-help, advocacy, transportation, equipment loan

initiation of self-help groups or in subsequent support of such groups. Nurses will also refer individual clients to groups as appropriate. Nurses should function as facilitators of the group process, not as "leaders" or active participants in the group unless they also experience the chronic condition involved.

Community health nurses can facilitate the work of self-help groups in several ways. These include monitoring and directing active involvement by group members; encouraging the sharing of experiences and solutions to common problems; encouraging provision of mutual aid; and encouraging utilization of professional assistance as needed. Other facilitative measures include emphasizing personal responsibility for and control over events; maintaining positive pressure for behavior change; and emphasizing the need for positive coping strategies. Finally, the nurse should facilitate group interaction by providing the least amount of personal input possible.[58]

Community health nurses can refer clients to self-help groups or other community agencies that provide assistance in dealing with problems arising from chronic health problems. Table 31–6 provides infor-

TABLE 31–7. GOALS FOR TERTIARY PREVENTION AND RELATED COMMUNITY HEALTH NURSING INTERVENTIONS IN THE CONTROL OF CHRONIC PHYSICAL HEALTH PROBLEMS

Tertiary Prevention Goal	Nursing Intervention
1. Prevent further loss of function in affected systems Decrease risk factors for recurrence, exacerbation, or development of crises	1. Motivate client to comply with treatment regimen Assist client to identify risk factors amenable to change Assist client to identify ways of decreasing risk factors
2. Prevent loss of function in unaffected systems	2. Assist client to maintain function in unaffected systems
a. Prevent physical disability	a. Prevent physical complications of illness through: i. Breathing exercises ii. Skin care iii. Range-of-motion exercises iv. Adequate nutrition and fluids Provide physical care as required Refer for assistance with physical care as needed
b. Prevent social disability	b. Accept client as a unique person Encourage interaction with others Assist significant others to deal with feelings about client's illness Assist client to maintain independence as much as possible Assist with identification of need for changes in family roles Work to change public attitudes toward the disabled Promote legislation to aid chronically ill to maintain their independence
3. Regain functional abilities when possible	3. Assist with planning and implementation of programs to regain function (bowel training, physical therapy) Teach client and others to carry out program and evaluate effects
4. Monitor health status	4. Monitor client health status Identify changes in client situation that affect health Refer for follow-up as appropriate
5. Promote adjustment to chronic disease	5. Assist client to adjust to presence of chronic disease
a. Deal with feeling about disease	a. Accept client at his or her level of development and acceptance of disease Encourage client to discuss fears and apprehensions Refer to self-help groups as appropriate
b. Adjust life-style to accommodate chronic disease and its effects	b. Assist client to identify needed changes in life-style Assist client to plan and carry out life-style changes
c. Adjust environment to meet changed needs	c. Identify need for self-help devices and help client obtain them Identify environmental changes needed to foster independence Assist client to make necessary environmental changes
d. Adjust self-image	d. Assist client to adjust to change in self-image Refer for counseling as needed
e. Adjust to expense of chronic care	e. Refer for financial aid as needed

TABLE 31–8. STATUS OF THE 1990 NATIONAL OBJECTIVES FOR CHRONIC PHYSICAL HEALTH PROBLEMS

Objective	Evaluative Data	Status
1. Achieve control of blood pressure in at least 60% of persons with high blood pressure	11% of those with B/P of 140/90 and 33% of those with B/P of 160/95 or higher had their B/P under control	Objective unmet
2. Reduce average daily sodium intake to 3–6 g per person	Daily average sodium (excluding salt added at the table) was 1100–3300 mg in 1986)	Objective met
3. Reduce prevalence of significant overweight to 10% of men and 17% of women	25% of men and 26% of women are overweight	Objective unmet
4. Increase awareness of risk factors for heart disease and stroke to include at least 50% of adults	61% to 91% of adults aware of various risk factors, 1985	Objective met
5. Increase knowledge of own blood pressure to 90% of adults	61% of adults knew their blood pressure, 1985	Objective unmet
6. Increase extent of food labeling for sodium and cholesterol to 50% of processed food sold in grocery stores	65% of processed food was labeled in 1988	Objective met
7. Increase to 75% the number of cars with automatic restraint protection	5% of cars equipped with automatic restraints in 1988	Objective unmet
8. Increase presence of smoke detectors in residential units to 75%	Functioning smoke detectors in homes of 60% of those over age 18	Objective unmet
9. Educate 80% of parents on three major accident risks for children	27% to 82% of parents knowledgeable about risks in various areas	Objective unmet
10. All primary-health-care providers educate parents about child car safety	45% of families with children under 5 reported education regarding seat belt use, 1985	Objective unmet
11. Provide emergency response services within 20 minutes in 75% of communities	Average response time: in urban areas, 5.8 min; in rural area, 11.7 min, 1987	Objective met
12. Provide regional poison control services to 90% of population	Regional poison control services available to 59% of population, 1988	Objective unmet
13. Reduce proportion of adults smoking to under 25%	28.8% of adults smoked in 1987	Objective unmet
14. Reduce the proportion of women who smoke during pregnancy to under half of the proportion of all women smokers	32% of pregnant women in 1985 reported smoking in 12 months before delivery; only 21% of these quit when told of pregnancy	Objective unmet
15. Reduce proportion of persons aged 12–18 years who smoke to under 6%	12% of those aged 12–17 smoked, 1988	Objective unmet
16. Reduce average tar yield of cigarettes to under 10 mg	Average tar yield per cigarette: 13.3, 1987	Objective unmet
17. Increase proportion of adults aware of hazards of smoking to 90%	90% of adults aware of hazards of smoking	Objective met
18. Display tar, nicotine, and carbon monoxide yields on all cigarette packages	Tar and nicotine disclosed on low-yield brands, not others; carbon monoxide not discussed on any brands	Objective unmet
19. Enact laws in all 50 states prohibiting smoking in enclosed public places and work sites	42 states and District of Columbia had such laws by 1987	Objective unmet
20. Provide for nonsmoker's differential rates for health and life insurance	Few companies offer discounts for nonsmokers	Objective unmet

(Source: U.S. Department of Health and Human Services[1])

mation on a number of such organizations. Community health nurses should determine the availability of such agencies within their own communities and identify the services provided and eligibility requirements for each type of service so as to make appropriate referrals.

Tertiary prevention related to individuals with chronic health problems focuses on assisting clients to adjust to their condition and on preventing additional problems. Tertiary prevention at the community level might involve planning and implementing programs to assist with client adjustment or political activity to ensure the availability of tertiary prevention programs. Tertiary prevention goals and related nursing interventions are summarized in Table 31–7.

EVALUATING INTERVENTION FOR CHRONIC HEALTH PROBLEMS

Evaluating care related to chronic health problems is done in terms of care outcomes. Evaluation of care may be conducted in relation to the individual client or to a population group. In the case of the individual client, the nurse would evaluate the status of the chronic condition as well as the client's adjustment to having a chronic health problem. If interventions, both medical and nursing, have been effective, the condition will be controlled or may even be improving or will provide the least disruption possible to the life of the client and his or her significant others. Evaluative criteria would reflect both the client's physiologic status and his or her quality of life.

When the recipient of care is a community or population group, evidence of success in controlling chronic health problems lies primarily in changes in morbidity and mortality figures. Are there fewer cases of hypertension or cardiovascular disease in the population now than before the initiation of control efforts? Are there fewer disabilities due to accidental injuries? Do those with diabetes live longer or have fewer hospitalizations for diabetic complications? Based on the evaluative data, decisions can be made regarding the need to attempt other control strategies or to continue with current measures.

Evaluation of control strategies for chronic conditions in the population may focus on the extent to which chronic disease objectives for 1990 have been achieved. Objectives related to hypertension control, overweight, knowledge of one's blood pressure, motor vehicle accidents, automatic restraint protection in cars, and smoke detectors in residential units have not been met. Objectives related to the number of people smoking and women who smoke during pregnancy, children who smoke, and average tar yield of cigarettes also remain unmet. Objectives related to knowledge of risk factors for heart disease and cancer and salt consumption have been met, whereas those related to cholesterol levels, food labeling, and breast-feeding have yet to be achieved. Specific information on objectives related to chronic health problems, available evaluative data, and current status of the objectives is presented in Table 31–8.

CHAPTER HIGHLIGHTS

- Community health nurses may be involved in efforts to control chronic physical health problems by identifying risk factors for individuals or communities; case finding and referral of persons with chronic health problems; role-modeling healthful behaviors; and political activity to promote access to health care and control of risk factors.
- Personal effects of chronic physical health problems include disability, changes in lifestyle, social isolation, and financial burden. Population effects include the financial costs, morbidity and mortality, and years of potentially productive life lost because of chronic health problems.
- Chronic health problems can occur in any age-group, but their effects tend to be more sever in older persons.
- Genetic inheritance, race, sex, and physiologic disorders may constitute risk factors for some chronic physical health problems.
- Pollution and safety hazards that may lead to accidents that result in chronic disability are factors in the physical environment that might contribute to chronic physical health problems.
- Stress can constitute a psychological risk factor for some chronic health problems. Chronic health problems can also create psychological problems for clients.

(continued)

- Social environmental factors that influence chronic physical health problems include the extent of a client's social support system, social norms for behaviors that influence health, and income and educational levels. Chronic health problems can also influence a client's social interaction.
- Prominent life-style factors related to chronic physical health problems include diet, tobacco and alcohol use, occupational exposure to health hazards, sedentary life-style, nonuse of safety devices, and failure to conduct breast or testicular self-examinations.
- Health system factors that impede control of chronic physical health problems include failure of health-care providers to educate people to prevent chronic conditions and failure to provide adequate screening, diagnosis, and treatment facilities.
- Primary preventive efforts for chronic physical health problems include health education and political activity to promote health and action to modify or eliminate risk factors such as smoking, obesity, hypertension, and safety hazards.
- Aspects of secondary prevention include screening for and early diagnosis and prompt treatment of chronic conditions. Considerations in treatment include stabilizing the client's condition, establishing a treatment regimen, motivating compliance, and monitoring the effects of treatment.
- Tertiary prevention in the control of chronic physical health problems focuses on preventing further loss of function in affected systems, preventing loss of function in unaffected systems, restoring function when possible, monitoring the client's health status, and promoting adjustment to the chronic condition.

Review Questions

1. Identify at least three major roles for community health nurses in controlling chronic physical health problems. Give an example of an activity that the community health nurse might perform in carrying out each role. (p. 811)
2. Describe at least three personal effects and four population effects of chronic physical health problems. (p. 811)
3. Identify at least three human biological factors that influence the development of chronic physical health problems. (p. 814)
4. Describe at least two factors related to the physical, psychological, and social environments that influence chronic physical health problems and their consequences. (p. 815)
5. Identify at least five life-style factors that contribute to the development of chronic physical health problems. (p. 817)
6. Describe three health system factors that impede efforts to control chronic physical health problems. (p. 819)
7. Describe at least four general approaches to primary prevention of chronic physical health problems. Give an example of an activity that a community health nurse might perform in relation to each. (p. 821)
8. Identify at least three aspects of the treatment of chronic physical health problems. What is the role of the community health nurse with respect to each? (p. 824)
9. Describe five considerations in tertiary prevention of chronic physical health problems. How might a community health nurse be involved in each? (p. 825)

APPLICATION AND SYNTHESIS

You have just started working as a community health nurse for the Wachita County Health Department in Mississippi. During your employment interview the nursing supervisor mentioned that one of your responsibilities would be to participate in developing plans for dealing with the high rate of hypertension in the county. The incidence rate for hypertension here is three times that of the state and twice that of the nation.

The population of the county is largely black with high unemployment rates and little health insurance. Folk health practices are quite common, one of them being drinking pickle brine for a condition called "high blood." While this condition is not related to high blood pressure, the two terms are frequently confused by both lay members of the community and professionals alike. Dietary intake is typical of the rural South, consisting of a variety of fried foods, beans and other boiled vegetables, and corn bread.

Few health services are available in the county itself, although there is a major hospital 50 miles away. There are two general practitioners in the area and one pediatrician. The health department holds well-child, immunization, tuberculosis, and family planning clinics regularly and all are well attended. Transportation is a problem for many community residents.

1. What are the human biological, environmental, life-style, and health system factors influencing the incidence and prevalence of hypertension?
2. Write two objectives for your efforts to resolve the community's problem with hypertension.
3. What primary, secondary, and tertiary activities might be appropriate in dealing with the problem of hypertension? Which of these activities might you carry out yourself? Which would require collaboration with other community members?
4. How would you evaluate the outcome of your interventions?

REFERENCES

1. United States Department of Health and Human Services. (1990). *Report of the expert panel on population strategies for blood cholesterol reduction*. Washington, DC: Public Health Service.
2. Blum, H. L., & Keranen, G. M. (1966). *Control of chronic diseases in man*. New York: American Public Health Association.
3. United States Department of Commerce. (1989). *Statistical Abstract of the United States* (109th ed.). Washington, DC: Government Printing Office.
4. Asthma—United States, 1980–1987. (1990). *MMWR, 39*, 493–497.
5. Economic costs of diabetes mellitus—Minnesota, 1988. (1991). *MMWR, 40*, 229–231.
6. Prevalence of arthritic conditions—United States, 1987. (1990). *MMWR, 39*, 99–102.
7. Prevalence and incidence of diabetes mellitus—United States, 1980–1987. (1990). *MMWR, 39*, 809–812.
8. Mortality trends—United States, 1986–1988. (1989). *MMWR, 38*, 117–118.
9. United States Department of Health and Human Services. (1987). *Setting nationwide objectives in disease prevention and health promotion: The United States experience*. Washington, DC: Government Printing Office.
10. Chronic disease reports: Mortality trends—United States, 1979–1986. (1989). *MMWR, 38*, 189–193.
11. Feinleib, M., & Wilson, R. W. (1985). Trends in health in the United States. *Environmental Health Perspectives, 62*, 267–276.
12. Update: Years of potential life lost before age 65—

United States, 1988 and 1989. (1991). *MMWR, 40,* 60–62.
13. Premature mortality due to malignant neoplasms—United States, 1983. (1986). *MMWR, 35,* 457–462.
14. Lung cancer among women—Tennessee. (1984). *MMWR, 33,* 586–587.
15. United States Department of Commerce. (1987). *Statistical Abstract of the United States* (107th ed). Washington, DC: Government Printing Office.
16. Progress toward achieving the national 1990 objectives for injury prevention and control. (1988). *MMWR, 37,* 138–140, 145–149.
17. Morrow, P. L., & Hudson, P. (1986). Accidental firearms fatalities in North Carolina, 1976–1980. *American Journal of Public Health, 76,* 1120–1123.
18. Gilliland, B. C., & Mannick, M. (1980). Rheumatoid arthritis. In K. J. Isselbacher, R. D. Adams, E. Braunwald, et al. (eds), *Principles of Internal Medicine* (9th ed.). New York: McGraw-Hill.
19. Regional variation in colon cancer mortality. (1986, April–June). *Statistical Bulletin,* 7–12.
20. Variations in mortality from cancer. (1986, January–March). *Statistical Bulletin,* 22–27.
21. Cancer patient survival by racial/ethnic group—United States, 1973–1979. (1985). *MMWR, 34,* 248–250, 255.
22. Premature mortality due to cerebrovascular disease. (1987). *MMWR, 36,* 316–317.
23. Ingram, R. H. (1980). Chronic bronchitis, emphysema, and chronic airways obstruction. In K. J. Isselbacher, R. D. Adams, E. Braunwald (eds), *Principles of Internal Medicine* (9th ed.). New York: McGraw-Hill.
24. Kovar, M. G., Harris, M. I., & Hadden, W. (1987). The scope of diabetes in the United States population. *American Journal of Public Health, 77,* 1549–1550.
25. Sugarman, J., & Percy, C. (1989). Prevalence of diabetes in a Navajo Indian community. *American Journal of Public Health, 79,* 511–513.
26. Williams, R. R., Hunt, S. C., Barlow, G. K., et al. (1988). Healthy family trees. *American Journal of Public Health, 78,* 1283–1286.
27. Schumacher, M. C., & Smith, K. R. (1988). Diabetes in Utah among adults: Interaction between diabetes and other risk factors for microvascular and macrovascular complications. *American Journal of Public Health, 78,* 1195–1201.
28. Johnson, J. V., & Hall, E. M. (1988). Job strain, work place social support, and cardiovascular disease. *American Journal of Public Health, 78,* 1336–1342.
29. McWhorter, W. P., & Mayer, W. J. (1987). Black/White differences in type of initial breast cancer treatment and implications for survival. *American Journal of Public Health, 77,* 1515–1517.
30. Havas, S. (1987, April). Prevention grant is the prime source for efforts against major causes of death. *The Nation's Health,* 20.
31. Viedma, C. (1988, May). A health and nutrition atlas. *World Health,* 2–31.
32. Patterson, B. H., & Block, G. (1988). Food choices and the cancer guidelines. *American Journal of Public Health, 78,* 282–286.
33. Centers for Disease Control. (1990a). The Surgeon General's report on the health benefits of smoking cessation: Executive summary. *MMWR, 39*(No. RR-12), 1–12.
34. Brownson, R. C., Chang, J. C., & Davis, J. R. (1987). Occupation, smoking, and alcohol in the epidemiology of bladder cancer. *American Journal of Public Health, 77,* 1298–1300.
35. New atlas of cancer in the U.S. shows that differences in death rates persist. (1987, July). *The Nation's Health,* 24.
36. Smoking and health: A national status report. (1986). *MMWR, 35,* 709–711.
37. Centers for Disease Control. (1990b). Behavioral risk factor surveillance, 1988. *MMWR, 39*(No. SS-2), 1–22.
38. Kraus, J. F., Morgenstern, H., Fife, D., et al. (1989). Blood alcohol tests, prevalence of involvement, and outcomes following brain injury. *American Journal of Public Health, 79,* 294–299.
39. Premature mortality from diabetes mellitus—Use of Sentinel Health Event Surveillance to assess causes. (1986). *MMWR, 35,* 711–714.
40. Wing, S., Casper, M., Riggan, W., et al. (1988). Socioenvironmental characteristics associated with the onset of decline of ischemic heart disease mortality. *American Journal of Public Health, 78,* 923–926.
41. Community-based exercise intervention: The Zuni diabetes project. (1987). *MMWR, 36,* 661–664.
42. Donahue, R. P., Abbott, R. D., Reed, D. M., & Yano, K. (1988). Physical activity and coronary heart disease in middle-aged and elderly men. *American Journal of Public Health, 78,* 683–685.
43. Shear, C. L., Freedman, D. S., Burke, G. L., et al. (1988). Secular trends of obesity in early life: The Bogalusa heart study. *American Journal of Public Health, 78,* 75–77.
44. Tucker, L. A., & Friedman, G. M. (1989). Television viewing and obesity in adult males. *American Journal of Public Health, 79,* 516–518.
45. Screening for cervical and breast cancer—Southeastern Kentucky. (1988). *MMWR, 36,* 845–849.
46. Survey of chronic disease activities in state and territorial health agencies. (1987). *MMWR, 36,* 565–568.
47. Provisional estimates from the National Health Interview Survey Supplement on cancer control—United States, January–March, 1987. (1988). *MMWR, 37,* 417–420, 425.
48. United States Department of Health and Human Services. (1991). *Healthy people 2000: National health promotion and disease prevention objectives.* Washington, DC: Government Printing Office.
49. Cigarette smoking in the United States, 1986. (1987). *MMWR, 36,* 581–585.
50. Warner, K. E. (1989). Effects of the antismoking campaign: An update. *American Journal of Public Health, 79,* 144–151.
51. Orleans, C. T., Schoenbach, V. J., Salmon, M. A., et al. (1989). A survey of smoking and quitting patterns among black Americans. *American Journal of Public Health, 79,* 176–181.

52. Byrd, J. C., Shapiro, R. S., & Schiedermayer, D. L. (1989). Passive smoking: A review of medical and legal issues. *American Journal of Public Health, 79,* 209–215.
53. Block, G., Rosenberger, W. F., & Patterson, B. H. (1988). Calories, fat and cholesterol: Intake patterns in the U.S. population by race, sex, and age. *American Journal of Public Health, 78,* 1150–1155.
54. Advancements in meeting the 1990 hypertension objectives. (1987). *MMWR, 36,* 144–151.
55. Treatment and perceived blood pressure control among self-reported hypertensives—Behavioral Risk Factor Surveillance System, 1986. (1987). *MMWR, 36,* 260–262, 267.
56. Redeker, N. S. (1988). Health benefits and adherence in chronic illness. *Image: Journal of Nursing Scholarship, 20,* 31–35.
57. Barry, P. D. (1989). *Psychosocial nursing assessment and intervention: Care of the physically ill person.* New York: J. B. Lippincott.
58. Cole, S. A., O'Connor, S., & Bennet, L. (1979). Self-help groups for clinic patients with chronic illness. *Primary Care, 6,* 325–341.

RECOMMENDED READINGS

Biegel, D. E., Sales, E., & Schulz, R. (1991). *Family caregiving in chronic illness.* Newbury Park, CA: Sage.

Provides insights into the care needed by families with members suffering from Alzheimer's disease, cancer, chronic mental illness, heart disease, and stroke.

Bronstein, K. S., Popovich, J. M., & Stewart-Amidei, C. (1990). *Promoting stroke recovery: A research-based approach for nurses.* St. Louis: C. V. Mosby.

Offers direction for nursing care of clients recovering from stroke. Also presents research findings related to nursing care for stroke victims.

Leahey, M., & Wright, L. M. (1987). *Family and chronic illness.* Springhouse, PA: Springhouse.

Addresses the needs of families dealing with chronic illnesses. Presents assessment techniques and intervention strategies for working with these families.

Lubkin, I. M. (1987). *Chronic illness: Impact and interventions* (2nd ed.). Boston: Jones and Bartlett.

Examines the experience of individuals and families confronted with chronic illnesses. Presents nursing interventions to deal with the problems of chronic conditions.

Majorowicz, K., & Hayes-Christiansen, C. V. (1989). *Cardiovascular nursing.* Springhouse, PA: Springhouse.

Sets forth care plans for nursing diagnoses related to cardiovascular diseases. Also addresses patient teaching in relation to cardiovascular disease.

Morse, J. M., & Johnson, J. L. (1991). *The illness experience: Dimensions of suffering.* Newbury Park, CA: Sage.

Presents insights into the human experience of chronic illness.

Otto, S. E. (1991). *Oncology nursing.* St. Louis: C. V. Mosby.

Looks at the nursing care of clients with cancer. Presents information on the epidemiology, prevention, screening, diagnosis, and treatment of various forms of cancer.

CHAPTER 32

Chronic Mental Health Problems: Schizophrenia and Affective Disorders

Kathleen Heinrich

KEY TERMS

affective disorders
chronic mental illness
delusions
enmeshed
hallucinations
illusions
mood history
recidivism
schizophrenia
stress theory

Working with individual clients and families coping with chronic mental illness is an increasingly important dimension of the community health nurse's role. Ever since the deinstitutionalization of mentally ill persons began in the 1960s, more and more people with chronic mental illness are living in the community. Community health nurses are one group of community-based professionals frequently called upon to follow clients after they have been discharged from a psychiatric facility. Sometimes community health nursing agencies employ psychiatric–mental-health clinical specialists to visit chronically mentally ill clients and their families; at other times they hire psychiatric–mental-health nurses or social workers to consult with staff nurses on specific cases. It is not uncommon, however, for community health nurses who follow chronically mentally ill clients to have little or no ongoing support from or communication with psychiatrists or mental health specialists. In these situations, community health nurses understandably feel uncertain about the nature and scope of their responsibility. A community health nurse who has limited experience with psychiatric disorders beyond his or her basic education is likely to feel unprepared to assess, evaluate, and intervene effectively with chronically mentally ill clients and their families.

This chapter is written for nurses working in the community who are expected to follow clients with chronic mental disorders like schizophrenia, or who discover that a client they are following for some other reason is displaying signs and symptoms of chronic mental illness. Two categories of chronic mental illness will be discussed: (1) schizophrenia and (2) the major affective disorders of bipolar manic depression and unipolar depression.

The community health nurse's role with clients who have a chronic mental disorder is a supportive one that can include ongoing assessment of clients' responses to medication and their adjustment to home, work, and social life. Community

(continued)

LEARNING OBJECTIVES

After reading this chapter you should be able to:

- Describe at least three biological theories related to the cause of schizophrenia.
- Describe three possible effects of the psychological environment on the development of schizophrenia.
- Identify at least five symptoms of schizophrenia.
- Identify three common thought disorders associated with schizophrenia.
- Describe four general principles in planning care for clients with schizophrenia.
- Identify at least three human biological factors that may influence the development of affective disorders.
- Describe at least five environmental factors that may contribute to the development of affective disorders.
- Identify three approaches to primary prevention of affective disorders.
- Describe at least three community health nursing activities related to secondary prevention of affective disorders.
- Identify at least two considerations in tertiary prevention of affective disorders.

health nurses are not educated as psychotherapists. Rather, they work most effectively as part of a treatment team of health-care providers who cooperate to develop treatment plans, establish clearly defined roles and expectations commensurate with educational preparation, and communicate regularly to coordinate care efforts.

Clients with chronic mental disorders may or may not be living with their families of origin. The word "family" will be used in the generic sense to refer to the group of significant others with whom the client lives or has consistent contact. For some clients, family may be an employer, a neighbor, or their fellow residents in a halfway house. It is important that clients' families be included in planning treatment. Families can be strong allies in preventing or controlling further episodes of chronic mental illness if they are educated about the nature of the illness, its prodromal symptoms, or the possible side effects of medications used to control it. Employing this knowledge, families can alert nurses and other health-care professionals to early manifestations of exacerbations.

THE IMPACT OF CHRONIC MENTAL ILLNESS

A ***chronic mental illness*** is a syndrome with specific symptoms that impairs an individual's cognition, perceptions, emotions, and/or behavior and that recurs over an extended period of time. In the case of schizophrenia, for example, the symptoms of the illness must last more than 2 years to be considered chronic.

Chronic mental illness not only takes a toll on an individual's quality of life but can also tax a family's emotional, physical, and financial resources. These family problems frequently become society's problems. As noted in Chapter 24, Care of Homeless Clients, chronic mental illness is a major contributing factor in the growing problem of homelessness. Mental illness also places many other stresses on individuals, families, and society as a whole.

In the largest study of its kind in North America, the National Institute of Mental Health (NIMH) surveyed 17,000 residents in five epidemiologic catchment areas (ECAs). Subjects were interviewed, and the diagnostic criteria of the American Psychiatric Association's *Diagnostic and Statistical Manual-III*, or *DSM-III* 1978,[1] were used to correlate and analyze the data. This work permitted the first estimates of *DSM-III* disorders in the general population of the United States. The data collected also enabled researchers to correlate sociodemographic factors such as age, sex, race, ethnicity, marital status, and socioeconomic status with the incidence of various mental illnesses.[2] Table 32–1 lists the prevalence of major categories of mental disorders as determined by this study. The NIMH-ECA findings will be cited throughout this chapter when referring to the incidence and prevalence of specific disorders.

The importance of chronic mental health problems in the United States is highlighted by the number of objectives related to these disorders in the national health objectives for the year 2000. These objectives are summarized in Box 32–1.

TABLE 32–1. PERCENT OF THE U.S. POPULATION AFFECTED BY SELECTED MENTAL DISORDERS ACCORDING TO THE NIMH-ECA STUDY

Type of Condition	Percent of Population Affected
Anxiety disorders (phobias)	8.9
Substance abuse disorders	6.0
Affective disorders	5.8
Dysthymia (mental distress)	3.3
Major depressive disorder	3.0
Schizophrenia	0.8
Bipolar disorder	0.5

BOX 32–1

National Health Objectives for the Year 2000 Related to Chronic Mental Health Problems

1. Reduce to less than 10% the prevalence of mental disorders among children and adolescents.
2. Reduce the prevalence of mental disorders (excluding substance abuse) to less than 10.7% of adults living in the community.
3. Reduce to less than 35% the proportion of people 18 years of age and older who experienced adverse effects of stress in the past year.
4. Increase to at least 30% the proportion of people 18 years of age and older with severe mental disorders who use community support programs.
5. Increase the proportion of people with major depressive disorders who obtain treatment to at least 45%.
6. Increase the proportion of people aged 18 and older who seek help in coping with personal and emotional problems to at least 20%.
7. Increase the proportion of primary-care providers who routinely assess client's emotional, cognitive, and behavioral functioning to at least 50%.

Source: United States Department of Health and Human Services. (1991). *Healthy people 2000: National health promotion and disease prevention objectives.* Washington, DC: Government Printing Office.

SCHIZOPHRENIA

The disorder called schizophrenia was described in Sanskrit writings as early as 1400 B.C. ***Schizophrenia*** is a psychotic condition that manifests itself in massive disruptions in perception, cognition, emotion, and behavior.[3] For many clients this illness results in lifetime psychological disability and disrupted family relationships. Over the last 100 years, between 1 percent and 2 percent of the United States population has been diagnosed as having schizophrenia. The NIMH-ECA study found that 6.4 of every 1000 people are afflicted. In the United States alone, the societal cost of schizophrenia is estimated to be between $10 billion to 20 billion annually, primarily because of the lack of productive employment of individuals with schizophrenia.[4]

The term "schizophrenia" is derived from the Greek, meaning "split mind." Although the term itself has existed since 1912, its definition has changed over time and is different is various parts of the world.[5] A common misconception is that a person who has schizophrenia has dual personalities, a Dr. Jekyll and Mr. Hyde. Rather than a dual personality, schizophrenia involves a disassociation of thinking from feeling and from actions. Schizophrenia may be defined as a severe emotional disorder marked by disturbances of thinking, mood, and behavior, with thought disorder (confused or bizarre thinking) as the primary feature.[6] According to the *DSM III-R* (1987), there are four basic markers of schizophrenia—psychotic symptoms including illusions, delusions, or hallucinations; deterioration from a previous level of function; onset before age 45; and a duration of at least 6 months.

To be considered chronic, schizophrenic symptoms must persist over a 2-year period. People with chronic schizophrenia who are in remission often appear "normal." It is only during exacerbations that they exhibit symptoms.

Diagnosis of schizophrenia is difficult. Because it encompasses such a nonspecific cluster of symptoms, some experts believe that schizophrenia is not a distinct disorder. Diagnosis is further complicated by the fact that people with schizophrenia are a heterogeneous group whose illness is marked by the presence of various symptoms and whose course of recovery differs. Some clinicians are concerned that schizophrenia is used more as an accusation than as a diagnosis. In fact, studies have shown that clients with the same symptoms will be diagnosed as having schizophrenia if they are of lower socioeconomic status and as having depression or some other less serious disorder if they are of higher socioeconomic status.[7]

Misunderstandings about schizophrenia and the wide variation in its course have led to its being understood by some physicians, including psychiatrists, and lay people as equivalent to a diagnosis of cancer in that it is incurable. While it is true that there is no cure for schizophrenia, comparing it to diabetes is more appropriate because both diseases are chronic, marked by exacerbations, and can be controlled by medication.[8]

THE EPIDEMIOLOGIC PREVENTION PROCESS MODEL AND CHRONIC SCHIZOPHRENIA

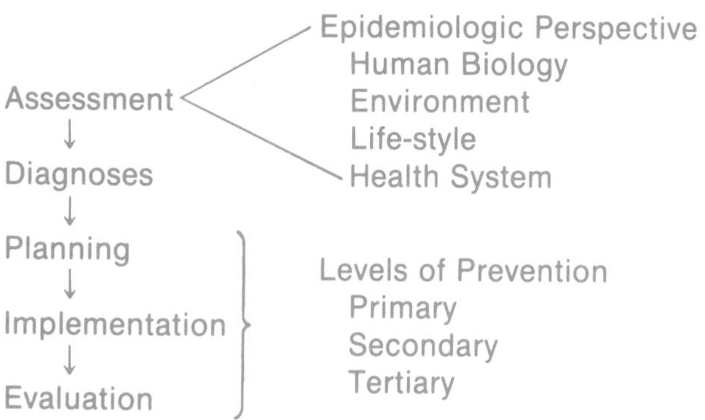

ASSESSING FACTORS ASSOCIATED WITH SCHIZOPHRENIA

Several factors in each of the four areas of the epidemiologic perspective have been associated with schizophrenia.

HUMAN BIOLOGY

Biological findings suggest a variety of explanations of schizophrenia including genetics and physiologic dysfunctions in the neurotransmitter systems of the brain.

Genetics

Various studies of families, twins, and adopted children provide strong evidence that some people have a genetic predisposition to develop schizophrenia. Relatives of persons with schizophrenia are more likely to develop the illness than those without a family history of the disease. Only 1 percent of the general population develops schizophrenia, but 10 percent of the parents, siblings, and children of people with schizophrenia also are diagnosed with the illness. Furthermore, the closer the relationship of an individual to a person with schizophrenia, the greater the chance of that individual developing the illness. When both parents are schizophrenic, they have two in three chances of producing schizophrenic children.[8,9]

Studies of twins show that both heredity and environment play a role in schizophrenia. The potential for schizophrenia developing in both members of identical twins is 75 percent higher than in the general public, and the risk of schizophrenia in both members of fraternal twins is 15 percent higher than in the general population.[9] Studies have indicated that 35 percent to 58 percent of identical twins separated at birth who grew up in two different households both developed schizophrenia later in life. Because the chance of identical twins both developing schizophrenia is not 100 percent, environmental influences may well play a part in the emergence of the disease.

How much of a role either heredity or environment plays in the etiology of schizophrenia remains unknown, but the weight of evidence suggests that the illness is genetically, rather than environmentally, induced.[10] However, there is no single biological marker consistently found in schizophrenic people that is not also found in people without.[11]

One way to assess whether family members are at risk for developing schizophrenia is to construct a genogram in an initial session with families. A genogram is a family tree that includes both sides of the family and identifies both physical illnesses and mental disorders that run in the family (Figure 32–1). It is most revealing to include at least three generations in the genogram.[12] If schizophrenia is noted in close relatives or in the parents themselves, family members are genetically more at risk for developing schizophrenia than the general public.

Physiologic Function

Researchers have investigated the action of the drugs that control the symptoms of schizophrenia in an attempt to understand the biochemical basis of the disease. It is known that the two classes of drugs used in the treatment of schizophrenia, phenothiazines (Thorazine) and butyrophenones (Haldol), both block dopamine receptors. On this basis, researchers suspect that schizophrenia may be related to excessive levels of dopamine linked to overactive neuronal activity. Both genetics and environmental factors like stress, nutrition, and exposure to viruses can influence biochemical states.[13] The dopamine hypothesis—that the amount of dopamine available at particular synapses is altered in people with schizophrenia—is the most promising explanation of schizophrenia.[14] The monoamine oxidase (MAO) explanation of schizophrenia, on the other hand, postulates that levels of a type of MAO (an enzyme that oxidizes monoamines such as epinephrine) are lower in people with schizophrenia than in the general population.[14]

Other physiologic phenomena have also been associated with schizophrenia. Brain ventricular size is significantly larger in chronic schizophrenic clients than in members of control groups,[15] while two types of schizophrenia have been proposed on the basis of dopamine receptors.[16] Type I is associated with the biological abnormality of increased dopamine receptors and is characterized by hallucinations, delusions, and thought disorders. Onset is acute and the client

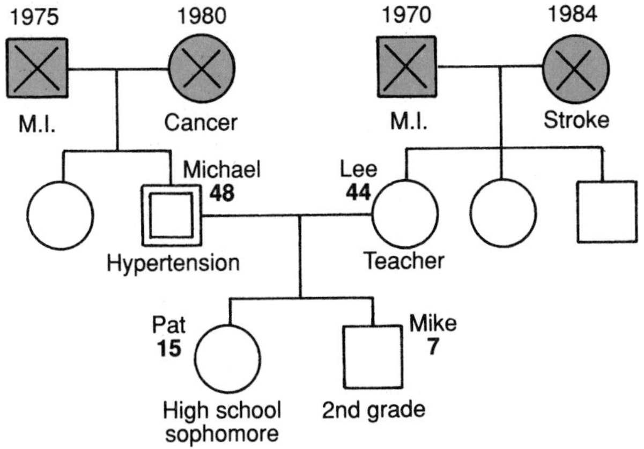

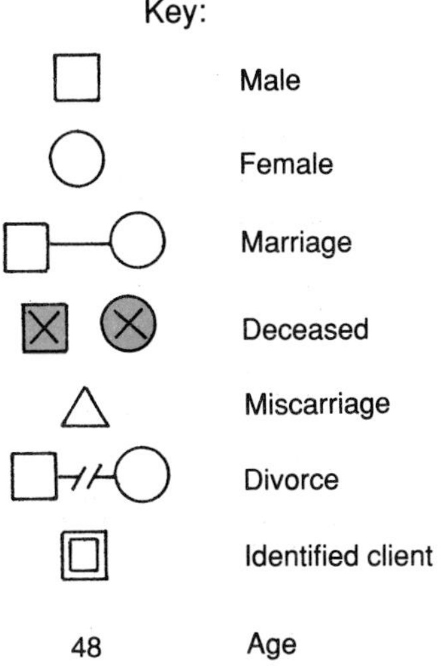

Figure 32–1. Family genogram. (*Adapted from Roth*[12])

responds well to medication. Type II schizophrenia is associated with flattened affect, loss of motivation, and poverty of speech, and it shows little response to treatment.[11] Another researcher has suggested that schizophrenia may be an autoimmune disease because of variable age of onset, a course characterized by exacerbations and remissions, and the low incidence of rheumatoid arthritis in persons with schizophrenia.[17]

Another aspect of assessing factors related to physiologic function in clients with schizophrenia is identification of physical illness. In general, psychiatric clients have higher rates of undiagnosed physical illness, particularly cardiovascular diseases and diabetes, than the general population.[18,19] Assessing the individual with schizophrenia for physical symptoms may be difficult because nonspecific behavior and mood changes may be the only signs of physical illness exhibited.[19] Or, physical illness may be manifested through psychological symptoms, leading the nurse to focus on the psychologic aspects of disease.[20] Finally, symptoms of physical illness may mimic symptoms of an earlier schizophrenic episode.[21]

Individuals with schizophrenia may exhibit four additional behaviors that could affect assessment of physiological problems. First, they seldom verbalize pain or discomfort. Second, they may display a propensity to self-mutilation by inserting objects into body cavities or removing body parts. Third, they exhibit a tendency to tolerate or exhibit lesions to get a response from others. Finally, clients with schizophrenia are frequently unwilling to tolerate medical care.[22] Keeping these factors in mind, the community health nurse assessing the physical symptoms of an individual with schizophrenia needs to be alert to small behavioral changes, explore physical as well as psychological explanations for illnesses, and encourage or arrange for periodic physical examinations.[18]

Maturation and Aging

Researchers who have studied people with schizophrenia over time[23–28] have demonstrated that these individuals are a heterogenous group ranging from those who are in complete remission and asymptomatic to those who are floridly psychotic. Older people with schizophrenia often evidence a "burn-out" effect in which symptoms like hallucinations and bizarre behavior seem to decrease with age.[29,30] However, other symptoms such as withdrawal, passivity, and poverty of speech may increase with age.[25] These shifts in symptomatology may result in better social adjustment as a result of fewer socially undesirable symptoms that provoke conflict with others.[18] There remains a small group of elderly people with schizophrenia who continue to exhibit florid symptoms and who are assaultive, destructive, and threatening throughout old age.[31]

It is important for the community health nurse to be aware that the number of older people afflicted with chronic mental illness is rising as the general population of the elderly increases in size. Nurses working with schizophrenic clients over the age of 65 should be aware that these clients are at greater risk of adverse reactions to medications used to control their disorder. They may develop tardive dyskinesia, involuntary rhythmic muscle movements that may occur as a side effect of antipsychotic drug therapy. Tardive dyskinesia is related to increased morbidity and mortality due to increased susceptibility to respiratory infections,[32] disturbed gag reflex leading to asphyxia; weight loss and malnutrition; and impaired gait leading to increased potential for falls.[33] Older clients may also experience chronic constipation as a side effect of the use of anticholinergic agents or metabolic changes due to neuroleptics.

ENVIRONMENT

Psychological Environment

The family has long been blamed for schizophrenia in children, and mothers specifically have been implicated. The "schizophrenogenic mother" was thought to be either overwhelmingly intrusive or coldly rejecting of the child.[34] Some research indicated that families that are ***enmeshed*** (emotionally overinvolved) are at risk for schizophrenia, whereas other research indicated that families that are critical and hostile, as well as overinvolved, may create schizophrenia in family members.[35]

A number of theories based on family communication research propose that schizophrenic families have characteristic dysfunctional patterns of communication.[34,36,37] One researcher suggested that dysfunctional family communication causes schizophrenia only in people with a genetic predisposition to the disease.[37] The biological findings to date suggest that there are multiple factors or one complex, multifacted factor responsible for the etiology of schizophrenia.

Family theories can serve as a reminder to the nurse that it is important to include the family in the assessment if the individual lives with or is in close contact with family members. Ongoing assessment with families at risk for schizophrenia includes assessing how they cope with major changes. Prominent family therapists like Jay Haley[38] believe that schizophrenia is one of the symptoms that can emerge when families are unable to make the transition from one stage of family development to another. The nurse and family can assess the stage of family development to see whether the family is, in

BOX 32–2

Questions for Assessing Individuals for Signs of Schizophrenia

- Have you noticed any changes in your sleeping patterns?
- Have you noticed that you are spending more time by yourself lately?
- Have you noticed any changes in the way you think? Have you had nagging thoughts that will not go away?
- Have you noticed you have less energy for keeping up your appearance—for example, putting on makeup, taking showers or baths?
- Have you been feeling more nervous lately? More anxious?
- Have you noticed any changes in your eating patterns? Have you suddenly gained weight? Lost weight?
- Have you noticed people reacting differently to you at home? At work?
- How are you liking yourself these days?

fact, "stuck" at a particular stage. Information on assessing family developmental stages was presented in Chapter 18, Care of the Family Client.

In addition to assessing families for risk factors that contribute to schizophrenia, the community health nurse may identify signs and symptoms of schizophrenia in individual clients. The best way to assess an individual for signs of schizophrenia is to observe and interview the client and family members. The family may be observing prodromal signs of schizophrenia including difficulty sleeping, changes in thought patterns, social withdrawal, deteriorating physical appearance due to self-care deficits, and impaired verbal communication reflecting changes in thought patterns. Other prodromal signs include heightened anxiety or fear; changes in nutrition; disturbances in self-concept and body image, self-esteem, role performance, or personal identity; changes in behavior toward family members; changes in behavior at school or work; and potential for violence.

The nurse also needs to interview the individual. This interview should take place in a quiet, private place away from other family members. The nurse will first assess whether the individual is oriented to time, place, and person by asking who they are, where they are, and what day, month, and year it is. After asking these questions, the nurse can use the questions included in Box 32–2. The nurse's observations during the interview can indicate that a client is experiencing schizophrenic symptoms. If the nurse had difficulty following what the client is saying, the individual may be experiencing disordered thought patterns, the most common of which are presented in Table 32–2.

If the person appears to have difficulty concentrating on the questions asked, he or she may be experiencing confusion or be preoccupied with illusions, delusions, or hallucinations. ***Illusions*** are perceptions that occur when ambiguous stimuli are misinterpreted. During an interview, for example, a client may say something like, "I was driving home yesterday, and someone was following me, and I knew they were from the F.B.I. because they had license plates from Washington, D.C." The person probably did see a car with a Washington, D.C., license plate, but it is probably a misinterpretation to conclude that the driver of the car is from the F.B.I.

TABLE 32–2. COMMON FORMS OF THOUGHT DISORDERS

Thought Disorder	Manifestation
Loose associations	One thought is barely connected to the next thought
Circumstantiality	Begins with one thought and leads "round the mulberry bush" before answering the question
Flight of ideas	Moves quickly from one idea to another with no connection between thoughts

Delusions are fixed false beliefs that are not open to change by reason or experience. Delusions may be paranoid (beliefs that others are persecuting one), somatic (beliefs that one's body is changing or responding in some unusual way), grandiose (beliefs that one is a prominent person like Napoleon or Jesus Christ), or religious (beliefs that one has some special mission given by God). There is no way to ask about delusions directly because the person believes them to be true, so it is important to explore all facets of the person's life during the interview. In the course of general conversation, the person may begin talking about relatives, supervisors, or neighbors who are trying to harm him or her in some way or about a God-given mission such as wiping out prostitution.

Hallucinations are sensory experiences that occur without sensory input. Although hallucinations can involve any of the five senses, auditory and visual hallucinations are the most common. If the person appears preoccupied because he or she seems to be focused on seeing something or is engaged in a conversation with someone the nurse cannot see, that individual may be experiencing a hallucination. To learn whether the person is experiencing a hallucination, the nurse can ask, "Do you see things other people do not see or hear things that other people do not hear?"

It is important for community health nurses to remember that schizophrenia is a disorder that can appear quite different in different people. If the person or the family reports significant disturbances in an individual's behavior, thoughts, perceptions, or feelings, the nurse may need to make a referral for further evaluation and treatment as needed. Nurses should also keep in mind that schizophrenia, like a number of physiologic diseases, includes a prodromal (pre-episode) phase, an active phase (the schizophrenic episode), and a recovery phase. Episodes can be prevented or their intensity reduced if individuals, family members, and the nurse identify the prodromal symptoms that preceded earlier episodes. The community health nurse should get a "baseline" assessment of the individual's personality prior to the onset of the disorder. This may need to be obtained from the client's significant others, because many clients with schizophrenia will already be affected by the disease before coming in contact with the community health nurse.

Another aspect of psychological assessment related to schizophrenia is the potential for suicide in the schizophrenic client. Suicide is the most devastating potential outcome of schizophrenia, and studies indicate that there is a 10 percent probability of suicide in the first 10 years after diagnosis and a 15 percent lifetime risk.[39] Community health nurses need to be particularly attentive to the potential for suicide when clients with schizophrenia experience depressive episodes.

Social Environment

Although sociocultural theories are difficult to test in research, one sociological theory of schizophrenia, the stress theory, bears mentioning. The ***stress theory*** suggests that schizophrenia results from exposure to major stressors including poor nutrition, inadequate housing, crime, and inadequate medical care experienced by those in poverty.[3,40] Indeed, international comparative studies show that there are greater numbers of schizophrenics in industrialized, urban areas than in rural, agrarian societies.[9] That social and emotional isolation may predispose one to schizophrenia is demonstrated by higher rates of the disorder among single, widowed, or divorced individuals.[15]

Because many experts believe that schizophrenia is caused by a genetic susceptibility combined with a stressful environment, it is important for community health nurses to assess the family environment with particular attention to the level of nurturing exhibited and the consistency, fairness, and age-appropriateness of limits set for children. The nurse should also assess the situation for economic and social stressors that may contribute to schizophrenia.

The homeless mentally ill population constitutes a growing social problem in the United States. Between 1955 and 1980, deinstitutionalization resulted in the release of 427,000 chronically mentally ill people from state mental hospitals.[41] During these years there were inadequate community-based facilities to care for them, so many of these people became homeless. Difficult to serve, the homeless mentally ill are unwilling to seek either medical or psychiatric care and are not based in any one place. It would seem that the best avenue for addressing the needs of this segment of the mentally ill population is to provide mental health services along with shelter, food, and physical health care in shelters for the homeless. Community health nurses working in shelters for the homeless can play an active role in assessing the mental health needs of shelter residents.

LIFE-STYLE

Particular life-style choices can precipitate the onset of an episode of schizophrenia. People who have had one or more episodes of schizophrenia do best when they minimize stress and live balanced lives. The community health nurse needs to assess leisure activities to ensure that the person exercises in a regular and balanced way.

With regard to consumption patterns, there is a growing awareness among health-care providers that many of the same people who abuse substances have underlying chronic mental disorders that they are attempting to mask with the use of mind-altering drugs.[9] This becomes evident when the person is weaned from the substance and the symptoms of schizophrenia become more prominent. It is also known that abuse of alcohol, marijuana, or hallucinogens can cause hallucinations in persons vulnerable to schizophrenia.

The nurse needs to assess the effects of occupational factors on clients with schizophrenia. Jobs with high levels of perceived stress or irregular hours that upset biorhythms may lead to schizophrenic episodes.

HEALTH SYSTEM

In most cases, the public mental-health-care delivery system of the 1990s is unable to provide more than custodial care to people suffering from chronic disorders like schizophrenia. The trend toward reimbursement systems favoring prospective payment means that hospital stays will be shorter and coverage for outpatient services will be decreased. As treatment for psychiatric problems is increasingly focused on short-term therapy for acute problems, clients with chronic mental health problems suffer.

While federal and state funding of mental health services is decreasing, treatment of chronic mental illness is becoming increasingly complex. At the same time, persons trained or interested in dealing with the chronically mentally ill are fewer. In the face of fewer treatment options for the chronically mentally ill, community health nurses are more likely to see clients with chronic mental illness in their caseloads.

Most of the mentally ill can live normally in the community if they receive outpatient care, rehabilitative services, and decent housing.[42] A system of half-way houses and day treatment facilities is needed to provide ongoing care, support, and treatment for the chronically mentally ill. Programs like "Training in Community Living," a model of community-based treatment for seriously mentally ill adults, have been shown to be effective in keeping clients out of the hospital and in the community and in helping them with employment, independent living, and social functioning.[43] At present there are too few of these facilities available and, although they are much less costly than inpatient facilities, their services are covered by few insurance companies.

Diagnostic Reasoning in Schizophrenia

Community health nurses may make a variety of nursing diagnoses related to schizophrenia. These diagnoses can reflect the health needs of an individual client, the client's family, or the needs of population groups. For example, the nurse might diagnose "impaired reality orientation due to schizophrenic episode" in an individual client or an "exacerbation of psychotic symptoms due to family stress" in a client with diagnosed schizophrenia. Another nursing diagnosis at this level might reflect "disruption of family function due to exhibition of symptoms of schizophrenia" on the part of one member.

Nursing diagnoses may also be made that reflect problems related to schizophrenia affecting population groups. For example, the community health nurse might diagnose an "increased incidence of schizophrenia in the homeless population." Or, a diagnosis of "inadequate treatment facilities for persons with chronic mental health problems due to reduced program funds" might be made.

Planning and Implementing Control Strategies for Schizophrenia

To develop a realistic psychological treatment plan for persons and families affected by schizophrenia, community health nurses need to establish ongoing communication with the mental health professionals involved. Both clients and families need to be involved in the planning, implementation, and evaluation phases to ensure the most favorable outcome. It is often difficult for both nurses and mental health professionals to match treatment goals with clients' rates of recovery. Nurses, as well as mental health care-givers and family members, can become overly enthusiastic when the client shows signs of recovery. They can inadvertently pressure the client with plans that are unrealistically optimistic or not matched to the client's pace of recovery. This is particularly true in the case of the client whose level of functioning shows deterioration after every exacerbation. The best plans are flexible and remove any added stressors by making steps small and easily accomplished so the client and family experience many small successes along the way to recovery.

The case of a 22-year-old male client recovering from his second psychotic episode illustrates this point. As a result of the client's steady progress, his psychiatrist, mental health care-givers, and family were encouraging him to begin looking for a job. The young man expressed concern that he was not ready and, in fact, began experiencing sleeplessness, extreme anxiety, and auditory hallucinations the week he was to begin looking in the newspaper for a job. The family alerted the community health nurse to these symptoms, and she reported these changes to the psychiatrist. They decided his behavior indicated that he was not ready to seek employment. The health-care team collaborated with the client and his family to revise the plan: (1) the client would cease looking for employment; (2) he would continue to attend an outpatient group that focused on job seeking; (3) when he felt ready, he could return to a volunteer job that he had held and enjoyed prior to this last psychotic episode; and (4) his long-term goal was to get and maintain a paying job.

This case underlines two general principles in planning care for individual clients with schizophrenia: (1) make the plan fit the client, rather than forcing the client to fit the plan, and (2) start with a plan that incorporates several small steps that ensure success at every level. Because the first plan was overly ambitious, the client experienced failure when he was not able to interview for a job. The revised plan incorporated group support, return to a volunteer position he had enjoyed and in which he had been successful, with a *long-term* goal of seeking gainful employment, and it actively included the family as allies in planning, implementing, and evaluating the plan.

When planning and implementing interventions for clients with schizophrenia, it is important for nurses to keep two additional principles in mind—they need continuously to involve the client and family in planning and they need to be flexible and creative in their approaches to implementing plans. Continuous involvement of the family strengthens the potential for open, honest communication between the nurse and all family members. It also increases the possibility that the nurse will be able to determine quickly whether all family members are committed to the plan or are unclear or sabotaging the treatment plan. Flexibility and creativity in implementation will assure that if plan implementation is not progressing smoothly there is openness on the part of the nurse to revise the plan or implement a new one.

Plans may also be made for programs to address

problems related to schizophrenia at the population level. Such plans will be based on the principles of program planning discussed in Chapter 19, Care of the Community or Target Group, but may require creativity in reaching underserved populations. As noted in Chapter 24, Care of Homeless Clients, plans to care for the homeless mentally ill will need to address the constraints imposed by their homelessness and the transient nature of this population.

Planning for control of schizophrenia can occur at primary, secondary, and tertiary levels of prevention. Primary prevention involves identifying families at risk and providing support and education around topics such as parent effectiveness. Secondary prevention includes the diagnosis and treatment of clients with schizophrenia. Preventing further episodes by monitoring compliance with medication and other treatment regimes falls under tertiary prevention.

PRIMARY PREVENTION

The community health nurse's role lends itself to primary prevention in the areas of family education, referral, and stress-factor or risk-factor reduction. To plan effectively for primary prevention, the nurse needs to keep in mind the current understanding of the major factors contributing to schizophrenia discussed earlier.

Education

Based on assessment of the family environment and the level of nurturing present; consistency, fairness, and age-appropriateness of limits set for children; and the quality of communication between and among family members, the nurse can plan appropriate teaching strategies. Based on the notion that "actions speak louder than words," the nurse can model effective parenting skills that may be lacking in the family repertoire. For example, the nurse may notice that parents neglect to praise their 4-year-old son for his accomplishments. Rather than address this directly, the nurse begins to compliment the child on things he does well. The nurse can also comment in general terms on the need for positive reinforcement of a healthy self-image to reinforce the behavior being modeled.

Since families with impaired communication may be at risk for schizophrenia, the nurse would want to plan to help the family avoid unhealthy communication patterns. For example, the nurse might notice a situation in which a father "double binds" his son. The father may first tell the son that if he does not take his insulin immediately he will ground him. As the son prepares his insulin injection, the father tells him that if he is not out of the house practicing soccer immediately he will ground him. The son is caught in a double bind and will be in the wrong no matter what he does. In this situation, the nurse might plan to speak to the father about how the son could become confused by two such contradictory messages, find out what the father really wants the son to do, and help him deliver his message clearly.

Referral

When teaching and modeling are not sufficient to help a family change potentially harmful child-rearing practices, the nurse may plan to refer the family for counseling. The nurse needs to plan carefully about how to bring up the topic of referral. Many families are comfortable with a community health nurse helping them with their problems but uncomfortable with the idea of seeking psychological counseling. After rapport has been established and it is clear that teaching and modeling are not achieving the desired result, the nurse may gently suggest that the family may want to "talk to someone skilled in dealing with the communication problems they are experiencing." Often the family is relieved and will want to begin to plan how to obtain treatment. If family members appear to be upset at the suggestion, but are not refusing, the nurse might outline reasons for suggesting counseling and explore why family members are upset by the suggestion. Frequently, when families understand that the problem is one for which help is available, they will accept the referral. If the family flatly refuses a referral, the nurse can drop the subject for the present and bring it up again at another time. The nurse may need to bring up the idea of counseling several times before the family is amenable to the suggestion.

Once the family is willing to accept a referral for counseling, the nurse will consider the family's financial resources and other factors that may affect the appropriateness of a specific source of care. For example, if the family is able to pay for services themselves, they may be referred to a private facility. If they have insurance, they may be able to be reimbursed for a portion of visits. If they belong to an HMO, they may be entitled to a specified number of sessions, but the providers to whom they may be referred will probably be restricted. If families have little funding for counseling services, they may be referred to agencies that will accept whatever the family is able to pay.

Risk-Factor Reduction

The third aspect of primary prevention in the control of schizophrenia is eliminating or reducing stress or risk factors for the disease. Families who are at risk for schizophrenia may need anticipatory guidance to cope with major changes and major life transitions. Some family therapists believe that schizophrenia is one of the symptoms that can emerge when families have difficulty moving from one stage of family development to another. Basing primary prevention efforts on this psychological developmental theory, the community health nurse can plan to give anticipatory guidance when the family is making the transition to a new stage of development that may be stressful—for example, when families with preadolescent children move into the stage of adolescence or when young adult children begin to leave home. Nurses can encourage families at risk to seek family counseling before or early in the process of undergoing disruptive transitions in their lives, including major geographic moves or divorce.

SECONDARY AND TERTIARY PREVENTION

In many instances, secondary and tertiary preventive measures for schizophrenia are very similar, so both categories of intervention will be discussed here. Secondary prevention may entail referral for diagnosis and treatment; educating both client and family about the disease and about medications and other aspects of treatment; motivating compliance; and monitoring the effects and possible side effects of treatment. Similarly, tertiary prevention involves referral for assistance with exacerbations of schizophrenia; educating clients and their families to prevent recurrent schizophrenic episodes and about the signs and symptoms of exacerbation; encouraging continued compliance with a treatment regimen; and monitoring the client's psychological health.

The community health nurse may be in the situation of following a person for a physical health problem who suddenly begins to show signs of schizophrenia discussed earlier in this chapter. The nurse's role in this case is to refer the client for further diagnosis and treatment. The community health nurse would also refer the client who is exhibiting signs of exacerbation of the disease.

Community health nurses may also be asked to follow clients with diagnoses of schizophrenia to provide support, encourage compliance, and monitor the effects of treatment. Prior to initial contact with the client, it is important for the community health nurse to consult with the referring mental health professional to determine whether the health professional has discussed the diagnosis with the individual and his or her family and the types and typical side effects of medications prescribed. Until about 15 years ago, many psychiatrists did not tell clients their diagnosis because they feared clients would lose all hope, since schizophrenia is incurable. More and more psychiatrists are beginning to share diagnoses with clients and their families and are actively involving them in the ongoing treatment process.

Daniel Patterson,[8] a prominent psychiatrist and early pioneer in the movement for full-disclosure and family-centered intervention, has developed an innovative, cost-effective, and pragmatic program for educating clients and their families. This program was designed to minimize hospitalization by preventing or quickly intervening when exacerbations occur. Dr. Patterson's common-sense approach to family education about schizophrenia can be applied by community health nurses to plan secondary and tertiary prevention for schizophrenia.

Early in the process of following a client with chronic schizophrenia, community health nurses will plan for several meetings with clients and their families to determine their level of knowledge about the disease. It is important for the nurse to explore with the client and family (1) what they understand about the diagnosis of schizophrenia and its treatment; (2) how they feel about the prescribed medication; and (3) what side effects, if any, the client is experiencing. This allows the nurse to evaluate any teaching needs that the client and family may have. Translating psychological jargon into everyday language is very important when discussing any form of chronic mental disorder with clients and families. In the initial session, the community health nurse tells the client and family that schizophrenia is a medical disease that tends to run in families. The nurse will also plan to complete a genogram with clients and families (if not done previously) to determine familial patterns of physical and emotional disorders.

In addition to finding out how the client feels about the prescribed medication and what side effects he or she may be experiencing, the nurse can ask whether the client has ever discontinued taking medication for any reason. It is common for clients, after the first, second, or even third schizophrenic episode, to put themselves at risk for exacerbation by discontinuing their medication without telling their family or mental-health-care providers. They may take themselves off medication to "prove" to themselves, their families, or mental health professionals that they do not have schizophrenia. They may also discontinue medications in order to drink alcohol or use some other mind-altering substance such as marijuana. It sometimes takes several psychotic episodes before the client truly believes he or she has schizophrenia, and the nurse should plan for frequent reinforcement of the need to continue taking medication as prescribed.

During the second session, the nurse can review with the client and family members the four best ways of staying in control of schizophrenia. These include developing a balanced, sensible life-style; use of medication to control symptoms; developing knowledge of the disease; and involvement in counseling and psychotherapy to reduce stress levels.

Community health nurses can assist clients to plan for a regular life-style that includes sufficient sleep, regular patterns of waking and sleeping (not rotating shifts), and limited or no use of stimulants such as coffee, tobacco, and decongestants that contain stimulants that may trigger schizophrenic episodes. Hallucinogens, amphetamines, and even marijuana can trigger episodes, and the nurse should plan to educate the client abut the risks involved in their use. Moderate use of alcohol does not seem to trigger episodes, but clients should be cautioned about overuse, particularly in conjunction with medication.

Nurses should also assist clients to plan ways of limiting their exposure to stressful situations. Some stressors occur without warning, but the client can plan to space out the occurrence of stressors over which he or she has some control such as buying a new house or changing jobs.

Clients and their families should be made aware of the prodromal signs that signal an episode of schizophrenia, and the nurse can help them to identify these signs specific to the individual client. The nurse should also encourage clients or family members to seek professional assistance when prodromal signs are noted. The plan for early notification of mental health professionals of the occurrence of prodromal signs should be openly discussed with the client to prevent feelings that they are being "spied on." It is very important to acknowledge and understand clients' feelings regarding these plans. Clients often feel more secure when they know that family members, the nurse, and mental health professionals will work with them as a team to help them stay well.

In the third session with the client and family, other ways of staying in control of the disorder can be discussed. One of these is medication. Most people who have schizophrenia continue on medication for the rest of their lives to keep symptoms under control. All medication has both beneficial effects and side effects. Some side effects are nuisances, annoying but not life-threatening.[8] Serious side effects, however, can be life-threatening. Nuisance side effects secondary to the major tranquilizers include dry mouth, blurred vision, skin sensitivity to sun, headaches, dizziness on standing or bending, and weight gain.

Health-care providers often fail to mention nuisance side effects that affect the client's sexuality. It is important that women know they may miss periods and men may experience difficulty ejaculating or be impotent. In addition, there are three nervous-system side effects that include parkinsonian side effects or "mummy" or "zombie" effects when the client shuffles his or her feet and cannot smile or swing arms when walking; acathisia, which is a condition characterized by restless legs where the person cannot sit still; and acute distonic reactions, which are severe muscle spasms of the neck and back. This last can occur within the first few days after starting medication. These spasms are frightening, but they can be eliminated quickly with an injection of anticholinergic medication. All these nuisance side effects can be treated with anticholinergics. Patients should be cautioned to be careful driving when they first begin the medication because of initial drowsiness.

Among the physically harmful side effects are liver disturbances that can lead to jaundice and bone marrow problems that decrease blood cell production and cause anemia. Tardive dyskinesia, an especially troublesome condition, involves involuntary movements of the face, tongue, or body muscles and is secondary to high doses of certain medications over a long period of time. The effects of tardive dyskinesia are reversible to a point, and the nurse should plan to monitor the client closely so medications can be changed or the condition treated if symptoms occur.

Clients and families need to know that depression often occurs sometime during or following a schizophrenic episode. Several types of depression are associated with schizophrenia. Stress can trigger depression, which can trigger a schizophrenic episode. In addition, some people experience recovery depression, normal feelings during recovery from what some people have called a "living hell." A third type of depression arises in response to knowledge of an incurable disease. Again, this is a normal response. Depression may also result from medication. Finally, there is a chronic depression that sometimes accompanies schizophrenia and is not treatable.[8] When nurses observe depression in clients, they need to alert the treatment team and monitor clients for suicidal behaviors.[39]

EVALUATING CONTROL STRATEGIES FOR SCHIZOPHRENIA

Evaluating the treatment plan for schizophrenia includes assessing clients and families for their understanding of schizophrenia and their ability to monitor client status and behaviors in response to the nursing interventions discussed above. The nurse's role often includes evaluating interventions to ensure that they focus on the behavioral, perceptual, cognitive, and emotional aspects of the client's functioning as evidenced by improved communication, self-care, and judgment.[11] These interventions and plans need to be realistic, reflecting the client's level of functioning and the course of the disorder.

Evaluation at the group or population level would focus on the incidence and prevalence of schizophrenia in the population. If primary prevention efforts are effective, these rates should decline. Other foci for evaluation at the group level include the adequacy of treatment facilities and the extent of ***recidivism***, or rehospitalization, as a result of recurrent episodes of schizophrenia. When secondary and tertiary interventions are effective, evaluation should indicate that hospitalization occurs less frequently.

AFFECTIVE DISORDERS

Some experts call this the "Age of Melancholy" because of the ominous threats of nuclear warfare, overpopulation, environmental pollution, and economic instability.[44] This state of affairs may be reflected in the fact that depression is the most prevalent psychiatric disorder in the United States, affecting as many as 20 percent of the adult population.[9] An estimated 15 million people suffer from clinical depression.[45] An ***affective disorder*** is a disturbance in mood that manifests mainly as depression but can also involve elation or mania. In the *DSM-III-R*[1] affective disorders include depressive disorder, which is referred to as unipolar disorder, and manic depression disorder, which is referred to as bipolar disorder. This chapter will use the terms *depressive disorder* and *manic-depressive disorder* to distinguish between the two types of depression.

Affect refers to emotional tone. Affect includes verbal descriptions of emotional states and nonverbal behaviors like facial expression, motor activity, or physiologic responses. Another way to think of affect is on a continuum from depression through "normal" to manic. *DSM III-R*[1] defines affective disorders as disorders of mood. People diagnosed as having major unipolar depression experience loss of interest in life and an unresponsive mood lasting for at least 2 weeks. Manic-depressive episodes include times when the person is depressed and periods where the person experiences elation, needs less sleep, and exhibits enormous capacity for activity. The manic phase begins suddenly and the depressive phase is briefer than in major depressive disorder.

While an estimated 15 percent to 30 percent of adults in the general population experience depressive episodes at some time in their lives, only a minority seek psychiatric or mental health care. Given this, community health nurses are likely to encounter many individuals suffering from various forms of affective disorders that have never been treated.

THE EPIDEMIOLOGIC PREVENTION PROCESS MODEL AND AFFECTIVE DISORDERS

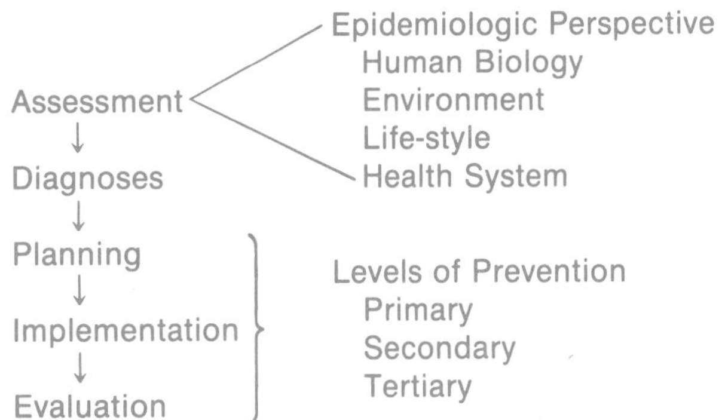

ASSESSING FACTORS ASSOCIATED WITH AFFECTIVE DISORDERS

A variety of factors are associated with the development of affective disorders. These factors occur in each of the four areas of the epidemiologic perspective.

HUMAN BIOLOGY

Human biological factors related to age and sex, genetic inheritance, and physiologic function have been associated with the incidence and course of affective disorders.

Age and Sex

Approximately 30 million to 40 million Americans suffer from depression. The lifetime risk of developing depression is approximately 20 percent for women and 10 percent for men.[46] The incidence of depression among children of depressed parents ranges from 14 percent to almost 50 percent. The rate of depression doubles in adolescence, and depression is more common in prepubertal boys and adolescent girls.[47]

Research findings are contradictory in terms of the interconnections of gender and age with depression. Some studies report patterns of higher prevalence of depression in younger women that plateau with age and increased prevalence in men with increasing age.[48] Other studies report a peak prevalence of depression in both older men and women.[49,50] Some authors report that the peak incidence of depression in women is between 45 and 55 years of age and between 65 and 86 years of age for men.[49]

Genetic Inheritance

Strong evidence exists for the role of genetic factors in mood disorders. It is highly possible that genetic factors make some individuals more susceptible to environmental stressors or styles of parenting that may contribute to depression. Evidence suggests that genetic etiologies play a role in both unipolar depression and bipolar manic-depressive disorder.

Genetic factors have been linked to the development of mood disorders. Close relatives of people with mood disorders face a 20 percent risk of developing these disorders compared to a risk of 5 percent to 10 percent for the general population. Longitudinal studies indicate that in 68 percent of identical twins and 23 percent of fraternal twins both develop affective disorders. These rates support the hypothesis of genetic etiology.[51] There is virtually unanimous agreement that the frequency of affective illness, particularly manic-depressive disorder, also increases in close relatives of the diagnosed client (10 percent to 25 percent versus 1 percent to 2 percent in the general population). Although it is not possible to say what causes bipolar mood disorder, it has been suggested that bipolar mood disorders are transmitted by an X-linked gene.[52]

A relatively new and promising area of research has to do with investigating the relationship between neurotransmitters and the affective disorders. One theory holds that monoamine oxidase secreted in the brain may be under genetic control. Another theory postulates that there is a genetic predisposition to a lower threshold for stress. Therefore, those with a low threshold are more susceptible to chemical changes that occur with stress, thus leading to depression.[47]

In assessing the potential for depression in individuals and families, the community health nurse can use a genogram to describe familial patterns of affective disorder. Evidence of a family history of depression would direct the nurse's attention to a more in-depth assessment for signs of depression in current family members. These signs and symptoms of affective disorder will be discussed later in this chapter.

Physiologic Function

Other physiologic theories have been advanced to explain depression. The endocrine model holds that endocrine changes that occur after exposure to stress result in the biophysical changes known as the "vegetative signs of depression." Hormones, particularly cortisol, growth hormone, thyroid-stimulating hormone, thyroid-releasing hormone, leutenizing hormone, and prolactin, have all been found in abnormal levels in depressed clients, supporting belief in a psychoendocrinologic mechanism for depression. In 1986 *Science News* reported that NIMH researchers postulated that high levels of cortisol, a steroid hormone, seen in depressed people, reflect abnormally high levels of corticotropin-releasing hormone released by the hypothalamus.[54] Community health nurses can assess clients at risk for depression for vegetative signs including psychomotor slowing, sleeping disorders, appetite disturbances, diminished libido (sexual desire), difficulty concentrating, and constipation. Vegetative signs of depression are summarized in Box 32–3.

One test used to diagnose endogenous depression (chronic depression not caused by external factors like grief or loss) is related to the psychobiologic theory of depression. The dexamethasone suppression test (DST) involves administering a single dose of dexamethasone followed by blood or urine monitoring of cortisol levels.[9] In depressed people, dexamethasone does not suppress adrenocortical functioning because of a failure of the normal inhibitory influence of the brain in release of ACTH and cortisol. This suggests that this limbic system dysfunction is not simply a response to stress. Rather, it is associated with disturbances in mood, affect, appetite, sleep, and autonomic nervous system activity. A related theory suggests that depressed people suffer from a failure of the central nervous system circadian inhibitory mechanism. Seasonal affective disorders (SADs) are being studied in people who live in the Northern Hemisphere and who suffer increased depressions

BOX 32–3

Vegetative Signs of Depression

Disturbances in sleep patterns
- Difficulty falling asleep
- Early morning awakening
- Difficulty waking up

Alterations in eating habits
- Significant weight gain
- Significant weight loss

Diminished energy level
Decreased interest in sex
Difficulty concentrating

(*Note:* The presence of one or more of these symptoms can indicate that a client is experiencing depression.)

during winter when there is less sunlight. When these people are exposed to sunlight for 8 hours a day, their depressive symptoms decreased markedly.[44]

Community health nurses should assess clients with possible depression for changes in biorhythms, mood, affect, and appetite. The nurse may also want to assess seasonal patterns to depressive episodes that suggest seasonal affective disorders.

In assessing individual clients with affective disorders, the nurse should conduct a head-to-toe physical examination. Organically caused depression is due to a person's changed biochemical condition and should not be confused with normal reactions to illness. Organically caused depression may result from hormonal or chemical imbalances and even from some physical disease such as infectious mononucleosis, hepatitis, or atherosclerosis.[9] Postpartum depression is a fairly common depressive response thought to be physiologically induced by changes in hormone levels and relationships as the body readjusts to a nonpregnant state. While most postpartum depression lasts a few days to a week, a small percentage of postpartum women may experience depression lasting for months and requiring treatment.

Because depression often precedes or results from physical illnesses, the nurse needs to be particularly sensitive to the powerful connections between mind and body when people with depression experience exacerbations of conditions such as eczema or psoriasis, asthma, ulcerative colitis, and Crohn's disease. AIDS, multiple sclerosis, systemic lupus erythematosus, thyroid and parathyroid disorders, adrenal insufficiency, carcinoid syndrome, and central nervous system tumors are among the disorders associated with depression.[53]

Some clients experience "iatrogenic depression" as a side effect of some medications taken for physical illnesses. Medications implicated in iatrogenic depression include opiates, antineoplastics, phenothiazines, digitalis, guanethidine, hydralazine, methyldopa, propranolol, reserpine, levodopa, sedatives, and steroids.[54–56] Community health nurses caring for clients who are on any of these medications should assess clients carefully for evidence of depression.

Clients who exhibit symptoms mimicking depressive or manic-depressive disorders may be experiencing serum electrolyte imbalance instead, and the community health nurse should assess the client for other signs of electrolyte imbalance and refer the client for serum electrolyte testing.

Because people who are depressed may lack the energy to tell the nurse what physical symptoms they are experiencing, and people in the manic state of manic-depressive disorder may be too anxious, scattered, or hostile to be good reporters, the nurse will need to expand his or her interviewing to include the family or significant others to do a thorough assessment. The nurse should also be alert to physical evidence of depression such as slow response, depressed affect, and listlessness.

ENVIRONMENT

As noted earlier, it is believed that lack of exposure to sunlight may be a contributing factor in seasonal depression, indicating that the physical environment may influence the occurrence of affective disorders. Elements of both the social and psychological environments also contribute to the development of depression.

Epidemiologic studies indicate populations most at risk for affective disorders include women; people in unhappy marriages; those who are separated, widowed, or divorced; low-income blacks; and the elderly (NIMH-ECA study). One particularly high-risk group is young unmarried women with young children.[57,58] High levels of maternal depression affect the well-being of children. Maternal depression has been linked to lower physical and mental health status as well as learning and behavioral problems among school children.[59–61] Community health nurses should assess young women with children for depression as well as assessing the offspring of women with depression for adverse physical, psychological, and behavioral problems.

Stressful life events can play a significant part in the development of an affective disorder. Marital dissatisfaction and unhappiness are highly correlated with depression. The effects of racism, sexism, and agism can also contribute to depression.[47] The social status theory holds that the way a person is viewed by society affects that person's propensity to be perceived as mentally ill or developing mental illness. Most writers and researchers agree that women's socialization in Western culture predisposes them to depression.[62,63] Research has indicated that the American definition of mental health has been equated with the "healthy" male qualities of assertiveness, logic, rationality, independence, and nonemotionalism. Women are traditionally expected to be passive, irrational, dependent, and emotional, and rigid role expectations for women predispose them to depression whether or not they fulfill traditional role expectations.

The social status theory can also be applied to older people. Because youth is desirable and old age is associated in American culture with uselessness, unimportance, and even repulsiveness, the social status of older people is low and their vulnerability to depression is increased.[47]

The interpersonal theory of affective disorders focuses on the effects of the psychological climate created by loss of interpersonal relationships, particularly in families with impaired parenting abilities. In this theory the large percentage of women and elderly persons who experience depression is explained by the loss of relationships to which they have been socialized. Women, for example, have been socialized to look to other people for approval and see the maintenance of relationships as a measure of their own worth. When a relationship is lost through divorce, death of a spouse, or loss of a boyfriend, a woman's self-esteem is diminished and depression may result. Similarly, older people who sustain many losses through the deaths of family members and friends are vulnerable to depression. Community health nurses working with individuals who have sustained the loss of one or more significant interpersonal relationships should assess the meaning of the loss for the client, its effects on client's self-esteem, and the adequacy of client's efforts to cope with the loss.

Another aspect of assessing the client with an affective disorder is to determine the potential for suicide. Depression and suicide are highly correlated, and the nurse should explore with the client any suicidal tendencies or thoughts of suicide. Suicide tends to occur most frequently when clients are recovering from an episode of depression; this is because the severely depressed client probably does not have the energy to commit suicide.

LIFE-STYLE

Life-style factors related to consumption patterns, employment, and leisure activities can also influence affective disorders.

Consumption Patterns

Consumption patterns in the form of substance abuse can mask the symptoms of affective illness. Substance abuse can be an attempt at self-medication to relieve the symptoms of affective disorders. For individuals with affective disorders, alcohol, barbiturates, and tranquilizers are the substances most often abused. Some experts estimate that as many as 70 percent of alcoholics, for example, may have a manic-depressive disorder.

The community health nurse should assess a client's consumption of alcohol and other substances that may mask or exacerbate affective disorders. The nurse should pay particular attention to tendencies to mix alcohol and medications as these may be lethal combinations.

Employment

Within urban centers and highly competitive settings are many overachieving professionals who capitalize on the manic side of their bipolar disorder. They may seek hypomania (the state preceding mania) to increase their productivity. When hypomania becomes full-blown mania, a person's carefully planned career can be lost in a few days as he or she becomes progressively more grandiose, more irritable and argumentative, or more prone to sexual excesses or extravagant buying. This is one of the tragic outcomes of untreated manic-depressive disorders.

In depression, the person may have difficulty finding the energy to go to work or to perform adequately when he or she is there. This state can also lead to difficulties with supervisors, increased stress, and deepening depression. The community health nurse should assess the effects of affective disorders on clients' employability and ability to perform their expected roles.

Leisure Activity

As was the case with schizophrenia, balance is the key in assessing leisure activity. In the case of depression, nurses need to determine whether the individual is including leisure activities into his or her schedule. Most people suffering from depression have very little energy, and they often lose their ability to enjoy life. Leisure activities for the person in the manic stage of manic-depressive disorder may pose safety hazards if excessive risks are taken during periods of grandiose thinking.

HEALTH SYSTEM

The major issue in affective disorders related to the health-care system is reaching those persons suffering from depression—many individuals do not seek treatment. Lack of attention to symptoms of depression by health-care providers may further decrease the opportunity to treat people with affective disorders. Primary-care providers are often inclined to ignore signs and symptoms of depression or attribute them to physical illnesses. They may also fail to warn clients of the potential for depression caused by many medications and to monitor them for evidence of depression.

Lack of access to care is another health system factor that may impede diagnosis and treatment of affective disorders. For example, some health insurance policies may not cover care for emotional disorders, particularly if they are not yet severe enough to warrant hospitalization. The nurse should assess clients' abilities to pay for care as well as the availability and accessibility of resources for care of affective disorders in the community.

DIAGNOSTIC REASONING AND AFFECTIVE DISORDERS

Nursing diagnoses related to affective disorders might reflect the presence or consequences of these diseases for individual clients or the existence of a high incidence of affective disorder or lack of care facilities in the community. Possible nursing diagnoses for an individual might be "depression due to recent divorce and financial stress" or "potential for loss of job due to manic manifestations of manic-depressive disorder." At the community level, the nurse might make a diagnosis of "increased incidence of depressive disorder due to economic instability" or "lack of facilities for care of affective disorders due to diminished tax revenues."

PLANNING AND IMPLEMENTING CONTROL STRATEGIES FOR AFFECTIVE DISORDERS

As was the case with schizophrenia, it is important that both client and family be actively involved in planning and implementing control strategies for affective disorders. Effective strategies can involve primary, secondary, and tertiary prevention measures depending on whether the disorder has already manifested itself in a particular client.

PRIMARY PREVENTION

The community health nurse is in an excellent position to engage in primary prevention of affective disorders. Because the number of people suffering from affective disorders far exceeds the number of those who seek treatment, the nurse is likely to encounter individuals with active disorders who are either unaware they are depressed or do not want to face it.

Primary preventive measures may include family teaching, referral, and risk-factor reduction. Prevention measures can be developed for individuals and families who are at risk for affective disorders owing to family history or situational stressors. Teaching them about the prevalence of depression in society, the genetic factors involved, and the potential for stressful life events that can cause depression can help clients and their families deal with feelings about the disorder. Teaching how to handle stress is another way of preventing depression in people who are at risk for affective disorders.

Because many chronically depressed people are socially isolated and do not seek help, community health nurses need to plan to increase the level of support available to clients. Community support groups exist for those who are adjusting to separation, divorce, or the death of a loved one, and nurses can make referrals to these and similar support groups for clients who are undergoing stressful life events. The nurse can also plan to refer parents to parenting groups that can provide them with opportunities for social interaction as well as parenting support.

Reducing or eliminating stressors and risk factors for depression is another way to lessen the feelings of helplessness and hopelessness that can lead to depression. For example, one study indicated that screening mothers for exposure to stressors could lead to the development of primary prevention measures for depression.[64] Working to improve the social conditions of persons at risk for depression may effectively reduce their exposure or vulnerability to socioeconomic stressors and associated higher risks of physical and mental illness.

SECONDARY PREVENTION

When the community health nurse suspects that an individual is suffering from a depressive or manic-depressive disorder, the nurse can plan to refer the client for further diagnosis and treatment. Again, the nurse would want to consider the type of referral that will be most appropriate to the client's circumstances. Areas to be considered include the client's financial resources, the acceptability of a particular source of services to the client, and any other circumstances that might influence the client's ability to follow through on the referral (for example, lack of transportation). Because depressed clients frequently do not have the energy to seek care, the nurse may plan to make an appointment for the client and help the client plan the logistics of getting there.

In caring for the client with a diagnosis of affective disorder, the nurse may plan to obtain a "mood history." Particularly useful in manic-depressive disorder, the ***mood history*** is a picture obtained from the client and family about the cyclical ups and downs of the client's moods over the last several years. When this picture is completed, the nurse, client, and family can often identify particular times of the year or particularly stressful events that precipitated either manic or depressive episodes. This knowledge can then be used to design strategies or minimize stress at expected periods of exacerbation, thus limiting response. In addition, the nurse and the family can plan for intensive observation of the client at these times to identify early signs of depression or manic behavior so treatment can be initiated or reinforced.

Antidepressant medications may be indicated and should be prescribed by a psychiatrist who is trained in the use of psychopharmacologic agents. Internists and family-practice physicians are generally not experts in psychopharmacology and should not be expected to prescribe medications or treat clients with affective disorders. Because depression and anxiety often go hand in hand, both symptoms can be treated pharmacologically. Several categories of antidepressant and antianxiety agents are commonly prescribed. Two classes of antidepressants have been prescribed since 1960, tricyclics like Elavil and Tofranil, and monoamine oxidase inhibitors (MAOIs) like Nardil and Parnate.

Although the reason for their effectiveness is not known, both types of antidepressants share one property—the ability to boost the action of serotonin and norepinephrine. While the tricyclics block reabsorption of these neurotransmitters, MAO-inhibitors interfere with enzymes that break them down. When a client is started on a traditional tricyclic, he or she spends several weeks taking progressively larger doses. The psychiatrist uses blood tests to determine the effective serum concentration, which is different for each individual. Because an overdose of tricyclics can be extremely toxic, resulting in low blood pressure, heart disturbances, blurred vision, constipation, dizziness, sluggishness, and weight gain, many doctors often prescribe too little. Because the therapeutic range is so narrow, too little medication is often ineffective. The MAOIs can cause a hypertensive response to foods containing retsin (for example, chocolate, cheese, wines). Many people chose depression over these side effects.

The community health nurse caring for clients on antidepressant medications would educate them about the medication and its therapeutic and toxic effects as well as potential side effects. Prozac (fluoxetine), a new classification of antidepressant introduced in 1987, is now America's leading antidepressant. Although Prozac costs 20 times as much as a generic antidepressant, an estimated 650,000 Prozac prescriptions are being written every month.[65] Prozac works like a tricyclic that focuses on serotonin. As one psychiatrist put it, "Instead of using a shotgun, you're using a bullet."[65] Although Prozac takes 3 weeks to become effective, there is no blood monitoring, because a dose of 20 to 40 mg is usually effective. There is less risk of overdose, and the most common side effects are nuisance effects such as headaches, nausea, insomnia, nervousness, weight loss, decreased sexual interest and loss or delay of orgasm, and a slight risk of seizures. In rare cases, suicidal thoughts and overtly violent behavior have been traced to Prozac. A small number of clients develop a "caffeine syndrome" in which they become restless and sometimes experience tremors. Because it is a new drug, the long-term effects of Prozac are unknown. There is concern that because administration of Prozac is so simple, the drug may be indiscriminately prescribed like Valium was in the 1970s. Psychiatrists are cautioned that Prozac may not be as effective as the tricyclics. Clients may not be helped if they are suffering depression associated with a hidden illness like cancer, hypothyroidism, or AIDS. Finally, because trials have been done exclusively on young, healthy adults, the effects on the less robust and the elderly remain unknown.

Antianxiety agents, sedatives and hypnotics, are often prescribed when symptoms of anxiety are related to depression. These classes of drugs share similar pharmacologic properties, and they can be effective in small doses to relieve anxiety and in larger doses to induce sleep. Meprobamate (Miltown, Equanil) was the first antianxiety agent released in the 1960s. Both its questionable level of effectiveness and its addictive and fatal overdose potential resulted in its obsolescence. The benzodiazepines are the most commonly used antianxiety agents today. These include Librium and Valium, both of which are widely prescribed and widely abused. Newer drugs in the benzodiazepine family include Ativan, Xanax, Clonopin, and Vestran. Drugs in the benzodiazepine family offer rapid, effective, and safe treatment for anxiety states.[11] They have a low addiction potential and do not affect the metabolism of medications taken concurrently, although caffeine interferes with their effectiveness. The major side effect of the benzodiazepines is drowsiness, and community health nurses should plan to warn clients not to drive when they feel drowsy.

The barbiturates (Secanol) are a group of sedative-hypnotic drugs. These are often contraindicated in treating anxiety states because they are very addictive, used in suicide attempts, depress the CNS and respiratory system, and depress REM sleep, possibly resulting in the insomnia these drugs are intended to control.

Many well-controlled clinical studies have found lithium to be the most effective agent for treating acute manic and hypomanic states.[11] Tegretol and valproic acid amide are being used to treat clients who cannot tolerate lithium. However, lithium continues to be the drug of choice for treating bipolar and cyclic unipolar depression as well as "rapid cyclers," persons who have bipolar episodes spaced unusually close together. Lithium is a salt whose ion can be detected in the blood. Lithium is given in divided doses with increases in the daily dose until, in the acute phase of an affective episode, the blood level is between 1.0 and 1.5 mEq/L, the effective level. After a week to 10 days, as the symptoms subside, the blood level should be maintained in the range of 1.0–1.2 mEq/L.

Because the gap between the therapeutic level

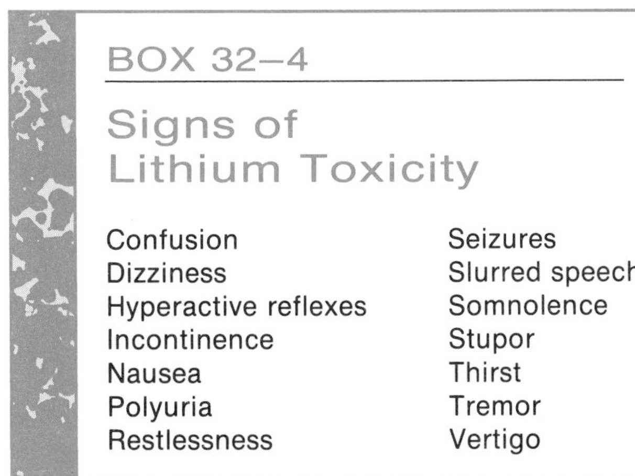

BOX 32–4

Signs of Lithium Toxicity

Confusion	Seizures
Dizziness	Slurred speech
Hyperactive reflexes	Somnolence
Incontinence	Stupor
Nausea	Thirst
Polyuria	Tremor
Restlessness	Vertigo

and the toxic level of lithium is the narrowest of any psychopharmacologic drug, blood levels must be monitored after each change. When first prescribed, daily blood tests may be necessary, decreasing to weekly and, finally, to monthly checks when the client is being maintained on lithium. Tests of kidney function must be done before putting a person on lithium. Significant side effects are correlated with blood levels above 1.5 mEq/L.

Community health nurses would plan to educate clients who are on lithium about the need to drink eight glasses of water a day, eat foods high in potassium (lithium can deplete potassium levels), and watch for early signs of toxicity. The nurse would also plan to monitor the client closely for the signs of lithium toxicity that are included in Box 32–4. The nurse would refer the client back to the psychiatrist if signs of toxicity are evident. The nurse would also plan to reinforce the need for periodic checks of blood levels of lithium to assure early identification of toxic levels.

TERTIARY PREVENTION

When a person has suffered repeated bouts of unipolar depression or bipolar disorder, tertiary prevention is an issue. As in schizophrenia, the entire family should be included in the treatment of both unipolar depression and bipolar disorder. Both depression and bipolar disorder are cyclical, and there are exacerbations and remissions. Seasonal patterns have been noted in both unipolar and bipolar disorders. In the first session with a client, it is enlightening to the family and helpful to the clinician to draw a time line that reflects the client's history of mood swings over several years. Trends might begin to appear. For example, for the last 5 years a client has experienced mood alterations in late summer or early fall. The nurse, client, and family would then be alerted that late September or early October is a time when the

TABLE 32–3. RESOURCES FOR CHRONIC MENTAL HEALTH PROBLEMS

Agency or Organization	Services
American Psychiatric Association 1400 K. St., NW, Suite 501 Dept. USN Washington, DC 20005	Information, literature
DEPRESSION/Awareness, Recognition, Treatment (D/ART) National Institute of Mental Health Rockville, MD 20857	Public information
Emotional Health Anonymous 2420 San Gabriel Blvd. Rosemead, CA 91770 (818) 573-5482	Self-help group
Emotions Anonymous P.O. Box 4245 St. Paul, MN 55104 (612) 647-9712	Self-help group
National Alliance for the Mentally Ill (NAMI) P.O. Box NAMI-Depression Arlington, VA 22216	Political advocacy, information
National Association for Research on Schizophrenia and Depression 60 Cutter Mill Rd., Suite 200 Great Neck, NY 11021	Research, public information
National Depressive and Manic Depressive Association 53 West Jackson Blvd. Box USN Chicago, IL 60604 (312) 993-0066	Research, advocacy, help for clients and families; public education
National Foundation for Depressive Illness P.O. Box 2257 New York, NY 10116	Research, information, literature
National Institute of Mental Health 5600 Fishers Lane Rockville, MD 20857 (301) 443-3673	Research, information
National Mental Health Association Information Center 1021 Prince St. Alexandria, VA 22314	Public information
Project Overcome 2735 Blaisdell Ave., South Suite 202 Minneapolis, MN 55408 (612) 870-0838	Advocacy for persons with mental illness; consultation on mental health systems; public education
Western Center for Behavioral and Preventive Medicine 208-125 E. 13th St. North Vancouver, BC V7L 2L3 Canada	Annoted bibliography on stress, printed information

client and family will need to pay special attention to the client's affective state. Nurses must rely heavily on family members' monitoring of the prodromal signs of mania because clients who have bipolar disorder are notoriously poor at identifying these signs in themselves. For this reason, the nurse should plan to make family members thoroughly conversant with prodromal signs of mania. Not sleeping is often the first sign of a person moving toward mania. If the client has difficulty sleeping for more than 2 nights, the nurse and the psychiatrist should be notified.

It is important that community health nurses learn to assess levels of depression and suicide risk and refer clients at risk to psychiatric treatment immediately if clients are not already involved in some ongoing therapy. Open lines of communication are imperative among nurse, psychiatric care-giver, and client at times when the client is deeply depressed or actively suicidal.

EVALUATING CONTROL OF AFFECTIVE DISORDERS

Evaluating the effectiveness of care for clients with affective disorders demands constant vigilance, given the changeable nature of affective disorders. A chilling example of this need for vigilance is the case of a 16-year-old boy who had been suffering from severe depression and suicidal thoughts for several months. His family and health-care providers were very relieved when he began to respond to medication, when his mood lifted, and his energy returned. One day his parents went to his room after he failed to respond to being called and found that he had hanged himself. Because of his recovery, he had regained sufficient energy to execute his plan for suicide. This true story is a stark reminder that nurses need constantly to evaluate clients and families who are at risk for or are suffering from affective disorders. However, it also points out the need for nurses to be aware of the very real limitations they have in "controlling" affective disorders—clients ultimately must take responsibility for their own lives, and the nurse and other mental health care-givers can only work with what clients tell them either verbally or nonverbally. Resources that may assist community health nurses working with clients with schizophrenia or affective disorders are presented in Table 32–3.

CHAPTER HIGHLIGHTS

- Community health nurses are one group of community-based professionals frequently called upon to care for clients who have chronic mental illnesses.
- Two common forms of chronic mental illness that community health nurses may encounter are schizophrenia and affective disorders.
- Although many theories have been advanced about the etiology of schizophrenia—ranging from genetic, neurotransmitter, and brain dysfunction theories to theories of dysfunctional family communication—no one knows for sure why some people become schizophrenic.
- Elderly people who have schizophrenia often exhibit fewer symptoms of the disease as they age.
- Psychotropic medications used in the treatment of schizophrenia have some "nuisance" side effects and some potentially serious side effects that the community health nurse needs to monitor.
- Psychiatric clients have a documented higher rate of undiagnosed physical illness than does the general population.
- Genograms can be used with families to assess their vulnerability to either schizophrenia or affective disorders.
- Many people suffer from depression related to physiological disorders or to medications taken for physiological disorders.
- Stressful life events can play a significant role in the development of affective disorders. For example, marital dissatisfaction and unhappiness are highly correlated with depression.
- A balanced life-style is important for people recovering from both schizophrenia and affective disorders.
- Prevention, planning, timely intervention, and evaluation are crucial with depressed people because of the potential for suicide.

Review Questions

1. Describe at least three biological theories advanced to explain the development of schizophrenia. (p. 842)
2. Describe at least three ways in which the psychological environment might contribute to the development of schizophrenia. (p. 844)
3. Identify at least five symptoms of schizophrenia for which the community health nurse might assess an individual client. (p. 844)
4. Identify three common thought disorders associated with schizophrenia. Give an example of each. (p. 845)
5. What are the four general principles to be considered in planning care for clients with schizophrenia? (p. 847)
6. Identify at least three human biological factors that may influence the development of affective disorders. (p. 851)
7. Describe at least five environmental factors that may contribute to the development of affective disorders. (p. 853)
8. Identify three approaches to primary prevention of affective disorders. Give an example of community health nursing involvement in each. (p. 855)
9. Describe at least three community health nursing activities related to secondary prevention of affective disorders. (p. 855)
10. Identify at least two considerations in tertiary prevention of affective disorders. Give an example of a community health nursing action related to each. (p. 857)

APPLICATION AND SYNTHESIS

You are the community health nurse assigned to see Jane for a well-baby visit several weeks after she delivered a healthy son. Jane is 39 and has been married to Jack, 48, for a year. Stephen is their first child. When you arrive at Jane's house you note that she and her family live in a comfortable home in an upper middle-class neighborhood. Jane answers the door, and you see that her eyes and nose are red as though she has been crying. You explain the purpose of your visit and examine the baby, who is in a freshly painted nursery with a bright mobile over the crib and plenty of stuffed animals and toys around. Stephen is neat, clean, and appears to be well-fed, happy, and healthy.

When you finish with the baby, you ask how Jane is doing. Jane bursts into tears. She tells you that she has been feeling desperately unhappy since her pregnancy began. She has been feeling so depressed, she reports, that she is not sure she will be able to get out of bed anymore to take care of her son. You say, "Tell me about this past year." Jane tells you that this is a first marriage for her and for Jack, and neither of them has children from previous relationships. In their discussions prior to marriage, she and Jack had never resolved their differences about having children. Jane was ambivalent about having a child; her husband was sure he did not want one. Because they are devout Catholics, they used the rhythm method of birth control. When Jane told Jack she was pregnant after 2 months of marriage, he became very angry and blamed Jane for tricking him into having a baby. Although she had not tricked him, Jane felt guilty and blamed herself for becoming pregnant. Terrified that Jack would leave her if she told him how she felt, she kept all her own feelings of sadness, anger, and depression inside. She did not want to be a single parent. Abortion was never considered because of their religious beliefs.

During the pregnancy, Jack was emotionally withdrawn, depressed, and refused to take part in any activity related to the upcoming birth. Jane's sister attended Lamaze classes with her and coached her during the birth because Jack would not attend. Jane felt jealous of the women whose husbands were so attentive during these classes. Ever since her son's birth, Jane says that she has had "postpartum depression." She has told no one how depressed she feels because she is afraid she will have to be hospitalized as she was several times in her late 20s and early 30s for episodes of clinical depression.

When you do a genogram with her, you discover a family history of depression. Both her grandmother and mother suffered bouts of deep depression, and her grandmother had been hospitalized for a year in a psychiatric institution following menopause. Jane's father is an emotionally withdrawn man whose only sister committed suicide when she was 40. Jane's sister has an eating disorder; she is bulimic.

Now that Jane has been home for 3 weeks with her son, she sees her sister twice a week. Jack is pleased that they have a son and he is beginning to spend time after he comes home from work playing with Stephen. Jane cannot understand why it makes her angry instead of happy that Jack is becoming involved with their child. Because Jack has refused to support them in a manner that would allow Jane to stay home with Stephen, Jane must return to work after her 6-week maternity leave. She is afraid she will be unable to function at work and has yet to find a day-care facility for Stephen. Jane worries about these things and has difficulty in both falling asleep and in getting up during the night to feed her son. She cries for "no reason" several times a day and has lost weight. She weighs less now than before she was pregnant. She has little interest in anything, including her baby, and she says that life does not really seem worth living anymore.

1. Does Jane have any vegetative signs of depression? If so, describe them.
2. How would you assess her potential for suicide?
3. How would you determine whether Jane's depression is "normal" postpartum depression or clinical depression requiring psychiatric assessment and treatment?
4. Based on your assessment, will you follow Jane yourself or refer her to a psychiatrist or mental health worker?
5. How will you involve Jane's husband and sister in the plan of care?

REFERENCES

1. American Psychiatric Association. (1987). *Diagnostic and statistical manual (3rd ed. revised)*. Washington, DC: American Psychiatric Association.
2. Talbott, J. A., Hales, R. E., & Yudofsky, S. C. (1988). *Textbook of psychiatry*. Washington, DC: American Psychiatric Association Press.
3. Tsuang, M. T., Faraone, S. V., & Day, M. (1988). Schizophrenic disorders. In A.M. Nicholi (Ed.), *The new Harvard guide to psychiatry*. Cambridge, MA: Belknap Press of Harvard University.
4. Baker, A. F. (1989). How families cope: Schizophrenia. *Journal of Psychosocial Nursing, 27*(1), 31–36.
5. Eaton, W. W. (1985). Epidemiology of schizophrenia. *Epidemiologic Reviews, 7,* 105–126.
6. Butler, R. N., & Lewis, M. I. (1982). *Aging and mental health*. St. Louis: C.V. Mosby.
7. Hollingshead, A. B., & Redlich, F. C. (1966). *Social class and mental illness: A community study*. New York: Wiley.
8. Patterson, D. (1979). Families living with schizophrenia. Unpublished paper.
9. Smith, W. (1989). *Epidemiology of mental disease*. New York: Facts on File.
10. Faraone, S. V., & Tsuang, M. T. (1985). Quantitative models of the genetic transmission of schizophrenia. *Psychological Bulletin, 98,* 41–66.
11. Wilson, H. S., & Kneisl, C. R. (1988). *Psychiatric Nursing* (3rd ed.). Menlo Park, CA: Addison-Wesley.
12. Roth, P. (1989). Family support systems. In P. Bomar (Ed.), *Nurses and family health promotion: Concepts, assessments, and interventions*. Baltimore: Williams & Wilkins.
13. Faraone, S. V., Curran, J. P., Laughren, T., et al. (1986). Neuroleptic availability, psychosocial factors, and clinical status: A one-year study of schizophrenic outpatients after dose reduction. *Psychiatry Residence, 19,* 311–322.
14. Schwartz, S. R., & Africa, B. (1984). Schizophrenic disorders. In H. H. Goldman (Ed.), *Review of general psychiatry*. Los Altos, CA: Lange Medical Publications.
15. Liberman, et al., (1984). The nature and problem of schizophrenia. In A.S. Bellack (Ed.), *Schizophrenia: Treatment, management, and rehabilitation*. New York: Grune & Stratton.
16. Crow, T. J. (1980, January). Molecular pathology of schizophrenia: More than one disease process? *British Medical Journal, 12,* 67.
17. Knight, C. (1985). Possible autoimmune response in schizophrenia. *Integrated Psychiatry, 3,* 134–143.
18. Strome, T. M. (1989). Schizophrenia in the elderly: What nurses need to know. *Archives of Psychiatric Nursing, 3*(1), 47–52.
19. Koranyi, E. K. (1979). Morbidity and rate of undiagnosed physical illness in a psychiatric clinical population. *Archives of General Psychiatry, 36,* 414–419.
20. Ouslander, J. G. (1982). Illness and psychopathology in the elderly. *Psychiatric Clinics of North America, 5*(1), 145–158.
21. Coyle, M. K. (1987). Organic illness mimicking psychiatric episodes. *Journal of Gerontological Nursing, 13*(1), 31–45.
22. Talbott, J. A., & Linn, L. (1978). Reactions of schizophrenics to life-threatening disease. *Psychiatric Quarterly, 50*(3), 218–227.
23. Ciompi, L. (1980a). Catamnestic long-term study on the course of life and aging of schizophrenics. *Schizophrenia Bulletin, 6,* 606–618.
24. Ciompi, L. (1980b). The natural history of schizophrenia in the long term. *British Journal of Psychiatry, 136,* 413–420.
25. Ciompi, L. (1985). Aging and schizophrenic process. *Acta Psychiatrica Scandinavica* (Suppl. 319), *71,* 93–105.
26. Huber, G., Gross, G., Schuttler, R., & Linz, M. (1980). Longitudinal studies of schizophrenic patients. *Schizophrenia Bulletin, 6,* 592–605.
27. Keefe, R. S., Mohs, R. C., Losonczy, M. F., et al. (1987). Characteristics of very poor outcome schizophrenics. *American Journal of Psychiatry, 144*(7), 889–895.
28. Watts, C. A. (1985). A long-term follow up of schizophrenic patients, 1946–1983. *Journal of Clinical Psychiatry, 46,* 210–216.
29. Belsky, J. (1984). *The psychology of aging*. Monterey, CA: Brooks/Cole.
30. Bridge, T. P., Cannon, H. E., & Wyatt, R. J. (1978). Burned out schizophrenics: Evidence for age effects on schizophrenic symptomatology. *Journal of Gerontology, 33,* 835–839.
31. Goodman, A. B., & Siegel, C. (1986). Elderly schizophrenics in the wake of deinstitutionalization. *American Journal of Psychiatry, 32*(1), 21–27.
32. Youssef, H. A., & Waddington, J. L. (1987). Morbidity and mortality in tardive dyskinesia: Associations in chronic schizophrenia. *Acta Psychiatrica Scandinavica, 75*(1), 74–77.
33. Yassa, R., & Jones, B. D. (1985). Complications of tardive dyskinesia: A review. *Psychosomatics, 26*(4), 305–313.
34. Lidz, R. W., & Lidz, T. (1952). Therapeutic considerations arising from the intense symbiotic needs of schizophrenic patients. In M.W. Brady & F. Redlick (Eds.), *Psychotherapy with schizophrenics*. New York: International University Press.
35. Falloon, I. R. H., Boyd, J. L., & McGill, C. W. (1984). *Family care of schizophrenia*. New York: Guilford Press.
36. Bateson, G. (1956). Toward a theory of schizophrenia. *Behavioral Science, 1,* 251–264.
37. Wynn, L. (1981). Current concepts about schizophrenia and family relationships. *Journal of Nervous Mental Disorders, 169,* 82–89.
38. Haley, J. (1967). *Uncommon therapy: The psychiatric technique of Milton H. Erickson*. New York: W.W. Norton.
39. Cohen, L. J., Test, M. A., & Brown, R. L. (1990). *American Journal of Psychiatry, 147,* 602–607.
40. Weiner, H. (1985). Schizophrenia: Etiology. In H.I. Kaplan & B.J. Shadock (Eds.), *Comprehensive testbook of psychiatry* (Vol. 1) (4th ed., pp. 669–679). Baltimore: Williams & Wilkins.

41. Riesdorph-Ostrow, W. (1989). Deinstitutionalization: A public policy. *Journal of Psychosocial Nursing, 27*(6), 4–8.
42. Torrey, E. F. (1989). *Nowhere to go: The tragic odyssey of the homeless mentally ill.* New York: Harper & Row.
43. Stein, L. I., & Test, M. A. (1980). An alternative to mental hospital treatment: Comprehensive model, treatment program and clinical evaluation. *Archives of General Psychiatry, 34,* 409–412.
44. Klerman, G. (1988). Depression and related diagnoses of mood. In A. M. Nicholi (Ed.), *The new Harvard guide to psychiatry* (pp. 309–366). Cambridge, MA: Belknap Press of Harvard University.
45. Cowley, G., & Springen, K. (1990, March 26). The promise of Prozac. *Newsweek, 115*(13), 38–41.
46. Kaplan, G. A., & Sadock, B. J. (1985). *Modern synopsis of the comprehensive textbook of psychiatry* (4th ed.). Baltimore: Williams & Wilkins.
47. Cook, J. S., & Fontaine, K. L. (1991). *Essentials of mental health nursing* (2nd ed.). Redwood City, CA: Addison-Wesley.
48. Weissman, M. M., & Myers, J. K. (1979). Depression in the elderly: Research directions in psychopathology, epidemiology, and treatment. *Journal of Geriatric Psychiatry, 12,* 187–201.
49. Weissman, M. M., & Klerman, C. K. (1977). Sex differences and the epidemiology of depression. *Archives of General Psychiatry, 34,* 98–111.
50. Freedman, E., Bucci, W., & Elkowitz, E. (1982). Depression in a family practice elderly population. *Journal of the American Geriatric Society, 30,* 372–377.
51. Schuckit, J. as cited in A.I. Green, J.J. Mooney, J.J. Schildkraut (1988). The biochemistry of affective disorders: An overview. In A.I. Nicholi, Jr. (Ed.), *The new Harvard guide to psychiatry.* Cambridge, MA: Belknap Press of Harvard University.
52. As cited in R.M.A. Hirschfeld, & F.K. Goodwin (1988). Mood disorders. In J.A. Talbott, R.E. Hales, & S.C. Yudofsky (Eds.), *Textbook of psychiatry.* Washington, DC: American Psychiatric Association Press.
53. Gold, M., & Herridge, P. (1988). The risk of misdiagnosis of physical illness as depression. In F. Flach (Ed.), *Affective Disorders* (No. 3), (pp. 64–76). New York: W.W. Norton.
54. Cohen, C. D. (1988). *The brain in human aging.* New York: Springer.
55. Ronsman, K. (1987). Therapy for depression. *Journal of Gerontological Nursing, 13*(12), 18–25.
56. Yates, W. R. (1987). Depression. In W.R. Yates (Ed.), *Psychiatric illness: Primary care* (pp. 657–668). Philadelphia: W.B. Saunders.
57. Zuckerman, B., & Beardslee, W. (1987). Maternal depression: An issue for pediatricians. *Pediatrics, 79* 110–117.
58. Belle, D. (1982). Introduction. In D. Belle (Ed.), *Lives in stress: Women and depression* (pp. 11–23). Beverly Hills, CA: Sage.
59. Weissman, M. M., Merikangas, K. R., & John, K. (1986). Depressed parents and their children: General health, social and psychiatric problems. *American Journal of Disabled Children, 140,* 801–805.
60. Weissman, M. M., John, K., & Gammon, D. (1987). Children of depressed parents: Increased psychopathology and early onset of major depression. *Archives of General Psychiatry, 44,* 837–853.
61. Weissman, M. M., Profoff, B. A., Gammon, G. D., et al. (1984). Psychopathology of children (ages 6–18) of depressed and normal parents. *Journal of the American Academy of Child Psychiatry, 23,* 78–84.
62. Fopma-Loy, J. (1988). The prevalence and phenomenology of depression in elderly women: A review of the literature. *Archives of Psychiatric Nursing, 2*(2), 74–80.
63. Kaas, M. J. (1984). Older women and mental health: A social policy perspective. In B.A. Hall (Ed.), *Mental health and the elderly* (pp. 65–81). New York: Grune & Stratton.
64. Orr, S. T., James, S. A., Burns, B. J., & Thompson, B. (1989). Chronic stressors and maternal depression: Implications for prevention. *American Journal of Public Health, 79,* 1295–1296.
65. Halikas, J. (1990, March 26). In The promise of Prozac. *Newsweek, 115*(13), 38–41.

RECOMMENDED READINGS

Cook, J. S., & Fontaine, K. L. (1991). *Essentials of mental health nursing* (2nd ed.). Redwood City, CA: Addison-Wesley.

Provides a clearly written introduction to psychiatric nursing. Translates psychological concepts and both physical and psychological assessment of psychological disorders into applicable terms for practitioners.

Fopma-Loy, J. (1988). The prevalence and phenomenology of depression in elderly women: A review of the literature. *Archives of Psychiatric Nursing*, 2(2), 74–80.

Reviews and critiques the extant research on women and depression. Makes recommendations for future investigation.

Murray, R. B., & Huelskoetter, M. M. (1991). *Psychiatric/mental health nursing: Giving emotional care* (3rd ed.). Norwalk, CT: Appleton & Lange.

Emphasizes the importance of the nurse-client relationship in intervening with individuals and families suffering from emotional disorders.

Strome, T. M. (1989). Schizophrenia in the elderly: What nurses need to know. *Archives of Psychiatric Nursing*, 3(1), 47–52.

Presents both the physical and psychological needs of elderly schizophrenic clients.

Wilson, H. S., & Kneisl, C. R. (1988). *Psychiatric nursing* (3rd ed.). Menlo Park, CA: Addison-Wesley.

Offers an in-depth discussion of psychological disorders. Provides a valuable resource for community health nurses working with clients with psychiatric disorders.

CHAPTER 33

Substance Abuse

KEY TERMS

anhedonia
co-dependent
counter-normative strategies
crack
drug abuse
drug tolerance
drug use
freebasing
intervention
intoxication
psychoactive substances
psychoactive substance abuse
psychoactive substance dependence syndrome
sinsemilla
teratogenic substances
withdrawal syndrome

Both drug use and drug abuse were known in ancient civilizations. Alcohol consumption in the form of fermented beverages used as recreational drinks or as medicinal preparations is recorded in early writings, and many herbal preparations, forerunners of today's drugs, were used in ancient Egypt, Greece, China, and the Arab lands.[1] Marijuana was smoked in ancient China, and although opium use is often associated with the Orient, its use probably began in Sumeria 4000 years before the birth of Christ and was also known to the Greeks. Opium was a frequent ingredient in patent medicines in the United States until the passage of the Harrison Narcotic Act in 1914.[1] In the Americas, Indian tribes used cocaine, peyote, and other substances in religious ceremonies.[2] Stimulants such as cocaine and amphetamines may have been used by the Vikings during their raids, and cocaine was an ingredient in early soft drinks in the United States. Tobacco use originated in the New World and was brought to Europe by returning explorers. Cigarettes became popular during the American Civil War, when they were issued to soldiers because they were easier to carry than pipes and tobacco. Barbiturates were discovered by a German chemist in 1884 and were first used medically in 1903. Barbiturates rapidly became widely used and abused and remain the primary pharmacologic means of committing suicide.[1]

Problems associated with these substances have also been known for centuries. The dangers of excessive alcohol consumption were recognized by the Sumerians, Babylonians, Egyptians, Greeks, Romans, and Hebrews. Some cultures and religious groups (for example, Moslems and some Protestant sects) completely prohibit the use of alcoholic beverages.[1]

Most drugs are used appropriately for medicinal purposes, but there is a growing tendency for these substances to be abused. The fact that many of the substances with potential for abuse also have legitimate use has made control of substance abuse

(*continued*)

LEARNING OBJECTIVES

After reading this chapter you should be able to:

- Identify at least three criteria for diagnosing psychoactive substance dependence.
- Distinguish between psychoactive substance dependence and abuse.
- Identify at least five psychoactive substances that lead to dependence and abuse.
- Describe at least two personal effects, two family effects, and two societal effects of substance abuse.
- Describe the five aspects of community health nursing assessment in relation to substance abuse.
- Identify two major approaches to primary prevention of substance abuse.
- Describe the components of the intervention process in secondary prevention of substance abuse.
- Identify at least four general principles in the treatment of substance abuse.
- Describe at least three treatment modalities in secondary prevention of substance abuse.
- Identify three considerations in treatment for substance abuse.

difficult. ***Drug use*** is the taking of a drug in the correct amount, frequency, and strength for its medically intended purpose. ***Drug abuse***, on the other hand, is the deliberate use of a drug for other than medicinal purposes in a manner that can adversely affect one's health or ability to function.[3]

Substance abuse is a growing problem worldwide. Areas of particular concern in the United States are the abuse of alcohol and other drugs and the use of tobacco products. The importance of these concerns is seen in the development of more than 30 national health-promotion and disease-prevention objectives for the year 2000 related to tobacco use and the abuse of alcohol and other drugs.[4] Selected objectives are included in Box 33–1.

In this chapter, trends in substance use and abuse are examined. Risk factors contributing to all forms of substance abuse, signs and symptoms of specific types of abuse, and community health nursing interventions in the control of substance abuse are addressed. The focus of the chapter is on the abuse of psychoactive substances addressed by the *Diagnostic and Statistical Manual of Mental Disorders-III* of the American Psychiatric Association as revised in 1987 (*DSM-III-R*).[5]

COMMUNITY HEALTH NURSING AND SUBSTANCE ABUSE

Because community health nurses interact with people in their homes, where most substance abuse occurs, they are in a unique position to identify persons with substance abuse problems.[6] Community health nurses assess individuals, families, and communities for risk factors that may contribute to substance abuse, and they engage in primary prevention efforts to eliminate risk factors. Nurses assess individuals and families for signs of problems related to substance abuse and refer clients for assistance. They also provide support to individuals and families in dealing with problems of substance abuse.

At the community level, community health nurses may be engaged in political activities to modify risk factors that contribute to substance abuse. For example, they might campaign for stricter enforcement of laws related to substance use by, and sales to, minors or driving while intoxicated. Or, they might work to promote increased taxes on tobacco and alcohol as a means of decreasing sales. In addition, community health nurses may educate individuals and their families, as well as groups of clients, on the hazards of substance use and abuse in an effort to prevent or minimize these practices.

PSYCHOACTIVE SUBSTANCES: DEPENDENCE AND ABUSE

Substance abuse involves the inappropriate use of psychoactive substances. ***Psychoactive substances*** are drugs or chemicals that alter ordinary states of consciousness including mood, cognition, or behavior.[7] The *DSM-III-R* recognizes abuse of several substances under umbrella diagnoses of psychoactive substance dependence and psychoactive substance abuse. The ***psychoactive substance dependence syndrome*** is a cluster of cognitive, behavioral, and physiologic symptoms that indicate impaired control over the use of a psychoactive substance and continued use despite adverse consequences.[8] Diagnosis of psychoactive substance dependence is based on the presence of three or more of the characteristic signs included in Box 33–2.

Psychoactive substance abuse involves maladaptive patterns of substance use that do not meet the criteria for dependence.[8] Criteria for a diagnosis of abuse include continued use of a substance (or sub-

BOX 33–1

Summary of Selected National Health Objectives for the Year 2000 Related to Substance Abuse

1. Reduce deaths due to alcohol-related motor vehicle crashes to no more than 8.5 per 100,000 population.
2. Reduce cirrhosis deaths to no more than 6 per 100,000 population.
3. Reduce drug-related deaths to no more than 3 per 100,000 population.
4. Reduce drug abuse-related emergency room visits by at least 20%.
5. Increase by at least 1 year the average age of first use of cigarettes, alcohol, and marijuana by persons aged 12 through 17.
6. Reduce recent use (in the past month) of
   a. alcohol to 12.6% of those aged 12 to 17 and 29% of those aged 18 to 20.
   b. marijuana to 3.2% of those aged 12 to 17 and 7.8% of those aged 18 to 20.
   c. cocaine to 0.6% of those aged 12 to 17 and 2.3% of those aged 18 to 20.
7. Reduce the proportion of young people engaging in heavy drinking of alcoholic beverages to no more than 28% of high school seniors and 32% of college students.
8. Reduce annual alcohol consumption by people aged 14 and older to no more than 2 gallons per person.
9. Establish in all 50 states programs to ensure access to alcohol and drug treatment programs for underserved populations.
10. Provide education on alcohol and other drugs in all primary and secondary school programs.
11. Extend adoption of alcohol and drug policies for the work environment to at least 60% of workplaces with 50 or more employees.
12. Increase to 50 the number of states that enact and enforce policies toreduce access to alcoholic beverages by minors.
13. Increase to at least 20 the number of states that restrict promotion of alcoholic beverage sales targeted to young audiences.
14. Extend to all 50 states legal blood alcohol tolerance levels of 0.04% for drivers aged 21 and older and 0.00% for those under age 21.
15. Increase to at least 75% the proportion of primary-care providers who screen for substance abuse problems and provide counseling and referral as needed.
16. Reduce the prevalence of cigarette smoking to no more than 15% of people aged 20 and older.
17. Reduce the initiation of smoking by children and youth so no more than 15% become regular smokers by age 20.
18. Increase the proportion of pregnant women smokers who quit smoking during their pregnancies to at least 60%.
19. Increase to at least 75% the proportion of workplaces with formal policies that prohibit or severely restrict smoking in the workplace.
20. Enact in all 50 states laws that prohibit or strictly limit smoking in the workplace and enclosed public places.
21. Enact and enforce in all 50 states laws prohibiting tobacco sales to persons under age 19.
22. Eliminate or severely restrict all forms of tobacco advertising to which people under age 18 are likely to be exposed.
23. Increase to at least 75% the proportion of primary-care providers who routinely counsel clients about smoking cessation.

(Source: United States Department of Health and Human Services. [1990]. Health United States 1989. Hyattsville, MD: Public Health Service.)

BOX 33–2.

Diagnostic Criteria for Psychoactive Substance Dependence

Three or more of the following:

- Increasing amounts of the substance used, or use extends over a longer period of time than intended
- Persistent desire for the substance or one or more unsuccessful attempts to control its use
- Increased time spent in obtaining, using, or recovering from the effects of the substance
- Frequent symptoms of intoxication or withdrawal interfering with obligations
- Elimination or reduction of important occupational, social, or recreational activities as a result of substance use
- Continued use of the substance despite recurrent problems caused
- Increased tolerance to the substance
- Experience of characteristic withdrawal symptoms
- Increased substance use to decrease withdrawal symptoms

AND

Consistent presence of at least three or more criteria over a period of 1 month or recurrent presence of criteria for more than 6 months.

(Source: Skodol[7]).

stances) despite persistent or recurrent physical, psychological, or social problems related to its use or recurrent use of the substance in physically dangerous situations (for example, driving while intoxicated). Evidence of abuse should have been consistently present for at least a month or have occurred periodically over a longer period of time.[7] Because substance abuse is a precursor to dependence, the term *substance abuse* will be used throughout this chapter in discussing the role of the community health nurse in its prevention and control.

PSYCHOACTIVE SUBSTANCES AND THEIR USE

It is estimated that 10 percent to 20 percent of the adult population in the United States uses some type of nonprescription psychoactive drug on a regular basis.[9] Psychoactive substances are abused because of their desirable initial effects. Some of these effects and the drugs associated with them are presented in Table 33–1. Unfortunately, psychoactive drugs with potential for abuse generally have rebound effects that are usually the opposite of their initial effects and that lead to repeated use to eliminate the undesirable symptoms created by the rebound.[10] These adverse effects will be discussed later in this chapter. Because of the phenomenon of tolerance, the user requires larger and larger doses of many drugs to combat rebound effects and to achieve the desired pleasurable effect. **Drug tolerance** is an adaptation of the body to a substance such that previous doses do not have the desired effect. Psychoactive substances that may be involved in either dependence or abuse are included in Box 33–3.

ALCOHOL

The alcohol contained in alcoholic beverages is ethyl alcohol created by the fermentation of grain mixtures or the juice of fruits and berries. After ingestion, alcohol is rapidly absorbed into the bloodstream through the gastrointestinal tract and functions as a central nervous system depressant.

Alcohol abuse is a serious problem in the United States and elsewhere in the world. During the years from 1977 to 1986, overall consumption of alcohol declined by 2.3 percent to less than 2.6 gallons of absolute alcohol per person over age 14.[11] Despite this decline, approximately 6.5 percent of the adult population of the United States drink half of the alcohol consumed.[12] Per capita consumption of alcohol is considerably higher than the average in some parts of the country. For example, the average annual per person sale of liquor is highest in Washington, DC, at 6.45 gallons, compared to 1.14 gallons in West Virginia. Beer sales are highest in Nevada (53.1 gallons per person per year) and lowest in Utah (22.5 gallons).[13] States with higher per capita sales of alcoholic beverages also tend to have higher prevalence of reported heavy drinking on the Behavioral Risk Factor Surveillance Surveys (BRFSS).[13,14] In the 1988 BRFSS, reports of "binge drinking" (five or more drinks on one occasion at least once in the past month) varied from 7.1 percent of the population in the District of Columbia to more than 25 percent in Wisconsin. Wisconsin residents also reported a high prevalence of

TABLE 33–1. SELECTED PSYCHOACTIVE SUBSTANCES, STREET NAMES, TYPICAL ROUTES OF ADMINISTRATION, AND EFFECTS PROMOTING ABUSE

Substance	Street Names	Typical Route of Administration	Effects Promoting Abuse
Alcohol	Beer, wine, spirits, booze, various brand names	Oral ingestion	Relaxation, decreased inhibitions, increased confidence, euphoria
Sedatives, hypnotics and anxiolytics		Oral ingestion, injected	Calming effect, decreased nervousness and anxiety, ability to sleep, relaxation, mild intoxication, loss of inhibition
Barbiturates			
Amytal	Blues, downers		
Nembutal	Yellows, yellow jackets		
Phenobarbital	Phennie, purple hearts		
Seconal	Reds, F-40s		
Tuinal	Rainbows		
Quaalude	Ludes, 714s, Q's		
Tranquilizers (minor)	Tranks, downs		
Dalmane			
Equinil/Miltown			
Librium			
Valium			
Serax			
Opiods			
Codeine	Schoolboy	Oral ingestion	Relief of pain, euphoria
Demerol	Demies	Injected	
Dilaudid	Little D	Injected	
Heroin	Smack, junk, downtown, H, black tar, horse	Injected, smoked, sniffed	
Methadone	Meth, dollies	Injected	
Morphine	M, Miss Emma, morph	Injected	
Opium	Blue velvet, black stuff, Dover's powder, paregoric	Oral ingestion, smoke, injected	
Percodan	Perkies	Oral ingestion	
Cocaine	Coke, snow, uptown, flake, crack	Nasal snorting, injected, smoked	Increased alertness and confidence, euphoria, reduced fatigue
Amphetamines		Oral ingestion	Increased alertness and confidence, decreased fatigue, euphoria
Benzedrine	Bennies		
Biphetamine	Black beauties		
Desoxyn	Co-pilots		
Dexedrine	Dex, speed		
Methedrine	Meth, crank		
Phencyclidine	Angel dust, krystal, DOA, hog	Smoke, oral ingestion, injected	Dreamlike state producing hallucinations
Hallucinogens		Oral ingestion, smoked, injected	Altered perceptions, mystical experience
LSD	Acid, microdot		
MDA	The love drug		
Mescaline	Cactus, mesc		
Peyote	Buttons		
Psilocybin	Magic mushrooms, shrooms		
Cannabis		Smoked, oral ingestion	Relaxation, euphoria, altered perceptions
Hashish	Kif, herb, hash		
Hashish oil	Honey, hash oil		
Marijuana	Grass, ganja, weed, dope, reefer, Thai sticks, pot, Acapulco gold		
Inhalants		Inhaled	Relaxation, euphoria, intoxication
Amyl nitrate	Poppers		
Butyl nitrate	Locker room, rush		
Nitrous oxide	Laughing gas		
Nicotine	Various brand names of tobacco products	Smoked, chewed	Relaxation, mild stimulation

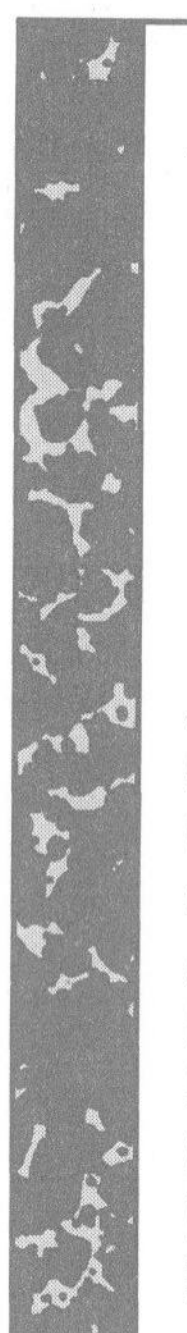

BOX 33–3.

Psychoactive Substances with Potential for Dependence and Abuse

Alcohol
Sedatives, hypnotics, and anxiolytics
Opioids
Cocaine
Amphetamines
Phencyclidine
Hallucinogens
Cannabis
Inhalants
Nicotine

drinking and driving (more than 6 percent of the population surveyed). The prevalence of "heavier drinking" (60 or more drinks in the past month) ranged from slightly over 3 percent of the population in North Dakota to almost 11 percent in New Hampshire.[15] While figures on the extent of alcohol abuse are alarming, the fact that only an estimated 10 percent of abusers receive treatment for their disorder[16] is even more disconcerting.

SEDATIVES, HYPNOTICS, AND ANXIOLYTICS

A second group of drugs frequently abused includes sedatives, hypnotics, and anxiolytics. Sedatives are used to calm nervousness, irritability, and excitement, while hypnotics induce sleep. Many drugs have sedative effects in lower doses and hypnotic effects in higher doses.[17] Anxiolytics (also known as antianxiety agents or minor tranquilizers) are used to reduce anxiety and tension and promote sleep. All three types of drugs are central nervous system (CNS) depressants.

These drugs are frequently prescribed for symptoms of nervousness, anxiety, or difficulty sleeping. Unfortunately, their prescription for legitimate use often creates a dependence. In low doses, these drugs produce a mild state of euphoria, reduce inhibitions, and create feelings of relaxation and decreased tension. Their major pharmacologic action is CNS depression. Drugs involved in this category of substance abuse include tranquilizers such as Librium and Valium, barbiturate sedatives, nonbarbiturates such as Atarax and Equanil, and hypnotics such as Quaalude, Nytol, Sleep-eze, and Sominex.[18] Because of their widespread use for both legitimate and illegitimate reasons and their easy availability, precise figures on the abuse of these drugs are difficult to obtain. However, in national surveys 1 percent or less of the American population engaged in nonmedical use of sedatives and tranquilizers in 1988 compared to use by 2 percent to 15 percent of people in various age groups in 1974.[19] In 1987, abuse of these psychoactive drugs accounted for only 1 percent of all admissions for treatment of substance-abuse disorders.[20]

OPIOIDS

Opioids are also CNS depressants and are derived naturally from the opium poppy or created synthetically. Opioids bind to CNS cell receptors to mimic the action of naturally produced endorphins that relieve pain. In addition to relief of pain, opioids create a psychological euphoria that prompts continued use.[18]

Opioid dependence (along with barbiturate dependence) was once a primary concern in relation to substance abuse, and its continued use is still of concern to health-care professionals. The proportion of people who have ever used heroin, the primary illicit form of opioid, declined from 1974 to 1988 for those under age 25, but doubled to just over 1 percent for those 26 and older,[19] and an estimated 800,000 people use heroin daily.[21] Current nonmedical use of narcotic analgesics (for example, morphine and codeine) was reported by 0.4 percent to 1.5 percent of people in various age groups in 1988.[19]

COCAINE

Cocaine is a stimulant derived from the leaves of the coca plant. Its use produces euphoria and a sense of competence. Other desired effects include increased energy and clarity of thought. Unlike many of the other drugs presented here, the pleasurable effects of cocaine are extremely short-acting (approximately 30 minutes) followed by an intense letdown and craving for another dose.[18] Use of cocaine may be accompanied by the practice of "freebasing." Normally, to maintain its stability, cocaine is combined with a hydrochloride base, creating a substance that is usually only about 25 percent cocaine. ***Freebasing*** involves the use of heat and ether to free the cocaine from its hydrochloride base, thus creating a purer product that produces a more intense effect. Because of the combination of heat and the highly volatile and explosive ether, freebasing is an extremely dangerous practice. To eliminate the need for freebasing, drug dealers created ***crack***, a stable form of cocaine without the hydrochloride base that can be smoked rather than inhaled, for a more rapid and more intense effect.

Next to alcohol, cocaine is the abusive substance of greatest concern because of the rapid escalation in its use and its severe adverse effects. It is estimated that more than 50 million Americans have used cocaine at some time,[9] and, in 1988, nearly 5 percent of people aged 18 to 25 years reported current cocaine use.[19] Cocaine use accounts for 5 of every 1000 deaths in the United States.[22]

AMPHETAMINES

Amphetamines are CNS stimulants manufactured chemically. Amphetamines have, on occasion, been prescribed to assist weight loss and relative fatigue, but they are not recommended for either condition. Amphetamines and similar drugs produce feelings of euphoria, energy, confidence, increased ability to concentrate, and improved physical performance. They are often used by truck drivers and students who wish to stay awake to study or by athletes desiring to improve their performance.[18]

Stimulant use was reported by as much as 2.4 percent of people aged 18 to 25 in 1988 compared to 3.7 percent of this population in 1974.[19] However, regular use of amphetamines and related drugs is much higher in some areas. Methamphetamine use, for example, is particularly prevalent in Southern California and accounts for 33 percent to 40 percent of all referrals to drug treatment centers in San Diego County[9] compared to only 1 percent of total admissions in the United States.[20]

PHENCYCLIDINE

Phencyclidine (PCP) was originally developed as an anesthetic, but its use was discontinued because of its many adverse side effects. The effects of PCP are variable and may include stimulation or depression of the CNS or hallucinations. Its more desirable effects include heightened sensitivity to stimuli, mood elevation, and a sense of omnipotence, and relaxation. Unfortunately, PCP has some serious adverse effects. PCP-induced psychosis constitutes a psychiatric emergency and requires immediate hospitalization.[18]

While PCP was considered a serious problem in the 1980s, its overall use has declined. In 1987, PCP abuse accounted for less than 1 percent of admissions for substance abuse compared to 79 percent for alcohol abuse and 6 percent for heroin abuse.[20]

HALLUCINOGENS

Hallucinogens or psychedelic drugs such as d-lysergic acid diethylamide (LSD), mescaline, peyote, or psilocybin mushrooms alter experience to create hallucinations. They also distort the distinction between self and the environment to make the user extremely vulnerable to environmental stimuli. Common effects of these drugs include changes in mood (euphoria or terror and despair), heightened sensation or synesthesia (merging of the senses so colors, for example, are experienced as odors or vice versa), changes in perceptions of time and objects, and changes in relations leading to depersonalization and feelings of merging with other people and objects.[18]

Like PCP use, the use of hallucinogens has declined somewhat in recent years. For example, in 1974, more than 16 percent of people 18 to 25 years of age reported ever using a hallucinogen, and 2.5 percent were current users, compared to 1.9 percent of this age group who were current users and 13.8 percent who had ever used this class of drugs in 1988.[19]

CANNABIS

Cannabis species of plants are the source of marijuana and hashish. The primary psychoactive substance in these drugs is delta-9-tetrahydrocannabinol (THC). THC may be inhaled by smoking marijuana or hashish or ingested and produces relaxation, euphoria, and occasionally altered perceptions of time and space. Marijuana use may contribute to exacerbation of other mental health problems such as schizophrenia or depression. ***Sinsemilla*** a form of marijuana consisting of dried flowers of female plants without seeds is approximately 10 times as potent as regular marijuana mixtures that also contain leaves and seeds. Use of sinsemilla may lead to hallucination or severe anxiety attacks.[18]

Reports of current marijuana use by people under age 25 have declined, while use by those 26 and older has increased. Between 1974 and 1988, for example, marijuana use by 12- to 17-year-olds decreased by 47 percent, and use by people aged 18 to

25 decreased by 39 percent. Marijuana use by those over 26 years of age nearly doubled in the same time period.[19]

INHALANTS

Inhalants are abused by sniffing products such as airplane model glue, nail polish remover, gasoline, aerosols, and anesthetics such as nitrous oxide. They usually produce a sense of euphoria, loss of inhibition, and excitement. Inhalants are often used by people who do not have the financial resources to support more expensive drug habits. In addition to a variety of adverse physical effects such as kidney and heart damage, there is the potential for suffocation while inhaling these substances from a plastic bag. Because of their volatile nature, explosion is another hazard presented by inhalants.[18]

The proportion of people who have ever used inhalants increased in all age groups from 1974 to 1988. In 1988, current use of inhalants was reported by 2 percent of people aged 12 to 17 and slightly less than 2 percent of those 18 to 25 years of age. Current use was reported by less than 1 percent of those 26 and older.[19]

NICOTINE

Nicotine, the last of the abusive substances included in the *DSM-III-R* categories of psychoactive substance dependence and abuse, is the psychoactive substance present in tobacco smoke. Nicotine produces feelings of well-being, increases mental acuity and ability to concentrate, and heightens one's sense of purpose. Nicotine may also exert a calming effect on the smoker.[10] Unfortunately, nicotine also contributes to a host of adverse physical effects including heart disease, several forms of cancer, and chronic respiratory diseases. While a great deal of progress has been made in efforts to limit tobacco use in the United States, its use among young people continues to be relatively prevalent. In fact, as social norms change and tobacco use becomes less socially acceptable, it has been suggested that tobacco use has assumed the defiant symbolism of rebellion against authority that influenced marijuana use in the 1960s.[10]

Because of the highly addictive nature of nicotine and its adverse health effects, all forms of tobacco use should be discouraged. Unlike moderate alcohol use, even moderate smoking produces negative effects on health. Nicotine, unlike many other abused substances, has no medical applications.

Efforts to eliminate smoking in the American population have been somewhat successful. For example, in 1988, just under 30 percent of people over age 25 smoked compared to 39 percent in 1974. Results of efforts to eliminate smoking among young people have also been effective, resulting in a 52 percent decrease in the proportion of smokers aged 12 to 17 between 1974 and 1988 and a 28 percent decrease in the 18- to 25-year-old group during the same time period.[19]

EFFECTS OF SUBSTANCE ABUSE

Substance abuse contributes to adverse effects for the abusing individual, for his or her family, and for society at large.

PERSONAL EFFECTS

The effects of substance abuse upon the individual are physical, psychological, and social. Physical effects include increased morbidity directly related to the effects of the drug or drugs abused as well as increased potential for exposure to diseases such as AIDS and hepatitis when abuse involves use of contaminated needles or results in sexual promiscuity as a means of financing a drug habit or because of lowered inhibitions. Other physical effects of substance abuse include physical deterioration due to malnutrition and poor hygiene.[8] Some drugs such as alcohol, nicotine, barbiturates, and others also result in withdrawal symptoms when the drug is removed from the client's system. The **withdrawal syndrome** caused by these and other drugs is a complex of symptoms usually including severe discomfort, pain, nausea, and vomiting, and may include convulsions.[23] Some drugs also produce chromosomal changes that cause congenital malformations in children as well as increased potential for spontaneous abortion. Death is the ultimate adverse effect of drug use and may result from a drug overdose, from withdrawal, or from the effects of long-term consequences of drug use such as cirrhosis, cancer, or cardiovascular disease. Assessment for both short-term and long-term physical effects of specific substances is discussed later in this chapter.

In addition to the desired effects that promote drug use and abuse, psychological effects of drug abuse can include personality disturbances, anxiety, and depression.[8] Organic mental disorders characterized by hallucinations, delusions, dementia, delirium, and disorders of mood or perception may also be caused by substance abuse. In addition, substance abuse may trigger exacerbations of existing schizophrenic or affective disorders.[7]

TABLE 33–2. MAXIMUM PENALTIES FOR ILLEGAL DRUG MANUFACTURE OR POSSESSION

Type of Drug	Schedule	Penalty for Sale or Manufacture	Penalty for Possession
Alcohol	N/A	N/A	N/A
Sedatives, hypnotics, anxiolytics	II, III, or IV	First offense: 3 to 5 years in prison and $10,000 to $15,000 fine Second offense: 6 to 10 years in prison, $10,000 to $30,000 fine	First offense: 1 year in prison and $5000 fine (may get probation only) Second offense: 2 years in prison, $10,000 fine
Opioids	I or II	First offense: 15 years in prison, $25,000 fine Second offense: 30 years in prison, $50,000 fine	First offense: 1 year in prison, $5000 fine Second offense: 2 years in prison, $10,000 fine
Cocaine	II	First offense: 5 years in prison, $15,000 fine Second offense: 10 years in prison, $30,000 fine	First offense: 1 year in prison, $5000 fine Second offense: 2 years in prison, $10,000 fine
Amphetamines	II	First offense: 5 years in prison, $15,000 fine Second offense: 10 years in prison, $30,000 fine	First offense: 1 year in prison, $5000 fine Second offense: 2 years in prison, $10,000 fine
Phencyclidine	I	First offense: 5 years in prison, $15,000 fine Second offense: 10 years in prison, $30,000 fine	First offense: 1 year in prison, $5000 fine Second offense: 2 years in prison, $10,000 fine
Hallucinogens	I	First offense: 5 years in prison, $15,000 fine Second offense: 10 years in prison, $30,000 fine	First offense: 1 year in prison, $5000 fine Second offense: 2 years in prison, $10,000 fine
Cannabis	I	First offense: 5 years in prison, $15,000 fine Second offense: 10 years in prison, $30,000 fine	First offense: 1 year in prison, $5000 fine Second offense: 2 years in prison, $10,000 fine
Inhalants	N/A	N/A	N/A
Nicotine	N/A	N/A	N/A

(Adapted from Reed & Lang[2])

Preoccupation with the abused substance can lead to a variety of social problems for the substance abuser. Impaired relationships with family and friends can occur, or abusers may become incapable of or disinterested in performing their jobs and may be fired. Unemployment can lead to difficulties in obtaining housing and can contribute to homelessness. The need to obtain money to support a drug habit or to obtain necessities may lead to criminal activity. Table 33–2 lists the possible legal penalties for the manufacture and distribution or possession of drugs regulated by the Comprehensive Drug Abuse and Control Act of 1970. The drugs are classified as Schedule I through V based on their abuse potential, with Schedule I drugs having the highest potential for abuse and Schedule V the lowest.[2] Legal penalties are also warranted for theft, violence, or prostitution committed in efforts to support a drug habit.

FAMILY EFFECTS

The effects of substance abuse on the family of the abuser can be many and severe. These families are characterized by frequent conflict, anger, ambivalence, fear, guilt, confusion, mistrust, and violence as a mode of conflict resolution. The family frequently becomes socially isolated in efforts to cover up the problem of abuse and so are not able to make use of sources of assistance that might be available to them.

In families in which one parent or the other is a substance abuser, the husband-wife coalition present in most families is frequently absent. Often it is replaced by a strong dyad of the nonabusing parent and a child. Such coalitions may require children to assume adult responsibilities, either as a "little mother" or as a parental confidant. The pressure caused by these responsibilities may be one of the contributing factors in later substance abuse by children of abusers.[24]

The effects of parental alcoholism on children has been widely studied. More than 28 million people in the United States were raised in homes where alcohol abuse was evident. These individuals tend to exhibit both physical and psychological effects of parental alcoholism both as children and as adults. They may experience feelings of guilt, premature responsibility, and a sense of being trapped by the situation. Approximately 80 percent of adolescent suicides occur in families where one or more parents abuse substances.[24] As adults, children of alcohol abusers tend to have frequent marital problems, psychosomatic illnesses, and experience high levels of guilt and anxiety.[24]

Some researchers have described stages of family response to alcohol abuse that are similar to responses to abuse of other substances by family members.[6,24] The first stage is usually characterized by denial of the problem and attempts to mitigate the social effects of abuse. For example, a spouse may call to explain the abuser's absence from work as illness when it is actually due to a drug hangover. In this stage, family members exhibit the phenomenon of "co-dependency." A ***co-dependent*** is a person in a continuing relationship with the substance abuser, whose behavior enables the abuser to continue his or her drug-dependent existence.[25] Co-dependents practice maladaptive behaviors to cope with the problem of abuse.[26] Characteristics of co-dependents are summarized in Box 33–4.

The second stage of family response to substance abuse involves unsuccessful attempts to eliminate the problem. For example, the family may conspire to prevent the alcohol abuser from having access to alcohol. In the third stage, the family becomes disorganized, control attempts are abandoned, and there is diminished support for the abuser in his or her family roles. The fourth stage of response is characterized by the attempt of the other spouse (or a child) to control the family and to function without the input of the abusing member. This is usually followed by an escape stage in which a separation may occur. In the sixth stage, the family reorganizes and redistributes family roles in the absence of the abuser. With effective treatment, families may also experience a seventh stage in which the family is again reorganized to reintegrate the recovered abuser into his or her previous family roles.[24] The stages of family response to substance abuse are summarized in Box 33–5.

BOX 33–4.

Characteristics of Co-dependence

- Assumption of responsibility for others' feelings or behaviors
- Difficulty in identifying and expressing feelings
- Excessive worry over the response of others to one's feelings
- Difficulty in forming or maintaining close relationships
- Fear of rejection by others
- Unrealistic expectations of self and others
- Difficulty making decisions
- Tendency to minimize or deny feelings
- Self-concept tied to others' responses to oneself
- Reluctance to ask for help
- Reluctance to share problems with others
- Though misplaced, steadfast loyalty to others
- Need to be needed

(Adapted from Zerwekh & Michaels[26])

BOX 33–5.

Stages of Family Response to Substance Abuse

Stage 1: Denial of the problem and attempts to mitigate the social effects of substance abuse

Stage 2: Unsuccessful attempts by family members to control or eliminate the problem

Stage 3: Disorganization, abandonment of control efforts, diminished support for substance abuser in prior family roles

Stage 4: Attempts by one or more family members to control the family and to function without the input of the abusing member

Stage 5: Separation or other attempts to escape the problem

Stage 6: Reorganization and redistribution of family roles without the abuser

Stage 7: Reintegration of the recovered substance abuser into the family and into prior family roles

(Source: Finley[24])

Direct exposure of children to psychoactive substances has a variety of adverse physical and psychological effects. Children with perinatal exposures to alcohol, nicotine, or other drugs may be lower in birth weight, be particularly irritable and difficult to comfort, and experience poor school performance later in life.[27–29] Drug use during pregnancy may also contribute to premature labor.[30] As noted earlier, despite educational efforts on the hazards of smoking during pregnancy, approximately 60 percent of pregnant women continue to smoke during pregnancy. In one study of women in labor in Rhode Island, almost 8 percent of the women had positive tests for at least one drug, primarily marijuana (3 percent) and cocaine (2.6 percent), followed by opioids (1.7 percent) and amphetamines (less than 1 percent). These figures from a sample of all women delivering in the state in a specified time period are significant because they indicate the widespread nature of drug use in the general population as well as in high-risk groups.[31]

Home exposure to tobacco smoke also affects the health status of children and may contribute to a variety of respiratory conditions as well as childhood cancers. According to one study, even among women smokers who quit smoking during their pregnancy, 70 percent resume smoking within a year after delivery.[32] The health effects of drug exposures for children are discussed in more detail later in this chapter.

SOCIETAL EFFECTS

Societal effects of substance abuse include increased morbidity and mortality, higher economic costs, and increased crime. Physical morbidity related to psychoactive substance abuse was addressed in relation to personal effects of substance abuse. At the societal level, abuse leads to increased incidence and prevalence of these conditions.

MORTALITY

As noted earlier, substance abuse also leads to increased mortality, either directly as a result of drug overdose or withdrawal, or indirectly due to other conditions related to abuse. The contribution of smoking to increased mortality was discussed Chapter 31, Chronic Physical Health Problems. The rate of deaths due to drugs other than nicotine and alcohol increased from 2.7 per 100,000 population in 1978[33] to 3.8 per 100,000 in 1987 despite efforts to reduce drug-related mortality. Age-adjusted mortality rates among opioid abusers remain almost seven times higher than those for the general population.[34]

Mortality related to alcohol abuse is of particular concern. In 1987, nearly 5 percent of all deaths were due to alcohol-related causes,[35] and in 1989 more than 22,000 alcohol-related traffic fatalities occurred in the United States.[36] In addition to motor vehicle accident fatalities, alcohol is a factor in other accidental deaths; these include homicide; suicide; deaths due to cancers of the lip, oral cavity, pharynx, esophagus, stomach, liver, and larynx; cardiovascular deaths; and deaths due to respiratory diseases, digestive diseases, and diabetes mellitus.[35]

COST

Substance abuse also affects society in terms of its economic costs. Alcohol abuse, for example, is considered the most expensive health problem in the United States, costing an estimated $90 billion in 1980. This figure exceeds the $80 billion in costs associated with circulatory problems, $45 billion for digestive system problems, and $43 billion for cancer.[37] In 1988, the economic costs of alcohol abuse in Wisconsin alone, which has a high prevalence of heavy drinking, were estimated at almost $1.5 billion. Alcohol-related health-care costs for treatment and rehabilitation of alcohol-caused diseases and injuries exceeded $150 million in Wisconsin during 1988, while more than $27 million was spent on residential treatment for mental retardation due to fetal alcohol syndrome.[38]

In addition to costs related to the effects of substance abuse, there are the costs of the substances involved and their production and marketing. Figures are not available on the overall costs of illicit drugs, but the average per person expenditure for alcoholic beverages nationwide in the 1987 Consumer Expenditure Survey was $289 annually.[19] Annual advertising expenses nationwide for alcoholic beverages amount to $20 billion.[10]

CRIME

One final social effect associated with the abuse of many substances (excluding nicotine) is increased crime. For example, drugs have been implicated in the commission of many crimes that are not strictly related to drugs (selling or possessing drugs; driving while intoxicated).[39] In one study of arrestees in 14 major U.S. cities, 15 percent to 38 percent of those arrested for nondrug-related offenses reported drug use at some time in their lives and more than half of the arrestees in some areas tested positive for drug use.[40]

Alcohol is also implicated in criminal activity. In one study, for example, alcohol use was involved in 55 percent of all arrests studied, 74 percent of homicides, 69 percent of beatings, 39 percent of sexually aggressive acts against women, and 67 percent of sexually aggressive acts against children.[41] In other studies, as many as 83 percent of homicides involved alcohol.[39]

THE EPIDEMIOLOGIC PREVENTION PROCESS MODEL AND CONTROL OF SUBSTANCE ABUSE

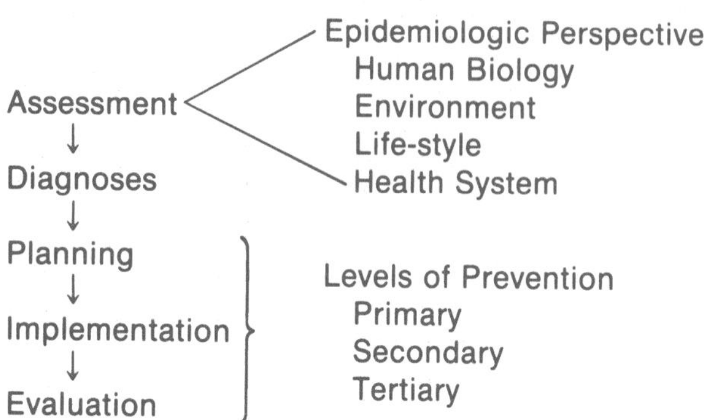

To engage in efforts to control problems of substance abuse, community health nurses must identify those persons and groups at risk for substance abuse and its adverse effects, as well as those who are actually experiencing problems of abuse. The epidemiologic prevention process model provides a framework for identifying these people and for planning, implementing, and evaluating interventions to assist them in controlling substance abuse.

ASSESSMENT

Several aspects of community health nursing assessment relate to problems of substance abuse. These include assessing for risk factors, for signs of abuse and dependence, for intoxication, for signs of withdrawal, and for long-term physical and psychological effects of substance abuse. Because of the negative connotations associated with substance abuse, the nursing assessment must be conducted with tact and with an accepting and a nonjudgmental, nonthreatening approach.[42] The nurse must first examine his or her own attitudes to substance abuse and work through any negative feelings that may interfere with nurse-client interactions. If clients sense a disparaging or judgmental attitude on the part of the nurse, they are less likely to respond truthfully to questions about their use of psychoactive substances.

ASSESSING FOR RISK FACTORS

The epidemiology of substance abuse indicates that there are contributing factors in each of the four components of Dever's epidemiologic perspective. Community health nurses should keep in mind that the interplay of biological, psychological, and social factors that lead to substance abuse are unique to each individual,[10] and all areas of clients' lives should be assessed in relation to the potential for substance abuse.

Human Biology

Human biological factors influencing substance abuse and its effects include genetic inheritance, maturation and aging, and physiologic function.

Genetic Inheritance. A growing body of evidence suggests that substance abuse may be associated with some form of genetic predisposition. Studies of adopted children, for example, indicate that alcohol abuse by one or both of the biological parents is associated with alcohol abuse by the child, even if the adoptive parents are nonabusers. Alcohol abuse by the adoptive parents, on the other hand, does not appear to be associated with later abuse by the child.[25] Further support for a genetic predisposition for alcoholism comes from the link between borderline personality disorder and alcoholism and the fact that persons with a family history of borderline personality disorder were two to three times as likely to be alcohol abusers as were members of the general population.[43]

Research indicating similar ways of processing alcohol and other drugs (for example, opioids) in the brain suggests that there may also be a genetic component in the abuse of drugs other than alcohol.[10] In assessing individuals and families for the level of risk for substance abuse, the community health nurse would obtain a detailed genogram that includes information about the family history of substance abuse as well as the presence of physical and emotional illnesses with a genetic component.

Maturation and Aging. Age influences one's risk of exposure to drugs and alcohol through social factors. For example, young people are more likely to be exposed to pressure to use drugs and alcohol or to smoke than are older people. Adolescents and preadolescents are particularly vulnerable to this type of pressure because of their developmental need to conform to peer expectations and to be part of a group. Often, being part of the group depends upon engaging in behaviors that place the individual at risk, such as sexual activity, smoking, and drug and alcohol use. Community heath nurses working with young people should assess the level of maturity of the youngsters and their ability to resist pressure to conform.

One's age also influences the effects of drug exposure, and perinatal exposures to drugs and alcohol have a variety of adverse effects on the fetus. As many

TABLE 33–3. FETAL, NEONATAL, AND DEVELOPMENTAL EFFECTS OF PERINATAL PSYCHOACTIVE SUBSTANCE EXPOSURE

Substance	Fetal Effects	Neonatal Effects	Developmental Effects
Alcohol	Growth deficiency, microcephaly, stillbirth, low birth weight (LBW), joint and facial anomalies, cardiac and kidney anomalies	Acute withdrawal with sedation, seizures, poor feeding	Developmental delay, low IQ, hyperactivity
Sedatives, hypnotics	Sedation at delivery	Tremors, hypertonicity, poor suck, high-pitched cry	Unknown
Opioids	Intrauterine growth retardation, prematurity, microcephaly, hyperactivity	Withdrawal with tremors, hypertonicity, poor feeding, diarrhea, seizures, irritability	Increased rate of sudden infant death syndrome (SIDS)
Cocaine	Spontaneous abortion	Tremors, hypertonicity, muscle weakness, seizures	Developmental delay, increased rate of SIDS
Amphetamines	Intrauterine growth retardation, biliary atresia, transposition of great vessels	Stillbirth, LBW, cardiac anomalies, withdrawal	Poor school performance
Phencyclidine	Agitation at delivery, microcephaly	Irritability, poor fine-motor coordination, sensory input problems	Unknown
Hallucinogens	Unknown	Unknown	Unknown
Cannabis	Bleeding problems in delivery	Sedation, tremors, excessive response to light	Unknown
Inhalants	Unknown	Unknown	Unknown
Nicotine	Intrauterine growth retardation, microcephaly	Jitteriness, poor feeding	Poor school performance, increased rate of SIDS

as 10 percent to 25 percent of neonates may be exposed to drugs in utero.[9,22] Some psychoactive substances, such as alcohol, amphetamines, and cocaine, have "teratogenic" effects when taken during pregnancy.[44] **Teratogenic substances** are those that cause physical defects in the developing embryo. Other drugs do not affect fetal development per se but have other adverse health effects for the neonate or long-term effects for the child. Specific fetal, neonatal, and developmental effects of selected psychoactive substances are presented in Table 33–3.

The elderly may also be at increased risk for substance abuse because of social factors that promote drug use such as loneliness or loss of significant others.[45] The elderly are also at risk for adverse effects of drugs because of decreased ability to metabolize drugs, a condition that occurs with advancing age. In addition, aging itself results in cell loss in target organs, thus increasing their sensitivity to the effects of alcohol and other drugs.[46]

Two general types of substance abuse have been noted among the elderly—early onset abuse and late onset abuse.[45] In early onset abuse, the abuser has developed a pattern of substance abuse over a lifetime and continues abuse in old age. The late onset abuser begins to abuse alcohol or other drugs in response to the stresses that occur as a result of aging. In one study, approximately 40 percent of alcohol abusers over age 65 were of the late onset type.[45]

Abuse of alcohol and sedatives, hypnotics, and anxiolytics is particularly prevalent among the elderly, whereas abuse of stimulants, cocaine, and cannabis is rare.[47] It has been suggested that more than half of all hospital admissions of older persons are due to alcohol-related problems.[46] In addition to alcohol abuse, 10 percent to 20 percent of elderly individuals in one Canadian study reported use of tranquilizers or sleeping pills.[47]

In working with newborns and young children the community health nurse would be alert to signs of perinatal drug exposure. He or she would also assess for risk factors that would make the child or older person particularly vulnerable to substance abuse and its effects.

Physiologic Function. Deterioration in physiologic function as the result of physical disability may be a contributing factor in substance abuse. For example, in one study of spinal-cord injured people, 62 percent had substance abuse problems.[48] In another study, 25 percent of people with physical or mental handicaps abused alcohol or other drugs.[49]

In many instances, disability is due to injuries caused by substance abuse (for example, in motor vehicle accidents that occur while one is intoxicated). At other times, the person with a disability may abuse drugs or alcohol as an escape from pain, depression, or stress related to the disability.[49] Or, substance abuse may stem from a desire for gratification when other avenues are denied or as a method of regaining control over one's choices and actions.[48] In working with disabled clients, community health nurses would assess clients' responses to disability and their vulnerability to substance abuse as a means of coping with disability.

Environment

Psychological Environment. Both personality traits and the presence of psychopathology may contribute to problems of substance abuse. There seem to be some commonalities in the personalities of substance abusers regardless of the type of substance abused. Personality traits that may place one at risk for substance abuse include rebelliousness and nonconformity that may lead to substance abuse as an expression of defiance or as an escape from the constraints and expectations of the adult world. Other common traits in abusers are a greater tolerance of deviant behavior, a poor self-concept, and passive surrender to their belief of their own inevitable failure in life. Abusers of psychoactive substances also tend to be impulsive, unable to value themselves, and have poor tolerance for frustration and anxiety. They may also have difficulty in acknowledging their feelings and in developing interests and deriving pleasure from them.[10] In addition, people who abuse psychoactive substances frequently feel alienated from those around them and are socially isolated. They may also feel powerless, and they usually have poor coping skills.[23]

Substance abusers also tend to display a common set of defense mechanisms that include denial, projection, rationalization, all-or-nothing thinking, conflict minimization and avoidance, narcissism, nonanalytic modes of thinking, passivity, and difficulty with compromise.[42,43] Abusers frequently deny that they have a problem with substance abuse and assert that they can change their behavior. They may exhibit inability to accept responsibility for their own behavior in other areas as well, and they frequently project or transfer the blame for their own behavior onto others. They also rationalize their behavior without developing true insights into the reason for that behavior. They tend to try to avoid conflict, and may turn to substance abuse as a means of escaping from the stress generated by conflict rather than engaging in positive modes of conflict resolution. Their thinking is characterized by an all-or-nothing quality, and they often make decisions that are inflexible and narrow in scope.

The presence of definite psychopathology also places many people at increased risk of substance abuse, and substance abuse is frequently an attempt to relieve or mask the symptoms of underlying psychiatric disorders. For example, the prevalence of alcohol abuse is higher among those with borderline personality disorder than among the general public.[43] Depressive disorders and a history of psychiatric treatment or hospitalization are also risk factors for alcohol abuse.[50] Similarly, mood disorders and attention-deficit disorder have been found to be associated with cocaine abuse.[22] Evidence also suggests that people with eating disorders are at higher risk for abuse of alcohol and other drugs.[51]

Psychological factors involved in smoking initiation are somewhat different from those involved in the abuse of other substances although there are some commonalities. Approximately one-third of smokers report that they smoke as a means of dealing with stress, fear, anxiety, or pressure,[18] indicating an absence of other effective coping skills. Smokers do not tend to display the psychopathology, alienation, or defense mechanisms typical of other substance abusers. As noted earlier, young people who begin smoking in the face of current social pressures not to smoke may be exhibiting the defiance that is typical of those who abuse other substances.[10]

Social Environment. Factors in the social environment may also contribute to problems of substance abuse. These factors can exist within the family unit, one's peer group, or in society at large. Within the family, research indicates that favorable parental attitudes toward marijuana use are associated with the use of marijuana by children. Similarly, the use of alcohol or drugs by parents or older siblings may influence drug use by children. Family tolerance of drunkenness may also contribute to alcohol use in children.[10] Families with low cohesion, high levels of conflict, few shared interests and activities, poor coping strategies, and marital dissatisfaction increase the risk of substance abuse in their members. Families encountering multiple stressors and who have inadequate resources are also at risk.[52] Episodes of violence within the family can also lead family members to use substance abuse as a means of escape from family tensions. Community health nurses should assess families for conditions that may contribute to substance abuse by family members.

Peer influence is another factor in the social environment that may contribute to substance abuse. In adolescents and preadolescents in particular, pressure from peers to smoke, drink, or use other psychoactive drugs is a powerful motivator for initiating these behaviors. For example, socialization with people who use or abuse psychoactive substances has been shown to contribute to cocaine use as well as the use of other drugs.[53] Peer influences also tend to determine the type of drug abused, particularly the influence of one's best friend.[10] In working with young people, in particular, the nurse would carefully assess peer attitudes to substance use and abuse as well as the degree to which the individual feels a need to conform to peer-dictated norms.

Social factors such as poverty, unemployment, and discrimination may create a sense of hopelessness and powerlessness that leads to substance abuse as an escape or in order to enhance one's own feelings of competence. These factors might explain the higher prevalence of some forms of substance abuse among members of minority groups and the poor. It has been suggested, for example, that the high incidence of alcohol abuse among Native Americans, for whom the top five causes of death are alcohol-related, is due to displacement from their traditions and culture as well as to poverty and other social factors.[23]

Culture also seems to play a part in the development of alcohol abuse. Cultural attitudes and modes of introducing alcohol use to young people can either contribute to or impede the development of alcohol abuse. In cultural groups where the introduction of alcohol is part of a family-centered activity or religious observance, the incidence of alcohol abuse is relatively low[23] compared to groups where alcohol use is perceived as evidence of adulthood or where alcohol use is considered totally unacceptable.

In assessing individuals, families, and communities for potential for substance abuse, the community health nurse would investigate both the influence of cultural norms and sources of stress on the use of psychoactive substances. In addition, the nurse would look for risk factors such as poverty and unemployment that increase stress and that might prompt substance abuse.

Other societal factors that contribute to substance abuse should also be assessed including general norms for abusive behaviors and the availability of psychoactive substances.[10] Media portrayals of drinking and smoking as desirable behaviors influence use of these substances. Ready availability of amphetamines in Southern California, where methamphetamine labs abound, make this a drug of choice in the area and increase its abuse relative to other psychoactive substances.[9]

Easy access to alcohol and cigarettes has also contributed to abuse of these substances. On the other hand, laws controlling access to alcohol through higher taxes on alcohol sales and by raising the minimum age of purchase have decreased both the use and misuse of alcohol.[16] In the same vein, social changes that include a ban on tobacco advertising and restrictions on sales promotion, new health warnings, and restricting smoking on commercial airlines, as well as economic assistance to tobacco growers to switch to other crops, have been credited with decreases in Canadian tobacco consumption.[54]

Life-style

Life-style factors that influence substance abuse are related to consumption patterns, occupation, and leisure activities. The community health nurse should assess individual and family consumption patterns related to tobacco, alcohol, and medications. The nurse should ascertain the frequency and amount of substance use as well as the appropriateness of its use. For example, the nurse might determine whether sedatives are in fact being used as prescribed, whether they are kept away from young people in the home, and whether they are ever used in conjunction with alcohol. Nurses should also determine the extent of alcohol use by families. Many people, for example, do not consider taking medications with an alcohol base as drinking, but may be receiving a hefty dose of alcohol through repeated use. Similarly, Mexican-American families might return to Mexico to obtain medications such as paregoric (an opioid preparation) for use for diarrhea without even knowing about its potential for abuse. The nurse would also want to ask about medicinal uses of alcohol, particularly with children, such as giving alcohol for teething pain or to quiet a fretful child.[6]

Some occupational groups are at increased risk for substance abuse. People whose work involves travel outside the United States may have access to illicit drugs that promote abuse. Similarly, there is a relatively high incidence of substance abuse among health-care providers because of easy access to controlled drugs.[55]

Employer sanctions against substance use and abuse have been shown to decrease these practices. For example, policies related to drug use in the U.S. military have led to reduced rates of drug abuse in this occupational group compared to the civilian population. On the other hand, lack of attention to alcohol use and smoking by military personnel has led to increased prevalence of these behaviors as compared to civilians.[56] Employer policies related to smoking in the workplace have also been shown to decrease smoking behaviors both on and off the job. In fact, in one study, 21 percent of employees who were smoking at the time of no-smoking policy implementation quit smoking altogether, and almost half reported quitting because of the policy.[57]

Recreational activities can contribute to the use of psychoactive substances in that alcohol and tobacco use are frequent adjuncts of such activities. People tend to drink and smoke when they socialize with others. Friday or Saturday night binges are a relatively common phenomenon, when people can "let go" and drink because they know they will have time to recover before returning to work on Monday. Next to alcohol, marijuana is the most widely used recreational drug, but cocaine is also used recreationally and has the connotation of high status, glamour, and excitement. PCP is also used for recreational purposes.[18]

Health System

Several aspects of the American health system have also contributed to the growing problem of substance abuse. Lack of attention to educating clients and the public about the hazards of substance abuse and failure to identify clients with substance-abuse problems have impeded efforts to control abuse. Practitioners have been particularly slow to identify pregnant women and older clients with problems of abuse.[45,50] At the same time, some health-care providers have actively fostered drug abuse by prescribing psychoactive drugs inappropriately or by not monitoring the extent of clients' use of these drugs.

The health-care system also impedes control of substance abuse by failing to provide adequate treatment for persons affected. For example, health insurance coverage for treatment for substance abuse is minimal at best. One study of health maintenance organizations, for example, revealed that only two-thirds of them provided coverage for treatment of alcohol or drug abuse.[58] Provision of adequate treatment of substance abuse may be further impeded by negative feelings on the part of health-care providers toward those who abuse psychoactive substances.

The health system may pose additional barriers to care that are particularly burdensome for some population groups. For example, most treatment programs are geared toward the needs of younger people and may not recognize the unique needs of the elderly substance abuser. Certainly Medicare, in the implementation of the DRG (diagnosis related group) system, does not take note of the extended time needed to safely detoxify the elderly substance abuser. In addition, because older people are considered nonproductive members of society, priority for placement in treatment facilities may be given to younger people.[45] Pregnant women have similar problems in that many treatment facilities will not admit them because their pregnancies place them in medically high-risk categories and because of the high potential for adverse maternal and fetal effects during detoxification.[50]

ASSESSING FOR SIGNS OF SUBSTANCE ABUSE

In addition to assessing individuals, families, and communities for risk factors that may contribute to substance abuse, the nurse should assess individual clients for general indications of existing abuse. General indicators that a person has a problem with abuse of a psychoactive substance include frequent intoxication, preoccupation with obtaining and using the substance, binge use, changes in personality or mood, withdrawal, problems with family members related to use of the substance, problems with friends or neighbors, problems on the job (absenteeism, poor performance, interpersonal difficulties), and conflicts with law enforcement officials. Additional indicators include belligerence, financial problems, inability to discontinue substance use despite attempts, continued use of the substance despite related health problems and other problems, and increasing tolerance to the substance.[18,49]

ASSESSING FOR INTOXICATION

Another aspect of the community health nurse's assessment related to substance abuse is assessing individuals for signs of intoxication. ***Intoxication*** is a state of diminished physical or mental control that occurs as a result of the current use of psychoactive drugs. Intoxication with different drugs may be reflected in differing symptoms. For example, cocaine intoxication is characterized by disinhibition, impaired judgment and impulsivity, grandiosity, and compulsively repeated actions. Other common symptoms include hypersexuality, hypervigilance, and hyperactivity.[22] Nicotine intoxication, on the other hand, is characterized by increased blood pressure, heart rate, and muscle tone.[10] Signs of intoxication with selected psychoactive substances are presented in Table 33–4.

ASSESSING FOR WITHDRAWAL

The physiological dependence engendered by some psychoactive substances leads to withdrawal or abstinence syndrome when the substance is withheld.[42] A withdrawal syndrome is a complex of symptoms that accompany abstinence from a psychoactive substance, usually characterized by severe discomfort, pain, nausea, vomiting, and, possibly, convulsions. The severity of withdrawal may vary with the abusive substance and the degree of dependence experienced by the client. The community health nurse working with clients who may abuse psychoactive substances would assess the client for signs of withdrawal. Typical withdrawal symptoms for selected psychoactive substances are presented in Table 33–5.

TABLE 33–4. SIGNS OF INTOXICATION WITH SELECTED PSYCHOACTIVE SUBSTANCES

Substance	Typical Indications of Intoxication
Alcohol	Decreased alertness, impaired judgment, slurred speech, nausea, double vision, vertigo, staggering, unpredictable emotional changes, stupor, unconsciousness
Sedatives, hypnotics, anxiolytics	Slurred speech; slow, shallow respiration; cold and clammy skin; weak and rapid pulse; drowsiness, blurred vision, unconsciousness
Opioids	Sedation, hypertension, respiratory depression, impaired intellectual function, constipation, pupillary constriction
Cocaine	Irritability; anxiety; slow, weak pulse; slow, shallow breathing; sweating; dilated pupils; increased blood pressure; insomnia; seizures; dysinhibition; impulsivity; compulsive actions; hypersexuality; hypervigilance; hyperactivity
Amphetamines	Sweating, dilated pupils, increased blood pressure, agitation, fever, irritability, headache, chills, insomnia, agitation, tremors, seizures
Phencyclidine	Flushing, fever, sweating, agitation, incoherent speech, aggression, coma
Hallucinogens	Dilated pupils, mood swings, elevated blood pressure, paranoia, bizarre behavior, nausea and vomiting, tremors, panic
Cannabis	Redened eyes; increased pulse, respirations, and blood pressure; laughter; confusion; panic
Inhalants	Giddiness, drowsiness, increased vital signs; headache, nausea, fainting, stupor, fatigue, disorientation
Nicotine	Headache; loss of appetite; nausea; increased pulse, blood pressure, and muscle tone

(*Source: Chychula & Okore*[22]*; McCorry*[10]*; Naegle, M. A. (1991). Utilizing the nursing process with patients who abuse drugs and alcohol. In M. M. Kuhn (Ed.),* Pharmacotherapeutics: A nursing process approach *(2nd ed.) (pp. 280–306). Philadelphia: F.A. Davis; and Reed & Lang*[2])

Withdrawal can be extremely dangerous and may even by life-threatening, especially for vulnerable clients. Withdrawal is a particularly serious event for pregnant women, when both mother and fetus are at risk,[50] and for the elderly,[45] and the community health nurse should be alert in assessing these clients for signs of withdrawal. Interventions during the withdrawal phase will be addressed later in this chapter.

TABLE 33–5. INDICATIONS OF WITHDRAWAL FROM SELECTED PSYCHOACTIVE SUBSTANCES

Substance	Indications of Withdrawal
Alcohol	Anxiety, insomnia, tremors, delirium, convulsions
Sedatives, hypnotics, anxiolytics	Anxiety, insomnia, tremors, delirium, convulsions (may occur up to 2 weeks after stopping use of anxiolytics)
Opioids	Restlessness, irritability, tremors, loss of appetite, panic, chills, sweating, cramps, watery eyes, runny nose, nausea, vomiting, muscle spasms, impaired coordination, depressed reflexes, constricted pupils
Cocaine	*Early crash:* agitation depression, anorexia, high level of craving *Middle crash:* fatigue, depression, no craving, insomnia *Late crash:* exhaustion, hypersomnolence, hyperphagia, no craving *Early withdrawal:* normal sleep and mood, low craving, low anxiety *Middle and late withdrawal:* anhedonia, anxiety, anergy, high level of craving exacerbated by conditioned cues *Extinction:* normal hedonic response and mood; episodic craving triggered by conditioned cues
Amphetamines	Fatigue, hunger, long periods of sleep, disorientation, severe depression
Phencyclidine	Short-term or long-term depression
Hallucinogens	Slight irritability, restlessness, insomnia, reduced energy level
Cannabis	Insomnia, hyperactivity, decreased appetite
Inhalants	None reported
Nicotine	Nervousness, increased appetite, sleep disturbances, anxiety

(*Source: Reed & Lang*[2]*; Sizer & Whitney*[3])

The physical and psychological discomfort and the deep depression that may occur with withdrawal from psychoactive drug use may lead to suicide. The community health nurse assessing clients for withdrawal symptoms should also carefully assess them for potential suicide. Clients should be monitored carefully and asked about suicidal thoughts.

Because of the duration and unique features of cocaine abstinence, the cocaine withdrawal syndrome merits specific discussion here. Cocaine abstinence occurs in three phases: crash, withdrawal, and extinction.[22] The crash phase occurs anywhere from 9 hours to 4 days after discontinuing the use of the drug and is characterized by agitation, depression, anorexia, and intense craving. This phase is also characterized by feelings of extreme exhaustion following a cocaine binge. During the withdrawal phase, the client first experiences normal sleep patterns, low anxiety levels, and low cravings for cocaine. Later in this phase, which may last up to 10 weeks, the client experiences **anhedonia** (an inability to experience pleasure), high anxiety, and high levels of craving. Cravings are exacerbated by conditioned cues associated with prior drug use such as seeing people with whom one used drugs or returning to places where drugs have been used. The extinction phase, which lasts for an indefinite period, is characterized by a normal hedonic experience, normal moods, and episodic cravings triggered by conditioned cues. Cravings occurring in both the withdrawal and extinction phases may lead to resumed drug use.[22]

ASSESSING FOR LONG-TERM EFFECTS OF SUBSTANCE ABUSE

In addition to assessing clients for signs and symptoms of intoxication and withdrawal, community health nurses should also assess individual clients for symptoms of long-term effects of substance abuse. These effects can be physical or psychological in nature and will vary among psychoactive substances. For example, long-term effects of alcohol abuse might include malnutrition, cirrhosis, or liver cancer, while typical effects of phencyclidine abuse include psychoses and insomnia. Typical long-term effects that should be considered with specific substances are presented in Table 33–6. The community health nurse assessing the health of population groups would assess morbidity and mortality related to these long-term effects of substance abuse in the population.

TABLE 33–6. LONG-TERM EFFECTS ASSOCIATED WITH ABUSE OF SELECTED PSYCHOACTIVE SUBSTANCES

Substance	Long-Term Effects of Abuse
Alcohol	Malnutrition; impotence; ulcers; cirrhosis; esophageal, stomach, and liver cancers; organic brain syndrome; deafness
Sedatives, hypnotics, anxiolytics	Potential for death due to overdose from increasing doses due to tolerance; impaired sexual function
Opioids	Lethargy, weight loss, sexual disinterest and dysfunction
Cocaine	Damage to nasal tissue, high blood pressure, weight loss, muscle twitching, paranoia, hallucinations
Amphetamines	Depression, paranoia, hallucinations, weight loss
Phencyclidine	Memory loss, inability to concentrate, insomnia, chronic or recurrent psychosis
Halucinogens	Flashbacks, psychosis
Cannabis	Chromosome changes, reduced sperm count, impaired concentration, poor memory, reduced alertness, inability to perform complex tasks
Inhalants	Organic brain syndrome, liver and kidney damage, bone marrow damage, anemia, hearing loss, nerve damage
Nicotine	Cardiovascular disease, lung cancer, bladder cancer, chronic disease, diabetic complications

(*Source: Levy, Dignan, & Shirreffs*[1]; *Reed & Lang*,[2])

DIAGNOSTIC REASONING AND SUBSTANCE ABUSE

Community health nurses make nursing diagnoses related to substance abuse at two levels. The first level is diagnoses related to individuals who have problems of substance abuse and their families. For example, the nurse might make a diagnosis for the individual client of "increased risk of substance abuse due to family history of alcohol abuse" or " abuse of sedatives due to increased life stress and poor coping skills." Nursing diagnoses related to the family of a substance abuser might include "co-dependency due to family feelings of guilt related to daughter's cocaine abuse" or "school behavior problems due to children's anxiety over mother's alcoholism."

At the second level, the community health nurse might make diagnoses of community problems related to substance abuse. For example, the nurse might diagnose an "increased incidence of motor vehicle fatalities due to driving under the influence of psychoactive drugs." Or, a diagnosis of "increased prevalence of drug abuse among minority group members due to discrimination and feelings of powerlessness." Another area in which community health nurses might make community-based diagnoses might be an "increased prevalence of fetal alcohol syndrome due to alcohol abuse among pregnant women."

PLANNING AND IMPLEMENTING CONTROL STRATEGIES FOR SUBSTANCE ABUSE

Strategies for controlling problems of substance abuse can involve primary, secondary, or tertiary prevention. In planning for interventions at all three levels, community health nurses and other health-care providers may find themselves in need of information and other assistance. Several resources for dealing with substance abuse are presented in Table 33–7.

PRIMARY PREVENTION

There are three major goals for primary prevention of substance abuse.[10] The first goal is to prevent nonusers from initiating use of psychoactive substances. The second goal is to prevent progression from experimentation to chronic use, and the third goal is to prevent expansion to the use of other substances. Using smoking as an example, primary prevention may be aimed at preventing the initiation of smoking in the first place, preventing movement from occasional smoking to regular use of tobacco, and preventing movement from tobacco use to the use of other drugs such as marijuana.

Effective primary prevention programs generally share several characteristics.[10] First, they involve peer programming. For example, a program to prevent drug use in junior high school would involve junior high students in program development. Second, the program will employ "counter-normative strategies." ***Counter-normative strategies*** are efforts to change the attitudes and norms related to the use of certain substances, thus reinforcing abstention as a group norm. The creation of student groups to reduce driv-

TABLE 33–7. RESOURCES FOR DEALING WITH SUBSTANCE ABUSE

Problem Area	Agency or Organization	Services
Alcohol abuse	Agency International (404) 266-2200	Conducts liquor-free vacation tours for alcoholics
	Al Anon Family Group Headquarters 1372 Broadway New York, NY 10018 (212) 302-7240	Support group for family members of alcoholics
	Alcohol Education for Youth and Community 362 State St. Albany, NY 12210 (518) 436-9319	Education for youth on alcoholism; advocacy; help with development of communication skills
	Alcohol Research Information Service 1106 E. Oakland Lansing, MI 48906 (517) 485-9900	Public education; information; teaching material for primary and secondary school programs; statistics
	Alcoholics Anonymous World Services P.O. Box 459 Grand Central Station New York, NY 10163 (212) 686-1100	Support group for alcoholics; advocacy
	American Council on Alcohol Problems 3426 Bridgeland Dr. Bridgeton, MO 63044 (314) 739-5944	Research; public education; advocacy; legislation
	Calix Society 7601 Wayzata Blvd. Minneapolis, MN 55426 (612) 546-0544	Self-help group for Catholic alcoholics
	Children of Alcoholics Foundation 200 Park Ave., 31st floor New York, NY 10166 (212) 949-1404	Public education; research; information on parent-child relations, development, abuse, and substance abuse in children of alcoholics
	National Association for Children of Alcoholics 31706 Coast Hwy., Suite 201 South Laguna, CA 92677 (714) 499-3889	Self-help groups; advocacy; public education

(*continued*)

TABLE 33–7. (*Continued*)

Problem Area	Agency or Organization	Services
Alcohol abuse (*continued*)	National Institute on Alcohol Abuse and Alcoholism 5600 Fishers Lane Rockville, MD 20857 (301) 443-3885	Research; information on treatment; rehabilitation training
	Recovery Adventures (213) 470-0606	Conducts liquor-free vacation tours for alcoholics
	Sober Adventures International (213) 837-4631	Conducts liquor-free vacation tours for alcoholics
	Sobriety Adventures (208) 983-2414	Conducts liquor-free vacation tours for alcoholics
	The Other Victims of Alcoholism P.O. Box 921 Radio City Station, New York, NY 10101 (212) 247-8087	Information on effects of alcoholism on family and business; advocacy
Drug abuse	American Council for Drug Education 5820 Hubbard Dr. Rockville, MD 20852 (301) 984-5700	Information and research on marijuana, cocaine, and other psychoactive drugs; resource information kits
	Drug-Anon Focus P.O. Box 9108 Long Island, NY 11103 (718) 361-2169	Self-help group for family and friends of drug abusers
	Drugs Anonymous P.O. Box 473 Ansonia Station New York, NY 10023 (212) 874-0700	Self-help group for drug abusers
	Ethos Foundation Three Skyline Place 5201 Leesburg Pike Suite 100 Falls Church, VA 22041 (703) 671-5335	Education of drug abusers, family, public; research; counselling and rehabilitation
	Families in Action National Drug Information Center 3845 N. Druid Hills Rd. Suite 300 Decatur, GA 30033 (404) 325-5799	Public education on adolescent drug use
	Families Anonymous P.O. Box 528 Van Nuys, CA 91408 (818) 989-7841	Self-help group for families with drug-abuse and related behavioral problems
	Narcotics Anonymous P.O. Box 9999 Van Nuys, CA 91409 (818) 780-3951	Self-help group for drug abusers
	National Association on Drug Abuse Problems 355 Lexington Ave. New York, NY 10017 (212) 986-1170	Job placement; rehabilitation of drug abusers; prevention

TABLE 33–7. (*Continued*)

Problem Area	Agency or Organization	Services
Drug abuse (*continued*)	National Institute on Drug Abuse 5600 Fishers Lane Rockville, MD 20857 (301) 443-6480	Research; information; training
	National Parents Resource Institute for Drug Education 100 Edgewood Ave., Suite 1002 Atlanta, GA 30303 (404) 658-2548	Information: help in developing support groups against drug use
	Potsmokers Anonymous 316 E. 3rd St. New York, NY 10009 (212) 254-1777	Information; 9-week course of quit marijuana use
	Straight, Inc. P.O. Box 21686 St. Petersburg, FL 33742 (813) 576-8929	Rehabilitation program for adolescent drug abusers
	Therapeutic Communities of America 131 Wayland Ave. Providence, RI 02906 (401) 331-4250	Self-help drug rehabilitation agencies; residential programs
	United States House of Representatives Select Committee on Narcotics Abuse and Control H2-234 House Office Bldg. Annex II Washington, DC 20515 (202) 226-3040	Policy formation
Dual agencies	Alcohol and Drug Problems Association of North America 444 N. Capitol St., NW Suite 181 Washington, DC 20001 (202) 737-4340	Public information; advocacy; policy formation
	Alcohol, Drug Abuse, and Mental Health Administration 5600 Fishers Lane Rockville, MD 20857 (301) 443-4797	Research; information; policy formation
	International Council for Prevention of Alcoholism and Drug Dependency 6830 Laurel St., NW Washington, DC 20012 (202) 722-6729	Research; public education; printed material
	Just Say No Clubs c/o Oakland Parents in Action 1404 Franklin St., Suite 610 Oakland, CA 94612 (415) 836-6078	Student clubs to prevent substance abuse; peer support; teaching aids for elementary grades
	United States Senate Committee on Labor and Human Relations Subcommittee on Children, Family, Drugs, and Alcoholism SH-639 Hart Bldg. Washington, DC 20510 (202) 224-5630	Policy formation

ing while intoxicated (for example, Students Against Drunk Drivers, or SADD) or drug-free dance clubs are examples of counter-normative strategies. For young people involved in these activities, nonuse of psychoactive substances is the norm of expected behavior.

A third characteristic of effective primary prevention programs, particularly among young people, is the inclusion of extracurricular activities or, possibly, mediation as an alternative mode of achieving a health "high." Finally, successful programs frequently make use of special events to highlight the focus of the program (for example, a health fair or a "smoke out").

Primary prevention efforts to control substance abuse usually focus on two approaches. These include education and action to modify risk factors for abuse.

Education

Education usually focuses on acquainting the public with the hazards of substance abuse. Both general public education campaigns and school-based educational programs have shown moderate success in limiting the use of psychoactive substances. However, they tend to be more effective in moderating the effects of substance abuse such as preventing drug-related motor vehicle fatalities. One of the criticisms of school-based programs is that they may not be reaching groups at greatest risk for substance abuse, those with a family history of abuse or who display characteristics associated with potential abusers.[16]

Community health nurses may be involved in educating individual clients and families or in providing substance-abuse education for groups of people. In either case, the nurse would employ the principles of teaching and learning discussed in Chapter 7, The Health Education Process.

Risk-Factor Modification

Risk-factor modification can occur with individuals, families, or in society at large. Community health nurses may assist individuals to plan to modify factors that put them at increased risk for substance abuse. For example, the nurse might assist clients experiencing stress to eliminate or modify sources of stress in their lives. Or, the nurse can assist clients to develop more effective coping skills.

Community health nurses might also assist families to develop more effective coping skills. In addition, the nurse may make referrals for social services to eliminate financial difficulties and other sources of stress. Or, the nurse might assist a harried single parent to obtain respite care. Nurses can also assist families to plan means of enhancing family communication and cohesion to minimize the risk of substance abuse among children.

At the societal level, community health nurses can engage in political activity to control access to and limit the availability of psychoactive substances as well as to modify societal factors that contribute to abuse. For example, the nurse might work to see that laws restricting the sale of alcohol and tobacco to minors are enforced. Or, the nurse might engage in efforts to reduce discrimination against members of minority groups or to ensure a minimal income for all families.

SECONDARY PREVENTION

Secondary prevention is employed when there is an existing problem with substance abuse. The goal in secondary prevention is early intervention aimed at those who have not yet developed irreversible pathological changes due to substance abuse.[16] Planning for secondary prevention necessitates mutual goal setting by the nurse and the family of the person experiencing a substance abuse problem.[52] Goals will relate to "intervention" and to treatment for substance abuse.

Intervention

Intervention, in terms of substance abuse, is the act of confronting the substance abuser with the intent of making a referral for assistance in dealing with the abuse.[50,59] The goal of the intervention is to elicit an agreement from the individual involved to be evaluated for a possible problem with substance abuse.[59]

Community health nurses may facilitate intervention by families of individual abusers but are not usually the interveners themselves. In this respect, the family, rather than the abuser, is the community health nurse's client.[59]

Many families may not see themselves as clients, and the community health nurse may need to reinforce the idea that substance abuse is a family disorder in order to motivate family members to engage in intervention.[52] To this end, the first step in preparing for intervention is providing the family or significant others with basic information about substance abuse and the defense mechanisms that are used by both the abuser and his or her significant others. In this way, family members can be helped to see their role as co-dependents or enablers of the abusive behavior. The nurse also educates family members about the intervention process, their responsibility for that process, and some of the feelings that they may experience during intervention.[59]

In assisting family members to prepare for intervention, the nurse will aid them to determine who should be involved. It may be that some members will not be able to follow through with confronting the individual with his or her behavior and should be asked not to participate in the intervention. Individuals who should be involved in the intervention include those who are close to and concerned for the abuser, those who may be able to influence his or her behavior in a positive way, and those who are able to engage in the intervention.

Next the nurse would assist those who will be involved in the intervention to identify in writing the causes for their concern and to describe how they felt when significant events related to substance abuse occurred.[59] Areas that the group should plan to address during the intervention are the problem as they perceive it, statements about the individual's behavior that indicate a problem of substance abuse, effects of the abuse problem, and their concern for the individual.[50]

Prior to the intervention, the group should arrange an appointment for an evaluation for substance abuse to take place immediately after the intervention session, since it is wise to follow through on the referral as soon as possible while the individual is motivated to seek help. It is suggested that appointments be made in more than one facility so the individual can exercise some choice in the matter and will feel less coerced.[59]

The group planning the intervention should also consider potential roadblocks to the success of the effort. For example, the individual might be concerned about the cost of care or about the need for child care while he or she is in treatment. If anticipated, these difficulties can be circumvented.[59]

The nurse can also assist family members to plan for their response to the individual's possible refusal to comply with a request for evaluation for substance abuse. If the wife plans to threaten divorce if the husband does not seek help, will she be able to carry through this threat in the face of his refusal? The nurse can help the family plan for these contingencies and work through feelings created by the proposed intervention by helping group members practice the intervention, who will say what, when, etc. Practice should also include who will sit nearest the individual (those with the greatest influence) and between the abuser and the door and who will initiate the intervention.[59]

Once the group is ready for the intervention, the individual should be brought to the place selected and the intervention initiated. Just prior to the intervention, while waiting for the individual to arrive, the nurse may remind family members why they are there and what is planned. The nurse is present to keep the intervention moving, but is not otherwise an active participant.[59]

If the individual agrees to be evaluated, one or more of the group members should accompany him or her to the evaluation appointment to prevent a potential suicide attempt. While this is occurring, the nurse may meet with the other members of the group to discuss their feelings about the process and its outcome. If the intervention has not been successful, the nurse can reassure group members and assist them to plan a subsequent intervention.[59]

Treatment

General Principles of Treatment for Substance Abuse. Treatment for problems of substance abuse will vary somewhat depending upon the type of substance involved. There are, however, some general principles that guide treatment for substance abuse.[8] First, a combination of modalities of treatment is usually more effective than a single mode. Second, treatment should be geared to individual problems, responses, and resources. For example, issues of aging related to retirement, physical loss, and loss of significant others leading to social isolation are issues that may need to be addressed with the elderly person but may not be factors in substance abuse by others. Similarly, the effects of physical disability must be dealt with in the handicapped person who abuses psychoactive substances, whereas this is not likely to be an issue with most other clients.

The third principle is that treatment should be administered by both professional and lay persons. For example, a combination of professional psychotherapy and participation in a self-help group such as Alcoholics Anonymous may be far more effective in dealing with alcohol abuse than either mode by itself. Family members or significant others should also be actively involved in treatment in order to refrain from enabling behaviors that allowed the individual to continue his or her substance abuse.[8]

Fourth, detoxification is necessary before any further treatment can be undertaken. Fifth, associated psychopathology requires psychiatric treatment not just the assistance of a self-help group.[8,43] Finally, social and vocational rehabilitation may be needed to reintegrate the person into the family and into society at large.[8] The principles of treatment for substance abuse are summarized in Box 33–6.

Treatment Modalities for Substance Abuse. Treatment modalities that may be employed include pharmacologic methods, psychosocial methods, sociotherapies, and self-help groups.[8] Pharmacologic methods use medication to help the abuser deal with the symptoms of withdrawal or to handle cravings for the substance involved. For example. Librium and Valium may be used to help the alcohol abuser relieve

BOX 33–6.

General Principles of Treatment for Substance Abuse

- A combination of modalities is usually more effective than a single treatment modality.
- Treatment should be tailored to the problems, responses, and resources of the individual abuser.
- Treatment should be provided by both professionals and lay persons.
- Detoxification and achievement of sobriety is the first step in treatment.
- Associated psychopathology requires psychiatric treatment.
- Social and vocational rehabilitation may be required to reintegrate the substance-abusing individual into the family and society.

(Source: Balis[8])

the anxiety caused by alcohol withdrawal, while disulfiram (Antabuse) may be given to modify the craving for alcohol. Similarly, methadone may be used to control cravings for heroin.[8] Psychosocial methods of treatment include individual, group, and family therapy; behavior modification; contracting; and aversion or relaxation therapies. Sociotherapy involves participation in therapeutic communities and residential programs where clients learn new life-styles consistent with sobriety. Finally, self-help groups consist of people who are abusers of the same substance and who provide for each other understanding and support in conquering their substance-abuse habit. For example, Alcoholics Anonymous is a self-help group for alcohol abusers, while Potsmokers Anonymous is a self-help group for marijuana abusers. Treatment modalities typically used for specific types of substance abuse are indicated in Table 33–8.

Community health nurses may plan for involvement in treatment for substance abuse in a number of ways. First, nurses might identify cases of substance abuse and plan to refer clients and their families to treatment resources in the community. Nurses may also educate the general public on the signs and symptoms of substance abuse as well as the availability of treatment facilities. In addition, community health nurses can monitor the use of medications during withdrawal (if this is done on a outpatient basis) or on a long-term basis.

Community health nurses might also be involved in psychosocial therapies in referring clients to sources of group, individual, or family therapy, or

TABLE 33–8. TREATMENT MODALITIES TYPICALLY USED FOR SELECTED FORMS OF PSYCHOACTIVE SUBSTANCE ABUSE

Substance	Typical Treatment Modalities
Alcohol	Detoxification; psychotherapy; group therapy; family therapy; self-help groups (Alcoholics Anonymous, Al-Anon); pharmacologic therapy (disulfiram, short-term use of tranquilizers or antidepressants); residential programs; referral for vocational rehabilitation and social services as needed
Sedatives, hypnotics, anxiolytics	Detoxification; psychotherapy and group therapy (for underlying psychiatric disorders)
Opioids	Pharmacologic therapy (methadone, opioid antagonists); therapeutic communities (Synanon, Odyssey House, Daytop, Phoenix House); group therapy; assistance with social skills, vocational training, and job placement; family therapy; self-help groups (Narcotics Anonymous, Chemical Dependency Anonymous); psychotherapy
Cocaine	Hospitalization; self-help groups; contingency contracting (client agreement to urinary monitoring and acceptance of aversive contingencies for positive results); pharmacologic therapy (tricyclic antidepressants)
Amphetamines	No established treatment guidelines; may be similar to treatment for cocaine abuse
Phencyclidine	Detoxification, psychotherapy (for underlying psychiatric disorders); group therapy; residential programs
Hallucinogens	Same as for phencyclidine
Cannabis	Same as for phencyclidines; self-help groups
Inhalants	Psychosocial interventions; psychotherapy (for underlying psychiatric disorder); sociodrama; vocational rehabilitation; family therapy, social support services
Nicotine	Aversive conditioning; desensitization; substitution; hypnotherapy; group therapy; relaxation training; supportive therapy; abrupt abstinence

(*Source: Balis*[8])

the nurse might reinforce contracts made for reducing the use of substances. This is particularly true in measures to help clients stop smoking. In this instance, community health nurses may initiate behavioral contracts with clients to enable them gradually to cut down on tobacco consumption or to quit smoking for gradually lengthened periods of time.

Community health nurses' involvement with therapeutic communities and self-help groups will usually occur in the form of referrals for these types of services. In some instances, however, community health nurses are actively involved in initiating support groups.

At the community level, nursing efforts to control substance abuse might include political activity to support the development of adequate treatment facilities, especially those geared to the needs of currently underserved population groups such as pregnant women and the elderly. Community health nurses might also be involved in political activity and advocacy to encourage insurance coverage of treatment for substance abuse.

The goals of treatment for substance abuse include early intervention for persons who have not yet become abusers but who use psychoactive substances; managing withdrawal and reducing cravings for the substance involved; and building a foundation for recovery.[16,53] Successful treatment efforts are usually characterized by patience, perseverance, and commitment by the helper; realistic goals; abstinence during treatment and as the ultimate goal; some degree of coercion involving the setting of limits, contracts, or substance-control measures; breaking through the abuser's denial to acceptance of the problem; bolstering his or her motivation to maintain abstinence; and development of alternate coping styles and enhanced self-esteem.[8]

Early Treatment. For some psychoactive substances, such as cocaine, use at any level almost always leads to abuse because of the vicious rebound cycle that occurs. For other substances like alcohol, sedatives, and tranquilizers, moderate use may be acceptable when these substances are used appropriately. Some authors suggest early intervention with people using these substances to allow them to use the substance in moderation. To this end, brief treatment is undertaken to stabilize and to moderate use of the substance in question so that it does not reach the level of abuse. Programs of this type involve teaching clients self-control skills and skills for decision making about responsible behavioral choices. Programs of this sort targeted to young people not fully enmeshed in substance abuse have shown promising results.[16]

Managing Withdrawal and Cravings. For clients who have already reached a level of substance abuse that does not admit of moderate use or for substances for which there is no level of moderate use, the goal of treatment is abstinence and long-term sobriety.[43] The first step to abstinence is detoxification, which often involves supporting the client through withdrawal. Community health nurses may be involved in referring clients to detoxification facilities and in supporting them during detoxification.

Persons who are at risk for serious consequences of withdrawal should always go through detoxification under medical supervision. Of particular concern are pregnant women and the elderly. Many of the drugs used to mitigate the adverse symptomatology of withdrawal from psychoactive substances are contraindicated in pregnancy. For example, Valium and Librium, both of which may be used to combat the anxiety and sleeplessness that may accompany withdrawal, may be teratogenic and should not be given to the pregnant substance abuser.[50] Similarly, detoxification procedures may need to be modified for older adults because of their tendency to be overmedicated by relatively small doses of medication.[45]

Community health nurses may monitor medication use during withdrawal or on a long-term basis, and they should be alert to the potential for use of medications for suicide purposes and to the potential for abuse of some of the substances used (for example, Valium). The nurse should assess clients on medications for suicide potential and should monitor mood changes closely. The nurse should also plan to educate clients and their families as to the adverse effects of combining medications with alcohol or other psychoactive drugs. Since disulfiram (Antabuse), in particular, is contraindicated in both pregnant women and clients with cardiac arrhythmias and pulmonary disease, the nurse should monitor clients for evidence of these conditions.

Other nursing considerations related to withdrawal and craving include maintaining levels of hydration and nutrition. Hydration is particularly important for the client who abuses alcohol because of the diuretic effects of alcohol. Nutrition is important for most drug abusers because substance abuse frequently leads to a disinterest in food in favor of consumption of the abusive substance. Decreased intake of stimulants such as caffeine is also advisable.[53] Treatment can also be enhanced by a regular program of exercise that will improve self-esteem, prevent excessive weight gain, and stimulate the release of endorphins.[53] Community health nurses can educate clients on the need for hydration and nutrition and suggest exercise. Vigorous aerobic exercise should not be undertaken before a thorough medical assessment of cardiovascular status has been conducted.[53] In the interim, however, the nurse can suggest a program of stretching exercises.

Building a Foundation for Recovery. Treatment for substance abuse is more than a matter of detoxification and modification of cravings for the drug in question. It is usually a total program of modification that results in changes in modes of thinking and acting. This may be achieved through professional therapy, participation in self-help groups, changes in environment and life-style, enhancing one's self-image, developing new coping skills, and developing new patterns of family interaction.

Community health nursing involvement in therapy and in self-help groups was addressed earlier. Nurses can also assist clients to plan changes in their environment to minimize stresses that may contribute to substance abuse. For example, the nurse can refer a client for help with financial difficulties or for respite from the care of a handicapped child or elderly parent. Socially isolated older persons who abuse substances can be linked to sources of social support, while unemployed persons can be assisted to find employment or to learn skills that enhance their employability.

Community health nurses can also help clients develop stronger self-images by reinforcing their successes and helping them realistically examine their failures and their expectations for themselves. In addition, nurses can help clients who abuse psychoactive substances to develop alternative ways of coping with stress by taking action to modify stressors or changing their perceptions of and responses to stressors.

Treatment efforts will also be needed for members of the abuser's family to enable them to recover from co-dependency.[26] Goals in the care of families of substance abusers include stabilizing the family system, making changes in family interactions, and developing mechanisms for maintaining those changes.[52] Family stabilization may be achieved by linking families to needed support services and engaging in the crisis intervention strategies described in Chapter 18, Care of the Family Client. The nurse can also make referrals for marital or family therapy as needed and can assist families to identify their use of defense mechanisms similar to those used by the substance abuser.

The community health nurse might also provide families with anticipatory guidance about the negative effects of life-change events and help them deal with these events without resorting to substance abuse. Family members may also need help in working through resentment related to substance abuse and subsequent behaviors by the abuser.

Building positive experiences in the life of the family also fosters cohesion and helps to stabilize the family. The community health nurse can assist the family to plan activities in which all members can participate. It is particularly important to integrate the substance-abusing member into these occasions to prevent further alienation.

TABLE 33–9. PRIMARY, SECONDARY, AND TERTIARY PREVENTION GOALS AND RELATED COMMUNITY HEALTH NURSING INTERVENTIONS IN THE CONTROL OF SUBSTANCE ABUSE

Goal of Prevention	Nursing Intervention
Primary Prevention	
1. Develop positive coping skills	1. Teach coping skills
2. Develop strong self-image	2. Foster and reinforce development of strong self-image
3. Public education on the hazards of substance abuse	3. Educate clients and public
4. Develop policies and programs to prevent abuse	4. Political activity and advocacy
Secondary Prevention	
1. Early detection of persons with substance-abuse problems	1. Case finding
2. Early intervention for persons with problems related to substance abuse	2. Assist families to plan and carry out intervention
3. Treatment of substance abuse	3. Referral for treatment Monitor client during treatment
4. Public education on signs of abuse and resources available	4. Educate clients and public
5. Provide treatment facilities	5. Political activity to support treatment facilities and programs
6. Ensure insurance coverage for treatment	6. Political activity and advocacy
Tertiary Prevention	
1. Provide support to abusers	1. Provide emotional support and encouragement Refer to support groups
2. Make life-style changes that discourage abusive behavior	2. Assist with life-style changes
3. Modify stressors that contribute to substance abuse	3. Assist with modification of stressors

TABLE 33–10. STATUS OF SELECTED 1990 NATIONAL OBJECTIVES RELATED TO SUBSTANCE ABUSE

Objective	Evaluative Data	Status
1. Reduce alcohol-related motor vehicle fatalities to under 9.5 per 100,000 population per year	9.5 deaths per 100,000 population 1988	Objective met
2. Reduce deaths from other alcohol-related accidents to under 5 per 100,000 population per year	4.3 deaths per 100,000 1983	Objective met
3. Reduce cirrhosis death rate to 12 per 100,000 population per year	10.8 per 100,000, 1987	Objective met
4. Reduce incidence of infants born with fetal alcohol syndrome by 25%	1–3 per 1000 live births in 1987 compared to 1 per 2000 births in 1977	Objective unmet
5. Reduce drug-related deaths to 2 per 100,000 population per year	4 per 100,000, 1987	Objective unmet
6. Contain per capita consumption of alcohol to 1978 levels	2.54 gallons per person per year in 1987 compared to 2.71 gallons in 1978	Objective met
7. Maintain the proportion of persons aged 12 to 17 who abstain from alcohol and drug use at 1977 levels	75% to 98% of adolescents abstained in 1988 compared to 69% to 99% in 1977	Objective met
8. Maintain the proportion of persons aged 18 to 25 reporting frequent drug use at 1977 levels	7% for marijuana and 1.3% for other drugs in 1988 compared to 19% and 0.8%, respectively, in 1977	Objective met for marijuana and unmet for other drugs
9. Maintain the proportion of persons aged 12 to 17 reporting frequent drug use at 1977 levels	2% for marijuana and 0.8% for other drugs in 1988 compared to 9% and <.05%, respectively, in 1977	Objective met
10. Reduce the proportion of adults with drinking problems to 8%	10% of adults continue to have drinking problems	Objective unmet
11. Increase awareness of hazards of drinking during pregnancy to 90% of women of childbearing age	62% to 87% of women of childbearing age aware of various risks in 1985	Objective unmet
12. Increase awareness of hazards of substance use to 80% of high school seniors	43% to 77% of seniors aware of risks of various behaviors in 1988	Objective unmet
13. Increase proportion of firms providing substance abuse prevention and referral programs to 70%	70% of firms, 1988	Objective met
14. Reduce the proportion of adults who smoke to less than 25%	28.8% of adults smoked in 1988	Objective unmet
15. Reduce the proportion of children age 12 to 18 years who smoke to less than 6%	12% of those aged 12 to 17 smoked in 1988	Objective unmet
16. Increase the proportion of workers who are offered smoking-cessation programs through the workplace to at least 35%	58% of the U.S. work force were offered cessation programs at work	Objective met
17. Pass legislation in all 50 states limiting smoking in enclosed public places and creating separate smoking areas at work	42 states had such legislation in 1987	Objective unmet

(*Source: United States Department of Health and Human Services. (1990).* Health United States 1989. *Hyattsville, MD: Public Health Service.*)

The community health nurse can also assist families to develop new patterns of interaction. For example, the nurse might help the family realign members into the more usual husband-wife coalition rather than parent-child coalitions by improving family communication and developing joint problem-solving skills. The nurse can also assist family members to identify and express feelings and learn negotiating strategies.[52]

TERTIARY PREVENTION

Tertiary prevention is aimed at preventing a relapse into prior substance-abusing behaviors by the individual or into enabling behaviors by family members and significant others. Community health nurses can contribute to these efforts by providing emotional support to recovering abusers and their families and by linking them with other support groups. Other tertiary prevention measures might include efforts to eliminate or modify stressors that contribute to relapse. For example, assisting the recovering abuser to find work can alleviate the stress of unemployment and financial worries.

The nurse can also reinforce the individual's motivation to abstain from drug use by commending and highlighting successes and periods of sobriety. Development of positive coping skills may also prevent relapse. Other tertiary prevention needs may involve providing information on resources, providing respite from onerous burdens of care, or helping individuals plan time for themselves.[60] Table 33–9 lists primary, secondary, and tertiary prevention goals in the control of substance abuse.

EVALUATING CONTROL STRATEGIES FOR SUBSTANCE ABUSE

Evaluating interventions with individual substance abusers and their families would focus on the extent to which problems of substance abuse have been resolved. Has the abuser been able to remain sober for extended periods of time? Have stresses contributing to substance abuse been modified?

At the level of the community, the nurse could evaluate the effects of intervention programs on the incidence and prevalence of substance abuse as well as indicators of morbidity and mortality related to abuse. The nurse evaluating the effects of programs directed at substance abuse might examine the extent to which the previous set of national health-promotion and disease-prevention objectives have been met in the community. Table 33–10 presents evaluative information on national efforts to meet the 1990 objectives, and similar information could be obtained by the nurse relative to one's own community.

CHAPTER HIGHLIGHTS

- Both the use and the abuse of psychoactive substances have been known from antiquity. Recently, however, both the incidence and the prevalence of problems related to substance abuse have increased and are of concern to community health nurses.
- The diagnosis of psychoactive substance dependence is based on the presence of three of nine criteria developed by the American Psychiatric Association. Diagnosis of substance hinges on continued use of a psychoactive substance despite related problems or recurrent use in physically dangerous circumstances and on the absence of sufficient criteria for a diagnosis of dependence.
- Psychoactive substances listed by the *DSM-III-R* as contributing to dependence or abuse include alcohol; sedatives, hypnotics, and anxiolytics; opioids; cocaine; amphetamines; phencyclidine; hallucinogens; cannabis; inhalants; and nicotine.
- Substance abuse has adverse personal, familial, and societal effects.
- Family members may be co-dependents in that they engage in behavior that enables the substance abuser to continue dependent behaviors.
- Societal effects of substance abuse include increased mortality as a direct result of substance use or as an indirect result of long-term effects of use. Other societal effects include the costs of substance abuse and its contribution to crime.
- Five areas of community health nursing assessment related to substance abuse include assessing for both risk factors and for signs of abuse, intoxication, withdrawal, and long-term effects of substance abuse.
- Human biological factors influencing substance abuse include the potential for genetic inheritance of a predisposition to abuse and the effects of abuse on the very young and the elderly. Physical disability can also be a biological risk factor for substance abuse.
- Elements of the psychological environment that may influence substance abuse include personality traits typical of abusers and the contribution of underlying psychopathology to problems of abuse.
- Social environmental factors that contribute to substance abuse may arise within the family, the peer group, or society at large. Family use of and attitudes toward psychoactive drug use may influence use in other members. Similarly, stress within families can lead to abuse.
- Peer groups influence psychoactive substance use or abstention by creating norms for use and exerting pressure on group members to conform to those norms.
- Societal influences on substance abuse may stem from sources of stress created by social factors such as poverty, unemployment, or discrimination; from societal attitudes to drug use and abuse; or from the availability of psychoactive substances.
- Life-style factors that may influence substance abuse include consumption patterns for psychoactive substances, employer sanctions for substance abuse, and leisure activities that involve use of psychoactive substances.
- Health-care providers contribute to substance abuse by failing to educate clients on the hazards of abuse or by prescribing psychoactive drugs inappropriately or failing to monitor their use. The health-care system also impedes control of substance abuse by failing to identify persons with substance-abuse problems and by not providing access to treatment and rehabilitative facilities that meet the needs of vulnerable population groups. In addition, individual health providers may impede control efforts through negative attitudes toward substance abusers.
- Primary prevention of substance abuse focuses on education about the hazards of abuse and risk-factor modification. Risk-factor modification may be undertaken with individuals, with families, or with society at large.
- Secondary preventive activities consist of intervention and treatment. Intervention is the act of confronting the substance abuser with the goal of getting him or her to agree to evaluation of the possible need for treatment.
- Treatment for substance abuse is based on several general principles, although treatment modalities used vary with the type of substance abuse. In general, combinations of four

(*continued*)

basic treatment modalities are used, including pharmacologic methods, psychosocial methods, sociotherapies, and self-help groups.
- Three considerations in treatment for substance abuse include early treatment of abusive behaviors, managing withdrawal and cravings, and building a foundation for recovery.
- Tertiary prevention focuses on preventing relapse into substance-abusing behaviors.
- Evaluating control strategies for substance abuse focuses on the extent to which problems of individuals and families related to substance abuse have been resolved and the incidence and prevalence of abuse and related health problems in the population.

Review Questions

1. Identify at least three criteria for diagnosing psychoactive substance dependence. Give examples of behaviors that might be performed by clients who meet these criteria. (p. 866)
2. Distinguish between psychoactive substance dependence and abuse. (p. 866)
3. Identify at least five psychoactive substance substances that lead to dependence and abuse. (p. 868)
4. Describe at least two personal effects, two family effects, and two societal effects of substance abuse. (p. 872)
5. What are the five aspects of community health nursing assessment in relation to substance abuse? (p. 876)
6. Identify two major approaches to primary prevention of substance abuse. How might community health nurses be involved in each? (p. 886)
7. Describe the components of the intervention process in secondary prevention of substance abuse. What might be the role of the community health nurse in the intervention process? (p. 886)
8. Identify at least four general principles in the treatment of substance abuse. (p. 887)
9. Describe at least three treatment modalities in secondary prevention of substance abuse. What is the role of the community health nurse with respect to each? (p. 887)
10. Describe three considerations in treatment for substance abuse. (p. 889)

APPLICATION AND SYNTHESIS

You have been working with the Martin family for the last several months. The youngest child, who is 18 months old, has multiple physical handicaps and has been in and out of the hospital numerous times for surgery. He is currently enrolled in physical and occupational therapy programs to promote his development. You have been following this child and working with the family to meet his needs. On your most recent home visit, Mrs. Martin voiced concern about her husband's drinking.

Since the birth of the baby, Mr. Martin has gone on periodic drinking binges. Initially, these occurred about once a month, but lately he has been getting drunk almost every weekend. This week Mrs. Martin had to call her husband's office, where he is employed as a civil engineer, to tell his employer that her husband was ill. Actually, he was too hung over to go to work. She has tried to talk to her husband about his drinking, but he becomes angry and storms out of the house. When he returns, he is drunk. Each time, after he sobers up, he is repentant and promises not to imbibe again. Mrs. Martin thinks her husband's drinking is the result of his worry about financial problems.

Since Mr. Martin's drinking problem has escalated, the older children have been reluctant to bring friends home because they are embarrassed by their father's drunken behavior. They have begun to ask Mrs. Martin rather pointed questions about their father, such as "Is Daddy an alcoholic?" They known that their grandfather, Mr. Martin's father, died of cirrhosis stemming from alcoholism. Mrs. Martin says she has told the children their father is not an alcoholic but is just tired and has been under a lot of stress at work.

Mr. Martin has always been a successful provider for the family and did not drink much before the baby was born. He did well in school, completing a master's degree in engineering, and was promoted to a new position with his engineering firm about 2 years ago. His job pays relatively well, but because their health insurance did not cover the baby when he was born, they have had to pay all of the new infant's medical expenses out of pocket. Mrs. Martin says they have exhausted their savings and indicates that they are having some difficulty meeting mortgage payments on their house. She would like to work but would have trouble finding someone to care for the baby, who has a tracheostomy and requires periodic suctioning. She has discussed her willingness to work with her husband, but he insists that he is not going to have his wife working when the children need her at home and that he will take care of things.

1. What are the human biological, environmental, life-style, and health system factors influencing these problems?
2. What are the health problems evident in this situation? Develop several nursing diagnostic statements related to these problems.
3. What evidence of co-dependence is present in this family situation?
4. What client-care objectives would you set in working with this family?
5. What primary, secondary, and tertiary intervention strategies should be employed with this family? Why?
6. How would you evaluate the effectiveness of your interventions with the Martin family? What evaluative criteria would you use? How would you obtain the evaluative data needed?

REFERENCES

1. Levy, M. R., Dignan, M., & Shirreffs, J. H. (1988). *Essentials of life and health* (5th ed.). New York: Random House.
2. Reed, R., & Lang, T. A. (1987). *Health behaviors* (2nd ed.). St. Paul: West Publishing Co.
3. Sizer, F. S., & Whitney, E. N. (1988). *Life choices: Health concepts and strategies.* St. Paul: West Publishing Co.
4. United States Department of Health and Human Services. (1991). *Healthy people 2000: National health promotion and disease prevention objectives.* Washington, DC: Government Printing Office.
5. American Psychiatric Association, Task Force on Nomenclature and Statistics. (1987). *Diagnostic and statistical manual of mental disorders* (3rd ed., revised). Washington, DC: American Psychiatric Association.
6. Fortin, M. L. (1983). Community health nursing. In G. Bennet, C. Vourakis, & D. S. Woolf (Eds.), *Substance abuse: Pharmacologic, developmental and clinical perspectives.* New York: Wiley.
7. Skodol, A. E. (1989). *Problems in differential diagnosis: From DSM-III to DSM-III-R in clinical practice.* Washington, DC: American Psychiatric Press.
8. Balis, G. W. (1989). Psychoactive substance use disorders. In W. H. Reid (Ed.), *The treatment of psychiatric disorders: Revised for the DSM-III-R* (pp. 131–145). New York: Brunner/Mazel.
9. Dixon, S. D. (1989). Effects of transplacental exposure to cocaine and methamphetamine on the neonate. *Western Journal of Medicine, 150,* 436–442.
10. McCorry, F. (1990). *Preventing substance abuse: A comprehensive program for Catholic educators.* Washington, DC: National Catholic Education Association.
11. Progress toward achieving the 1990 national objectives for the misuse of alcohol and drugs. (1990). *MMWR, 39,* 256–258.
12. Apparent per capita ethanol consumption—U.S., 1977–1986. (1989). *MMWR, 38,* 800–803.
13. Where liquor sells best. (1989). *U.S. News & World Report, 106*(8), 75.
14. Sex- and age-specific prevalence of heavier drinking in selected states in 1985—The Behavioral Risk Factor Surveys. (1987). *MMWR, 36,* 66, 71–74.
15. Anda, R. F., Waller, M. N., Wooten, K. G., et al. (1990). Behavioral risk factor surveillance. *MMWR, 39*(No. SS-2), 1–21.
16. Nathan, P. E. (1988). Alcohol dependency prevention and early intervention. *Public Health Reports, 103,* 683–689.
17. Schneider, F. C. (1991). Sedatives and hypnotics. In M. M. Kuhn (Ed.), *Pharmacotherapeutics: A nursing process approach* (2nd ed., pp. 605–631). Philadelphia, F. A. Davis.
18. Edlin, G., & Golanty, E. (1988). *Health and wellness: A holistic approach.* Boston: Jones and Bartlett.
19. United States Department of Commerce. (1991). *Statistical abstract of the United States, 1990* (110th ed.). Washington, DC: Government Printing Office.
20. Thombs, D. L. (1989). A review of PCP abuse trends and perceptions. *Public Health Reports, 104,* 325–328.
21. Kulberg, A. (1986). Substance abuse: Clinical identification and management. *Pediatric Clinics of North America, 33,* 325–357.
22. Chychula, N. M., & Okore, C. (1990). The cocaine epidemic: A comprehensive review of use, abuse and dependence. *Nurse Practitioner, 15*(7), 31–39.
23. Dintiman, G. B., & Greenberg, J. S. (1989). *Health through discovery* (4th ed.). New York: Random House.
24. Finley, B. G. (1983). The family and substance abuse. In G. Bennet, C. Vourakis, & D. S. Woolf (Eds.), *Substance abuse: Pharmacologic, developmental, and clinical perspectives.* New York: Wiley.
25. Insel, P. M., & Roth, W. T. (1988). *Core concepts in health.* Moutain View, CA: Mayfield.
26. Zerwekh, J., & Michaels, B. (1989). Co-dependency: Assessment and recovery. *Nursing Clinics of North America, 24,* 109–120.
27. Petitti, D. B., & Coleman, C. (1990). Cocaine and the risk of low birth weight. *American Journal of Public Health, 80,* 25–28.
28. Piazza, S. F., Lanza, B., & Dweck, H. S. (1989). Neurological abnormalities and developmental delays in infants of substance abusing mothers. *Pediatric Research,* 260A.
29. Smith, J. E. (1988). The dangers of prenatal cocaine use. *MCN, 13,* 174–179.
30. Chasnoff, I. J., Burns, W. J., Schnoll, S. H., & Burns, K. A. (1985). Cocaine use in pregnancy. *The New England Journal of Medicine, 313,* 666–669.
31. Statewide prevalence of illicit drug use by pregnant women—Rhode Island. (1990). *MMWR, 39,* 225–227.
32. Fingerhut, A., Kleinman, J. C., & Kendrick, J. S. (1990). Smoking before, during, and after pregnancy. *American Journal of Public Health, 80,* 541–544.
33. Status of the 1990 objective on misuse of alcohol and drugs. (1987). *MMWR, 36,* 720–723.
34. Joe, G. W., & Simpson, D. D. (1987). Mortality rates among opioid addicts in a longitudinal study. *American Journal of Public Health, 77,* 347–348.
35. Alcohol-related mortality and years of potential life lost—United States, 1987. (1990). *MMWR, 39,* 173–178.
36. Alcohol-related traffic fatalities—United States, 1982–1989. (1990). *MMWR, 39,* 889–891.
37. Harwood, H. (1987). The high cost of alcohol abuse and associated injuries. *Public Health Reports, 102,* 645–646.
38. Alcohol-related disease impact—Wisconsin, 1988. (1990). *MMWR, 39,* 185–187.
39. Lightfoot, L. O., & Hodgins, D. (1988). A survey of alcohol and drug problems in incarcerated offenders. *International Journal of the Addictions, 23,* 687–706.
40. Urine testing for drug use among male arrestees—United States, 1989. (1990). *MMWR, 38,* 780–783.
41. Weston, J. T. (1980). Alcohol's impact on man's activities: Its role in unnatural death. *American Journal of Clinical Pathology, 74,* 755–758.
42. Tweed, S. H. (1989). Identifying the alcoholic client. *Nursing Clinics of North America, 24,* 13–31.

43. Vaccani, J. M. (1989). Borderline personality disorder and alcohol abuse. *Archives of Psychiatric Nursing, 3*(2), 113–119.
44. Bingol, N., Fuchs, M., Diaz, V., et al. (1987). Teratogenicity of cocaine in humans. *Journal of Pediatrics, 110*, 93–96.
45. Johnson, L. K. (1989). How to diagnose and treat chemical dependency in the elderly. *Journal of Gerontological Nursing, 15*(12), 22–26.
46. Parette, H. P., Hourcade, J. J., & Parette, P. C. (1990). Nursing attitudes to geriatric alcoholism. *Journal of Gerotological Nursing, 16*(1), 26–31.
47. Smart, R. G., & Adlaf, E. M. (1988). Drug and alcohol use among the elderly: Trends in use and characteristics of users. *Canadian Journal of Public Health, 79*, 236–242.
48. Bozzacco, V. (1990). Vulnerability and alcohol and substance abuse in spinal cord injury. *Rehabilitation Nursing, 15*, 70–72.
49. Kircus, E., & Brillhart, B. A. (1990). Dealing with substance abuse among people with disabilitites. *Rehabilitation Nursing, 15*, 250–253.
50. Jessup, M., & Green, J. R. (1987). Treatment of the pregnant alcohol dependent woman. *Journal of Psychoactive Drugs, 19*, 193–203.
51. Killen, J. D., Taylor, C. B., Telch, M. J., et al. (1987). Depressive symptoms and substance abuse among adolescent binge eaters and purgers: A defined population study. *American Journal of Public Health, 77*, 1539–1541.
52. Captain, C. (1989). Family recovery from alcoholism. *Nursing Clinics of North America, 24*, 55–67.
53. Nuchols, C. C., & Greeson, J. (1989). Cocaine addiction: Assessment and intervention. *Nursing Clinics of North America, 24*, 33–43.
54. Kaiserman, M. J., & Rogers, B. (1991). Tobacco consumption declining faster in Canada than in the U.S. *American Journal of Public Health, 81*, 902–904.
55. McAuliffe, W. E., Rohman, M., Santangelo, S., et al. (1986). Psychoactive drug use among practicing physicans and medical students. *New England Journal of Medicine, 315*, 805–810.
56. Bray, R. M., Marsden, M. E., & Peterson, M. R. (1991). Standardized comparisons of the use of alcohol, drugs, and cigarettes among military personnel and civilians. *American Journal of Public Health, 81*, 865–869.
57. Sorenson, G., Rigotti, N., Rosen, A., et al. (1991). Effects of a worksite nonsmoking policy: Evidence for increased cessation. *American Journal of Public Health, 81*, 202–204.
58. Levin, B. L., Glasser, J. H., & Jaffee, C. L. (1988). National trends in coverage and utilization of mental health, alcohol, and substance abuse services. *American Journal of Public Health, 78*, 1222–1223.
59. Williams, E. (1989). Strategies for intervention. *Nursing Clinics of North America, 24*, 95–107.
60. Free, T., Russell, F., Mills, B, & Hathaway, D. (1990). A descriptive study of infants and toddlers exposed prenatally to substance abuse. *MCN, 15*, 245–249.

RECOMMENDED READINGS

Balis, G. W. (1989). Psychoactive substance use disorders. In W. H. Reid (Ed.), *The treatment of psychiatric disorders: Revised for the DSM-III-R.* (pp. 131–145). New York: Brunner/Mazel.

Describes the general principles of treatment of substance abuse. Details treatment modalities typically used with specific forms of substance abuse.

Bennet, G., Vourakis, C., & Woolf, D. S. (Eds.). (1983). *Substance abuse: Pharamcologic, developmental, and clinical perspectives.* New York: Wiley.

Addresses the role of the nurse in preventing and treating substance abuse. Examines the effects of abuse and its treatment on both the individual involved and his or her family.

Chychula, N. M., & Okore, C. (1990). The cocaine epidemic: A comprehensive review of use, abuse and dependence. *Nurse Practitioner, 15*(7), 31–39.

Presents a concise overview of cocaine abuse, contributing factors, and its effects. Contains a very detailed and useful account of the course of cocaine withdrawal.

Johnson, L. K. (1989). How to diagnose and treat chemical dependency in the elderly. *Journal of Gerontological Nursing, 15*(12), 22–26.

Details some of the factors that contribute to substance abuse by older persons. Also addresses barriers experienced by the elderly in obtaining help for problems of substance abuse.

Kinney, J. (1991). *Clinical manual of substance abuse.* St. Louis: Mosby Yearbook.

Examines the role of health-care providers in assessing for and treating substance abuse. Presents information on substance abuse and its control in special population groups such as the elderly, clients with dual diagnoses, infants, and members of minority groups.

Nursing and substance abuse. (1989). *Nursing Clinics of North America, 24*, 1–125.

This journal issue includes several well-written and informative articles on nursing roles in the control of substance abuse. Deals with alcohol abuse and several forms of drug abuse, interventions, and a family focus for care.

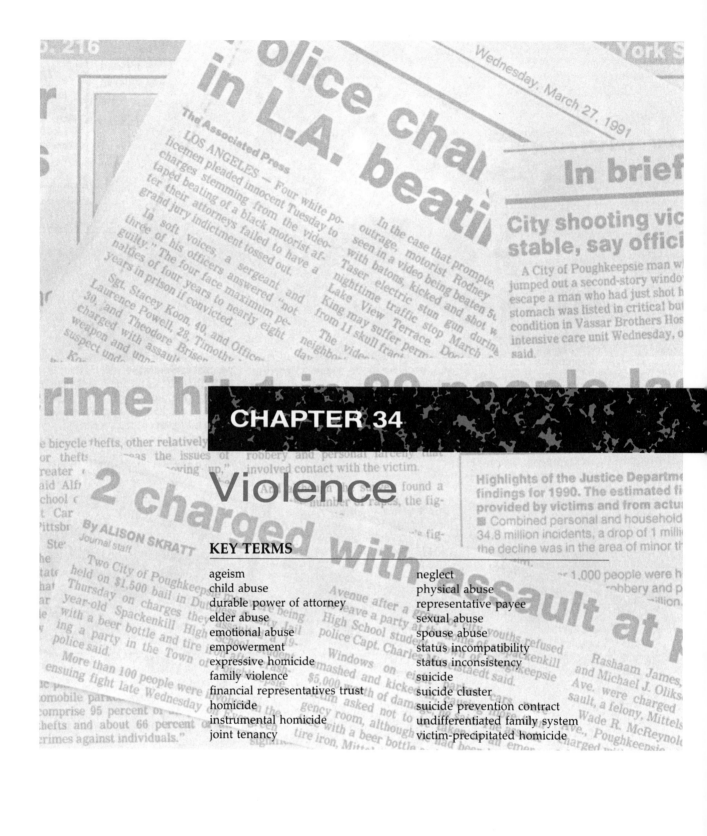

CHAPTER 34

Violence

KEY TERMS

ageism
child abuse
durable power of attorney
elder abuse
emotional abuse
empowerment
expressive homicide
family violence
financial representatives trust
homicide
instrumental homicide
joint tenancy
neglect
physical abuse
representative payee
sexual abuse
spouse abuse
status incompatibility
status inconsistency
suicide
suicide cluster
suicide prevention contract
undifferentiated family system
victim-precipitated homicide

Violence is a pervasive phenomenon in American society. In part, this is a function of the American heritage and the activities required to carve a nation from a wild and uncivilized land. Violence has historically been seen as a mode of resolving conflict and even of ensuring support of law and order. The vigilante approach to justice on the Western frontier is one example of the use of violence to protect society.

In societies in which survival is subjected to physical threats that must be countered by physical force, violent behavior may be more or less of a necessity. However, some authorities contend that humankind has failed to adapt to changes in survival needs and has continued to exercise proclivities to violence that are not warranted in today's society.

Family violence, homicide, and suicide are forms of violence that are of particular concern to society and, hence, to community health nurses who are charged with promoting the health of the population. The need for concern for problems associated with violence is seen in conditions that prompted the development of 18 national objectives for the year 2000 related to violent and abusive behaviors. Some of these objectives are summarized in Box 34–1. Violence contributes to a variety of physical and psychological health problems that can be prevented by community health nursing efforts to modify factors that contribute to violence against self or others.

LEARNING OBJECTIVES

After reading this chapter you should be able to:

- Describe four types of child abuse.
- Describe the three stages of spouse abuse.
- Identify at least five forms of elder abuse.
- Describe the influence of at least three human biological factors in family violence.
- Identify at least four environmental factors that influence family violence.
- Describe at least three areas of focus in primary prevention of family violence.
- Identify at least two approaches to the secondary prevention of family violence.
- Describe at least two factors in each of the four components of the epidemiologic perspective related to homicide.
- Describe at least two factors in each of the components of the epidemiologic perspective related to suicide.
- Identify at least three primary prevention measures for homicide and suicide.

FAMILY VIOLENCE

Family violence involves actions taken by one family member with the intent to inflict harm on another member. In 1984, 4 million cases of family violence were identified by the Surgeon General's Workshop on Violence and Public Health.[1] For the most part, violence occurring within family constellations is a hidden phenomenon, so the actual frequency of family violence is probably far higher. Targets of family violence may be children, spouses, or the elderly.

> BOX 34–1
>
> **National Objectives for the Year 2000 Related to Family Violence**
>
> 1. Reverse the incidence of maltreatment of children under age 18 to less than 25.2 per 1000 children.
> 2. Reduce physical abuse of women by male partners to no more than 27 per 1000 couples.
> 3. Extend protocols for identifying, treating, and referring victims of spouse abuse, child abuse, and elder abuse to 90% of hospital emergency departments.
> 4. Extend implementation of unexplained child death review systems to at least 45 states.
> 5. Increase to at least 30 the number of states in which at least 50% of children identified as abused receive physical and mental evaluation and appropriate follow-up.
> 6. Reduce to less than 10% the proportion of battered women and their children turned away from emergency housing due to lack of space.
> 7. Increase to at least 50% the proportion of elementary and secondary schools that teach nonviolent conflict-resolution strategies.
>
> (Source: U.S. Department of Health and Human Services[6])

CHILD ABUSE

As defined by Public Law 93-247, ***child abuse*** is any physical or mental injury, sexual abuse, or negligent treatment of a child that harms or threatens the child's health or welfare.[2] Child abuse is manifested at the level of individual abusive families. It is potentiated, however, by institutional policies that permit children to be abused, and by social mores and policies that foster circumstances leading to abuse.[3]

Four categories of child abuse are recognized: neglect, physical abuse, emotional abuse, and sexual abuse. ***Neglect*** occurs when things necessary to the child's health and development are withheld. In instances of physical neglect, for example, the child might be deprived of food, clothing, or housing, or be exposed to hazardous environmental conditions. Neglect can also be emotional, occurring when the child is denied the emotional nurturance and support that would foster normal psychosocial development. ***Physical abuse*** occurs when a child is intentionally subjected to physical injury. ***Emotional abuse*** involves continual active efforts to erode the child's self-esteem and feelings of self-worth. ***Sexual abuse*** consists of any involvement of a child in involuntary sexual activity, including fondling, exposure, and exploitation, in addition to actual sexual intercourse.

The problem of child abuse seems to be escalating

in the United States. From 1976 to 1986, overall reports of child abuse rose from 101 to 328 per 10,000 children.[4] In 1986, 2.2 million cases of child abuse and neglect were reported throughout the United States.[5] In part, these increases are attributable to better recognition and reporting of the problem, but there is also a definite increase in the actual number of instances of abuse occurring.

The incidence of some forms of child abuse in the United States is declining while the incidence of others has increased. Many reports of child abuse are concerned with instances of neglect. However, reports of neglect actually decreased between 1976 and 1986, as did reported instances of physical abuse and emotional abuse. Unfortunately, during this same period, reports of sexual abuse of children increased almost fivefold.[4] Despite decreases in the actual incidence of child neglect, in 1986 roughly 16 of every 1000 children under the age of 18 were victims of neglect, while almost 6 children in every 1000 was subjected to physical abuse. Emotional abuse in 1986 was reported at a rate of 3.4 cases per 1000 children, and the incidence of reported sexual abuse was 2.5 per 1000 children.[6]

The effects of abuse on children are many and varied. Abused youngsters are more likely than their age-mates to have problems with discipline and fighting at home and at school. They are also more likely to engage in vandalism or theft, develop problems related to drug or alcohol abuse, and get arrested than are children who are not abused.[7] In addition, childhood abuse predisposes these youngsters to become abusive parents in later years.

SPOUSE ABUSE

Spouse abuse is also a problem in this country. ***Spouse abuse*** involves violent or nonviolent aggression between partners in an intimate relationship, who may or may not be legally married. In spouse-abuse situations, nonviolent aggression involves the expression of feelings, the goal of which is to force or control the partner's behavior.[8] Nonviolent aggression may involve face-to-face confrontation in which fear is the motivating force that influences the behavior of the victim, or it can involve instilling feelings of guilt in order to manipulate the behavior of the other person.

Spouse abuse involving overt physical violence is a cyclical phenomenon that occurs in three stages.[9,10] The first stage is one of rising tension in which the abuser is irritated by minor events or behavior on the part of the abused spouse. The second stage is that of the acute battering episode in which the tension explodes in anger manifested in physical violence. The third phase consists of a period of calm and loving reconciliation in which the abuser expresses contrition, tries to make amends, and vows to change.

Actual reports of spouse abuse occur in 16 percent to 25 percent of sample populations.[10–12] However, some estimates of spousal abuse are placed as high as 50 percent of couples in intimate relationships, involving as many as 2 million to 4 million persons annually.[10] In 1985, the rate of reported cases of abuse of women by male partners was 30 out of every 1000 women, and it is estimated that 21 percent to 30 percent of all women in the United States have been beaten by a partner at least once.[6] Intimate violence is a leading cause of injuries to women. In one study, violence directed at women by their partners accounted for more injuries than motor vehicle accidents, rape, and mugging combined.[13]

Spouse abuse can result in a variety of both physical and psychological effects. Abused women, for example, have been found to experience poor health and symptoms of psychological distress such as headaches, nervousness, depression, and feelings of worthlessness and hopelessness. They are also more likely than women who are not abused to contemplate or attempt suicide.[7]

ELDER ABUSE

Elder abuse is purposeful physical or psychological harm directed toward elderly persons. Elder abuse can occur within families or in institutional settings such as nursing homes and other residential facilities for the elderly. The focus of this chapter, however, is on abuse of older persons by family members.

As is the case with child abuse, elder abuse takes several forms including physical abuse, emotional abuse, financial abuse, active and passive neglect, denial of civil rights, and self-abuse and neglect.[14] Physical abuse can involve inflicting physical pain or injury, sexual molestation, or involuntarily and inappropriately restraining the individual. Overmedicating older people to keep them quiescent is another form of physical abuse. Emotional abuse is intended to cause mental suffering and may consist of name-calling, insults, humiliation, intimidation, or threats directed at the older person. Intentional, illegal, or unethical confiscation or use of money or personal property belonging to an older person constitutes financial neglect.[14] Passive neglect usually involves unintentional failure to engage in needed care or leaving the older person alone and socially isolated. In active neglect, items necessary for daily life such as food, medication, or assistance are deliberately withheld.[14,15] Older people may also be abused by intentional denial of their personal rights, particularly their right to self-determination. Overprotection, denial of the older person's need for independence, and removal from active participation in personal decisions also constitute denial of the individual's civil rights. Finally, older people may engage in self-injurious behaviors or neglect, either by self-inflicted injury, failure to eat, or failure to take reasonable safety precautions. Self-abuse can be either intentional or unintentional.[14]

The extent of elder abuse in the United States is largely unknown. Estimates of abuse of older persons vary from 1 percent to 10 percent of those over age 65,[14,16,17] with as many as 700,000 to 1 million cases of elder abuse occurring each year.[18] In one study, 60 percent of police, physicians, nurses, social workers, protective services and mental health personnel, lawyers, clergy, and coroners participating reported dealing with elder neglect on a regular basis. In the same study, 8 percent of the respondents reported dealing regularly with serious physical abuse of the elderly.[15]

The figures cited here represent only a small portion of the actual cases of elder abuse. It is estimated that only 1 of 4 to 1 out of 14 cases of elder abuse are actually reported.[17,19,20] Reasons for this failure to report instances of abuse may include the reluctance of older person to admit that they raised a child who could abuse them (because most abusers are family members), love of the abuser, dependence on the abuser and fear of further injury, and a lack of alternatives.[17]

The physical effects of neglect and abuse in elderly persons can lead to malnutrition, mobility limitations due to injuries, or skin breakdown due to poor hygiene. Psychological effects can include fear, anxiety, and depression, as well as feelings of hopelessness and helplessness that may lead to substance abuse or suicide as attempts to escape the situation.

Societal consequences of all forms of family violence are also of concern. Naturally, there are the economic costs of medical care for physical injury, but there are also other costs. These include the cost of counseling services, legal and social services, and the cost of imprisoning convicted abusers, in addition to the pain and suffering experienced by the victims of abuse. When abuse leads to substance abuse, there are the additional costs related to these problems, which were discussed in Chapter 33, Substance Abuse.

THE EPIDEMIOLOGIC PREVENTION PROCESS MODEL AND FAMILY VIOLENCE

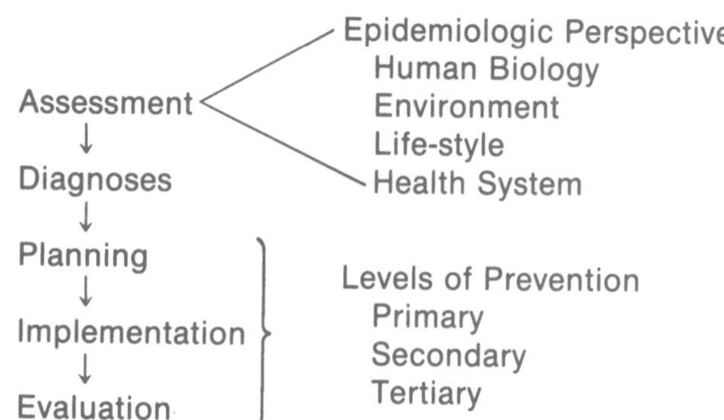

ASSESSMENT

Nursing assessment related to family violence focuses on two major areas. First, the nurse assesses families for risk factors that may contribute to violence. The second aspect of the community health nurse's assessment is related to indicators of abuse actually occurring within families. Both aspects of assessment would also be applied to population groups. Nurses could assess communities for risk factors for family violence as well as for the actual incidence of cases of abuse.

Prior to engaging in either aspect of assessment for family violence, community health nurses should examine their own feelings with respect to violence and their commitment to nursing intervention related to family violence.[21] There is a need for early identification of families with potential for violence or in which actual abuse is occurring. To intervene effectively, community health nurses will need to be able to deal with their own emotional responses to the fact of abuse.

ASSESSING RISK FACTORS

For family violence of any kind to occur, three conditions must exist. There must be motivation for abuse on the part of the abuser, acquiescence on the part of the victim, and a situation conducive to abuse. Various factors related to human biology, environment, life-style, and the health system contribute to the existence of these conditions.

Human Biology

Maturation and Aging. Generally speaking, reports of child abuse tend to involve younger children more often than older ones. This may be because younger children are physically more fragile and more likely to suffer injuries requiring medical treatment than are older children. Some of the differences in reports of abuse of children of different ages may also stem from perceptions of older children, particularly adolescents, as provoking instances of violence. An exception to the tendency to more frequent reports of abuse among younger children occurs with respect to girls. Older girls tend to be more likely to suffer abuse than younger girls.[17]

The age of the abuser can also influence the incidence of child abuse. It has often been purported that adolescent parents are more likely than older parents to engage in child abuse because of their emotional immaturity. These beliefs, however, are not supported by controlled research.[22,23] Researchers have surmised that adolescent parents are under closer surveillance than other potential child abusers and that cases of child abuse are more readily identified in this group, thus accounting for prior associations of adolescent parenthood with child abuse.[23]

Age is also a factor in elder abuse. Abuse of older people most often occurs in the "old elderly," those over 75 years of age.[14,16,24] The age and developmental level of the abuser can also be a contributing factor in elder abuse. As one author points out, the most frequent perpetrators of elder abuse are daughters of the victims. At the point when the older person usually becomes dependent, the daughter is frequently experiencing menopause, which is accompanied by changing physical appearance and, possibly, by illnesses that may remind her of her own aging. At the same time, the daughter is usually immersed in developmental tasks related to family and career with multiple role demands that deplete energy reserves, thus leading to increased stress that may be manifested in abuse of the older person.[25]

Sex. Both boys and girls are at risk for child abuse. Despite the common belief that girls are more often victims of sexual abuse than boys, members of both genders appear to be at equal risk of this form of abuse.

Spouse abuse is usually directed toward women. However, men are also occasionally subjected to violence perpetrated by females.[10] In one study, for example, women were the assailants and men the victims of purposefully inflicted burn injuries, most of which occurred in the course of domestic altercations.[26] In the United States in 1984, 1310 wives were killed by their husbands, whereas 806 husbands were killed by their wives.[17] Over a decade ago, Steinmetz,[27] a leading researcher in family violence, concluded that men were as likely as women to be the victims of spousal assault and women were as likely as men to be the assailants. These conclusions have largely been ignored because of a lack of interest by researchers and the reluctance of men to admit to victimization by women.[26] In addition, because of their larger size, greater strength, and better access to social resources, men are less likely to suffer adverse physical or social effects of abuse.[17]

Victims of elder abuse are more likely to be female than male.[14,16] Gender differences in the incidence of abuse among older persons may be a function of age; women typically live longer than men and are therefore older and more vulnerable.

Physiologic Function. The health of both the victim and the abuser can be influencing factors in child abuse. Children who are born prematurely, who are the result of a multiple pregnancy, who have physical or mental handicaps, who are hyperactive, or who experience feeding or sleep problems have been found to be at somewhat higher risk of abuse than other children.[22,28] Diminished parental health has also been associated with child abuse.[29]

The physiologic condition of pregnancy can be a contributing factor in spouse abuse.[10] In one study, 8 percent of pregnant women admitted being battered during their pregnancy and another 9 percent demonstrated behaviors suggesting abuse, but could not be brought to admit to abuse. An additional 4 percent of the women had been threatened with physical violence during the pregnancy.[30]

There is some question of the role of physical disability in the abuse of older persons. Several authors have suggested that abused elders are likely to suffer from a variety of physical impairments or be physically dependent upon the abuser.[14,16,17,25,31] Other research, however, suggests that abused older persons are no less healthy or more debilitated than their nonabused counterparts. In fact, in some areas, the abused elders were found to be more self-sufficient than were those not abused.[32]

Environment

Factors in both social and psychological environments contribute to all forms of family violence.

Social Environment. Social environmental factors can influence family violence in four primary ways. First, social definitions of abuse and violence influence societal responses to abusive behaviors. Second, myths regarding family violence impede efforts to control it. Third, the socialization of individuals may contribute to the use of violence as a mode of conflict resolution. Finally, the social environment may create stressors that contribute to violence in families.

The concept of abuse presumes that one individual is acting toward another in a manner that violates societal norms.[19] In this respect, then, family violence is socially defined. A permissive societal attitude toward family violence contributes to abuse within families.[3] Several researchers have noted that in societies where family life is a relatively public matter and where neighbors and friends actively interfere with abusive behavior, the incidence of family violence is limited.[33–35] Until fairly recently, however, violence within families was an accepted way of life in the United States and few people, including health-care providers and law enforcement officials, intervened to curtail violent episodes.[36,37]

Societal attitudes toward and definitions of violence influence legal sanctions that are employed to prevent or curtail family violence. In the United States, legal action to protect children and the elderly from abuse are more extensive than those designed to protect spouses.

Community health nurses assessing community responses to the problems of family abuse should familiarize themselves with relevant legislation in their own jurisdictions. They should also assess the extent to which legislation is enforced in their communities. This type of information might be obtained from domestic court personnel, from law enforcement officials, or from protective services personnel in the area.

In the past, physical and emotional mistreatment of children was perceived by some people as in the best interests of the child and as an appropriate form of socialization. Mistreatment has occasionally been defended on religious grounds of teaching children right from wrong.[24] More recently, however, such behavior is perceived as abuse, and reporting of suspected child abuse is mandated in all 50 states and the District of Columbia.

Some cultural groups define child abuse somewhat differently from that of the legal system. In some cultures, behaviors that would be defined as abusive by the majority culture are perceived as beneficial to the child. These culturally prescribed behaviors were described in Chapter 15, Cultural Influences on Community Health, and include practices such as pinching to release harmful gases, coining (abrasion of the skin with a coin), and burning with a lighted cigarette or a wisp of burning cotton to treat diarrhea.[38–40] The community health nurse should assess the prevalence of these and similar practices, particularly among Asian clients.

Although physical abuse of spouses is a criminal offense, enforcement of legislation is frequently predicated on the victim pressing charges, which many abused women are reluctant to do for fear of repercussions for themselves, their children, or for the abuser. In some jurisdictions, for example, both victims and perpetrators of family violence have been arrested.[37]

States vary greatly in their approach to protecting the abused spouse. In some states, courts may order eviction of the abuser or counseling for the abuser, the victim, or both. However, in 1986, seven states had no provisions for protection of spouses and two had legislation pending. At that same time, only 17 states made legal provision for protection of people living as spouses but who were not legally married, and 18 states specified no penalties for violating a court protection order.[41] Even when legislation does exist protecting potentially abused spouses, it is not always enforced.[37] Or, if the abuser is arrested, he or she is often released in a short period of time to return to exact retribution.

Most states have laws mandating reporting of abuse of older persons[20] and have penalties for the failure of health professionals to report suspected abuse.[16] In 1985, however, nine states still did not have laws for reporting elder abuse.[42] State statutes differ greatly in their definitions of elder abuse and the types of abuse covered.[16] For example, only 19 states included financial abuse of older persons as a form of abuse covered under the law.[43]

Strongly held myths about family violence are another social environmental factor influencing abusive behavior within families. These myths may dissuade members of society, including health-care professionals, from interfering in abusive situations. Some common myths and related realities in family violence are presented in Box 34–2. Community health nurses can assess the extent to which these myths prevail in their community by talking with health-care providers, social services personnel, and other members of the community. The nurse should also assess for belief in these myths among potential perpetrators or victims of abuse. Victims, in particular, may internalize societal beliefs that they are somehow to blame for or deserving of abuse.[44,45]

Socialization to violence as an acceptable means of resolving conflict is the third type of social environmental factor influencing family violence. Violence as a way of resolving conflict is a learned behavior that tends to be communicated from one generation to the next. Child abusers, for example, have frequently been found to have been abused children themselves. It is believed, in these instances, that abusive parenting roles enacted by the abuser's

BOX 34–2

Common Myths and Realities Regarding Family Violence

Myth: Family violence is rare.
Reality: Family violence is a common occurrence and its incidence is increasing.

Myth: Family violence is confined to families in which there is mental illness.
Reality: Family violence occurs in many families without psychopathology.

Myth: Family violence occurs more frequently in certain racial and cultural groups.
Reality: Family violence occurs in all socioeconomic groups and among all racial and ethnic groups.

Myth: Social factors do not influence family violence because it occurs in all societies.
Reality: Social factors that tax family coping abilities do contribute to family violence.

Myth: Abused children invariably become abusers.
Reality: Abused children may become abusive adults if the cycle of violence is not broken.

Myth: Substance abuse is the real cause of family violence.
Reality: Substance abuse may trigger an abusive episode or may be used as an excuse for abusive behavior, but does not *cause* abuse.

Myth: Violence and love do not coexist in abusing families.
Reality: Abusive family members frequently love each other, but may have difficulty expressing that love or controlling other emotions.

Myth: Abused women must like being abused or they would leave.
Reality: Abused women do not like being abused, but may feel like they deserve abuse. They may also be unable to leave an abusive situation because of economic, cultural, or religious constraints or because they fear for the safety of themselves or their children.

Myth: Violence among family members is a private matter, and they have a right to privacy.
Reality: No one has a right to abuse another. Early intervention by family, friends, or outsiders can prevent family violence.

Myth: Abused women deliberately provoke attacks.
Reality: Abused women go to great lengths to avoid confrontation with the abuser.

Myth: Abusers are uneducated people who are unable to cope with the world.
Reality: Abusers are frequently successful and respected citizens.

Myth: Children need their parents even if they are abusive.
Reality: Child abuse or witnessing other family violence can have lasting effects on young children, and removal of victims from an abusive situation may be necessary.

Myth: Once an abused wife, always an abused wife.
Reality: Violent families can be rehabilitated, and many women who escape abusive situations are careful not to enter others.

Myth: Once an abuser, always an abuser.
Reality: Abusive family members can be helped and families can be reconstructed with assistance.

(*Sources: Collier*[9]*; Gelles & Cornell*[17]*; and King & Ryan*[44]).

parents are interpreted as normal parenting behavior. Children who witness violence in the home come to view violence as an acceptable means for conflict resolution that may lead to abuse of their own children, their spouses, or their parents in later life.[1]

Abused spouses, particularly women, have also frequently been socialized to violence in their own families. In one study, for example, more than half of abused women came from families characterized by recurrent strife or violent behavior compared to less than one-fourth of women who were not abused. In this same study, half of the abused women had been abused by their partners in previous relationships.[46]

It has also been suggested that elder abuse is a function of prior socialization to violence in one's family of origin.[31,42] In fact, one researcher alluded to a family history of violence as evidence of an ***undifferentiated family system***, which is a family that is closed to the surrounding environment and unable or unwilling to use environmental resources to resolve problems. Undifferentiated family systems have been found to be at higher risk for elder abuse than differentiated systems.[25]

In assessing families for risk factors contributing to family violence, the community health nurse would ask about family patterns of conflict resolution and observe for evidence of verbal aggression, threats of violence, or inability to resolve conflicts successfully without resorting to violence. The nurse would also assess forms of discipline used to socialize children, their appropriateness, and who administers disciplinary action. Child abuse tends to occur more often in homes where one parent is responsible for discipline than when both parents participate.[21] In addition, the nurse should inquire about conflict-resolution strategies and modes of discipline used when adult family members were growing up. Again, construction of a genogram detailing a family history of violence may be helpful in identifying families at risk.[21]

The last way in which the social environment may contribute to family violence is through stressful circumstances that tax family members' coping abilities. Stress-producing factors are similar for all forms of family violence and include restricted family resources related to unemployment, poverty, and poor social support systems. Other social factors that may create stress within the family include intolerance of differences of opinion, and rigid or unsatisfactory role allocation.[21] The nurse would explore with family members their economic status and the existence and use of support systems that can provide emotional as well as material support. In addition, the nurse would examine the appropriateness of role allocation and family members' satisfaction with roles allocated. Patterns of decision making within the family can also be assessed because family violence tends to occur more often in families where one partner is the exclusive decision-maker.[17]

Other social factors that may contribute to stress and, thereby, to family violence include "status inconsistency" and "status incompatibility."[17] ***Status inconsistency*** exists when one member of the family has a job inconsistent with his or her educational level (for example, the aerospace engineer who drives a taxicab or the wife with a doctorate who is expected to stay home with the children or an elderly parent). ***Status incompatibility*** occurs when one member of a spousal dyad (usually the wife) has more education or a better job than the other spouse. The community health nurse could obtain information about status inconsistency and status incompatibility by asking about family members' educational levels and their employment. When discrepancies are apparent, the nurse would explore their effects on the family and their potential for creating stress that might lead to abuse.

One social factor that may contribute to abuse of older persons is "ageism." ***Ageism*** is a generally negative attitude toward the elderly held by members of a society.[14] Ageism promotes stereotypes of older persons as senile, demanding, or debilitated, thus increasing their vulnerability to exploitation.

Social, cultural, and economic factors may also result in decisions to care for elderly family members in the home when this may not be in the best interests of either the older person or the caretaker. For example, the family may not be able to afford nursing home care or may perceive social expectations that they will care for their elderly members at home.[25] The increase in the average age of the American population is also a factor in that, as a greater proportion of the population becomes elderly, the responsibility for their care falls to a diminishing number of younger people, thus increasing the burden of caretaking for these younger people.

Social factors not only influence the potential for abuse within families but may also pose barriers to escaping an abusive situation for the victim of abuse. Victims of family violence may be economically dependent upon the abuser or have no other alternative.[17,44] Culture and religious beliefs may also make it difficult for abused women to leave an abusive relationship.[44] In addition, the woman may fear loss of her children if she leaves an abusive situation. Abused elders may be the economic support of the abuser and may be reluctant to abandon that individual or any grandchildren in the home.[32]

Psychological Environment. Factors in the psychological environment that may contribute to family violence include poor coping skills, the emotional climate in the family, personality traits of the abuser or the victim, or the presence of psychopathology. Families with poor coping skills have difficulty dealing with situational stressors that create tension, resulting in violence. Constant family crises or upheavals indicative of poor coping abilities are characteristic of abusive families.[47]

The emotional climate in the family can also contribute to abuse. Families that exhibit increased emotional tension and anxiety, with little display of visible affection or emotional support, are considered emotionally impoverished and are at risk for violence. Similarly, family communication patterns that are non-nurturing, destructive, or ambiguous may also indicate risk for family violence.[21]

The distribution of power within the family is another element of the emotional climate that may lead to abuse. Abusive families are characterized by autocratic decision making and power struggles between members.[21] Abusers tend to abuse the power they have over other family members when they feel their power is threatened.[45] Various studies of elder abuse, for example, have indicated that some abusers are economically dependent on the victims of abuse, and abuse may be an indication of frustration over their helplessness.[17,32]

Personality traits of either the abuser or the victim can influence the incidence of family violence. Abusers and victims alike tend to have poor self-esteem. Abusers may also be emotionally immature, hostile, and unable to cope with problems in a healthy manner. They frequently feel personally insecure and inadequate,[17] although they often appear successful to others.

Child abusers tend to have unrealistic expectations of children, particularly as sources of warmth and love. When they are disappointed in these expectations, abuse may occur.[48] For example, children who are irritable, who cry often, or who do not care to be cuddled may be perceived as rejecting the parent. For parents with low self-esteem, this perceived rejection can set the stage for abuse.

Abused women tend to be dependent, passive, and reluctant to make changes. Grief and guilt are other frequent feelings exhibited by victims of spouse abuse. Furthermore, an abused woman may respond to abuse by adopting what is termed a "hostage response."[49] This adaptive behavior is characterized by feelings of responsibility for the abuse, feeling unworthy of help, fearing one will be disbelieved, and wariness of the motivation of others.

Depression is also frequently encountered in abused females. In one study the presence of depressive and other psychiatric symptoms differentiated women who escaped abusive situations from those who did not.[46]

Psychological traits can also lead to decisions to care for older individuals in the family home, resulting in the potential for abuse. Feelings of obligation or responsibility or even of personal satisfaction may be involved in these decisions.

Psychological traits exhibited by the older person might also contribute to abuse. For example, the older person may have difficulty adjusting not only to physical and emotional losses but also to the loss of autonomy associated with age and the need to move in with family members. This difficulty in adjusting can make people querulous and difficult to live with, adding to the stress experienced by family caretakers and, possibly, leading to abuse.[25] In one study of abused elders, 65 percent of the abusers perceived the victim as a source of stress.[31]

The presence of psychopathology can also contribute to family violence. Mental illness on the part of the abuser has been found to be associated with elder abuse.[32] This association seems to be stronger for emotional abuse than for physical abuse.[14] Mental retardation on the part of the caretaker can also be a factor in abuse.[50]

In assessing families for potential for violence, the nurse would explore family coping methods and observe for evidence of an emotional climate that might contribute to violence. Families experiencing stress and who demonstrate poor coping skills, poor communication patterns, or lack of affection and cohesion are at risk for abusive behaviors. The nurse would also be alert to evidence of personality traits that might place some family members at greater risk for victimization (for example, passivity or whining and complaining). The nurse may also note personality traits such as immaturity and feelings of insecurity and personal inadequacy on the part of family members who might become abusive.

Life-style

Life-style factors may be associated with all forms of family violence. For example, life-styles experienced by single parents produce stressors not encountered by two-parent families.[17] Single parents must assume the roles of both mother and father and function as the family's primary wage earner. Because single-parent families more often experience economic difficulties, the single parent is typically under considerably more stress than parents in the average two-parent household. Single parents may also have little outside emotional or material support and may have little or no respite from the responsibilities of parenthood.

The use of both alcohol and drugs has received mixed reviews in terms of contributing to family violence. Some studies indicate that alcohol and drug use plays a significant role in abusive families.[46] Other researchers contend that alcohol and drugs are used as a justification or rationalization for abusive behavior. Psychoactive substances such as alcohol and other drugs do diminish inhibitions against violence. However, sober abusers often inflict more damage than their intoxicated counterparts.[44]

Research has established a link between spouse abuse and abuse of alcohol by the victim.[46] However, it may be that alcohol use by the abused woman may be an attempt to escape from the realities of her situation.[17,44] Whatever the causal relationship between substance abuse and family violence, substance abuse is an indication of an undifferentiated family that may be at risk for violence.[25] For this reason, the nurse should be alert to indications of substance abuse discussed in Chapter 33, Substance Abuse, as a possible risk factor for, or an effect of, family violence.

For abused women, a life-style that involves cohabitation, frequently with a substance-abusing male, may contribute to abuse. In one study, abused women cohabited with significantly more partners than did women who were not abused, and they were also less likely to be married. In the same study, half of the abused women had been abused in a previous relationship—again, frequently with a substance abuser.[46]

Health System

The nation's health-care system tends to ignore the problem of family violence. Victims of abuse are seen in a variety of health-care settings such as well-child and prenatal clinics, schools, and emergency rooms, yet the diagnosis of abuse is frequently overlooked because of provider inattention to significant cues. In one study of pregnant abused women, for example, a third of the women sought medical attention for problems resulting from or related to abuse, yet none of the women were assessed for battering or provided with information on relevant community services.[30]

The average health-care provider's index of suspicion for abuse due to family violence is relatively low. One study demonstrated that, in the routine practice of an emergency room, less than 6 percent of female trauma patients were diagnosed as victims of abuse. However, when a specially designed protocol for identifying abuse was employed, the percentage of these same women diagnosed as abused rose to 30 percent.[11] In another similar study, physicians identified less than 3 percent of women seen in an emergency room as abused, when closer examination indicated that closer to 25 percent of the women exhibited indications of abuse.[51] Lack of attention to the possibility of family violence is also demonstrated by other studies indicating that few physicians routinely make direct inquiries regarding possible abuse[12] and that of referrals made to a shelter for battered women, few are made by physicians.[41]

Part of the inattention to problems of family violence stems from lack of education of health-care providers regarding this phenomenon. In one study, 90 percent of health-care personnel reported that they had had no training in assessing elderly persons for potential abuse.[18] The absence of standardized written guidelines for assessing for violence has also been suggested as a reason for health-care providers' reluctance to address problems of violence.[19]

Other reasons for nonintervention by health-care providers might include concerns about the potential for litigation, time constraints, and difficulties in determining that abuse is actually taking place.[14] Ethical considerations can also surface relative to the potential for damage to the abuser, further injury to the victim, or violation of a client's confidence. The potential for depression and suicide by the victim of abuse is another ethical concern. With adult clients there may be the additional issue of going counter to the victim's wishes in reporting an instance of abuse.[16] For example, a community health nurse may need to decide whether to report an instance of abuse when the victim prefers, for whatever reasons, that it not be reported. Finally, the health-care provider may fear that he or she will not be able to intervene successfully, that dealing with abusive situations will evoke painful memories, that the provider's concern and efforts will be rejected, or that the provider might be in danger from the abuse.[44]

Health-care providers may also impede efforts to control family violence by exhibiting attitudes and values that can prevent victims of abuse from seeking help. For example, failure to believe clients or intimating that they are exaggerating the problem might be interpreted as rejection. Similarly, expressing value judgments that the person is weak or could have prevented the abuse is not helpful. Abused adults may be reluctant to make changes or to initiate legal proceedings, and their feelings and decisions should be respected.[9]

Health-care providers who address the problem of violence in the families with whom they work typically take a militant attitude toward intervention. Militancy may involve recommendations for the arrest of the abuser, legal protection of the victim, or removal of the victim from the situation. While these actions might protect the victim from further abuse, they might also serve to increase the danger to the victim.[36] In fact, in one study one-fifth of instances of spouse abuse involved partners from a relationship that had been terminated.[13] Militancy may also violate the victim's desires or needs and may further impair the health-care professional's ability to assist the client. In addition, militancy merely treats the symptoms of family violence rather than getting at the underlying causes of the problem and rehabilitating both the abuser and the family.[36]

It has also been suggested that the health-care system itself perpetrates abuse of older persons when they are discharged from hospitals and other institutions before they are sufficiently recovered. The point has been made that the Medicare reimbursement system based on diagnosis related groups (DRGs) does not account for the longer recovery periods frequently required by older people.[14]

Factors in the epidemiology of family violence are summarized in Box 34–3.

ASSESSING FOR EVIDENCE OF FAMILY VIOLENCE

The second aspect of community health nursing assessment related to family violence is observing for actual evidence of abuse. To this end, the nurse should routinely include questions related to possible abuse in taking health histories from all clients. In addition, the nurse should check for physical signs and symptoms of abuse and observe for behaviors on the part of either the client or significant others that might indicate abuse.

The behavior of both parents and children should be observed on each encounter with the community health nurse. Children who are withdrawn, fearful, or particularly clinging may be victims of abuse, while parents who give vague or conflicting histories for child injuries may be perpetrators of abuse. Abusive parents may exhibit excessive concern given the nature of the child's injuries or display little or no concern.

Physical examination of a child can provide a variety of indicators of abuse. Of particular concern are bruises in unlikely locations for the child's age or in various stages of resolution, indicating multiple injury incidents, fractures sustained in suspicious circumstances, burns in unusual places or with characteristic outlines (for example, of a cigarette touched to the skin; burns in the shape of an iron or heater grill; immersion burns), and abdominal injuries in the absence of a history of major trauma.[5] Additional physical and psychological signs of child abuse are included in Table 34–1.

The nurse should also assess children exposed to abuse of other family members for adverse effects. Generally speaking, children from homes where violence is a frequent occurrence respond with withdrawal, anxiety, or aggression. These effects seem to be most pronounced in boys under the age of 10, although they are also seen in girls. There may also be a difference in the types of responses exhibited by boys and girls. In one study, boys were more prone to externalize symptoms including short attention spans, argumentativeness, cruelty, bullying, and temper tantrums. Girls, on the other hand, more often displayed internalizing behaviors such as anxiety, depression, clinging behavior, and perfectionism.[1]

In a similar fashion, the nurse would assess spouses, especially women, for physical and psychological evidence of abuse. A history of nonspecific complaints, frequent hospitalizations, and frequent emergency room visits for injuries are suggestive of abuse. Abused women may also exhibit anxiety, substance abuse, or eating disorders, or attempt suicide in response to abuse. Women who are assaulted by their spouses attempt suicide five times more often than women who are not abused.[7] Similarly, women who respond overly casually to serious injuries or are overly emotional regarding relatively minor injuries may be victims of abuse.[44]

Again, injuries that are inconsistent with the explanation given are possible indicators of abuse. Particularly suspicious injuries include lacerations of the face; injuries to the chest, breasts, back, abdomen, and genitalia; symmetrical injuries; and distinctive burn patterns. Frequent illness is another indicator of possible abuse because abused women spend twice as many days in bed for illness as do other women.[7] Typical signs and symptoms of spouse abuse are presented in Table 34–2.

Assessment of the older adult for possible abuse should focus on a general assessment, physical assessment, life-style patterns, social interaction, and medical assessment.[18] The general assessment would include observation of hygiene, confusion that may be due to overmedication or to anxiety, emotional state, and appropriateness of dress for the weather. Physical manifestations of abuse in older people can include bruises and other injuries.[16,20] Life-style patterns would reflect the client's nutritional level and possible substance abuse or self-neglect. Information on life-style might also indicate a lack of assistance

BOX 34–3

Factors Associated with Family Violence

Human Biology

- Younger children are more physically vulnerable to abuse.
- Older girls are more frequently abused than younger girls.
- Adolescent parents do not seem to be more abusive than older parents.
- The "old" elderly are more often abused than younger persons.
- Abusers of older persons are often women experiencing menopause and associated developmental stresses of that time of life.
- Abused older persons may have difficulty adjusting to the effects of age, becoming querulous and adding to caretaker stress.
- Male and female children are equally subject to child abuse.
- Both men and women engage in spouse abuse, but women are more vulnerable to the physical and social effects of abuse.
- Children born prematurely, who are the result of a multiple pregnancy, who have physical or mental handicaps, who are hyperactive, or who have feeding or sleep problems may be more likely to be abused than other children.
- Pregnancy may be a precipitating factor in abuse of women.
- Physical or mental disability may place older persons at greater risk for abuse.
- Diminished health on the part of the abuser may also be a factor in family violence.

Environment

Social environment

- Social definitions and attitudes may contribute to family violence.
- Myths regarding family violence impede control efforts.
- Prior socialization to family violence contributes to the problem.
- Social environmental factors such as unemployment, poverty, and poor social support that create stress for families may contribute to family violence.
- Status inconsistency and status incompatibility may contribute to family violence.
- Agism in society may contribute to abuse of older persons.
- Social environmental factors may also pose barriers to escape from an abusive situation.

Psychological environment

- Poor coping skills may result in family violence.
- The emotional climate within the family may also foster abuse.
- The emotional climate of the family may be influenced by the distribution of power within the family.
- Personality traits of abusers that promote violence include poor self-esteem, immaturity, hostility, inability to cope with problems effectively, and feelings of personal insecurity and inadequacy.
- Victims of abuse also tend to have poor self-esteem and exhibit guilt, grief, and depression.
- Abusers may have unrealistic expectations of themselves and others.
- Psychopathology in the abuser can also result in violence.

Life-style

- Single parenthood may lead to increased stress and result in family violence.
- Substance abuse may complicate family violence or be used as an excuse for abusive behavior.
- Substance abuse may be used as an escape mechanism by victims of family violence.
- Abused women are more likely to have cohabited with several men than women who are not abused.

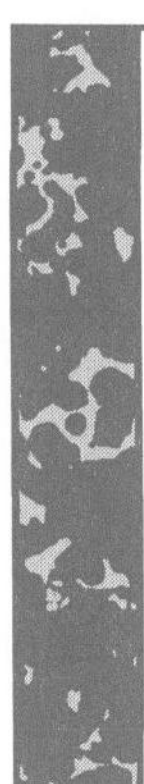

BOX 34–3 (*continued*)

Health System

- Failure to identify potential abusers and victims of family violence impedes control efforts.
- Health-care providers may be reluctant to intervene in abusive situations.
- Health-care providers' attitudes to victims of abuse may interfere with help-seeking behaviors on the part of victims.
- Militancy by health-care providers may lead to short-term solutions to problems of family violence but does nothing to rehabilitate families.
- Elder abuse may be perpetrated by health-care providers in rigid adherence to DRGs and early discharge of clients.

TABLE 34–1. PHYSICAL AND PSYCHOLOGICAL INDICATIONS OF CHILD ABUSE

Type of Abuse	Physical Indications	Psychological Indications
Neglect	• Persistent hunger • Poor hygiene • Inappropriately dressed for the weather • Constant fatigue • Unattended physical health problems • Poor growth patterns	• Delinquency due to lack of supervision • School truancy • Begging or stealing food
Physical abuse	• Bruises or welts in unusual places or in several stages of healing; distinctive shapes • Burns (especially cigarette burns; immersion burns of hands, feet, or buttocks; rope burns; or distinctively shaped burns) • Fractures (multiple or in various stages of healing, inconsistent with explanations of injury) • Joint swelling or limited mobility • Long-bone deformities • Lacerations and abrasions to the mouth, lip, gums, eye, genitalia • Human bite marks • Signs of intracranial trauma • Deformed or displaced nasal septum • Bleeding or fluid drainage from the ears or ruptured eardrums • Broken, loose, or missing teeth • Difficulty in respirations; tenderness or crepitus over ribs • Abdominal pain or tenderness • Recurrent urinary tract infection	• Wary of physical contact with adults • Apprehension when other children cry • Behavioral extremes of withdrawal or aggression • Appears frightened of parents • Inappropriate response to pain
Emotional abuse	• Nothing specific	• Overly compliant, passive, and undemanding • Extremely aggressive, demanding, or angry • Behavior inappropriate for age (either overly adult or overly infantile) • Developmental delay • Attempted suicide
Sexual abuse	• Torn, stained, or bloody underwear • Pain or itching in genital areas • Bruises or bleeding from external genitalia, vagina, rectum • Sexually transmitted disease • Swollen or red cervix, vulva, or perineum • Semen around the mouth or genitalia or on clothing • Pregnancy	• Withdrawn • Engages in fantasy behavior or infantile behavior • Poor peer relationships • Unwilling to participate in physical activities • Wears long sleeves and several layers of clothes even in hot weather • Delinquency or running away • Inappropriate sexual behavior or mannerisms

TABLE 34–2. PHYSICAL AND PSYCHOLOGICAL INDICATIONS OF SPOUSE ABUSE

Physical Indications	Psychological Indications
• Chronic fatigue • Vague complaints, aches, and pains • Frequent injuries • Recurrent sexually transmitted diseases • Muscle tension • Facial lacerations • Injuries to chest, breasts, back, abdomen, or genitalia • Bilateral injuries of arms or legs • Symmetrical injuries • Obvious patterns of belt buckles, bite marks, fist, or hand marks • Burns of hands, feet, buttocks, or with distinctive patterns • Headaches • Ulcers	• Casual response to a serious injury or excessively emotional response to a relatively minor injury • Frequent ambulatory or emergency room visits • Insomnia • Nightmares • Depression • Anxiety • Anorexia or other eating disorder • Drug or alcohol abuse • Poor self-esteem • Suicide attempts

with necessary functions. The extent and quality of the client's social interaction might indicate passive neglect or suggest depression or withdrawal due to abuse or neglect. Finally, the medical assessment, focusing on signs and symptoms of existing disease, might disclose unattended medical needs indicative of neglect or sexually transmitted diseases suggesting sexual abuse. Specific signs and symptoms of elder abuse for which the community health nurse should assess older clients are presented in Table 34–3. The nurse should be particularly careful in assessing the older client to differentiate signs of abuse from signs and symptoms that accompany aging or that reflect existing chronic conditions.[14] Assessment for the effects of aging and chronic disease in the elderly was discussed in Chapter 23, Care of Older Clients.

DIAGNOSTIC REASONING AND FAMILY VIOLENCE

Community health nurses use the information obtained during client assessments to derive nursing diagnoses related to family violence for individual families or population groups. At the group level, nursing diagnoses would most likely reflect the prevalence of or potential for family violence in the community. For example, the nurse might make a diagnosis of "potential for increased child abuse due to an increase in single-parent families." Another diagnosis reflecting the needs of a population group might be "increased incidence of elder abuse due to lack of residential facilities for the elderly and increased stress on family caretakers."

Nursing diagnoses may also be made relative to violence in families with whom the nurse is working. Examples of diagnoses at this level might be "potential for emotional neglect due to lack of parental recognition of affective needs of children" or "excessive physical punishment due to unrealistic parental expectations of children."

PLANNING AND IMPLEMENTING CONTROL STRATEGIES FOR FAMILY VIOLENCE

Control of violence may be undertaken with communities or target groups or with individuals and their families. Control efforts may also be employed at the primary, secondary, or tertiary level of prevention.

Community health nurses may find themselves in need of information or other assistance in order to plan effective interventions for problems of family violence. Some sources of assistance for nurses dealing with family violence are presented in Table 34–4.

Planning to resolve problems of family violence is based on three general principles.[21] First, the nurse and the family should establish mutually acceptable goals that are put in writing. When the goals of individual family members are contradictory or inconsistent with those of the nurse, discrepancies should be discussed and compromises achieved. Second, the nurse and family members should set concrete achievable objectives that lead to accomplishment of identified goals. Finally, the nurse should refrain from imposing solutions on the family.

PRIMARY PREVENTION

Primary prevention for family violence can be aimed at potential abusers, potential victims of abuse, or at society in general.

Interventions Directed toward Potential Abusers

When the nurse identifies a family in which factors that may lead to violence are present, the nurse can plan efforts to modify those factors. Areas of emphasis include increasing the potential abuser's coping skills, improving his or her self-esteem and sense of competence and decreasing dependence, treating existing psychopathology or substance abuse, discussing development issues and expectations, providing

TABLE 34–3. PHYSICAL AND PSYCHOLOGICAL INDICATIONS OF ELDER ABUSE

Type of Abuse	Physical Indications	Psychological Indications
Neglect	• Constant hunger or malnutrition • Poor hygiene • Inappropriate dress for the weather • Chronic fatigue • Unattended medical needs • Poor skin integrity or decubiti • Contractures • Urine burns/excoriation • Dehydration • Fecal impaction	• Listlessness • Social isolation
Emotional abuse	• Hypochondria	• Habit disorder (biting, sucking, rocking) • Destructive or antisocial conduct • Neurotic traits (sleep or speech disorder, inhibition of play) • Hysteria • Obsessions or compulsions • Phobias
Physical abuse	• Bruises and welts • Burns • Fractures • Sprains or dislocations • Lacerations or abrasions • Evidence of oversedation	• Withdrawal • Confusion • Fear of caretaker or other family members • Listlessness
Sexual abuse	• Difficulty walking • Torn, stained, or bloody underwear • Pain or itching in genital area • Bruises or bleeding on external genitalia or in vaginal or anal areas • Sexually transmitted disease	• Withdrawal
Financial abuse	• Inappropriate clothing • Unmet medical needs	• Failure to meet financial obligations • Anxiety over expenses
Denial of rights	• Nothing specific	• Hesitancy in making decisions • Listlessness and apathy

emotional support and relief from stress, and changing attitudes toward violence.

Improving Coping Skills. The community health nurse can plan to assist a potential abuser to improve his or her coping abilities by exploring with the client currently used coping strategies and their effectiveness. The nurse can then assist the client to develop more effective and more appropriate coping strategies. For example, the nurse might assist the client to change his or her perceptions of circumstances that create stress and that lead to abuse. Or, the client might be assisted to change his or her response to stressors. The nurse can also assist clients to learn how to modify or eliminate stress by teaching them the process of problem solving. In teaching this process, the nurse would assist the client to identify desired outcomes of action, to determine and evaluate alternative means of achieving outcomes, and to implement selected alternatives and evaluate their effectiveness in achieving the desired outcomes.

Enhancing Self-esteem. Community health nurses can also assist potential abusers to create a more positive self-image. To this end, the community health nurse might plan to praise and reinforce positive qualities displayed by the client, foster self-reliance, and use problem-solving skills to help the client decrease his or her dependence on others. For example, if the client is economically dependent on an older person living in the home, the nurse might assist the client to obtain employment or show the person how to budget for his or her own needs. The client could also be encouraged to contribute to the support of the household either monetarily or through activities in the home such as making repairs around the house.

Treating Psychopathology and Substance Abuse. If treatment is required for existing psychopathology or for substance abuse by a potentially violent family member, the nurse can plan to make referrals for a variety of treatment services. For example, the nurse might assist the potential abuser to enter a program

TABLE 34–4. RESOURCES FOR DEALING WITH FAMILY VIOLENCE

Agency or Organization	Services
Batterers Anonymous 1269 North E St. San Bernardino, CA 92405 (714) 383-2972	Self-help group for abusers of women
Child Abuse Listening Mediation P.O. Box 718 Santa Barbara, CA 93116 (805) 682-1366	Advocacy, information
Emerge 280 Green St. Cambridge, MA 02139 (617) 547-9870	Public education, referral for counseling for abusive men
Feminist Alliance Against Rape P.O. Box 21033 Washington, DC 20009 (202) 686-9463	Education on rape and self-defense
National Coalition Against Domestic Violence 2401 Virginia Ave., NW, Suite 306 Washington, DC 20037 (202) 293-8860	Information, referral, statistics
National Coalition Against Sexual Assault c/o Volunteers of America 8787 State St., Suite 202 East St. Louis, IL 62203 (618) 398-7764	Information, advocacy for rape victims, statistics
National Committee for Prevention of Child Abuse 332 S. Michigan Ave., Suite 950 Chicago, IL 60604 (312) 663-3520	Advocacy, public education
National Council on Child Abuse & Family Violence 1050 Connecticut Ave., NW, Suite 300 Washington, DC 20036 (202) 429-6695	Public education
Parents Anonymous 6733 S. Sepulveda, Suite 270 Los Angeles, CA 90045 (213) 410-9732	Self-help group for abusive parents

of psychotherapy or might refer the person to a self-help group. Community health nursing involvement in treatment for psychiatric disorders and substance abuse was discussed in Chapter 32, Chronic Mental Health Problem, and Chapter 33, Substance Abuse.

Creating Realistic Developmental Expectations. Another aspect of primary prevention of family violence is educating potential abusers about developmental expectations at various stages of life. For example, the potentially abusive parent can be acquainted with expected behavior as children mature and can be given anticipatory guidance in dealing with these behaviors. Anticipatory guidance and information about parenting skills may even be given before couples have children. In this way they can make decisions about starting a family with a clear idea of the expectations of parenthood. In families that already have children the nurse can refer potentially abusive parents to parenting programs that focus on skills needed to deal effectively with the expectations and stresses of parenthood.

Similarly, family members may need to be acquainted with the difficulties that older persons might experience in adjusting to aging and changed circumstances and that may make them querulous and difficult to live with. The nurse can also suggest to family members ways in which the older person's adjustment can be made easier. For example, the nurse can suggest that the older person be afforded as much privacy as possible, given the home situation, and that he or she be allowed to keep cherished possessions, even if it means that the home becomes somewhat crowded.

The nurse might also educate the potential abuser about personal developmental changes that he or she can expect. For example, if the primary caretaker of an older adult is a woman entering menopause, the nurse can discuss with her the psychological effects of menopause and strategies for minimizing them. The nurse can also refer the client for assistance as needed.

Providing Emotional and Material Support. Nurses can also plan to provide emotional support to clients who are under stress, which may cause them to engage in violence. In addition, the nurse can help the client modify or eliminate sources of stress that contribute to family tension and, potentially, to violence. For example, the nurse might refer the family for financial assistance or assist them to obtain respite care for a handicapped child or an older member.

Changing Attitudes Toward Violence. The final aspect of primary prevention directed toward the potential abuser is changing his or her perceptions of violence as an acceptable mode of conflict resolution. This is particularly needed for clients who come from a family in which violence was common. In working with these families, the nurse might discuss with parents the purposes of disciplining children and help them to develop appropriate forms of discipline to accomplish those purposes without the risk of physical or psychological damage to the child. (See Chapter 20, Care of Children, for a discussion of considerations related to discipline). Similarly, the nurse can assist families to develop positive conflict-resolution strategies similar to those presented in Chapter 11, The Change, Leadership, and Group Processes.

Interventions Directed Toward Potential Victims

Many of the primary prevention strategies directed toward potential victims of abuse are similar to those for potential abusers. For example, the nurse might work with women who grew up in violent families to change their perceptions of violence as an acceptable form of family interaction. To this end, the nurse might educate children, spouses, and older persons about abuse and some of the factors that contribute to family violence.

Similarly, community health nurses can help family members develop strong self-images that will prevent them from accepting abusive situations. The nurse might also assist potential victims to develop good coping, problem-solving, and conflict-resolution skills so that they can look for ways of circumventing potential violence. In addition, the nurse can plan to assist family members to develop effective communication skills that are assertive but do not prompt others to perceive them as whining or demanding.

Another primary prevention strategy directed toward potential victims of abuse is empowerment. ***Empowerment*** is the process of creating within the individual the ability to care for and protect oneself from imposition by others. Children can be empowered by being educated about abuse and what constitutes abuse. They can also be taught, in health-care settings or in schools, what to do if they are being abused. Similarly, adults at risk for abuse can be educated about their options and ways of protecting themselves. Teaching both children and adults that no one has a right to abuse them, no matter what, is another form of empowerment.

Empowerment can also come from encouraging potential victims of abuse to maintain relationships with people outside of the family situation who could spot signs of possible abuse. It is particularly important to encourage family members to invite outside friends into the home. Family members who may be at risk for abuse should also be encouraged to participate in groups and activities outside the home and to ask for help when needed.[50]

One final primary prevention measure that is particularly relevant to older persons in potentially abusive situations is to make arrangements to prevent financial abuse. There are four financial arrangements that can be made to safeguard the funds and property of older people. These include creating a financial representatives trust, providing a durable power of attorney, designating a representative payee, or providing for joint tenancy.[43]

In a ***financial representative trust***, the older person transfers to a trustee, selected by themselves, responsibility for managing his or her property. In this type of arrangement the trustee is required to manage the older person's assets in a particular manner for the benefit of the older person or others designated (for example, grandchildren).

A ***durable power of attorney*** is a written document in which the older person grants another person the authority to act in his or her stead. The durable power of attorney only comes into force when the older person (the "principal") chooses to relinquish control of his or her affairs to the designated person or when the principal becomes incapacitated.

A ***representative payee*** is a person or organization that receives payments as a substitute for the beneficiary. For example, an older person may make arrangements for his or her Social Security benefits to be paid to a specific family member who uses that money to meet the beneficiary's financial obligations. This type of arrangement is restricted to payments to veterans, recipients of Social Security and supplemental security income, and retirees from railroad companies or state agencies. The agreement only covers that one source of the older person's income. The person receiving the money is required by law to use the funds for the care of the beneficiary, and the agency remitting the checks may demand an accounting of expenditures.

In ***joint tenancy***, the person is co-owner of the assets covered with one or more designated others. All parties involved have the use of funds or property covered under joint tenancy. In the event of the death of one party, ownership automatically devolves on other members of the joint tenancy agreement. Advantages and disadvantages of these four methods of preventing financial abuse of older people are summarized in Table 34–5. The community health nurse can plan to assist older clients at risk for financial abuse to evaluate these financial management options and select those best suited to their needs. If the older person needs help in implementing the alternative suggested, the nurse could refer the individual to a source of assistance.

Interventions Directed Toward Society

Community health nurses may also be involved in primary prevention measures at the community or societal level. For the most part, these measures would involve advocacy and political activity. For example, nurses might be active in promoting nonviolence at a societal level by teaching people more effective strategies for conflict resolution, or they might

TABLE 34–5. ADVANTAGES AND DISADVANTAGES OF FINANCIAL ARRANGEMENTS TO PREVENT FINANCIAL ABUSE OF THE ELDERLY

Type of Financial Arrangement	Advantages	Disadvantages
Financial representatives trust	• Legal accountability for use of funds • Ability to specify use of funds and beneficiaries	• Cost of establishing and administering trust
Durable power of attorney	• Financial needs met if older person becomes incapacitated • Ability to designate person to control funds • Retention of control of funds by older person until he or she chooses to relinquish it or becomes incapacitated.	• Limited measures to safeguard older person if designee does not use funds as intended
Representative payee	• Limited control of funds by designated payee • Legal responsibility to use funds for the benefit of the stated beneficiary • Mechanism for demanding accounting of use of funds	• Restrictions on types of funds covered
Joint tenancy	• Ability of older person to designate recipient of funds • Automatic right of survivorship eliminates inheritance taxes	• Both parties have access to and use of property, and the joint tenant may use them for his or her own benefit and not that of the older person

work to decrease the level of violence portrayed on television and in films. Nurses might also be involved in teaching positive conflict-resolution strategies and effective coping skills to school populations.

Activity is also warranted to promote positive attitudes toward the elderly and to reduce the effects of agism in society. Community health nurses might be involved in advocacy efforts that encourage older people to remain involved in the community and to become politically active. In a similar vein, nurses might support changes in the DRG system to account for the effects of age on recovery from a variety of health problems.

Community health nurses may also be involved in political activity to promote legal sanctions for family violence that will serve as deterrents to abuse. Nurses may also need to engage in community organization activities to ensure that law enforcement officials and judges enforce legislation.

Political activity may also be needed to eliminate societal conditions that contribute to family violence. Nurses may campaign, for example, for access to alternative forms of care for older adults for families already experiencing high levels of stress, or they might advocate respite care for family members caring for handicapped children or debilitated elders. Action may also be warranted to ensure adequate income for families in need.

Finally, community health nurses can engage in research related to family violence and its contributing factors. They can then convey their findings to policymakers to promote efforts aimed at preventing family violence.

SECONDARY PREVENTION

Secondary prevention takes place when violence and abuse are identified within a family. Secondary prevention of family violence is guided by three general principles.[45] First, the health-care provider should reject the violence and the abuser's (or victim's) justifications for it. Second, the provider should support the victim and validate the correctness of one's action in seeking help. Third, the abuser should be brought to face the consequences of his or her behavior.

Two major goals in secondary prevention of family violence are protecting the victim from further abuse and breaking the cycle of violence. Protecting the victim may require treatment for serious injuries, reporting the abuse (or suspected abuse) to the proper authorities, and/or removal of the victim from the abusive situation. Breaking the cycle of violence will involve treatment of the abuser, the victim, and the family.

Reporting Confirmed or Suspected Abuse

Health-care providers and some other personnel (for example, teachers or child caretakers) are required by law in all 50 states and the District of Columbia to report all confirmed or suspected instances of child abuse. Usually the report would be made immediately by telephone to the local child protection agency or similar government bureau, followed by a written report within 24 hours. If a provider encounters a suspected or confirmed case of child abuse during nonbusiness hours, he or she should report the incident to the local law enforcement agency at that time and follow with a report to the child protection agency on the next business day. The nurse should ascertain the agency designated to receive reports of potential cases of abuse in his or her jurisdiction and obtain copies of the forms to be used in submitting reports. An example of a reporting form used in one jurisdiction is included in Appendix R, Suspected Child Abuse Report.

In many states, health-care providers are also required to report suspected abuse of older individuals, and the community health nurse should determine the status of reporting laws in his or her state as well as the procedures to be followed. The nurse should also determine the agency to which cases of abuse should be reported. Unfortunately, there are no requirements for reporting spouse abuse. The community health nurse can, however, report instances of spouse abuse (and elder abuse in those states without reporting legislation) to law enforcement agencies, family courts, or other agencies that may be concerned with family violence. While these agencies may not be required to take any action, they will at least be alert to the possibility of violence in the particular family. Another possible resource to which the nurse may report cases of abuse are ombudsman organizations that function as advocates for the elderly or for abused women (or occasionally men).

In addition to making the report, the nurse should inform the abuser that he or she will be reporting the incident to the appropriate authorities. Even if the agencies involved take no action, the fact of having been reported may deter future abuse in some situations.

The question of reporting possible abuse of adults or even older children may pose some ethical dilemmas for the nurse. These include the possibility that reporting instances of abuse may place the victim at greater risk for subsequent abuse, questions of violating client confidentiality, and questions of violating a client's autonomy and right of self-determination. Victims may not want the abuse reported for fear of the consequences for themselves or for the abuser. Reporting of self-neglect or self-abuse by elderly clients may violate their right of self-determination, as can decisions to report abuse when the victim does not want it reported.[50] The nurse will need to make a determination as to what is really in the client's best interest based on the ethical principles discussed in Chapter 14, Ethical Influences on Community Health.

Removing the Victim from an Abusive Situation

Promoting the safety of the victim may necessitate his or her removal from the abusive situation. This may mean placement of an abused child in foster care or arranging for an abused spouse or older person to go to a temporary shelter until more permanent arrangements can be made.

Forcibly removing a child from his or her home may pose ethical questions for health-care providers and social services personnel. While community health nurses are not usually directly responsible for the decision for foster placement, their assessments of family situations often figure prominently in decisions by child-protection services personnel. In removing a child from the home, there is the possibility that removal from familiar surroundings and people that the youngster loves may cause more trauma for the child than leaving him or her in the abusive situation.

Adults cannot be removed involuntarily from an abusive situation unless they are mentally incompetent to make their own decisions. However, the nurse can encourage the spouse or older person who seems to be in danger to go to a shelter or other source of care. In general, three guidelines can assist the nurse and client to determine whether removal is warranted.[16] First, the person should be encouraged to leave if he or she is experiencing a life-threatening medical condition that is not being treated. Second, removal may be warranted by hazards within the environment (for example, lack of heat, food, or water). Third, the client should be encouraged to leave if there is unimpeded access to the client by an individual who has previously harmed that person.

It may be very difficult for abused women or older clients to leave an abusive situation. For the woman, she is leaving a home and a relationship into which she has put considerable time and energy. In addition, the woman may not have any source of economic support should she leave. Or she may fear the loss of her children. Older clients may be reluctant to leave a familiar place or fear going to a nursing home as the only alternative to remaining in an abusive situation. Moreover, the older client may fear complete isolation from family members or the effects of their removal on others in the family (for example, grandchildren).

The nurse should help the client explore the advantages and disadvantages of leaving the situation. If the client decides to leave, he or she should be encouraged to take along personal valuables or place them for safekeeping with a responsible friend or family member. Important personal documents (for example, children's birth certificates and health records, wills) should also be taken. If the woman has young children, she should take the children and a small amount of clothing (as well as important toys) with her. Once the client has been placed in a shelter there may be a need to assist in planning further action such as permanent housing, employment, or legal action. The community health nurse can either help the client with these matters or make referrals for appropriate services.

The client may also require assistance in helping children cope with the upheaval created in their lives. The community health nurse can help the client understand that children are apt to act out their fear and frustration in the situation by being disobedient or quarrelsome with the parent or at school. The nurse can help the client deal with frustrations stemming from these behaviors by children and can also make referrals for counseling for both client and children as needed.

If either abused women or older clients decide not to leave an abusive situation, the community health nurse must accept that decision without conveying disgust for the client or abandoning the person. The nurse can also provide the client with shelter information and suggest contingency plans that the client might make for reaching the shelter should this become necessary at a later time.

Treating the Abuser

The abusive family member usually will also require assistance from the community health nurse. As noted earlier, the militant approach to family violence taken by some health-care providers may (or may not) result in the accomplishment of short-term goals but does nothing to restore the "personhood" of the abuser or the victim.[36] Treatment of the abuser should focus not only on strategies to cope or to manage anger but also on reconstructing a whole person who has dealt with the psychological factors that may have contributed to the abuse. The goals of treatment for the abuser are cessation of violence, expanding the abuser's emotional repertoire beyond anger to acknowledge other positive and negative feelings, and providing an environment in which violence is *not* reinforced and nonviolence *is* reinforced.[36] To achieve these goals, the community health nurse should make referrals for counseling, for psychotherapy for underlying psychopathology, and for treatment for problems of substance abuse if these exist. The nurse may also make referrals to residential programs in which families can learn new patterns of interaction in a nonviolent environment. In addition, the community health nurse would provide emotional support while the abuser learns a new way of thinking and acting and new attitudes toward interpersonal interactions.

The nurse can also help bolster the abuser's self-esteem and sense of personal competency and assist the client to eliminate or modify situational stresses that contributed to abuse. For example, the nurse might assist the abuser to find employment or obtain financial assistance.

Treating the Victim

Victims of abuse will also require treatment. Treatment may be needed for both the physical and psychological effects of abuse, and the community health nurse may make referrals for both types of services. When extensive medical care is needed for severe injuries, the nurse may also need to make referrals for financial assistance. In addition, the nurse can also make referrals for counseling to deal with the emotional effects of abuse.

The nurse should also support the victim emotionally through the treatment of physical defects resulting from abuse. Clients may need assistance adjusting to the long-term consequences of abuse (for example, permanent deformity or other disability). Victims of abuse should be encouraged to ventilate and work through their fears and anxieties about future abuse and to develop strategies for coping with their changed life circumstances. Clients may also need assistance in obtaining financial support, housing, and other necessities.

Treating the Family

Family members other than the direct victim of abuse also suffer the effects of family violence. As noted earlier, children exposed to family violence, even when they are not the target of that violence, tend to accept violence as an appropriate way of resolving differences. In addition, these children may exhibit symptoms related to the increased tension caused by family violence. Community health nurses should assist these youngsters and other family members to deal with their feelings about violence and its effects on their lives. They should be encouraged to develop adaptive responses toward previous abuse and to learn effective strategies for resolving interpersonal conflict without resorting to violence.[1] Community health nurses can assist family members in developing these skills and refer them to sources of additional help as needed.

Families may also need to be assisted to reconstruct themselves along lines that do not include violence. It is particularly important for families that maintain their structure (including the abuser) to plan activities that will enhance family cohesion.[21] To this end, the community health nurse might help the family plan social activities in which all can engage.

TERTIARY PREVENTION

Many of the activities discussed as primary prevention measures can also be used in tertiary prevention, preventing the recurrence of abuse once an abusive situation unfolds. For example, abusive parents can be assisted to develop parenting skills and more realistic expectations of their children. Abusers of all types can be helped to develop more appropriate ways of dealing with stress. Both abusers and victims can be assisted to develop more positive self-concepts. This is particularly important for victims of child abuse if the intergenerational cycle of abusive behavior is to be broken.

Elimination of social environmental and life-style factors contributing to abuse may also prevent recurrence. Community health nurses can work to reduce long-term vulnerability factors such as poor social support networks, historical patterns of abuse, and poor coping abilities. Nurses can also plan to reduce short-term stresses such as unemployment, and increase long-term and short-term protective factors.[28] Furthermore, nurses need to increase the independence of abusers of older persons as a means of min-

TABLE 34–6. GOALS FOR PRIMARY, SECONDARY, AND TERTIARY PREVENTION OF FAMILY VIOLENCE AND RELATED COMMUNITY HEALTH NURSING INTERVENTIONS

Goal of Prevention	Nursing Intervention
Primary Prevention	
1. Development of effective coping skills	1. Teach coping skills
2. Development of strong self-image	2. Foster and reinforce development of strong self-image; foster independence of potential abusers
3. Treatment of psychopathology or substance abuse	3. Refer abusers for counseling or therapy; refer to self-help groups
4. Development of realistic expectations of self and others	4. Educate parents on child development; educate caretakers on developmental needs of the elderly; assist clients to recognize own limitations
5. Development of parenting skills	5. Teach parenting skills
6. Provision of emotional and material support	6. Assist clients to modify sources of stress; refer to outside assistance; provide emotional support; engage in political activity to change conditions conductive to abuse
7. Change in attitudes toward violence	7. Teach nonviolent modes of conflict resolution; teach problem-solving and decision-making skills; discuss attitudes and approaches to discipline; discourage societal glorification of violence
8. Development of policies that discourage violence and protect potential victims	8. Engage in political activity and advocacy
9. Empowerment of potential victims	9. Foster self-esteem; teach coping, communication, and problem-solving skills; educate clients about abuse; encourage clients to maintain relationships outside the family; assist older clients to make appropriate financial arrangements
10. Elimination of negative attitudes to potential victims of abuse	10. Engage in advocacy; convey a positive attitude toward the elderly; educate the public on abuse and dispell myths
Secondary Prevention	
1. Reporting of confirmed and suspected cases of abuse	1. Engage in case finding; report potential cases of abuse
2. Removal of victims from abusive situations	2. Refer to shelters; arrange for foster home placement of abused children
3. Treatment of abusers	3. Refer for counseling; foster self-esteem; provide emotional support; engage in political activity to ensure availability of treatment services
4. Treatment of victims	4. Refer for physical care; refer for counseling; provide emotional and material support
5. Treatment of families	5. Refer for counseling; provide emotional support; encourage activities that foster family cohesion; assist family members to deal with feelings about abuse
Tertiary Prevention	
1. Provision of support to abusers	1. Provide emotional support; teach parenting skills; assist with the development of realistic expectations; foster self-esteem
2. Provision of support to victims	2. Foster self-esteem, foster independence;
3. Reduction of sources of stress	3. Refer for financial help and other material support; assist in obtaining respite care; increase social support networks

imizing elder abuse.[32] Other potential tertiary strategies for elder abuse include providing alternatives to home care of the elderly and increasing community support services for persons who are caring for older family members. For example, respite services or adult day-care centers might reduce the burden on caretakers and prevent recurring incidents of abuse. Intervention goals for family violence and related community health nursing actions at the primary, secondary, and tertiary levels of prevention are summarized in Table 34–6.

EVALUATING CONTROL STRATEGIES FOR FAMILY VIOLENCE

Evaluating interventions to control violence within specific families will focus on the occurrence of abuse in those families as well as other aspects of family behavior. Is the parent more realistic in his or her expectations of children's behavior? Have any further instances of physical abuse of an older person been reported? Is the husband better able to cope with his feelings of jealousy and low self-esteem rather than project them onto his wife?

Evaluation of population-based control strategies would reflect the extent to which incidence rates for all forms of family violence have increased or decreased. For example, if rates of child abuse by adolescent parents declines following mandatory inclusion of parenting education in high school curricula, the education program has been a successful control measure.

Community health nurses can also examine the extent to which national objectives related to abuse have been achieved. The primary objective in this area is to reduce the rate of injury and death to children resulting from parental abuse. Unfortunately, rates of abuse have increased from 9.8 per 1000 children in 1980 to 16.3 in 1986.[52] As noted earlier, this increase may, in part, be due to greater public awareness of abuse and subsequent increases in reporting.

HOMICIDE AND SUICIDE

Family violence is not the only form of violence evident in today's society. Homicide and suicide are two other forms of violence that are of particular concern.

Homicide, as addressed in this chapter, involves death resulting from injury purposefully inflicted by another person.[53] Overall annual incidence rates for homicide have fluctuated somewhat in recent years, rising from slightly more than 8 per 100,000 population in 1970 to peak at 10.7 per 100,000 in 1980, then dropping to almost 8.4 per 100,000 people in 1988.[4] In 1987, homicide was the twelfth leading cause of death in the United States.[54] Despite somewhat lower rates in recent years, the number of years of potential life lost (YPLL) as a result of homicide has risen dramatically (44 percent from 1968 to 1985). In part, the increase in YPLL is due to a steady decrease in the average age of victims. Homicide is occurring at younger and younger ages among persons who have considerably more years of life ahead of them were they not killed prematurely.[55] In fact, homicide is one of the five leading causes of death among children 1 to 18 years of age.[17]

The number of homicides that occur each year would appear to be only the tip of the iceberg in terms of the extent of societal violence. For example, the incidence of forcible rape reported to police officials in 1988 was nearly 38 cases per 100,000 population, while the incidence of aggravated assault was 370 per 100,000 population.[4] These figures represent violent crimes reported to law enforcement agencies. Approximately four times as many cases of assault are seen in emergency rooms as are reported to police officials.[56] While not specifically related to homicide, these figures indicate the growing problem of violence in American society.

Homicide is of particular concern for some segments of the population, particularly black males 15 to 24 years of age. From 1978 to 1987, for example, homicide rates for young black males were four to five times higher than those for black females and five to eight times higher than for white males in the same age group.[54] Despite the focus of the national health objectives for 1990 on reducing homicides in the population of young black males, incidence rates for this population rose from between 22 percent to 76 percent in some states between 1984 and 1987.

Suicide is another area of concern to community health nurses. ***Suicide*** is the voluntary taking of one's own life. Generally speaking, suicide rates have remained relatively stable since the turn of the century with the exception of two peaks in 1910 and during the 1930s.[57] In 1988, the age-adjusted mortality rate for suicide in the United States was 11.3 per 100,000 population.[4]

Despite the overall stability of suicide rates in the United States, there have been rather marked differences for certain population groups. For example, the 1987 rate of suicide for men 20 to 34 years of age was more than twice that for the general population, while the rate for white men over the age of 65 was four times higher.[6]

While problems of homicide and suicide are often thought to be the province of law enforcement agencies, community health nurses and other community health professionals are concerned to the extent that these problems of societal violence can be prevented. The extent of this concern is seen in the number and scope of national objectives for the year 2000 that relate to homicide and suicide. Several of these objectives are presented in Box 34–4. The main focus of community health intervention in these two areas is primary prevention, although nurses may also be involved in preventing recurrent suicide attempts in people who have already made at least one attempt and in assisting the families of homicide or suicide victims to deal with their grief.

> **BOX 34–4**
>
> **National Health Objectives for the Year 2000 Related to Homicide and Suicide**
>
> 1. Reduce homicides to no more than 7.2 per 100,000 population.
> 2. Reduce suicides to no more than 10.5 per 100,000 population.
> 3. Reduce weapon-related violent deaths to no more than 12.6 per 100,000 population.
> 4. Reduce by 15% the incidence of injurious suicide attempts among adolescents aged 14 through 17.
> 5. Reduce by 20% the incidence of weapon-carrying by adolescents aged 14 through 17.
> 6. Extend protocols for identifying, treating, and referring possible suicide victims to at least 90% of hospital emergency departments.
> 7. Increase to at least 50% the proportion of elementary and secondary schools that teach nonviolent conflict-resolution strategies.
> 8. Extend coordinated, comprehensive violence-prevention programs to at least 80% of local jurisdictions with populations over 100,000.
>
> (Source: U.S. Department of Health and Human Services[6])

THE EPIDEMIOLOGIC PREVENTION PROCESS MODEL AND CONTROL OF HOMICIDE AND SUICIDE

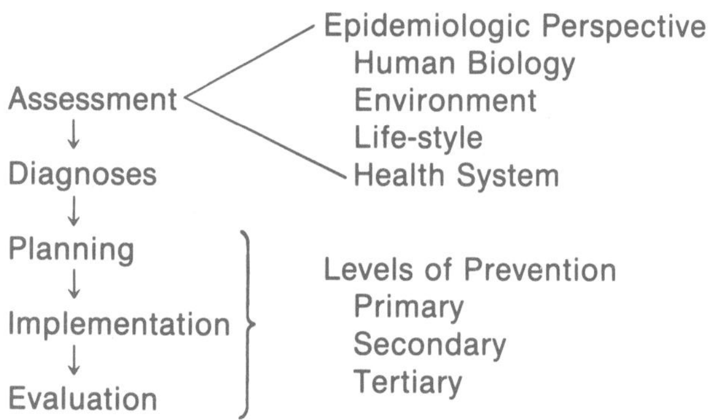

COMMUNITY HEALTH NURSING ASSESSMENT RELATED TO HOMICIDE AND SUICIDE

Community health nurses may be involved in assessing risk factors that contribute to homicide and suicide for both individuals and for communities. Factors related to human biology, environment, life-style, and the health system are associated with both homicide and suicide. Because factors associated with each of these conditions may differ somewhat, each will be addressed separately before interventions related to both are discussed.

ASSESSING RISK FACTORS FOR HOMICIDE

Human Biology

As noted earlier, differences exist in the incidence of homicide in different age and ethnic groups. There are also gender differences in homicide rates. For the most part, these differences are the result of differential exposure to social factors that contribute to homicide. However, they should be addressed here because knowledge of the age, race, and sex composition of the population affected will enable the community health nurse to identify communities at risk for higher rates of homicide.

In 1987, the homicide rate for young black males was more than 90 cases per 100,000 population compared to 8.5 cases per 100,000 for the general population. The increase in homicides among black adolescents (ages 15 to 19 years) from 1984 to 1987 was even more dramatic than that experienced by young adult black males (a 55 percent increase compared to a 33 percent increase for the 20- to 24-year-old group).[54] Black females are also at higher risk for homicide than either Caucasian males or females.[58]

Younger Hispanic males also have rates of homicide three times those of non-Hispanics in the Southwestern United States.[59] Hispanic females, on the other hand, have homicide incidence rates comparable to those of Anglo females.[60] Although more men than women are victims of homicide, more women than men (43 percent versus 15 percent) are killed by a family member or intimate acquaintance.[61]

Environment

Factors in both the psychological and social environments contribute to homicide. Psychological environmental factors associated with homicide are similar to those discussed in relation to family violence and include poor coping strategies and perceptions of violence as an acceptable means of resolving conflict. Other psychological factors associated with homicide include poor impulse control and, on occasion, psychopathology. The feelings of hopelessness and powerlessness that may occur with poverty and discrimination may also lead to defiance that erupts in the form of violence and homicide.

One other aspect of the psychological environment is the state of mind of the victim at the time of the homicide. Homicides often occur as a result of arguments (frequently when both parties have been drinking). In fact, in 1988, more than one-third of all homicides were preceded by an argument.[4] It has been suggested that a fair number of these altercations are provoked by the victims in an effort to motivate another person to kill them. This phenomenon is referred to as ***victim-precipitated homicide*** and has been noted in persons with AIDS who desire death but are unwilling to commit suicide.[62]

Social environmental factors that contribute to homicide include societal acceptance of personal violence, stress due to a variety of underlying factors, crime and gang membership, and the availability of weapons. Many of the societal factors that influence family violence also contribute to homicide. The use of force to settle conflicts and the failure of members of society to interfere in the face of escalating violence contribute to homicide as well as to other forms of violence. In addition, media portrayal of violence without elucidating its consequences glamorizes violence.

Stress due to social conditions appears to be a contributing factor in homicide although its contribution is somewhat unclear.[63] Poverty, poor job opportunity, education, movement from rural to urban settings, changes in family structure, increased population mobility, drug trafficking, and racial discrimination have all been cited as sources of stress that may influence the risk of homicide.[54,64] There appears to be a differential effect of these stressors on the type of homicide involved, in which poverty and related stressors are more closely related to ***expressive homicides*** (those motivated by interpersonal conflict), and stress due to inequality and discrimination are more closely associated with ***instrumental homicides*** (those that occur in the process of committing a crime such as robbery).[63]

Levels of stress experienced and the poverty and other social factors that contribute to stress may partially explain the difference in homicide rates noted between urban and rural areas. Significant differences in urban and rural homicide rates are seen even among segments of the population already at risk. Black males living in urban areas, for example, are twice as likely to be victims of homicide as black males of the same age living in rural areas.[58] Urban areas are frequently characterized by poverty, high population density, and poor housing, which create stress that may lead to violence. Homicide rates tend to be particularly high in cities where economic status contributes to interpersonal confrontations of either the expressive or instrumental variety.[63] Cities with homicide rates in excess of 25 per 100,000 population are included in Table 34–7.

Crime and gang activity in urban areas also place residents at greater risk of homicide. Homicides may be committed in the process of other criminal activity, particularly robbery and the sale of illegal drugs. Cities, for example, with high rates of crime related to robbery and drug trafficking also tend to have high homicide rates.[63] Although much attention is given in the media to homicide connected with criminal be-

TABLE 34–7. U.S. CITIES WITH HOMICIDE RATES GREATER THAN 25 PER 100,000 POPULATION, 1988

City	Homicide Rate
Washington, DC	59.5
Detroit	57.9
Atlanta	48.8
Denver	43.4
New Orleans	42.4
Dallas	36.0
Newark, NJ	36.0
St. Louis	32.9
Baltimore	30.6
Oakland	30.5
Kansas City, MO	29.9
Memphis	26.0
New York	25.8
Houston	25.5
Cleveland	25.2

havior, the proportion of total homicides related to crime is less than one might expect. In 1988, for example, slightly under 19 percent of all homicides occurred during the commission of a felony, and an additional 1.3 percent occurred during a suspected felony.[4] Unfortunately, many of the victims of crime-related homicides are innocent bystanders.

The availability of weapons is a significant social environmental contribution to homicide.[54] Weapons used to commit homicide vary, but in the majority of cases the weapon used is some type of firearm.[54,59,60] This choice of weapon is probably influenced by the lethality of the method as well as the ease of access to guns. According to a National Rifle Association study, 38 states required no permit to purchase a gun in 1987, and 31 states did not require a license to openly carry a gun.[65] Other weapons used include cutting implements and bludgeons.[64]

Life-style

Two aspects of life-style may increase one's risk of homicide. The first is drug and alcohol use and abuse, and the second is occupation.

Drug and alcohol use may contribute to one's propensity to commit homicide as well as the probability of being a victim of homicide. Use of psychoactive substances frequently decreases a person's inhibitions against violent behavior and may lead to homicide, particularly as the culmination of an argument.[66] Studies of alcohol and drug intake among perpetrators are understandably few; this is because the arrest of a murder suspect frequently does not occur until some time after the crime when blood and urine levels of psychoactive substances are likely to be quite different from those that might be obtained earlier. In one study of suspects arrested during or immediately after the homicide, however, 67 percent had urine alcohol concentrations greater than 100 mg%.[66]

Use of alcohol and drugs can also contribute to a person's likelihood of becoming a victim of homicide. In one study, for example, 30 percent of homicide victims had blood alcohol levels exceeding legal limits for most states. Again, the relationship of alcohol use to homicide was stronger for homicides that occurred as a result of arguments than for those that did not (two-thirds versus one-third, respectively). It has even been suggested that just being present in places where alcohol use occurs may increase one's risk of being a homicide victim.[66]

Drug use and abuse may also contribute to homicides both while one is under the influence of the drug and during activities performed to support a drug habit (for instance, robbery). Narcotics-related crimes, for example, accounted for almost 6 percent of all homicides in 1988.[4]

A person's occupation can also increase his or her risk of being a homicide victim. From 1980 to 1985, over 13 percent of work-related fatalities were attributed to homicide. American women seem to be at greater risk of occupational homicide than men. Homicide accounted for 42 percent of occupational fatalities for women and only 12 percent of fatalities for men. Jobs that require frequent contact with the public or the exchange of money increase one's risk for homicide. Working at night in a high crime area is another occupational risk factor for homicide. The risk of homicide can be reduced, however, by factors within the work setting itself. Examples of risk-reduction strategies include training employees in conflict management, limiting the amount of money available or access to that money by employees, increasing employee visibility to the general public, and controlling access to the premises.[53]

Health System

The major contribution of the health system to homicide lies in failure to engage in primary preventative efforts to control the problem. For example, in 1987 less than 1 percent of more than 300 state injury programs included a focus on homicide. Similarly, only one of more than 550 award-winning community programs for health promotion since 1986 has dealt with homicide.[54]

Other health system factors may also contribute to homicide. Emergency facilities in many cities with high homicide rates are sometimes ill equipped to deal with the sheer numbers of people seriously injured in assaults, and many of these people become part of the statistical picture of homicide. In addition, less than one quarter of nonfatal assault cases seen in emergency rooms are reported to police.[56] If health-care providers were more consistent in reporting cases of nonfatal assault, more of the perpetrators of these assaults might be apprehended by law enforcement authorities before they eventually kill someone. Epidemiologic factors associated with homicide are summarized in Box 34–5.

ASSESSING RISK FACTORS FOR SUICIDE

Human Biology

Human biological factors that may be related to suicide include effects of maturation and aging and physiologic function. Some age groups have higher suicide rates than others, and differences in suicide rates for different age groups vary with gender. For women, the incidence of suicide peaks in mid-life and then declines. For example, the highest incidence of

BOX 34–5

Factors Associated with Homicide

Human Biology
- Younger persons are at greater risk of homicide than older persons.
- Males are at greater risk than females, but more women are killed by a family member or intimate acquaintance.
- Black and Hispanic males have higher rates of homicide than do white males.

Environment

Psychological environment
- Poor coping strategies may lead to homicide.
- Perceptions of violence as a means of resolving interpersonal conflicts can lead to homicide.
- Victims may provoke homicidal attacks in an effort to die.

Social environment
- Societal acceptance of violent behavior contributes to homicide.
- Societal factors that lead to stress (for example, poverty, discrimination, unemployment, migration) may contribute to homicide.
- Crime and gang-related activity can increase the incidence of homicide.
- Easy access to weapons is associated with higher rates of homicide.

Life-style
- Drug and alcohol use can contribute to homicide by lowering one's inhibitions to violent behavior.
- Drug and alcohol use may also lead to arguments that result in homicide.
- Frequenting places where drugs and alcohol are used and where there is interpersonal conflict is likely to increase one's risk of being murdered.
- Criminal activities to support a drug habit are associated with homicide.
- Occupational factors such as working with the public, handling money, or working in high crime areas increase one's risk of being a homicide victim.

Health System
- Failure to develop programs to promote nonviolent behavior adds to the homicide rate.
- Lack of facilities to care for victims may increase the rate of fatalities due to assault.
- Failure of health-care providers to report cases of assault impedes control of homicide.

suicide among women in 1986 occurred among those who were 45 to 54 years of age (8.8 per 100,000 women). For men, on the other hand, the incidence of suicide rises with increasing age, with the highest rates experienced by men 85 years of age and older (over 61 cases per 100,000 men in 1986).[4]

Age-gender differences in suicide may be explained, in part, by maturational events that occur at these times for men and women. Women at mid-life usually experience menopause accompanied by hormonal changes that may lead to severe depression and consequent suicide. At the same time, women may be experiencing social factors, such as children leaving home, that may contribute to depression. Men, on the other hand, may be responding to the effects of age on physical and mental abilities and social interaction, again leading to depression and, possibly, to suicide.

Although objectively not as high as rates for older people, suicide rates for individuals 15 to 24 years of age are also of concern because of their rapid escalation in recent years. For example, suicide rates for this age group increased by 200 percent from 1950 to 1978, at which time they peaked. Suicide rates for this group have remained relatively stable at about 12 to 13 cases per 100,000 persons through 1988.[4,67] Again, this is a period in one's life that is characterized by rapid hormonal and social changes with which the individual may have difficulty coping, thus leading to increased potential for suicide. When working with people in age groups at particular risk for suicide, the community health nurse would be careful to assess for other suicidal risk factors as well as specific indicators of suicidal intent.

There is also some evidence that physiologic function may contribute to suicide. Research has indicated rather consistently that lower levels of the biochemical neurotransmitter serotonin, also linked to depressive illness, is associated with suicide. Less consistent associations have also been demonstrated between suicide and other neurotransmitters such as norepinephrine, dopamine, and acetylcholine.[57,68] Racial differences in suicide rates are consistent with these findings since both depressive illness and suicide occur more often in Caucasians as in blacks and other racial groups.[57,69] In 1986, for example, the overall suicide rate for whites was twice as high as that for blacks.[4]

Environment

Psychological Environment. Some authors assert that most victims of suicide suffer from some type of mental disorder.[57,70] In one study of factors influencing adolescent suicide, adolescents who had attempted suicide were four times as likely to report prior psychiatric hospitalization as were physically ill adolescents in a control group.[71] In a similar study, Navajo adolescents who had attempted suicide were more than three times as likely to have a history of mental health problems.[72] As noted in Chapter 32, Chronic Mental Health Problems, both schizophrenics and persons with depressive disorders have higher incidence rates for suicide than does the general population.

In some cases of suicide associated with mental illness it is unclear whether the suicide is a result of the illness or the effects of psychotropic drugs used in treatment of mental illness. Antidepressants, in particular, can reverse depression sufficiently to give severely depressed clients the energy they lacked to commit suicide.

The hopelessness that may accompany severe debilitating or terminal illness is another psychological factor that may lead to suicide. Clients with terminal cancers or AIDS, for example, may see suicide as an escape from a painful and lingering illness for which there is no cure.[62] Community health nurses working with clients with either mental or serious physical illness or disability should carefully assess them for suicide potential, focusing particularly on inability to cope with the effects of the illness or its treatment and on the presence of signs of depression discussed in Chapter 32.

People who commit suicide frequently exhibit several common personality traits. For example, in one study suicidal adolescents showed less impulse control than did their nonsuicidal counterparts. Suicidal adolescents also exhibited higher 3-month stress scores than did nonsuicidal teens.[71]

Exposure to suicide by others may create a psychological climate that encourages suicide in vulnerable individuals. Both direct knowledge of someone who has committed suicide and indirect knowledge via media presentations of suicide have been found to be associated with subsequent suicide.[57,67,68,70] For example, adolescents who had a friend who committed suicide are almost three times more likely to attempt suicide as those who have not. Similarly, those with a family history of suicide or a suicide attempt are more than twice as likely to attempt suicide.[72] Community health nurses would obtain information related to suicide and attempted suicide as well as other conditions in constructing family genograms early in their interactions with individuals and families. This information might help to identify people exposed to prior suicides. The nurse would then explore with the client his or her resolution of grief related to the prior suicide.

A previous attempt at suicide is a particularly significant risk factor for successful suicide.[57,71,72] In one study, 15 percent of suicidal adolescents had a history of previous suicide attempts, often more than one attempt.[72] In another similar study, 39 percent of suicidal adolescents reported previous attempts compared to only 10 percent of a group of physically ill adolescents.[71] Community health nurses assessing clients for suicide potential should be particularly alert to a past history of suicide attempts by the individual, and they should ask about any prior attempts.

Other psychological signs of suicide potential for which the nurse should assess clients include a sudden change in mood, particularly from agitation and depression to calm, and expression of suicidal thoughts. Generally speaking, the more persistent the thoughts of suicide, the more likely the event. Also, the more detailed the plan for suicide and the more lethal the method described in the plan, the more likely the person is actually to attempt suicide. Finally, clients who make few references to the future in terms of plans or goals are at risk for suicide.[73]

The nurse should ask clients if they have ever thought about committing suicide. If the response is yes, the nurse should ask the client about the frequency and persistence of these thoughts and also inquire as to what plans, if any, have been made for

BOX 34–6

Indications of Potential for Suicide

- Family history of suicide
- History of prior suicide attempt(s)
- Recent loss (particularly in the last 6 months)
- Signs of depression
- Feelings of hopelessness and helplessness expressed
- Feelings of anxiety, irritability, or panic exhibited
- Lack of references to future goals or activities
- Frequent or persistent thoughts of committing suicide
- Carefully thought-out plan for suicide
- Method planned for suicide is lethal
- Reduced likelihood of rescue, given method planned and other aspects of suicide plan
- Specific time frame planned for suicide
- Suicide planned for the near future
- Behaviors designed to "put one's house in order" (making a will, giving away prized possessions, making a final contact with significant others)

(Source: Assey[73])

a potential suicide. Indicators of potential suicide for which the nurse should assess are summarized in Box 34–6.

Social Environment. Social environmental factors that influence the incidence of suicide may arise from the personal social environment or from the larger environment. Within the personal social environment, poor interpersonal relationships, particularly family relationships, have been associated with suicide. In one study, for example, adolescents whose parents were separated were one and a half times more likely to attempt suicide as were those whose parents were living together.[72] In another study, the parents of 73 percent of suicidal adolescents were divorced or separated, compared to 59 percent of a control group.[71] A history of running away[71] or physical or sexual abuse[72] was also more common among suicidal subjects.

Suicide among adults has also been linked to changes in interpersonal relationships, particularly to divorce or death of a spouse,[67] while marriage appears to be a protective factor against suicide for men and, to a lesser extent, for women as well. Widowed and divorced men have suicide rates nearly four times higher than those for married men, whereas rates for single men are twice as high as for their married counterparts. Divorced women commit suicide three times more often than do married women, and single women have suicide rates 40 percent higher than those of married women.[57,74]

Suicidal adolescents are also more likely than their nonsuicidal counterparts to exhibit poor school performance. Poor school performance and poor attitudes toward school were twice as likely to be exhibited by suicidal adolescents in one study,[72] and six times more likely in another study.[71]

Societal factors that have been associated with increased incidence of suicide include the easy availability of firearms and drugs, joblessness, and media coverage of suicide. Firearms are the most frequently used mode of committing suicide. In 1986, for example, nearly two-thirds of suicides were committed using firearms, while drug ingestion accounted for another 14 percent of suicides.[4] Hanging, strangulation, and suffocation are less frequently used methods of suicide.

The relationship of joblessness to suicide is not completely clear.[57,75] However, it is a reasonable conjecture that joblessness contributes to hopelessness and depression, which may culminate in suicide as a means of escape from an unbearable situation. It may also be that people with psychiatric disorders that can culminate in suicide are unemployed as a result of their disease rather than depressed because of their unemployment. Suicide victims do exhibit more frequent job changes and periods of unemployment than does the general population,[57] which may be evidence of general mental instability.

Prominent coverage of suicides in the news media is another societal factor that has been shown to be associated with suicide, particularly among young people.[68] This is particularly true of "cluster suicides." A ***suicide cluster*** is a group of suicides or suicide attempts that occur closer together in time and space than would otherwise be expected.[76] Suicide clusters account for only 1 percent to 5 percent of all suicides, but they are especially traumatizing to communities in which they occur. There is some evidence that such events arise from imitative behavior due to exposure to suicide by knowing the victim or through media coverage of the event.

Life-style

The major life-style factors associated with suicide are drug and alcohol abuse. Psychoactive substance abuse may lead to depression that culminates in suicide. In addition, the use of both alcohol and drugs results in disinhibition and may minimize the effects of religious and ethical strictures against suicide.[62] Adolescents who engage in weekly use of hard liquor have been found to be almost three times more likely to attempt suicide as their nondrinking counterparts, while weekly users of beer and wine were almost one-and-a-half times more likely to attempt suicide.[72] In one study, suicidal adolescents were more likely to have used cigarettes, marijuana, and other drugs (cocaine, phencyclidine, amphetamines, barbiturates, tranquilizers, and heroin) than nonsuicidal teenagers.[71]

Alcohol use among adults has also been linked to suicide. In one study, for example, 76 percent of Alaskan Native suicide victims were found to have detectable blood alcohol levels. In the same study, 48 percent of suicides among Caucasians in Alaska involved elevated blood alcohol levels.[77] Community health nurses should be alert to evidence of suicide potential among persons who abuse alcohol or other psychoactive substances.

Health System

Health system factors that contribute to suicide include lack of attention to persons at high risk and failure to identify potential suicide victims. Lack of access to a regular source of health care may also be a contributing factor because it limits the opportunity of health-care professionals to identify persons at risk. The results of one study, for example, indicated that suicidal teenagers were less likely to identify a regular provider of primary health care than were members of a control group, and they were significantly more likely to report use of emergency rooms for routine health care.[71] Epidemiologic factors associated with suicide are summarized in Box 34–7.

DIAGNOSTIC REASONING, HOMICIDE, AND SUICIDE

Nursing diagnoses related to homicide and suicide may reflect existing or potential health problems for individuals, families, or population groups. For example, nursing diagnoses for individual clients might be "potential for homicide due to night work in a high crime area" or "potential for suicide due to depression following father's death." The nurse working with a family might make a diagnosis of "unresolved grief due to suicide of eldest child."

Similar diagnoses at the community level might also reflect either existing problems related to homicide and suicide or potential for increased incidence of either. For example, the nurse might diagnose a "potential for increased incidence of teenage suicide due to media coverage of a group suicide pact" or "increased incidence of homicide due to relaxation of gun control laws."

PLANNING AND IMPLEMENTING CONTROL STRATEGIES FOR HOMICIDE AND SUICIDE

Control of homicide and suicide may require primary, secondary, or tertiary prevention measures. At each of these levels, intervention may be directed toward the individual or family experiencing the problem or to the population as a group. Nurses designing primary, secondary, or tertiary interventions can contact the organizations included in Table 34–8 for information and assistance.

PRIMARY PREVENTION

Primary prevention for homicide and suicide is similar to that for family violence and substance abuse and involves promoting a positive self-image and developing adequate coping abilities among clients, particularly those at high risk for suicide or homicide. Educating individual clients and the public with respect to stress management and coping is one means of limiting the incidence of both homicide and suicide. In addition, teaching conflict-management strategies can help to prevent homicide. Community health nurses can also encourage clients not to frequent places where homicides occur frequently (for example, a bar in a high crime area) and not to use alcohol or drugs in circumstances where interpersonal conflict is likely to occur.

At the aggregate level, limiting accessibility to firearms and other weapons employed in suicide and homicide can contribute to prevention, and community health nurses can plan for political activity related to control of guns and other weapons. Nurses can also advocate control of alcohol and drugs that contribute to suicide and homicide or that may be used as a method of suicide.

School-based education about suicide has been suggested as a means of decreasing the incidence of suicide in young people. However, there is a possibility that discussion of suicide may lead to imitative behavior on the part of vulnerable individuals within the group. For this reason, caution is suggested in the implementation of such programs. Any programs that are instituted should make provision for coun-

BOX 34–7

Factors Associated with Suicide

Human Biology

- Suicide incidence is highest among middle-aged women and elderly men, but is increasing dramatically among young men.
- Increased suicide in specific age groups may be related to maturational events such as adolescence, menopause, and aging.
- Suicide is more prevalent among Caucasians than among other groups.
- Suicide is more common among males than females.
- Suicide may be related to lower levels of serotonin and other neurotransmitters found to be associated with depressive illness.

Environment

Psychological environment

- Suicide may be associated with psychopathology.
- Medications used to treat psychiatric illness may contribute to suicide.
- Hopelessness associated with terminal or debilitating illness may lead to suicide.
- Impulsivity and higher levels of stress are associated with suicide.
- Exposure to suicide by others may result in suicide.
- Previous attempts increase one's risk for successful suicide.
- Depression, persistent thoughts of suicide, and detailed plans for suicide are indicators of potential suicide.

Social environment

- Poor interpersonal and family relationships may lead to suicide.
- A history of abuse may result in taking one's life.
- Attempts to run away are an indicator of suicide potential.
- Changes in interpersonal relationships (divorce, death of a spouse) may precipitate suicide.
- Poor school performance is associated with suicide in adolescents.
- Easy access to methods of suicide may foster suicide attempts.
- Joblessness and other social factors that create stress may result in suicide. Or self-selected unemployment may indicate instability and risk for suicide.
- Media coverage of suicide may lead to imitative behavior.

Life-style

- Drug and alcohol use and abuse are associated with suicide.

Health System

- Failure to identify and treat persons at risk for suicide impedes control efforts.
- Lack of a source of regular health care may impede recognition of persons at risk for suicide.

seling of those students who seem unduly disturbed by discussion of suicide.

SECONDARY PREVENTION

Secondary prevention involves the early identification of persons who are contemplating suicide and intervention to prevent the act or limit the consequences. Nurses, school teachers, and counselors may recognize the signs of impending suicide and should take immediate action. Such action might include counseling, referral, or hospitalization if the danger of suicide appears imminent. Community health nurses may also be involved in educating individuals who work with young people, the elderly, and others at risk for suicide to recognize indicators of a potential suicide attempt.

There is at present no evidence to suggest that providing suicide "hotlines" decreases the incidence

TABLE 34–8. SOURCES OF INFORMATION AND ASSISTANCE IN CONTROLLING SUICIDE

Agency or Organization	Services
American Association of Suicidology 2459 S. Ash Denver, CO 80222 (303) 692-0985	Information
International Association for Suicide Prevention c/o Charlotte P. Ross Suicide Prevention & Crisis Center 1811 Trousdale Dr. Burlingame, CA 94010 (415) 877-5604	Information, public education
National Committee on Youth Suicide Prevention 67 Irving Place, South New York, NY 10003 (212) 677-6666	Public education, information, and referral; assistance in the development of local programs; advocacy
National Save-a-Life League 4520 Fourth Ave., Suite MH3 New York, NY 11220 (212) 492-4067	Suicide prevention; crisis intervention; aid to families; public education
Parents of Suicides c/o Bergen/Passaic TCF P.O. Box 373 Englewood, NJ 07631 (201) 894-0042	Support for parents and siblings of suicide victims
Samaritans 500 Commonwealth Ave. Kenmore Square Boston, MA 02215 (617) 247-0220	Information on suicide and its prevention
Season: Suicide Bereavement c/o Joan Clark 1358 Sunset Dr. Salt Lake City, UT 84116 (801) 596-2341	Support group for families of suicide victims, public education
Youth Suicide National Center 1825 Eye Street, NW, Suite 400 Washington, DC 20006 (202) 429-2016	Public education, development of model prevention programs

of suicide. However, there is also no evidence that such services are harmful, so they may at least be worth a try as a secondary prevention strategy.

Community health nurses and other health-care providers can employ a suicide prevention contract with an individual client who has expressed thoughts of committing suicide. A ***suicide prevention contract*** is a mutual agreement between the nurse and the client that specifies the contributions of each party in preventing the client's self-destruction.[73] These contracts are characterized by three features: balance, open expression of caring, and continual reinforcement. Balance is required between coercive measures that forcibly protect the client from harm and trusting the client with a certain level of freedom of action. An effective contract is also characterized by the expression of concern for the client by the nurse and evidence of the nurse's willingness to do what is necessary to protect the client. Finally, the nurse reinforces the contract by making it clear and specific. The exact nature of what is or is not to be done should be spelled out clearly and simply. For example, the nurse might get the client to agree not to kill himself or herself without first talking to the nurse.

Because clients are reluctant to commit themselves to giving up the notion of suicide permanently, the contract may need to be time-limited at first. For example, the nurse might be able to get the client to agree not to kill oneself until after completing at least a month of therapy. Whatever agreement is reached, the nurse witnesses the client's verbal statement of the terms of the contract. This verbalization seems to increase the reality of the contract for the client and strengthens the contract's chances for success. Contracts made in a group setting appear to have even more influence than those made only in the presence of the nurse.[73]

TERTIARY PREVENTION

Tertiary prevention is particularly relevant in the prevention of cluster suicides. Because of the traumatic nature of such occurrences, a working group has developed specific guidelines for preventing and controlling cluster suicides. These guidelines include community development of a response plan in the event of the onset of a suicide cluster, involvement of all concerned segments of the community (especially the media so as to prevent overdramatization of instances of suicide), and coordination of the planned response by one designated agency. Specific elements of a community response plan for preventing suicide clusters are presented in Box 34–8.

Tertiary prevention of suicide and homicide may also involve working with families of victims. The community health nurse can assist family members to work through their grief over the death of a loved one. They can also assist families to deal with any feelings of guilt that they may be suffering. In addition, the nurse can assist violence-prone families to find ways of coping with their loss that will prevent further suicide or homicide. Primary, secondary, and tertiary control measures for suicide and homicide are summarized in Table 34–9.

BOX 34–8

Recommendations for a Community Plan to Prevent Suicide Clusters

- The community should develop a response plan before the onset of a suicide cluster.
- The response should involve all concerned segments of the community and should be planned by representatives of all concerned agencies.
- One agency should be designated to coordinate response planning and be responsible for:
  - Calling the initial meeting of the planning committee
  - Establishing a mechanism for notification of a potential suicide cluster
  - Convening the group when a suicide cluster appears to be occurring
  - Maintaining the response plan and seeing that the planning group reviews and updates it periodically.
- Relevant community resources should be identified including hospitals and emergency services, local academic resources, clergy, parent groups, suicide crisis centers or hotlines, survivor groups, students, police, media personnel, representatives of local government, etc.
- The plan should be implemented when a suicide cluster occurs or when one or more trauma-related deaths occur that may influence others to commit suicide.
- Plan implementation should include:
  - Contacting agencies involved
  - A review of responsibilities and tasks to be accomplished
  - Preparation for dealing with the problems and stresses encountered by those responding to the crisis.
- The response should be conducted in a manner that avoids glorifying the victims and minimizes sensationalism by:
  - Having the spokesperson present as accurate a picture of the victim as possible to students, parents, family, media, and others
  - Announcing suicides among persons of school age in a manner that will maximize support and minimize hysteria
- Persons at risk for suicide should be identified and have at least one screening with a trained counselor. These individuals include relatives of victims, boy friends or girl friends, close friends, fellow employees, or students. Identification may be accomplished by:
  - Identifying people present at funerals who seem particularly upset
  - Asking teachers to identify students who seem to be at risk
  - Identifying those associated with the victim who themselves have attempted suicide.
  - Identifying and referring depressed persons
  - Identifying those with poor social support systems.
- The community may establish a suicide hotline or a walk-in crisis center.
- Counselors should be provided at a particular site and their availability made known to community residents.
- The assistance of local media should be sought to disseminate information on sources of help.
- Counseling services should also be made available to those responding to the crisis.
- Plans should be made for a timely flow of accurate and appropriate information to the media, including:
  - Designating a single spokesperson or one spokesperson from each agency involved in the response
  - Providing accurate information without whitewashing or sensationalism
  - Providing information on positive steps being taken
  - Not disclosing the precise mode of suicide employed

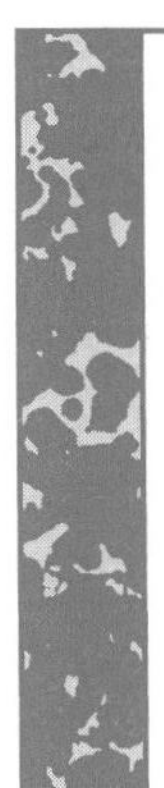

BOX 34–8 (continued)

- Enlisting the help of the community in referring all requests for information to the spokespersons.
- Elements in the initial suicide that might increase the likelihood of other suicides should be identified and changed (for example, erecting barriers along a cliff where suicide has occurred).
- Long-term issues suggested by the nature of a suicide cluster should be addressed (for example, if all those committing suicide were unemployed, action can be taken to reduce unemployment levels).

(Source: Centers for Disease Control. [1988]. CDC recommendations for a community plan for the prevention and containment of suicide clusters. MMWR, 37[suppl. no. S-6], 1–12.)

EVALUATING CONTROL STRATEGIES FOR HOMICIDE AND SUICIDE

Whether intervention takes place at the primary, secondary, or tertiary level of prevention, there is a need to evaluate its effectiveness in solving problems of violence. Evaluation of interventions directed toward individuals and their families is assessed in terms of whether or not the factors underlying a problem have been modified in such a way that the problem is controlled. If the individual is suicidal, have interventions contributed to better abilities to cope with stress?

Programs designed to resolve problems of violence at the community or group level are also evaluated in terms of their outcomes. However, the outcome would be measured in terms of the extent of the problem in the population. Several of the 1990 objectives dealt with societal violence and can be used as a basis for evaluating control strategies for homicide and suicide. By and large, these objectives have not been met.

Because of a high rate of homicide among black males 15 to 24 years of age, one of the objectives specifically targeted this group for a reduction in homicide rates. Unfortunately, rather than decreasing, the homicide rate in this group has increased. Similarly, rates for suicide for this age group within the total population have also increased.[52]

TABLE 34–9. GOALS FOR PRIMARY, SECONDARY, AND TERTIARY PREVENTION OF HOMICIDE AND SUICIDE AND RELATED COMMUNITY HEALTH NURSING INTERVENTIONS

Goals of Prevention	Nursing Intervention
Primary Prevention	
1. Development of effective coping skills	1. Teach coping skills and stress-management skills
2. Development of self-esteem	2. Foster self-esteem, advocate school programs to foster self-esteem in young people
3. Promotion of nonviolent conflict resolution	3. Teach nonviolent conflict-management strategies
4. Reduction of risk behaviors	4. Encourage clients not to frequent places where homicides occur and not to use drugs and alcohol in circumstances in which interpersonal conflict is likely
5. Decreased availability of weapons, drugs, and alcohol	5. Engage in political activity to promote control of weapons and limit access to drugs and alcohol
Secondary Prevention	
1. Identification of persons contemplating suicide	1. Case finding; teach teachers and counselors to recognize signs of possible suicide
2. Provision of counseling for persons at risk for suicide or who express suicidal thoughts	2. Refer for counseling, use a suicide prevention contract to motivate the client not to commit suicide
3. Provision of treatment for homicide and suicide victims	3. Engage in political activity and advocacy to ensure adequate treatment facilities
Tertiary Prevention	
1. Prevention of suicide clusters	1. Assist in the development of community response plans
2. Provision of care to families of homicide and suicide victims	2. Assist family members to work through feelings of grief and guilt; assist families to find positive ways to cope with loss

CHAPTER HIGHLIGHTS

- Violence is a pervasive phenomenon in American society, stemming in part from the historical need to counter threats of physical harm with force. Areas of particular concern to community health nurses include family violence, homicide, and suicide.
- Family violence involves action taken by one family member with the intent to inflict harm on another member and may include child abuse, spouse abuse, or elder abuse.
- Child abuse can be perpetrated in four ways: neglect, physical abuse, emotional abuse, and sexual abuse.
- Spouse abuse usually occurs in a three-stage cycle beginning with rising tensions in the family and irritation of the abuser, followed by an explosive manifestation of violence and then by a period of calm and loving reconciliation.
- Elder abuse can involve physical abuse, emotional abuse, financial abuse, active or passive neglect, denial of civil rights, and self-abuse and neglect.
- Human biological factors of age, sex, and physiologic function may influence the incidence of family violence. The very young and the elderly are the most vulnerable to family violence. Women and men engage equally in abusive behaviors toward each other, but women are more vulnerable to the physical and social effects of abuse. Physical disability may also make one more vulnerable to abuse.
- Social environmental factors that influence family violence include social definitions of and attitudes toward violent behaviors, and the extent of protection afforded victims of abuse, myths about family violence, family history of violence, and social circumstances that create stress and tax family members' coping abilities.
- Psychological environmental factors contributing to family violence include poor coping skills on the part of abusers, impoverished emotional climates in families, personality traits of abusers and victims, and the presence of psychopathology.
- Life-style factors influencing the incidence of family violence include single-parenthood, abuse of psychoactive substances, and cohabitation.
- Health system factors contributing to family violence include failure to identify families at risk for abuse and to diagnose abuse when it occurs. Health-care providers may also choose not to intervene in an abusive situation for a variety of reasons. In addition, providers may display negative attitudes toward victims of abuse based on social myths. The health-care system itself may perpetrate elder abuse in early discharge of older people from health-care facilities.
- Abused family members may exhibit both physical and psychological signs and symptoms of abuse and should be carefully assessed for indicators in both areas.
- Primary prevention of family violence may be directed toward the potential abuser, the potential victim, or society at large. Interventions directed toward the abuser include improving coping skills, enhancing self-esteem, treating psychopathology and substance abuse, creating realistic developmental expectations, providing emotional and material support, and changing attitudes toward violence as a means of resolving conflict.
- Interventions directed toward the potential victim include changing perceptions of the acceptability of violence, enhancing self-esteem, and strengthening empowerment.
- Interventions directed toward society include advocacy and political activity to promote nonviolence and effective conflict resolution, reducing agism, promoting legal sanctions for violent behavior, and eliminating societal conditions that create stress for vulnerable families.
- Secondary prevention of family violence is directed toward two goals—protecting the victim and breaking the cycle of violence. This involves reporting cases of abuse, removing victims from abusive situations, and treating the abuser, the victim, and the family.
- Tertiary prevention of family violence may involve providing emotional and material support, providing respite, and referral to self-help groups.
- Homicide involves death resulting from injury purposefully inflicted by another person; suicide is the voluntary taking of one's own life.

- Groups at particular risk for homicide include children and young black and Hispanic males.
- Psychological environmental factors that may contribute to homicide include poor coping strategies, views of violence as an appropriate means of resolving conflict, poor impulse control, and possible psychopathology. Homicide may also be purposefully provoked by the victim.
- Social environmental factors that contribute to homicide include societal acceptance of violence; stress due to societal circumstances such as poverty and discrimination; crime and gang membership; and the availability of weapons.
- Life-style factors of psychoactive substance use and abuse and occupation may contribute to homicide.
- Human biological factors that may influence suicide include low levels of biochemical neurotransmitters and maturational events such as adolescence, menopause, and aging.
- Psychological environmental factors in the incidence of suicide can include psychopathology, hopelessness engendered by a terminal or debilitating disease, poor impulse control, response to stress, feelings engendered by the suicide of others, previous suicide attempts, and persistent thoughts about suicide.
- Social environmental factors related to suicide include poor interpersonal relationships, poor school performance, easy availability of means of suicide, joblessness, and media coverage of suicides.
- Alcohol and drug abuse are the primary lifestyle factors associated with suicide.
- Health system factors contributing to suicide include lack of attention to persons at risk for suicide and failure to identify potential suicide victims. Lack of access to a regular source of health care can also be a contributing factor.
- Primary prevention of suicide and homicide involves teaching coping skills and enhancing clients' self-esteem, assisting in the development of stress-management skills, and teaching conflict-management strategies. Other measures include limiting accessibility to weapons and other modes of suicide and homicide. The effects of school-based education about suicide are questionable at present.
- Secondary prevention of homicide and suicide includes identifying persons at risk for suicide, referral for treatment, and/or use of a suicide prevention contract. Secondary prevention also involves providing adequate care to victims of assault and suicide.
- Tertiary prevention of suicide involves the prevention of suicide clusters through the development of community response plans. Tertiary prevention may also involve working with the families of homicide and suicide victims.

Review Questions

1. Describe the four types of child abuse. (p. 900)
2. Describe the three stages of spouse abuse. (p. 901)
3. Identify at least five forms of elder abuse. (p. 901)
4. Describe the influence of at least three human biological factors in family violence. (p. 902)
5. Identify at least four environmental factors that influence family violence. (p. 903)
6. Describe at least three areas of focus in primary prevention of family violence. How might the community health nurse be involved in each? (p. 912)
7. Identify at least two approaches to the secondary prevention of family violence. What community health nursing activities might be related to each? (p. 916)
8. Describe at least two factors in each of the four components of the epidemiologic perspective related to homicide. (p. 921)
9. Describe at least two factors in each of the components of the epidemiologic perspective related to suicide. (p. 923)
10. Identify at least three primary prevention measures for homicide and suicide. How might the community health nurse be involved in each? (p. 927)

APPLICATION AND SYNTHESIS

On a routine postpartum visit, your client, Mrs. Thompson, mentions that she is very concerned about her next-door neighbor, Mrs. Drew, who is pregnant. Mrs. Thompson tells you that she thinks Mr. Drew beat his wife last night. She heard shouting during the night, and this morning she noticed that Mrs. Drew had a black eye that she said she got when she ran into the bedroom door in the dark. Before leaving the apartment complex, you knock on the Drews' door, but no one answers. You leave your card asking Mrs. Drew to call you.

When Mrs. Drew phones the next day, you explain that you were responding to the concern of a friend for her safety and ask if she is in need of assistance. Mrs. Drew tells you that there is nothing wrong. When you mention that Mrs. Thompson described some injuries, she denies that her husband is abusive. She states that she is receiving prenatal care from a private physician, will contact him if she has any problems with the pregnancy, and is not in need of your services. You accept her refusal of help, but you inform her that you are available and can be reached by phone if she needs assistance at some time in the future.

A month later you receive a call from Mrs. Drew, who asks to see you. She indicates that she is afraid to have you come to her home lest her husband return while you are there. She agrees to meet you at the health department when she comes to get a copy of her daughter's immunization record for school entry.

When you see Mrs. Drew, she admits that her husband beat her the previous day. This is the second time he has assaulted her since she became pregnant. She has several bruises on her face and one particularly large bruise on her abdomen where her husband hit her. Mrs. Drew says that her husband is very jealous and does not believe the baby is his. She insists that she has been faithful to her husband and has tried to convince him of this. She says her husband gets angry because she "shows herself off to other men and gives them a come-on." She comments, "I guess he's right. I do wear shorts a lot, because they're comfortable in this hot weather. I really should try to respect his wishes more."

Mrs. Drew has tried to convince her husband that the baby is his. She has stopped going out with female friends and even tries to avoid talking to the mailman and other males who come to the house. She has not even been to see her family because her husband refuses to go with her and accuses her of meeting her lover on these excursions.

Since the beating yesterday, Mrs. Drew says she is afraid for her own safety as well as that of her unborn child. She says that her husband loves their daughter and would not hurt her. Mrs. Drew has never worked although she completed nursing school before she got married. She feels as though she should get away from her husband even though she still loves him. However, she has no money to support herself and her daughter. She does not feel she can go to relatives because her husband would be able to find her there and bring her back home. She is also afraid that if she leaves him, her husband will attempt to get custody of their daughter.

1. What are the health problems evident in this situation? What are the human biological, environmental, life-style, and health system factors influencing these problems?
2. What considerations are important in planning care for Mrs. Drew?
3. What secondary prevention measures would be warranted to deal with existing health problems? Describe specific actions that you would take to resolve these problems.
4. What could be done in terms of tertiary prevention to prevent further consequences or recurrence of health problems in this situation?
5. What primary prevention measures might have prevented the development of the health problems in this situation? How might you, as a community health nurse, be involved in such measures?

REFERENCES

1. Gage, R. B. (1990). Consequences of children's exposure to spouse abuse. *Pediatric Nursing, 16*, 258–260.
2. Broome, M. E., & Daniels, D. (1987). Child abuse: A multidimensional phenomenon. *Holistic Nursing Practice, 1*(2), 13–24.
3. Gil, D. G. (1975). Unraveling child abuse. *American Journal of Orthopsychiatry, 45*, 346–356.
4. United States Department of Commerce. (1991). *Statistical abstract of the United States*. Washington, DC: Government Printing Office.
5. Cupoli, J. M. (1988). Is it child abuse? *Patient Care, 22*(15), 28–51.
6. United States Department of Health and Human Services. (1991). *Healthy people 2000: National health promotion and disease prevention objectives*. Washington, DC: Government Printing Office.
7. Straus, M., & Gelles, R. J. (1987). The costs of family violence. *Public Health Reports, 102*, 638–641.
8. Symonds, M. (1978). The psychodynamics of violence-prone marriages. *The American Journal of Psychoanalysis, 38*, 213–222.
9. Collier, J. A. (1987). When you suspect your patient is a battered wife. *RN, 50*(5), 22–25.
10. Tilden, V. P., & Shepherd, P. (1987). Battered women: The shadow side of families. *Holistic Nursing Practice, 1*(2), 25–32.
11. McLeer, S. V., & Anwar, R. (1989). A study of battered women presenting in an emergency department. *American Journal of Public Health, 79*, 65–66.
12. Nuttall, S. E., Greaves, L., & Lent, B. (1985). Wife battering: An emerging problem in public health. *Canadian Journal of Public Health, 76*, 297–299.
13. Family and other intimate assaults—Atlanta, 1984. (1990). *MMWR, 39*, 525–529.
14. Baumhover, L. A., Beall, S. C., & Pieroni, R. E. (1990). Elder abuse: An overview of social and medical indicators. *Journal of Health and Human Resources Administration, 12*, 414–433.
15. Hickey, R., & Douglass, R. (1981). Mistreatment of the elderly in the domestic setting: An exploration study. *American Journal of Public Health, 71*, 500–507.
16. Fulmer, T. T., & O'Malley, T.A. (1987). *Inadequate care of the elderly: A health perspective on abuse and neglect*. New York: Springer.
17. Gelles, R. J., & Cornell, C. P. (1990). *Intimate violence in families* (2nd ed). Newbury Park, CA: Sage.
18. Fulmer, T., & Ashley, J. (1989). Clinical indicators of elder neglect. *Applied Nursing Research, 2*, 161–167.
19. Ashley, J., & Fulmer, T. T. (1988). No simple way to determine elder abuse. *Geriatric Nursing, 9*, 286–288.
20. Spence, D. M. (1990). The elder assessment team: Protecting elders from abuse and neglect. *Nursing Administration Quarterly, 14*(2), 24–28.
21. Campbell, J. (1984). Nursing care of families using violence. In J. Campbell & J. Humphreys (Eds.), *Nursing care of victims of family violence*. Reston, VA: Reston.
22. Benedict, M. I., & White, R. B. (1985). Selected perinatal factors and child abuse. *American Journal of Public Health, 75*, 780–781.
23. Jason, J., Andereck, N. D., Marks, J., & Tyler, C. W. (1982). Child abuse in Georgia: A method to evaluate risk factors and reporting bias. *American Journal of Public Health, 72*, 1353–1358.
24. Mowbray, C. A. (1989). Shedding light on elder abuse. *Journal of Gerontological Nursing, 15*(10), 20–24.
25. Hamilton, G. P. (1989). Using a prevent elder abuse family systems approach. *Journal of Gerontological Nursing, 15*(3), 21–26.
26. Krob, M. J., Johnson, A., & Jordan, M. H. (1986). Burned-and-battered adults. *Journal of Burn Care Rehabilitation, 7*, 529–531.
27. Steinmetz, S. (1980). Women and violence: Victims and perpetrators. *American Journal of Psychotherapy, 34*, 334–349.
28. Cicchetti, D., & Toth, S. L. (1987). The application of a transactional risk model to intervention with multirisk maltreating families. *Zero to Three, VII*(5), 1–8.
29. Zuravin, S. (1985). Housing and child maltreatment: Is there a connection? *Children Today, 14*(6), 9–13.
30. Helton, A. S., McFarlane, J., & Anderson, E. T. (1987). Prevalence of battering during pregnancy: Focus on behavioral change. *Public Health Nursing, 4*(3), 166–174.
31. Delunas, L. R. (1990). Prevention of elder abuse: Betty Neuman health care systems approach. *Clinical Nurse Specialist, 4*(1), 54–58.
32. Pillemer, K. (1985). The dangers of dependency: New findings on domestic violence against the elderly. *Social Problems, 33*(2), 146–157.
33. Erchak, G. M. (1984). Cultural anthropology and spouse abuse. *Current Anthropology, 25*, 331–332.
34. Gibbs, J. L. (1984). On cultural anthropology and spouse abuse. *Current Anthropology, 25*, 533.
35. Levinson, D. (1985). On wife-beating and intervention. *Current Anthropology, 26*, 665–666.
36. Ewing, W. A. (1987). Domestic violence and community care ethics: Reflections on systemic intervention. *Family and Community Health, 10*(1), 54–62.
37. Kjervik, D. H. (1990). Ethical and legal dilemmas of battered women. *Journal of Professional Nursing, 6*, 253.
38. Louie, K. B. (1985). Providing health care to Chinese clients. *Topics in Clinical Nursing, 7*(3), 18–25.
39. Rosenberg, J. A. (1986). Health care for Cambodian children: Integrating treatment plans. *Pediatric Nursing, 12*(2), 118–125.
40. Muecke, M. A. (1983). Caring for Southeast Asian refugee patients in the U.S.A. *American Journal of Public Health, 73*, 431–438.
41. Blair, K. A. (1986). The battered woman: Is she a silent victim? *Nurse Practitioner, 11*(6), 38–47.
42. Janz, M. (1990). Clues to elder abuse. *Geriatric Nursing, 11*, 220–222.
43. Weiler, K. (1989). Financial abuse of the elderly: Recognizing and acting on it. *Journal of Gerontological Nursing, 15*(8), 10–15.
44. King, M. C., & Ryan, J. (1989). Abused women: Dispelling myths and encouraging interventions. *Nurse Practitioner, 14*(5), 47–58.

45. Straus, M. B. (1988). Introduction. In M. B. Straus (Ed.), *Abuse and victimization across the life span.* Baltimore: Johns Hopkins University Press.
46. Bergman, B., Larsson, G., Brismar, B., & Klang, M. (1989). Battered wives and alcoholic females: A comparative social and psychiatric study. *Journal of Advanced Nursing, 14,* 727–734.
47. Snyder, C., & Spietz, A. (1977). Characteristics of abuse: A report of five families. *Nurse Practitioner, 2*(8), 23–27.
48. Wegmann, M. P., & Lancaster, J. (1981). Child neglect and abuse. *Family & Community Health, 4*(2), 11–17.
49. Limandri, B. J. (1987). The therapeutic relationship with abused women: Nurses' response that facilitate or inhibit change. *Journal of Psychosocial Nursing, 25*(2), 9–16.
50. Fulmer, T. T. (1989). Mistreatment of elders: Assessment, diagnosis, and intervention. *Nursing Clinics of North America, 24,* 707–716.
51. Bullock, L., McFarlane, J., Bateman, L. H., & Miller, V. (1989). The prevalence and characteristics of battered women in a primary care setting. *Nurse Practitioner, 14*(6), 49–56.
52. United States Department of Health and Human Services. (1990). *Health United States 1989.* Hyattsville, MD: Public Health Service.
53. Occupational homicides among women—United States, 1980–1985. (1990). *MMWR, 39,* 544–545, 551–552.
54. Homicide among young black males—United States, 1978–1987. (1990). *MMWR, 39,* 869–873.
55. Premature mortality due to homicides—United States, 1968–1985. (1988). *MMWR, 37,* 543–545.
56. Prothrow-Stith, D. (1987). Violence prevention. *Public Health Reports, 102,* 615–616.
57. Monk, M. (1987). Epidemiology of suicide. *Epidemiologic Reviews, 9,* 51–69.
58. Homicide among young black males—United States, 1970–1982. (1985). *MMWR, 34,* 629–633.
59. Homicide surveillance: High-risk racial and ethnic groups—Blacks and Hispanics, 1970 to 1983. (1987). *MMWR, 36,* 634–636.
60. Smith, J. C., Mercy, J. A., & Rosenberg, M. L. (1988). Comparisons of homicides among Anglos and Hispanics in five southwestern states. *Border Health, IV*(1), 2–15.
61. Homicide—Los Angeles, 1970–1979. (1986). *MMWR, 35,* 61–65.
62. Hall, J. M., & Stevens, P. E. (1988). AIDS: A guide to suicide assessment. *Archives of Psychiatric Nursing, 1,* 115–120.
63. Rose, H. M. (1987). Homicide and minorities. *Public Health Reports, 102,* 613–615.
64. O'Carroll, P. W. (1988). Homicides among black males 15–24 years of age, 1970–1984. *CDC Surveillance Summaries, 37*(SS-1), 53–60.
65. Have gun, will carry. (1987). *U.S. News & World Report, 103*(25), 76.
66. Goodman, R. A., Mercy, J. A., Loya, F., et al. (1986). Alcohol use and interpersonal violence: Alcohol detected in homicide victims. *American Journal of Public Health, 76,* 144–149.
67. Progress toward achieving the national 1990 objectives for injury prevention and control. (1988). *MMWR, 37,* 138–140.
68. Shaffer, D. (1987). Strategies for prevention of youth suicide. *Public Health Reports, 102,* 611–613.
69. Suicide—United States, 1970–1980. (1985). *MMWR, 34,* 353–357.
70. Barraclough, B., & Hughes, J. (1987). *Suicide: Clinical and epidemiological studies.* London: Croom Helm.
71. Slap, G. B., Vorters, D. F., Chaudhuri, S., & Centor, R. M. (1989). Risk factors for attempted suicide during adolescence. *Pediatrics, 84,* 762–772.
72. Grossman, D. C., Milligan, B. C., & Deyo, R. A. (1991). Risk factors for suicide attempts among Navajo adolescents. *American Journal of Public Health, 81,* 870–874.
73. Assey, J. L. (1985). The suicide prevention contract. *Perspectives in Psychiatric Care, XXIII,* 99–103.
74. Smith, J. C., Mercy, J. A., & Conn, J. M. (1988). Marital status and risk of suicide. *American Journal of Public Health, 78,* 78–80.
75. Saltzman, L. E., & Levenson, A. (1988). Suicide among persons 15–24 years of age, 1970–1984. *CDC Surveillance Summaries, 37*(SS-1), 61–68.
76. O'Carroll, W., Mercy, J. S., & Steward, J. A. *CDC recommendations for a community plan for the prevention and containment of suicide clusters.* (1988). *MMWR, 37*(Suppl. S-6), 1–12.
77. Hlady, W. G., & Middaugh, J. P. (1988). Suicides in Alaska: Firearms and alcohol. *American Journal of Public Health, 78,* 179–180.

RECOMMENDED READINGS

Assey, J. L. (1985). The suicide prevention contract. *Perspectives in Psychiatric Care, XXIII,* 99–103.

Describes the use of a suicide prevention contract between nurse and client to motivate clients to refrain from killing themselves. Also presents indicators of impending suicide for which nurses can assess clients.

Barraclough, B., & Hughes, J. (1987). *Suicide: Clinical and epidemiological studies.* London: Croom Helm.

Presents an overview of the epidemiology of suicide. Describes the findings of research studies on factors associated with suicide.

Baumhover, L. A., Beall, S. C., & Pieroni, R. E. (1990). Elder abuse: An overview of social and medical indicators. *Journal of Health and Human Resources Administration, 12,* 414–433.

Offers a concise overview of elder abuse, etiological theories, clinical signs and symptoms of abuse, and interventions.

Campbell, J. C. (1989). A test of two explanatory models of women's responses to battering. *Nursing Research, 38,* 18–24.

Sets forth two theoretical models explaining the differing responses of women to battering. Also presents findings of a research study testing the two models.

Fulmer, T. T. (1989). Mistreatment of elders: Assessment, diagnosis, and intervention. *Nursing Clinics of North America, 24,* 707–716.

Contains an overview of the phenomenon of elder abuse, theoretical explanations, difficulties in assessing older clients for abuse, and interventions to prevent abuse.

Gelles, R. J., & Cornell, C. P. (1990). *Intimate violence in families* (2nd ed.). Newbury Park, CA: Sage.

Presents an overview of violence occurring within family constellations. Addresses child abuse, spouse abuse, and elder abuse.

Hamilton, G. P. (1989). Using a prevent elder abuse family systems approach. *Journal of Gerontological Nursing, 15*(3), 21–26.

Discusses four patterns of family systems interaction that may indicate abuse of older clients.

King, M. C., & Ryan, J. (1989). Abused women: Dispelling myths and encouraging interventions. *Nurse Practitioner, 14*(5), 47–58.

Examines myths that create barriers to effective intervention with abused women. Also discusses nursing responses that facilitate change in abusive situations.

Leahey, M., & Wright, L. M. (1987). *Families and psychosocial problems.* Springhouse, PA: Springhouse.

Focuses on nursing assessment and intervention with families experiencing a variety of psychosocial problems including family violence.

Limandri, B. J. (1987). The therapeutic relationship with abused women: Nurses' responses that facilitate or inhibit change. *Journal of Psychosocial Nursing, 25*(2), 9–16.

Looks at factors that influence the behavior of abused women in seeking help and nursing responses that facilitate or inhibit help-seeking behavior.

Monk, M. (1987). Epidemiology of suicide. *Epidemiologic Reviews, 9,* 51–69.

Discusses epidemiologic factors contributing to the incidence of suicide.

Scherb, B. J. (1988). Standardized care plans: Suspected abuse and neglect of children. *Journal of Emergency Nursing, 14*(1), 44–47.

Describes subjective and objective data suggestive of child abuse and possible nursing diagnoses related to abuse. Also presents a standardized plan of care for abused children.

UNIT SEVEN

Other Models for Community Health Nursing

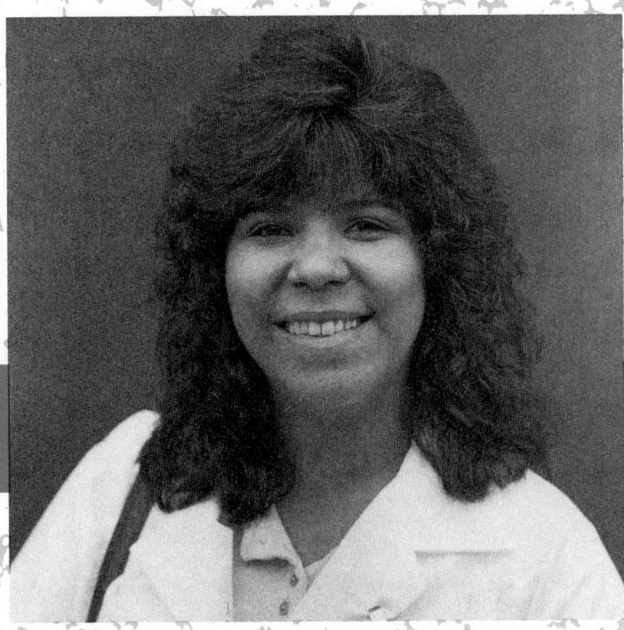

The epidemiologic prevention process model around which this book is organized may not meet the needs of every community health nurse in every situation. For that reason, this unit is devoted to a discussion of several other models that may be useful in community health nursing practice.

A number of nursing models have been described in the literature over the years. However, many of these were developed exclusively for use with individual clients and are not easily adapted for use with families or communities. In Chapter 35, Nursing Models for Community Health Practice, several nursing models that can be adapted to meet the needs of the variety of clients served by community health nurses are explored. The models to be addressed include the Roy Adaptation Model, Levine's Principles of Conservation, Orem's Self-Care Model, Johnson's Behavioral Systems Model, Neuman's Health Systems Model, and Pender's Health Promotion Model.

For each of the models discussed, underlying concepts of the model and their interrelationships are presented. Each model is also applied to the care of individuals, families, and communities.

From the Community: A Nurse's Voice

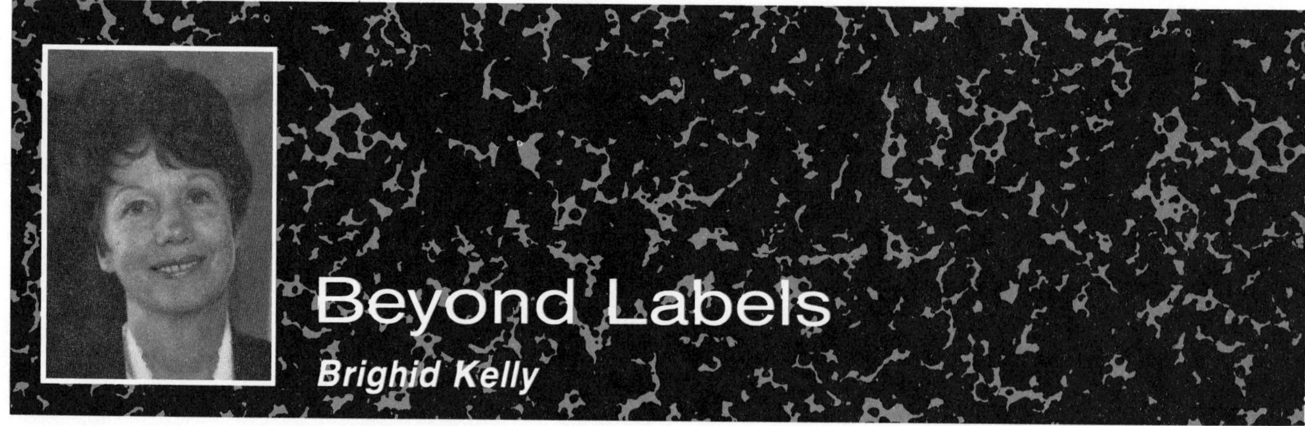

Beyond Labels

Brighid Kelly

In our work as community health nurses, what we believe is best for a client sometimes conflicts with the client's right to self-determination. All too frequently, when a client does not adhere to our "care plan," we are apt to label the client as being "noncompliant." True, as nurses we have spent years learning about health and illness and have a professional service to provide. Nevertheless, we poorly serve our clients' needs when we yield to the temptation to affix labels rather than to take the time to inquire into clients' concerns.

Ruth, a student of mine, was serving her community health practicum with a local home health agency. On her first visit, the agency nurse accompanying Ruth was quick to point out that the client they would see that day was constantly "noncompliant." The client, an elderly woman, was being followed for hypertension, the treatment plan involving a series of relaxation exercises in conjunction with diet and medication. During the visit, Ruth noticed that the client was trying to tell the agency nurse about a family concern, but the nurse showed little interest. Prior to leaving, the nurse dutifully went over all the points of the plan and informed the client that Ruth would be visiting her for several weeks.

On subsequent visits, Ruth learned that the client was upset about her granddaughter, who was apparently being physically abused by the grandchild's stepfather. On several occasions, the granddaughter had shown up at the client's home in the middle of the night, pounding on the front door and screaming in terror. Ruth listened, investigated the situation, and—with my help—notified the proper authorities. As a result, a social worker was assigned to the granddaughter and the frantic nighttime visits soon stopped. Would it surprise you to learn that the client's hypertension showed remarkable improvement? Ruth learned that a "label" (in this case "noncompliant") was obscuring the complete picture of the client's circumstances.

Or consider another case in which a woman with a medical diagnosis of diabetes had become intensely belligerent with the nurses at the agency. The nurses working with this client claimed she was not maintaining her proper level of insulin nor was she eating properly. Eventually, the client refused to talk to them. The agency had just about decided to terminate services to the client on the basis that she was "noncompliant." I persuaded the agency to assign the client to one of my students, and together we paid her a visit. I was immediately aware of the client's hostility by her expression and tone of voice. Questions about her health status were curtly answered and often accompanied by remarks about how "nobody really cares anyhow."

I asked her, "What do *you* think is your biggest problem?" Her expression softened. After a moment of silence she said that her biggest problem was the loss of her Social Security check because of some misunderstanding about her widow's status. She had spent weeks on the phone trying to sort it out, but to no avail. The local Social Security office had sent a number of forms that she couldn't understand. I asked to see them and soon realized our client was functionally illiterate. I told her we would look into the problem for her, and in the meantime my student would assist her in filling out the forms. As it turned out, her benefits were reinstated. Although the client's health status did not improve dramatically, her attitude did, and she showed a renewed interest in maintaining her health.

How often, then, is a diagnosis of "noncompliance" really attributable to poor communication or even to lack of caring on the nurse's part? While the ability to communicate well is the greatest skill a nurse can possess, it is useless without caring. Caring is taking the extra time to look beyond the "record" in order to get to know the client. Caring is listening and watching for what is not being said and seeing a client as someone with unique strengths, priorities, and goals. A caring community health nurse can facilitate enormous change simply by looking beyond labels.

CHAPTER 35

Nursing Models for Community Health Practice

KEY TERMS

adaptation
adaptation level
basic structure
behavioral system
behavioral subsystem
conservation of energy
contextual stimuli
developmental self-care
flexible line of defense
focal stimuli
health deviation self-care
individual perceptions
lines of resistance
modifying factors
normal line of defense
nursing model
nursing theory
perseverative set
personal integrity
preparatory set
reconstitution
regulatory mechanisms
residual stimuli
social integrity
stressor
structural integrity
universal self-care
zone of adaptation

One of the hallmarks of a scientific profession is the unique body of knowledge that it uses to direct professional practice. This body of knowledge is the result of systematic, scientific inquiry involving the formulation and testing of theory. As is the case with other scientific disciplines, professional nursing practice needs a sound theoretical foundation that describes the interrelationships among four key concepts: client, society, health, and nursing.

A ***nursing theory*** is a set of interrelated concepts explaining events of interest to nursing.[1] Many nurses regard nursing theory and practice as separate professional dimensions that are only vaguely interrelated. In reality, theory and practice are inseparably intertwined. Theory arises out of practice to direct or explain practice.[1]

As noted in Chapter 10, The Research Process, community health nursing research often lacks a theoretical basis. This professional shortcoming has been attributed in part to the lack of a community or aggregate focus in many nursing models developed to date.[2] There are, however, some theoretical models in nursing that can be adapted for use in community health nursing.

LEARNING OBJECTIVES

After reading this chapter you should be able to:

- Describe three major concepts of the Roy Adaptation Model.
- Describe four major concepts of Levine's Principles of Conservation.
- Describe three major concepts of Orem's Self-Care Model.
- Describe five major concepts of Johnson's Behavioral Systems Model.
- Describe five major concepts of Neuman's Health Systems Model.
- Describe three major concepts of Pender's Health Promotion Model.

NURSING MODELS

For it to be systematic rather than haphazard, nursing practice requires a framework that arises from a specific approach to the client. This framework is supplied by a nursing model. A ***nursing model*** is a systematic and logically related set of concepts incorporating the essential components of nursing practice and the scientific theories on which practice is based.[3] A model may encompass several theories and give rise to others.

Think of a model in terms of building a house. The model is similar to the blueprint according to which the house is constructed. The blueprint provides the basic outline or framework around which the structure is erected. The materials from which the house is constructed (for example, the bricks and wood) are analogous to the concepts involved in nursing, such as self-image or oxygenation. Theories are the cohesive bond that joins the materials into a unit—nursing practice—just as the mortar and nails join bricks and wood in a house.

To direct practice, nursing models must incorporate three basic components: the client, the goal of nursing intervention, and the activities involved in nursing intervention. First, a nursing model must define who is the client or recipient of nursing action. Is the nursing client always someone who is ill or can the client be a healthy individual? Furthermore, can the recipient of care be a family or a community rather than an individual? Second, the model must specify the expected outcome of nursing intervention. Different nursing models use different terms to express outcomes; for instance, "adaptation," "reconstitution," or "self-care." The final requisite for a nursing model is a description of the nurse's activities in providing care. Again, depending on the nursing model, these activities may be educative, curative, restorative, supportive, or preventative in nature.

NURSING MODELS FOR COMMUNITY HEALTH NURSING

Most of the chapters in this book have applied one nursing model, the Epidemiologic Prevention Process Model, to community health nursing. This chapter presents six other nursing models developed by Roy, Levine, Orem, Johnson, Neuman, and Pender. All of these models were developed for use with individual clients but can be adapted for use with families, groups, or communities.

THE ROY ADAPTATION MODEL

The Adaptation Model of Callista Roy conceives of the client as a system adapting to changes in the environment. Within the environment, the client interacts with others, including the nurse, and this interaction influences adaptive capabilities.

CONCEPTS OF THE ROY MODEL

Three concepts are basic to the Roy model: person or client, adaptation, and nursing. The person or client is viewed as a totality, as a "biopsychosocial unit" interacting with the environment. In adapting the model for use in community health nursing, the "person" or client who receives nursing care can be an individual, a family, a group, or a community.

The goal of the client in interactions with the environment is ***adaptation***, a positive response to changes in the internal and/or external environment.[4] The client's ability to adapt is related to the extent of the change experienced and to the ability to cope with the change.[5] For example, everyone is exposed to various forms of stress each day. Stress causes changes in one's internal psychological environment as well as physiologic changes. Moderate levels of stress keep one alert and motivated, whereas too much stress causes maladaptation. One's ability to cope with stress also influences one's response. Suppose that two people are exposed to the same level of stress, but that one has good coping skills and one does not. The person with good coping skills will probably be able to adapt positively to the stress encountered; the other person will not.

Families and groups of people can also vary in their ability to adapt to changes in the environment. For example, a family may adapt positively or negatively to a move to another town, whereas a community adapts positively or negatively to the establishment of a new industry in town.

The client's ability to cope, or ***adaptation level***, is influenced by three categories of stimuli: focal stimuli, contextual stimuli, and residual stimuli.[4] ***Focal stimuli*** include the environmental change to which the client must adapt. ***Contextual stimuli*** are those other stimuli in the situation that influence the client's adaptive response. In the stress example, the focal stimulus might be a dead auto battery, the current source of stress, while other factors such as fatigue and worry about being late for work would be contextual stimuli affecting the client's response to the focal stimulus. ***Residual stimuli*** are the result of past experiences that affect current responses to focal stimuli. For example, one might have painful memories about a time when a dead car battery caused one to miss an important appointment.

Adaptation occurs when the total stimuli impinging on the client fall within the ***zone of adaptation***, or the limits of the client's adaptive capacity. For the individual, the amount of stress related to the focal stimulus of a dead battery and the contextual and residual stimuli operating in the situation may result in a negative response or maladaptation. Similarly, if unemployment is the reason for the family's move to another locale, that factor, coupled with the move itself, may place events beyond the family's zone of adaptation. In the same way, a community that is coping with other stressors may not be able to adapt effectively to the advent of a new industry. For example, if roadways are already heavily congested with traffic, the addition of a major new industry may move the traffic problem beyond the community's zone of adaptation.

Adaptation takes place in four modes: physiologic, self-concept, role function, and interdependence.[4] The physiologic mode involves adaptation to maintain physical integrity. The detoxification of alcohol by the liver is an example of this mode. Maintenance of psychological integrity is the function of the self-concept mode. For example, the husband who attributes his wife's anger to her having a bad day at work rather than to his own behavior is adapting in the self-concept mode to maintain psychological integrity. The self-concept mode includes the physical self, the personal self, and the interpersonal self.[4]

The role-function mode involves adaptation in interpersonal interactions to maintain social integrity. A client who successfully accomplishes the parenting role after the birth of a child is adapting in the role-function mode. Adaptation in the interdependence mode involves maintaining a balance between dependence and independence. Adaptation in this mode may take the form of seeking help, seeking affection, or initiative taking.[4] A client with a new baby, for example, who seeks advice on child care from his or her mother while continuing to accept primary responsibility for the child's welfare is adapting in the interdependence mode.

Nursing intervention, in the Roy model, attempts to alter stimuli to fall within the client's zone of adaptation or to alter the client's response to stimuli.[6] Nursing action begins with assessment at two levels. First-level assessment involves looking for evidence of maladaptive behaviors. Second-level assessment involves determining the focal, contextual, and residual stimuli influencing the maladaptive behavior.[4] The nurse then engages in activity designed to promote adaptive behaviors. Nursing intervention might involve manipulating the client system, manipulating the environment, or both.[4]

APPLYING THE ROY MODEL TO COMMUNITY HEALTH NURSING

The Roy model can be used to direct nursing care for an individual, a family, or a community as client. All three levels of client must adapt to changes in the environment in order to survive. Table 35–1 describes

TABLE 35–1. CLIENT ASSESSMENT IN THE ROY ADAPTATION MODEL

	Assessment		
Model Concept	***Individual***	***Family***	***Community***
Situation requiring adaptation	Unwed pregnancy	Teenage daughter's pregnancy	Increased incidence of teenage pregnancy
Focal stimulus	Pregnancy	Pregnancy of teen	Increased incidence rate for teenage pregnancy
Contextual stimuli	Overall health status Extent of family support Attitude toward pregnancy Relationship with baby's father Access to prenatal care	Age of teenage daughter Family attitude to teen sexual activity Presence or absence of other family stressors	Availability of contraceptive services Community attitudes toward teen sexual activity
Residual stimuli	Age and maturity of teen Family and cultural attitude toward illegitimacy Attitudes to children Personal ambitions and goals Income level Educational level	Cultural and religious background Family income Educational level	Extent of teen population Availability of prenatal and child health services Community attitudes toward illegitimacy and sex education for teens Income levels Educational levels

a situation involving adolescent pregnancy in which an individual, a family, and a community must engage in adaptive behaviors. This example is used throughout the chapter and is addressed from the perspective of the adolescent client who plans to continue the pregnancy and keep the baby.

Table 35–1 presents an assessment of the potential focal, contextual, and residual stimuli involved for the individual, the family, and the community. The focal stimulus for the individual is the fact of her pregnancy. Their daughter's pregnancy is also the focal stimulus for the family. In the case of the community, the focal stimulus is a recent rise in the number of teenage pregnancies. Contextual stimuli for the individual include her overall health status, the extent of family support available, her attitude to the pregnancy, her relationship with the baby's father, and the availability of prenatal care. All of these factors will influence the way in which the teen will respond to the fact of pregnancy.

Contextual stimuli for the family include the age of their daughter, family attitudes to teen sexual activity, and the extent of other stressors in the family. If the girl is quite young, parents might argue for abortion or adoption rather than keeping the baby. Or, if family members have strong feelings against sexual activity by teens, they might feel compelled to force the girl to leave home. Additional stressors within the family will also affect the family's ability to adapt effectively. For example, if parents are unemployed, the addition of another family member will be more difficult than if family income is adequate.

In the case of the community, contextual stimuli might include the availability of contraceptive services and community attitudes toward adolescent sexual activity. Communities with adequate facilities for contraceptive services for teens will have less difficulty adapting to the problem of teenage pregnancy than those with inadequate services. Similarly, community resistance to sexual activity by teens will make it more difficult to deal realistically with the problem.

From the point of view of Roy's model, residual stimuli are less amenable to change than are focal or contextual stimuli. For the individual, residual stimuli include the age and maturity level of the teen, family and cultural attitudes to illegitimacy, attitudes toward children, personal ambitions and goals, and income and educational levels. A very mature teenager will adapt to the reality of pregnancy more readily than an immature girl. Adaptation will also be easier in situations in which illegitimacy carries little stigma and in which children are welcomed and cherished. On the other hand, personal goals for college and a career might influence decisions in favor of abortion or adoption. Income and educational levels will also affect the ease of adaptation by influencing the resources at hand for dealing with the pregnancy.

Residual stimuli for the family are similar to those for the individual client and include the family's cultural and religious background and income and educational levels. These factors will influence family adaptation in much the same way that they influence the adaptation of the individual. For the community, residual stimuli include the extent of the teenage population, the availability of prenatal and child health services to meet increased demands for care, community attitudes toward illegitimacy and sex education, and community income and educational levels. If there are relatively few teens in the total population, the problem is more easily dealt with than if teens constitute a large percentage of the population. Similarly, the existence of adequate health-care services will allow the community to deal with the problem of increased demands for prenatal and child health care with greater ease than would otherwise be the case. Community attitudes and income and educational levels influence community adaptation in much the same way that these factors influence the adaptation of the individual and family.

In Roy's model, when the total of focal, contextual, and residual stimuli falls within the client's zone of adaptation, adaptation occurs. Table 35–2 presents examples of possible adaptive behaviors on the part of the individual, family, and community in each of the adaptive modes. Again, the situation requiring adaptive behavior is adolescent pregnancy.

Adaptation in the physiologic mode involves maintaining appropriate internal functioning to deal with the problem. For the individual, the body's response to pregnancy includes increased hunger, fatigue, and changes in hormonal levels. These responses stimulate behaviors of eating and rest designed to meet the body's heightened needs during pregnancy. For the family, adaptation in this mode involves activities to provide for the physical needs of the teen and the new baby. In the community, adaptation may necessitate expansion of existing prenatal and well-child services to meet increased needs.

Within the self-concept mode, the individual client who is adapting effectively adjusts to the pregnancy without perceiving herself as "bad." Parents must also adapt by accepting the situation without blaming themselves. For the community, adaptation in the self-concept mode entails recognition that a serious problem exists and that action must be taken to resolve it. The community that is not adapting well in this mode might continue to display the attitude that adolescent pregnancy does not occur despite evidence to the contrary.

TABLE 35–2. SAMPLE ADAPTIVE BEHAVIORS IN THE ROY MODEL

Model Concept	Adaptive Behaviors		
Modes of Adaptation	*Individual*	*Family*	*Community*
Physiologic mode	Increased hunger to meet baby's need for food Increased fatigue Changes in hormonal levels	Provision for meeting physical needs of teen and baby	Health-care delivery system expands prenatal care and well-child services to meet increased need
Self-concept mode	Client perceives self as good, deals with guilt over pregnancy	Parents deal with feelings of guilt and do not see themselves as "failures" Family adjusts to advent of new member	Community recognizes problem and begins to take action for resolution
Role-function mode	Client begins to learn maternal role Client makes adjustments in student, family, and social roles to accommodate motherhood	Family recognizes daughter in mother role Family members prepare for new roles as grandparents, aunts, uncles, etc.	Community expands its role in provision of sex education by mandating sex education in school curricula
Interdependence mode	Client seeks advice or assistance (e.g., seeks prenatal care, help from parents, etc.)	Family seeks help in adjusting to pregnancy and advent of new member	Community seeks outside help (e.g., federal funds for family planning, prenatal services)

Changes in the role-function mode must be made by clients at all three levels. The individual must begin to learn the mother role and must make adjustments within other roles (for example, student, daughter, single person) to accommodate additional role functions. For example, the girl might enroll in a school that provides child-care services on the premises. Dating activities might also be curtailed and scheduled around the baby's needs.

Family members must acknowledge the assumption of the mother role by the teen and must adjust relationships with her in relation to this role. It is sometimes difficult for parents to see their daughter as a mother with responsibility for a child, and parents may need to be encouraged to allow the girl to care for the baby herself. Family members must also adopt new roles as grandparents, aunts, uncles, and so on, which may necessitate other changes in relationships.

The community may need to reshape perceptions of its role in providing sex education and contraceptive services for teens. If these activities have been relegated to families and the private medical sector in the past because of community attitudes toward adolescent sexuality, the community may need to assume a more active role in these efforts. One way to accomplish this might be to mandate the inclusion of sex education in junior high and high school curricula.

In terms of the Roy model, adaptive behaviors in the interdependence mode for all three levels of client would involve seeking assistance. For the individual, these behaviors include seeking prenatal care and seeking assistance from parents. The family may seek counseling to adjust to the pregnancy or may seek help in finding prenatal care for the teen or well-child care for the baby. The community may seek outside assistance in the form of federal funding for special services for teens.

Using the Roy Adaptation Model, the nurse dealing with the individual, family, or community assesses the client's adaptive capabilities in each of the four modes and examines the focal, contextual, and residual stimuli involved, Nursing intervention is indicated whenever the total stimuli lie outside the client's zone of adaptation. Intervention may involve manipulation of the client or the environment, or both, directed toward a positive response to the situation. Table 35–3 presents sample nursing interventions with the individual client, family, and community in each of the four adaptive modes.

Working with the individual client and family in the physiologic mode, the nurse can aid adaptation by acquainting the teen and her family with the nutritional needs of a pregnant adolescent and, later, of a new baby and breast-feeding mother. The nurse might also encourage the teen to get adequate exercise and may provide suggestions for dealing with the discomforts of pregnancy. The nurse will also assess the client's ability to care for the child and educate her and the family to meet the baby's physiologic needs. Manipulation of the environment could

TABLE 35–3. NURSING INTERVENTIONS IN THE ROY MODEL

Model Concept	Nursing Interventions: Individual	Family	Community
Physiologic mode	*Manipulation of client:* Provide adequate nutrition; Maintain hydration; Encourage exercise; Deal with discomforts of pregnancy; Educate client to meet baby's physiologic needs. *Manipulation of environment:* Promote rest to allow redirection of energy; Refer to WIC as needed	*Manipulation of client:* Review family diet to ensure adequate nutrition for mother and baby; Educate family to meet nutritional needs of both teen and baby. *Manipulation of environment:* Refer for food supplement programs as needed	*Manipulation of client:* Help expand prenatal and child health services to meet needs of both teens and babies. *Manipulation of environment:* Solicit federal funds for programs such as WIC, etc.
Self-concept mode	*Manipulation of client:* Allow client to ventilate regarding pregnancy; Help client to deal with guilt over pregnancy; Help client to adjust to bodily changes	*Manipulation of client:* Allow family members to ventilate regarding difficulty posed by pregnancy; Help parents deal with feelings of guilt; Help family adjust to advent of new member	*Manipulation of client:* Help community to recognize existence of problem; Educate community to extent of problem
Role-function mode	*Manipulation of client:* Assist client to learn maternal role; Assist client to adjust school, family, and social roles to accommodate motherhood	*Manipulation of client:* Encourage family to allow teen to exercise mother role; Assist family to adapt to changing roles of other members	*Manipulation of environment:* Encourage view of community as having responsibility for sex education for teens; Help establish contraceptive services for teens
Interdependence mode	*Manipulation of client:* Encourage client to become independent of parents but seek their help as needed. *Manipulation of environment:* Assist client to get prenatal care; Assist client to find financial assistance; Make referrals for other assistance as needed	*Manipulation of client:* Encourage family to make use of external supports; Encourage family to allow teen independence. *Manipulation of environment:* Make referrals for outside assistance as needed; Encourage family to grant teen some independence	*Manipulation of environment:* Serve as resource person or liaison between community and outside agencies

include encouraging arrangements for the teen to get adequate rest and assisting in exploring safe sleeping arrangements for the new baby. Other activities in this area include referral of the individual or family for food supplement programs such as the Women, Infants, and Children (WIC) program. Manipulation of the community client in the physiologic mode might include the participation of the nurse in plans to expand existing prenatal and child-health services to meet increased demands.

Intervention in the self-concept mode might involve allowing the individual client and family to ventilate their feelings about the pregnancy and the difficulties it poses. The nurse can also help the teen and her parents deal with any feelings of guilt related to the pregnancy. In addition, the teen may need help in adjusting to bodily changes that occur with pregnancy, and the nurse can help her to explore and deal with her feelings regarding these changes. Both individual and family may need help in thinking of themselves in new ways necessitated by the assumption of new roles.

For the community client, nursing intervention in the self concept-mode might involve making the community aware of the growing problem of adolescent pregnancy. The nurse might accomplish this by educating the community and policymakers about the extent of the problem and its consequences for those involved and for the community at large. If the community continues to regard itself as not having a problem, adaptation will not occur.

Assistance in the role-function mode would include helping the client to learn the maternal role and suggesting ways of modifying old roles to accommodate the assumption of new role functions. For example, the nurse might teach the teen to feed, bathe, and dress the baby or make a referral for a special educational program for teens with children. The nurse may also need to encourage the family to allow the teen to exercise her role as the baby's mother and assist family members to learn new roles as grandparents. In the community, the nurse can foster a sense of community responsibility for providing sex education and contraceptive services for teenagers.

In the interdependence mode, both individual and family may require referral for outside assistance to adjust to the pregnancy and the advent of a new family member. The nurse might provide referrals for prenatal care, financial assistance, food supplement programs, and child care. The nurse may also need to function as an advocate for the teen, encouraging the family to let her function as the mother of a young child. For the community, the nurse may serve as a liaison between the community and outside sources of assistance in dealing with the teen pregnancy problem.

LEVINE'S PRINCIPLES OF CONSERVATION

The nursing model proposed by Myra Levine also addresses the necessity of adaptation to ensure survival. In this model, however, adaptation involves the conservation of energy and the integrity of the client.

CONCEPTS OF LEVINE'S MODEL

Health, in Levine's model, is defined as structural, personal, and social integrity, and energy.[7] Disruption in any of these areas results in health problems. Nursing care is directed toward conservation of these four elements of health, thereby maintaining the unity and integrity of the client. Nursing intervention is based on four principles of conservation: conservation of energy, conservation of structural integrity, conservation of personal integrity, and conservation of social integrity.[8]

Levine maintained that the ability of the individual to function depends on his or her energy potential and the energy available.[7] In the ***conservation of energy***, the nurse assesses the extent of the client's energy expenditure in relation to energy resources. Energy must be channeled into those functions most vital to survival when energy demands exceed resources. When the client is unable to conserve energy, the nurse must institute measures to assist in energy conservation.

Changes in structure lead to functional changes. ***Structural integrity*** reflects normal physiologic structure and function. The structural integrity of the client must be maintained so as to ensure adequate function. For instance, when a client loses an arm, the structural change results in loss of function. The client must adapt and relearn activities of daily living such as dressing and tying shoes. Similarly, a family must adapt to the structural change involved in death of the mother, while a community must adapt to destruction of part of the town by fire. When structural integrity is threatened, the nurse intervenes to assist the client to maintain integrity or to adapt to the change.

Personal integrity relates to the client's self-respect, identity, and individuality. Personal integrity is maintained when clients are assured their rights as unique entities and participate in decisions regarding health care. Maintenance of personal integrity also involves consideration of the client's values and social patterns.[7]

The last of Levine's principles, conservation of ***social integrity***, is concerned with the effectiveness of the client's interactions with other people. Ethnic and subcultural considerations as well as interpersonal relationships are elements of social integrity. Maintenance of social integrity involves fostering positive interactions with others.

Nursing, in Levine's model, involves assessing the degree of clients' adaptation to changes in the internal or external environments. Whenever structural, personal, or social integrity or energy use is threatened, the nurse intervenes. Intervention can be either supportive or therapeutic in nature. Supportive interventions may maintain the client at the current level of integrity or fail to prevent progressive loss of integrity. Therapeutic intervention influences adaptation to renewed integrity.

APPLYING LEVINE'S MODEL TO COMMUNITY HEALTH NURSING

Myra Levine's principles of conservation can be applied to all levels of client. Table 35–4 presents possible activities by an individual client, a family, and a community for each of the four principles of conservation related to the problem of adolescent pregnancy.

Activities of the individual directed toward conservation of energy in Levine's model would include increasing caloric intake to provide for the needs of a growing fetus and maintaining a good balance between rest and exercise. For the family, efforts in the area of energy conservation might involve redirection

TABLE 35–4. SAMPLE CONSERVATION ACTIVITIES

Model Concept	Conservation Activities: *Individual*	*Family*	*Community*
Problem	Pregnancy	Pregnancy of teenage daughter	Increased incidence of adolescent pregnancy
Conservation Principles: Conservation of energy	Increase dietary intake to provide needed energy sources Maintain balance between energy resources and expenditures	Redirect family energy to deal with pregnancy and advent of new family member	Redirect community energy and resources to provide sex education and contraceptive services for teenagers
Conservation of structural integrity	Prevent complications of pregnancy Maintain bodily functions	Maintain family function in spite of pregnancy Restructure family roles	Maintain vital community functions related to teenage pregnancy (e.g., prenatal and family planning services) Revise community structure to accommodate role in sex education
Conservation of personal integrity	Maintain self-concept as a productive person	Maintain family cohesion	Promote community participation in health-care decisions
Conservation of social integrity	Maintain interpersonal contacts in spite of pregnancy	Maintain relations with external support system Deal with guilt related to daughter's pregnancy	Maintain relations with the outside world Promote cooperation of various groups in dealing with the problem

of family energies to deal with the pregnancy and planning for the advent of a new family member. For example, the family might decide to use its savings to build an extra room on the house. Because savings can be considered an expendable commodity, it might be considered a source of family energy. The community might choose to conserve energy by redirecting resources to provide sex education and contraceptive services for teens.

In terms of Levine's model, preventing complications of pregnancy would be one way of conserving structural integrity for the individual teen. The family might take steps to be sure that the daughter's pregnancy did not cause a division of husband and wife, thus threatening the structural integrity of the family. For the community, conservation of structural integrity might involve revising the health-care structure to meet the demands of teen pregnancies, or preventing the problem from becoming a divisive issue within the community.

For the individual client, conservation of personal integrity involves maintaining one's self-concept as a productive individual, which may be impaired by guilt feelings regarding the pregnancy. Dealing positively with such feelings will help the individual to maintain personal integrity. Maintaining family cohesion by working as a group to resolve the problems of a teen pregnancy can promote the personal integrity of the family. Promotion of citizen participation in health-care decisions can serve the same function for the community.

Conservation of social integrity in the case of the individual client involves maintaining interpersonal relationships and contacts in spite of the pregnancy. Too often, adolescent girls who become pregnant are removed from school and lose the contact with peers necessary for the accomplishment of adolescent developmental tasks. If this is a local policy, other opportunities for interpersonal contact will need to be provided. Families, likewise, often shut themselves off from others in such situations, fearing the stigma of an illegitimate birth. Dealing with these feelings openly and maintaining external relationships, particularly with support networks, can assist the family to conserve social integrity. Social integrity within the community can be maintained by promoting the cooperation of various groups in the resolution of the teen pregnancy problem. When some groups work in isolation or in opposition to each other, the social integrity of the community is threatened.

Using Levine's model, the nurse working with an individual, family, or community must assess the degree of client adaptation achieved in each of the four areas of conservation. Wherever problems are identified, the nurse plans and implements supportive or therapeutic interventions as appropriate. Table 35–5 lists several nursing interventions with each level of client designed to conserve energy or structural, personal, or social integrity.

Nursing interventions that promote conservation of energy for the individual client include providing an environment conducive to rest, teaching about adequate nutrition, and encouraging an appropriate balance between rest and exercise. The family client can be encouraged to problem-solve with respect to the pregnancy and related problems, rather than to waste time and energy on recriminations. The nurse can help the family focus on the desire to protect the health of the teen and the unborn child. The nurse might also assist the family to reallocate resources to meet the needs of a new baby. Similarly, the nurse might assist the community to allocate resources in order to provide needed prenatal and child-health services. Conservation of community energy might also entail coordinating health personnel and their activities to ensure efficient use of resources in the delivery of care.

Conservation of the structural integrity of the individual in terms of Levine's model might include preventing complications of pregnancy. The nurse would closely monitor the course of the pregnancy, encourage the client in regular prenatal visits, and teach and encourage healthful behaviors such as moderate exercise, adequate nutrition, and not smoking or drinking. The structural integrity of the family could be maintained by encouraging family members to discuss problems and feelings related to the pregnancy and by providing referrals to minimize the stress of the pregnancy on the family. For example, if family income is limited, the nurse might refer the family to an agency providing low-cost prenatal care. At the community level, nursing efforts to lower the teen birth rate, such as providing sex education and contraceptive services for teens, would help to prevent overloading local health resources, thereby maintaining the structural integrity of the community.

From the perspective of Levine's model, activities designed to conserve the personal integrity of the individual might include encouraging ventilation of

TABLE 35–5. NURSING INTERVENTIONS IN THE LEVINE MODEL

	Nursing Interventions		
Model Concept	***Individual***	***Family***	***Community***
Conservation of energy	Provide environment conducive to rest Provide adequate nutrition with sufficient energy sources Encourage appropriate exercise	Encourage family to deal realistically with pregnancy and not waste energy on recriminations Help family explore location of resources to meet needs of new member	Coordinate activities of health personnel to ensure efficient delivery of prenatal, child-health, family planning, and sex education services Assist community to allocate resources to meet demands of teen pregnancies
Conservation of structural integrity	Prevent complications of pregnancy	Assist family to meet all necessary functions Refer for outside help as needed Encourage family to discuss problems presented by pregnancy	Work to lower teen birth rate to prevent overload of community resources
Conservation of personal integrity	Encourage ventilation of anxiety regarding changes in self-image, fears of labor and delivery, etc. Praise demonstration of appropriate parenting behaviors	Encourage family to discuss problems and plan to meet needs of the situation Reinforce positive efforts to deal with problems	Encourage participation of community members in health services planning Reinforce positive accomplishments in dealing with problem
Conservation of social integrity	Provide for interpersonal contacts (e.g., return to school, dating, etc.)	Function as liaison with outside sources of help Make referrals to other agencies as needed Help family maintain normal relationships with outside world as much as possible	Facilitate cooperate efforts among groups within community Function as resource and/or liaison with outside agencies

feelings about the pregnancy such as guilt feelings or fears about labor. The teen may need assistance in adjusting to the bodily changes that occur as the pregnancy advances, maintaining a positive self-image despite an ungainly figure. The personal integrity of the family can be enhanced by encouraging family members to discuss their problems and to plan to meet situational needs. Both the individual and the family can be assisted to conserve personal integrity by praising positive efforts to deal with problems. For the community client, active participation by community members in health-care planning and reinforcing positive accomplishments in dealing with the teen pregnancy problem can help to conserve personal integrity.

The social integrity of the individual and family can be conserved by promoting interpersonal contacts with persons outside the family. In terms of Levine's model, both teen and family should be encouraged to maintain as normal a social life as possible. The nurse can also help maintain relationships with the outside world by making referrals and acting as a liaison with other health-care agencies and providers. The nurse can also function as a liaison between the community and other sources of assistance. For example, the nurse might contact a nearby city for information on a successful program to lower the teen pregnancy rate. In addition, the nurse can facilitate cooperative efforts in the community to resolve the problem, thus assisting the community to maintain its social integrity.

OREM'S SELF-CARE MODEL

Dorothea Orem's model is based on the premise that human beings engage in self-care activities that serve to maintain a state of well-being. Self-care may be performed by the client or by a self-care agent, as when a mother cares for a young child.

CONCEPTS OF OREM'S MODEL

According to Orem,[9] self-care takes place in two phases. The first phase involves decisions about self-care that necessitate an awareness of a problem and the various factors involved, as well as knowledge of alternative solutions and their consequences. The second phase of self-care consists of actions taken to promote well-being. The action phase requires knowledge sufficient to carry out the action, motivation, commitment to the goal of action, and the ability and sufficient energy to carry out the action. The ability to engage in self-care depends on several factors, including the age of the client, the general state of health, the client's usual pattern of response to stimuli, values and goals, available resources, and the extent of health-care knowledge.[9]

Self-care actions can be divided into three categories: universal self-care, developmental self-care, and health deviation self-care.[6] ***Universal self-care*** includes activities designed to meet the needs of everyday life related to: (1) the need for air, food, and water; (2) excretion of body wastes; (3) rest and activity needs; (4) the need for both solitude and social interactions; (5) elimination of physical, social, or psychological hazards to health; and (6) being normal.[10] Table 35–6 depicts typical universal self-care activities by the individual, family, or community client.

Developmental self-care involves activities designed to foster achievement of developmental tasks. For example, a mother will engage in certain activities designed to help her child achieve the developmental task of becoming toilet-trained.

Health deviation self-care is required to combat illness or injury. Health deviation self-care can occur in several forms including: (1) adjusting ways of meeting universal needs; (2) establishing new self-care techniques; (3) modifying self-image; (4) revising the daily routine; (5) developing a new life-style consistent with the deviation; and (6) coping with the effects of the deviation or its diagnosis and treatment.[10]

Nursing intervention is indicated whenever the client experiences impairment of the ability to engage in either universal or health deviation self-care. Nursing intervention constitutes therapeutic care that contributes to the achievement of four goals: (1) support of life processes and normal functioning; (2) maintenance of normal growth and development; (3) prevention, control, and cure of disease; and (4) prevention of or compensation for disability.[9]

The nurse intervenes within one of three systems depending upon the needs of the client. In the "wholly compensatory system," the client is unable to engage in self-care and the nurse carries out self-care activities for the client. In the "partly compensatory system," the nurse and client share responsibility for self-care activities, whereas in the "supportive/educative system," the client carries out self-care activities with assistance from the nurse as needed.[10]

Nursing intervention consists of an intellectual phase and a practical phase. The intellectual phase involves identification of difficulties in self-care and the extent of the client's needs for assistance, as well as planning to meet those needs. The practical phase consists of action to implement the plan and evaluate its effectiveness. Action may be directed toward (1) compensation for self-care inability, (2) elimination of self-care limitations, and/or (3) protection of self-care abilities and prevention of new limitations.[10]

TABLE 35–6. SAMPLE UNIVERSAL SELF-CARE ACTIVITIES

Model Concept	Self-Care Activities		
Universal Self-Care	***Individual***	***Family***	***Community***
Air, food, and water	Ingest food and water needed for life Maintain oxygen source	Purchase, preparation and consumption of food	Maintain pure food, air, and water supplies
Excrement	Maintain elimination processes	Remove family trash Dispose of unwanted items	Dispose of community wastes (e.g., sewage, solid waste)
Rest/activity	Maintain a balance between rest and activity	Provide resources for adequate rest for all family members Provide adequate sleeping arrangements	Direct community activity into productive channels Provide avenues for community members to be active in decision making
Solitude/social interaction	Maintain harmonious interpersonal relations Develop ability to be comfortable alone	Maintain harmonious relationships within the family Provide for both joint and individual activities Maintain harmonious relationships with those outside the family	Maintain harmonious relationships among groups in the community and with the outside world
Elimination of hazards	Repair a broken stair	Child-proof the house	Purify water supplies Control noise patterns

Nursing interventions consist of both general methods of helping and specific helping techniques. Methods of helping include: (1) acting for the client, (2) guiding, (3) supporting, (4) providing an environment conducive to meeting needs, and (5) teaching the client. Specific helping techniques include:

1. communicating with the client
2. establishing and maintaining interpersonal, intragroup, and intergroup relations
3. giving assistance to meet specific needs
4. controlling the physical environment and the client's relations with it for therapeutic purposes
5. assistance with maintenance of life processes
6. promoting growth and development
7. assessing, changing, or controlling psychophysical modes of functioning, and
8. establishing and maintaining therapeutic relations based on psychosocial modes of functioning.[10]

APPLYING OREM'S MODEL TO COMMUNITY HEALTH NURSING

Orem's self-care model can easily be adapted for application to the care of individuals, families, or communities. Table 35–7 presents ways in which an individual, a family, and a community might meet health deviation self-care needs. The area of deviation is that of adolescent pregnancy.

In accordance with Orem's model, the individual client might adjust ways of meeting universal needs in keeping with pregnancy by increasing her dietary intake, while family members might change their approaches to eating to be sure that the teen receives an adequate prenatal diet. After the birth of the baby, both teen and family will need to adopt new ways of meeting the needs of the infant. The community may need to revise its health-care structure to meet the needs of pregnant teens and their babies.

The teenager will probably need to learn new self-care skills in order to care for her baby. She might also learn exercises involved in prepared childbirth. Family members may need to review or learn child-care skills and may need to learn how to function as the teenager's coach during delivery. The community may find that new clinics are required for family planning and prenatal services to cope with the teen pregnancy problem.

From the perspective of Orem's model, modification of self-image would occur for the individual and family when both are able to accept the fact of pregnancy without giving or accepting blame for its occurrence. Again, the teen will need to adjust to bodily changes occurring with the pregnancy. Self-image is also modified for the teen and other family members as they take on new roles and adjust relationships in existing roles. For instance, the teen must accept the new role of mother and the family must allow her to do so. The community must also modify

TABLE 35–7. HEALTH DEVIATION SELF-CARE ACTIVITIES

Model Concept	Self-Care Activities: Individual	Self-Care Activities: Family	Self-Care Activities: Community
Area of health deviation	Unwed pregnancy	Pregnancy of teenage daughter	Increased incidence of teenage pregnancy
Adjustment of ways of meeting universal needs	Increase dietary intake	Other family members help meet universal needs of teen and baby	Modify health-care system to provide prenatal, and child-health care, WIC services, etc.
Establishment of new self-care techniques	Take prenatal vitamins Learn child-care skills	Review feeding, diapering techniques, etc.	Establish prenatal and family planning clinics
Modification of self-image	Accept mother role	Recognize teen in mother role and other family members in support roles	View community as having a problem Seek outside help
Revision of daily routine	Adjust schedule to meet needs of pregnancy After birth, adjust schedule to meet needs of infant	Revise family routines to accommodate pregnancy Adjust family schedules to accommodate new baby	Redirect community resources to deal with problem of teen pregnancies
Establish new life-style consistent with deviation	Date less Change educational plans to accommodate baby	Change family-member interactions to reflect new roles	Establish planning group to deal with problem
Coping with effects of deviation and/or diagnostic and treatment measures	Adjust to changes in life-style necessitated by parenthood	Continue to adjust family routines to accommodate growth and development of child	Allocate funds for sex education campaign Expand contraceptive, prenatal, and well-child services to meet need

its self-image to acknowledge the existence of a problem and to accept outside help in its resolution.

The individual may revise her daily routine to accommodate the demands of pregnancy and, later, the needs of the baby. For example, early in the pregnancy, the teen may need to take a light breakfast or change the foods usually eaten to minimize the discomforts of morning sickness. After the baby is born, she may need to revise her school or social schedule to care for the child adequately. During the pregnancy, the family might need to adjust its schedule somewhat to obtain prenatal care for the teen. Routine schedules will probably also be disrupted by the advent of a newborn into the home. The community might need to redirect resources to meet the needs of pregnant teens. For example, it may be necessary to initiate an after-school prenatal clinic, as well as evening clinics for contraceptive services.

In terms of the model, teenage pregnancy will require life-style adaptations on the part of the individual, family, and community. The teen may need to date less frequently so as to care for her infant or delay or alter plans for her education. The family will need to change family member interactions to accommodate new roles. For example, mother and dad may not be able to go out as often should they be called upon to babysit for their grandchild. The community might also need to make some long-term changes in the ways in which it addresses the health-care needs of the adolescent population. It may be necessary to establish a special task force to explore the problem and oversee its solution.

The last task of health deviation self-care is coping with the effects of the deviation and with the effects of diagnostic and treatment measures. From Orem's perspective, pregnancy will have far-reaching consequences or effects that need to be dealt with by each level of client. The individual must adjust to long-term changes in her life necessitated by parenthood, whereas the family will continue to adjust family routines to the growth and development of the child. The teen will face the prospect of labor and delivery, a somewhat fearful experience, and the family will need to deal with the inroads of the pregnancy on their budget. The community will need to allocate funds for sex education and other services to deal with the problem, thus necessitating cuts in expenditures in other areas.

According to Orem's model, whenever the client is unable to engage in effective self-care, nursing intervention is required. Table 35–8 presents possible nursing interventions with the individual, family, and community in each of the three nursing systems. In the *wholly compensatory system*, the nurse acts for the client. If the teen has had a particularly difficult delivery or experienced complications during the pregnancy, the nurse may need to carry out universal and health deviation self-care activities for her—feeding, bathing, and dressing both client and baby.

If the family is likewise disabled by the crisis of the teen's pregnancy, the nurse may need to refer the family to others for help with self-care needs. For example, the nurse might assist the family to obtain a homemaker aide to cook, clean house, or shop for food. The nurse can also arrange for child care, transportation, and other family needs if family members are unable to deal with these needs themselves. At the community level, health-care personnel may find the teen pregnancy problem warrants mandating sex education in all junior and senior high schools. This can be done, of course, only when such action lies within the jurisdiction of the local health authority.

Once the teen has recovered somewhat from the delivery experience, nursing intervention will move into the *partly compensatory system*, with the client carrying out most self-care activities with some help from the nurse. For example, the client might feed the baby and then dress the infant after the nurse has demonstrated how to give a baby bath. In the family situation, most functions may be executed by the family, but the nurse may be called upon to make a referral for child care. With the community, the nurse will facilitate activity to resolve the teen pregnancy problem and may be involved in establishing or expanding family planning and prenatal services or sex education programs. The nurse would also encourage active involvement of other segments of the community in resolving the problem. For example, the nurse might organize and instruct school teachers in providing a sex education program.

In the *supportive/educative system*, the nurse provides support while the client engages in self-care activities. With the individual client, such support might take the form of instruction in child-care techniques, and information about contraception or immunizations. The nurse might also assist the family to adjust to a new member, providing emotional support and practical suggestions for dealing with problems that arise. For the community client, the nurse may need to educate community members regarding the extent of the teen pregnancy problem and the necessity for sex education and contraceptive ser-

TABLE 35–8. NURSING INTERVENTIONS IN THE OREM MODEL

	Nursing Interventions		
Model Concept	***Individual***	***Family***	***Community***
Wholly compensatory system	Nurse carries out all universal and health-care functions for the client (e.g., feeds and bathes client and baby, etc.)	Nurse carries out or arranges for others to carry out family functions related to universal and deviation self-care needs (e.g., sends homemaker to cook, care for children, clean house; arranges transportation for visit to physician)	Nurse initiates mandatory sex education in schools
Partly compensatory system	Client carries out self-care activities with assistance by nurse as needed (e.g., client feeds and dresses baby, nurse assists with bath)	Family carries out most of its functions; nurse arranges for child care so teen can return to school	Nurse assists community in planning to resolve problems Helps set up family planning and prenatal clinics Encourages other systems in the community to participate as appropriate (e.g., schools provide sex education)
Supportive/educative system	Nurse instructs client in self-care and child-care measures and provides support as needed	Nurse assists family to adjust to new member Provides suggestions for child care Reinforces positive approach to problems	Nurse educates community on need for sex education and contraceptive services for teens

vices. The community, once alerted, could then take steps to deal with the problem with additional supportive input from the nurse as needed.

JOHNSON'S BEHAVIORAL SYSTEMS MODEL

Dorothy Johnson defined nursing's contribution to client welfare as "the fostering of efficient and effective behavioral functioning in the patient to prevent illness and during and following illness."[11] The focus of Johnson's model is the client's behavior—what is done, why it is done, and its consequences.

CONCEPTS OF JOHNSON'S MODEL

A ***behavioral system*** is "the patterned, repetitive, and purposeful ways of living which characterize each man's life."[11] One's behavioral system determines the character of one's interaction with the environment. For example, one person's usual behavioral response to stress may be aggression. This will undoubtedly result in continual conflict between the individual and his or her environment.

The behavioral system is comprised of several ***behavioral subsystems*** or sets of responses organized around specific drives. These subsystems are reasonably stable in nature, occur with regularity, and are capable of a certain degree of modification. Each subsystem consists of four structural elements: (1) a drive that motivates behavior, (2) "set," (3) the repertoire of behavioral choices available, and (4) the behavior itself.[11] The drive results from a need that is not being met. For example, hunger is a drive resulting from a need for food. "Set" is a predisposition to act in certain ways. For instance, one person will typically satisfy the hunger drive by cooking a meal, whereas another may habitually eat in a restaurant. The totality of the behavioral repertoire relates to the alternative choices available to achieve a goal. With respect to the hunger drive, for example, the behavioral repertoire of one person included the ability to cook. Other alternatives might include stealing food or going home to mother's cooking. The behavior is the implementation of the alternative selected from the repertoire.

The behavioral subsystems common to humanity are: (1) the affiliative subsystem, (2) the dependency subsystem, (3) the ingestive subsystem, (4) the sexual subsystem, (5) the aggressive subsystem, and (6) the achievement subsystem. Instability in any of these subsystems is demonstrated by disorderly, purposeless, or unpredictable behavior.[11] Table 35–9 describes the goals of behavioral subsystems for an individual, a family, and a community.

Nursing assessment in Johnson's model involves consideration of the effectiveness of client behaviors in achieving subsystem goals. First-level assessment includes identifying problem areas and the client's ability to cope with them. Second-level assessment is undertaken when problematic behavior exists. This level involves a more detailed analysis of the structure and function of the subsystem involved.[12] The first consideration in the second-level assessment is the behavior itself. The nurse would examine when the behavior occurs, what triggers the behavior, and what terminates it. The behavior is also considered in terms of its function and purpose.

"Set" is a further consideration in the analysis of problematic behaviors and consists of both preparatory and perseverative set. The ***preparatory set*** is the stimuli on which the client tends to focus. For example, in dealing with children who hit classmates, a teacher may habitually focus on the behavior involved rather than on the reasons for the behavior. This focus will make a difference in the teacher's response to the situation. ***Perseverative set*** refers to the client's preferred behavior in a situation. One teacher, for example, might prefer to deal with classroom violence by giving out detention, while another usually sends the offender to the principal's office.

The choice of behaviors open to the client in a given situation and the degree of client awareness of choice are other factors that can influence one's response to a situation. Clients might use maladaptive behaviors because they are not aware of other options. The final consideration in the second-level assessment of problematic behavior is that of regulatory mechanisms that influence the behavior.[12] ***Regulatory mechanisms*** are constraints operating in the situation that promote certain behaviors and inhibit others. For example, if the principal has a policy that teachers should handle classroom behavior themselves, an individual teacher's response to classroom violence will be regulated by that policy.

Following the detailed assessment of problem areas, the nurse develops a nursing diagnosis. Nursing intervention is then planned to establish regular behavior patterns that better fulfill subsystem goals. Nursing intervention can involve any of four categories of action: (1) restricting or controlling behavior, (2) defending the client from exposure to unnecessary stressors, (3) inhibiting ineffective behaviors through nurturing activities, and (4) facilitating incorporation of new behaviors.[12]

APPLYING JOHNSON'S MODEL TO COMMUNITY HEALTH NURSING

Johnson's behavioral systems model provides a framework for nursing care to individuals, families,

TABLE 35–9. BEHAVIORAL SUBSYSTEM GOALS IN JOHNSON'S MODEL

Model Concept	Subsystem Goals		
Subsystem	***Individual***	***Family***	***Community***
Affiliative subsystem	Achieve satisfactory interpersonal relations with family, friends, co-workers, etc.	Maintain harmonious relationships among family members Meet family members' needs for affection Maintain satisfactory relationships with kin and others	Maintain satisfactory and harmonious relationships among community groups Develop productive relations with outside world
Achievement subsystem	Achieve mastery and control of one's body and its functions (e.g., toilet training, learning to ride a bike, etc.)	Achieve family goals (e.g., college education for children, a new house, etc.)	Maintain appropriate community functions and mastery of environment (e.g., educate members about health; dam a nearby river for power, etc.)
Aggressive/protective subsystem	Protect self or others from hazards (e.g., take care in crossing streets; prevent others from imposing guilt on oneself)	Protect family members from hazardous circumstances (e.g., know where children are, meet their friends; install smoke detectors in the home, etc.)	Protect community members from hazardous influences (e.g., prevent air pollution by local industry, noise control, etc.) Protect the community from infringement by outside groups (e.g., prevent graft and corruption in a food supplement program)
Dependency subsystem	Maintain environmental resources necessary for survival (e.g., food, clothing, housing, etc.)	Provide family needs to ensure survival (e.g., arrange housing, purchase and prepare food, etc.)	Maintain community resources to ensure survival (e.g., provide for pure air, provide access to health care, maintain adequate housing, etc.)
Ingestive subsystem	Provide energy resources adequate for survival function (e.g., eat a balanced diet)	Provide adequate family nutrition resources (e.g., prepare well-balanced meals)	Provide community resources for survival and function (e.g., provide adequate funds for health programs, establish a food bank, etc.)
Eliminative subsystem	Eliminate bodily wastes (e.g., urinate and defecate)	Eliminate family wastes (e.g., arrange for trash removal, etc.)	Eliminate community wastes (e.g., sewage treatment or disposal of industrial wastes, noise control, etc.)
Restorative subsystem	Relieve fatigue or redistribute energy (e.g., take an afternoon nap)	Redistribute family energy to meet situational needs (e.g., father fixes dinner when mother works late)	Redistribute energy to meet situational needs (e.g., draw health personnel from other activities to care for the injured in a disaster)
Sexual subsystem	Provide for personal gratification and procreation (e.g., use contraceptives as needed)	Maintain satisfactory sexual relationships Meet family planning needs	Provide services related to sexuality (e.g., family planning) Provide for community expansion and growth (e.g., recruit new industry)

and communities. Employing the model, the community health nurse assesses each behavioral subsystem to identify specific problems then plans interventions of those problem behaviors. Table 35–10 describes a second-level analysis of problematic behavior in the aggressive/protective subsystem. Problematic behavior exhibited by the individual and the family is failure to seek prenatal care for the pregnant teen. For the community, the problematic behavior is the failure to provide sex education for teens.

TABLE 35–10. SECOND-LEVEL ANALYSIS OF PROBLEM BEHAVIOR IN JOHNSON'S MODEL

Model Concept	Second-Level Analysis		
	Individual	***Family***	***Community***
Problem area: aggressive/protective subsystem	Unwed pregnancy	Pregnancy of teen daughter	Increased teen pregnancy rate
Behavior	Failure to get prenatal care	Failure to get prenatal care for teen	Failure to provide sex education for teens
Function of behavior	Attempt to deny pregnancy and associated guilt	Attempt to deny pregnancy and need to deal with it	Prevent criticism of condoning teen sexual activity
Preparatory set	Belief that pregnancy reflects "bad" behavior Knowledge of family disappointment Fear of unknown related to pregnancy, labor and delivery	Belief that pregnancy reflects failure as parents	Belief that sex education increases sexual behavior Belief that pregnancy is just punishment for illicit sexual activity
Perseverative set	Continued failure to follow up on referral for prenatal care	Failure to follow up on referral for prenatal care for teen	Resistance to inclusion of sex education in school curricula
Choice of behaviors	Going to family physician, prenatal clinic, teen clinic, or nurse midwife	Take teen to family doctor, prenatal clinic, teen clinic, or nurse midwife	Provision of sex education by schools, families, or churches
Other variables	Lack of money, transportation, etc. Educational level	Family income Educational level Family attitudes toward illegitimacy	Community attitudes to teen sexual activity Religious and cultural composition of community Lack of qualified educators
Regulatory mechanisms	Insistence of nurse Pressure from school	Advocacy by nurse	Advocacy by nurses

In Johnson's model, the behavior exhibited by each client is intended to accomplish a specific function. For example, the teen may delay seeking prenatal care in an effort to deny the pregnancy and avoid feelings of guilt. The purpose of family behavior in failing to seek care may also be a wish to deny the problem and the need to deal with it. The community may not provide sex education for teens for fear of appearing to condone or encourage adolescent sexual activity.

Preparatory and perseverative "sets" can also influence clients' behaviors in this situation. From the perspective of the model, for example, the teen might be reacting to a belief that pregnancy reflects "bad" behavior on her part, or to a fear of what will happen to her as a result of pregnancy. The family might be focusing on what others will think of them if they acknowledge their daughter's pregnancy. Preparatory "set" for the community might include beliefs that sex education increases sexual activity or that pregnancy is a fitting punishment for sexual activity by adolescents.

For the individual and the family, the perseverative "set" or preferred behavior seems to be to ignore the problem, resulting in the failure to seek prenatal care. Perseverative "set" in the case of the community also involves ignoring adolescent sexual activity.

With respect to the available repertoire of behaviors, neither family nor individual may be aware of the range of options for obtaining prenatal care open to them. Similarly, community members might not have considered the possibility of encouraging sex education by training parents or church members to educate teens in a more acceptable atmosphere than the school. Other behavioral options may, of themselves, be either adaptive or maladaptive and their potential consequences should be considered. For example, if the community were to rely exclusively on parents to educate their children regarding sexuality, many youngsters would receive no sex education at all.

Other variables involved in the problematic behavior of the individual and the family, from the perspective of Johnson's model, might include lack of money for prenatal care, lack of awareness of the importance of prenatal care, lack of transportation, or attitudes to illegitimacy. Other factors in community behavior might include community attitudes to ad-

TABLE 35–11. NURSING INTERVENTIONS IN THE JOHNSON MODEL

Model Concept	Nursing Interventions		
Categories of Action	***Individual***	***Family***	***Community***
Restriction	Withhold WIC vouchers until client obtains prenatal care	Withhold WIC vouchers until prenatal care is provided to teen	Work for legislative mandate for sex education in schools
Protection	Advocacy for baby by encouraging teen to get prenatal care	Advocacy for teen and baby within family Report neglect as needed	Political involvement to advocate sex education for teens
Inhibition of ineffective behaviors by nurturance	Educate client about need for prenatal care Focus on desire for healthy baby	Educate family about need for prenatal care Focus on desire to protect teen	Encourage participation of resistant groups in planning Point out research findings on sex education and sexual activity by teens
Facilitation of new behaviors	Assist to make appointment for prenatal care Give positive reinforcement for seeking care Arrange transportation for prenatal visit Refer for financial aid	Assist family to make appointment for care Give positive reinforcement for seeking care Arrange transportation Refer for financial aid	Develop compromise plan for sex education employing church leaders, etc.

olescent sexual activity, the religious and cultural composition of the community, or a lack of qualified persons to implement an effective sex education program.

In Johnson's model, regulatory mechanisms affecting the situation can also influence clients' behavior. For example, pressure from the nurse or school may eventually motivate the individual or family to seek prenatal care. The opinions of others can also serve a regulatory function, either encouraging the current behavior or a more adaptive one. Regulatory mechanisms in the community situation might include advocacy by concerned nurses or the fact that the community's budget can no longer support the added expense of prenatal and child care for pregnant teens and their offspring.

From the perspective of the model, once the factors contributing to the problematic behavior have been identified, the nurse can proceed to plan interventions that restrict or control behavior, protect the client from exposure to stressors, inhibit undesirable behavior through nurturing, or facilitate performance of new behaviors. Table 35–11 presents sample nursing interventions in each of these categories for the individual, the family, and the community.

Restrictive action by the nurse, in terms of Johnson's model, might involve withholding WIC vouchers from the individual or family until prenatal care is obtained. This restriction might encourage both the individual and the family to seek care, because the need for WIC can be certified by the provider of prenatal care. At the community level, the nurse might push for legislation mandating sex education in all state-supported schools.

A protective intervention with the individual client might involve explaining the benefits of prenatal care in protecting the baby from potential harm. If the teen is concerned about her baby, such knowledge might encourage her to obtain care. A similar intervention might be employed with the family by explaining the higher risk of complications of pregnancy in teenagers and the need for prenatal care to protect the teen. It might even be necessary, if the teen is a minor, for the nurse to report as child neglect the family's failure to obtain prenatal care for their daughter. In the case of the community, the nurse can become politically involved to advocate sex education in schools, presenting to policymakers the dangers in unprotected sexual activity.

In Johnson's model, nurturance can also encourage both family and individual to seek care. The nurse who exhibits concern for the teen and seems genuinely interested in protecting her welfare may be more effectively in educating client and family regarding the need for prenatal care. Again, the nurse might want to focus on client's desires to benefit the baby and the teen herself. Individuals within the community at odds with these aims can be nurtured by being encouraged to participate in the planning of a sex education program that would be acceptable to them. The nurse can also defuse fears about sex education by pointing out research findings that show a positive effect on teen sexual activity.

The last mode of nursing intervention in Johnson's model is facilitating new behaviors. The nurse can accomplish this with the individual and family client by assisting them to make an appointment for prenatal care, making referrals for financial assistance to pay for care, or by arranging transportation. Helping to develop a compromise plan for sex education in the community that includes church leaders and other influential persons can facilitate effective community behavior in providing sex education for teens.

NEUMAN'S HEALTH SYSTEMS MODEL

The model for nursing intervention developed by Betty Neuman involves a client system striving to prevent "penetration" or disruption of the system by a variety of stressors. The client's state of health is dependent on the degree of success achieved in preventing penetration of the client system by stressors or in effecting "reconstitution" of the system after penetration by stressors. Nursing intervention is indicated whenever the client is unable to prevent penetration or accomplish reconstitution without assistance.

CONCEPTS OF NEUMAN'S MODEL

A ***stressor*** is a problem or condition capable of causing instability in the system.[13] Exposure to bacteria, for example, is a stressor that might affect the health status of an individual, whereas unemployment might be a stressor for individuals, families, or communities.

In Neuman's model, the client is viewed as a composite of several elements including a basic structure, lines of resistance, and normal and flexible lines of defense.[14] These elements of the client are depicted in Figure 35–1. The client system is protected from penetration by the flexible line of defense. The ***basic structure*** is the inner core of the client that must be maintained to ensure survival. For example, elements of the basic core of the individual would be a functioning brain and heart. Penetration of the basic structure results in death. Using the example of an individual client, a cardiac arrest would constitute penetration of the basic structure, much like the ghost towns of the Old West were the victims of stressor penetration of their basic structures.

The ***normal line of defense*** is the client's usual state of wellness or the normal range of response to stressors. For example, a client with diabetes and a client without any specific medical problem both have a normal state of health represented by their normal lines of defense. For the client with diabetes, that normal state of health includes the presence of a chronic disease.

The ***flexible line of defense*** is a dynamic state of wellness that changes over time and is composed of factors that fluctuate. The flexible line of defense provides a protective cushion that prevents stressors from penetrating the normal line of defense. An in-

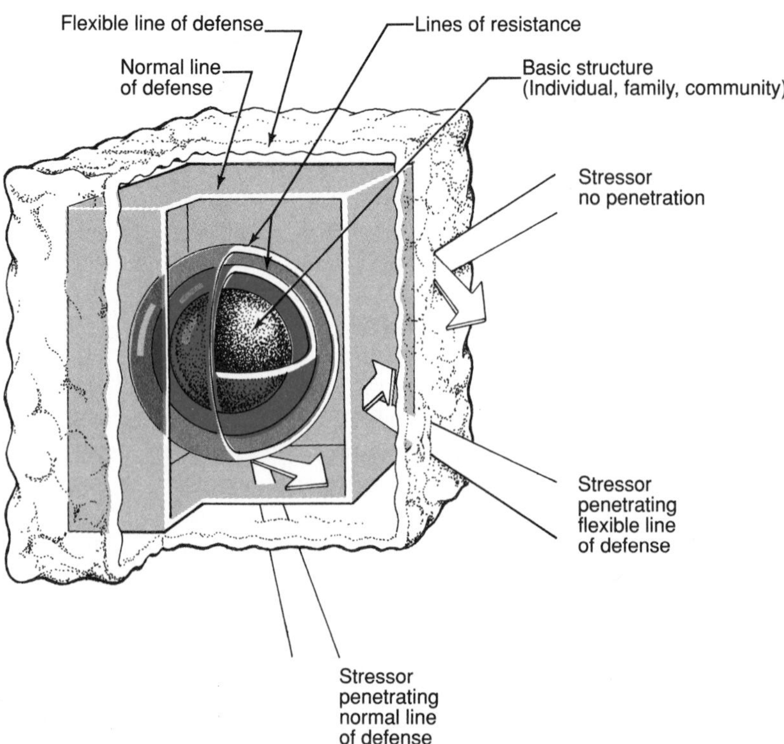

Figure 35–1. Elements of client in the Neuman model. (Adapted from Neuman[14])

dividual's flexible line of defense, for example, might include his or her level of fatigue at any given time. If the individual is well rested, he or she may be able to deal effectively with the stress of a noisy child without problems. If the client is tired, on the other hand, exposure to a noisy child might lead to penetration of the normal line of defense and result in a headache. Similarly, unemployment levels might be a factor in a community's flexible line of defense. When unemployment levels are low, the community will be better able to withstand the onslaught of a stressor like a flood because people will be more likely to possess the resources to rebuild both their homes and their lives.

When the flexible line of defense is incapable of protecting the system, penetration of the normal line of defense occurs. The extent of penetration and the degree of reaction to penetration are influenced by the strength of the normal line of defense and the lines of resistance. ***Lines of resistance*** are internal factors that protect the client against penetration of the basic structure by stressors. The strength of the lines of resistance influence the degree of the client's reaction to stressor penetration of the lines of defense. Using the example of someone exposed to a noisy child, if this person can employ relaxation techniques, he or she might be less affected by the stress than might otherwise be the case. The ability to use relaxation techniques minimizes the effects of stressor penetration. Without the use of this element of the lines of resistance, the person might end up in bed with a migraine headache.

The degree of client reaction to stressor penetration is also affected by developmental, physiological, psychological, and sociocultural variables impinging on both client and stressor and by intrapersonal, interpersonal, and extrapersonal (or intracommunity, intercommunity, and extracommunity) factors.[14] Developmental variables relate to the age or developmental level of the client. For example, a new community would probably have fewer resources for dealing with a stressor like a flood than would a well-established community. Physiologic variables reflect physical structure and function. For example, the fact that a client has diabetes will affect his or her response to a stressor such as exposure to a communicable disease. Psychological variables include such factors as self-concept and attitudes to health. Individuals, for example, who have positive attitudes to health and engage in health-promoting behaviors like exercise and not smoking will be less likely to develop cardiovascular disease than those who do not engage in healthful behaviors. Sociocultural variables are factors such as culture, educational level, and income. For instance, the client who is better educated usually has greater knowledge of healthful behaviors that can prevent stressor penetration than someone who is not as well educated.

Intraclient factors are influences within the client that affect reaction to a stressor—for example, good coping strategies that allow the client to deal effectively with a noisy child. Interclient factors reflect interactions between the client and significant others in the environment. For example, the family that has an effective social support network among extended family members will be better able to minimize the effects of a parent's unemployment than will a family with a poor support network. Extraclient factors are those outside of the client that influence the situation and the client's response to the situation. Again, using the family with a recently unemployed member as an example, the availability of financial support through community agencies will influence the effects of this stressor on the health of the family.

Once penetration of the client system occurs, the system engages in activities aimed at reconstitution. ***Reconstitution*** involves stabilization of the system and movement back toward the normal line of defense. The normal line of defense may be stabilized at either a higher or lower level than that prior to penetration. For the client system to survive stressor penetration, reconstitution must take place before penetration of the basic structure can occur. For instance, when an individual has a heart attack, reconstitution can be accomplished if cardiovascular function can be reestablished (for example, through cardiopulmonary resuscitation) and maintained.

Whenever a client system is unable to prevent penetration by a stressor or to accomplish reconstitution following penetration, nursing intervention is indicated. The nurse assesses the client to identify stressors, the factors involved, and the degree of reaction to penetration. Nursing intervention occurs at three levels—primary, secondary, and tertiary.[14]

Primary prevention involves action taken before stressor penetration occurs and is aimed at preventing penetration by strengthening the lines of defense or decreasing the potential for exposure to the stressor. Secondary prevention takes place after penetration of the lines of defense by the stressor. Activities at this level are geared toward problem resolution and minimization of reaction to the stressor. Tertiary prevention is directed toward reestablishing equilibrium and preventing complications or recurrences of the problem.

APPLYING NEUMAN'S MODEL TO COMMUNITY HEALTH NURSING

Components of Neuman's model revolving around the stressor of an unwed teen pregnancy as applied

TABLE 35–12. CLIENT ASSESSMENT IN THE NEUMAN MODEL

Model Concept	Client Assessment		
	Individual	*Family*	*Community*
Stressor	Unwed pregnancy	Pregnancy of teenage daughter	Increased incidence of teen pregnancy
Basic structure	Physical body, vital functions, age	Composition of family Typical family roles	Age composition of population, vital community functions
Normal line of defense	Presence or absence of other acute or chronic disease Nutritional level Usual life-style and habits (e.g., smoking, drinking, exercise, etc.) Attitude toward health	Family attitude toward teen sexual activity Family composition Family cohesion	Extent of teen population Educational levels Income levels Availability of contraceptive services Usual teen pregnancy rate
Flexible line of defense	Fatigue level Presence or absence of other stressors	Presence or absence of other family stressors	Availability of funding for health programs
Lines of resistance	Attitude toward child Extent of child-care skills	Flexibility of family Availability of support system Family income Family educational level	Availability and adequacy of health-care facilities and services Educational and income levels Adequacy of transportation to health-care facilities
Developmental variables	Age and developmental stage	Age and developmental stage of family members	Age composition of population History of action taken in similar situations
Physiologic variables	Current health status Nutritional status Immunization status	Health of other family members	Community nutritional levels
Psychological variables	Self-image Attitudes toward parenthood Personal goals	Family's feelings about pregnancy Religious beliefs and practices Willingness of other family members to assume other role functions	Community attitudes toward teen sexual activity
Sociocultural variables	Religious or cultural influences Income level Extent of child-care knowledge	Cultural attitudes toward teen sexuality and illegitimacy Family income	Ethnic and religious composition of population Income and educational levels Political structure Sources of funding for health care
Intraclient factors	Presence of juvenile diabetes	Grandmother living in home	Available prenatal and child-care services
Interclient factors	Assistance from other family members	Assistance from neighbors and extended family	Existing program for pregnant teens in neighboring city
Extraclient factors	Possession of health insurance	Availability of family counseling to assist in adjusting to daughter's pregnancy	Assistance from federal government with funds for prenatal and contraceptive services for teens
Goal of reconstitution	Healthy mother and baby Development of sound parenting skills Future use of effective contraceptive method	Adjustment of family to new member and related role changes	Provision of sex education and contraceptive services for teens Decrease in teen pregnancy rate

to an individual, a family, and a community are presented in Table 35–12. For the individual, the basic structure consists of the physical body and its characteristics (age, race, sex, etc.), while the basic structure of the family involves its continued existence as a social unit. In terms of the community client, the basic structure would consist of the physical structure of the community; the locale; community history; the age, race, and sex composition of the population; and vital community functions.

The normal line of defense of the individual might include the presence or absence of other health problems. For instance, a juvenile diabetic who becomes pregnant is at higher risk for complications of pregnancy than a nondiabetic juvenile. Other factors in the normal line of defense for the individual include nutritional level and life-style habits. Again, the undernourished or overweight teen or the teen who smokes is at higher risk during pregnancy.

Factors in the normal line of defense for the family might include family attitudes to teenage sexual activity and illegitimacy; family composition; and the degree of family cohesion. From the perspective of Neuman's model, a cohesive family should be better able to adapt to the pregnancy of the teen without threatening its basic structure as opposed to a family that lacks cohesion. If the teen is the only daughter, family response to her pregnancy may be different had she several sisters. For instance, pregnancy in an older daughter might lead parents to be overly strict with younger girls, driving them to rebellion. Families with decided feelings against illegitimacy are more likely than other families to fail to support the teen in her decision to keep the baby.

Components of the normal line of defense for the community are the extent of the teenage population, community income and educational levels, the availability of contraceptive services for teens, and the usual teen pregnancy rate. If the teen population is small, the community will be better able to deal with it than if the problem is extensive. In terms of the model, the availability of sex education and contraceptive services could be seen as part of the community's normal state of health, preventing teens from becoming pregnant, and thereby preventing the problem of adolescent pregnancy for the community.

Examples of factors influencing the individual's flexible line of defense are the degree of fatigue experienced by the pregnant teen and the presence or absence of other stressors. If the teen has recently broken up with her boyfriend, her pregnancy may be more stressful than would otherwise be the case. If the girl's father is unemployed this might be an additional stressor that would weaken the family's flexible line of defense and make adaptation to the pregnancy more difficult. The availability of funding for health programs, on the other hand, would strengthen the community's flexible line of defense.

The lines of resistance for the pregnant teenager might include her attitude to the baby, and the extent of her child-care skills. According to the model, both factors should affect how well she adapts to pregnancy and motherhood. Flexibility and adaptability within the family as well as the availability of support systems and income and educational levels are part of the lines of resistance that affect the family's response to the pregnancy.

For the community, the availability and adequacy of health-care services and facilities will determine how effectively the community can deal with the problem of teenage pregnancies. Other factors in the lines of resistance for the community include community educational and income levels and the adequacy of transportation to health care-facilities. All of these factors will influence the degree to which pregnancy disrupts normal client function and threatens the basic structure of the individual, family, or community.

Developmental variables for the individual client include her age and developmental stage. From the perspective of Neuman's model, an adolescent who has accomplished most of the developmental tasks of adolescence could more easily move on to the tasks of motherhood than one who has not. Similarly, the age and developmental stage of family members could affect family response to the pregnancy. For the community, the age composition of the population and a history of action taken in similar situations in the past would affect the community's ability to deal with the problem.

According to the Neuman model, physiological variables are those related to the physical structure and function of the client. Physiological variables for the individual would include her current health, nutrition, and immunization status. The health of other family members will influence family reaction to the pregnancy, and community nutritional levels will affect the extent of problems caused by widespread teenage pregnancy.

Psychological variables, in terms of the model, would include factors such as the client's self-concept and attitude toward health. For the individual, psychological variables might include the teenager's self-image, her attitudes toward parenthood, and her personal goals. If she has always wanted to be a mother, her response to the pregnancy is likely to be more positive than if she views the pregnancy as interfering with personal career goals. Family feelings about the pregnancy, religious beliefs and practices, and the willingness of other family members to assume new roles with respect to the teen and her baby are psychological factors influencing the response of the family to the stressor. Community attitudes to adolescent sexual activity are a psychological factor for the community. Cultural influences and income and educational levels are sociocultural variables that may affect the reaction of the individual, family, or community to the stress of teen pregnancy.

Client reaction to stressor penetration is also influenced by intraclient, interclient, and extraclient factors. Intraclient factors are influences within the individual, family, or community that affect reaction to the stressor. In terms of the model, intraclient factors for the individual teen might include the presence of juvenile diabetes. The presence of a grandmother living in the home might be an intrafamily factor that would influence the family's response to the pregnancy. Availability of prenatal and child-care services would be an intracommunity factor that could limit reaction to the stressor of teenage pregnancy.

Assistance from other family members, neighbors, and extended family might be interclient factors limiting reaction of the individual and family to stressor penetration, whereas the existence of a successful program for pregnant teens in a neighboring city might aid the community in responding to the situation. Extraclient factors for the individual might include possession of health insurance to pay for prenatal care, while the availability of counseling to help the family deal with the problem of the pregnancy is an extraclient factor for the family. For the community, an extraclient factor might be the availability of federal funding for prenatal and contraceptive services for teens.

Reconstitution is required for each of the three levels of client. From the perspective of Neuman's model, the primary goals of reconstitution for the individual are a healthy mother and baby and development of sound parenting skills by the teen. An additional goal is the prevention of subsequent pregnancy by the use of an effective contraceptive. Reconstitution for the family entails positive adjustment to the presence of a new member and the role changes involved. For the community, the goal of reconstitution would be sex education and contraceptive services for teens resulting in a decrease in the teen pregnancy rate.

Nursing intervention related to the problem of adolescent pregnancy could take place at levels of primary, secondary, or tertiary prevention for each of the three types of clients. Table 35–13 provides examples of nursing interventions in the Neuman model for an individual, a family, and a community at each of the three levels of prevention.

Primary prevention for the individual client would include general health promotion and encouraging the use of effective contraception to prevent pregnancy. Primary prevention in terms of Neuman's model might also include promotion of a strong self-image to foster resistance to peer pressure for sexual activity. For the family, primary prevention might

TABLE 35–13. NURSING INTERVENTIONS IN THE NEUMAN MODEL

	Nursing Interventions		
Model Concept	***Individual***	***Family***	***Community***
Primary prevention	Promote health through adequate nutrition, rest, exercise, etc. Encourage use of effective contraceptive by sexually active teens	Educate parents to provide sex education for children Assist development of a climate in which children can discuss sexuality issues with parents	Provide sex education and contraceptive services for teens
Secondary prevention	Refer for prenatal care Monitor course of pregnancy and prevent complications Prepare for delivery and parenthood	Assist family to adjust to advent of new member and related role changes	Assist in development of prenatal and child-care services to meet demands
Tertiary prevention	Encourage use of effective contraception after delivery to prevent recurrence of pregnancy	Discuss prevention of subsequent pregnancies Discourage family from overprotection of other daughters	Educate pregnant teens for future contraceptive use to prevent recurrence of pregnancy Provide adequate sex education to prevent recurrence

entail preparing parents to provide sex education to their children and offering assistance in developing communication patterns that foster communication among family members. Such communication will encourage teens to come to parents to discuss sexuality issues and may help to prevent later pregnancy. Primary prevention at the community level would involve providing sex education and contraceptive services for teens.

From the perspective of the model, secondary prevention for the individual client would include referral for prenatal care, monitoring the course of the pregnancy, and preventing complications of pregnancy. The nurse will also educate the client in preparation for labor and delivery and for parenthood. For the family client, secondary prevention might entail activities to assist the family to adjust to a new member, such as helping the family plan role changes, reviewing child-care skills, and dealing with feelings about the pregnancy. Secondary prevention for the community involves developing programs for prenatal and child-health care to meet increased demands for service.

For the individual client, nursing intervention at the tertiary-prevention level would involve education and encouraging the use of effective contraception to prevent a subsequent pregnancy. The family might also need education regarding contraception. The community health nurse may also find that he or she needs to discourage parents from becoming overly protective or restrictive of other girls in the family in response to their own daughter's pregnancy. At the community level, the nurse might develop programs for contraceptive education and services for pregnant teens to prevent subsequent pregnancies.

PENDER'S HEALTH PROMOTION MODEL

Nola Pender has described a nursing model that directs nursing intervention for health promotion. Because health promotion is a major emphasis in community health nursing, Pender's model is presented here even though it only addresses one aspect of community health nursing.

CONCEPTS OF PENDER'S MODEL

The health promotion model has three basic components: individual perceptions, modifying factors, and variables that affect the likelihood of health-promoting action. ***Individual perceptions*** are beliefs and values that facilitate health-promoting behavior. Perceptions considered in the model are: (1) the importance of health, (2) perceived control, (3) desire for competence, (4) self-awareness, (5) self-esteem, (6) definition of health, (7) perceived health status, and (8) perceived benefits of action.[15]

Pender contended that people placing a high value on health would seek health-related information that would result in healthful behaviors.[15] Similarly, people who see themselves as able to control their environment, and who have a strong desire to do so, are more likely than those who do not take action to enhance their health. Competence is one's ability to interact effectively with the environment.[15] Clients who desire to achieve competence are more likely to engage in health-promoting behaviors than are clients who are less concerned with competence.

Increased self-awareness is another individual perception that influences health-related behaviors. People who are more self-aware tend to be more likely to take positive health action than are those who are not self-aware.[15] Self-esteem also affects the likelihood of a person taking health-promoting action. Clients who have a high self-regard are more likely than others to be involved in health-promoting behavior.

When clients define health as adaptation or stability, they are likely to engage in more health-protecting than health-promoting behaviors. The client who views health as the actualization of potential, however, is more likely to be concerned with health promotion.[15] Clients' perceptions of their health status also influence the probability of their engaging in health-promoting behaviors. Clients who view themselves as basically healthy will take steps to maintain and enhance their health.[15] The last client perception addressed in the health promotion model is the benefits accruing from action. One is unlikely to engage in health-promoting activities unless one can see some benefit deriving from them.

The second element in the health promotion model is that of ***modifying factors*** that influence the performance of healthful behavior. These modifying factors are grouped into three categories: demographic variables, interpersonal variables, and situational variables. Demographic variables include the age, race, sex, ethnicity, and income and educational level of the client. Interpersonal variables that influence healthful behavior include the expectations of significant others, family health patterns, and past interactions with health professionals. Research has discovered that the expectations of others are highly influential in the behavioral choices of many people. Previous interactions with and perceptions of health-care professionals can also influence healthful behavior.

Situational variables addressed in the health promotion model include the options available to the client and prior experience with health-promoting behaviors. Clients will act on the basis of the types of behavioral options open to them. These options may be limited by factors within the client situation, thus inhibiting healthful behavior. On the other hand, prior experience and familiarity with health-promoting behaviors can also favorably influence the client's willingness to act.

The final element of the health promotion model is the likelihood of action, which is influenced by both perceived barriers and cues to action. Barriers may be real or imagined and involve perceptions of the unavailability, inconvenience, or difficulty of a specific behavior. Cues to action are the other factors that affect the likelihood of action. Even when all other factors are in favor of healthful behavior, clients may need some event to trigger performance of that behavior.

APPLYING PENDER'S MODEL TO COMMUNITY HEALTH NURSING

Pender's model is applicable to individuals, families, and groups or communities. Using the model, the community health nurse would first identify perceptions that are influencing clients' behavior. Once again using a case of adolescent pregnancy, examples of such perceptions and their influence on health behaviors of an individual, a family, and a community are provided in Table 35–14. From the perspective of the model, if the individual client values health and desires a healthy baby, she is more likely to seek pre-

TABLE 35–14. EXAMPLES OF PERCEPTIONS PROMOTING HEALTHFUL BEHAVIORS

Model Concept	Healthful Behavior		
Perception	*Individual*	*Family*	*Community*
Importance of health	Client desires healthy baby, seeks prenatal care	Family values teen's health, seeks prenatal care for teen	Community values health of teen population, takes steps to prevent teen pregnancy
Control	Client sees self as able to influence delivery; does exercises to tone muscles and ease delivery	Family sees opportunity for choice in health care; takes teen to nurse midwife	Community believes sex education will help control teen pregnancy problem; starts program in schools
Desire for competence	Client desires to be "good parent," learns child-care skills	Parents desire to be good parental role models; practice and encourage good family communication patterns	Community wishes to be seen as forerunner in dealing with teen pregnancy; seeks innovative ideas for prevention program
Self-awareness	Client aware of own social interaction needs; plans schedule to meet own needs as well as baby's needs	Parents aware of guilt feelings over daughter's pregnancy; able to deal with them openly	Community recognizes teen pregnancy as a problem; takes steps toward resolution
Self-esteem	Client sees self as good person; able to deal with guilt over pregnancy and move on	Parent view themselves as good parents; able to deal effectively with daughter's pregnancy	Community has history of dealing effectively with similar problems; approaches teen pregnancy problem positively
Definition of health	Client defines health as achievement of potential; continues with plans to go to college despite pregnancy	Family defines health as achievement of potential of each family member; supports daughter's plans for college despite her pregnancy	Community defines health as ability to be productive; provides educational alternatives for pregnant teens
Health status	Client sees self as healthy; doesn't allow pregnancy to interfere with life activities	Family sees itself as healthy; deals with daughter's pregnancy in active problem-solving approach	Community sees itself as healthy; takes steps to maintain health status
Benefits of health-promoting behavior	Client sees prenatal care as enhancing likelihood of healthy baby; seeks prenatal care	Family sees prenatal care as benefiting teen and baby; pays for prenatal services	Community sees sex education as means to control teen pregnancy problem; allocates resources to fund program

natal care than one who has a low value for health. Similarly, a family that values the health of the teenager will also be encouraged to obtain prenatal care for her. With a high value for the health of its teen population, the community is likely to take steps to prevent teen pregnancy as a threat to the health of young people. Such steps might include sex education in school curricula and provision of contraceptive services to adolescents.

Clients' perceptions of their ability to control the environment will also influence behavior. For example, in terms of the model, the individual teen who believes she is able to control the course of her delivery to some extent is likely to engage in exercises to tone muscles and ease delivery. A sense of control of circumstances by the family, seen as an opportunity for choice among health-care alternatives, might lead family members to seek prenatal care for the teen from a nurse midwife rather than from the traditional obstetrician. In the case of the community, a belief that sex education will help to control the problem of adolescent pregnancy will lead to the establishment of such programs.

According to the model, the individual who desires to function competently as a parent will endeavor to learn child-care and other skills involved in effective parenting. Similarly, parents who desire competence in their parental role will encourage patterns of family communication that will influence the healthful behaviors of members. A community that wishes to be viewed as a forerunner in the prevention of teen pregnancy will seek innovative solutions to the problem and not be bound by traditional ideas.

Self-awareness may also influence behavior. An example of self-awareness in the individual client might be recognition of her own needs for social interaction. In terms of Pender's model, the adolescent mother who is self-aware in this regard will probably arrange her life to meet her own needs as well as those of the baby, thereby improving her own emotional health. The teen who has no awareness of her own needs may be so caught up in trying to be a "good mother" that she fails to meet personal needs and provides no outlet for relieving stress.

Whether or not it is warranted, most parents would experience some degree of guilt were their daughter to become pregnant out of wedlock. From the perspective of Pender's model, those parents who are aware of their feelings and can deal with them effectively are doing more to promote their own health and that of the total family than are parents who are not self-aware and do not deal with their underlying guilt. Likewise, the community that is aware of the problem of teenage pregnancy and its effects on the health of the community is more likely to take action to control it than a community that denies the existence of a problem.

According to the model, the teen with strong self-esteem, who sees herself as a basically good person, will be able to deal with any guilt engendered by her pregnancy and move on to deal effectively with other problems presented by the situation. On the other hand, the teen who sees her pregnancy as an indication of her failure as a person may try to "punish" herself by not taking adequate care of her health. Similarly, parents who have a strong self-image will be able to deal with guilt feelings arising from their daughter's pregnancy and take action to help the girl through the situation. For the community, a history of having dealt effectively with similar problems in the past will create a willingness to approach the problem of teenage pregnancy positively.

The individual client who defines health as achievement of her full potential will probably proceed with plans to go to college and develop a career while coping with the demands of parenthood. Also from the perspective of the model, family members who hold the same beliefs will encourage their daughter in her plans and provide her with the emotional (and perhaps financial) support needed to implement those plans. A community that defines health as actualization of the potential to be a productive citizen might provide educational alternatives for teenage parents that allow them to complete their education while caring for their children.

According to Pender's model, clients' perceptions of their own health status may contribute to efforts to protect and promote health. For instance, the individual who sees herself as healthy is less likely to allow her pregnancy to interfere with her normal activity. One who sees herself as unhealthy is more likely to take to her bed and restrict her own activities for the duration of the pregnancy. Similarly, the family that views itself as healthy is more likely to deal positively with problems posed by their daughter's pregnancy than is a family that considers itself unhealthy. For example, a family that perceives itself as able to cope effectively (an element of health) will look for solutions to problems, whereas a family with less confidence in its ability to cope may assume that problems are insoluble and take no action. In the same vein, a community that perceives itself as healthy is likely to take steps to maintain that health. Conversely, from the perspective of Pender's model, a community that sees itself as in decline may view the problem of teenage pregnancies as one more indication of its demise and fail to take action to control the problem.

Clients' perceptions of the benefits of health-related actions may also influence their willingness to act. From the perspective of Pender's model, for example, the teen who believes that prenatal care is unlikely to alter the course of the pregnancy and the health of the baby will be less likely to obtain care than one who believes that prenatal care can enhance the outcome of the pregnancy. Seeking prenatal care could be similarly influenced by the beliefs of the family regarding its efficacy. For the community, the belief that sex education helps to prevent teen pregnancy will motivate the community to provide funding for sex education in the schools.

Modifying factors may also influence the health-related behaviors of individuals, families, and communities. Table 35–15 presents examples of the effects of modifying factors on the behavior of the pregnant adolescent, her family, and a community

TABLE 35–15. EXAMPLES OF MODIFYING FACTORS INFLUENCING HEALTHFUL BEHAVIORS

Model Concept	**Behavior**		
Modifying Factor	***Individual***	***Family***	***Community***
Demographic variables:			
Age	Client old enough to seek prenatal care without parental consent; obtains care	Other children grown, so parents can afford prenatal care for teen	Older, well-established community has sufficient tax base to expand prenatal services to meet needs
Ethnicity	Client is Hispanic and plans to keep baby	Family is of Hispanic culture; accepts baby as unique and contributing member of family	Community has large Hispanic population resistant to family planning services for teens
Education	Client aware of need for prenatal care; seeks services in prenatal clinic	Family aware of need for prenatal care; insists that daughter obtain care	Community aware of risks of teen pregnancy; is committed to action to reduce pregnancy rate
Income	Client unable to afford prenatal care; does not seek care until time of delivery	Family has health insurance; obtains prenatal care for teen	Community has no funds for health educators; adds sex education program to school nurse's duties
Interpersonal variables:			
Expectations of significant others	Client's family expect teen to care for baby herself; teen arranges school schedule to accommodate baby	Extended family expects parents to keep baby, so parents arrange sleeping arrangements to accommodate teen with baby	Federal family planning sources expect services will be provided to sexually active teens, so services are made available without parental consent
Family health patterns	Client's family has always gone to private physician; teen seeks care from physician rather than nurse midwife	Mother has always seen family-practice physician for pregnancies; makes appointment with him for teen	Large segment of community has no private source of health care; community provides publicly funded clinics to meet health-care needs
Interactions with health professionals	Client afraid physician will tell parents of pregnancy; delays seeking prenatal care	Family has been satisfied with private medical care; is critical of care provided in public clinics	Community members seek professional help only with serious illness; prenatal clinics poorly attended
Situational variables:			
Options available	Client lives in small town with only one health-care provider who does deliveries	Family belongs to a health maintenance organization with physician and nurse-midwife options available for prenatal care	Community is in large metropolitan area with several options available for prenatal care; most teens receive care from first trimester
Prior experience with health-promoting behaviors	Client accompanied mother on prenatal visits during last pregnancy; feels comfortable seeking prenatal care	Family is new in town and knows of no reputable source of prenatal care; delays seeking care until late in second trimester	Community previously attempted comprehensive sex education program in high schools; discontinued due to parental complaints

experiencing a high rate of adolescent pregnancies. Demographic variables of race and sex are not particularly relevant to the problem of teen pregnancy and have not been included in Table 35–15.

The age of the teen may affect her ability to obtain prenatal care. If she is old enough to do so without parental consent, she may do so. If she is not, she will be dependent on her parents to arrange for care. The age composition of the family may also affect the ability to obtain prenatal care. If other children are grown and away from home, parents may be better able to provide prenatal care for the teen than if there were still several young children at home. The developmental history of the community may similarly affect its ability to deal with the problem of teen pregnancy. A relatively new community may not have a sufficiently large tax base to pay for prenatal services for teens. In this case, community members may have to rely on services provided outside the community. In an older, well-established community such services may already be in place.

Ethnicity can also influence individual and family decisions regarding the pregnancy. According to the model, if the teen and her family come from a culture that values children whatever their parentage, they may decide to keep the baby. If not, abortion or adoption may be the alternatives selected. The ethnic and cultural composition of the community can influence its ability to take action regarding the problem. For example, a community with a large Hispanic Catholic population may encounter resistance to contraceptive services for teens.

Individual, family, and community educational and income levels will affect abilities to engage in healthful behaviors in similar ways. Lower educational levels may involve a lack of awareness of the need for prenatal and other services, while lower income levels will influence the accessibility of such services.

For the individual, interpersonal variables related to the expectation of her parents that she will care for the child herself might lead the pregnant teen to learn child-care skills and to arrange her school and social schedules to accommodate the child's needs. If extended family members expect the family to keep the child, parents may be influenced to do so rather than choose the alternatives of abortion or adoption. Finally, if the community is aware that the expectation attached to federal funding for family planning services is the provision of such services to teens, such services are likely to be provided.

Prior interaction with health-care providers might also influence clients' actions. In terms of Pender's model, the teen who is fearful that a health-care provider will inform her parents of her pregnancy is unlikely to seek care early in the pregnancy. The family that has always received private medical care may be critical of the long wait involved in obtaining services from a public prenatal clinic. In the community situation, if community members seek professional assistance only in serious illness, prenatal clinics are likely to be poorly attended and many clients will go without prenatal care.

According to the model, situational variables may limit behavioral options available to clients. If the individual or family, for example, live in a small town with few available resources, there may be a delay in seeking prenatal care or the choice of the source of care may be extremely limited. If, on the other hand, the family belongs to a health maintenance organization (HMO) that provides alternatives for prenatal care, members may choose to seek care from a nurse midwife rather than a physician. If the community is in a large metropolitan area with several options for care available, it is more likely that a large number of teens will receive prenatal care early in the pregnancy than would otherwise be the case.

The client's prior experience with health-promoting behaviors may result in health-related action. For instance, if the teen has accompanied her mother to prenatal visits or has had a previous vaginal exam she may be less frightened of seeking prenatal care. On the other hand, if the family is new in town and has no previous experience with any of the health-care providers there, the family may delay seeking prenatal care. Similarly, if the community has experienced an unsuccessful attempt at sex education in the schools, one that raised a public outcry, leaders may be less willing to attempt another such program despite the rise in teen pregnancies.

Perceived barriers and cues to action might also influence health-promoting behaviors by the teenager, the family, and the community. Examples of possible barriers and cues for each level of client are presented from the perspective of Pender's model in Table 35–16. The teen who sees her regularly scheduled prenatal visits as interfering with her social life is likely to miss appointments because of perceived barriers posed by health-related actions. Similarly, the family that views prenatal care as too expensive is not likely to obtain care for a pregnant daughter. A community that anticipates parental opposition to sex education for teens is less likely to implement such a program than is a community where sex education is supported by parent groups.

Finally, according to the model, there may or may not be cues to action present in the situation that motivate the individual, family, or community to take health-promoting actions. For example, the teen may see a presentation by the March of Dimes on pre-

TABLE 35–16. EXAMPLES OF FACTORS INFLUENCING LIKELIHOOD OF ACTION

	Likelihood of Action		
Model Concept	***Individual***	***Family***	***Community***
Perceived barriers to action	Client sees prenatal care as interfering with social life; frequently misses appointments	Family views prenatal care as too expensive; fails to provide care for teen	Community anticipates parental opposition to sex education for teens, so does not initiate needed program
Cues to action	Client sees March of Dimes presentation on preventing birth defects; seeks prenatal care	Family learns of friend's daughter who died of childbirth complications; seeks prenatal care for teen	Community receives statistics on the societal costs of teen pregnancy; votes funds for sex education program

venting birth defects that motivates her to seek prenatal care. Likewise, the family may be motivated to seek care for their daughter by news of the death of a friend's daughter from toxemia. A cue to action for the community might be the findings of a study on the societal costs of teen pregnancy.

Nursing interventions in Pender's health promotion model involve modifying the variables that influence client behavior. These interventions might be similar for individual, family, and community clients. Examples of interventions related to each of the model variables are presented in Table 35–17.

From the perspective of the model, the community health nurse may need to change the client's perception of the importance of health. One way to accomplish this is to link health to another highly valued variable. For example, the teen might be encouraged to exercise during pregnancy if she thought this would help her regain her figure after delivery. Or the family or community might be encouraged to permit teen contraceptive use by underscoring the financial and social costs of teen pregnancy.

In keeping with the model, clients' perceptions of control of events might be enhanced by including them in health-care decision making and planning nursing interventions. Desire for competence might be enhanced by praising clients' current abilities and presenting opportunities for further enhancement of skills. For example, the teen might be praised for her care of younger brothers and sisters and asked if she would like to attend child-care classes to broaden her skills. Desire for competence might also be increased by decreasing negative aspects of the mastery of skills. For instance, parents could be referred to free counseling services to help them improve communication skills in the family, thereby eliminating the financial barrier to the enhancement of competence in this area. Setting short-term attainable goals and reinforcing their accomplishment can also increase the desire for competence. The community that can see some progress in its efforts to control teen pregnancy problems, for example, is likely to continue action in this direction.

The community health nurse can also influence the client's self-awareness by reflecting on his or her perceptions of the meaning of client behavior. For example, the nurse might say to the teen, "It sounds like you don't want to get prenatal care because you are afraid your parents will find out about your pregnancy." Such reflection allows the client to examine the underlying cause of behavior and to make an effort to change it. Similarly, the nurse might say to community members, "It seems as though you believe that sex education for teens will increase their desire to engage in sexual activity." The nurse can then assist community members to explore the lack of a factual basis for such beliefs.

According to Pender's model, enhancing the client's self-esteem may also lead to a greater tendency to engage in healthful behavior. The community health nurse may accomplish this by praising previous client accomplishments and refraining from destructive criticism of client behavior. The nurse can also point out the positive aspects of behavior and the areas that need change. For example, the nurse might say to the family, "It's wonderful to see how concerned you are about your daughter's health. You can really help her by encouraging her to eat more fruits and vegetables and getting more exercise. Perhaps you and she could exercise together." In this way, the nurse reinforces positive behaviors and provides concrete suggestions to improve those behaviors even further.

Clients' definitions of health may be modified by first getting clients to verbalize their definitions. Many people have never consciously thought about what health means to them. The community health nurse can then assist clients to explore the ramifications of expanded definitions of health, saying, for example, "Wouldn't it be better if you just were not

TABLE 35–17. NURSING INTERVENTIONS INFLUENCING SELECTED VARIABLES IN THE PENDER HEALTH PROMOTION MODEL

Model Variable	Nursing Intervention
Importance of health	Enhance value of health to client by linking it to other closely held values
Perceived control	Enhance client's perceptions of control of events by including in planning of health care
Desire for competence	Enhance client desire for competence by praising present abilities and offering opportunities to enhance competence even more Decrease negative aspects of mastery of skills Set short-term attainable goals and point out achievement
Self-awareness	Increase client self-awareness by reflecting on meaning of client behavior as interpreted by the nurse
Self-esteem	Enhance client's self-esteem by praising previous accomplishments Refrain from destructive criticism of client behavior Point out positive aspects of behavior as well as avenues for improvement
Definition of health	Assist client to verbalize personal definition of health Encourage client to explore ramifications of more expanded definition of health
Perceived health status	Reflect accurate perceptions of client's actual state of health by pointing out specific signs, symptoms, or behaviors
Perceived benefits of health-promoting behaviors	Educate client on actual benefits of healthful behaviors
Education	Educate client where necessary with respect to healthful behaviors
Income	Refer client as needed for financial support
Ethnicity	Explore with client the implications of ethnicity for health Encourage healthful cultural behavior Discourage unhealthful behavior and give rationale
Expectations of significant others	Work with significant others to change expectations May need to encourage client to be more assertive
Family patterns of health care	Explore adequacy of previous health-care patterns for current situation Assist client to identify more appropriate health-care patterns
Interactions with health professionals	Develop rapport with client Treat client as worthwhile individual with personal dignity Include client in all phases of nursing process
Available options	Educate client regarding behavioral options available, their benefits, and consequences Provide referral for other options as needed
Prior experience with health-promoting behaviors	Explore client's previous experience with health-promoting behaviors Determine how previous situation compares and contrasts with current situation Help client to recognize similarities and differences in situations
Perceived barriers to action	Identify potential barriers to healthful behavior Attempt to eliminate or modify barriers
Cues to action	Assist client to recognize cues to action in own situation Provide cues to action through client education

ill, but actually felt good? What could you do to make yourself feel good?"

Accurately reflecting clients' health status may assist in modifying their perceived status. For example, the nurse might present figures that indicate the magnitude of the teen pregnancy problem and its effects on the community as a means of developing community awareness of the problem. Or the client's elevated blood pressure might be cited as evidence that she needs to take better care of herself and keep her prenatal appointments. Similarly, gently pointing out instances of poor communication may help the family recognize that there are problems in family communication patterns.

Education regarding healthful behaviors and their consequences is another way in which the community health nurse can influence the likelihood of client action in terms of Pender's model. Many clients are not aware of the need for or efficacy of health-promoting behaviors. Nurses can also be active in educating the general public in such matters, so that healthful behavior becomes the norm rather than the exception. Success for this type of approach has already been noted in areas such as smoking and dietary habits in the public at large.

When income is a deterrent to healthful behavior, the nurse can provide referrals for financial assistance. The nurse can also assist clients to find less expensive ways of meeting health needs or ways of reducing expenditures in other areas to provide more funds for health care.

Community health nurses need to assess the implications of culture and ethnicity for health-promoting behaviors. Healthful cultural practices should be encouraged, while unhealthful practices are tactfully discouraged or modified, and the reasons for modification given. (The implications of culture and ethnicity for health were addressed in Chapter 15, Cultural Influences on Community Health.)

Expectations of significant others can be modified to promote health by including them in planning health care. When this is not possible, or when significant others are resistant to change, the community health nurse may need to encourage greater assertiveness on the part of the client. For example, if members of the teen's family are encouraging her to offer the baby up for adoption when she wants to keep the child and seems mature enough to do so, the nurse might function as an advocate for the adolescent mother and support her in her decision. The nurse can also assist her in implementing that decision by helping her find housing and a source of financial support if these are not forthcoming from the family.

The community health nurse can also explore the adequacy of previous health-care patterns in dealing with the current situation. For example, if the community has always relied on outside funding to meet health-care needs, the community may need to be shown how internal funds can be freed to meet health needs. Similarly, if family members have always used a private physician for health care but can no longer afford to do so, the nurse can refer them to a public prenatal clinic, or assist them to obtain Medicaid to pay for care.

The effects of previous negative interactions with health-care professionals that interfere with healthful behaviors might need to be overcome. The nurse can do this initially by establishing rapport with the client (individual, family, or community) and treating the client with respect. Another nursing intervention that might help to overcome negative attitudes toward health-care providers is including the client in all phases of the nursing process.

From Pender's perspective, clients might need to be educated regarding options available to them. They also need to be apprised of the benefits and consequences of action. The individual or family client may not be aware of the availability of nurse midwives to provide prenatal care. Similarly, the community may need to be made aware of sources of funding to establish programs for preventing teenage pregnancy.

The nurse can also intervene to modify the effects of clients' previous experience with health-promoting behaviors. If the community has had a bad experience with trying to provide sex education in schools, the nurse can assist in circumventing resistance to a new program by incorporating opponents in the planning stages. Or the client may have heard horror stories from friends about labor and delivery. In this case, the nurse can provide factual information about the labor process and refer the client for prepared childbirth classes if desired.

The nurse can also be effective in removing perceived barriers to action and in providing cues to action. First, the nurse must identify barriers and then work toward their elimination. For example, if the barrier to getting prenatal care is cost, the nurse can refer the teen and her family to sources of financial assistance. The nurse can also provide cues to action by educating clients about the need for healthful behaviors and pointing out the consequences of nonhealthful behaviors. For example, the nurse might cite statistics on teenage pregnancy and its costs to the community to motivate action dealing with the problem.

CHAPTER HIGHLIGHTS

- Nursing models other than the epidemiologic prevention process model can be used to direct community health nursing practice.
- In the Roy Adaptation Model, health is the ability of the client to adapt to changes in the environment. Clients' responses to environmental changes are influenced by focal, contextual, and residual stimuli operating in the situation.
- Adaptation in the Roy model takes place in four modes—the physiologic mode, the self-concept mode, the role-function mode, and the interdependence mode. Whenever the client cannot adapt without assistance, nursing intervention is warranted.
- Nursing intervention in the Roy model entails manipulation of the environment or the client to modify stimuli operating in a given situation.
- In Levine's Principles of Conservation, health consists of structural, personal, and social integrity and energy. Health is maintained by conservation of these four components. Whenever the client is not capable of engaging in conservation without assistance, nursing intervention is warranted.
- In Orem's Self-Care Model, health is the ability to engage in self-care activities to promote well-being. There are three types of self-care: universal self-care, developmental self-care, and health deviation self-care.
- Universal self-care needs in Orem's model include providing air, food, and water; eliminating bodily wastes; rest and activity; solitude and social interaction; and eliminating hazards.
- Health deviation self-care needs in Orem's model include finding new ways of meeting universal needs, establishing new self-care techniques, modifying self-image, revising one's daily routine, establishing a life-style consistent with the deviation, and coping with the effects of the deviation and with diagnostic and treatment measures required.
- Nursing in Orem's model may occur in the wholly compensatory system, the partially compensatory system, or the supportive/educative system.
- In Johnson's Behavioral Systems Model, health involves effective functioning in eight behavioral subsystems: the affiliative, achievement, aggressive/protective, dependency, ingestive, eliminative, restorative, and sexual subsystems.
- Nursing assessment in Johnson's model takes place at two levels. First-level assessment involves identifying problems in behavioral subsystems. In second-level assessment, emphasis is on identifying the drive, preparatory and perseverative sets, behavioral repertoire, and regulatory mechanisms contributing to malfunction in a behavioral subsystem.
- Nursing intervention in Johnson's model may involve restricting or controlling behavior, protection from exposure to stressors, inhibiting ineffective behavior through nuturance, and facilitating new behaviors.
- In Neuman's Health Systems Model, health is absence of stressor penetration. The client is composed of an inner core protected by normal and flexible lines of defense and lines of resistance.
- In Neuman's model, the lines of defense attempt to prevent stressor penetration, while the lines of resistance moderate the client's response to stressor penetration and attempt to prevent penetration of the inner core.
- Nursing intervention in Neuman's model is directed toward reconstitution and may involve primary, secondary, or tertiary prevention measures.
- In Pender's Health Promotion Model, health-promoting behaviors are influenced by clients' perceptions, modifying factors, and factors affecting the likelihood of action.
- In Pender's model, client perceptions influencing action include the importance of health, perceptions of control, desires for competence, self-awareness, self-esteem, one's definition of health, one's perceived health status, and perceived benefits of health-promoting behaviors.
- Modifying factors that influence behavior in Pender's model include demographic variables, interpersonal variables, and situational variables.
- Factors that affect the likelihood of action in Pender's model include perceived barriers to action and cues action.

Review Questions

1. Describe three major concepts of the Roy Adaptation Model. Give an example of how each concept might be applied to an individual, a family, or a community. (p. 944)
2. Describe four major concepts of Levine's Principles of Conservation. Give an example of how each concept might be applied to an individual, a family, or a community. (p. 949)
3. Describe three major concepts of Orem's Self-Care Model. Give an example of how each concept might be applied to an individual, a family, or a community. (p. 952)
4. Describe five major concepts of Johnson's Behavioral Systems Model. Give an example of how each concept might be applied to an individual, a family, or a community. (p. 956)
5. Describe five major concepts of Neuman's Health System Model. Give an example of how each concept might be applied to an individual, a family, or a community. (p. 960)
6. Describe three major concepts of Pender's Health Promotion Model. Give an example of how each concept might be applied to an individual, a family, or a community. (p. 965)

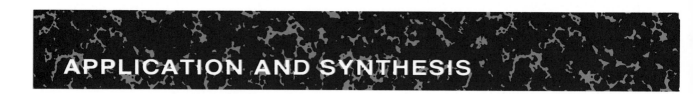

APPLICATION AND SYNTHESIS

Clarksville is a small rural town. Agriculture is the primary industry, and those residents of the area who are not farmers are involved in support services for the farming community. There are a few businesses in town including a grocery store, a hardware store, a grain elevator, a farm machinery dealership, two gas stations, and a bank.

The area recently suffered a severe drought. Several farmers defaulted on loans, and the mortgages on their farms have been foreclosed. Others are barely able to make a living. Because of the failing economy, the businesses in town have also suffered, and the grocery store will close at the end of the month.

Most families have gardens, so they are able to obtain fresh vegetables. Fruits are also available from area orchards, but the yield is small because of the drought. Many of the remaining farm families have been able to raise enough livestock to feed themselves and to have some left over for sale. Chickens have also continued to lay and eggs are plentiful.

Over the years, many young people have left the area and moved to nearby cities where work is available. Last year, the high school was closed because there were not enough students to keep it open. Those few students of high school age are now transported to a school in a nearby town. The grade school is currently open, but several grades have been combined because of the small numbers of students. Elderly residents have remained in their homes, and people over the age of 65 now comprise 60 percent of the population.

Health problems common in the community include hypertension, cardiovascular disease, anemia, and alcoholism. Tuberculosis and suicide are also prevalent among the elderly. There is one older doctor in town, but he plans to retire in a year or two. There is no hospital in town and no dentist. Consequently, hospital and dental services must be obtained in the nearest city, which is 50 miles away.

1. Select one of the models presented in the chapter and use the model to assess the community as a client for community health nursing services.
2. Describe the community's problems in terms of the model.
3. What nursing interventions would be appropriate in this situation? How would this intervention be carried out in terms of the model chosen?

REFERENCES

1. Barnum, B. J. S. (1990). *Nursing theory, analysis, application, evaluation.* (3rd ed.) Boston: Little, Brown.
2. Highriter, M. E. (1984). Public health nursing evaluation, education, and professional issues: 1977 to 1981. In H. H. Werley & J. J. Fitzpatrick (Eds.), *Annual review of nursing research* (Vol. 2). New York: Springer.
3. Riehl, J. P., & Roy, C. (1980). Theory and models. In J. P. Riehl & C. Roy (Eds.), *Conceptual models for nursing practice.* New York: Appleton-Century-Crofts.
4. Roy, C. (1984). *Introduction to nursing: An adaptation model* (2nd ed.). Englewood Cliffs, NJ: Prentice-Hall.
5. Galbreath, J. G. (1980). Sister Callista Roy. In The Nursing Theories Conference Group, *Nursing theories: The base for professional nursing practice.* Englewood Cliffs, NJ: Prentice-Hall.
6. Hanchett, E. S. (1990). Nursing models and community as client. *Nursing Science Quarterly, 3*(2), 67–72.
7. Levine, M. E. (1967). The four conservation principles of nursing. *Nursing Forum, VI* (1), 45–59.
8. Esposito, C. H., & Leonard, M. K. (1980). Myra Estrin Levine. In the Nursing Conference Theories Group, *Nursing theories: The base for professional nursing practice.* Englewood Cliffs, NJ: Prentice-Hall.
9. Orem, D. E. (1985). *Nursing: Concepts of practice* (3rd ed.). New York: McGraw-Hill.
10. Foster, P. C., & Janssens, N. P. (1980). Dorothea E. Orem. In The Nursing Theories Conference Group, *Nursing theories: The base for professional nursing practice.* Englewood Cliffs, NJ: Prentice-Hall.
11. Johnson, D. E. (1980). The behavioral system model for nursing. In J. P. Riehl & C. Roy (Eds.), *Conceptual models for nursing practice.* New York: Appleton-Century-Crofts.
12. Grubbs, J. (1980). An interpretation of the Johnson Behavioral Systems Model for nursing practice. In J. P. Riehl & C. Roy (eds.), *Conceptual models for nursing practice.* New York: Appleton-Century-Crofts.
13. Venable, J. F. (1980). The Neuman Health Care Systems Model. In J. P. Riehl & C. Roy (Eds.), *Conceptual models for nursing practice.* New York: Appleton-Century-Crofts.
14. Neuman, B. (1980). The Neuman Health Care Systems Model. In J. P. Riehl & C. Roy (Eds.), *Conceptual models for nursing practice.* New York: Appleton-Century-Crofts.
15. Pender, N. J. (1982). *Health promotion in nursing practice.* Norwalk, CT: Appleton-Century-Crofts.

RECOMMENDED READINGS

Barnum, B. J. S. (1990). *Nursing theory: Analysis, application, evaluation* (3rd ed.). Glenview, IL: Scott, Foresman, Little, Brown.

Describes the use of theory in nursing practice. Presents an overview of nursing practice based on theoretical foundations.

Bower, F. N. & Patterson, J. (1986). A theory-based assessment of the aged. *Topics in Clinical Nursing, 8*(1), 22–32.

Details the application of Orem's Self-Care Model to the care of older clients.

Davidhizar, R. (1990). The use of Orem's model in psychiatric rehabilitation assessment. *Rehabilitation Nursing, 15*(1), 39–41.

Sets forth the use of Orem's Self-Care Model to the care of clients with psychiatric illnesses.

Delunas, L. R. (1990). Prevention of elder abuse: Betty Neuman health care systems approach. *Clinical Nurse Specialist, 4*(1), 54–58.

Discusses the application of Neuman's Health Care Systems Model to the care of abused older persons and their families.

Derdiarian, A. K. (1990). The relationships among the subsystems of Johnson's behavioral systems model. *Image: The Journal of Nursing Scholarship, 22,* 219–225.

Presents the results of a research study testing the relationships among the behavioral subsystems of Johnson's model.

Hanchett, E. S. (1990). Nursing models and the community as client. *Nursing Science Quarterly, 3*(2), 67–72.

Describes the application of the nursing models of Roy, Orem, King, and Rogers to community health nursing practice.

Hanucharurnkul, S. (1989). Comparative analysis of Orem's and King's theories. *Journal of Advanced Nursing, 14,* 365–372.

Compares the nursing models of Dorothea Orem and Imogene King in the terms of their scope, usefulness, and contribution to nursing.

Knight, J. B. (1990). The Betty Neuman systems model applied to practice: A client with multiple sclerosis. *Journal of Advanced Nursing, 15,* 447–455.

Examines the application of Neuman's Health Systems Model in assessing the health-care needs of a client with multiple sclerosis. Also discusses use of the model to derive a nursing care plan.

Limandri B. J. (1986). Research and practice with abused women: Use of the Roy adaptation model as an explanatory framework. *Advances in Nursing Science, 8*(4), 52–61.

Focuses on the use of the Roy Adaptation Model as a framework for research and practice with abused women.

Schaefer, K. M. & Pond, J. B., with Levine, M. E. & Fawcett, J. (1991). *Levine's conservation model: A framework for nursing practice.* Philadelphia, F. A. Davis.

Enumerates and evaluates Levine's Principles of Conservation model. Presents research testing the model and discusses the application of the model to several different client populations.

APPENDICES

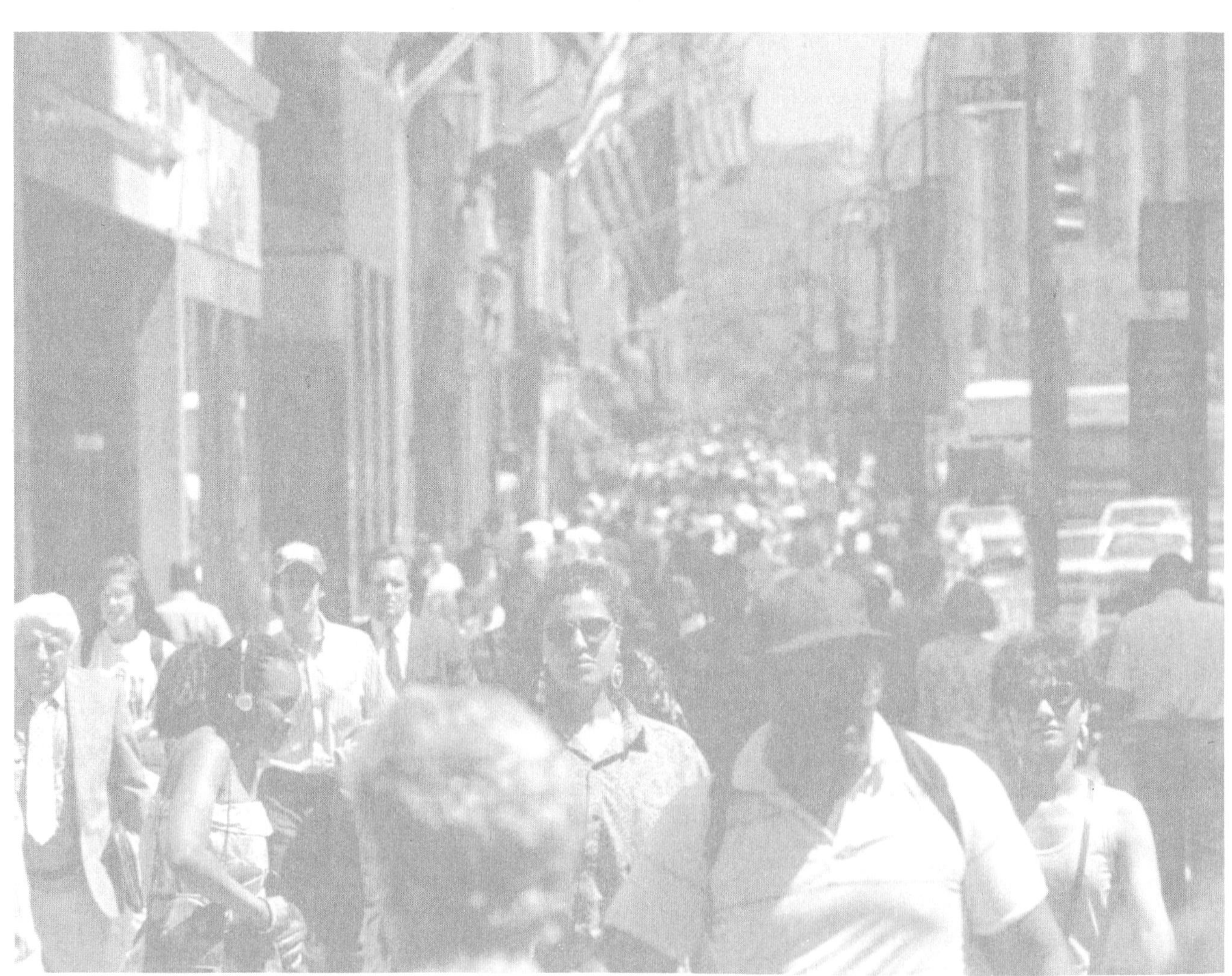

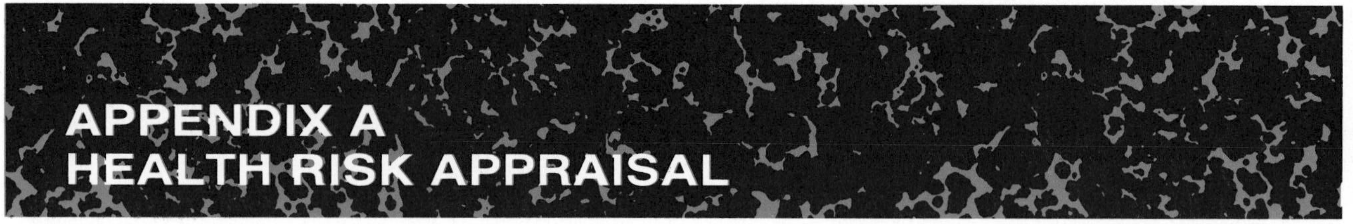

APPENDIX A HEALTH RISK APPRAISAL

The questions provided here are from the University of Minnesota *Health Risk Appraisal*, a computer-based tool for health assessment and education designed by John R. Raines and Lynda B. Ellis. The questions attempt to determine the health interventions or behavior changes most appropriate to the individual in a way that motivates change. The program presents questions related to the top 10 causes of death for the user based on information about the user's age, race, and sex. The program then computes the user's probability of death from these causes in comparison with the probability of death for that general age, race, and sex group. Suggestions for changes in behavior are then made to decrease the probability of death. Both risk factors addressed and behavioral changes suggested are supported by research findings. The tool is a useful one for indicating to clients their need to change health-related behaviors, but, because of the potential for misinterpretation, the community health nurse should interpret the results of the *Health Risk Appraisal* for the client. Copies of the computer program for Apple (2e and Macintosh), IBM (5-¼″ or 3-½″ diskettes), or TRS 80 computers may be obtained from Queue, Inc., 338 Commerce Drive, Fairfield, CT 06430—(800) 232-2224 or (203) 335-0908—at a cost of $99 per copy.

HEALTH RISK APPRAISAL

1. Are you male or female?
2. What is your first name?
3. What is your race?
   (W)hite (B)lack (N)ative American (O)ther
4. How old are you? (Range accepted: 10–99.)
5. What is your weight in pounds? (Range accepted: 30–500 lb.)
6. What is your height in inches? (Range accepted: 57–79.)
7. How regularly do you exercise?
   a. Little or not at all
   b. Occasionally
   c. Regularly (at least 3 times per week)
8. Did either of your parents die of a heart attack before age 60?
   a. No
   b. Yes, one of them
   c. Yes, both of them
   d. Not sure
9. Has any member of your immediate family (parents, brothers, sisters, or children) ever had diabetes?
   a. No
   b. Yes
   c. Don't know
10. Have you ever been told that you have diabetes (too much sugar in your blood)?
    a. No
    b. Controlled
    c. Not controlled
    d. Don't know
11. How many miles per year do you ride in a car, truck, or bus—either as the driver or a passenger? (Range accepted: 100–150,000 miles.)
12. How much of the time do you use a seat belt?
    a. Always
    b. About 25% to 74%
    c. About 15% to 24%
    d. Less than 15%
13. How often do you use drugs or medications that affect your mood or help you to relax?
    a. Rarely or never
    b. Sometimes
    c. Almost every day
14. How much do you drink each week?
    a. Nondrinker
    b. Stopped drinking
    c. 1–2 drinks
    d. 3–6 drinks
    e. 7–24 drinks
    f. 25–40 drinks
    g. Over 40 drinks
15. How often in the past year did you witness or become involved in a violent or potentially violent argument?
    a. Once or never
    b. 2 or 3 times
    c. 4 or more times
    d. Not sure
16. How many of the following things do you usually do?
    - Hitchhike or pick up hitchhikers
    - Carry a gun or knife for protection
    - Keep a gun at home for protection

    a. None
    b. One
    c. Two or more
    d. Not sure
17. How many of the following things do you usually do?
    - Criticize or argue with strangers
    - Live or work in a high crime area
    - Seek entertainment in high-crime areas or bars

    a. None
    b. One
    c. Two or more
    d. Not sure
18. Have you ever had polyps or growths in your rectum (not hemorrhoids)?
    a. No
    b. Yes
    c. Don't know
19. Have you ever had any bleeding from your rectum?
    a. No
    b. Yes
    c. Don't know
20. Do you have an annual rectal exam?
    a. Yes
    b. No
    c. Don't know
21. Considering your age, how would you describe your overall health?
    a. Excellent
    b. Good
    c. Fair
    d. Poor

22. In general, how satisfied are you with your life?
    a. Mostly satisfied
    b. Partly satisfied
    c. Mostly disappointed
    d. Not sure
23. In general, how strong are your social ties with friends and family?
    a. Very strong
    b. About average
    c. Weaker than average
    d. Not sure
24. How many hours of sleep do you usually get at night?
    a. 6 hours or less
    b. 7 hours
    c. 8 hours
    d. 9 hours or more
25. Have you suffered a serious personal loss or misfortune in the past year? (Examples: job loss, disability, divorce, death of a close person.)
    a. No
    b. Yes, one serious loss
    c. Yes, two or more serious losses
26. What is your marital status?
    a. Single (never married)
    b. Married
    c. Separated
    d. Widowed
    e. Divorced
    f. Other
27. Do you smoke?
    a. No
    b. Cigarettes
    c. Cigars or pipe
28. Did you smoke in the past?
    a. No
    b. Cigarettes
    c. Cigars or pipe
29. How many years ago did you stop? Enter 1 if it was less than a year.
30. How much do (did) you smoke each day?
    a. 40 or more cigarettes
    b. 20 to 39 cigarettes
    c. 10 to 19 cigarettes
    d. 1 to 9 cigarettes
31. How much do you smoke each day?
    a. 5 or more cigars or pipes (inhaled)
    b. Less than 5 cigars or pipes (inhaled)
    c. 5 or more cigars or pipes (not inhaled)
    d. Less than 5 cigars or pipes (not inhaled)
32. Have you ever been told that you have emphysema or chronic bronchitis?
    a. No
    b. Yes
    c. Don't know
33. Have your sisters, mother, or daughters ever had breast cancer?
    a. No
    b. Yes
    c. Don't know
34. How often do you examine your breasts for lumps?
    a. Monthly
    b. Once every few months
    c. Rarely or never
35. Have you ever had a hysterectomy?
    a. No
    b. Yes
    c. Don't know
36. How often do you have a Pap smear?
    a. At least once a year
    b. At least once every 3 years
    c. More than 3 years apart
    d. Never had one
    e. Not sure
37. Do you know your blood pressure?
    a. No
    b. Yes
38. What is your systolic blood pressure? (The systolic is the larger number and is written before the /.) Just type one number now.
39. What is your diastolic blood pressure (the other number)?
40. Do you know your cholesterol value?
    a. No
    b. Yes
41. What is you cholesterol value? (Range accepted: 40–3000.)

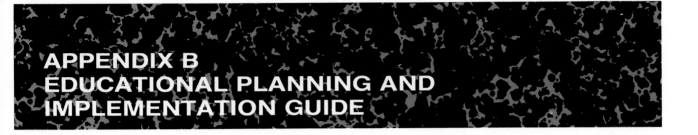

APPENDIX B EDUCATIONAL PLANNING AND IMPLEMENTATION GUIDE

The tool presented here is designed to assist the community health nurse to plan health education for individual clients, families, or groups. It is based on the epidemiologic prevention process model and can be used by the community health nurse to assess and diagnose client educational needs as well as to plan, implement, and evaluate a health education encounter.

The first and second pages of the tool list assessment of the learner and the learning situation. Nursing diagnoses of learning needs and the intervention plan for the health education encounter are documented on the third page of the tool. The intervention plan includes identification of learning tasks, learning objectives, teaching strategies to be used, and plans for evaluation. On the final page of the tool there is space to document evaluation of the health education encounter and to enter any recommendations for revisions for future encounters.

EDUCATIONAL PLANNING AND IMPLEMENTATION GUIDE

Client: ______________________ Phone: __________

Address: ______________________

Contact person (for group encounters): ______________________

Assessment of Learning Situation

Human Biology

Client age(s): __________ Sex: __________ Race: __________

Possible influence of physical maturation on learning: ______________________

Physical conditions giving rise to health educational needs: ______________________

Physical conditions that might influence ability to learn: ______________________

Environment

Physical environment

- Physical environmental conditions giving rise to health education needs: ______________________
- Physical environment for learning (*noise, light levels, distractions*): ______________________

Psychological environment

- Readiness and motivation to learn: ______________________
- Psychological factors that may impede learning (*stress, anxiety, depression, confusion, disorientation*): ______________________
- Coping abilities: ______________________

Social environment

- Educational level: ______
- Socioeconomic level: ______
- Religion: ______
- Ethnicity: ______
- Primary language: ______
- Facility with English: ______
- Cultural influences on the learning situation: ______
- Social support for healthy behavior (*peer interactions, role models*): ______

______

Life-style

Occupation(s): ______

Nutrition (*food consumption, preferences, preparation*): ______

______

Other consumption patterns: ______

______

Health-promotive behaviors: ______

- Immunizations: ______
- Exercise: ______
- Dental hygiene: ______
- Seat-belt use: ______
- Other safety precautions: ______
- Contraceptive use: ______

Health System

Access to health care: ______

Knowledge of health-care resources: ______

Use of promotive health services: ______

Use of restorative/rehabilitative services: ______

Planning and Implementing the Health Education Encounter

Educational Diagnoses	Learning Tasks	Learning Objectives	Teaching Strategies	Evaluation Plan

Evaluation of Health Education Encounter

Evaluation of learning outcomes:

Objective	Status Met/Unmet	Evidence

Process evaluation: ______________________________

Revisions needed: ______________________________

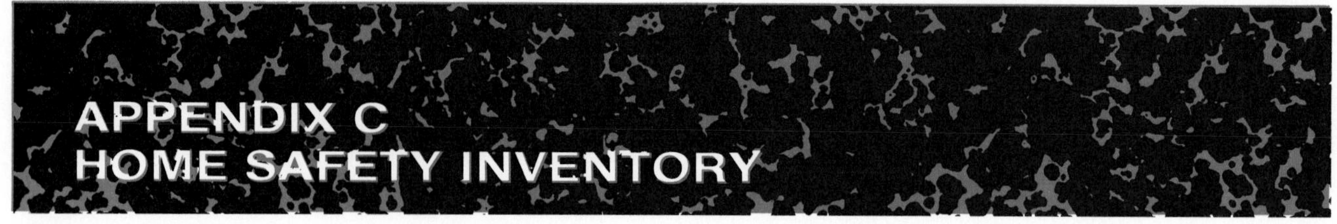

APPENDIX C HOME SAFETY INVENTORY

The two tools included in this appendix are designed to aid in the assessment of home safety for families with children and homes where older adults live. Relevant portions of tools may also be used to assess the safety of the home for other clients.

HOME SAFETY INVENTORY—CHILD

Age	Safety Consideration	Yes	No
Infant	1. Safe sleeping arrangements made for infant?	☐	☐
	2. Parents aware of bathing safety (not leaving child unattended, water temperature)?	☐	☐
	3. No loose parts on toys?	☐	☐
	4. Approved car restraint used consistently?	☐	☐
	5. Infant seat left on elevated surfaces?	☐	☐
	6. Infant restraint straps consistently used in infant seat, stroller, high chair, car seat?	☐	☐
	7. Small objects kept out of reach?	☐	☐
Toddler/preschool child	1. Poisons, sharp objects, etc., kept locked away?	☐	☐
	2. Poisonous substances stored in appropriate containers?	☐	☐
	3. Child-proof lids correctly placed on medications and other toxins?	☐	☐
	4. Medications stored in locked area?	☐	☐
	5. Gates/barriers placed on stairs?	☐	☐
	6. Safety locks present on doors and upstairs windows?	☐	☐
	7. Child closely supervised at play?	☐	☐
	8. Child supervised at all times during bath?	☐	☐
	9. Toys have no small parts?	☐	☐
	10. Electrical outlets covered?	☐	☐
	11. Electrical cords left dangling?	☐	☐
	12. Pots and pans placed toward back of stove with handles turned toward rear?		
	13. Play equipment in good repair?	☐	☐
	14. Outdoor play area is fenced and gates locked?	☐	☐
	15. Poisonous plants present in home or yard?	☐	☐
	16. Car seat-belt used consistently?	☐	☐
	17. Caution used and taught in crossing streets?	☐	☐
School-age child	1. Child supervised in sports and outdoor play?	☐	☐
	2. Play equipment free of safety hazards?	☐	☐
	3. Outdoor play area floored with sand, shavings, or wood chips?	☐	☐
	4. Firearms kept locked with key inaccessible?	☐	☐
	5. Bicycle helmet worn consistently?	☐	☐
	6. Children taught not to open door to strangers?	☐	☐
	7. Car seat-belt used consistently?	☐	☐
Adolescent	1. Firearms safety taught?	☐	☐
	2. Firearms stored unloaded with safety lock on?	☐	☐
	3. Teen cautioned not to admit being home alone?	☐	☐
	4. Car seat-belt used consistently?	☐	☐

HOME SAFETY INVENTORY—OLDER PERSON

Safety Consideration	Yes	No
1. Lighting adequate on stairs?	☐	☐
2. Stair rails present and in good repair?	☐	☐
3. Nonskid surfaces on stairs?	☐	☐
4. Throw rugs present safety hazard?	☐	☐
5. Crowded living area present safety hazard?	☐	☐
6. Tub rails installed?	☐	☐
7. Tub has nonslip surface?	☐	☐
8. Space heaters present safety hazard?	☐	☐
9. Adequate provision made for refrigeration of food?	☐	☐
10. Medications kept in appropriately labeled containers with readable print?	☐	☐
11. Toxic substances have labels with readable print and are stored well away from food?	☐	☐
12. Home is adequately ventilated and heated?	☐	☐
13. Neighborhood is safe?	☐	☐
14. Fire and police notified of older person in home?	☐	☐

APPENDIX D
CLIENT DISCHARGE INVENTORY

This inventory is intended to be used to identify client discharge needs and to direct planning to meet those needs. It may be used for clients being discharged from an acute-care setting to community health nursing services, or for clients being discharged from community health nursing services to other agencies or to self-care. It is designed around the components of the epidemiologic prevention process model.

CLIENT DISCHARGE INVENTORY

Human Biology

Name: ______________________ Age: ____ Sex: ____ Ethnicity: __________

Indicate the extent to which the client needs assistance and the type of assistance needed with each of the following functions:

Area of Function	Type of Assistance Needed	To be Provided By
Bathing		
Dressing		
Eating		
Elimination		
Mobility		

Does the client have medical diagnoses that require follow-up?

Medical Diagnosis	Type of Follow-up Needed	To be Provided By

Is the client on any medications? Do these medications give rise to needs for care?

Medication	Care Needed	To be Provided By

Does the client have physical impairments that affect self-care abilities? ______________________

____

Does the client have other physical needs that necessitate care? ______________________

____

Environment

Discharge address: ____________________

Will there be physical hazards in the discharge environment? Describe them. ____________________

____

Does the client's emotional/mental state give rise to needs for care? ____________________

____

Is the client able to cope effectively? ____________________

Describe the client's social support network. ____________________

____

Are there cultural influences affecting client needs for care? ____________________

____

Does the client have needs related to the following socioeconomic concerns?

Area of Need	Type of Assistance Needed	To be Provided By
Finances		
Transportation		
Social interaction		
Shopping		
Child care		

Life-style

Do any of the following life-style factors give rise to needs for care?

Life-style Factor	Type of Assistance Needed	To be Provided By
Alcohol use		
Diet		
Drug use		
Leisure activity		
Occupation		
Safety precautions		
Smoking		

Health System

What level(s) of services are needed from the health-care system?

Level of Prevention	Type of Services Needed	To be Provided By
Primary		
Secondary		
Tertiary		

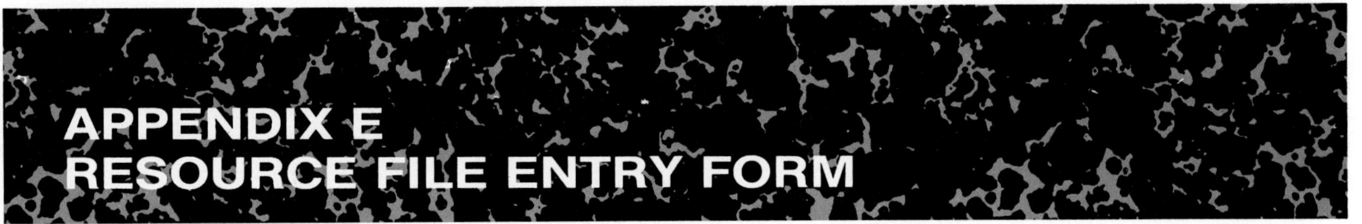

APPENDIX E RESOURCE FILE ENTRY FORM

The form presented here is intended for use by community health nurses in exploring the available resources of a community. Information contained in the entry will allow the nurse to identify resources that will best meet clients' needs. Information about community agencies will also allow the community health nurse to make appropriate referrals for services. Information obtained about a particular agency or referral resource should be updated frequently.

RESOURCE FILE ENTRY FORM

Resource category: ______________________ Funding source: ______________________

Agency name: ____

Address: ____

Phone number: ______________________ Business hours: ______________________

Contact person: ______________________ Title: ______________________

Source of referral: ____

Eligibility: ____

____

Fee: ____

Services: ____

____

____

____

____

____

____

____

Access: ____

Other comments: ____

____

____

____

____

____

____

____

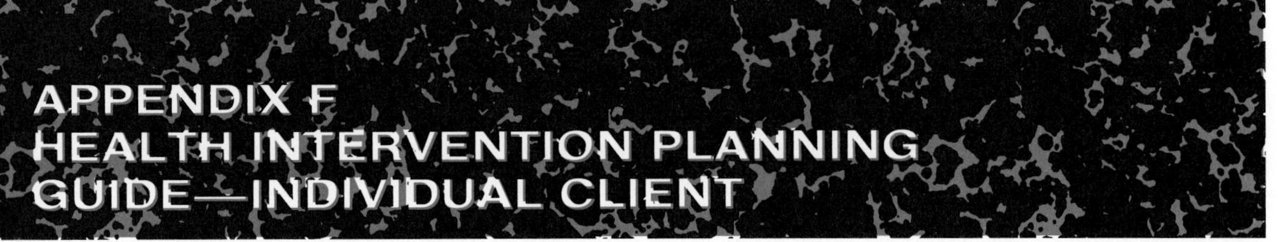

APPENDIX F HEALTH INTERVENTION PLANNING GUIDE—INDIVIDUAL CLIENT

This tool is intended to assist the community health nurse to use the epidemiologic prevention process model to assess the health-care needs of the individual client and to plan, implement, and evaluate interventions to meet those needs.

HEALTH INTERVENTION PLANNING GUIDE—INDIVIDUAL CLIENT

Client's name: ______________________ Phone: ____________

Address: ______________________________________

Assessment

Human Biology

Age: ____ Date of birth: ________ Sex: ____ Race/ethnic group: ____________

Significant family health history (*include a genogram*): ____________

____

Current acute or chronic illnesses (*describe problem, status, treatment if any*): ____________

____

Current signs or symptoms of physical health problems: ____________

____

Areas of physical disability or limitation of function: ____________

____

Significant past illnesses, injuries, hospitalizations (*describe what, when, outcomes*): ____________

____

Developmental assessment (*based on developmental tasks appropriate to the client's age*): ________

____

____

Review of systems

Head (*headache [how often, quality, treatment, outcome], syncope, head trauma*): ____________

____

Eyes (*vision problems, tearing, burning eyes, glasses, last eye exam*): ____________

____

Ears (*difficulty hearing, discharge, earache*): ____________

____

Mouth and throat (*sore throat, lesions, toothache, caries, last dental visit*): ____________

____

Respiratory system (*frequent colds, nosebleeds, cough, pneumonia, asthma, shortness of breath, sinusitis, hay fever*): ____

____

Cardiovascular system (*heart problems, hypertension, chest pain, cyanosis, shortness of breath, murmurs, edema*): ____

____

Gastrointestinal system (*nausea, vomiting, diarrhea, constipation, flatulence, abdominal pain, loss of appetite, increased appetite, weight loss or gain, rectal pain or bleeding*): ____________________

____

Urinary tract (*dysuria, urinary frequency, urgency, nocturia, difficulty voiding, urinary retention, back pain in costovertebral angle*): ____

____

Reproductive system (*edema of labia or vulva, vaginal or penile discharge, use of oral or other contraceptives, pregnancies [past or current] and outcome, age at menarche, last menstrual period, dysmenorrhea, irregular menses, sexual satisfaction, breast discharge, self-breast exam, breast lumps, changes in breast contour, prostatitis, history of sexually transmitted disease*):

____

Musculoskeletal system (*joint pain, swelling, tremor, history of fractures, muscle weakness*):

____

____

Integumentary system (*lesions [describe character, locale, color], changes in skin color, itching, hair loss, discoloration or pitting of nails, swollen glands*): ____________________________

____

Hematopoietic system (*anemia, bleeding tendencies, bruise easily, transfusions [when, why]*):

____

____

Physical examination

Vital signs (*T P R Ht Wt B/P*): ____

General appearance (*posture, gait, deformities, hygiene*): ____________________________

Skin (*including nails and hair*): ____

Head and neck (*lymph nodes, face*): ______

Eyes: ______

Ears: ______

Nose and sinuses: ______

Mouth and throat (*lips, gums, tongue, palate, larynx, teeth*): ______

Chest:

- Breast exam: ______
- Heart: ______
- Lungs: ______

Abdomen: ______

Genitalia (*including anus and rectum*): ______

Musculoskeletal system (*spine, extremities, joints, muscles*): ______

Nervous system (*cranial nerves, DTRs, temperature, kinesthetic sense*): ______

Results of screening and other laboratory tests: ______

Immunization status: ______

Environment

Physical environment

Where does the client live? Is there adequate space and privacy in the home? ______

Are safety hazards present in the home? (See Appendix C and the Home Safety Assessment guides.)

______

Are there pets in the home? (*What kind? How many? Inside or outside?*) ______

What is the neighborhood like? (*Describe safety, services and facilities available, pollutants.*)

Psychological environment

Does the client have a history of mental illness? (*Describe what, when, treatment, outcome.*)

What is the client's emotional state or mood? Have significant changes been noted recently?

What is the client's level of orientation?

What coping strategies does the client use? How effective are they?

What is the client's level of self-esteem?

Does the client talk of committing suicide?

Does the client communicate well with others? How satisfying are the client's interpersonal relationships?

Has the client experienced a recent significant loss? What is the effect of this loss on the client?

Does the client report high levels of stress? What are the sources of this stress?

Social environment

What is the client's educational level? What is the client's level of health knowledge? Does the client have special learning needs related to health? (See Appendix B, Educational Planning and Implementation Guide.) Is the client literate?

What is the client's source of income? Is the client's income adequate to meet his or her needs? Does the client appropriately budget for expenses? ____________________

____

Describe the client's social support network. Is the network adequate to meet needs? Is the network effectively utilized? ____________________

____

Do any cultural practices influence the client's health? ____________________

____

What is the client's religion? What effect does religion have on health? ____________________

____

Life-style

Consumption patterns

What is the client's usual diet? (*Describe number of meals per day, food preferences, usual mode of preparation, adequacy, special dietary needs and level of compliance, cultural restrictions.*)

____

____

Does the client smoke, drink alcohol, or use drugs? (*How much? How often?*) ____________________

____

How much caffeine does the client consume? ____________________

____

What medications does the client use? Is use appropriate? ____________________

____

Occupation

Is the client employed? (*Specify occupation, employer, occupational hazards, frequent job changes.*)

____

____

Leisure

What leisure pursuits does the client engage in? How much exercise does the client get?

____

____

Other

Is the client sexually active? (*Describe sexual preference, multiple partners, use of condoms and other contraceptives, sexual practices.*) ____________________

____

Does the client use seat belts and other safety devices regularly? ____________________

____

Health System

What is the client's attitude toward health and health care? ____________________

____

What is the client's usual source of health care? ____________________

____

How does the client finance health care? ____________________

____

Are there barriers to obtaining health care? ____________________

____

Is the client's use of health-care services appropriate to health-care needs? ____________________

____

Diagnosis, Planning, Implementation, and Evaluation

Identified Health Need	Objective	Intervention	Evaluative Criteria

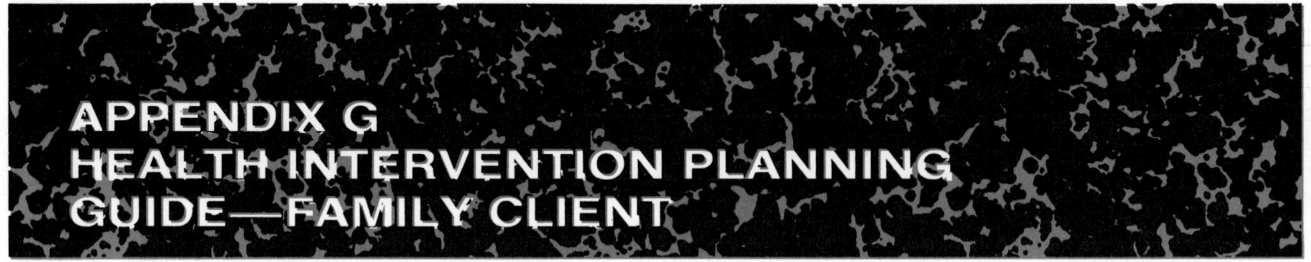

APPENDIX G HEALTH INTERVENTION PLANNING GUIDE—FAMILY CLIENT

The tool presented in this appendix is designed to assist the community health nurse to apply the epidemiologic prevention process model to the care of families. The assessment portion of the tool is offered here. For the diagnosis, planning, implementation, and evaluation sections of the model, use page A–25 of Appendix F, Health Intervention Planning Guide—Individual Client.

HEALTH INTERVENTION PLANNING GUIDE—FAMILY CLIENT

Family surname(s): ______________________ Phone: ______________

Address: ____

____

Human Biology

Name	Age	Sex	Physical Health Status

Maturation and aging

Individual family member's developmental tasks met? ______________________

____

Effects of individual development on family health: ______________________

____

Significant past health problems of family members: ______________________

____

Physiologic function

Treatment for current family health problems (*type, effects, source*): ______________________

____

Significant family history of hereditary conditions: ______________________

____

Immunization status of family members: ______________________

____

Environment

Physical environment

Family home (*location, adequacy for family size*): ______________________________

____

Safety hazards present in home: ______________________________

____

Neighborhood (*safety, services and facilities available, pollutants*): ______________________________

____

Psychological environment

Family strengths and weaknesses: ______________________________

____

Family communication (*typical patterns, effectiveness, purposes, tone, rules*): ______________________________

____

Family stage of development: ______________________________

____

Status of developmental tasks of this and previous stages: ______________________________

____

Extent of emotional support for family members: ______________________________

____

____

Coping strategies used (*type, effectiveness*): ______________________________

____

____

Discipline (*type, source, consistency, appropriateness*): ______________________________

____

____

History of mental illness in family members: ______________________________

____

Family roles:

Role	Performed by	Adequacy	Role model
Leader			
Child care			
Sexual			
Breadwinner			
Confidant			
Disciplinarian			
Homemaker			
Repairperson			
Financial manager			

Presence of role conflict or role overload: ______________________________

____

Family goals (*congruence with individual and societal goals*): ______________________________

____

Social environment

Religious affiliations of family members and their influence on health: ______________________________

____

Family cultural affiliations and influences on health: ______________________________

____

Family income (*source, adequacy, effectiveness of management*): ______________________________

____

Educational level of family members: ______________________________

____

External resources available to family: ______________________________

____

Life-style

Consumption patterns

Family dietary patterns (*amount, food preferences, preparation, adequacy, special needs*): ______

______

Use of other substances (*tobacco, alcohol, other drugs*): ______

______

Use of prescription and nonprescription medications: ______

______

Rest and exercise patterns: ______

______

Occupation and leisure

Family Member	Occupation	Employer	Leisure Activities

Occupational health hazards for family members: ______

______

Health hazards posed by family leisure pursuits: ______

______

Use of recreational activities to enhance family cohesion: ______

______

Other behaviors

Use of safety devices and practices: ______

______

Family planning (*need for, type, effectiveness*): ______

______

Health System

Family attitudes toward health: ______________________________

____

Family response toward illness: ______________________________

____

Use of folk remedies and self-care practices: ______________________________

____

Usual source of health care: ______________________________

____

Means of financing health care: ______________________________

____

Barriers to obtaining health care: ______________________________

____

APPENDIX H HEALTH INTERVENTION PLANNING GUIDE—COMMUNITY CLIENT

The tool presented here can be used by the community health nurse to apply the epidemiologic prevention process model to the care of communities as clients. The assessment portion of the tool is included here. For the diagnostic, planning, implementation, and evaluation aspects of the model, use page A–25 of Appendix F, Health Intervention Planning Guide—Individual Client.

HEALTH INTERVENTION PLANNING GUIDE—COMMUNITY CLIENT

Human Biology

Births (*annual rate, extent of illegitimacy, abortion*): __________

Composition of population:

Age	Total	Male	Female	White	Black	Hispanic	Asian	Native American
<1 yr								
1–5 yrs								
6–12 yrs								
13–20 yrs								
21–30 yrs								
31–50 yrs								
51–65 yrs								
66–80 yrs								
>80 yrs								

Mortality rates (*overall, age specific, cause specific*): __________

Morbidity:

Disease	Incidence	Prevalence

Disease	Incidence	Prevalence

How do morbidity and mortality rates compare with previous years? With state and national rates?

____

Environment

Physical environment

Community location (*boundaries, urban/rural*): ____________________

____

Size and density: ____________________

____

Prominent topographical features: ____________________

____

Housing (*type, condition, adequacy, number of persons per dwelling, sanitation*): ____________________

____

Safety hazards present in the environment: ____________________

____

Source of community water supply: ____________________

____

Sewage and waste disposal: ____________________

____

Nuisance factors: ____________________

____

Potential for disaster: ____________________

____

Psychological environment

Future prospects for the community: ____________________

____

Significant events in community history: ____________________

____

Interaction of groups within the community (*racial tension, etc.*): ____________________

____

Protective services (*adequacy, local crime rate, insurance rates*): ______

______

Communication network (*media, informal channels, links to outside world*): ______

______

Sources of stress in the community: ______

______

Extent of mental illness in the community: ______

______

Social environment

Government (*type, effectiveness, community officials*): ______

______

Unofficial leaders (*significant informants*): ______

______

Political affiliations of community members: ______

______

Status of minority groups (*influence, length of residence*): ______

______

Languages spoken by community members: ______

______

Community income levels (*poverty, coverage by assistance programs*): ______

______

Education (*prevailing levels, attitudes, facilities*): ______

______

Religion (*major affiliations, programs and services, influence on health*): ______

______

Culture (*affiliation, influence on health*): ______

______

Employment level: ____________________

____

Transportation (*type, availability, cost, adequacy*): ____________________

____

Shopping facilities (*type, availability, cost, use*): ____________________

____

Social services (*type, availability, adequacy, use*): ____________________

____

Life-style

Consumption patterns

Nutrition (*general levels, preferences, preparation, special needs, prevalence of anemia, obesity*):

____

Alcohol (*consumption patterns, extent of abuse*): ____________________

____

Drug use (*licit and illicit*): ____________________

____

Smoking (*extent, cessation program availability*): ____________________

____

Exercise (*extent, type*): ____________________

____

Occupation

Primary occupations of community members: ____________________

____

Major employers (*occupational health programs*): ____________________

____

Occupational hazards: ____________________

____

Leisure pursuits

Primary leisure pursuits of community members: ____________________

Recreational facilities (*availability, adequacy, cost*): ____________________

Health hazards posed by recreation: ____________________

Other behaviors

Use of safety devices: ____________________

Contraceptive use: ____________________

Health System

Community attitudes toward health (*definitions, support of services*): ____________________

Health services and resources (*type, availability, cost, adequacy, utilization*): ____________________

Prenatal care (*availability, use*): ____________________

Emergency services (*availability, adequacy*): ____________________

Health education services (*availability, adequacy*): ____________________

Health-care financing (*extent of insurance coverage, Medicaid, Medicare, tax support*): ____________________

APPENDIX I HEALTH INTERVENTION PLANNING GUIDE—TARGET GROUP

For the most part, assessing the health needs of a target group from the perspective of the epidemiologic prevention process model is similar to assessing a community. For most of the information needed, the community health nurse can use the assessment guide provided in Appendix H, Health Intervention Planning Guide—Community Client. There are, however, some specific assessment considerations for a target group that differ from those in assessing a community. These special considerations are presented here. Again, this tool only addresses the assessment of a target group's health needs. Page A–25 of Appendix F, Health Intervention Planning Guide—Individual Client, should be used to guide the diagnostic, planning, implementation, and evaluation phases in the use of the epidemiologic prevention process model.

HEALTH INTERVENTION PLANNING GUIDE—TARGET GROUP

Target group: ______

Human Biology

What is the age, sex, and racial or ethnic composition of the target group? ______

Are there any special maturational or developmental concerns for group members? ______

What health problems are commonly experienced by group members? ______

Are group members particularly vulnerable to any particular illnesses? ______

Are there any special immunization concerns for group members? ______

Environment

Physical environment

Where is the target group located? ______

Are there any special environmental considerations for group members (*wheelchair access, ramps*)? ______

Are group members particularly vulnerable to environmental conditions (*pollutants, temperature changes*)? ______

Do group members have special housing needs? ______

Psychological environment

What effect does group membership have on members' self-image? ______

What coping skills do group members display? Are they adequate? ______

______

What is the incidence and prevalence of psychological problems among group members?

______

What psychological stressors are experienced by group members? ______

______

Social environment

What are the attitudes of the larger society toward group members? ______

______

What is the extent of group members' social status and influence? ______

______

Are there special economic concerns for group members? ______

______

Are there special educational concerns for group members? ______

______

Does the group have an official spokesperson or group to represent its interests? ______

______

Do group members have particular protective services needs? ______

______

Do group members have unique transportation needs? ______

______

Life-style

Consumption patterns

Do group members have special nutritional needs? ______

______

What is the extent of drug or alcohol abuse among group members? ______

______

Does smoking pose any special problems for group members? ________________

____

Does exercise pose any special problems for group members? ________________

____

Occupation

Are group members employable? ________________

____

Are there particular occupational concerns for group members? ________________

____

Leisure pursuits

Do certain leisure pursuits pose problems for group members? ________________

____

Do group members have access to recreational opportunities open to other members of society?

____

Other behaviors

Are special safety precautions warranted for group members? ________________

____

Does contraception pose special problems for group members? ________________

____

Health Services

What health services are needed by group members? Are they available and accessible?

____

What is the attitude of health-care professionals toward group members? ________________

____

How do group members finance health care? Are there problems with financing such care?

____

Do group members experience barriers to obtaining health care? ________________

____

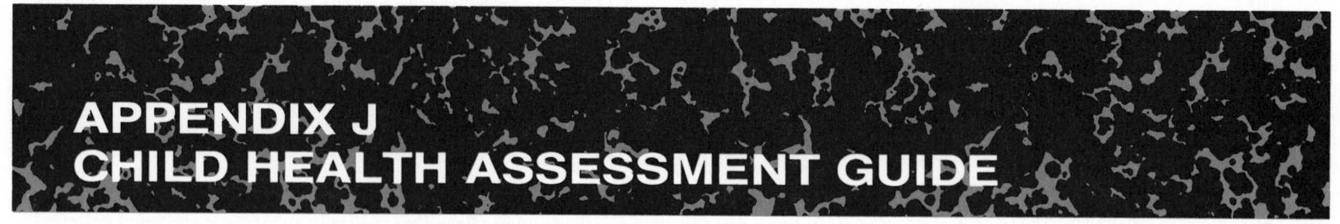

APPENDIX J CHILD HEALTH ASSESSMENT GUIDE

Generally speaking, the health status of a child can be assessed using the tool in Appendix F, Health Intervention Planning Guide—Individual Client. There are, however, some assessment considerations unique to the child client. These additional considerations are addressed here.

CHILD HEALTH ASSESSMENT GUIDE

Human Biology

Maturation and aging

Birth weight and length: ______________________________

____

Pattern of growth (*compared to norms and to previous pattern*): ______________________________

____

Accomplishment of developmental milestones (DDST *or other appropriate test*): ______________________________

____

Parental knowledge of child development and its implications: ______________________________

____

Physiologic function

Significant events during the pregnancy: ______________________________

____

Significant events during delivery: ______________________________

____

Congenital defects: ______________________________

____

Review of symptoms

Respiratory system (*colds and ear infections [frequency and outcome]*): ______________________________

____

Cardiovascular system (*murmur, cyanosis when crying*): ______________________________

____

Gastrointestinal system (*quality of stool, frequency*): ______________________________

____

Urinary tract (*frequency of urination, strength of urinary stream, odor*): ______________________________

____

Reproductive system (*breast development in girls, vaginal discharge, menarche; wet dreams in boys, extent of sex education*): ______

Integumentary system (*eczema, diaper rash*): ______

Physical examination

Height, weight, head and chest circumference: ______

Eyes (*ability to focus on and follow objects*): ______

Ears (*ability to localize sound*): ______

Mouth and throat (*monilial patches, number of teeth, dental hygiene, caries*): ______

Genitalia (*undescended testes, vaginal tears, discharge*): ______

Gastrointestinal (*imperforate anus, anal tears*): ______

Musculoskeletal (*equal movement of extremities, spina bifida, congenital hip dislocation*): ______

Nervous system (*newborn reflexes*): ______

Integumentary (*diaper rash, eczema, bruises, burns, hygiene*): ______

Screening test results (PKU, T4, *hematocrit, sickle cell test, serum lead,* TB, *urinalysis as appropriate*): ______

Immunization status (*up-to-date for age*): ____________________

____

Environment

Physical environment

Safety hazards (see Appendix C for Home Safety Assessment guides): ____________________

____

Psychological environment

Reactivity patterns and parental responses: ____________________

____

Parental expectations (*appropriateness*): ____________________

____

Discipline (*type, consistency, appropriateness*): ____________________

____

Parental coping skills: ____________________

____

Parent–child interactions: ____________________

____

Self-image: ____________________

____

Evidence of abuse or neglect: ____________________

____

Social environment

Interaction with others ____________________

____

Life-style

Nutrition

Infant (*formula or breast, frequency, amount, formula preparation, feeding and burping techniques*):

____

____

Other age groups (*well-balanced diet, amount of "junk food"*): ______

Parental knowledge of nutritional needs: ______

Rest and exercise

Sleeping patterns: ______

Type and amount of exercise: ______

Childrearing and socialization

Child care outside the home (*where, by whom, adequacy*): ______

School performance: ______

Health System

Use of primary prevention services (*general and dental*): ______

Source of illness care: ______

Parental knowledge of illness care and need for medical assistance: ______

APPENDIX K NURSING INTERVENTIONS FOR COMMON HEALTH PROBLEMS IN CHILDREN

The interventions presented here are general guidelines that the community health nurse can use to educate parents for home-care of minor health problems commonly encountered among young children.

NURSING INTERVENTIONS FOR COMMON HEALTH PROBLEMS IN CHILDREN

Organ System	Problem	Interventions
Gastrointestinal	Spitting up	Burp baby more frequently Keep infant upright for short time after feeding Check size of nipple hole Change to soy formula
	Colic	Give small amounts of warm water Exert gentle pressure on abdomen with infant's legs and thighs bent
	Diarrhea or vomiting (mild)	Begin oral rehydration to prevent dehydration Do not discontinue feedings Seek medical help if condition continues or worsens
	Constipation	Increase fluid intake Add bulk to diet Encourage regular toileting habits Discourage postponing defecation Avoid use of laxatives or enemas
Respiratory	Mild respiratory infection	Increase fluid intake Use a cold mist humidifier to ease breathing Do not use Vicks or other aromatic substances Seek medical help for severe or persistent cough, difficulty breathing, stridor, nasal flaring
Integumentary	Diaper rash	Wash diapers with mild soaps and rinse thoroughly Add ¾ cup vinegar to last rinse to remove ammonia If using disposable diapers, use ones that allow air circulation Frequent diaper change and cleansing of diaper area Do not use powders or lotion in diaper area Leave diaper area exposed when possible
	Allergic dermatitis	Explore changes in foods or soaps Eliminate possible causative substances Seek medical help for severe rashes or secondary infection
	Cradle cap	Scrub scalp with soap and soft washcloth during bath Brush scalp with soft brush after bath Do not use oil or lotion on scalp
	Abrasions and lacerations	Wash with soap and water Keep clean
Urinary tract	Urinary tract infection	Seek medical assistance

Organ System	Problem	Interventions
Urinary tract (*continued*)	Bedwetting	Limit fluid intake after dinner Empty bladder before bed Awaken child to urinate before parents go to bed Do not make an issue of the problem If problem is severe or continues beyond age 6, seek medical attention
Musculoskeletal	Sprains and fractures	Perform basic first aid and immobilize injured area Seek medical attention
	Leg cramps	Increase calcium intake If severe or persistent, seek medical attention
Neurological	Headache	Give non-aspirin analgesic according to child's age and size If severe or recurrent, seek medical attention
	Hearing problem	Seek medical attention
	Vision problem	Seek medical attention
	Delayed speech	Discourage older children and parents from talking for child Encourage child to verbalize needs before meeting them Seek medical attention for prolonged delay
	Speech defect	Seek medical attention
Other	Fever	For temperature over 102°F, give non-aspirin antipyretic For high or persistent fever, seek medical attention
	Suspected abuse	Refer to child protective services
	Night terrors	Use a night light or leave bedroom door open Use bedtime rituals of checking for "monsters" if helpful Use a "guardian" stuffed animal to scare away monsters Comfort the child after waking and stay until child returns to sleep Seek assistance for persistent terrors or those related to a real traumatic event
	Jealousy of new baby	Prepare siblings for birth of another child Have child assist with care of newborn Emphasize positive aspects of being older Accept regressive behavior and do not belittle Spend time with just the older child Encourage friends and relatives to pay attention to older child as well as new baby

Organ System	Problem	Interventions
Other (*continued*)	Sibling rivalry	Mediate arguments Encourage children to work out own differences Encourage compromise Give reasons for differences in privileges Use role-play with older children to give insight into feelings and behaviors of others
	Tantrums	Ignore behavior if possible Remove child to bedroom if disturbing others Do not give in to child's demands
	Bed-time	Complete bedtime rituals and put child in bed Ignore crying for 15 to 20 minutes. If the child does not stop, see what is wrong If child gets up, put him or her back to bed Place several safe toys in bed with child and allow play until the child falls asleep
	Poor self-esteem	Praise child for accomplishments Correct mistakes without denigrating child Help child identify and strengthen talents Assist child to accept limitations Seek assistance for severe depression or low self-esteem on the part of child

APPENDIX L HEALTH ASSESSMENT GUIDE—ADULT CLIENT

Assessment of the health needs of adult clients can be undertaken using the assessment tool for individual clients included in Appendix F, Health Intervention Planning Guide—Individual Client. There are, however, some considerations unique to adult men and women that are presented here.

HEALTH ASSESSMENT GUIDE—ADULT CLIENT

Human Biology

Accomplishment of adult developmental tasks: ______________________

____

Past illnesses, hospitalizations, surgery, injuries: ______________________

____

Review of systems

Eyes (*use of glasses, contacts*): ______________________

____

Cardiovascular (*history of heart disease, hypertension, chest pain, shortness of breath*): __________

____

Urinary tract (*frequent urinary tract infection, difficulty voiding*): ______________________

____

Reproductive (*sexual satisfaction, extent of sexual activity*): ______________________

____

Male (*prostatitis, history of STDs, penile discharge, lesions on penis, testicular self-examination, testicular pain, lumps, impotence*):

____

Female (*breast self-examination, breast lumps, discharge from breasts or vagina [color, character, odor], menarche, last menstrual period, changes in menses, pregnancy history, abortions, dysmenorrhea, dyspareunia*):

____

Environment

Psychological

Self-image, coping abilities: ______________________

____

Potential for suicide: ______________________

____

Sources of psychological stress: ______________________

____

Evidence of physical or emotional abuse: ______

Social

Extent of social support system: ______

Extent of social support for healthy behaviors: ______

Adequacy of adult role models: ______

Life-style

Consumption patterns

Use of alcohol (*frequency, amount, adverse effects on client or significant others*): ______

Use of drugs (*type, frequency, effects*): ______

Use of medications (*type, frequency, appropriateness*): ______

Use of tobacco (*type, amount, frequency, number of years*): ______

Occupation

Employment history (*type of occupation, length of time in jobs*): ______

Occupational hazards: ______

Other

Extent of sexual activity: ______

Sexual preference (*male or female partner*): ______________________________

____

Number of sexual partners: ______________________________

____

Contraceptive use (*need, type, effectiveness*): ______________________________

____

Sexual practices (*oral or anogenital intercourse*): ______________________________

____

Use of condoms and other barrier devices: ______________________________

____

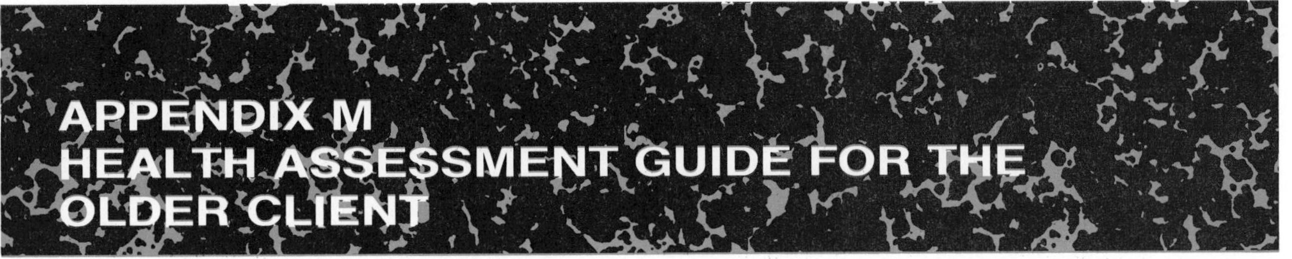

APPENDIX M HEALTH ASSESSMENT GUIDE FOR THE OLDER CLIENT

Generally speaking, Appendix F, Health Intervention Planning Guide—Individual Client, can be used to assess the health-care needs of older clients as well as those of persons in other age groups. Remember, though, that there are some assessment considerations unique to older clients. These unique considerations are presented here.

HEALTH ASSESSMENT GUIDE FOR THE OLDER CLIENT

Human Biology

Physiologic function

Perceptions of personal health: ______________________________

____

Review of systems (include effects of aging)

Eyes (*visual impairment, use of glasses*): ______________________________

____

Ears (*hearing impairment, use of hearing aid*): ______________________________

____

Mouth and throat (*dentures [fit, use], dry mouth, bleeding gums*): ______________________________

____

Integumentary (*skin integrity, fragility, dryness, itching, lesions, bruises, bleeding, skin color changes, hair distribution, thickened nails; hair, nail, and skin-care practices; temperature of extremities, decreased perspiration*):

____

____

Respiratory (*shortness of breath with exertion, cyanosis, emphysema, cough*): ______________________________

____

Cardiovascular (*history of heart disease, palpitations, hypertension, effect of activity on heart rate; edema, fatigue, orthostatic hypotension, varicosities, venous ulcers*): ______________________________

____

Gastrointestinal (*flatulence, constipation, heartburn, rectal bleeding, incontinence dysphagia, appetite, ability to chew*): ______________________________

____

Musculoskeletal (*mobility, joint swelling, pain, use of cane or other device, history of fractures, kyphosis*): ______________________________

____

Neurological (*diminished sense of smell, touch, heat sensation, taste, numbness or tingling*):

Reproductive (*decreased libido*):

Male (*difficulty in achieving erection, prostatitis, impotence*):

Female (*onset of menopause, last Pap smear, mammogram, breast self-examination*):

Urinary (*frequency, urgency, incontinence, color, odor, nocturia*):

Hematopoietic (*anemia, epistaxis, bleeding tendencies*):

Existence of acute and chronic health problems (*diagnosis, status, treatment, effects*):

Functional abilities related to:

Bathing:

Dressing:

Toileting:

Mobility:

Eating:

Bowel and bladder function:

Communicating: ______________________________

____

Immunization status (*tetanus, pneumonia, influenza*): ______________________________

____

Environment

Physical environment

Safety hazards in home (See Appendix C for Home Safety Assessment guides): ______________________________

____

Presence of safety features in home: ______________________________

____

Availability of resources in neighborhood: ______________________________

____

Neighborhood safety: ______________________________

____

Driving: ______________________________

____

Home maintenance and repair: ______________________________

____

Pets: ______________________________

____

Adequacy of heating, lighting, ventilation: ______________________________

____

Psychological environment

Mental status/orientation: ______________________________

____

Changes in self-image due to aging, retirement: ______________________________

____

Adjustment to retirement: ______________________________

____

Coping abilities: ______________________________

____

History of mental illness: ______________________________

____

Provision for privacy: ______________________________

____

Loss of loved ones: ______________________________

____

Life satisfaction: ______________________________

____

Preparation for death: ______________________________

____

Evidence of depression: ______________________________

____

Evidence of abuse or neglect: ______________________________

____

Social environment

Social interaction and support network: ______________________________

____

Income (*source, adequacy, ability to budget*): ______________________________

____

Relationships with family: ______________________________

____

Educational level: ______________________________

____

Religion and importance in client's life: ______________________________

____

Ethnicity and influence on client's health: ______________________________

____

Possibility of institutionalization and client response: ______________________________

____

Life-style

Consumption patterns

Nutrition (*adequacy for needs, special needs, appetite, meal pattern, food preferences and modes of preparation, food supplements, food storage, shopping practices*): ______________________________

____

Use of alcohol or other drugs: ______________________________

____

Use of medications (*type, appropriateness, effectiveness*): ______________________________

____

Exercise: ______________________________

____

Sleep patterns: ______________________________

____

Occupation

Current employment: ______________________________

____

Previous occupation: ______________________________

____

Leisure activity

Preferred leisure pursuits: ______________________________

____

Opportunity for leisure activities: ______________________________

____

Sexuality

Opportunity for intimacy: ____________________

____

Alternative modes of meeting sexual needs: ____________________

____

Independence

Ability to care for self: ____________________

____

Ability to make independent decisions: ____________________

____

Health System

Source of health care: ____________________

____

Health care financing (*Medicare, insurance*): ____________________

____

Use of health services: ____________________

____

Barriers to obtaining health care: ____________________

____

APPENDIX N SAMPLE FORMS FOR DOCUMENTING HOME NURSING CARE

The forms included here are examples of the types of forms that may be used to document home nursing care. The first form is a two-page Home Health Nursing Assessment that can be used by the community health nurse to identify the health-care needs of the client seen in the home setting. The second form, Patient Progress Notes, can be used to record subsequent observations of the client's status and progress toward desired outcomes. The final two forms are the Home Health Certification and Plan of Treatment form (HCFA-485) and the Medical Update and Patient Information form (HCFA-486). Both of these forms are required to document home nursing care for reimbursement under Medicare.

HOME HEALTH
NURSING ASSESSMENT

Patient Name ______________________________

MR# ____________ Birth Date ____________

Primary Diagnosis:

Past Medical History:

General Appearance:

Vital Signs: Temp ________ Pulse: Apical ________ Radial ________ Respirations ________

Weight ________ Height ________

Blood Pressure: 1) Right arm - Supine ________ Sitting ________ Standing ________

2) Left arm - Supine ________ Sitting ________ Standing ________

Communication: No Problems ________ Difficulty understanding spoken communication ________

Difficulty producing speech ________ Difficulty reading ________ Difficulty writing ________

Language used is: English ________ other (Specify) ________________

Interpreter ________________ Phone (if other than patient's) (   ) ________________

Hearing: Normal ________ Hearing impaired ________ Deaf ________ Uses hearing aid R ________ L ________

Vision: Normal ________ Blind ________ Limited ________ Uses glasses: Sometimes ________ Always ________

Medications	Venous Access. Good ________ Fair ________ Poor ________
	Telephone ________ Refrigerator ________ Electric ________
	Comments
Allergies: ________________	

NEUROLOGICAL: ____ No Problems ____ Oriented x ____________ Headache ____ Vertigo ____ Tremors ____ Seizures ____
____ Syncope ____ Parathesias ____ Weakness

LOC: ______________________________ Activity Limitation: ______________________________

Comments:

CARDIOVASCULAR: ____ No Problems ____ Palpitations ____ Fainting ____ Dizziness ____ Edema ____ Cyanosis
____ Neck Vein Distention ____ Chest Pain ____ Pulse Irregularity ____ Syncope ____ Circumoral Pallor

Comments:

RESPIRATORY: ____ No Problems ____ Dyspnea ____ SOB ____ SOBOE ____ Orthopnea ____ Cough ____ Cyanosis ____ Pain
____ Sputum ____ IPPB ____ 02

Lung Sounds:

Comments:

GASTROINTESTINAL: ____ No Problems ____ Nausea ____ Vomiting ____ Anorexia ____ Bleeding ____ Pain ____ Diarrhea
____ Constipation ____ Incontinent ____ Distension ____ Aphagia ____ NGT ____ GT ____ JT

Bowel Sounds:

Comments:

GENITO/URINARY: ____ No Problems ____ Frequency ____ Urgency ____ Pain ____ Burning ____ Nocturia ____ Hematuria
____ Difficulty Urinating ____ Incontinent ____ Retention ____ Catheter

Comments:

SKIN: ____ No Problems ____ Cool ____ Warm ____ Rash ____ Bruises ____ Diaphoresis ____ Pallor ____ Cyanosis ____ Flushing
____ Jaundice ____ Pruritis ____ Petechiae ____ Dry ____ Pressure Areas ____ Wound/Incision ____ Decubitus

Turgor:

Comments:

PAIN: ____ No Problems **Description** ______________________________

Intensity: ____ 1+(mild) ____ 2+(discomfort) ____ 3+(distressing) ____ 4+(severe) ____ 5+(excruciating)

Analgesics taken ______________________ Frequency ____________ Effectiveness ____________

Comments:

PSYCHOSOCIAL: ____ No Problems ____ Depressed ____ Uncooperative ____ Anxious ____ Restless ____ Forgetful ____ Dependent
____ Other (Specify) ______________________________

Comments:

PATIENT PROGRESS NOTES

CIRCLE ALL APPLICABLE:

1. Nursing Assessment
2. Medication
   a. administration
   b. instruction
   c. review compliance
   d. review side effects
3. Infusion device
   a. instruction
   b. insertion
   c. maintenance care
   d. discontinue
4. IV hydration
   a. instruction
   b. review compliance
   c. review side effects
5. Chemotherapy
   a. administration
   b. instruction
   c. review compliance
   d. review side effects
6. TPN
   a. instruction
   b. administration
   c. review compliance
   d. review side effects
7. Enteral feedings
   a. insert tube
   b. instruction
   c. review compliance
   d. review side effects
8. Pain Management
   a. instruction
   b. review compliance
   c. review side effects
9. Lab Specimen drawn
10. Nutrition assessment
12. Equipment
    a. delivered
    b. returned
    c. inventoried
11. Instruction
    a. patient
    b. caregiver
    c. staff-informal

OBSERVATIONS:	TEMPERATURE	APICAL PULSE	RADIAL PULSE	RESPIRATIONS	BLOOD PRESSURE	WEIGHT

NEUROLOGICAL: ☐ Oriented x________ ☐ Level of Alertness ☐ Headache ☐ Vertigo ☐ Tremors ☐ Seizures ☐ Syncope ☐ Coordination ☐ Parathesias ☐ Weakness ☐ Mobility ☐ No Problems

Comments:

CARDIOVASCULAR: ☐ Palpitations ☐ Fainting ☐ Dizziness ☐ Edema ☐ Cyanosis ☐ Neck Vein Distention ☐ Chest Pain ☐ Peripheral Pulses ☐ Pulse Irregularity ☐ Syncope ☐ Circumoral Pallor ☐ No Problems

Comments:

RESPIRATORY: ☐ Dyspnea ☐ SOB ☐ SOBOE ☐ Orthopnea ☐ Cough ☐ Cyanosis ☐ Pain ☐ Lung Sounds ☐ Sputum ☐ Used IPPB ☐ 02 Used ☐ No Problems

Comments:

GASTROINTESTINAL: ☐ Nausea ☐ Vomiting ☐ Anorexia ☐ Bleeding ☐ Pain ☐ Diarrhea ☐ Incontinent ☐ Nutritional Problem ☐ Bowel Sounds ☐ Distension ☐ Aphagia ☐ NGT ☐ GT ☐ JT ☐ No Problems

Comments:

GENITO/URINARY: ☐ Frequency ☐ Urgency ☐ Pain ☐ Burning ☐ Nocturia ☐ Hematuria ☐ Difficulty Urinating ☐ Incontinent ☐ Retention ☐ Catheter Plugged ☐ No Problems

Comments:

SKIN: ☐ Rash ☐ Bruises ☐ Diaphoresis ☐ Pallor ☐ Cyanotic ☐ Flushing ☐ Jaundice ☐ Pruritis ☐ Petechiae ☐ Dry ☐ Pressure Areas ☐ Wound/Incision ☐ Cool ☐ Warm ☐ Decubitus ☐ No Problems

Comments:

PAIN: No Problems ______ Description ________________ Location ________

Intensity: 1+ mild ______ 2+ discomfort ______ 3+ distressing ______ 4+ severe ______ 5+ excruciating ______

Analgesics taken: ________________ Frequency ________ effectiveness ________

Comments:

INFUSION: ☐ Peripheral ☐ Sub Q ☐ Central Line ☐ VAD Type ________ ☐ Intermittant ☐ Continuous ☐ Pump Type ________

Comments:

PSYCHOSOCIAL: ☐ Depressed ☐ Uncooperative ☐ Anxious ☐ Restless ☐ Forgetful ☐ Dependent ☐ Other (Specify) ☐ No Problems

Comments:

NARRATIVE

SIGNATURE

NAME: ________________ MR # ________ DATE ________ TIME: ________

Department of Health and Human Services
Health Care Financing Administration

Form Approved
OMB No. 0938-0357

HOME HEALTH CERTIFICATION AND PLAN OF TREATMENT

1. Patient's HI Claim No.	2. SOC Date	3. Certification Period From: To:	4. Medical Record No.	5. Provider No.

6. Patient's Name and Address

7. Provider's Name and Address.

8. Date of Birth: 9. Sex ☐ M ☐ F

10. Medications: Dose/Frequency/Route (N)ew (C)hanged

11. ICD-9-CM	Principal Diagnosis	Date
12. ICD-9-CM	Surgical Procedure	Date
13. ICD-9-CM	Other Pertinent Diagnoses	Date

14. DME and Supplies

15. Safety Measures:

16. Nutritional Req.

17. Allergies:

18.A. Functional Limitations

1 ☐	Amputation	5 ☐	Paralysis	9 ☐	Legally Blind
2 ☐	Bowel/Bladder (Incontinence)	6 ☐	Endurance	A ☐	Dyspnea With Minimal Exertion
3 ☐	Contracture	7 ☐	Ambulation	B ☐	Other (Specify)
4 ☐	Hearing	8 ☐	Speech		

18.B. Activities Permitted

1 ☐	Complete Bedrest	6 ☐	Partial Weight Bearing	A ☐	Wheelchair
2 ☐	Bedrest BRP	7 ☐	Independent At Home	B ☐	Walker
3 ☐	Up As Tolerated	8 ☐	Crutches	C ☐	No Restrictions
4 ☐	Transfer Bed/Chair	9 ☐	Cane	D ☐	Other (Specify)
5 ☐	Exercises Prescribed				

19. Mental Status:	1 ☐ Oriented	3 ☐ Forgetful	5 ☐ Disoriented	7 ☐ Agitated	
	2 ☐ Comatose	4 ☐ Depressed	6 ☐ Lethargic	8 ☐ Other	
20. Prognosis:	1 ☐ Poor	2 ☐ Guarded	3 ☐ Fair	4 ☐ Good	5 ☐ Excellent

21. Orders for Discipline and Treatments (Specify Amount/Frequency/Duration)

22. Goals/Rehabilitation Potential/Discharge Plans

23. Verbal Start of Care and Nurse's Signature and Date Where Applicable:

24. Physician's Name and Address

25. Date HHA Received Signed POT

26. I ☐ certify ☐ recertify that the above home health services are required and are authorized by me with a written plan for treatment which will be periodically reviewed by me. This patient is under my care, is confined to his home, and is in need of intermittent skilled nursing care and/or physical or speech therapy or has been furnished home health services based on such a need and no longer has a need for such care or therapy, but continues to need occupational therapy.

27. Attending Physician's Signature (Required on 485 Kept on File in Medical Records of HHA)

Date Signed

Form HCFA-485 (U4) (4-87)

PROVIDER

Department of Health and Human Services
Health Care Financing Administration

Form Approved
OMB No. 0938-0357

MEDICAL UPDATE AND PATIENT INFORMATION

1. Patient's HI Claim No.	2. SOC Date	3. Certification Period From: To:	4. Medical Record No.	5. Provider No.

6. Patient's Name	7. Provider's Name

8. Medicare Covered: ☐ Y ☐ N | 9. Date Physician Last Saw Patient: | 10. Date Last Contacted Physician:

11. Is the Patient Receiving Care in an 1861 (J)(1) Skilled Nursing Facility or Equivalent? ☐ Y ☐ N ☐ Do Not Know | 12. ☐ Certification ☐ Recertification ☐ Modified

13. Specific Services and Treatments

Discipline	Visits (This Bill) Rel. to Prior Cert.	Frequency and Duration	Treatment Codes	Total Visits Projected This Cert.

14. Dates of Last Inpatient Stay: Admission Discharge | 15. Type of Facility:

16. Updated Information: New Orders/Treatments/Clinical Facts/Summary from Each Discipline

17. Functional Limitations (Expand From 485 and Level of ADL) Reason Homebound/Prior Functional Status

18. Supplementary Plan of Treatment on File from Physician Other than Referring Physician: ☐ Y ☐ N
(If Yes, Please Specify Giving Goals/Rehab. Potential/Discharge Plan)

19. Unusual Home/Social Environment

20. Indicate Any Time When the Home Health Agency Made a Visit and Patient was Not Home and Reason Why if Ascertainable

21. Specify Any Known Medical and/or Non-Medical Reasons the Patient Regularly Leaves Home and Frequency of Occurrence

22. Nurse or Therapist Completing or Reviewing Form | Date (Mo., Day, Yr.)

Form HCFA-486 (C3) (4-87)

PROVIDER

APPENDIX O SPECIAL ASSESSMENT CONSIDERATIONS IN THE SCHOOL SETTING

Assessing the health needs of groups of people within a school setting requires attention to some specific assessment considerations. This tool is designed to assist the community health nurse to apply the epidemiologic prevention process model to the care of groups of clients in schools. The tool addresses only the assessment component of the model. For the diagnosis, planning, implementation, and evaluation components of the model, the community health nurse can use page A–25 of Appendix F, Health Intervention Planning Guide—Individual Client.

SPECIAL ASSESSMENT CONSIDERATIONS IN THE SCHOOL SETTING

Human Biology

Age, sex, and racial/ethnic composition of the school population: ______

Presence of handicapping conditions: ______

Incidence and prevalence of disease: ______

Immunization status: ______

Environment

Physical environment

Traffic patterns around the school: ______

Safety hazards in the neighborhood: ______

Use of pesticides and other poisons in the neighborhood: ______

Pollutants in the area of the school: ______

Fire or safety hazards in the school environment: ______

Use of toxic chemicals in labs, art classes, cleaning and maintenance: ______

Use of hazardous equipment in home economics or "shop" classes: ______

Broken glass in play areas: ______

Play equipment in poor repair: ____________________

____

Hard surfaces below play equipment: ____________________

____

Animals in the school environment: ____________________

____

Plant allergens or poisons in the school environment: ____________________

____

Adequacy of heating, lighting, cooling: ____________________

____

Noise levels: ____________________

____

Food sanitation practices: ____________________

____

Toilet facilities (*adequacy, state of repair*): ____________________

____

Cleaning of shower facilities: ____________________

____

Isolation facilities for children with communicable diseases: ____________________

____

Facilities and access for handicapped children or staff: ____________________

____

Psychological environment

Organization of the school day (*appropriateness to needs, effects on health*): ____________________

____

Aesthetic quality of environment: ____________________

____

Relationships among students (*quality, appropriateness of adult monitoring*): ______

______

Teacher–student relations (*quality, extent*): ______

______

Teacher-to-teacher relations: ______

______

Discipline (*type, extent, appropriateness, consistency, fairness*): ______

______

Grading practices (*consistency, fairness*): ______

______

Parent–school relations (*quality, extent*): ______

______

Social environment

Community attitudes toward education and toward school: ______

______

Community support of school program: ______

______

Crime in neighborhood (*extent, effect on school and student health*): ______

______

Funding (*extent, adequacy, priorities*): ______

______

Home environment of students: ______

______

Availability of before- and after-school care: ______

______

Socioeconomic status of students, staff: ______

______

Presence of intergroup conflicts: ____________________

Cultural background of staff, students: ____________________

Educational level of families and extent of health knowledge: ____________________

Life-style

Consumption patterns

Quality of school meal programs: ____________________

Student/staff nutritional levels: ____________________

Nutrition knowledge (*extent among students, staff, parents*): ____________________

Extent of alcohol or drug use by students, staff, family members: ____________________

Extent of smoking by students, staff, family members: ____________________

Rest and exercise patterns of school population: ____________________

Leisure

Recreational opportunities (*type, age-appropriateness*): ____________________

Use of appropriate safety equipment: ____________________

Other

Sexual activity by students (*extent, use of contraceptives, use of condoms and other barrier devices*):

____

Use of safety devices (seat belts): ______________________________

____

Health System

Health services offered by school: ______________________________

____

Availability of other health services: ______________________________

____

Use of health services by school population: ______________________________

____

Financing of health services: ______________________________

____

Support of school health program by health professionals in the community: ______________________________

____

School and community attitudes toward health and health care: ______________________________

____

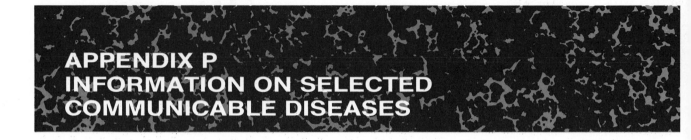

APPENDIX P INFORMATION ON SELECTED COMMUNICABLE DISEASES

CHLAMYDIAL INFECTION

Agent: Chlamydia trachomatis
Reservoir: man
Incubation: probably 7–14 days
Communicability: unknown
Modes of transmission: sexual contact
Immunization: none
Prophylaxis: antibiotics following sexual exposure or for infants born to infected mothers
Treatment: tetracycline, doxycycline, or erythromycin
Contact notification: sexual contacts

Symptoms: Frequently asymptomatic. *Males* may have urethritis with burning on urination, urethral itching, penile discharge. *Females* may have purulent vaginal discharge.

Prevention: Monogamy, condom use.

DELTA HEPATITIS

Agent: Hepatitis Delta Virus (HDV)
Reservoir: man
Incubation: 2–10 weeks
Communicability: during active infection
Modes of transmission: sexual contact, direct inoculation
Immunization: none
Prophylaxis: none
Treatment: symptomatic
Contact notification: none

Symptoms: Jaundice, fatty food intolerance, dark urine, clay-colored stool, pruritis.

Prevention: Avoid exposure to blood via drug use or needle-stick injury; condom use; monogamy.

DIPHTHERIA (pharyngotonsillar, laryngeal)

Agent: Corynebacterium diphtheriae
Reservoir: man
Incubation: 2–5 days
Communicability: usually 2 weeks
Modes of transmission: airborne, raw milk; contact with articles soiled with discharge from lesions (rare)
Immunization: routine use of DTP vaccine
Prophylaxis: antitoxin for children under age 10
Treatment: diphtheria antitoxin and penicillin or erythromycin
Contact notification: none

Symptoms: Sore throat with patchy, grayish membrane over pharynx, tonsils, uvula, and soft palate; cervical lymphadenopathy.

Prevention: Immunization of susceptible individuals.

GONORRHEA

Agent: Neisseria gonorrhoea
Reservoir: man
Incubation: usually 2–7 days
Communicability: until treated
Modes of transmission: sexual contact
Immunization: none
Prophylaxis: antibiotics after exposure
Treatment: ceftriaxone and doxycycline
Contact notification: sexual contacts

Symptoms: Vary with site of infection. Usually associated with penile discharge and burning on urination in urethritis; anal discharge, tenesmus, and pruritis in rectal infection. May be associated with vaginal discharge and foul odor in females; sore throat in oral infection.

Prevention: Monogamy, use of condoms.

HEPATITIS A

Agent: hepatitis A virus (HAV)
Reservoir: man
Incubation: average 28–30 days
Communicability: latter half of incubation period to a few days after onset of jaundice
Modes of transmission: fecal-oral, sexual contact (homosexual males), contaminated food or water, direct inoculation (?)
Immunization: none
Prophylaxis: immune globulin (IG)
Treatment: symptomatic
Contact notification: household contacts

Symptoms: Abrupt onset of fever, malaise, anorexia, nausea and vomiting, abdominal discomfort followed by jaundice.

Prevention: Sanitation, personal hygiene (handwashing)

HEPATITIS B

Agent: hepatitis B virus (HBV)
Reservoir: man
Incubation: average 60–90 days
Communicability: several weeks before and after symptom onset. May be lifelong carrier
Modes of transmission: sexual contact, direct inoculation
Immunization: hepatitis B vaccine
Prophylaxis: hepatitis B immune globulin and/or immunization
Treatment: symptomatic
Contact notification: household or sexual contacts, drug partners

Symptoms: Insidious onset of anorexia, abdominal discomfort, nausea and vomiting, followed by jaundice.

Prevention: Immunization of persons in high-risk groups; monogamy, condom use, blood donor screening, drug-abuse treatment; avoid needle sharing.

HIV INFECTION

Agent: Human immunodeficiency virus (HIV)
Reservoir: man
Incubation: 2 months to 10 years
Communicability: unknown; presumed lifelong
Modes of transmission: sexual contact, direct inoculation, transplacental inoculation
Immunization: none
Prophylaxis: antiviral agents (effects ?)
Treatment: antiviral agents (effects ?)
Contact notification: sexual partners, drug-use partners who share needles, clients of infected health professionals, recipients of blood or tissue from infected donors

Symptoms: Fatigue, malaise, recurrent and sustained opportunistic infections.

Prevention: Monogamy, condom use, drug treatment; avoid needle sharing; screen blood and organ donors.

HSV INFECTION

Agent: Herpes simplex virus (HSV) type 2
Reservoir: man
Incubation: 2–12 days
Communicability: 7–12 days, initial lesion; 4–7 days, recurrent lesions
Modes of transmission: sexual contact
Immunization: none
Prophylaxis: none
Treatment: symptomatic, acyclovir
Contact notification: pregnant women

Symptoms: Painful genital lesions.

Prevention: Monogamy, condom use.

INFLUENZA

Agent: Influenza viruses A, B, C
Reservoir: man (animals for new subtypes)
Incubation: 1–5 days
Communicability: 3–7 days after onset of symptoms
Modes of transmission: airborne
Immunization: annual use of influenza vaccine for high-risk individuals
Prophylaxis: amantadine in high-risk persons (type A only)
Treatment: symptomatic
Contact notification: none

Symptoms: Fever, headache, myalgia, prostration, coryza, sore throat, cough, nausea, vomiting, diarrhea.

Prevention: Immunization of persons at risk; general health promotion.

MEASLES

Agent: Measles virus
Reservoir: man
Incubation: average 10 days
Communicability: beginning of prodrome to 4 days after onset of rash
Modes of transmission: airborne
Immunization: routine use of measles, mumps, rubella vaccine (MMR)
Prophylaxis: MMR within 72 hours of exposure. Measles immune globulin for children under 1 year within 3 days of exposure
Treatment: symptomatic
Contact notification: none

Symptoms: Prodrome of fever, conjunctivitis, cough, coryza, and Koplik's spots, followed by rash on face and spreading downward.

Prevention: Routine immunization of all susceptible individuals.

MUMPS

Agent: mumps virus
Reservoir: man
Incubation: usually 18 days
Communicability: 6–7 days before swelling to 9 days after
Modes of transmission: airborne
Immunization: routine use of measles, mumps, rubella (MMR) vaccine
Prophylaxis: none
Treatment: symptomatic
Contact notification: none

Symptoms: Pain and swelling in parotid area accompanied by difficulty swallowing. Redness and swelling around Stensen's duct.

Prevention: Immunization of susceptible individuals.

NON-A, NON-B HEPATITIS

Agent: unidentified
Reservoir: man
Incubation: 26–42 days
Communicability: unknown
Modes of transmission: fecal-oral, direct inoculation
Immunization: none
Prophylaxis: none
Treatment: symptomatic
Contact notification: household contacts

Symptoms: Insidious onset of jaundice and malaise.

Prevention: Sanitation, handwashing, drug-abuse treatment; avoid needle sharing.

PERTUSSIS

Agent: Bordetella pertussis
Reservoir: man
Incubation: 7–10 days
Communicability: early catarrhal stage to 3 weeks after cough begins
Modes of transmission: airborne
Immunization: routine use of DTP vaccine
Prophylaxis: DTP booster and erythromycin
Treatment: erythromycin may reduce communicability
Contact notification: nonimmune children

Symptoms: Initial catarrhal stage followed by paroxysmal whooping cough.

Prevention: Immunization of susceptible individuals.

POLIOMYELITIS

Agent: poliovirus, types 1, 2, 3
Reservoir: man
Incubation: 7–14 days
Communicability: unknown, possible 36–72 hours after exposure to 10 days after symptoms occur
Modes of transmission: airborne, contaminated milk and food
Immunization: routine use of trivalent oral polio vaccine (OPV)
Prophylaxis: none
Treatment: symptomatic
Contact notification: close contacts

Symptoms: Fever, headache, gastrointestinal disturbance; stiffness of neck and back with or without paralysis.

Prevention: Immunization of susceptible children; sanitation.

RUBELLA

Agent: rubella virus
Reservoir: man
Incubation: 16–18 days
Communicability: 1 week before to 4 days after onset of rash
Modes of transmission: airborne, transplacental inoculation
Immunization: routine use of measles, mumps, rubella vaccine (MMR)
Prophylaxis: immune globulin (IG) for pregnant women (value ?)
Treatment: symptomatic
Contact notification: pregnant women

Symptoms: Prodrome of mild fever, headache, and malaise, followed by discrete maculopapular rash, occipital node enlargement.

Prevention: Immunization of susceptible individuals, especially women of child-bearing age.

SYPHILIS

Agent: Treponema pallidum
Reservoir: man
Incubation: 10–90 days (usually 3 weeks)
Communicability: in stages with lesions
Modes of transmission: sexual contact, direct inoculation, transplacental inoculation

Immunization: none
Prophylaxis: antibiotics after exposure
Treatment: penicillin
Contact notification: sexual contacts to primary, secondary, and early latent syphilis; persons sharing needles

Symptoms: Vary with stage of disease.

Primary: Painless chancre or lesion at site of infection (usually genitalia, lips, etc.). May be accompanied by localized lymphadenopathy in the area of the lesion.

Secondary: Coppery, macular rash (may be found in all areas but particularly on palms and soles.) May be accompanied by malaise and generalized lymphadenopathy.

Latent: Asymptomatic.

Late: Depends on organ system affected.

Congenital: Hutchinson's teeth and raspberry molars, saddle nose, snuffles, rash if in secondary stage.

Prevention: Monogamy, condom use, drug-abuse treatment; avoid needle sharing; screening of blood donors.

TETANUS

Agent: Clostridium tetani
Reservoir: man and animals
Incubation: 3–21 days
Communicability: not directly communicable
Modes of transmission: introduction via wound in skin or unhealed umbilicus

Immunization: routine use of DTP vaccine
Prophylaxis: Td booster for immunized persons. Tetanus immune globulin (TIG) or tetanus antitoxin and Td for unimmunized individuals.
Treatment: tetanus immune globulin (TIG) or antitoxin and penicillin
Contact notification: N/A

Symptoms: Painful muscular contractions with progressive rigidity, especially in muscles of neck and shoulders.

Prevention: Immunization of susceptible individuals; prevent injury, cleanse injuries thoroughly, control animal feces; asepsis during deliveries.

TUBERCULOSIS

Agent: Mycobacterium tuberculosis
Reservoir: man, cattle
Incubation: 4–12 weeks
Communicability: during periods of respiratory expulsion of bacteria
Modes of transmission: airborne, contaminated milk

Immunization: BCG for selected individuals
Prophylaxis: isoniazid
Treatment: antituberculin agents
Contact notification: close contacts

Symptoms: Cough, hemoptysis, unexplained weight loss, night sweats.

Prevention: Improve social conditions, promote general health.

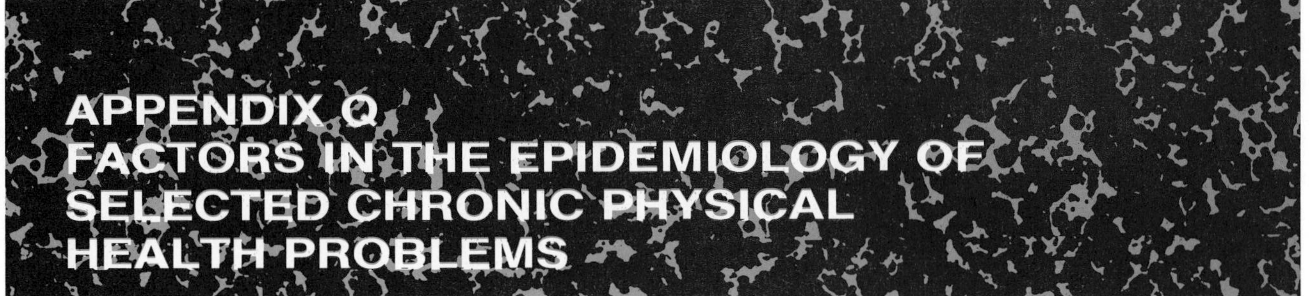

APPENDIX Q FACTORS IN THE EPIDEMIOLOGY OF SELECTED CHRONIC PHYSICAL HEALTH PROBLEMS

Information presented here includes epidemiologic factors associated with the incidence of selected chronic physical health problems. The health problems discussed are arthritis, cancer, cardiovascular and cerebrovascular disease, chronic obstructive pulmonary disease (COPD), diabetes mellitus, obesity, and conditions resulting from accidental trauma. Factors related to each condition are organized in terms of the epidemiologic prevention process model.

Epidemiologic Factors Associated with Arthritis

Human Biology

There may be a genetic predisposition to arthritis

Asians and Native Americans have low incidence rates for arthritis

The onset of arthritis usually begins in the 4th decade of life

Older persons usually have greater disability from arthritis

Women are more likely than men to develop arthritis

Previous injury to bones and joints may predispose one to arthritis

Obesity increases stress on joints and may exacerbate arthritis

Life-style

Occupational or recreational factors that contribute to injury may lead to arthritis in later life

Overeating may lead to obesity and increased severity of arthritis

Health System

Many people with arthritis engage in self-care rather than seek medical help

Medical treatment for arthritis has limited effects

Epidemiologic Factors Associated with Cancers

Human Biology

Genetic inheritance may predispose one to cancer

Incidence and survival rates for cancer vary among ethnic and racial groups

Males have higher mortality rates for most forms of cancer than do females

Environment

Cancer incidence is higher in urban than in rural areas

Environmental pollutants can contribute to cancer incidence

Life-style

Smoking increases one's risk of several forms of cancer

Lack of dietary fiber and increased fat in the diet have been linked to increased risk of colon cancer

Alcohol consumption can be associated with increased cancer risk (especially liver cancer)

Occupational exposures can contribute to cancer

Self-screening health practices such as breast self-examination and testicular self-examination increase one's chances of cancer survival

Health System

Lack of emphasis on screening has contributed to cancer mortality

Aggressiveness of treatment influences cancer survival rates

Epidemiologic Factors Associated with Cardiovascular and Cerebrovascular Disease

Human Biology

Genetic inheritance may predispose one to cardiovascular or cerebrovascular disease

Cardiovascular disease is more common in young blacks and older whites

Females have lower mortality rates for cardiovascular and cerebrovascular disease than do males

Racial differences in incidence of cardiovascular and cerebrovascular disease probably reflect differences in the prevalence of other biological risk factors such as hypertension, increased serum cholesterol, and diabetes

Environment

Stress in the environment can contribute to cardiovascular and cerebrovascular disease

High-income and educational levels are associated with decreased mortality due to cardiovascular and cerebrovascular disease

Life-style

Sedentary life-style increases the risk of cardiovascular and cerebrovascular disease

Smoking increases the risk of cardiovascular and cerebrovascular disease

Overeating and increased fat and cholesterol consumption contribute to cardiovascular and cerebrovascular disease

White-collar occupations are associated with decreased mortality from cardiovascular and cerebrovascular disease

Health System

Attention to elimination of risk factors has decreased the incidence of cardiovascular and cerebrovascular disease

Access to emergency services reduces mortality due to cardiovascular and cerebrovascular disease

Epidemiologic Factors Associated with COPD

Human Biology

Some evidence supports a genetic predisposition to COPD

Recurrent respiratory infections early in life can contribute to COPD later in life

Respiratory allergies and asthma can increase the risk of COPD

Environment

Environmental pollution can contribute to or exacerbate COPD

COPD is more prevalent in highly industrialized urban areas than in rural areas

Exposure of nonsmokers to tobacco smoke exacerbates COPD

Life-style

Occupational exposure to dusts or gases increases the risk of COPD

Smoking increases the risk of COPD and interacts with other contributing factors to increase the risk still more

Health System

Lack of emphasis on primary prevention contributes to COPD

Treatment of COPD is minimally effective

Epidemiologic Factors Associated with Diabetes Mellitus

Human Biology

Genetic predisposition is a contributing factor in diabetes

Native Americans and blacks have higher incidence rates of diabetes than do other racial groups

The presence of hypertension complicates diabetes

Diabetes is a risk factor for heart disease and stroke

Environment

Diabetes is more prevalent in industrialized countries

Life-style

Affluence increases incidence rates of diabetes

Smoking interacts with diabetes to increase the risk of heart disease and stroke

Overeating and consequent overweight contribute to diabetes

Alcohol use contributes to diabetes mortality

Exercise can contribute to diabetes control

Health System

Lack of emphasis on screening leads to later diagnosis and poor control of diabetes

Lack of access to health care influences diabetes control

Failure to monitor treatment effects can contribute to increased diabetes mortality

Epidemiologic Factors Associated with Obesity

Human Biology

There may be a slight genetic predisposition to obesity

Obesity occurs in all age groups, both sexes, and all ethnic groups

Environment

Prevalence of junk food contributes to obesity

Fast-paced life leads to poor nutrition and obesity

Life-style

Consumption of excess calories, especially fats, contributes to obesity

Sedentary life-style and lack of exercise contribute to obesity

Occupations that contribute to a sedentary life-style also contribute to obesity

Health System

Lack of emphasis on nutrition education contributes to poor dietary habits and obesity

Treatment of obesity is less effective than it might be because of high rates of noncompliance

Epidemiologic Factors Associated with Trauma Due to Accidents

Human Biology

Drowning, poisoning, and suffocation are common among young children

Firearms injuries are common among preadolescents and adolescents

Motor vehicle accidents affect all age groups, but occur most often among adolescents and young adults

The elderly are particularly susceptible to the effects of falls and fires

The presence of physical disability increases the risk of accidental injury

Environment

Improper storage of hazardous materials increases accident risk

Use of space heaters contributes to fires and burn injuries

Absence of smoke detectors in buildings contributes to fire injuries

Road conditions and automobile crashworthiness influence motor vehicle accidents and their effects

Easy access to firearms contributes to accidental injuries

Life-style

Alcohol and drug use and abuse contribute to accidents

Recreational activities pose a variety of accident hazards

Occupations involving heavy labor increase the risk of accidents

Failure to use safety devices increases the risk of injury

Common use and improper storage of medications contribute to poisoning

Health System

Lack of emphasis on safety education has contributed to accidental injuries

Access to emergency services influences accident survival rates

Long-term consequences of accidents are affected by the availability of rehabilitation services

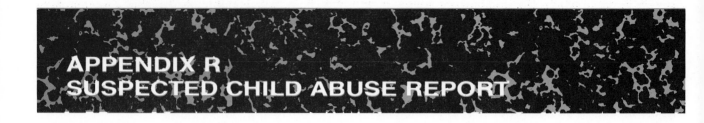

APPENDIX R SUSPECTED CHILD ABUSE REPORT

The form included here is an example of the type used to report suspected child abuse. In jurisdictions where reporting of elder abuse is mandated by law, similar forms would be used. Generally, cases of suspected or confirmed abuse are reported immediately by telephone and followed with a completed reporting form within 24 hours. Whenever feasible, specific events leading to suspicion of abuse should be described as fully as possible, including information about specific behavior observed or exact words of those describing events.

SUSPECTED CHILD ABUSE REPORT

To Be Completed by Reporting Party
Pursuant to Penal Code Section 11166

A. CASE IDENTI-FICATION — *TO BE COMPLETED BY INVESTIGATING CPA*

VICTIM NAME: ______

REPORT NO./CASE NAME: ______

DATE OF REPORT: ______

B. REPORTING PARTY

NAME/TITLE		
ADDRESS		
PHONE ( )	DATE OF REPORT	SIGNATURE OF REPORTING PARTY

C. REPORT SENT TO

☐ POLICE DEPARTMENT ☐ SHERIFF'S OFFICE ☐ COUNTY WELFARE ☐ COUNTY PROBATION

AGENCY	ADDRESS	
OFFICIAL CONTACTED	PHONE ( )	DATE/TIME

D. INVOLVED PARTIES

VICTIM

NAME (LAST, FIRST, MIDDLE)	ADDRESS	BIRTHDATE	SEX	RACE
PRESENT LOCATION OF CHILD		PHONE ( )		

SIBLINGS

	NAME	BIRTHDATE	SEX	RACE		NAME	BIRTHDATE	SEX	RACE
1.					4.				
2.					5.				
3.					6.				

PARENTS

NAME (LAST, FIRST, MIDDLE)	BIRTHDATE	SEX	RACE	NAME (LAST, FIRST, MIDDLE)	BIRTHDATE	SEX	RACE
ADDRESS				ADDRESS			
HOME PHONE ( )	BUSINESS PHONE ( )			HOME PHONE ( )	BUSINESS PHONE ( )		

E. INCIDENT INFORMATION

IF NECESSARY, ATTACH EXTRA SHEET OR OTHER FORM AND CHECK THIS BOX. ☐

1. DATE/TIME OF INCIDENT — PLACE OF INCIDENT — *(CHECK ONE)* ☐ OCCURRED ☐ OBSERVED

IF CHILD WAS IN OUT-OF-HOME CARE AT TIME OF INCIDENT, CHECK TYPE OF CARE:

☐ FAMILY DAY CARE ☐ CHILD CARE CENTER ☐ FOSTER FAMILY HOME ☐ SMALL FAMILY HOME ☐ GROUP HOME OR INSTITUTION

2. TYPE OF ABUSE: *(CHECK ONE OR MORE)* ☐ PHYSICAL ☐ MENTAL ☐ SEXUAL ASSAULT ☐ NEGLECT ☐ OTHER

3. NARRATIVE DESCRIPTION:

4. SUMMARIZE WHAT THE ABUSED CHILD OR PERSON ACCOMPANYING THE CHILD SAID HAPPENED:

5. EXPLAIN KNOWN HISTORY OF SIMILAR INCIDENT(S) FOR THIS CHILD:

SS 8572 (REV. 7/87)

INSTRUCTIONS AND DISTRIBUTION ON REVERSE

DO NOT submit a copy of this form to the Department of Justice (DOJ). A CPA is required under Penal Code Section 11169 to submit to DOJ a Child Abuse Investigation Report Form SS-8583 if (1) an active investigation has been conducted and (2) the incident is **not** unfounded.

Blue and Green Copies to: Social Services Dept.
P.O. Box 11341
San Diego, CA 92111

Police or Sheriff-WHITE Copy; County Welfare or Probation-BLUE Copy; District Attorney-GREEN Copy; Reporting Party-YELLOW Copy

INDEX

A

B

C

D

F

G

H

J

K

L

N

O

P

Q

R

S

T

U

V

W

Z